# Health Information Management

## Concepts, Principles, and Practice

**Seventh Edition**

AHIMA
PRESS

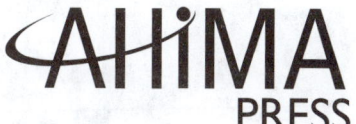

Copyright ©2025 by the American Health Information Management Association. All rights reserved. Except as permitted under the Copyright Act of 1976, no part of this publication may be reproduced, stored in a retrieval system, or transmitted, in any form or by any means, electronic, photocopying, recording, or otherwise, without the prior written permission of AHIMA, 35 West Wacker Ste. 1600, Chicago, Illinois, 60601-5809 (https://www.ahima.org/reprint).

ISBN: **978-1-58426-968-7**
eISBN: **978-1-58426-969-4**
AHIMA Product No.: AB103323

AHIMA Staff:
Jasmine T. Agnew, DHPE, MHIIM, RHIA, CPHIMS, Senior Vice President of Academic Affairs and
    Professional Credentials
Jessica Ervin, MA, Senior Production Development Editor
Christine Scheid, Content Development Manager

Cover image: ©Rach27, iStock

Limit of Liability/Disclaimer of Warranty: This book is sold, as is, without warranty of any kind, either express or implied. While every precaution has been taken in the preparation of this book, the publisher and author assume no responsibility for errors or omissions. Neither is any liability assumed for damages resulting from the use of the information or instructions contained herein. It is further stated that the publisher and author are not responsible for any damage or loss to your data or your equipment that results directly or indirectly from your use of this book.

The websites listed in this book were current and valid as of the date of publication. However, webpage addresses and the information on them may change at any time. Users are encouraged to perform their own general web searches to locate any site addresses listed here that are no longer valid.

CPT® is a registered trademark of the American Medical Association. All other copyrights and trademarks mentioned in this book are the possession of their respective owners. AHIMA makes no claim of ownership by mentioning products that contain such marks.

For more information, including updates, about AHIMA Press publications, visit **https://www.ahima.org /education-events/education-by-product/books/**.

American Health Information Management Association
35 West Wacker Ste. 1600
Chicago, Illinois 60601-5809
ahima.org

# Health Information Management

## Concepts, Principles, and Practice

### Seventh Edition

**Pamela K. Oachs,** MA, RHIA, CHDA, FAHIMA

**Lisa M. Delhomme,** MHA, RHIA

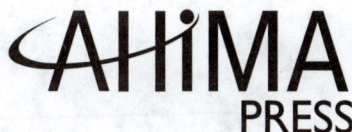

# Contents

| | |
|---|---|
| Contents | iv |
| Detailed Contents | vi |
| About the Volume Editors | xxii |
| About the Authors | xxiii |
| Acknowledgments | xxix |
| Online Resources | xxx |
| Introduction | xxxi |

## Part I — Data Content, Standards, and Governance — 1

**Chapter 1** — The US Healthcare Delivery System — 3
*David L. Gibbs, PhD, CHDA, CHPS, CISSP, CPHI, CPHIMS, FHIMSS, and Karen A. Gibbs, PhD, PT, DPT, MSPT, CWS*

**Chapter 2** — Governing Data and Information Assets — 37
*Joseph C. Brown, DHA, CHDA*

**Chapter 3** — Health Record Content and Documentation — 61
*Katie Kerr, EdD, RHIA*

**Chapter 4** — Clinical Classifications, Vocabularies, Terminologies, and Standards — 93
*Brooke Palkie, EdD, RHIA, CPHIMS, FAHIMA*

**Chapter 5** — Data Management — 121
*Marcia Y. Sharp, EdD, MBA, RHIA, FAHIMA, and Charisse Madlock-Brown, PhD, MLS*

## Part II — Revenue Management and Organizational Compliance — 147

**Chapter 6** — Reimbursement Methodologies — 149
*Anita C. Hazelwood, EdD, RHIA, FAHIMA*

**Chapter 7** — Revenue Cycle Management — 177
*Lauree Handlon, MHA, RHIA, CCS, CHCRS, CRCR, CSAF, FAHIMA, FHFMA*

**Chapter 8** — Clinical Documentation Integrity and Coding Compliance — 205
*T. J. Hunt, PhD, RHIA, CHDA, FAHIMA, and Megan Tober, MBA, RHIA*

**Chapter 9** — Legal Issues in Health Information Management — 233
*Laurie A. Rinehart-Thompson, JD, RHIA, CHP, FAHIMA*

**Chapter 10** — Data Privacy, Confidentiality, and Security — 259
*Danika Brinda, PhD, RHIA, CHPS, FAHIMA, and Amy Watters, EdD, RHIA, FAHIMA*

**Chapter 11** — Clinical Quality Management — 295
*Rosann M. McLean, DHSc, MS, RHIA, CDIP*

## Part III — Informatics, Analytics, and Data Use — 323

| | | |
|---|---|---|
| Chapter 12 | Health Information Technologies<br>*Scott B. Lee-Eichenwald, MSDD* | 325 |
| Chapter 13 | Health Information Systems Planning<br>*Braden Tabisula, MBA, RHIA, CHDA* | 365 |
| Chapter 14 | Public Health and Consumer Engagement<br>*Ryan H. Sandefer, PhD* | 397 |
| Chapter 15 | Healthcare Statistics<br>*Cindy Edgerton, MEd, MHA, RHIA* | 417 |
| Chapter 16 | Healthcare Data Analytics<br>*Susan White, PhD, RHIA, CHDA* | 441 |
| Chapter 17 | Data Visualization<br>*David T. Marc, PhD, CHDA* | 465 |
| Chapter 18 | Research Methods<br>*Shannon H. Houser, PhD, MPH, RHIA, FAHIMA* | 485 |
| Chapter 19 | Biomedical and Clinical Research Support<br>*Shannon H. Houser, PhD, MPH, RHIA, FAHIMA* | 515 |

## Part IV — Organizational Management and Leadership — 539

| | | |
|---|---|---|
| Chapter 20 | Leadership and Management Theories and Strategies<br>*Pamela K. Oachs, MA, RHIA, CHDA, FAHIMA, and Amy Watters, EdD, RHIA, FAHIMA* | 541 |
| Chapter 21 | Strategic Management<br>*Ryan H. Sandefer, PhD* | 575 |
| Chapter 22 | Human Resources Management<br>*Madonna M. LeBlanc, MA, RHIA, FAHIMA* | 599 |
| Chapter 23 | Employee Training and Development<br>*Barbara A. Glondys, MA, RHIA, CHPS* | 623 |
| Chapter 24 | Work Design and Process Improvement<br>*Pamela K. Oachs, MA, RHIA, CHDA, FAHIMA* | 651 |
| Chapter 25 | Financial Management<br>*Rick Revoir, EdD, MBA, CPA* | 685 |
| Chapter 26 | Project Management<br>*Brandon D. Olson, PhD, PMP* | 721 |
| Chapter 27 | Ethical Issues in Health Information Management<br>*Eric S. Swirsky, JD, MA, MHPE* | 753 |

| | | |
|---|---|---|
| **Appendix A** | Odd-Numbered Answer Key | 781 |
| **Glossary** | | **835** |
| **Index** | | **887** |

# Detailed Contents

| | |
|---|---|
| Contents | iv |
| Detailed Contents | vi |
| About the Volume Editors | xxii |
| About the Authors | xxiii |
| Acknowledgments | xxix |
| Online Resources | xxx |
| Introduction | xxxi |

## Part I  Data Content, Standards, and Governance — 1

### Chapter 1  The US Healthcare Delivery System — 3

| | |
|---|---|
| History of Western Medicine | 4 |
|   *Standardization of Medical Practice* | 4 |
|   *Standardization of Hospital Care* | 5 |
|   *Expansion of Health Professions* | 6 |
|   *Interprofessional Education* | 6 |
| Modern Healthcare Delivery in the US | 7 |
|   *Effects of the Great Depression* | 7 |
|   *Postwar Efforts Toward Improving Healthcare Access* | 7 |
|   *Influence of Federal Legislation* | 7 |
|   *Biomedical and Technological Advances in Medicine* | 9 |
| Healthcare Providers and Settings | 11 |
| Organization and Operation of Modern Hospitals | 11 |
|   *Types of Hospitals* | 12 |
|   *Organization of Hospital Services* | 13 |
| Organization of Ambulatory Care | 17 |
|   *Private Medical Practice* | 18 |
|   *Hospital-Based Ambulatory Care Services* | 18 |
|   *Ambulatory Care Services* | 18 |
|   *Public Health Services* | 19 |
|   *Home Healthcare Services* | 19 |
|   *Voluntary Agencies* | 19 |
| Post-Acute Care | 20 |
| Long-Term Care | 20 |
|   *Long-Term Care and the Continuum of Care* | 21 |
|   *Delivery of Long-Term Care Services* | 21 |
|   *Behavioral Health Services* | 21 |
| Integrated Delivery Systems | 22 |
| Forces Affecting Healthcare Organizations | 23 |
|   *Development of Peer Review and Quality Improvement Programs* | 23 |
|   *Malpractice* | 24 |
|   *Efforts at Healthcare Reengineering* | 24 |
|   *Value-Based Care* | 24 |
|   *Licensure and Certification of Healthcare Facilities* | 24 |
|   *Accreditation* | 25 |

Detailed Contents    vii

|  |  |
|---|---|
| Reimbursement of Healthcare Expenditures | 26 |
|    *Evolution of Third-Party Reimbursement* | 26 |
|    *Government-Sponsored Reimbursement Systems* | 26 |
|    *Insurance* | 28 |
|    *Managed Care* | 28 |
|    *Continued Rise in Healthcare Costs* | 30 |
| Future of Healthcare in the US | 30 |
| **References** | **32** |

## Chapter 2   Governing Data and Information Assets    37

|  |  |
|---|---|
| Navigating Emerging Terms in Data and Information Governance | 38 |
| Governance | 39 |
| Data Governance and Information Governance | 40 |
|    *Data Governance Background* | 42 |
|    *Information Governance Background* | 42 |
| Data Management Domains | 45 |
|    *Data Life Cycle Management* | 45 |
|    *Data Architecture Management* | 46 |
|    *Metadata Management* | 46 |
|    *Master Data Management* | 46 |
|    *Content Management* | 47 |
|    *Data Security Management* | 47 |
|    *Business Intelligence Management* | 47 |
|    *Data Quality Management* | 48 |
|    *Terminology and Classification Management* | 49 |
| Governance Program Planning | 49 |
| Data and Information Governance Implementation and Stewardship | 51 |
|    *Data Governance Implementation Frameworks* | 51 |
|    *Information Governance Implementation Frameworks* | 56 |
| **References** | **58** |

## Chapter 3   Health Record Content and Documentation    61

|  |  |
|---|---|
| Evolution of the Health Record | 62 |
|    *Historical Overview* | 62 |
|    *Factors Influencing the Content of the Health Record* | 63 |
|    *Documentation and Maintenance Standards for the Health Record* | 63 |
|    *Today's Health Record* | 64 |
|    *Responsibility for Quality Documentation* | 66 |
| Content and Format of the Health Record | 68 |
|    *Administrative Information* | 68 |
|    *Clinical Data* | 69 |
|    *Conclusions at Termination of Care* | 75 |
|    *External Records Filed with the Health Record* | 76 |
|    *Specialized Health Record Content* | 76 |
| Management of Health Record Content | 80 |
|    *Document Creation* | 80 |
|    *Incomplete Record Control* | 81 |
|    *Template (Forms) Design and Management* | 84 |
| Health Record Life Cycle | 85 |
|    *Health Record Creation and Identification* | 85 |
|    *Health Record Storage and Retrieval* | 87 |
|    *Health Record Retention and Disposition* | 88 |
| **References** | **91** |

## Chapter 4: Clinical Classifications, Vocabularies, Terminologies, and Standards — 93

- Development of Classification Systems, Vocabularies, and Terminologies for Healthcare Data — 94
- Common Healthcare Classifications and Code Sets — 96
  - *International Classification of Diseases* — 96
  - *International Classification of Diseases for Oncology, Third Edition, Second Revision* — 98
  - *International Classification on Functioning, Disability, and Health* — 100
  - *Healthcare Common Procedure Coding System* — 101
  - *Current Procedural Terminology* — 101
  - *Diagnostic and Statistical Manual of Mental Disorders* — 102
  - *International Classification of Primary Care* — 102
  - *Current Dental Terminology* — 103
  - *National Drug Codes* — 103
- Other Healthcare Terminologies, Vocabularies, and Classification Systems — 104
  - *Systematized Nomenclature of Medicine Clinical Terminology* — 105
  - *Logical Observation Identifiers Names and Codes* — 106
  - *Clinical Care Classification* — 107
  - *RxNorm* — 107
  - *MEDCIN* — 108
  - *Specialty Healthcare Terminologies, Vocabularies, and Classifications* — 108
- Data Standardization — 112
  - *Interoperability* — 114
  - *National Library of Medicine's Role in Healthcare Terminologies* — 114
  - *Artificial Intelligence* — 115
- **References** — **116**

## Chapter 5: Data Management — 121

- Data and Data Sources — 122
- Indices — 123
  - *Master Patient Index* — 123
  - *Disease and Operation Indices* — 123
  - *Physician Index* — 123
- Registries — 124
  - *Cancer Registries* — 124
  - *Trauma Registries* — 126
  - *Diabetes Registries* — 127
  - *Transplant Registries* — 127
  - *Immunization Registries* — 128
  - *Other Registries* — 129
- Database Management and Design — 130
  - *Relational Databases* — 130
  - *Entity Relationship Modeling* — 130
  - *Structured Query Language* — 132
  - *Database Implementation* — 132
  - *Common Data Models for EHR Data Warehouses* — 133
- Healthcare Databases — 134
  - *National and State Administrative Databases* — 134
  - *National, State, and County Public Health Databases* — 135
  - *Vital Statistics* — 136
  - *Clinical Trials Databases* — 137
  - *Health Services Research Databases* — 137
  - *National Library of Medicine* — 137
- Processing and Maintenance of Secondary Databases — 138
  - *Automated versus Manual Methods of Data Collection* — 138

## Detailed Contents

|  |  |
|---|---|
| *Vendor Systems Versus Facility-Specific Systems* | *138* |
| *Data Security and Confidentiality Issues* | *139* |
| *Trends in Collecting Secondary Data* | *139* |
| Data Quality | 140 |
| *Data Quality Standards* | *140* |
| *Data Quality Requirements for Information Systems* | *142* |
| *Types of Data Dictionaries* | *142* |
| *Development of Data Dictionaries* | *143* |
| **References** | **143** |

## Part II — Revenue Management and Organizational Compliance — 147

### Chapter 6 — Reimbursement Methodologies — 149

|  |  |
|---|---|
| Healthcare Reimbursement Systems | 150 |
| *Commercial Insurance* | *150* |
| *Not-for-Profit Insurance Companies* | *151* |
| *Types of Healthcare Savings Accounts* | *151* |
| *Government-Sponsored Healthcare Programs* | *152* |
| *Managed Care* | *157* |
| Healthcare Reimbursement Methodologies, Accountable Care Organizations, and Risk Adjustment | 161 |
| *Fee-for-Service Reimbursement Methodologies* | *161* |
| *Episode-of-Care Reimbursement Methodologies* | *162* |
| *Reimbursement for Telehealth* | *163* |
| *Accountable Care Organizations* | *163* |
| *Risk Adjustment Models* | *164* |
| Medicare's Prospective Payment Systems | 164 |
| *Medicare's Acute-Care Prospective Payment System* | *165* |
| *Hospital-Acquired Conditions and Present on Admission Indicator Reporting* | *166* |
| *Inpatient Psychiatric Facilities Prospective Payment System* | *167* |
| *Resource-Based Relative Value Scale System* | *168* |
| *Medicare and Medicaid Outpatient Prospective Payment System* | *169* |
| *Ambulatory Surgery Center Prospective Payment System* | *170* |
| *Ambulance Fee Schedule* | *171* |
| *Medicare Skilled Nursing Facility Prospective Payment System* | *171* |
| *Home Health Prospective Payment System* | *172* |
| *Inpatient Rehabilitation Facility Prospective Payment System* | *173* |
| *Long-Term Care Hospital Prospective Payment System* | *174* |
| **References** | **175** |

### Chapter 7 — Revenue Cycle Management — 177

|  |  |
|---|---|
| Revenue Cycle Front-End Process | 179 |
| *Patient Access Components* | *180* |
| *Pre-encounter Services* | *183* |
| Revenue Cycle Middle Process | 184 |
| *Clinical Services* | *184* |
| *Clinical Documentation* | *184* |
| *Case Management and Utilization Management* | *184* |
| *Health Information Management and Clinical Coding* | *185* |
| *Charge Capture* | *186* |
| *Charge Description Master* | *188* |
| Revenue Cycle Back-End Process | 192 |

## Detailed Contents

|  |  |
|---|---|
| *Billing System* | *192* |
| *Claims Preparation* | *192* |
| *Claims Editing* | *193* |
| *Claims Submission* | *194* |
| *Payment Posting* | *194* |
| *Collections and Account Follow-Up* | *194* |
| *Denial Management* | *195* |
| *Remittance Management* | *196* |
| Revenue Cycle Support Services | 197 |
| *Payer Relations and Health Plan Contracts* | *197* |
| *Payer Relations and Physician Credentialing* | *198* |
| *Patient Relations and Customer Service* | *199* |
| Performance Measures for Improvement | 199 |
| **References** | **201** |

### Chapter 8 — Clinical Documentation Integrity and Coding Compliance — 205

| | |
|---|---|
| Clinical Documentation Integrity | 206 |
| *Documentation for Coded Data* | *207* |
| *Clinical Documentation Integrity Goals* | *207* |
| *Operational Considerations* | *208* |
| *Query Process* | *215* |
| *Technology Considerations in CDI* | *218* |
| Corporate Compliance | 221 |
| *Coding Compliance* | *222* |
| *Regulation* | *222* |
| *Governmental Audit Programs* | *223* |
| *Exclusion from Federal Programs* | *223* |
| *Auditing* | *223* |
| *Office of the Inspector General Compliance Guidance* | *224* |
| *Developing a Coding Compliance Plan* | *225* |
| *Fraud Surveillance* | *226* |
| *Key Clinical Documents* | *227* |
| *Coding Compliance Education* | *227* |
| *Medical Identity Theft* | *228* |
| *Anti-Kickback Statute* | *229* |
| *Stark Law* | *229* |
| *Emergency Medical Treatment and Labor Act* | *229* |
| **References** | **230** |

### Chapter 9 — Legal Issues in Health Information Management — 233

| | |
|---|---|
| Legal Foundations and Proceedings | 235 |
| *Branches of Government* | *235* |
| *Sources of Law* | *235* |
| *Public Law versus Private Law* | *236* |
| *Civil Law versus Criminal Law* | *236* |
| *The Court System* | *237* |
| *Civil Litigation* | *237* |
| *Criminal Proceedings* | *239* |
| Healthcare Causes of Action | 239 |
| *Torts* | *240* |
| *Contract* | *244* |
| Legal Aspects of Health Information Management | 245 |
| *Form and Content of the Health Record* | *245* |

| | |
|---|---|
| *The Health Record as a Business Record* | *247* |
| *Retention of the Health Record* | *247* |
| *Ownership of and Access to the Health Record* | *248* |
| The Health Record as Evidence | 249 |
| *Admissibility of the Health Record* | *249* |
| *The Electronic Health Record* | *249* |
| *Consent and Advance Directives* | *250* |
| *E-Discovery* | *251* |
| *Privilege* | *252* |
| *Government Right of Access to Health Records* | *252* |
| Release of Information | 253 |
| *Handling Highly Sensitive Information* | *253* |
| *Wrongful Disclosure* | *254* |
| Medical Identity Theft | 254 |
| Confidentiality of Quality Improvement Activities | 255 |
| *Incident Reports* | *255* |
| **References** | **256** |

## Chapter 10 — Data Privacy, Confidentiality, and Security — 259

| | |
|---|---|
| The Health Insurance Portability and Accountability Act (HIPAA) of 1996 | 260 |
| *The Privacy Rule* | *261* |
| *The Security Rule* | *262* |
| *The HITECH-HIPAA Omnibus Privacy Act* | *263* |
| Privacy and Security Requirements for Disclosure Management | 266 |
| *Use and Disclosure of Patient Information with Patient Authorization* | *266* |
| *Use and Disclosure of Patient Information without Patient Authorization* | *268* |
| *Use and Disclosure Requiring an Opportunity to Object* | *269* |
| *Use and Disclosure for Reproductive Health Care* | *270* |
| *Patient Identity Management for Use and Disclosure of PHI* | *270* |
| *Confidentiality of Alcohol and Drug Abuse Patient Records* | *271* |
| 21st Century Cures Act and Information Blocking | 273 |
| State Privacy and Security Laws | 274 |
| Managing an Effective Security Program | 275 |
| *Risk Analysis and Risk Management* | *276* |
| *Audit Logs and Monitoring* | *278* |
| *Contingency Planning* | *278* |
| *Data Security Methods* | *280* |
| Management of Privacy and Security in Health Information Exchange | 284 |
| Mobile Health Technology and HIPAA | 286 |
| Workforce Training | 287 |
| *HIPAA Training Components* | *288* |
| *HIPAA Training Principles and Strategies* | *289* |
| **References** | **290** |

## Chapter 11 — Clinical Quality Management — 295

| | |
|---|---|
| Historical Perspectives in Healthcare Quality | 296 |
| *Patient Safety Concerns Emerge* | *296* |
| *Legal Implications Related to Quality of Care* | *297* |
| *Toward Systematic Quality and Performance Initiatives* | *297* |
| Today's Drivers of Healthcare Quality | 299 |
| *Accreditation Standards* | *300* |
| *Regulatory Requirements* | *300* |

| | |
|---|---|
| *Quality Indicator Reporting and Transparency* | *301* |
| *Value-Based Care Reforms* | *302* |
| *The Patient as a Consumer* | *302* |
| Organizational Influence on Healthcare Quality | 303 |
| *Organizational Mission and Vision* | *303* |
| *Influence of Leadership* | *303* |
| *Organizational Culture* | *304* |
| *Interprofessional Education and Practice* | *304* |
| *Change Management* | *304* |
| *Risk Management* | *305* |
| *Business Continuity and Contingency* | *305* |
| Quality Management Tools and Processes | 306 |
| *Performance Measures* | *306* |
| *Quality and Knowledge Generation* | *307* |
| *Plan-Do-Check-Act Cycle* | *308* |
| *Peer Review* | *309* |
| *Tracer Methodology* | *310* |
| Assessing Outcomes and Effectiveness of Healthcare | 311 |
| *Healthcare Quality Measures* | *311* |
| *The Role of the Agency for Healthcare Research and Quality* | *312* |
| Systematic and Process-Driven Focus to Improve Performance | 313 |
| *Evidence-Based Care and Treatment* | *313* |
| *Clinical Pathways* | *314* |
| *Case Management* | *314* |
| *Care Coordination* | *315* |
| *Effective Deployment and Use of Information Technology* | *315* |
| Professional Designations and Roles in Healthcare Quality | 316 |
| *Certifications Related to Quality Management* | *316* |
| *The Health Information Manager Role in Healthcare Quality* | *316* |
| *Data Stewardship and Information Governance* | *317* |
| *Data Analytics* | *317* |
| *Regulatory Compliance* | *317* |
| Trends Impacting Healthcare Quality | 318 |
| *Reputation, Identity, and Social Media* | *318* |
| *Telehealth Services* | *318* |
| *Learning Health Systems* | *318* |
| **References** | **319** |

## Part III — Informatics, Analytics, and Data Use — 323

### Chapter 12 — Health Information Technologies — 325

| | |
|---|---|
| The Field of Informatics | 326 |
| Current and Emerging Information Technologies in Healthcare | 328 |
| Technologies Supporting the Capture of Different Types of Data and Formats | 329 |
| *Speech Recognition Technology* | *329* |
| *Natural Language Processing Technology* | *330* |
| *Electronic Document and Content Management Systems* | *331* |
| Technologies Supporting Efficient Access to and Flow of Data and Information | 333 |
| *Automatic Recognition Technologies* | *333* |
| *Enterprise Master Patient Indices and Identity Management* | *334* |
| *Cloud-Based Technologies and Applications* | *334* |
| Technologies Supporting the Diagnosis, Treatment, and Care of Patients | 337 |

| | |
|---|---|
| *Physiological Signal Processing Systems* | *337* |
| *Point-of-Care Information Systems* | *337* |
| *Mobile and Wireless Technology and Devices* | *337* |
| *Automated Clinical Care Plans, Practice Guidelines, Pathways, and Protocols* | *338* |
| *Telehealth Systems* | *338* |
| *Electronic Health Record Systems* | *339* |
| EHR Functionality and Technology | 341 |
| *Source Systems* | *341* |
| *Core Clinical EHR Applications* | *342* |
| Health Information Exchange | 348 |
| Interoperability and Its Challenges | 349 |
| *Medication Variability* | *349* |
| *Document Structure and Format* | *349* |
| *Protocols and Standards* | *349* |
| *Commitment and Trust* | *350* |
| Models for Health Information Exchange | 351 |
| *The Centralized Health Information Exchange Architecture* | *351* |
| *The Decentralized Health Information Exchange Architecture* | *351* |
| *The Hybrid Health Information Exchange Architecture* | *352* |
| *The Health Record Banking Health Information Exchange Architecture* | *353* |
| Legal Issues in the Exchange of Electronic Protected Health Information | 355 |
| Exchange Methodologies | 355 |
| *Directed Exchange* | *356* |
| *Query-Based Exchange* | *356* |
| *Consumer-Mediated Exchange* | *356* |
| Health Information Exchange Initiatives | 357 |
| *The Sequoia Project* | *357* |
| *Trusted Exchange Framework and Common Agreement* | *357* |
| Health Information Exchange Implementation Considerations | 359 |
| *Identification of a Trust Community* | *359* |
| *Development of Governance Committees* | *359* |
| *Identification of the Technology Platform* | *359* |
| *Contracts and Participant Agreements* | *359* |
| *Operational Policies* | *359* |
| *Development of Vendor and Participant Project Teams* | *360* |
| *Data Governance* | *360* |
| *The Creation of the Sandbox for System Testing* | *360* |
| Stages of HIE Implementation | 360 |
| *Stage 1 of Implementation* | *360* |
| *Stage 2 of Implementation* | *361* |
| *Stage 3 of Implementation* | *361* |
| Health Information Management in HIE | 361 |
| **References** | **362** |

**Chapter 13** — **Health Information Systems Planning** — **365**

| | |
|---|---|
| A Systems View | 367 |
| System Development Life Cycle | 369 |
| Strategic Planning for Health Information Systems | 370 |
| *Purpose of HIS Planning* | *370* |
| *Designing a Health Information Systems Plan* | *372* |
| Strategic Plan Execution | 377 |
| *Project Management* | *377* |

| | | |
|---|---|---|
| | *Requirements Analysis* | *378* |
| | *Acquisition* | *379* |
| | *Implementation* | *382* |
| | *Continued Information System Review and Support* | *384* |
| | Planning for Health Information System Optimization | 387 |
| | *EHR System Implementation Level of Maturity* | *387* |
| | *EHR System Adoption Level of Maturity* | *387* |
| | *EHR System Optimization Level of Maturity* | *388* |
| | Planning for Ongoing Management of Health Information | 388 |
| | *Health Data and Information Governance Plan* | *388* |
| | *Types of Health Data and Information* | *389* |
| | *Metadata* | *390* |
| | *Data Quality Management* | *391* |
| | **References** | **393** |
| **Chapter 14** | **Public Health and Consumer Engagement** | **397** |
| | Consumer Health Informatics and Consumer Engagement | 399 |
| | *The Evolution of Consumer Engagement in Healthcare* | *400* |
| | *Consumer Assessment of Healthcare Providers and Systems* | *400* |
| | *Patient-Centered Medical Home* | *401* |
| | *Promoting Interoperability Programs* | *401* |
| | *Hospital Value-Based Purchasing Program* | *401* |
| | Social Determinants of Health | 402 |
| | *HealthyPeople 2030* | *402* |
| | *Health Literacy* | *403* |
| | Health Information Online Resources | 404 |
| | *Healthcare-Focused Websites* | *404* |
| | *Internet Forums* | *404* |
| | *Patient Activation Measure* | *405* |
| | Patient Portals, Personal Health Records, and Telehealth | 405 |
| | *Patient Portals* | *406* |
| | *Personal Health Records* | *406* |
| | *Telehealth* | *408* |
| | Patient-Generated Health Data | 409 |
| | Precision Medicine | 410 |
| | Consumer Health Informatics and Next Steps | 411 |
| | **References** | **412** |
| **Chapter 15** | **Healthcare Statistics** | **417** |
| | Introduction to Healthcare Statistics | 418 |
| | *Use of Statistics* | *418* |
| | *Sources of Data* | *419* |
| | *Descriptive versus Inferential Statistics* | *419* |
| | Basic Calculations and Descriptive Statistics | 420 |
| | *Ratio* | *420* |
| | *Rate* | *420* |
| | *Average* | *421* |
| | Terminology Related to Healthcare Statistics | 422 |
| | Statistics Related to Volume of Service and Utilization | 423 |
| | *Inpatient Census* | *423* |
| | *Occupancy Data* | *425* |
| | *Hospital Bed Turnover* | *426* |
| | *Length of Stay* | *427* |

| | | |
|---|---|---|
| | Statistics Related to Clinical Services and Patient Care | 429 |
| | *Death Rates* | *429* |
| | *Autopsy Rates* | *431* |
| | *Hospital Infection Rates* | *432* |
| | Ambulatory Care Statistics | 434 |
| | Statistics in Revenue Cycle Management | 434 |
| | Case-Mix Analysis | 434 |
| | *Example One of Case-Mix Analysis* | *435* |
| | *Example Two of Case-Mix Analysis* | *435* |
| | Public Health and Epidemiology Data | 436 |
| | *Epidemiology Statistics* | *436* |
| | *Community-Based Disease Tracking* | *436* |
| | Finding and Using Healthcare Statistics | 437 |
| | **References** | **438** |
| **Chapter 16** | **Healthcare Data Analytics** | **441** |
| | Healthcare Initiatives and the Impact on Data Analytics | 442 |
| | Types of Data | 443 |
| | Descriptive versus Inferential Statistics | 444 |
| | *Impact of Sampling* | *445* |
| | *Tools for Sampling and Design* | *446* |
| | Analyzing Continuous Data | 449 |
| | *Measures of Central Tendency* | *449* |
| | *Measures of Spread* | *450* |
| | *Inferential Statistics for Continuous Data* | *450* |
| | *Normal Distribution* | *452* |
| | Analyzing Rates and Proportions | 453 |
| | *Descriptive Statistics for Rates and Proportions* | *453* |
| | *Inferential Statistics for Rates and Proportions* | *453* |
| | Analyzing Relationships between Two Variables | 455 |
| | *Correlation* | *455* |
| | *Simple Linear Regression* | *456* |
| | Analytics in Practice | 458 |
| | Data Mining | 458 |
| | *Predictive Modeling* | *459* |
| | *Risk-Adjusted Quality Indicators* | *459* |
| | *Real-Time Analytics* | *460* |
| | Opportunities for Health Information Management Professionals in Healthcare Data Analytics | 461 |
| | **References** | **462** |
| **Chapter 17** | **Data Visualization** | **465** |
| | Data Visualization Related to Perception and Decision-Making | 466 |
| | Charts versus Tables | 468 |
| | Considerations for Adopting Visualization Techniques | 469 |
| | *Context of the Situation* | *469* |
| | *Experience of the User* | *470* |
| | *Presentation Method* | *470* |
| | *Complexity of the Data* | *477* |
| | Using Data Visualization to Guide Decisions under the Inpatient Psychiatric Facility Quality Reporting Program | 479 |
| | **References** | **484** |

## Chapter 18  Research Methods — 485

- Research Methodology — 486
- Research Process — 488
  - *Defining the Research Problem and Research Question* — 488
  - *Conducting a Literature Review* — 490
  - *Selecting the Research Design* — 492
  - *Collecting Data* — 497
  - *Analyzing the Data* — 506
  - *Disseminating Results* — 507
- **References** — **511**
- **Resources** — **513**

## Chapter 19  Biomedical and Clinical Research Support — 515

- Clinical and Biomedical Research — 516
- Ethical Treatment of Human Subjects — 517
  - *The Nuremberg Code and the Declaration of Helsinki* — 517
  - *The US Public Health Services Syphilis Study* — 518
- Protection of Human Subjects — 519
  - *Institutional Assurances of Compliance* — 519
  - *Institutional Review Board* — 520
  - *Informed Consent* — 523
- Vulnerable Subjects — 525
- Role of HIM Professionals in Research — 526
  - *Privacy Considerations in Clinical and Biomedical Research* — 526
  - *Oversight of Clinical and Biomedical Research* — 527
  - *Types of Clinical and Biomedical Research Designs* — 528
  - *Risk Assessment* — 532
- Use of Comparative Data in Outcomes Research — 533
  - *Comparative Effectiveness Research* — 534
  - *Patient-Centered Outcomes Research Institute (PCORI)* — 534
- **References** — **535**

# Part IV  Organizational Management and Leadership — 539

## Chapter 20  Leadership and Management Theories and Strategies — 541

- Landmarks in Management as a Discipline — 542
  - *Scientific Management (1880–1920)* — 542
  - *Administrative Management (Circa 1920s)* — 543
  - *Humanistic Management (Circa 1924)* — 545
  - *Operations Management (1941–Present)* — 545
  - *Contemporary Management (1960–Present)* — 545
- Functions and Principles of Management — 548
  - *Managerial Functions* — 548
  - *Levels of Management* — 551
  - *Managerial Skills* — 552
  - *Managerial Activities* — 553
  - *Trends in Management Theory* — 554
- Trends in Leadership Theory — 555
  - *Classical Approaches to Leadership Theory* — 555
  - *Behavioral or Task-Relationship Theories of Leadership* — 556
  - *Contingency and Situational Theories of Leadership* — 557
  - *Values-Based Leadership* — 559
  - *Complexity Leadership and Systems Thinking* — 560

Detailed Contents xvii

Diffusion of Innovations .................................................................... 562
   *Categories of Adopter Groups* .................................................... 562
   *Dynamics Affecting Innovation Diffusion* ................................... 563
   *Innovator Roles* ........................................................................... 564
Change Management ........................................................................ 564
   *Differences between Leaders and Managers* ............................... 565
   *Organization Development Change Agent Functions* ................. 565
   *Internal and External Change Agents* ......................................... 565
   *Stages of Change* ........................................................................ 566
   *Leading through Cultural Change* .............................................. 569
   *Response to Change* ................................................................... 569
**References** ........................................................................................ **571**

### Chapter 21  Strategic Management — 575

From Strategic Planning to Strategic Management and Thinking ...... 576
Skills of Strategic Managers ............................................................... 577
Elements of Strategic Planning .......................................................... 578
Phase I: Environmental Assessment: Internal and External ............... 580
   *Understand Environmental Assessment Trends* ........................... 580
   *Assess and Manage Risk and Uncertainty* ................................... 582
Phase II: Identifying Organizational Direction from Vision to Strategy ... 583
   *Create a Commitment to Change with the Vision* ....................... 584
   *Define Areas of Excellence* ......................................................... 585
   *Formulate Key Strategies* ............................................................ 585
Phase III: Strategy Formulation ......................................................... 586
   *Use Techniques and Tools for Strategic Thinking* ........................ 586
   *Determine Impact of Competition* ............................................. 587
   *Identify a Future Strategic Profile* ............................................... 587
   *Create a Platform for Strategic Innovation* ................................. 588
   *Develop Final Strategic Findings and Conclusions* ..................... 588
Phase IV: Implementation ................................................................. 589
   *Roles of Strategic Goals and Strategic Objectives* ........................ 589
   *Importance of Implementation Plans* ........................................ 590
Support for the Change Program ...................................................... 592
   *Take a Systems Approach* ........................................................... 592
   *Create the Structure for Change* ................................................. 592
   *Manage the Politics of Change* ................................................... 592
   *Create a Sense of Urgency* .......................................................... 593
   *Engage with Communication* .................................................... 593
Implement Strategic Change ............................................................. 594
   *Create and Communicate Short-Term Wins* .............................. 594
   *Pace and Refine Change Plans* ................................................... 595
   *Maintain Momentum and Stay the Course* ................................ 595
   *Measure Your Results* ................................................................. 595
**References** ........................................................................................ **597**

### Chapter 22  Human Resources Management — 599

Role of the Human Resources Department ....................................... 600
   *Human Resources Planning and Analysis* .................................. 600
   *Equal Employment Opportunity Practices* ................................. 601
   *Rights of Employees and Employers* .......................................... 602
   *Staffing* ....................................................................................... 603
   *Compensation and Benefits Program* ......................................... 603

| | |
|---|---:|
|     *Health and Safety Program* | 603 |
|     *Labor Relations* | 603 |
| Role of the HIM Manager in Human Resources | 604 |
|     *Human Resources Planning* | 606 |
|     *Recruitment and Retention* | 607 |
|     *Effective Communication* | 611 |
|     *Employee Empowerment* | 611 |
| Compensation Systems | 614 |
|     *Compensation Surveys* | 615 |
|     *Job Evaluations* | 615 |
| Performance Management | 615 |
|     *Performance Counseling and Disciplinary Action* | 617 |
|     *Termination and Layoff* | 618 |
|     *Conflict Management* | 618 |
|     *Grievance Management* | 619 |
| Maintenance of Employee Records | 619 |
| Human Resources Trends and Practices | 619 |
| **References** | **621** |

## Chapter 23 — Employee Training and Development — 623

| | |
|---|---:|
| Training Program Development | 624 |
| Departmental Employee Training and Development Plan | 625 |
|     *Training and Development Model* | 625 |
| Elements of Workforce Training | 627 |
|     *New Employee Orientation and Training* | 628 |
|     *On-the-Job Training* | 631 |
|     *Staff Development through In-Service Education* | 633 |
| Adult Learning Strategies | 636 |
|     *Characteristics of Adult Learners* | 636 |
|     *Education of Adult Learners* | 637 |
|     *Learning Styles* | 638 |
|     *Special Considerations for Staff Development* | 638 |
| Delivery Methods | 640 |
|     *Delivery Methods: Instructor-Directed* | 640 |
|     *Delivery Methods: Self-Paced* | 641 |
| Artificial Intelligence in Training and Development | 644 |
| Positioning Employees for Career Development | 645 |
|     *Preparing the HIM Staff for Future Roles* | 645 |
|     *Continuing Education* | 645 |
|     *Soft Skills* | 646 |
|     *Promotion and Succession Planning* | 646 |
|     *Developing a Personal Career Plan* | 646 |
|     *Employment Laws and Regulations Impacting Training* | 647 |
| **References** | **648** |

## Chapter 24 — Work Design and Process Improvement — 651

| | |
|---|---:|
| Functional Work Environment | 652 |
|     *Departmental Workflow* | 652 |
|     *Space and Equipment* | 652 |
|     *Aesthetics* | 654 |
|     *Ergonomics* | 654 |

| | |
|---|---:|
| Methods of Organizing Work | 655 |
| *Work Division Patterns* | *655* |
| *Work Distribution Analysis* | *656* |
| *Work Scheduling* | *657* |
| *Work Procedures* | *660* |
| Performance and Work Measurement Standards | 662 |
| *Criteria for Setting Effective Standards* | *662* |
| *Types of Standards* | *662* |
| *Methods of Communicating Standards* | *663* |
| *Methods of Developing Standards* | *663* |
| Performance Measurement | 665 |
| *Performance Controls* | *665* |
| *Variance Analysis* | *666* |
| *Assessment of Departmental Performance* | *666* |
| Performance Improvement | 669 |
| *The Role of Customer Service* | *669* |
| *Identification of Performance Improvement Opportunities* | *669* |
| *Principles of Performance Improvement* | *670* |
| *Continuous Quality Improvement* | *671* |
| *Business Process Reengineering* | *678* |
| *Workflow Analysis and Process Redesign* | *679* |
| **References** | **684** |

## Chapter 25  Financial Management — 685

| | |
|---|---:|
| Healthcare Financial Management | 686 |
| Accounting | 688 |
| *Accounting Concepts and Principles* | *688* |
| *Authorities* | *689* |
| *Financial Organization* | *690* |
| *Sources of Financial Data* | *692* |
| *Uses of Financial Data* | *693* |
| Basic Financial Accounting | 694 |
| *Assets* | *694* |
| *Liabilities* | *696* |
| *Equity or Net Assets* | *696* |
| *Revenue* | *697* |
| *Expenses* | *697* |
| *Recording Transactions* | *699* |
| *Financial Statements* | *701* |
| *Ratio Analysis* | *702* |
| Basic Management Accounting | 706 |
| *Describing Costs* | *706* |
| *Cost Reports* | *707* |
| Internal Controls | 709 |
| *Preventive* | *709* |
| *Detective* | *709* |
| *Corrective* | *709* |
| Budgets | 710 |
| *Types of Budgets* | *711* |
| *Operational Budgets* | *711* |
| *Management of the Operating Budget* | *713* |
| *Capital Budget* | *715* |
| *Capital Projects* | *716* |
| **References** | **719** |

xx Detailed Contents

## Chapter 26 Project Management — 721

- The Project — 722
  - *Definition of a Project* — 722
  - *Determining a Project's Purpose* — 723
- Project Management — 724
  - *Project Management Process* — 724
  - *Alternative Project Methodologies* — 724
  - *Project Management Constraints* — 726
  - *Project Members* — 727
  - *Organizational Structures* — 729
  - *Team Structures* — 733
- The Project Manager — 735
  - *Roles of a Project Manager* — 736
  - *Project Management Competencies* — 737
  - *Project Manager Talent Triangle* — 739
- The Project Management Process Groups — 741
  - *Initiating* — 741
  - *Planning* — 743
  - *Executing* — 747
  - *Monitoring and Controlling* — 747
  - *Closing* — 747
- Managing Project Change — 748
  - *Types of Change* — 748
  - *Benefits of Change* — 748
  - *Negotiating Change and Managing Expectations* — 749
  - *Change Management Process* — 749
- Beyond Project Management — 751
  - *Project Selection* — 751
  - *Program Management* — 751
  - *Project Portfolio Management* — 751
- **References** — **752**

## Chapter 27 Ethical Issues in Health Information Management — 753

- Morality and Ethics in Health Information Management — 754
  - *Morality* — 754
  - *Moral Distress* — 755
  - *Ethical Theories, Principles, and Concepts* — 756
- Ethical Foundations of Health Information Management — 760
  - *Protection of Privacy, Maintenance of Confidentiality, and Assurance of Data Security* — 761
  - *Professional Code of Ethics* — 761
  - *Professional Values and Obligations* — 763
  - *Ethical Decision-Making* — 763
  - *Breach of Healthcare Ethics* — 766
- Important Health Information Ethical Problems — 768
  - *Ethical Issues Related to Documentation and Privacy* — 768
  - *Ethical Issues Related to the Release of Information* — 768
  - *Ethical Issues Related to Coding* — 769
  - *Ethical Issues Related to Public Health and Sensitive Health Information* — 769
  - *Ethical Issues Related to Research* — 769
  - *Ethical Issues Related to Diversity, Equity, and Inclusion* — 770
  - *Ethical Issues Related to Electronic Health Record Systems* — 771
  - *Ethical Issues Related to End-of-Life Care* — 773

| | |
|---|---:|
| *Ethical Issues Related to Disparities and Literacy* | *773* |
| *Ethical Issues Related to Social Media Use* | *774* |
| *Ethical Issues Related to Artificial Intelligence* | *775* |
| **References** | **776** |

**Appendix A**  Odd-Numbered Answer Key         781

**Glossary**                                    **835**
**Index**                                       **887**

## Online Appendices

**Appendix B**  Sample Documentation Forms and Research Sources

**Appendix C**  AHIMA Code of Ethics, Standards of Ethical Coding, and Ethical Standards for Clinical Documentation Improvement Professionals

# About the Volume Editors

**Pamela K. Oachs, MA, RHIA, CHDA, FAHIMA**, is an assistant professor and director of the health information management undergraduate program in the College of St. Scholastica's health informatics and information management department. She teaches courses related to health information technology, US healthcare, healthcare management, and clinical quality improvement. She has more than 15 years of healthcare experience. Her career includes a variety of positions, both managerial and professional, in the areas of utilization management, quality improvement, medical staff credentialing, Joint Commission coordination, information technology, project management, and patient access. She served on the board of directors of the Minnesota Health Information Management Association and the Northeastern Minnesota Health Information Management Association, was a commissioner on the Commission on Certification for Health Informatics and Information Management, and is a peer reviewer for the Council on Accreditation for Health Informatics and Information Management Education. Ms. Oachs was the recipient of AHIMA's 2023 Triumph Award in the educator category.

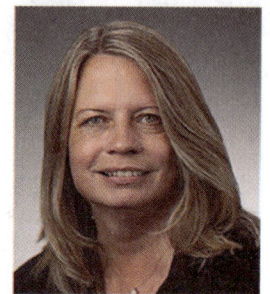

**Lisa M. Delhomme, MHA, RHIA**, is the program director of the health information management program at the University of Louisiana at Lafayette. She teaches courses in privacy and security, data analytics, and database management. Mrs. Delhomme is an active AHIMA volunteer and served on AHIMA's Council for Excellence in Education. She has served several volunteer roles with AHIMA and is a former president of the Louisiana Health Information Management Association. She is a frequent presenter at state and national conferences in her areas of expertise.

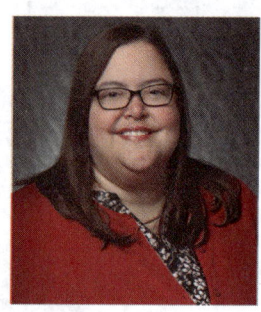

# About the Authors

**Danika E. Brinda, PhD, RHIA, CHPS, FAHIMA**, is the owner of TriPoint Healthcare Solutions and Planet HIPAA, where she specializes in advising, educating, and implementing privacy and security requirements in healthcare. With over 20 years of experience in healthcare privacy and security, Dr. Brinda is passionate about simplifying HIPAA concepts to help others understand them through practical, accessible processes. She also serves as the Privacy and Security Officer at NeuroPace in Mountain View, CA. Dr. Brinda earned her bachelor's degree in health information management and computer science/information systems and a master's degree from the College of St. Scholastica. She completed her doctor of philosophy in information technology with a focus in information governance and security in 2015.

**Joseph C. Brown, DHA, CHDA**, is the department chair for the allied health and health information management programs at Davenport University. He has 20 years of experience in the healthcare field, which includes being a distinguished adjunct at Davenport. His background includes working in insurance, technology, software management, data analytics, quality improvement, and the urgent care setting. Academically, Dr. Brown has obtained a bachelor's degree in telecommunications and mass media, a master's degree in science in administration, and a doctorate in healthcare administration. Most recently, he obtained the AHIMA's Certified Health Data Analyst (CHDA) credential. His healthcare career allowed him to visit Switzerland's World Healthcare Organization, the United Nations, and the Red Cross' offices. In addition to his academic and professional accomplishments, Dr. Brown has taught at the collegiate level for 10 years.

**Cindy Edgerton, MEd, MHA, RHIA**, is the health information management (HIM) program director at Charter Oak State College. Her professional background includes 30 years of experience as an educator and program director in HIM degree programs, including the development of one of the first online HIM associate degree programs. Currently, Ms. Edgerton has created and designed curriculum for countless residential and online courses. This experience has been instrumental in many successful HIM program accreditations. She has been very involved in both AHIMA and the Minnesota Health Information Management Association (MNHIMA). She was an elected board member for MNHIMA and an appointed member of the AHIMA Council for Excellence in Education. She has presented at the national AHIMA Assembly on Education conference for several years and was a presenter for the Train-the-Trainer Personal Health Record initiative. Ms. Edgerton graduated with a bachelor's degree in health information administration with a minor in management from the College of St. Scholastica. In 2007, she obtained her master of education degree with a specialization in leadership in higher education from Capella University. She earned a second master's degree, in healthcare administration, from Kaplan University in 2015. She has been a Registered Health Information Administrator (RHIA) since 1987.

**David L. Gibbs, PhD, CHDA, CHPS, CISSP, CPHIMS, CPHI, FHIMSS**, is the chair and an associate professor in the health informatics and information management department at Texas State University. He develops and delivers graduate and undergraduate courses online and on campus in the areas of health informatics, health information systems, and leadership. His research agenda combines the interrelated areas of health informatics and interprofessional education. He has written articles for various scholarly journals and textbook chapters. Dr. Gibbs earned a bachelor of science in computer science, a master of science in online teaching and learning, a doctorate in adult, professional, and community education, and a master's degree in applied biomedical informatics. He transitioned to academia from corporate and government consulting in 2015, with over 30 years of information systems experience. This included multi-year assignments with Hewlett Packard and Lockheed Martin, supporting enterprise-level projects for the Defense Health Agency and the Oak Ridge National Laboratory and National Security Complex. His most recent decade of consulting focused on federal healthcare information systems and solutions architecture. For his significant and sustained professional contributions, scholarly achievements, and leadership, Dr. Gibbs is recognized as a Senior Member of the Institute of Electrical and Electronics Engineers (IEEE) and a Fellow of the Healthcare Information and Management Systems Society (HIMSS).

**Karen A. Gibbs, PhD, PT, DPT, MSPT, CWS**, has been a faculty member in the department of physical therapy at Texas State University since 2004. Previously, she was on the faculty at the University of the Pacific and taught courses for East Tennessee State University. Dr. Gibbs served as chair of the College of Health Professions' curriculum committee and as a member of the university curriculum committee since 2013. She is the past president of the Academy of Clinical Electrophysiology and Wound Management, a component of the American Physical Therapy Association, and was instrumental in establishing the first profession-recognized national specialty certification for physical therapists in wound management through the American Board of Physical Therapy Specialties. Dr. Gibbs is well published and has given numerous local, state, national, and international presentations related to wound management and physical therapist education. Her professional service and academic contributions earned induction to the East Tennessee State University College of Clinical and Rehabilitative Health Sciences "Hall of Fame" in 2021. Dr. Gibbs holds a doctorate in adult, professional, and community education from Texas State University, a doctorate of physical therapy and master of science in physical therapy from University of the Pacific, and a bachelor of science in health education from East Tennessee State University. She is also a certified wound specialist through the American Board of Wound Management. Dr. Gibbs maintains her physical therapist license in Texas and Tennessee. Before entering higher education, she practiced as a physical therapist at Santa Clara Valley Medical Center, Los Gatos Community Hospital, and University Medical Center at Brackenridge with extensive experience in wound management.

**Barbara A. Glondys, MA, RHIA, CHPS**, is a clinical assistant professor in the health information management (HIM) program at the University of Illinois at Chicago. Her career in the HIM field includes work as a subject matter expert at AHIMA, management in both inpatient and outpatient HIM departments, sales, process-improvement consulting, education, and cost management. Ms. Glondys' work with the AHIMA VLab® in its early stages of development, coupled with experience using the applications in practice, enabled her to apply the technology available in the VLab with hands-on activities tailored to demonstrate the full functionality of these applications in HIM.

**Lauree Handlon, MHA, RHIA, CCS, CHCRS, CRCR, CSAF, FAHIMA, FHFMA**, is the vice president of reimbursement policy at the Craneware Group. She primarily leads the strategic development and implementation of consulting services for optimizing financial performance and regulatory compliance. With over two decades of experience in healthcare finance, revenue cycle management, coding, and reimbursement, she is committed to driving the industry's operational efficiency and financial sustainability. Currently pursuing a doctor of health administration (DHA) at the Medical University of South Carolina, she continues to leverage her experience to advance healthcare financial management through education, advocacy, and innovative policy development. Ms. Handlon received her master of health administration from the University of Cincinnati in 2017. She received a master's degree in allied health management through the School of Health and Rehabilitation Sciences from The Ohio State University in 2008. She received her bachelor's in health information management and systems from The Ohio State University in 2000. Ms. Handlon was a part-time instructor and a clinical site preceptor for the HIMS Department in the School of Health and Rehabilitation Sciences at The Ohio State University for more than fifteen years. She has presented numerous educational sessions for the Healthcare Financial Management Association (HFMA), Central Ohio Patient Account Managers, Ohio Health Information Management Association (OHIMA), and other HIM-related professional organizations. She has written several articles regarding provider payment issues and revenue cycle topics. She pilot tested many of CMS's Medicare Learning Network courses and has served as technical reviewer of various AHIMA textbooks. Ms. Handlon is a past-president and past two-term delegate for OHIMA. She is past president of the Central Ohio chapter of HFMA, the University of Cincinnati MHA Alumni Council, and The Ohio State University School of Health and Rehabilitation Sciences Alumni Society.

**Anita C. Hazelwood, EdD, RHIA, FAHIMA**, is a professor and the department head for health sciences in the College of Nursing and Health Sciences at the

University of Louisiana at Lafayette. She has written numerous articles, coauthored several textbooks, and authored chapters in a number of HIM textbooks. Dr. Hazelwood received the AHIMA Legacy Award and is a Fellow of the American Health Information Management Association. Dr. Hazelwood conducted numerous coding workshops at the local, state, and national levels.

**Shannon Houser, PhD, MPH, RHIA, FAHIMA**, is a professor in the health services administration department and graduate program in health informatics, school of health professions; a senior scientist in the Center for Clinical and Translational Science; a scholar of the Sparkman Center for Global Health; and an associate scientist in the Center for AIDS Research at the University of Alabama at Birmingham. With over 30 years of experience, Dr. Houser is a highly respected educator, researcher, and scholar who has made significant contributions to the fields of health information and informatics, healthcare administration, and public health at local, national, and international levels. As president of the Alabama Association of Health Information Management (AAHIM) and chair of the AHIMA Data Analytics and Data Use Practice Council, Dr. Houser is a renowned leader in the field. In addition to her teaching role, she has authored *Health IT and EHRs*, Seventh Edition, numerous textbook chapters and peer-reviewed articles, and served as a technical reviewer for many major textbooks. Dr. Houser is a mentor to countless students, faculty members, and peers, and her work has been recognized with several prestigious awards, including AHIMA's Triumph Research Award, Mentor Award, and Influencer Award, and the Distinguished Leadership Award of AAHIM. Dr. Houser's vast knowledge, experience, and unwavering commitment to the field make her an invaluable resource to the health services administration and health informatics communities. She is an inspiration to students and aspiring professionals alike.

**Thomas (T. J.) Hunt, PhD, RHIA, CHDA, FAHIMA**, is an assistant professor in the Department of Health Informatics at Rutgers University. He was previously associate dean and professor in the College of Health Professions at Davenport University. Before working in higher education Dr. Hunt served in leadership roles with Sparrow Health System, ProMedica Health System, and Mercy Health Partners. He is a past-president of the Michigan Health Information Management Association (MHIMA) and the Lake Huron Health Information Management Association. He is an elected commissioner of the Commission on Certification for Health Informatics and Information Management, previously served on the AHIMA Nominating Committee, and led the AHIMA Communities of Practice Committee as chairperson. Dr. Hunt is a Registered Health Information Administrator (RHIA) and Certified Health Data Analyst (CHDA) and was recognized as a Fellow of AHIMA and MHIMA Distinguished Member for service and contribution to the HIM profession.

**Katie Kerr, EdD, RHIA**, is director of the master in health information management (HIM) program and an associate professor in the department of health informatics and information management at the College of St. Scholastica. She also the academic coordinator of the professional practice experience program for undergraduate HIM students. She earned her doctor of education degree in leadership in higher education from Bethel University, and both her master's and bachelor's degrees in health information management from the College of St. Scholastica.

**Madonna M. LeBlanc, MA, RHIA, FAHIMA**, is an assistant professor in the health informatics and information management program at the College of St. Scholastica (CSS) in Duluth, MN, and a graduate of CSS's initial master of arts in health information management (HIM) program. Prior to her teaching role, she managed HI services at St. Mary's/Duluth Clinic Health System in Superior, WI. Her responsibilities included a broad spectrum of acute care HIM functions, from physician education to Joint Commission survey coordination. LeBlanc's field experience also includes cancer registry and physician peer administration. She was co-faculty for six years in the SHS Interdisciplinary Health Science Leadership course at CSS designed to provide transdisciplinary collaboration and problem solving in the healthcare setting. LeBlanc served for six years on the Minnesota Health Information Management Association's (MNHIMA) Board of Directors as director delegate and president, was a component state association community education coordinator for the AHIMA myPHR campaign, and volunteered on the AHIMA Council for Excellence in Education Community workgroup and the AHIMA Scholarship Committee.

**Scott Lee-Eichenwald, MSDD**, has diverse professional experience in social sciences and medical technologies. In addition, he taught online for more than 15 years. The bulk of his more than 20-year professional career has been spent working for medical devices companies. He managed research and development projects and many large-scale technology implementation projects on a global scale. Mr. Lee-Eichenwald received his Six Sigma Green Belt certification from the University of St. Thomas in 2012, and an information systems security certificate from Colorado Technical University in 2005. He earned a bachelor of arts degree in psychology from the College of St. Scholastica in 1992, and a master of software design and development from the University of St. Thomas in 2001. Mr. Lee-Eichenwald gained his professional experience working for Guidant, Boston Scientific, Medtronic, and Smiths Medical.

**Charisse Madlock-Brown, PhD, MLS**, is a faculty member in health informatics at the University of Iowa College of Nursing. She received her master of library science and doctor of philosophy degrees in health informatics from the University of Iowa. Dr. Madlock-Brown has expertise in data management, data mining, and visualization. She has a broad background in health informatics with a current focus on social determinants of health, COVID-19, health disparities, obesity trends, and multimorbidity. Her other areas of interest are network analysis and emerging topic detection in biomedicine. Dr. Madlock-Brown uses machine learning and biostatistics to analyze large electronic health record data warehouses. She authored several book chapters and journal articles and continues to keep up to date on data integration, data architecture, database management, and analytic methods.

**David Marc, PhD, CHDA**, is an associate professor, the health informatics and information management department chair, and the health informatics graduate program director at the College of St. Scholastica in Duluth, MN. Dr. Marc has a master's degree in biological sciences and a doctorate in health informatics from the University of Minnesota, and is a Certified Health Data Analyst (CHDA). He served as the former chair of the AHIMA foundation research network and as a member of the AHIMA Council for Excellence in Education, where he co-chaired the Educational Programming Workgroup. Dr. Marc also served on the Healthcare Information and Management Systems Society (HIMSS) Informatics Scholars Workgroup and the HIMSS Student and Early Careerists Committee. Dr. Marc is a frequent speaker at state and national meetings and workshops where he addresses topics related to healthcare data analytics. He is an accomplished researcher and author on topics related to health informatics and information management workforce trends.

**Rosann M. McLean, DHSc, MS, RHIA, CDIP**, is chair of the health information management (HIM) department at the University of Kansas School of Health Professions. In addition to her administrative role, she serves as a clinical assistant professor, teaching healthcare management, classifications and terminologies, and information governance courses. She is active in campus leadership, serving in a variety of capacities. Her scholarly activities include providing expert reviews of scholarly articles, textbook chapters, and a textbook on the topic of electronic health records. She was also the lead author of a textbook on the topic of ICD-10-CM and ICD-10-PCS and authored a chapter in prior editions of this textbook. Her service to the HIM profession has included volunteer roles as a commissioner of the Commission on Certification for Health Informatics and Information Management, member on the AHIMA Consumer Engagement and Clinical Terminology and Classification practice councils, service on the AHIMA Foundation Research and Periodicals Workgroup, and various elected roles through her component state association. Prior to her academic career, she primarily worked in acute care hospitals, managing HIM operations and serving on institutional committees such as HIPAA privacy, HIPAA security, oncology services, and clinical ethics.

**Brandon D. Olson, PhD, PMP**, is a professor and director of the master of science in applied data analytics at the College of St. Scholastica. Dr. Olson holds a doctor of philosophy in information technology with a specialization in project management and a master's degree in computer information resource management. His research interests include project management, data analytics, knowledge management, and IT strategy. Prior to entering academia, Dr. Olson worked as a project manager in the pharmaceutical, healthcare, and business services industries. Dr. Olson also consults in the areas of project management, data analytics, and governance.

**Brooke Palkie, EdD, RHIA, CPHIMS, FAHIMA**, is the health sciences and technology department chair and program director for the master of health informatics and master of healthcare administration programs at Charter Oak State College. Dr. Palkie is an AHIMA-approved ICD-10-CM/PCS trainer and has led numerous educational programs and grant-funded initiatives. Her teaching expertise spans clinical classifications and data standards, health informatics, healthcare quality assessment, and corporate compliance. She is a frequent author and speaker, contributing extensively to professional publications and conferences. Dr. Palkie actively serves in leadership roles within state, regional, and national professional associations.

**Rick Revoir, EdD, MBA, CPA**, is dean of strategic development at the College of St. Scholastica. He holds a doctor of education from the University of Minnesota–Duluth and a master of business administration from Arizona State University. He currently serves as president of the Duluth Seaway Port Authority Board of Commissioners. Prior to joining higher education, he worked for 11 years in a variety of healthcare finance positions.

**Laurie A. Rinehart-Thompson, JD, RHIA, CHP, FAHIMA**, is a professor and the director of the Health Information Management and Systems program at The Ohio State University. She earned both her bachelor of science degree in medical record administration and her juris doctor degree from The Ohio State University. In addition to HIM education, her professional experiences span the behavioral health, home health, and acute care arenas. Dr. Rinehart-Thompson has served as an expert witness in civil litigation, testifying as to the privacy and confidentiality of health information. She served as the chair of the AHIMA Professional Ethics Committee, on the Council on Excellence in Education, and in multiple AHIMA workgroups. She serves on the Ohio Health Information Management Association Board of Directors. A speaker on the HIPAA Privacy Rule, she is the author of AHIMA's *Introduction to Health Information Privacy and Security*, a co-editor and author of AHIMA's *Fundamentals of Law for Health Informatics and Information Management*, and a contributing author to *Ethical Challenges in the Management of Health Information*, and AHIMA's *Health Information Management Technology: An Applied Approach*, *Documentation for Health Records*, and *Introduction to Healthcare Informatics*. She has been published in the *Journal of AHIMA* and *Perspectives in Health Information Management*. She has received both the Ohio Health Information Management Association's Distinguished Member Award and the AHIMA Legacy Award.

**Ryan Sandefer, PhD**, is the vice president for Academic Affairs at the College of St. Scholastica. He is also an associate professor in the health informatics and information management department at the College of St. Scholastica. He is responsible for coordinating and integrating planning efforts around new and expanding academic programs. Using data analytics and metrics, Dr. Sandefer deepens the college's culture of evidence and the use of data for strategic decision-making. He ensures the alignment of initiatives with the college's mission and values, especially the challenge of creating community among online and extended site learners. Dr. Sandefer completed his doctor of philosophy in health informatics at the University of Minnesota and has a master's degree in political science from the University of Wyoming. Dr. Sandefer served as the chair of the AHIMA Council for Excellence in Education, was a presenter for the AHIMA data analytics workshops, and acted as an instructor for the Certified Health Data Analytics (CHDA) exam preparation workshops. He served on the AHIMA Board of Directors from 2022 to 2024. Dr. Sandefer has extensive experience working with large healthcare datasets and analytic procedures.

**Marcia Sharp, EdD, MBA, RHIA, FAHIMA**, is an associate professor and program director at the University of Tennessee Health Science Center in the health informatics and information management program. She teaches leadership, information technology, statistics, quality, and knowledge management. Prior to teaching, Dr. Sharp served in HIM leadership roles for over 15 years. She also has human resources (HR) experience as an HR director and retired from the US Navy Reserve. Previously, Dr. Sharp served as member of AHIMA's Council for Excellence in Education (CEE). Additionally, she served on the CEE's faculty development workgroup and as a delegate for the Tennessee Health Information Management Association (THIMA). Currently, Dr. Sharp is a reviewer for AHIMA's *Perspectives in Health Information Management* journal. She holds a doctorate in higher and adult education from the University of Memphis, a master of business administration from Webster University, and a bachelor of science in health information management from the University of Tennessee.

**Eric S. Swirsky, JD, MA, MHPE**, is a clinical associate professor and the director of graduate studies in the biomedical and health information sciences department. He also serves as associate director of the BA/MD program and co-lead for the health humanities curriculum in the College of Medicine's Department of Medical Education at UIC. Mr. Swirsky has created applied ethics and professionalism curricula across disciplines from the undergraduate through the post-doctoral levels. He has received numerous awards and distinctions related to teaching excellence including appointments as a UIC Master Teaching Scholar and chair of UIC's Teaching Recognition Program. Mr. Swirsky is past chair of the board of directors of the Commission on Accreditation for Health Informatics and Information Management Education (CAHIIM). He currently serves on the board of directors of the Council on Accreditation of Nurse Anesthesia Educational Programs and on the editorial board of the *American Journal of Bioethics*. His scholarly interests have focused on ethical conundrums attendant to the use of digital and information technologies in healthcare. In particular, he is interested in impacts upon clinical relationships, the delivery of health services, and end of life decision-making. His areas of expertise reside in topics related to ethical use of data, medical technologies, moral distress, and the sociotechnical milieu in which they converge. He received a bachelor of arts in religious studies from Ithaca College, a master of arts in South Asian Studies from the University of Wisconsin–Madison, a juris doctor from American University, and a master's degree in health professions education at UIC. He completed a fellowship in clinical medical ethics at the University of Chicago MacLean Center.

**Braden Michael Tabisula, MBA, RHIA, CHDA**, is the program coordinator of the master's-level health informatics program at Loma Linda University, where he is also an assistant professor. He earned a master of business administration degree from the University of Redlands and a bachelor's degree in health information management from Loma Linda University. He is currently pursuing a doctorate in computer information systems and technology from Claremont Graduate University.

**Megan R. Tober, MBA, RHIA**, is an assistant professor, associate department chair, and program director of the health information management and cancer tumor registry undergraduate programs in the College of Health Professions at Davenport University's allied health and information management department. She teaches courses related to health information technology, healthcare management, and information management. She has more than 20 years of experience in healthcare and HIM education. Her career includes a variety of positions, both managerial and professional, in the areas of external peer review, quality improvement, medical staff credentialing, human resources, Joint Commission coordination, information technology and coding. She has served as an AHIMA scholarship reviewer since 2022. She won the mentor of the year award from the Michigan Health Information Management Association in 2022.

**Amy L. Watters, EdD, RHIA, FAHIMA**, is a professor at the College of St. Scholastica. She teaches courses related to health information technology, best practices in HIM, management and leadership, and applied research and writing. She has more than 25 years of HIM experience in a variety of areas, such as release of information, HIM and admitting management in acute-care settings, product management at a software and consulting firm, and HIPAA security at a multispecialty physician group. In addition to serving as coeditor of the 5th and 6th editions of this textbook, Dr. Watters has coauthored chapters related to privacy and security in two other textbooks, and published work in various peer-reviewed publications. She served on the board of directors of the Minnesota Health Information Management Association and the Minnesota Healthcare Information and Management Systems Society, has been president of the Northeastern Minnesota Health Information Management Association, and previously served on the Commission on Accreditation for Health Informatics and Information Management Education HIM Accreditation Council. In addition to both a bachelor's and master's degree in HIM, she has a doctorate in education. Dr. Watters' research focuses on community and its impact on online learning.

**Susan White, PhD, RHIA, CHDA**, was the 2014 recipient of the Literary Legacy Award for her text *A Practical Approach to Analyzing Healthcare Data*. Dr. White is the chief analytics officer (CAO) at The Ohio State University Wexner Medical Center. As the CAO, she has responsibility for the enterprise analytics function for The Ohio State University health system. Dr. White served on AHIMA's National Board of Directors from 2015 to 2018. She is the author of AHIMA's *A Practical Approach to Analyzing Healthcare Data*, *Principles of Finance for Health Information and Informatics Professionals*, *Certified Health Data Analytics Exam Preparation*, *Calculating and Reporting Healthcare Statistics, Sixth Edition*, and many peer- and editor-reviewed articles. Dr. White is a regular presenter at the state and national level on healthcare data analytics, alternative payment models, and big data. She earned her doctor of philosophy in statistics from The Ohio State University. In 2016, Dr. White was honored with the Ohio Health Information Management Association (OHIMA) Professional Achievement Award.

# Acknowledgments

The volume editors and AHIMA Press staff would like to acknowledge Kathleen LaTour, MA, RHIA, FAHIMA, and Shirley Eichenwald-Maki, MBA, RHIA, FAHIMA, as the founding editors of this textbook. Their vision led to the creation of a practical, comprehensive resource written by industry experts for the education of future leaders in healthcare. We would like to express appreciation to the many authors who contributed chapters to this textbook. They willingly shared their expertise, met tight deadlines, accepted feedback, and contributed to building the body of knowledge related to health information management. Writing a chapter is a time-consuming and demanding task, and we are grateful for the authors' contributions.

We would also like to thank authors who contributed to previous editions of this textbook:

- Margret K. Amatayakul, MBA, RHIA, CHPS, CPEHR, FHIMSS
- Rita K. Bowen, MA, RHIA, CHPS, SSGB
- Elizabeth D. Bowman, RHIA, FAHIMA
- Bonnie S. Cassidy, MPA, RHIA, FAHIMA, FHIMSS
- Nadinia Davis, MBA, RHIA, CCS, CHDA, FAHIMA
- Chris R. Elliott, MS, RHIA
- Mehnaz Farishta, MS
- Susan H. Fenton, PhD, MBA, RHIA, FAHIMA
- Margaret M. (Maggie) Foley, PhD, RHIA, CCS
- Elizabeth Forrestal, PhD, RHIA, CCS, FAHIMA
- Sandra R. Fuller, MA, RHIA, FAHIMA
- Kathy Giannangelo, RHIA, CCS, CPHIMS, FAHIMA
- Leslie L. Gordon, MS, RHIA, FAHIMA
- Morley L. Gordon, RHIT
- Michelle A. Green, MPS, RHIA, CPC, FAHIMA
- Matthew J. Greene, RHIA, CSS
- J. Michael Hardin, PhD
- Laurinda B. Harman, PhD, RHIA, FAHIMA
- Loretta A. Horton, MEd, RHIA, FAHIMA
- Merida Johns, PhD, RHIA
- Diana Lynn Johnson, PhD
- Kathleen M. Kirk, PhD, RHIA
- Linda L. Kloss, MA, RHIA, FAHIMA
- Deborah Kohn, MPH, RHIA, CPHIMS, FACHE, FHIMSS
- Mary Cole McCain, MPA, RHIA
- Phillip McCann, MSC, MS, RHIA, CISSP
- Susan E. McClernon, PhD, FACHE
- Angela Morey, PhD, RHIA, CPHIMS
- Carol E. Osborn, PhD, RHIA
- Susan L. Parker, MEd, RHIA, FAHIMA
- Karen R. Patena, MBA, RHIA, FAHIMA
- Carol Ann Quinsey, MS, RHIA, CHPS
- Uzma Raja, PhD
- Rebecca B. Reynolds, EdD, RHIA, CHPS, FAHIMA
- Lynda A. Russell, EdD, JD, RHIA, CHP
- Rita Scichilone, MHSA, RHIA, CCS, CCS-P, CHC-F
- Patricia B. Seidl, RHIA
- Kam Shams, MA
- C. Jeanne Solberg, MA, RHIA, FAHIMA
- Carol Marie Spielman, MA, RHIA
- Cheryl Stephens, MBA, PhD
- David X. Swenson, PhD, LP
- Carol Venable, MPH, RHIA, FAHIMA
- Karen Wager, DBA
- Valerie J. M. Watzlaf, PhD, RHIA, FAHIMA
- Janelle A. Wapola, MA, RHIA
- Andrea Weatherby White, PhD, RHIA
- Frances Wickham Lee, DBA, RHIA
- Vicki Zeman, MA, RHIA

We also would like to thank the following reviewers who lent a critical eye to this edition: Amber Cucumber Sutton, MHA, RHIA, CHDA, PMEC, AIPEC; Brandy V. Gustavus, DHSc, MHA, RHIA, CSBI; Memory Ndanga, PhD, RHIA; and Kathleen Peterson, MS, RHIA, CCS, CPHI.

# Online Resources

## For Students

This book provides access to online learning tools and supplements to aid in mastering the subjects presented in each chapter. On the companion website you will find an online student workbook with assignments, activities, and a review quiz for each chapter, as well as the online appendices listed in the table of contents. To access the student resources, please follow the instructions behind the inside front cover of this book.

## For Instructors

Instructor materials for this book are provided only to approved educators. Materials include an instructor manual with a variety of activities and assignments, a test bank and chapter review questions with answer keys, full answer key for the Check Your Understanding questions, Microsoft PowerPoint slides, and a transition guide. Access to all student-facing resources is also included. Please visit https://www.ahima.org/education-events/education-by-product/books/ for further instruction on accessing instructor materials.

# Introduction

*Pamela K. Oachs, MA, RHIA, CHDA, FAHIMA, and Lisa M. Delhomme, MHA, RHIA*

As the healthcare industry recognized the importance of clinical recordkeeping and its impact on patient care and delivery, the health information management (HIM) profession emerged. Originally referred to as medical record science, the field of HIM has been a recognized profession for nearly 100 years. Today, HIM is described as the practice of acquiring, analyzing, and protecting digital and traditional medical information vital to providing quality patient care (AHIMA n.d.).

The role of the HIM professional, once known as medical record librarian, has evolved significantly over time. Changes in healthcare reimbursement systems, development of new healthcare delivery models, and advancements in medicine and technology have all contributed to the array of skills that HIM professionals must possess, and the diversity of jobs and settings in which they work. These professionals affect the quality of healthcare by linking clinical, administrative, technological, and operational functions. With expertise in advanced technology and a deep understanding of healthcare workflows, they play a crucial role in managing patient health information (AHIMA n.d.).

Although the core of the HIM profession has always been to collect and maintain high-quality health data, the methods to do so have changed as healthcare has become technology-driven. The HIM professional's knowledge and skills have transitioned manual management of paper-based records systems to a focus on managing electronic content. This transition has created an information-rich environment requiring a unique mix of clinical, management, and information technology competencies. Subsequently, HIM roles have grown to increasingly include data reporting and analysis.

The dynamic landscape of healthcare, marked by evolving regulations and technologies, necessitates the commitment of HIM professionals to ongoing learning and professional development. Health information professionals play a crucial role in navigating these changes by providing essential patient data that is accurate, complete, and readily accessible (AHIMA n.d.). When it comes to improving healthcare, they analyze data to identify trends and patterns to assist in developing targeted interventions to improve population health, track and report on quality indicators to enhance quality improvement efforts, streamline administrative tasks to reduce the burden on healthcare providers, accurately code and bill for services to optimize revenue while eliminating waste and abuse, and help to identify disparities in health outcomes to help clinicians address them (Nundy et al. 2022, 521).

Research studies conducted in 2019 and 2022 showed a demand for HIM professionals to possess a higher-education degree, technical proficiency in data analytics, in-depth knowledge of revenue cycle, current knowledge of compliance regulations, and an understanding of the overall flow of information within the healthcare industry (Nordgren et al. 2023). Professional credentials, such as the Registered Health Information Administrator (RHIA®), demonstrate that an individual has this sought-after competence. RHIA credential holders are valued in the healthcare industry and are prepared to offer their knowledge and skills to ensure in the proper collection, management, and use of health information.

While content expertise is undeniably critical to success as a HIM professional, the academic community and healthcare industry also recognize the importance of soft skills such as critical thinking, communication, and effective problem solving when developing a leader in the field. All of these skills are embedded in the HIM discipline and are core components of HIM leadership—communication skills, professionalism, and the concept of understanding organizational culture—all of which are critical for new and current HIM professionals alike (see figure 0.1).

**Figure 0.1.** Components of HIM leadership

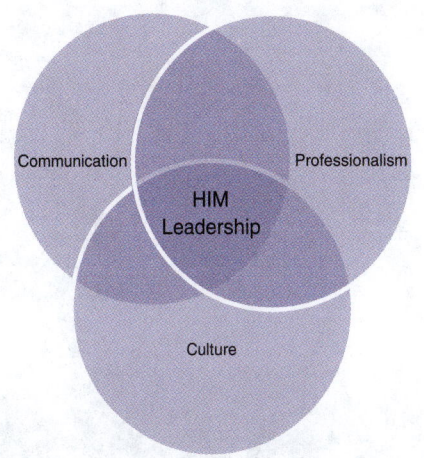

Communication skills include not only being able to write and speak clearly, but also to listen carefully. At its most basic level, communication is the exchange of information, which is central to health information management; effective communication is the foundation for quality care, efficient processes, strong relationships, collaboration, and a positive work environment. Communication skills are a key component of professional behavior as well as an organizational culture based on respect.

Professionalism is as integral to gaining respect in a chosen field as technical or content expertise. The ability to respectfully achieve results, meet goals, build relationships and network with others, adapt to change, be open to new ideas, and offer creative solutions are all characteristics of a strong leader. One can be a leader in their role or area of expertise by being confident in their knowledge, being honest and thoughtful, dependable, and collaborative. Being professional in all situations instills confidence and trust from others, which is essential for HIM professionals who serve as a bridge among people, systems, and concepts.

Understanding the workplace culture, and what impacts it, is another critical proficiency for the HIM leader. Thoughtful and effective communication skills along with consistent professional behavior create a culture of creativity, respect, and openness in the workplace. An environment where individuals are encouraged to share ideas, gain new skills, experience opportunities outside of their usual routine, and feel comfortable stating their opinions supports the development of strong leaders in HIM who can effect change (Mancilla et al. 2015). It is the efforts of these leaders who will make lasting contributions to the transformation of the healthcare industry.

# References

AHIMA (American Health Information Management Association). n.d. "Health Information 101." Accessed September 22, 2024. https://www.ahima.org/certification-careers/certifications-overview/career-tools/career-pages/health-information-101/.

Mancilla, D., C. Guyton-Ringbloom, and M. Dougherty. 2015 (June). Ten skills that make a great leader. *Journal of AHIMA* 86(6):38–41.

Nordgren, E., K. Kerr, and D. Marc. 2023. In an evolving industry, HI professionals must also grow and change. *Journal of AHIMA*. https://journal.ahima.org/page/in-an-evolving-industry-hi-professionals-must-also-grow-and-change.

Nundy, S., L. Cooper, and K. S. Mate. 2022. The quintuple aim for health care improvement. *Journal of the American Medical Association* 327(6):521. https://doi.org/10.1001/jama.2021.25181.

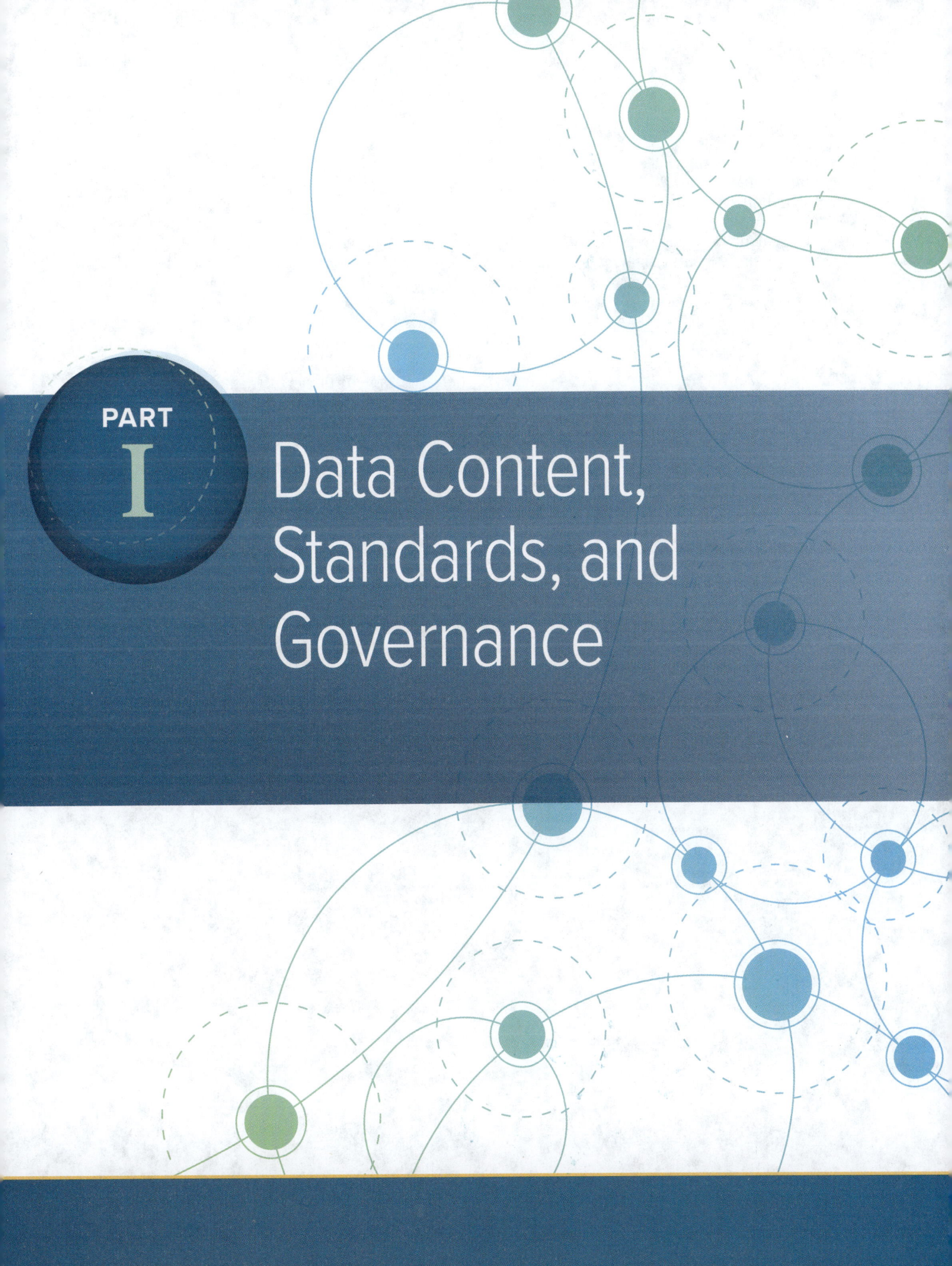

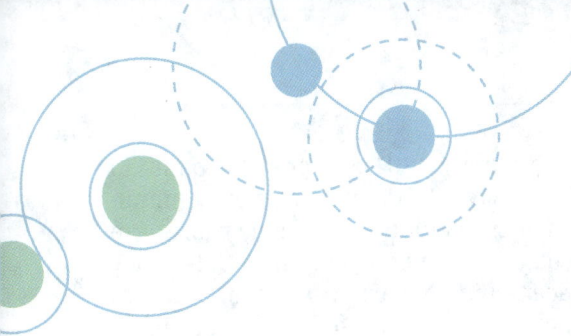

# chapter 1

# The US Healthcare Delivery System

*David L. Gibbs, PhD, CHDA, CHPS, CISSP, CPHI, CPHIMS, FHIMSS*
*Karen A. Gibbs, PhD, PT, DPT, MSPT, CWS*

## Learning Objectives

- Explain the evolution of US healthcare from its origins to the modern day
- Compare the basic organization of the various types of hospitals and healthcare organizations
- Differentiate a hospital-based healthcare organization from an integrated delivery system
- Evaluate the impact of external forces on the healthcare industry
- Discuss the systems used for reimbursement of healthcare services
- Assess the role of government in healthcare services

## Key Terms

Accountable care organization (ACO)
Accreditation
Acute care
Allied health professions
Ambulatory care
Biotechnology
Centers for Medicare and Medicaid Services (CMS)
Certification
Chief executive officer (CEO)
Clinical privileges
Continuum of care
Deemed status
For-profit healthcare organizations
Health maintenance organizations (HMOs)
Health reimbursement account (HRA)
Health savings account (HSA)
Home healthcare
Hospice
Hospital
Hospital outpatient
Inpatient
Integrated delivery system (IDS)
Interprofessional education (IPE)
Investor-owned hospital chain
Licensure
Long-term care
Managed care
Managed care organizations (MCOs)
Medicaid
Medical device
Medical staff
Medical staff bylaws
Medical staff classification
Medicare
Mission
Multihospital system
Network
Not-for-profit healthcare organizations
Peer review
Point of service (POS) plans
Post-acute care
Preferred provider organizations (PPOs)
Retail clinics
Skilled nursing facility (SNF)
Surgeon general
Value-based purchasing
Values
Vision
Workers' compensation

A broad array of healthcare services is available in the US today, ranging from simple preventive measures, such as vaccinations, to complex lifesaving procedures, such as heart transplants. An individual's contact with the healthcare delivery system may begin with family planning and prenatal care before birth and often continues through end-of-life planning and, potentially, hospice care.

Healthcare services are provided by an integrated interprofessional team of physicians, nurses, and other clinical providers who work in ambulatory care, acute care, rehabilitative and psychiatric care, and long-term care facilities. Healthcare services are also provided in the homes of hospice and home care patients. Additionally, assisted living centers, occupational health clinics, and public health department clinics provide services to many Americans.

While most healthcare is experienced locally and individually, healthcare is the single largest part of the US economy, consuming 17.3 percent of the gross domestic product (GDP) in 2022 (CMS 2023a). It is delivered by an ever-expanding variety of providers, from large multi-institutional integrated delivery networks (IDNs) to nurse practitioners within neighborhood drug stores, to providers visiting patients at home. Healthcare spending in the US grew to $4.5 trillion in 2022, and it is expected to grow 1.3 percentage points faster than the GDP over the next decade (CMS 2024f).

In 2024, there were 6,120 registered hospitals in the US (AHA 2024). Over 5,100 of those were community hospitals, which include nonfederal, short-term general hospitals and other specialty hospitals. They also include academic medical centers and teaching hospitals not owned by the federal government. About 24 percent of the community hospitals were for-profit and investor-owned, and over 3,500 were part of a system (AHA 2024). **Multihospital systems** include two or more hospitals owned, leased, sponsored, or contracted by a central organization. Hospitals can also be part of a **network**, which comprises hospitals, physicians, and other providers and payers that collaborate to coordinate and deliver services to their community (AHA 2024).

In addition to hospital systems and networks, there are other forms of organized healthcare delivery. US healthcare delivery involves a complex system of private and public institutions operating "in cooperation with, but largely independent of, each other" (Knickman and Elbel 2024, 16). These institutions face increasing pressure to provide high quality care from birth to death while reducing costs and improving access. This chapter discusses the origin and history of the healthcare industry in the US. Included in this history is the impact of external forces that have shaped the healthcare system of today.

## History of Western Medicine

Modern Western medicine can be traced to the ancient Greeks. However, it was not until the late 1800s that medicine became a scientific discipline. More progress occurred during the 20th century than over the preceding 2,000 years, with the past few decades including dramatic developments in the way diseases are diagnosed and treated and how healthcare is delivered.

Prior to the 1700s, people were largely treated at home, but population growth gave rise to hospitals. In Philadelphia, Benjamin Franklin and other colonists persuaded the legislature to develop the Pennsylvania Hospital, which provided care for physical and mental illness in the local community (Penn Medicine n.d.). The Pennsylvania Hospital, established in Philadelphia in 1752, was a model for the organization of hospitals with the New York Hospital opening in 1771 and Boston's Massachusetts General Hospital in 1821. A significant factor in the growth of Western medicine, the proliferation of hospitals created a locus for the standardization of medical practice and hospital care as well as the development of other health professions.

### Standardization of Medical Practice

The discovery of germ theory in the 19th century eventually led to more effective treatments for many diseases. However, there was very little standardization in the training or practice of medicine. The first attempts at regulation took the form of licensure. The first licenses to practice medicine were issued in New York in 1760. As the US population grew, the demand for medical practitioners far exceeded the supply. To staff new hospitals, many private medical schools appeared almost overnight. However, these programs did not follow established courses of study, with some requiring only six months of training before graduating. The result was poorly prepared physicians. The American Medical Association (AMA) was established in 1847, to represent the interests of US physicians (AMA n.d.). In 1876, the Association of American Medical Colleges (AAMC) was established to standardize US medical school curricula and to increase the public's awareness of the need to license physicians (AAMC n.d.).

Early in the 20th century, the push for medical school curricula reform and physician licensure was reinvigorated. In 1910, findings from Abraham Flexner's four-year curriculum study showed the poor quality of medical training. Reforms based on the Flexner Report required medical school applicants to hold a college degree, that medical training be founded on science, and that students receive practical hospital-based training. These changes resulted in about half of US medical schools closing in the subsequent 10 years (Cooke et al. 2006).

Today, medical school graduates must pass a standardized state-administered medical board exam before they can obtain a license to practice medicine. However, passing test scores vary by state. Most physicians also complete several years of residency training in addition to medical school.

Specialty physicians also complete extensive postgraduate medical education. Board certification for the various specialties requires the completion of postgraduate training and additional standardized testing. Common medical specialties include internal medicine, pediatrics, family practice, preventative medicine, and cardiology. Common surgical specialties include anesthesiology, orthopedics, and neurology. Some medical and surgical specialists undertake further graduate training to qualify to practice subspecialties. For example, some internal medicine subspecialties include endocrinology, geriatrics, hematology, pulmonary medicine, and rheumatology. Since 2013, physicians with specialization from the American Board of Pathology or the American Board of Preventative Medicine have been eligible to achieve a subspeciality in clinical informatics created in conjunction with the American Medical Informatics Association (AMIA n.d.). Additionally, physicians such as rheumatologists, endocrinologists, and podiatrists may limit their practices to the treatment of specific illnesses. Likewise, surgeons can work as general surgeons or in specialty or subspecialty areas such as orthopedics, cardiology, and neurology. For example, an orthopedic surgeon may limit their practice to surgery of the hand, knee, ankle, or spine.

Some physicians and healthcare organizations employ physician associates and assistants (PAs) and surgical assistants (SAs) to meet patient care demands. PAs require a master's degree to be licensed and practice under the supervision of licensed physicians. They may perform routine clinical assessments, provide patient education and counseling, prescribe medications, and perform simple therapeutic procedures. Most PAs work in primary care settings (AAPA 2024). SAs typically require a certificate or associate's degree but may receive on-the-job training. SAs assist surgeons with procedures during surgery, such as placing and holding clamps and closing surgical incisions (BLS 2024a). SAs work in hospitals and ambulatory surgery clinics (AAPA 2024).

## Standardization of Hospital Care

In 1910, Dr. Franklin H. Martin, the first editor of the *Journal of the American College of Surgeons*, suggested surgical care needed to pay better attention to patient outcomes (Townsend 2016). Martin learned these concepts from Dr. Ernest Codman, a British physician who thought that patient outcomes should be tracked over time to determine what treatment delivered the best results (Hazelwood et al. 2005).

At that time, Martin and other American physicians were concerned about the conditions in US hospitals. It was thought that the lack of an organized medical staff and lax professional standards contributed to the problems. In the early 20th century, hospitals were used mainly for performing surgery. Most nonsurgical medical care was still provided in the home. It was natural, then, for the force behind improved hospital care to come from surgeons.

The push for hospital reforms eventually led to the formation of the American College of Surgeons in 1913. In 1917, the leaders of the college asked the Carnegie Foundation for funding to plan and develop a hospital standardization program. The college then formed a committee to develop a set of minimum standards for hospital care and published the formal standards under the title of the Minimum Standards.

Adoption of the Minimum Standards was the basis of the Hospital Standardization Program and marked the beginning of the modern accreditation process for healthcare organizations. To this day, accreditation standards are developed to reflect reasonable quality standards, and the performance of each participating organization is evaluated annually against the standards. The accreditation process is voluntary. Healthcare organizations choose to participate to improve the care they provide to patients.

The American College of Surgeons continued to sponsor the hospital accreditation program until the early 1950s. In 1952, a new organization called the Joint Commission on Accreditation of Hospitals was formed by the American College of Physicians, the AMA, the American Hospital Association, and the Canadian Medical Association. The Joint Commission began performing accreditation surveys in 1953 (Joint Commission 2020).

Today, the Joint Commission surveys several types of healthcare organizations, including acute-care hospitals, long-term care facilities, ambulatory care facilities, psychiatric facilities, and home health agencies. Several other organizations also perform accreditation of healthcare organizations, including the American Osteopathic Association (AOA), the Commission on Accreditation of Rehabilitation Facilities, and the Accreditation Association for Ambulatory Health Care.

## Expansion of Health Professions

After World War I, many of the roles healthcare personnel played began to change. With the advent of modern diagnostic and therapeutic technology in the middle of the 20th century, the complex skills required of ancillary medical personnel necessitated specialized training programs and professional accreditation and licensure.

The term allied health professions appeared in 1966 with the Allied Health Professions Personnel Training Act, describing the expanding team of health professionals who work with physicians, nurses, dentists, and pharmacists. The Association of Schools of Allied Health Professions (ASAHP), established in 1967, further popularized the term for licensed or credentialed health professions distinct from medicine and nursing (ASAHP 2020).

These health professionals comprise nearly 60 percent of today's healthcare workforce and include health information management (HIM) professionals, dental hygienists, diagnostic medical sonographers, medical laboratory scientists, medical technologists, occupational therapists (OTs), physical therapists (PTs), radiographers, respiratory therapists (RTs), radiation therapists, audiologists, speech-language pathologists, and others (ASAHP 2020). All 50 states require licensure for some allied health professionals, such as OTs and PTs, while other professions may require licensure only in some states (AOTA n.d.). HIM professionals are certified rather than licensed.

In 2019, ASAHP was renamed to the Association of Schools Advancing Health Professions, dropping the term *allied* and reflecting further integration of health professions into one cohesive healthcare delivery team (Elwood 2019). The organization remains a driving force in healthcare education and a champion of interprofessional education and collaboration (ASAHP 2020).

## Interprofessional Education

Healthcare is increasingly delivered by interprofessional teams, so effective communication and collaboration among team members across disciplines is critical. Interprofessional education (IPE) has become an important element of education across all healthcare disciplines, including health information management (Peterson et al. 2023).

The World Health Organization (WHO) defines IPE as occurring when students from "two or more professions learn about, from, and with each other to enable effective collaboration and improve health outcomes" (WHO 2010, 13). It is important to emphasize that IPE involves learning *from* each other, which usually incorporates the other two factors of *with* and *about* each other. Healthcare professionals across all disciplines must have sufficient leadership ability to teach and learn together.

The Health Professions Accreditors Collaborative (HPAC) was established in 2014 to coordinate and provide guidance for IPE. HPAC now includes 25 accrediting organizations that represent almost all major healthcare professions. The Commission on Accreditation for Health Informatics and Information Management Education is one of the HPAC members that demonstrates commitment to IPE and the importance of HIM professionals engaging strongly as participants on the healthcare team (HPAC 2024).

IPE practices are significantly influenced by the Interprofessional Education Collaborative (IPEC), which formed in 2009. IPEC released the *Core Competencies for Interprofessional Collaborative Practice* in 2011, followed by version 2 in 2016, and version 3 in 2023. The primary IPEC competency areas remain (1) values and ethics, (2) roles and responsibilities, (3) communication, and (4) teams and teamwork (IPEC 2024). These competencies apply equally to all members of the healthcare team, including HIM.

### Check Your Understanding 1.1

**Answer the following questions in a separate document.**

1. Construct the timeline from the development of the first hospital in the late 1700s, to initial hospital reform efforts in 1910, to accreditation of healthcare organizations as it exists today by noting key milestones. Evaluate how these milestones have affected current Western medicine.

2. What issues in the early practice of medicine did the Flexner Report address? What actions resulted from it?

3. What educational path and examinations are required to become a pediatrician?

4. Determine why the push for hospital reform came from surgeons.

5. What elements are required to meet the WHO definition of interprofessional education? Why is it an important component of training across healthcare disciplines?

# Modern Healthcare Delivery in the US

20th century advances in medical science promised better outcomes and increased the demand for healthcare services in the US. However, even in the best economic times, many Americans have been unable to take full advantage of what medicine has to offer because they cannot afford it.

Concern over access to healthcare was especially evident during the Great Depression of the 1930s. During the Depression, US leaders were forced to consider how the poor and disadvantaged could receive the care they needed. Before the Depression, medical care for the poor and elderly had been handled as a function of social welfare agencies. During the 1930s, however, few people were able to pay for medical care. The problem of how to pay for the healthcare needs of millions of Americans became a public and governmental concern. Working Americans turned to employer-prepaid health plans to help them pay for healthcare, but the unemployed and the unemployable needed help from a different source.

## Effects of the Great Depression

The concept of prepaid healthcare, or health insurance, began with the Great Depression financial problems of one hospital—Baylor University Hospital in Dallas, Texas (Thomasson 2003). In 1929, the hospital's administrator arranged to provide 21 days of hospital services to Dallas's schoolteachers for a fixed six-dollar payment. Before that time, a few large employers had set up company clinics and hired company physicians to care for their workers, but the idea of a prepaid health plan purchasable by individuals had never been tried before.

The idea of public funding for healthcare services dates to the Great Depression. The decline in family income during the 1930s curtailed the use of medical services by the poor. In 10 working-class communities studied between 1929 and 1933, the proportion of families with incomes under $150 per capita had increased from 10 to 43 percent. A 1938 Gallup poll asked people whether they had put off seeing a physician because of the cost, and the results showed that 68 percent of lower-income respondents put off medical care, compared with 24 percent of respondents in upper-income brackets (Starr 1982, 271).

The decreased use of medical services and many patients' inability to pay meant lower incomes for physicians. Hospitals were in similar trouble. Beds were empty, bills went unpaid, and contributions to hospital fundraising efforts tumbled. As a result, private physicians and charities could no longer meet the demand for free services. For the first time, physicians and hospitals asked state welfare departments to pay for the treatment of people on relief.

The push for government-sponsored health insurance continued in the late 1930s, during the administration of President Franklin D. Roosevelt. However, compulsory health insurance (required by law) stood on the margins of national politics. It was not made part of the new Social Security program, and it was never fully supported by President Roosevelt.

## Postwar Efforts Toward Improving Healthcare Access

After World War II, the issue of healthcare access finally moved to the center of national politics. In the late 1940s, President Harry Truman expressed unreserved support for a national health insurance program. However, the issue of compulsory health insurance became entangled with America's fear of communism. Opponents of Truman's healthcare program labeled it "socialized medicine," and the program failed to win legislative support.

The idea of national health insurance did not resurface until President Lyndon Johnson's administration and the Great Society legislation of the 1960s. The Medicare and Medicaid programs were legislated in 1965. **Medicare** is a federally funded program that helps pay the cost of providing healthcare services to those 65 years of age and older as well as eligible individuals with disabilities. **Medicaid** is a joint federal and state program that assists with medical costs for those with low income. The issues of healthcare reform and national health insurance were again given priority during the first four years of President Bill Clinton's administration in the 1990s. However, the complexity of American healthcare issues at the end of the 20th century doomed reform efforts. Significant healthcare reform legislation was proposed by President Barack Obama and passed in 2010. The Patient Protection and Affordable Care Act (ACA) addresses healthcare costs, coverage, and quality. Effective in 2019, Congress repealed the ACA provision requiring Americans to have healthcare coverage by passing the Tax Cuts and Jobs Act in 2017.

## Influence of Federal Legislation

During the 20th century, Congress passed many pieces of legislation that had a significant impact on the delivery of healthcare services in the US. Many of these legislative efforts are described in table 1.1.

**Table 1.1.** Federal healthcare legislation

| Title | Date of enactment | Key provisions | Impact |
|---|---|---|---|
| Biologics Control Act | 1902 | Regulated the vaccines and serums sold via interstate commerce | Launched the research laboratories that later became the National Institutes of Health (NIH) |
| Social Security Act | 1935 | Provided states matching funds for maternal and infant care, rehabilitation of crippled children, general public health work, and aid for dependent children | Extended the federal government's role in public health |
| Hospital Survey and Construction Act (also known as the Hill-Burton Act) | 1946 | Authorized grants for states to construct new hospitals | Created a boom in hospital construction; hospitals grew from 6,000 in 1946 to a high of 7,200 |
| Public Law 89-97 | 1965 | Amendments to Social Security Act that created Medicare and Medicaid | Medicare provides healthcare benefits to citizens over the age of 65. Medicaid supports medical and hospital care for the medically indigent |
| Public Law 92-603 | 1972 | Expanded initial Medicare and Medicaid requirements for utilization review to include concurrent review; established the professional standards review organization (PSRO) program | Efforts to curtail the rising costs of the Medicare and Medicaid programs by evaluating patient care services for necessity, quality, and cost-effectiveness |
| Health Planning and Resources Development Act | 1974 | Created a system of local organizations called health systems agencies to make service and technology decisions | Along with other legislation of this type, unsuccessful in slowing cost increases and was repealed in 1986 |
| Utilization Review Act | 1977 | Required hospitals to conduct continued stay reviews to determine medical necessity of hospitalization for Medicare and Medicaid cases, also included fraud and abuse regulations | An additional effort to control growing healthcare costs |
| Peer Review Improvement Act | 1982 | Redesigned the PSRO program | Hospitals began to review medical necessity and appropriateness of hospitalizations prior to admission; in 2002, they were given a new name of Quality Improvement Organizations (QIOs) |
| Tax Equity and Fiscal Responsibility Act (TEFRA) | 1982 | Introduced the prospective payment system for Medicare reimbursement to control the rising cost of providing healthcare services to Medicare beneficiaries | Changed Medicare reimbursement from a fee-for-service model to a predetermined level of reimbursement |
| Prospective Payment Act/ Public Law 98-21 | 1982/1983 | Defined the prospective payment system and the use of diagnosis-related groups (DRGs) as the methodology for inpatient care | Prospective payment was successful at slowing the rate of growth of healthcare spending, so it was expanded to other service modalities like outpatient services in 2000 |
| Consolidated Omnibus Budget Reconciliation Act (COBRA) | 1985 | Allowed the federal government to deny reimbursement for substandard services provided to Medicare and Medicaid beneficiaries | Began establishing a link between quality and reimbursement for services in the Medicare and Medicaid programs |
| Healthcare Quality Improvement Act | 1986 | Established the National Practitioner Data Bank (NPDB) | Provides a clearinghouse for medical practitioners who have a history of malpractice suits and other quality problems |
| Omnibus Budget Reconciliation Act | 1989 | Instituted the Agency for Health Care Policy and Research now known as the Agency for Healthcare Research and Quality (AHRQ) | AHRQ mission is developing outcome measures to evaluate quality of healthcare services |

Continued

Table 1.1. Federal healthcare legislation (continued)

| Title | Date of enactment | Key provisions | Impact |
|---|---|---|---|
| Health Insurance Portability and Accountability Act (HIPAA) | 1996 | Addressed issues related to the portability of health insurance after leaving employment and administrative simplification of healthcare | Reduced the barriers to changing employers due to existing health conditions and created a federal floor for healthcare privacy |
| Mental Health Parity Act | 1996 | If mental health benefits are provided by an employer, it sets the annual and lifetime benefits equal to those for medical and surgical benefits provided | Began the discussion of equating mental health benefits with other health benefits; provided increased coverage for those with severe, disabling brain disorders |
| American Recovery and Reinvestment Act and the Health Information Technology for Economic and Clinical Health (HITECH) | 2009 | Accelerated the adoption of and use of information technology in healthcare through economic incentives and planned future financial penalties Expanded HIPAA privacy protections and established regional extension centers | In 2009, 12% of hospitals and 22% of physicians had electronic health record systems (EHRs). By 2017, that number had grown to 96% and 82% respectively (ONC 2018) |
| Patient Protection and Affordable Care Act (ACA) | 2010 | Enacted to provide insurance coverage to more Americans by helping small businesses afford insurance for their employees and extending the age limit for children to be covered by their parents' insurance. It also extended coverage for pre-existing conditions. Mandatory coverage repealed by the Tax Cuts and Jobs Act of 2018 (Galan 2023) | Number of people with ACA health insurance marketplace coverage in 2024 was a record high of 21.3 million, adding almost 5 million over the previous year (CMS 2024a) |
| 21st Century Cures Act | 2016 | Provided funding for accelerated cancer research and neurologic and precision medicine research. It also included funding to help address the national opioid crisis and mental health issues. Support for streamlining drug and medical device approvals by the US Food and Drug Administration is part of this act along with the promotion of increased EHR use and further implementation of telehealth. | Brought about concerns over the type and quality of information used to support approval of products, prohibited information blocking, and encouraged interoperability (Orlousky 2024; Cures Act 2016) |

As the largest payer of healthcare services, the US government has a dual role of the population's health and ensuring federal money is well spent. Beyond the legislative activities outlined previously, the Department of Health and Human Services (HHS) is responsible for just over 20 percent of all federal spending. Its mission is to "enhance the health and well-being of all Americans, by providing for effective health and human services and by fostering sound, sustained advances in the sciences underlying medicine, public health, and social services" (HHS n.d.). Updated every four years, HHS's strategic plan for the years 2022 to 2026 contains five strategic goals:

- Protect and strengthen equitable access to high quality and affordable healthcare
- Safeguard and improve national and global health conditions and outcomes
- Strengthen social well-being, equity, and economic resilience
- Restore trust and accelerate advancements in science and research for all
- Advance strategic management to build trust, transparency, and accountability (HHS 2022)

In setting these goals, HHS advances its mission and establishes strategic direction for programs over this time period. These priorities are demonstrated in research and policy initiatives.

## Biomedical and Technological Advances in Medicine

Rapid progress in medical science and technology during the late 19th, 20th, and early 21st centuries revolutionized the way healthcare is provided. One of the most important scientific advancements was the discovery of bacteria as the cause of infectious disease. Another important technological development was the use of anesthesia for surgical procedures.

These 19th-century advances formed the basis for the development of antibiotics and other pharmaceuticals and the application of sophisticated surgical procedures in the 20th century. Research using messenger ribonucleic acid (mRNA) began in the 1960s with significant advances in vaccine science and technology early in the 21st century. These scientific innovations laid the foundation for the quick production of mRNA-based vaccines in response to the global COVID-19 pandemic in 2020 (NIH 2023).

Table 1.2 offers a timeline of key biological and technological advances. These advances continue today through research and development in the diverse discipline of biotechnology. **Biotechnology** is "the manipulation (as through genetic engineering) of living organisms or their components to produce useful usually commercial products (such as pest resistant crops, new bacterial strains, or novel pharmaceuticals)" (Merriam-Webster n.d.). Two categories of companies in the field of biotechnology are pharmaceutical and medical device companies. These companies conduct research on, develop, market, and distribute drugs for the healthcare industry.

A **medical device** is "any instrument, apparatus, implement, machine, appliance, implant, reagent for in vitro use, software, material or other similar or related article, intended by the manufacturer to be used, alone or in combination for a medical purpose" (WHO 2023).

**Table 1.2.** Key biological and technological advances in medicine

| Time | Event |
| --- | --- |
| 1842 | First recorded use of ether as an anesthetic |
| 1860s | Louis Pasteur laid the foundation for modern bacteriology |
| 1865 | Joseph Lister was the first to apply Pasteur's research to the treatment of infected wounds |
| 1880s–1890s | Steam first used in physical sterilization |
| 1895 | Wilhelm Roentgen made observations that led to the development of x-ray technology |
| 1898 | Introduction of rubber surgical gloves, sterilization, and antisepsis |
| 1940 | Studies of prothrombin time first made available |
| 1941–1946 | Studies of electrolytes; development of major pharmaceuticals |
| 1957 | Studies of blood gas |
| 1961 | Studies of creatine phosphokinase |
| 1961–2000s | Studies of mRNA and foundation for structure-based vaccine design |
| 1970s | Surgical advances in cardiac bypass surgery, surgery for joint replacements, and organ transplantation |
| 1971 | Computed tomography first used in England |
| 1974 | Introduction of whole-body scanners |
| 1980s | Introduction of magnetic resonance imaging |
| 1990s | Further technological advances in pharmaceuticals and genetics; Human Genome Project |
| 2000s | NIH creates roadmap to accelerate biomedical advances, creates effective prevention strategies and new treatments, and bridges knowledge gaps in the 21st century |
| 2010s | First transcatheter aortic valve replacement (TAVR) device<br>First artificial pancreas or closed-loop insulin delivery system |
| 2020s | COVID-19 pandemic<br>Rise of augmented intelligence |

 **Check Your Understanding 1.2**

In a separate document, match the descriptions with the appropriate legislation and respond to the listed questions.

1. _____ Hospital Survey and Construction (Hill-Burton) Act
2. _____ Tax Equity and Fiscal Responsibility Act
3. _____ Public Law 89-97 of 1965
4. _____ Omnibus Budget Reconciliation Act of 1989
5. _____ Public Law 92-603 of 1972
6. _____ Healthcare Quality Improvement Act of 1986
7. _____ Patient Protection and Affordable Care Act of 2010

8. \_\_\_\_\_ 21st Century Cures Act of 2016
   a. Created the Medicare and Medicaid programs to pay the cost of healthcare for the elderly and the poor
   b. Authorized grants for states to construct new hospitals
   c. Required concurrent review for Medicare and Medicaid patients
   d. Established the National Practitioner Data Bank
   e. Provided insurance to more Americans by helping small businesses afford coverage for employees
   f. Changed Medicare reimbursement from a fee-for-service basis to a predetermined level of reimbursement to control rising costs
   g. Instituted the Agency for Health Care Policy and Research (now the Agency for Healthcare Research and Quality) to develop patient outcome measures
   h. Encouraged health data interoperability and prohibited information blocking

9. Analyze the impact of federal legislation on healthcare over time. Determine at least one trend and discuss whether it is positive or negative.

10. Assess the role that legislation and federal policy have in US healthcare. Do you agree this role is appropriate for the well-being of all US citizens? Why or why not?

11. Explain how biotechnological research from the 1960s positively impacted global public health in the 21st century.

## Healthcare Providers and Settings

According to the US Department of Labor, a healthcare provider or health professional is an organization or a person who professionally delivers proper healthcare in a systematic way to any individual in need of healthcare services (29 CFR 825.118). Healthcare delivery can be viewed as a continuum that spans services delivered in ambulatory, acute, sub-acute, long-term, residential, and other care environments (such as home health, school system, prison system, freestanding emergency or urgent care centers, and primary practice). There are several alternatives for healthcare delivery along this continuum.

## Organization and Operation of Modern Hospitals

The term **hospital** can be applied to any healthcare facility that has an organized medical staff, permanent inpatient beds, around-the-clock nursing services, and diagnostic and therapeutic services. Most hospitals provide acute-care services to inpatients. **Acute care** is the short-term care provided to diagnose and treat an illness or injury. Individuals who receive acute-care services in hospitals are considered inpatients. An **inpatient** is a person who is provided with room, board, and continuous general nursing services in an area of an acute-care facility where patients generally stay at least overnight.

Physicians with admitting privileges at a hospital are responsible for deciding whether a patient should be admitted as an inpatient. The admission decision is a complex medical judgment requiring consideration of several factors, including the patient's medical history, current medical needs, resources available to inpatients and to outpatients, the hospital's admissions policies, and the relative appropriateness of treatment in each available setting. Factors to be considered include the following:

- The severity of the signs and symptoms exhibited by the patient;
- The medical predictability of something adverse happening to the patient;
- The need for diagnostic studies that appropriately are outpatient services (i.e., their performance does not ordinarily require the patient to remain at the hospital for 24 hours or more) to assist in assessing whether the patient should be admitted; and
- The availability of diagnostic procedures at the time when and at the location where the patient presents. (CMS 2021, 7)

The average length of stay (ALOS) in an acute-care hospital is 30 days or fewer. Post-acute care hospitals such as long-term care hospitals (LTCHs), with patient stays over 25 days, provide acute care–level services to support patients with intensive treatment such as respiratory therapy, health trauma treatment, and pain management in order for patients to return home. Other healthcare facilities that have ALOSs longer than 25 days are considered long-term care facilities. With ongoing advances in surgical technology, anesthesia, and pharmacology, the ALOS in an acute-care hospital was 4.6 days in 2016 (Freeman et al. 2018). During the COVID-19 pandemic, ALOS increased due to deferred care leading to sicker patients (AHA 2022). In addition, many diagnostic and therapeutic procedures that once required inpatient care can now be performed on an outpatient basis. For example, before the development of laparoscopic surgical techniques, a patient might have been hospitalized for 10 days after a routine appendectomy (surgical removal of the appendix). Today, a patient undergoing a laparoscopic appendectomy might spend only a few hours in the hospital's outpatient surgery department and go home the same day. The influence of managed care and the emphasis on cost control in the Medicare and Medicaid programs also resulted in shorter hospital stays.

In large acute-care hospitals, hundreds of clinicians, administrators, managers, and support staff must work closely together to provide effective and efficient diagnostic and therapeutic services. Most hospitals provide both inpatient and outpatient services. Outpatient care is considered ambulatory care. A hospital outpatient is a patient who receives hospital services without being admitted for inpatient care.

## Types of Hospitals

Modern hospitals are complex organizations. Much of the clinical training for physicians, nurses, and other health professionals is conducted in hospitals. Medical research is another activity carried out in hospitals. Hospitals are often classified according to the number of beds, type of services provided, type of patients served, for-profit or not-for-profit status, and type of ownership.

### Number of Beds

A hospital's capacity is based on the number of beds licensed, equipped, and staffed for patient care. The term *bed capacity* is sometimes used to reflect the maximum number of inpatients the hospital can treat. Hospitals with fewer than 100 beds are usually considered small. Most US hospitals fall into this category, but some large, urban hospitals have more than 500 beds. The number of beds is usually broken down by adult and pediatric beds. The number of maternity beds and other special categories (such as a burn unit) may be listed separately.

### Type of Services Provided

Some hospitals specialize in certain types of services and treat specific illnesses:

- *Rehabilitation hospitals* provide long-term care services to patients recuperating from debilitating or chronic illnesses and injuries such as strokes, head and spine injuries, and gunshot wounds. Patients often stay in rehabilitation hospitals for several weeks to months.
- *Psychiatric hospitals* provide inpatient care for people with mental and developmental disorders. In the past, the ALOS for psychiatric inpatients was longer than it is today. Rather than months or years, most patients now spend a few days or weeks per stay. However, many patients require repeated hospitalization for chronic psychiatric illnesses.
- *General acute-care hospitals* provide a wide range of medical and surgical services to diagnose and treat most illnesses and injuries.
- *Specialty hospitals* provide diagnostic and therapeutic services for a limited range of conditions (for example, burns, cancer, obstetrics and gynecology).

### Type of Patients Served

Some hospitals specialize in serving specific types of patients. For example, children's hospitals provide specialized pediatric services in many medical specialties. Cancer centers offer diagnosis and integrated treatment regimens for cancer. There are also hospitals that specialize in surgical care with even further specialization for cardiac or orthopedic surgeries.

### For-Profit or Not-for-Profit Status

Hospitals also can be classified based on their ownership and profitability status. Not-for-profit healthcare organizations use excess funds to improve their services and finance educational programs and community services. For-profit healthcare organizations are privately owned. Excess funds are paid back to the managers, owners, and investors in the form of bonuses and dividends.

### Type of Ownership

The most common ownership types for hospitals and other kinds of healthcare organizations in the US include the following:

- *Government-owned hospitals* are operated by a specific branch of federal, state, or local government as not-for-profit organizations. Government-owned hospitals are sometimes called public hospitals. They are supported, at least partially, by tax dollars. Examples of federally owned and operated hospitals include those operated by the Department of Veterans Affairs to serve retired military personnel. The Department of Defense operates facilities for active military personnel and their dependents, and federal and state-owned prisons supply healthcare for incarcerated inmates. Many states also own and operate psychiatric hospitals. County and city governments often operate public hospitals to serve the healthcare needs of their communities, especially those residents who are unable to pay for their care.

- *Proprietary hospitals* may be owned by private foundations, partnerships, or investor-owned corporations. Large corporations may own several for-profit hospitals, and the stock of several large US hospital chains is publicly traded.
- *Voluntary hospitals* are not-for-profit hospitals owned by universities, churches, charities, religious orders, unions, and other not-for-profit entities. They often provide free care to patients who otherwise would not have access to healthcare services.

## Organization of Hospital Services

The organizational structure of every hospital is designed to meet its specific needs. For example, most acute-care hospitals are made up of an executive administrative staff, a board of directors, a professional medical staff, nursing (patient care) services, diagnostic and laboratory services, and support services (for example, nutritional services, environmental safety, and HIM services).

### Administrative Staff

The leader of the administrative staff is the **chief executive officer (CEO)**. The CEO is responsible for implementing the policies and strategic direction set by the hospital's board of directors. The CEO is also responsible for building an executive management team and coordinating hospital services. Most executive management teams include a chief financial officer (CFO), chief operating officer (COO), and a chief information officer (CIO). The team is responsible for managing hospital finances and ensuring compliance with federal, state, and local regulations, standards, and laws governing the delivery of healthcare services.

Depending on hospital size, the CEO's staff may include healthcare administrators with job titles such as vice president, associate administrator, department director or manager, or administrative assistant. Department-level administrators manage and coordinate activities of the highly specialized and multidisciplinary units that perform clinical, administrative, and support services in the hospital. Healthcare administrators may hold advanced degrees in health administration, nursing, public health, or business management. A growing number of hospitals are hiring physician executives to lead their executive management teams. Many healthcare administrators have master's degrees in health administration and are fellows of the American College of Healthcare Executives.

### Board of Directors

The board of directors has primary responsibility for setting the overall direction of the hospital. In some hospitals, the board of directors is called the governing board or board of trustees. The board works with the CEO and the leaders of the organization's medical staff to develop the hospital's strategic direction as well as its mission, vision, and values:

- *Mission:* A statement of the organization's core purpose and philosophies
- *Vision:* A description of the organization's desired future that sets direction and rationale for change
- *Values:* A descriptive list of the organization's fundamental principles or beliefs

Other specific responsibilities of the board of directors include the following:

- Establishing bylaws in accordance with the organization's legal and licensing requirements
- Selecting qualified administrators
- Approving the organization and makeup of the clinical staff
- Monitoring the quality of care

The board's members are elected for specific terms of service (for example, five years). Most boards also elect officers—commonly a chair, vice chair, president, secretary, and treasurer—but the size of governing boards varies considerably. Individual board members are called directors, board members, or trustees. Individuals serve on one or more standing committees such as the executive committee, joint conference committee, finance committee, strategic planning committee, and building committee.

The board's makeup depends on the type of hospital and the form of ownership. For example, the community hospital's board is likely to include local business leaders, representatives of community organizations, and others interested in the community's welfare. Likewise, a teaching hospital's board is likely to include medical school alumni and university administrators, among others. Boards of directors face strict accountability in terms of cost containment, performance management, and integration of services to maintain fiscal stability and ensure the delivery of high-quality patient care.

### Medical Staff

The medical staff consists of physicians with advanced training in various medical disciplines (for example, internal medicine, pediatrics, cardiology, obstetrics and gynecology, orthopedics, and surgery). The medical staff's primary objective is to provide high-quality patient care. Medical staff physicians diagnose illnesses and develop patient-centered treatment regimens. Physicians may also serve on the hospital's governing board, where they provide critical insight relevant to strategic and operational planning and policy making.

The **medical staff** is the aggregate of physicians and other approved practitioners who have been granted permission by a healthcare organization's governing board to provide patient services in the organization within specific practice limits. This permission is called **clinical privilege**. For example, an internal medicine physician would be permitted to diagnose and treat a patient with pneumonia but not to perform a surgical procedure. Most members of the medical staff are not employees of the hospital. However, there are exceptions as many hospitals employ radiologists, anesthesiologists, and hospitalists. Additionally, hospitals may contract with companies that provide physicians for specific services like emergency department physicians or radiologists.

**Medical staff classification** refers to the organization of physicians according to clinical assignment. Typical medical staff classifications include active, provisional, honorary, consulting, courtesy, and medical resident assignments. Depending on the size of the hospital and on the credentials and clinical privileges of its physicians, the medical staff may be separated into departments such as medicine, surgery, obstetrics, pediatrics, and other specialty services.

Officers of the medical staff usually include a president or chief of staff, a vice president or chief of staff elect, and a secretary. These offices are authorized by a vote of the entire active medical staff. The president presides at all regular medical staff meetings and is an ex officio member of all medical staff committees. The secretary ensures that accurate and complete minutes of medical staff meetings are maintained and that correspondence is handled appropriately.

The medical staff operates according to a predetermined set of policies called the **medical staff bylaws**. Bylaws spell out specific qualifications that physicians must demonstrate before they can practice medicine in the hospital. The bylaws are considered legally binding, and any changes to the bylaws must be approved by a vote of the medical staff and the hospital's governing body.

### Nursing Services

Nurses are responsible for providing continuous treatment and support for hospital inpatients. The quantity and quality of nursing care available to patients are influenced by several factors, including the nursing staff's educational preparation and specialization, experience, and skill level. There are various education levels in the field of nursing. These range from certificate programs for nursing assistants, one- to two-year programs for licensed practical or vocational nurses, bachelor's degree-prepared registered nurses, and graduate and doctoral-level training for nurse practitioners, midwives, and nurse specialists (Morris 2024). As nursing services are delivered around the clock, most direct patient care delivered in hospitals is provided by nurses.

Modern nursing requires a diverse skill set, advanced clinical competencies, and postgraduate education. Today's nurses play a wide role in treatment planning and case management. They identify timely and effective interventions in response to an extensive range of problems related to the patients' treatment, comfort, and safety. Responsibilities include performing patient assessments, creating care plans, delivering patient treatment, and evaluating the appropriateness of treatment and effectiveness of care. Nurses offer personal care that recognizes the patients' health concerns as well as the emotional needs of patients and their families. While registered nurses (RN) work in conjunction with physicians, advanced education and training provide nurses with opportunities for autonomous (independent) practice (Morris 2023). For example, nurse practitioners (NP) evaluate, diagnose, treat, and prescribe medication for patients independent of physician involvement in a variety of settings including acute care, adult health, oncology, pediatrics, and neonatal health (AANP n.d.). Certified nursing assistants (CNAs) work under the supervision of registered nurses. CNAs perform tasks such as taking vital signs, basic hygiene care, and supporting patient mobility (Munday 2022). Patient care technicians (PCTs) have similar skills and may receive advanced training and certification (HealthJob 2024). In almost every hospital, patient care services constitute the largest clinical department in terms of staffing, budget, specialized services offered, and clinical expertise required.

### Diagnostic and Therapeutic Services

Diagnostic and therapeutic services patients receive in hospitals go beyond the clinical services medical and nursing staff provide. Many diagnostic and therapeutic services involve the work of health professionals who receive specialized education and training, whose qualifications are registered or certified by discipline-specific specialty organizations, and who are licensed by the state.

Diagnostic and therapeutic services are critical to the success of every patient care delivery system. Diagnostic services include medical laboratory, radiology, and nuclear medicine. Therapeutic services include communication sciences and disorders, occupational therapy, physical therapy, radiation therapy, and respiratory therapy.

***Medical Laboratory Science*** The medical laboratory is divided into two sections: anatomic pathology and clinical pathology. Anatomic pathology deals with human tissues and provides surgical pathology, autopsy, and cytology services. Clinical pathology deals mainly with the analysis of body fluids, principally blood, but also urine, gastric contents, and cerebrospinal fluid. Laboratory results assist physicians in clinical decision-making regarding patient diagnosis and treatment planning, as well as monitoring disease progression or regression over time. Physicians who specialize in performing and interpreting the results of pathology tests are called pathologists. Medical laboratory scientists (MLSs) who complete four-year bachelor's degrees perform advanced laboratory procedures and analyses, interpret findings, and work collaboratively with medical teams in problem solving. Medical laboratory technicians, typically completing two-year training programs and supervised by an MLS, collect, process, and analyze biological specimens (for example, blood, tissue, body fluids) and document results in medical records (ASCLS n.d.; BLS 2024b).

***Radiology*** Radiology involves the use of radioactive isotopes, fluoroscopic and radiographic equipment, and computed tomography (CT), magnetic resonance imaging (MRI), and positron emission tomography (PET) equipment to diagnose disease (ACR n.d.). Physicians who specialize in radiology are called radiologists. They are experts in the medical use of radiant energy, radioactive isotopes, radium, cesium, and cobalt as well as x-rays and other radioactive materials. Radiologists interpret x-ray, MRI, CT, and PET scan diagnostic images and recommend treatment based on results (ACR n.d.). Interventional radiologists deliver site-specific treatments internally using guided instruments. Radiology technicians are allied health professionals trained to operate radiological equipment and perform radiological tests under the supervision of a radiologist.

***Nuclear Medicine and Radiation Therapy*** Radiologists also may specialize in nuclear medicine and radiation therapy. Nuclear medicine involves the use of ionizing radiation and small amounts of short-lived radioactive tracers to treat disease, specifically neoplastic disease (that is, nonmalignant tumors and malignant cancers). Radiation oncologists manage, prescribe, and monitor the care of patients with cancer (ACR n.d.). Radiation therapy uses high-energy x-rays, cobalt, electrons, and other sources of radiation to treat human disease. In current practice, radiation therapy is used alone or in combination with surgery, chemotherapy, or immunotherapy to treat many types of cancer. Radiation therapy may be delivered through external beam therapy or applied internally through radioactive implants (brachytherapy) placed in or near the target area (ACR n.d.). Radiation therapists, who complete four-year bachelor's degrees, work with radiation oncologists and administer prescribed radiation treatments and assist in monitoring patient responses to therapy (ARRT n.d.; Mayo Clinic College of Medicine and Science n.d.). Some states require radiation therapists to be licensed.

***Communication Sciences and Disorders*** Communication sciences and disorders include audiologists and speech-language pathologists. Audiologists, who complete doctoral-level degrees, prevent, diagnose, and treat hearing loss and associated auditory disorders and balance issues for patients across the lifespan. Audiologists treat patients with a variety of hearing loss etiologies including medications and medical procedures, traumatic injury, anatomical abnormality, and noise exposure (AAA 2024). Speech-language pathologists (SLPs) also work with patients of all ages. With a minimum of a master's degree required for licensure, their scope of practice focuses on the diagnosis and treatment of patients with speech, language, swallowing/feeding, or cognitive disorders and may include patients with traumatic brain injury, stroke, stuttering, or autism (ASHA n.d.).

***Occupational Therapy*** OTs use a variety of everyday activities and creative problem solving to develop, improve, and restore functional independence in patients' daily lives. Therapy includes evaluation of the patient, joint selection of therapeutic goals, and the development of highly individualized intervention plans targeting quality of life activities such as bathing, dressing, feeding and swallowing, or return to work activities (AOTA n.d.). OTs treat functional impairments related to developmental deficits, birth defects, learning disabilities, traumatic injuries, burns, neurological conditions, orthopedic conditions, mental deficiencies, and psychiatric disorders (AOTA n.d.a.). OTs practice in a variety of settings including inpatient, outpatient, rehabilitative, and school-based systems, and may treat patients independently or as part of an interdisciplinary team. The educational requirement for OTs is a master's or doctoral degree (AOTA n.d.b.). Occupational therapy assistants (OTA), who are supervised by and may assist OTs in the delivery of care, are required to complete an associate's level degree.

*Physical Therapy* PTs provide patient-centered care focused on improving quality of life through injury prevention and wellness, improved functional movement, and pain reduction. PTs treat patients across the lifespan directly or through referral and provide rehabilitative and preventative services as part of interprofessional healthcare teams in various settings (for example, inpatient, outpatient, home health, industrial, emergency, schools, sports teams, and private practice). Through comprehensive examination and evaluation, PTs develop individualized, evidence-based plans of care that may include targeted exercise, balance and functional mobility, debridement and other wound management techniques, manual therapy, and the application of physical energies (for example, compression, electrical stimulation, negative pressure, and ultrasound) with an emphasis on patient education and self-care. Since 2016, PTs have been required to have a doctoral degree to enter the field. Physical therapist assistants (PTA), who are trained at the associate's degree level, may assist in the delivery of care under the supervision of a licensed PT (APTA n.d.). The profession offers clinical specialist certifications for PTs in cardiovascular and pulmonary physical therapy, clinical electrophysiology, geriatrics, neurology, oncology, orthopaedics, pediatrics, sports, women's health, and wound management (ABPTS 2024).

*Respiratory Therapy* Respiratory therapy is a healthcare profession dedicated to improving the lives of individuals with breathing and cardiopulmonary disorders. RTs provide comprehensive care to patients of all ages, ranging from premature infants with underdeveloped lungs to older adults with chronic respiratory diseases. Their responsibilities encompass a wide spectrum of activities, including assessment and diagnostic testing, therapeutic intervention and mechanical ventilation support, patient education, emergency care and resuscitation, and pulmonary rehabilitation. RTs may specialize in practice areas such as neonatal and pediatrics, adult critical care, sleep medicine, or pulmonary diagnostics and work in diverse settings (for example, hospitals, clinics, home health, and long-term care). They collaborate with physicians and other healthcare professionals to provide comprehensive care for patients with respiratory and cardiopulmonary challenges. RTs may have associate's, bachelor's, or master's level degree and may obtain either or both Certified Respiratory Therapist (CRT) or Registered Respiratory Therapist (RRT) certifications to be licensed (AARC n.d.).

## Ancillary Support Services

The ancillary units of the hospital provide vital clinical and administrative support services to patients, medical staff, visitors, and employees.

*Clinical Support Services* Clinical support units provide the following services:

- Pharmaceutical services
- Food and nutrition services
- HIM services
- Social work and social services
- Patient advocacy services
- Environmental (housekeeping) services
- Purchasing, central supply, and materials management services
- Engineering and plant operations

The pharmacy is staffed by registered pharmacists and pharmacy technicians. Food and nutrition services are managed by registered dietitians (RDs), who develop general menus, special-diet menus, and nutritional plans for individual patients. HIM services are managed by HIM professionals, typically those who hold credentials such as the Registered Health Information Administrator (RHIA®) or Registered Health Information Technician (RHIT®). Social work services are provided by licensed social workers and licensed clinical social workers. Patient advocacy services may be provided by several types of healthcare professionals; most commonly, RNs and licensed social workers.

*Administrative Support Services* In addition to clinical support services, hospitals need administrative support services to operate effectively. Administrative support services provide business management and clerical services in several key areas, including admissions and central registration, claims and billing (business office), accounting, information services, human resources, public relations, fund development, and marketing.

## Check Your Understanding 1.3

**Answer the following questions in a separate document.**

1. A 35-year-old patient was diagnosed with meningitis and received antibiotics each day during her three days in the hospital. This type of short-term care is considered _____.
   a. Outpatient care
   b. Ambulatory care
   c. Acute care
   d. Long-term care

2. The hospital provided shareholders with dividends from the profits of the previous fiscal year. This hospital is _____.
   a. For-profit
   b. Not-for-profit
   c. Privately owned
   d. Research-based

3. The Veterans Affairs hospital is considered a _____ hospital.
   a. Government-owned
   b. Voluntary
   c. State-owned
   d. Proprietary

4. The hospital's CEO is retiring at the end of the year. Selecting a new qualified CEO is the responsibility of _____.
   a. The board of directors
   b. Hospital administration
   c. The medical staff
   d. The nursing staff

5. A patient with a recent traumatic brain injury now has difficulty with talking, swallowing, and feeding. The healthcare professional specifically trained to help patients with these types of issues is _____.
   a. An audiologist
   b. A speech-language pathologist
   c. A registered nurse
   d. An occupational therapist

6. A patient who had a stroke must regain strength and coordination in the affected side to walk again. The patient is seen by a _____ for rehabilitation.
   a. Nurse
   b. Health information manager
   c. Physician
   d. Physical therapist

7. The hospital was recently cited during a Joint Commission survey for not having a comprehensive strategic plan. The _____ is responsible for taking action to resolve this issue.
   a. Chief financial officer
   b. Chief executive officer
   c. Chief nursing officer
   d. Chief information officer

8. A patient with cardiovascular disease is receiving an image-guided procedure where a small instrument is snaked through a vessel to deliver targeted, internal treatment. The healthcare provider that would deliver this treatment is a _____.
   a. Radiation technician
   b. Interventional radiologist
   c. Radiation oncologist
   d. Nurse practitioner

## Organization of Ambulatory Care

**Ambulatory care** is the provision of preventative or corrective healthcare services on a nonresident basis in a provider's office, clinic setting, or hospital outpatient setting. Ambulatory care encompasses all the health services provided to individual patients who are not residents in a healthcare facility. Such services include the educational services provided by community health clinics and public health departments. Primary care, emergency care, and ambulatory specialty care (including ambulatory surgery) can all be considered ambulatory care. Ambulatory specialists include gastroenterologists, neurologists, and cardiologists and others who perform a variety of diagnostic tests, procedures, and therapies in the ambulatory setting. Ambulatory care services are provided in a variety of settings including urgent care centers, free-standing emergency centers, school-based clinics, public health clinics, and neighborhood and community health centers.

Current medical practice emphasizes performing healthcare services in the least costly setting possible. This change in thinking has led to decreased utilization of emergency services, increased utilization of nonemergency ambulatory facilities, decreased hospital admissions, and shorter hospital stays. The need to reduce the cost of healthcare also has led primary care physicians (PCPs) to treat conditions they once would have referred to specialists. The need to reduce cost and to provide access led facilities to increase the use of PAs and NPs as these providers can offer both primary care to patients and specialized technical assistance to physicians.

Physicians who provide ambulatory care services fall into two major categories: physicians working in private practice and physicians working for ambulatory care organizations. Physicians in private practice are self-employed. They work in solo, partnership, and group practices set up as for-profit organizations. Alternatively, physicians who work for ambulatory care organizations are employees of those organizations. Ambulatory care organizations also employ other healthcare providers including nurses, PTs, medical laboratory scientists, psychologists, and social workers. In addition to private medical practices, there are a wide range of ambulatory care organizations including health maintenance organizations; hospital-based and freestanding surgery, emergency, and urgent care centers; health department clinics; home health agencies; and school, workplace, and prison health services agencies.

## Private Medical Practice

Private medical practices are physician-owned entities that provide primary care or medical and surgical specialty care services in a freestanding office setting. The physicians may have medical privileges at local hospitals and surgical centers but are not employees of those healthcare entities.

## Hospital-Based Ambulatory Care Services

In addition to providing inpatient services, many acute-care hospitals provide various ambulatory care services. These services include emergency services; trauma care; and outpatient surgical, diagnostic, and therapeutic services.

### Emergency Services and Trauma Care

A hospital-based emergency department (ED) provides specialized care for victims of traumatic accidents and life-threatening illnesses. In urban areas, many also provide walk-in services for patients with minor illnesses and injuries who do not have access to regular PCPs. Many physicians on the hospital staff also use the ED as a setting to assess patients with problems that may either lead to an inpatient admission or require equipment or diagnostic imaging facilities not available in a private office or nursing home. Emergency services function as a major source of unscheduled admissions to the hospital.

### Outpatient Surgical Services

Ambulatory surgery refers to any surgical procedure that does not require an overnight stay in a hospital. It can be performed in the outpatient surgery department (often referred to as "day surgery") of a hospital or in a freestanding ambulatory surgery center. Hospitals report that a growing number of all surgeries are performed in the ambulatory surgery setting (Steiner et al. 2020). The increased number of procedures performed in ambulatory settings can be attributed to improvements in surgical technology and anesthesia and the utilization management demands of third-party payers.

### Outpatient Diagnostic and Therapeutic Services

Outpatient diagnostic and therapeutic services are provided in a hospital or one of its satellite facilities. Diagnostic services are those services performed by a physician to identify a patient's specific disease or condition. Therapeutic services are services performed by a physician to treat the identified disease or condition.

Hospital outpatients fall into different classifications according to the type of service they receive and the location of the service. For example, emergency outpatients are treated in the hospital's ED for conditions that require immediate care. Clinic outpatients are treated in one of the hospital's clinical departments (such as physical therapy and medical laboratory) on an ambulatory basis. Referral outpatients receive special diagnostic or therapeutic services in the hospital on an ambulatory basis, but responsibility for their care remains with the referring physician.

## Ambulatory Care Services

Community-based ambulatory care services refer to services provided in freestanding facilities that are not owned by or affiliated with a hospital. Facilities can range in size from a small medical practice with a single physician to a large clinic with an organized medical staff. Among the organizations that provide ambulatory care services are specialized treatment facilities such as birthing, cancer treatment, dialysis, retinal care, diagnostic imaging, medical laboratory, and rehabilitation centers.

### Freestanding Ambulatory Care Centers

Freestanding ambulatory care centers provide emergency services and urgent care for walk-in patients. Urgent care centers provide diagnostic and therapeutic care for patients with minor illnesses and injuries. They do not serve seriously ill patients, and most do not accept ambulance cases.

Three groups of patients find these centers attractive. The first group consists of patients seeking the convenience and access of emergency services without the delays and other forms of negative feedback associated with using hospital services for non-life-threatening problems. The second group consists of patients whose insurance treats urgent care centers preferentially compared with physicians' offices. As they have increased in number and become familiar to more patients, many of these centers now offer a combination of walk-in and appointment services. The third group of patients are willing to pay a slightly higher copayment to use urgent care center physicians as their PCP for the added convenience of weekend and extended or 24-hour medical services.

In 2000, the first retail clinics opened and by 2016, the number had grown to more than 2,000 (Barnes et al. 2023). By 2024, due to a variety of reasons (PCP shortages, extended hours, and upfront pricing and convenience), that number has grown to more than 3,000. In 2019, 25 percent of children and nearly 33 percent of adults visited a retail clinic or urgent care center (AHA 2024b). Retail clinics treat non-life-threatening acute illnesses and offer routine wellness services such as vaccinations, sports physicals, and prescription refills. While most retail clinics are housed in pharmacies such as CVS and Walgreens, they are also located in grocery stores and large discount retail chains such as Walmart and Target (MarkWideResearch 2024). Visits to retail clinics are covered by most insurers, including Medicare.

### Freestanding Ambulatory Surgery Centers

Generally, freestanding ambulatory surgery centers provide surgical procedures that take anywhere from 5 to 90 minutes to perform and that require less than a four-hour recovery period. Patients must schedule their surgeries in advance and be prepared to return home on the same day. Patients who experience surgical complications and require a longer period of care are sent to an inpatient facility.

Most ambulatory surgery centers are for-profit entities. They may be owned by individual physicians, managed care organizations (MCOs), or entrepreneurs. Generally, these centers can provide surgical services at lower cost than hospitals because their overhead expenses are lower.

## Public Health Services

Although states have constitutional authority to implement public health programs, a wide variety of federal programs and laws assist them. HHS is the principal federal agency for ensuring health and providing essential human services. All of its agencies have some responsibility for prevention. Through its 10 regional offices, HHS coordinates closely with state and local government agencies, and many HHS-funded services are provided by these agencies as well as by private-sector and nonprofit organizations.

The Office of the Secretary of HHS has two units important to public health: the Office of the Surgeon General of the United States and the Office of Disease Prevention and Health Promotion (ODPHP). ODPHP has an analysis and leadership role for health promotion and disease prevention.

The surgeon general is appointed by the US president and provides leadership and authoritative, science-based recommendations about the public's health. The surgeon general has responsibility for the public health service workforce (HHS 2024).

## Home Healthcare Services

Home healthcare is a wide range of healthcare services that can be delivered in the home. These services include nursing services (such as catheter insertion, wound care, and well-being checks) and PT care (such as rehabilitation, strengthening and exercise, and wound care). The US home healthcare market was a $142.9 billion industry in 2022 and is projected to grow to $253.4 billion by 2030 (Grand View Research 2022). The two main reasons for explosive growth are the increased number of seniors as the large number of babies born after World War II reach 65, and the lower cost of home healthcare when compared to other post-acute services. Moreover, patients generally prefer to be cared for in their own homes, no matter how complex their medical problems.

In 1989, Medicare rules for home healthcare services were clarified to make it easier for Medicare beneficiaries to receive such services. Patients are eligible to receive home healthcare services from a qualified Medicare provider when they are homebound; when they are under the care of a specified physician who will establish a home health plan; and when they need physical or occupational therapy, speech therapy, or intermittent skilled nursing care. Many hospitals have formed their own home healthcare agencies to increase revenues and allow earlier hospital discharge.

## Voluntary Agencies

Voluntary agencies provide healthcare and healthcare planning services, usually at the local level and to low-income patients. Their services range from giving free immunizations to offering family planning counseling. Funds to operate such agencies come from a variety of sources, including local or state health departments, private grants, and different federal bureaus.

Common examples of voluntary agencies are neighborhood and community health centers, which offer comprehensive, primary healthcare services to patients who might otherwise not have access to healthcare. Often patients pay for these services on a sliding scale based on income or according to a flat rate, discounted fee schedule supplemented by public funding.

Some voluntary agencies offer specialized services such as counseling for victims of domestic abuse. Typically, these are set up within local communities. An example of a voluntary agency that offers services on a much larger scale is the Red Cross.

### Check Your Understanding 1.4

Answer the following questions in a separate document.

1. A 29-year-old person wakes up on Saturday morning with a very sore throat and a low-grade fever. What is the most appropriate setting to seek healthcare services? Explain why.
2. A 52-year-old person experiences severe chest pain, dizziness, and nausea on a Sunday afternoon. What is the most appropriate setting to seek healthcare services? Explain why.
3. A patient is scheduled for a routine colonoscopy, a procedure that requires general anesthesia, but takes less than two hours to complete. Where would this patient expect to be seen? Explain why.
4. Which of the various healthcare settings is(are) appropriate for completing sports physicals for three active teenagers involved in winter sports? Explain why.
5. A person just had a hip replacement and will be recuperating at a family member's house. The person will be alone during the day while everyone else in the household is at work. What options are there for physical therapy rehabilitation?
6. Which local or community-level healthcare facility typically provides sliding scale or free immunizations to low-income patients and families?

## Post-Acute Care

**Post-acute care** supports patients who require ongoing medical management or therapeutic, rehabilitative, or skilled nursing care (AHA 2019). Patients require frequent physician oversight and advanced nursing care but no longer require the acute interventions and diagnostic services of acute-care settings. It is delivered in a variety of environments, including LTCHs, skilled nursing facilities (SNFs), rehabilitation centers, and through home health services (AHA 2019). Some hospitals have special units for patients needing less monitoring and interventions than acute care, labeled subacute care (Knickman and Elbel 2024). In 2024, there were more than 420 LTCHs in the US (CMS 2024d). Covered by Medicare, LTCHs provide intensive long-term services for patients with complex medical problems. Medicare requires an LTCH to meet the same conditions of participation as an acute-care hospital; however, the ALOS must be greater than 25 days (Medicare.gov 2019).

## Long-Term Care

**Long-term care** is the healthcare rendered in a non-acute-care facility to patients who require inpatient nursing and related services for more than 30 consecutive days. SNFs, nursing homes, long-term care facilities, and rehabilitation hospitals are the principal facilities that provide long-term care. Rehabilitation hospitals provide recuperative services for patients who have suffered strokes, traumatic injuries, and other serious illnesses. Specialized long-term care facilities serve patients with chronic respiratory disease, permanent cognitive impairment, and other incapacitating conditions.

Long-term care encompasses a range of health, personal care, social, and housing services provided to people of all ages with health conditions that limit their ability to carry out normal daily activities without assistance. People who need long-term care often have multiple physical and mental disabilities. Moreover, their need for the mix and intensity of long-term care services can change over time.

Long-term care is mainly rehabilitative and supportive rather than curative. Moreover, healthcare workers other than physicians can provide long-term care in the home or in residential or institutional settings. For the most part, long-term care requires little or no clinical technology; however, there is growing adoption of electronic health records as essential technology in long-term care facilities (Dayama et al. 2024).

## Long-Term Care and the Continuum of Care

The availability and cost of long-term care is one of the most important health issues facing the US and the world today. In the US, by 2060, people over the age of 65 will double from 50 to 100 million (Haseltine 2018).

As discussed earlier, healthcare is now viewed as a **continuum of care**. That is, patients are provided care by different caregivers at several different levels of the healthcare system. In the case of long-term care, the patient's continuum of care may have begun with a primary provider in a hospital and then continued with home care and eventually care in an SNF. That patient's care is coordinated from one care setting to the next.

Moreover, the roles of the different care providers along the patient's continuum of care are continuing to evolve. Health information managers play a key part in providing consultation services to long-term care facilities with regard to developing systems to manage information from a diverse number of healthcare providers.

## Delivery of Long-Term Care Services

Long-term care services are delivered in a variety of settings. Among these settings are SNFs or nursing homes, residential care facilities, hospice programs, and adult day care programs.

### Skilled Nursing Facilities

The most important providers of formal, long-term care services are **skilled nursing facilities (SNFs)**, commonly called nursing homes. SNFs provide medical, nursing, and, in some cases, rehabilitative care around the clock. The majority of SNF residents are over age 65 and quite often are classified as the "frail elderly."

Many nursing homes are owned by for-profit organizations. However, SNFs may also be owned by not-for-profit groups and local, state, and federal governments. Nursing homes are no longer the only option for patients needing long-term care. Various factors play a role in determining which type of long-term care facility is best for a particular patient, including cost, access to services, and individual needs.

### Residential Care Facilities

New living environments such as assisted living and memory care centers are more homelike, less institutional, and are a focus in the current long-term care market. Residential care facilities now play a growing role in the continuum of long-term care services. Having affordable and appropriate housing available for older adults and people with disabilities can reduce the level of need for institutional long-term care services in the community. Institutionalization can be postponed or prevented when individuals live in safe and accessible settings where assistance with daily activities is available.

### Hospice Programs

**Hospice** is an interdisciplinary program of palliative care and supportive services that addresses the physical, spiritual, social, and economic needs of the terminally ill and their families. Hospice is based on a philosophy of care imported from England and Canada that holds that during the course of terminal illness, the patient should be able to live life as fully and as comfortably as possible but without artificial or mechanical efforts to prolong life. Hospice services are mainly provided in the patient's home with the goals of controlling pain, maintaining independence, and minimizing the stress and trauma of death. The number of hospices is likely to continue to grow because this philosophy of care for people at the end of life has become a model for the nation.

### Adult Day Care Programs

Adult day care programs or day health centers offer a wide range of health and social services to adults during daytime hours. These centers are typically used by older adults in families where their regular caregivers work during the day. Many older adults who live alone also benefit from participating in programs designed to keep them active. The goals of adult day care programs are to delay the need for institutionalization and to provide respite for caregivers.

## Behavioral Health Services

From the mid-19th century to the mid-20th century, psychiatric services in the US were based primarily in long-stay institutions supported by state governments, and patterns of practice were relatively stable. Over the past 50 years, however, remarkable changes have occurred. These changes include a reversal of the balance between institutional and community care, inpatient and outpatient services, and individual and group practice.

The shift to community-based settings began in the public sector, and community settings remain dominant. The private sector's bed capacity increased in the 1970s and 1980s, including psychiatric units in nonfederal general hospitals, private psychiatric hospitals, and residential treatment centers for adults and children. Substance abuse centers and child and adolescent inpatient psychiatric units grew particularly quickly in the 1980s, as investors recognized their profitability. In the 1990s, the growth of inpatient private mental health facilities leveled off and the number of outpatient and partial treatment settings increased sharply. The number of mental health organizations providing 24-hour services (hospital inpatient and residential treatment) increased significantly over the 32-year period from 1970 to 2002 (Foley et al. 2004). Community hospitals are the primary source of inpatient psychiatric care delivered in either designated psychiatric units or in scatter beds throughout the medical units due to the closure of public psychiatric hospitals (Mark et al. 2010). However, in the last decade the number of nonfederal psychiatric hospitals has grown to 659 (AHA 2024a).

Residential treatment centers for children with behavioral health issues provide inpatient services to children under 18 years of age. The programs and physical facilities of residential treatment centers are designed to meet patients' daily living, schooling, recreational, socialization, and routine medical care needs.

Day hospital or day treatment programs occupy one niche in the spectrum of behavioral healthcare settings. Although some provide services seven days a week, many programs provide services only during business hours. Day treatment patients spend most of the day in structured therapeutic activities and return to their homes until the next day. Day treatment services include psychotherapy, pharmacology, occupational therapy, and other types of rehabilitation services. These programs provide alternatives to inpatient care or serve as transitions from inpatient to outpatient care or discharge. They also may provide respite for family caregivers and a place for rehabilitating or maintaining chronically ill patients. The number of day treatment programs has increased in response to pressures to decrease the length of hospital stays.

Insurance coverage for behavioral healthcare continues to lag behind coverage for other medical care. Although treatments and settings have changed, rising healthcare costs and insurers' continuing fear of the potential cost of this coverage have maintained the differences between medical and behavioral healthcare benefits. Most individuals covered by health insurance have some outpatient psychiatric coverage, however, many plans have restrictions including limits on the number of outpatient visits, higher copayment charges, and higher deductibles.

There have been significant changes in behavioral healthcare since 1955 when inpatient admissions to state mental hospitals were highest. Psychopharmacologic treatment has made possible the shift away from long-term custodial treatment. Psychosocial treatments continue the process of care and rehabilitation in community settings. Many large state hospitals have been replaced by psychiatric units in general hospitals, outpatient clinics, community mental health centers, day treatment centers, and mental health housing or residential recovery houses (formally referred to as halfway houses). Treatment has become more effective and specific based on our growing understanding of the brain and behavior (APA 2022).

## Integrated Delivery Systems

Many hospitals have responded to financial pressures by rapidly merging, acquiring, and entering into affiliations and various risk-sharing reimbursement agreements with other acute and nonacute providers, hospital-based healthcare systems, physicians and physician group practices, and MCOs. Transactions have included mergers of nonprofit organizations into either investor-owned or other nonprofit entities.

An **integrated delivery system (IDS)** combines the financial and clinical aspects of healthcare and uses a group of healthcare providers across facilities within the same system, selected according to quality and cost management criteria, to furnish comprehensive health services throughout the continuum of care.

The goal of an IDS is to organize the entire continuum of care, from health promotion and disease prevention to primary and secondary acute care, tertiary care, long-term care, and hospice care, to maximize its effectiveness across episodes of illness and pathways of wellness.

The ACA created a new model of IDS called the **accountable care organization (ACO)**. An ACO is a group of service providers who work together to manage and coordinate care of Medicare fee-for-service beneficiaries. The ACO receives incentive payments for delivering and coordinating care efficiently and effectively while focusing on preventative care and education. Guidelines for the establishment of an ACO are under the purview of the secretary of HHS, but they may include quality reporting, e-prescribing, and the use of electronic health records. In 2024, nearly half of traditional Medicare patients, totalling about 13.7 million, were served by one of the 480 ACOs participating in the Shared Savings Program. This represents a three percent increase over the previous year (CMS 2024e).

---

### Check Your Understanding 1.5

**Answer the following questions in a separate document.**

1. A terminally ill patient is being cared for by his son for several months. The patient, who wishes to remain in the son's home for palliative care, needs help with pain management and spiritual support. Which type of long-term care service would be best for the patient and family and why?

2. A 65-year-old female diagnosed with stage III breast cancer has been undergoing chemotherapy. Two hours after her latest treatment, she noted a potential urinary tract infection. The infection rapidly developed into cellulitis, which is a life-threatening condition. The patient's infection was treated successfully, but she was very weak from the intense treatment and lack of activity and could not care for herself at home. Differentiate the levels of care (settings) this patient likely encountered throughout her continuum of care.

3. How does an IDS maximize effectiveness across episodes of illness and wellness?

4. Evaluate how the behavioral care settings have changed since the mid-20th century. Compare the advantages and disadvantages of these changes.

---

## Forces Affecting Healthcare Organizations

Several developments in healthcare delivery have had far-reaching effects on the operation of hospitals in the US. Many of these developments focus on quality of care and organizational review.

### Development of Peer Review and Quality Improvement Programs

Healthcare quality was defined by the Institute of Medicine (IOM) as "the degree to which health care services for individuals and populations increase the likelihood of desired health outcomes and are consistent with current professional knowledge" (AHRQ 2020). The IOM framework for quality calls for safe, effective, patient-centered care with efficient, timely, and equitable delivery (AHRQ 2022). To meet this quality healthcare framework, the **Centers for Medicare and Medicaid Services (CMS)** and other organizations have implemented programs that require internal review and external reporting of a wide variety of procedural and outcome measures. CMS is the federal agency overseeing Medicare, Medicaid, Children's Health Insurance Program, and the Health Insurance Marketplace and setting standards for healthcare quality.

### Peer Review

In **peer review**, a member of a profession assesses the work of colleagues within that same profession. Peer review has traditionally been at the center of quality assessment and assurance efforts. The medical profession's peer review efforts have emphasized the scientific aspects of quality, such as appropriate use of pharmaceuticals, postoperative infection rates, and accuracy of diagnosis. Peer review is a requirement of both CMS and the Joint Commission.

### Quality Improvement

Quality improvement (QI) programs have been in place in hospitals for years and are required by Medicare and Medicaid programs and accreditation standards. QI programs have covered medical staff as well as nursing and other departments or processes. Efforts to encourage the delivery of high-quality care take place at the local and national levels. Such efforts are geared toward assessing the efforts of both individuals and institutions. Professional associations, healthcare education programs, healthcare organizations, government agencies, private external quality review associations, consumer groups, MCOs, and group purchasers of care all play a role in trying to promote high-quality care.

### Quality Reporting

The Hospital Inpatient Quality Reporting Program was mandated in 2003 by the Medicare Prescription Drug, Improvement, and Modernization Act (CMS 2023c). The program financially rewards hospitals for reporting data about quality that is then made available to the public. The program's goal is to improve quality through measurement and transparency. These comparative data are intended to assist consumers in making informed decisions about their healthcare and to encourage providers to improve the quality and cost of inpatient care. The data for selected measures are also used to evaluate performance in several value-based purchasing programs. Data are made available to the public on the Care Compare website (CMS 2024b).

## Malpractice

The federal government became involved in the quality-of-care and malpractice issues through the establishment of the National Practitioner Data Bank (NPDB) under the Healthcare Quality Improvement Act of 1986. Congress enacted this legislation to do the following:

- Moderate the incidence of malpractice
- Allow the medical community to demonstrate new willingness to weed out incompetence
- Improve the base of timely and accurate information on medical malpractice

The act required hospitals to request information from the data bank whenever they hire, grant privileges, or conduct periodic reviews of a practitioner.

## Efforts at Healthcare Reengineering

During the 1980s and 1990s, healthcare organizations attempted to adopt continuous quality improvement (CQI) processes, such as focused process improvement, major business process improvement and innovation, total quality management (TQM), and CQI. The drivers of this reengineering included cost reduction, staff shortages, patient satisfaction, and implementation of technology. Healthcare organizations attempted to look inside and think "process" as opposed to traditional "department" thinking and formed cross-functional collaborative teams to solve problems. At the same time, the Joint Commission reengineered the accreditation process to increase its focus on process and systems analysis. Gone were the days of thinking in a "silo" as healthcare teams learned about, with, and from each other implementing the guidance of interprofessional education.

## Value-Based Care

The federal government is beginning to focus on value-based care and is introducing programs that achieve better quality of care, improvement in population health, and reduction in healthcare costs by paying providers for value (that is, quality and cost outcomes) rather than a fee for every service provided (CMS 2023d).

As an example, Medicare launched the **value-based purchasing** program in 2013 as required by the ACA. The intent is to pay for care that rewards better value, patient outcomes, and innovation rather than just the volume of care provided. The Hospital Inpatient Quality Reporting measure infrastructure is used to identify quality care. Hospitals are evaluated and assigned points based on their performance compared to peer groups and their own performance improvement over time. Clinical process and patient experience criteria are both included in the evaluation. Because funding for the incentive increase is taken out of the overall pool of prospective payment funds, hospitals that do not qualify for payment increases may experience reductions in payment. Data collection, management, and reporting are important parts of successful compliance.

## Licensure and Certification of Healthcare Facilities

Under the 10th Amendment of the US Constitution, states have the primary responsibility for public health, which includes disease and injury prevention, sanitation, water and air pollution, vaccination, isolation and quarantine, inspection of commercial and residential premises, food and drinking water standards, extermination of vermin, fluoridation of municipal water supplies, and licensure of physicians and other healthcare professionals. Each state has a division or agency dedicated to promoting high-quality patient care and safety in healthcare facilities and outpatient services by conducting regular on-site surveys. State and federal licensing and certification programs require that high-performance standards be met in the provision of medical care and in the construction and maintenance of the healthcare facility.

### State Licensure

**Licensure** gives legal approval for a facility to operate or for a person to practice within his or her profession. States require that hospitals, nursing homes, and pharmacies be licensed to operate; although the requirements and standards for licensure may differ from state to state, state licensure is mandatory. Federal facilities such as those of the Department of Veterans Affairs do not require licensure.

Although licensure requirements vary, healthcare facilities must meet certain basic standards as determined by state regulatory agencies. These standards address such concerns as adequacy of staffing, personnel employed to provide services, physical aspects of the facility (such as equipment and buildings), and services provided, including management of health records. Licensure typically is performed annually, and facilities must usually meet the minimum acceptable standards for operation.

### Certification for Medicare Participation

Medicare is administered by CMS and provides national healthcare insurance coverage for individuals starting at age 65. Today, Medicare also covers individuals with disabilities regardless of age and patients requiring renal dialysis or transplant due to end stage renal disease (CMS 2023e). Medicare, under the Social Security Administration, and Medicaid, under the Social and Rehabilitation Service, were created in 1965 by amendments to the Social Security Act. The Health Care Financing Administration (HCFA), established in 1977 to manage both Medicare and Medicaid, became CMS in 2001.

CMS maintains oversight of the survey and certification of nursing homes and continuing care providers (including hospitals, nursing homes, home health agencies, end-stage renal disease facilities, hospices, and other facilities serving Medicare and Medicaid beneficiaries) and makes information about these activities available to beneficiaries, providers and suppliers, researchers, and state surveyors. In November 2002, CMS began the national Nursing Home Quality Initiative. The initiative website provides information about the quality of nursing home care through the Minimum Data Set and quality measures shared through Medicare's Care Compare website (CMS 2023b).

To be eligible for Medicare and Medicaid reimbursement, providers must become Medicare-certified by demonstrating compliance with the conditions of participation. **Certification** is the process by which government and nongovernment organizations evaluate educational programs, healthcare facilities, and individuals as having met predetermined standards. The certification of healthcare facilities is the responsibility of the states. However, Section 1865(a)(1) of the Social Security Act specifies that facilities accredited by the Joint Commission and the AOA must be deemed in compliance with the Medicare conditions of participation for hospitals. Those accredited are said to have *deemed status* (CMS 2024c).

## Accreditation

**Accreditation** is a voluntary process of organizational review in which an independent body created for this purpose periodically evaluates the quality of the entity's work against preestablished written criteria. Accreditation agencies create standards for medical care, construct measurements of quality, and determine which organizations meet their standards. Provider organizations seek accreditation to prove they meet the standards of legitimate and appropriate medical practice.

The Joint Commission operates voluntary accreditation programs for hospitals and other healthcare services. It certifies hospitals as having met the conditions of participation required for reimbursement under the federal Medicare program. The definition of federal **deemed status** is as follows:

> In order to participate in and receive federal payment from Medicare or Medicaid programs, a healthcare organization must meet the government requirements for program participation, including a certification of compliance with the health and safety requirements called Conditions of Participation (CoPs) or Conditions for Coverage (CfCs), which are set forth in federal regulations. (Joint Commission n.d.)

Most state governments also recognize Joint Commission accreditation as a condition of licensure and receiving Medicaid reimbursement. Inspections are typically triannual with accreditation and survey findings made publicly available. The standards are based on the premise that healthcare organizations exist to maximize the health of the people they serve while using resources efficiently. When an organization is found to be in substantial compliance with the Joint Commission standards, accreditation may be awarded for up to three years. Hospitals must undergo a full survey at least every three years. The Joint Commission publishes accreditation manuals with standards for hospitals, non-hospital-based psychiatric and substance abuse organizations, long-term care organizations, home care organizations, ambulatory care organizations, and organization-based pathology and clinical laboratory services.

### Check Your Understanding 1.6

Answer the following questions in a separate document.

1. What is the difference between licensure and accreditation in a healthcare organization? How does that difference impact standards development?
2. What is the relationship between peer review and QI?
3. Explain the impact of the Healthcare Quality Improvement Act of 1986 on malpractice.
4. What are some reasons facilities seek voluntary accreditation? Why would a facility choose not to seek accreditation?
5. How can organizations qualify for Medicare reimbursement?
6. How does quality reporting impact the quality of care?

## Reimbursement of Healthcare Expenditures

In the US, healthcare is paid for by the government, employers, and individuals. As healthcare technology and treatments have advanced and become more expensive, the payment systems have evolved. Originally dominated by fee-for-service payment systems, now Medicare and Medicaid programs and the managed care insurance industry have virtually eliminated fee-for-service reimbursement arrangements.

### Evolution of Third-Party Reimbursement

The evolution of third-party reimbursement systems for healthcare services began in the 1940s. The evolution created a need for systematic and accurate communications between healthcare providers and third-party payers. Commercial health insurance companies (for example, Aetna) offer medical plans similar to Blue Cross Blue Shield plans. Traditionally, Blue Cross organizations covered hospital services and Blue Shield covered inpatient physician services and a limited amount of office-based care. Today, Blue Cross plans and commercial insurance providers cover a full range of healthcare services, including ambulatory care services and drug benefits.

Most commercial health insurance is provided in the form of group policies offered by employers as part of their employee benefit packages. Unions also negotiate health insurance coverage during contract negotiations. In most cases, both employees and employers pay a share of the cost. Individual health insurance plans can be purchased through the health insurance marketplace created through the ACA. Initially, the ACA required individuals not covered by any of these options to pay a healthcare tax. This federal mandate for coverage was repealed as of 2019.

Commercial insurers also sell major medical and cash payment policies. Major medical plans are directed primarily at catastrophic illness and cover all or part of treatment costs beyond those covered by basic plans. Major medical plans are sold as both group and individual policies. Cash payment plans provide monetary benefits and are not based on actual charges from healthcare providers. For example, a cash payment plan might pay the beneficiary $150 for every day he or she is hospitalized or $500 for every ambulatory surgical procedure. Cash payment plans are often offered as a benefit of membership in large associations such as AARP.

### Government-Sponsored Reimbursement Systems

Until 1965, most of the poor and many of the elderly in the US could not afford private healthcare services. As a result of public pressure calling for attention to this growing problem, Congress passed Public Law 89-97 as an amendment to the Social Security Act. The amendment created Medicare (Title XVIII) and Medicaid (Title XIX). Medicare and Medicaid are not issuers of health insurance. They are public health plans through which individuals obtain health coverage.

#### Medicare

Medicare was first offered to retired Americans in July 1966. Today, Americans aged 65 years and older, as well as Americans living with certain disabilities eligible for Social Security benefits, qualify for Medicare coverage without regard to income. Coverage is offered under two coordinated programs: hospital insurance (Medicare Part A) and medical insurance (Medicare Part B).

Medicare Part A is financed through payroll taxes. Initially, coverage applied only to hospitalization and home healthcare. Subsequently, coverage for extended care in SNFs was added. Coverage for individuals eligible for Social Security disability payments for over two years and those who need kidney transplantation or dialysis for end-stage renal disease also was added.

Medical insurance under Medicare Part B is optional. It is financed through monthly premiums paid by eligible beneficiaries to supplement federal funding. Part B helps pay for physicians' services, outpatient hospital care, medical services and supplies, and certain other medical costs not covered by Part A. At the present time, Medicare Part B does not provide coverage of prescription drugs. In January 2006, Medicare Part D was implemented to provide prescription drug coverage for Medicare beneficiaries who select this option. Commercially offered Medicare plans, called Medicare Advantage plans, are sometimes referred to as Medicare Part C. Medicare Part C offers Medicare Part A and B coverage, and often includes vision, dental, hearing, and prescription drug coverage (CMS n.d.b).

## Medicaid

Medicaid is a medical assistance program for low-income Americans. The program is funded partially by the federal government and partially by state and local governments. The federal government requires that certain services be provided and sets specific eligibility requirements. Medicaid covers the following benefits:

- Early and periodic screening, diagnosis, and treatment services
- Family planning and rural health clinic services
- Inpatient and outpatient hospital care
- Laboratory and x-ray services
- Physicians' services
- SNF and home health services for persons over 21 years old

Individual states sometimes cover services in addition to those required by the federal government.

## Services Provided by Government Agencies

Federal health insurance programs cover health services for several additional specified populations including active and retired military and their families and American Indians. In partnership with state governments, additional insurance coverage is provided to children whose families cannot afford medical coverage although they do not qualify for Medicaid (Benefits.gov n.d.).

TRICARE provides healthcare benefits for eligible uniformed service members and their families, National Guard and Reserve members and their families, retired service members and their families, Medal of Honor recipients, and others who are registered in the Defense Enrollment Eligibility Reporting System (DEERS). The Department of Defense administers the TRICARE program (TRICARE 2024).

The Veterans Health Administration (VHA), the healthcare component of the Department of Veterans Affairs (VA), provides healthcare services to 9 million enrolled veterans of military service. The VA hospital system was established in 1930 to provide hospital, nursing home, residential, and outpatient medical and dental care to veterans of World War I. Today, the VA operates more than 1,321 sites of care including medical centers, clinics, counseling centers, and other medical facilities throughout the US (VA 2023). The Civilian Health and Medical Program of the Department of Veterans Affairs (CHAMPVA) provides health insurance to eligible spouses or surviving spouses or children of disabled or deceased veterans who are not eligible for TRICARE (VA 2024).

Through the Indian Health Service (IHS), HHS also finances healthcare services provided to individuals who are federally recognized as an American Indian or Alaska Native. Healthcare services are provided either at an IHS facility or through contracted services. IHS, like other federally funded healthcare programs, must submit an annual report to Congress on the quality of care provided (IHS n.d.).

State governments often operate healthcare facilities to serve citizens with special needs, such as people living with developmental disabilities and mental illnesses. Some states also offer health insurance programs to those who cannot qualify for private healthcare insurance. Many county and local governments also operate public hospitals and clinics to meet the medical needs of their communities with these facilities providing services regardless of the patient's ability to pay.

## Workers' Compensation

Workers' compensation is an insurance system operated by individual states. Each state has its own law and program to provide covered workers with some protection against the costs of medical care and the loss of income resulting from work-related injuries and, in some cases, illnesses. The first workers' compensation law was enacted in New York in 1910. By 1948, every state had enacted such laws. The theory underlying workers' compensation is that all accidents that occur at work, regardless of fault, must be regarded as risks of industry and that employer and employee should share the burden of loss (Knickman and Elbel 2024, 264).

## Insurance

Healthcare insurance was created to spread risk over a large pool of people and to protect assets in the event of a catastrophic illness or injury. Health insurance guards against financial devastation in the face of serious health problems. In 2022, 92.21 percent of Americans (304 million people) had health insurance (Keisler-Starkey et al. 2023). The US has public and private providers of health insurance. Medicare, Medicaid, IHS, TRICARE, and the VHA are examples of public health insurance programs funded by taxpayers. Private insurance companies sell insurance policies to consumers and collect payment through premiums. The economy of scale enables insurance companies to negotiate discounts with healthcare providers and compete for business. As part of the ACA, healthcare marketplaces were created by the federal and some state governments to facilitate consumer purchase of private health insurance at lower costs (Knickman and Elbel 2024). By the end of 2023, more than 15 million Americans signed up for a plan through ACA, and new options such as dental coverage are available as of 2024 (CMS 2023f).

## Managed Care

**Managed care** is a generic term for a healthcare reimbursement system that manages cost, quality, and access to services. Managed care refers to prepaid health plans that integrate the financial aspects and delivery of healthcare. Most managed care plans do not provide healthcare directly. Instead, they enter into service contracts with the physicians, hospitals, and other healthcare providers who provide medical services to enrollees in the plans.

The development of managed care was an indirect result of the federal government's enactment of the Medicare and Medicaid amendments in 1965. Medicare and Medicaid legislation stimulated the growth of university medical centers and prompted the development of **investor-owned hospital chains**, publicly traded for-profit groups of hospitals.

Managed care systems control costs primarily by presetting payment amounts and restricting patient access to healthcare services through precertification and utilization review processes. Managed care delivery systems also attempt to manage cost and quality by implementing various forms of financial incentives for providers, promoting healthy lifestyles, identifying risk factors and illnesses early in the disease process, and by providing patient education.

Restructured initiatives and increased use of technology have streamlined operations and improved operational efficiencies over recent years for the managed care industry. There are three types of managed care plans: **health maintenance organizations (HMOs)**, **preferred provider organizations (PPOs)**, and **point of service (POS) plans**. The more flexible a plan, the higher the cost. An HMO is a prepaid voluntary health plan that provides healthcare services in return for the payment of a monthly membership premium and usually only pays for care within its own network and the primary care doctor coordinates care. A PPO represents contractual agreements between healthcare providers and a self-insured employer or a health insurance carrier and usually will pay for care delivered outside the network, but it may cost the individual more. A POS plan lets the beneficiary choose between the HMO or PPO model each time care is accessed. Subscribers must select a PCP from a network of participating physicians to coordinate their care but are allowed to obtain care from outside the network potentially at a higher cost.

### Impact of Managed Care Organizations

Americans increasingly receive their health insurance through **managed care organizations (MCOs)**, where healthcare organizations assume the financial risk as well as provide healthcare services for a defined population of patients. The responsibilities of primary care providers have changed. In the fee-for-service model, the primary care provider is responsible only for the patients seen in their office, and a practice is viewed as being made up of individual patients. In a fully capitated managed care setting, however, particularly when the provider is paid through a capitation system rather than by a modified fee-for-service system, he or she is responsible for providing care to a defined population of patients assigned by the MCO. The MCO may audit the provider's practice to determine whether standards of care are being met. In the capitated MCO setting, providers are often held responsible for each patient on their panels, whether the patient ever comes to the office to be seen (Knickman and Elbel 2024).

The advent of managed care appeared to tame healthcare cost inflation during the early and mid-1990s, but costs are once again rising rapidly. In particular, the total cost of pharmaceuticals has increased dramatically since the 1980s (as shown in figure 1.1). In 2023, Americans spent $722.5 billion on prescription drugs, up 13.6 percent from 2022. Spending was expected to grow by 10 to 13 percent in 2024 (Tichy et al. 2024).

**Figure 1.1.** Rise in prescription drug spending

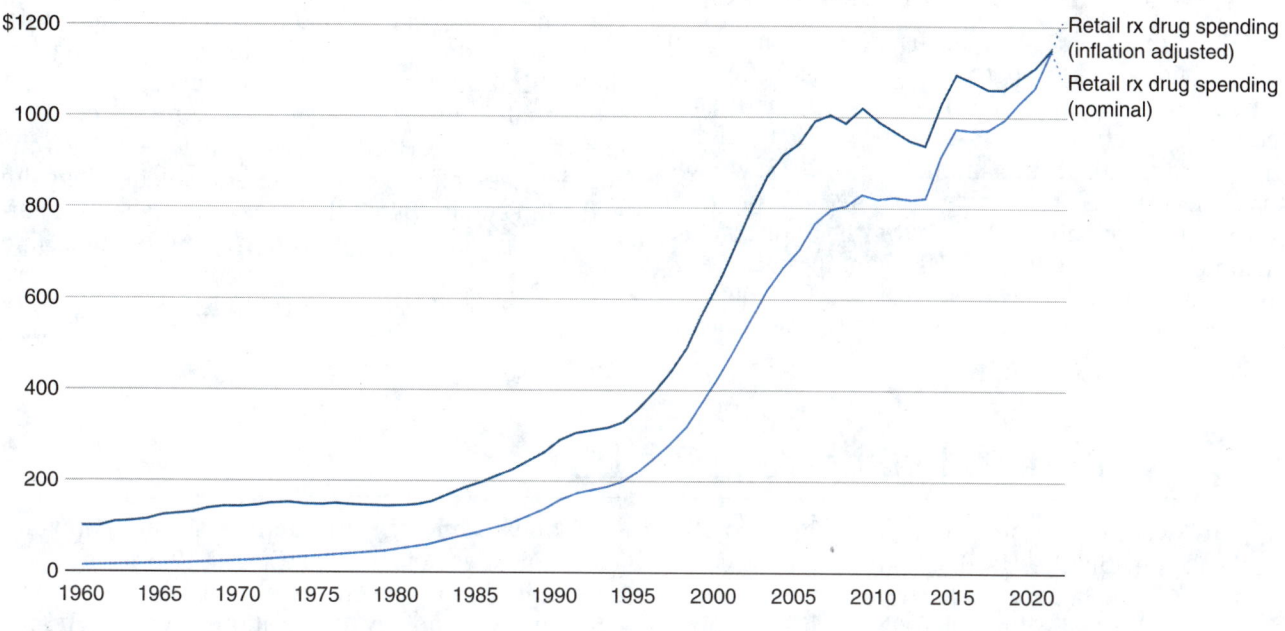

Source: KFF analysis of National Health Expenditures Accounts (NHEA)

Peterson-KFF
**Health System Tracker**

*Source:* Wager et al. 2023.

In addition to managing costs, the managed care industry faces the challenge of uncertain federal and state healthcare regulations. As politicians consider alternatives to the ACA, managed care executives must look beyond suggested legislation and develop programs that benefit both payers and providers. These programs focus on demonstrating improved clinical and financial outcomes. Analytics that combine clinical and financial data to align incentives and data sharing that supports decision-making and reduces waste are both critical to success (Knickman and Elbel 2024).

### Consumer-Directed Healthcare

An evolving option in the private insurance market is that of consumer-directed healthcare. This strategy seems to be gaining momentum to allow employees more choice in their healthcare decisions and to stabilize healthcare costs. The design of consumer-directed plans varies, but, essentially, it focuses on making consumers more price conscious by having lower premiums while setting a large deductible before individuals receive insurance benefits. High deductible health plan enrollment increased over 14 percent, from 25.3 percent to 39.4 percent, between 2010 and 2016. This approach is very different than managed care in that people have more choice but face sizeable personal financial risk (Knickman and Elbel 2024).

### Health Savings Accounts

**Health savings accounts (HSAs)** allow eligible individuals more control over how their healthcare dollars are spent. HSAs are a pretax way to save for future qualified medical and retiree health expenses. An HSA member pays for eligible expenses with pretax dollars. In 2023, 36 million Americans had an HSA (CFPB 2024).

### Health Reimbursement Accounts

**Health reimbursement accounts (HRAs)** are like HSAs but with a few significant differences. Like HSAs, they are typically offered with a deductible-based health plan and encourage employees to control their healthcare costs as there is a fixed number of resources available to the employee during the year. HRAs are completely funded by the employer, whereas the employee and the employer can fund HSAs (CMS n.d.c). The employer funds and owns the account, and money remaining at the end of the year

## Continued Rise in Healthcare Costs

In 2023, the average health insurance premium for an individual rose 7 percent while wages grew 5.2 percent (Claxton et al. 2023). Since 2013, the average cost of health insurance rose 17 percent for individuals (Kaiser Family Foundation 2018). In 2023, workers paid an average of 17 percent of the total premium for single coverage, a number that has not changed significantly since then (as shown in figure 1.2). However, due to the overall increase in premiums, the average monthly out-of-pocket cost for family coverage has increased from $380 in 2013 to $548 in 2023 (as shown in figure 1.3). In addition to increased premiums, the proportion of workers who pay deductibles has risen to 90 percent in 2023, up from 78 percent in 2013 and 55 percent in 2006 (as shown in figure 1.4).

Although the growth in healthcare spending has flattened in the last few years, it is unsustainable for individuals and employers (Kacik 2018). New benefit offerings like HSAs and HRAs may be part of the solution, as are new access solutions like telehealth and retail clinics. But without tackling high-cost pharmaceuticals and the administrative burden built into healthcare, spending is likely to continue to increase faster than the Consumer Price Index (Kacik 2018).

## Future of Healthcare in the US

Many factors influenced the evolution of healthcare in the US. Looking ahead, some old and some new factors are likely to shape continued change in the US health system. New clinical knowledge and technology are among the most obvious. The rapid development of COVID-19 vaccines and effective use of telehealth are examples of new knowledge and technology applications (Knickman and

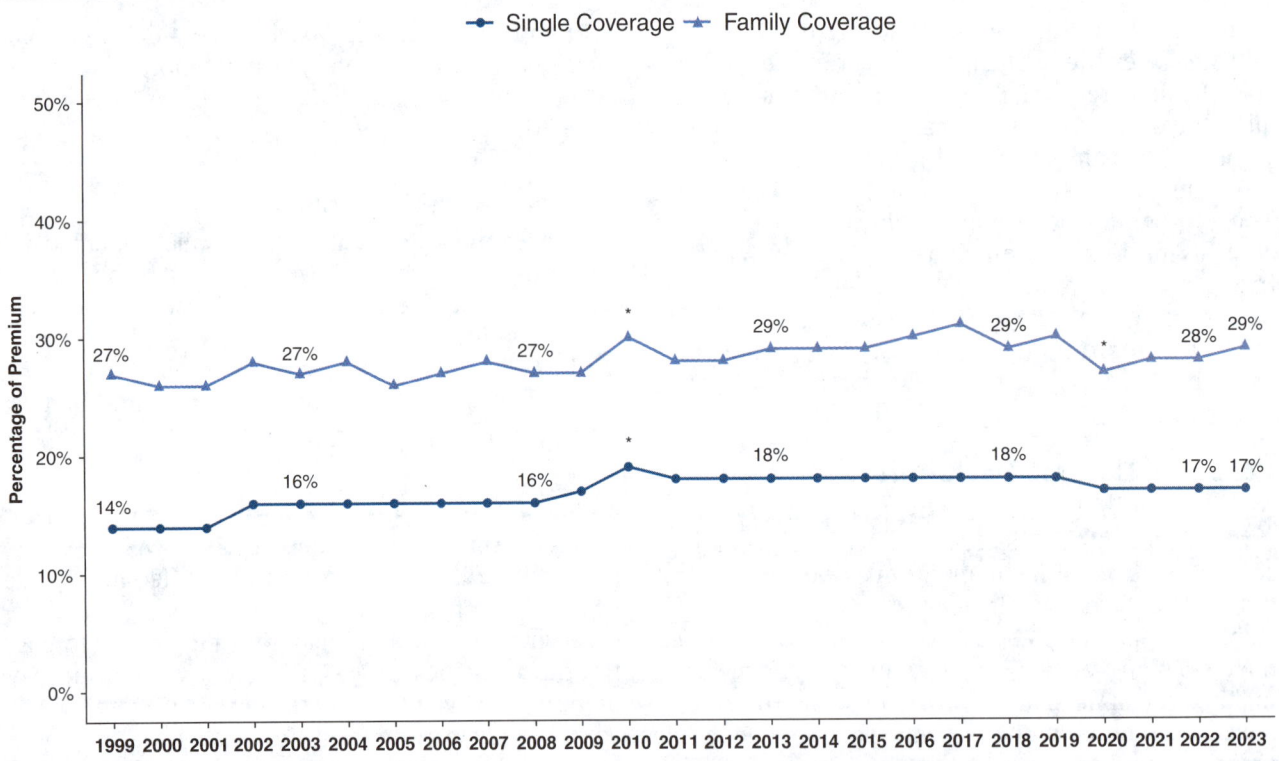

**Figure 1.2.** Average percentage of insurance premium paid by covered workers for single and family insurance coverage, 1999–2023

\* Estimate is statistically different from estimate for the previous year shown (p < .05).
SOURCE: KFF Employer Health Benefits Survey, 2018–2023; Kaiser/HRET Survey of Employer-Sponsored Health Benefits, 1999–2017

*Source:* Claxton et al. 2023. Reprinted with permission.

Future of Healthcare in the US 31

**Figure 1.3.** Average monthly employee contribution for single and family insurance coverage, 1999–2023

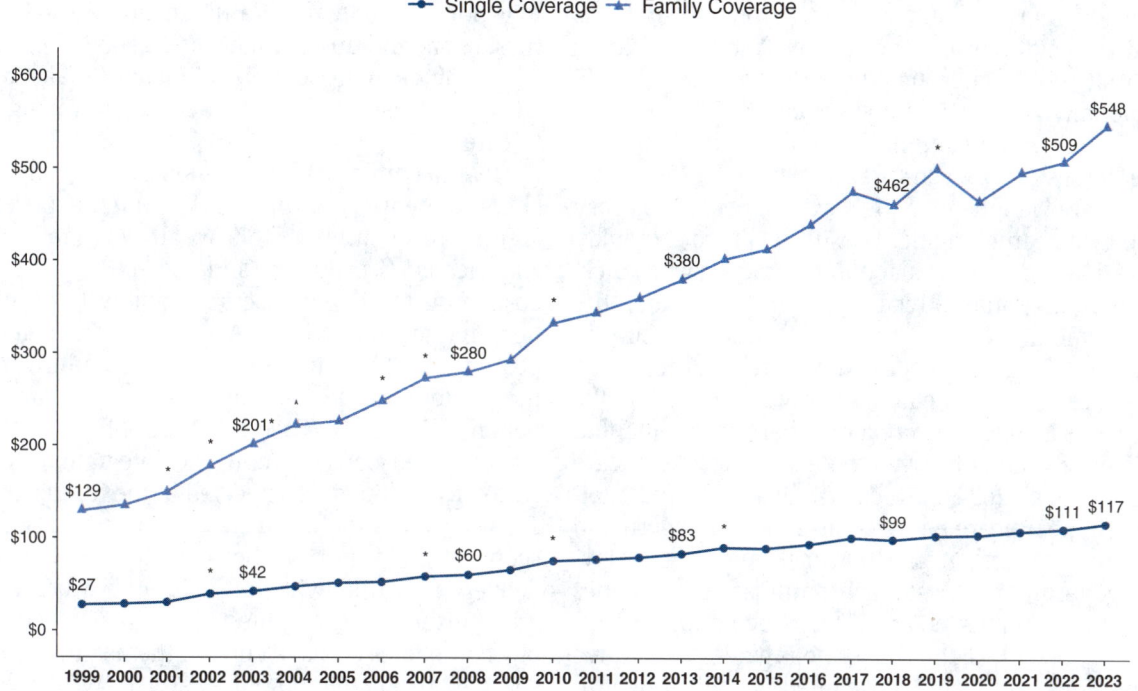

* Estimate is statistically different from estimate for the previous year shown (p < .05).
SOURCE: KFF Employer Health Benefits Survey, 2018–2023; Kaiser/HRET Survey of Employer-Sponsored Health Benefits, 1999–2017

*Source:* Claxton et al. 2023. Reprinted with permission.

**Figure 1.4.** Percent of workers with insurance coverage with a general annual deductible for single coverage, 2006–2023

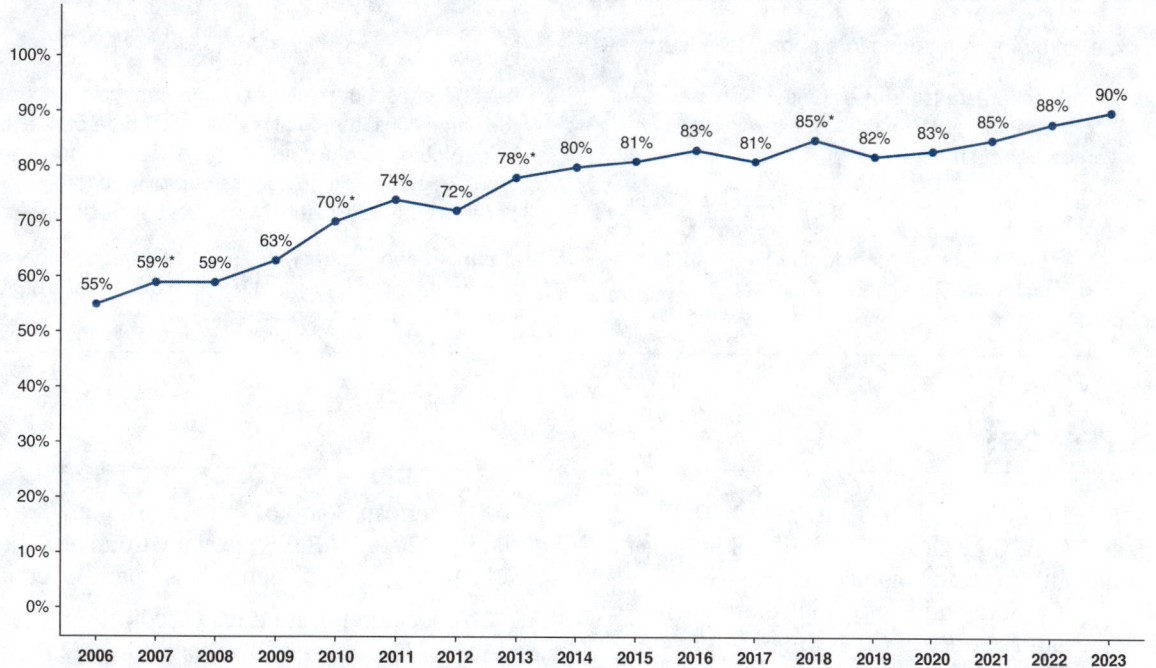

* Estimate is statistically different from estimate for the previous year shown (p < .05).
NOTE: Average general annual deductibles are for in-network providers.
SOURCE: KFF Employer Health Benefits Survey, 2018–2023; Kaiser/HRET Survey of Employer-Sponsored Health Benefits, 2006–2017

*Source:* Claxton et al. 2023. Reprinted with permission.

Elbel 2024). While the circumstances of the pandemic were devastating, the ability of the healthcare system to quickly innovate and adapt was proven and has raised expectations for the future. Another tectonic shift that will change healthcare delivery in the US and globally is artificial intelligence.

ChatGPT became publicly available in 2022 and immediately drew fresh attention to machine learning and large language models, which became as easy to use as a search engine. Uses in healthcare quickly emerged as did concerns about accuracy, governance, accountability, and ethical use. In healthcare, the term augmented intelligence is preferred by many to reinforce that algorithms and data are used to assist, not replace, licensed healthcare professionals to make clinical decisions. Many experts believe augmented intelligence is already driving the future of healthcare (Goldberg et al. 2024). Ethical use of augmented intelligence in healthcare has become a major concern and motivated working groups and task forces at all levels of government to establish boundaries and codes of conduct (Adams et al. 2024). Regulations needs to catch up with technology. Meanwhile, generative AI solutions are being developed to solve healthcare problems such as medication research and new diagnostic tools. Augmented reality adds immersive visualization to aid clinicians (Mesko 2024). Wearable technologies will become more sophisticated as will portable and remote diagnostic devices. Driven by sensors and augmented intelligence, these devices will provide data to help clinicians make accurate clinical decisions more quickly, improving access to care.

Health equity will continue to be a major factor shaping healthcare in the US. Life expectancy is significantly higher for wealthy than for poor Americans (Knickman and Elbel 2024). Reducing costs and improving access to quality healthcare will help reduce disparities. Augmented intelligence appears poised to be an important force multiplier to help the limited number of clinicians provide care to more patients (Sahni and Carrus 2023; Goldberg et al. 2024).

Continued consolidation and integration of healthcare organizations are expected in the future. Organizations expanding through increased volume and expanding scope of services have become the norm. Integrated delivery networks will continue to be watched closely while insurance companies, retail chains, and technology companies all have entered the healthcare delivery space (Knickman and Elbel 2024). While there are many unknowns about the future of healthcare delivery in the US, one certainty is continual change.

### Check Your Understanding 1.7

**Answer the following questions in a separate document.**

1. Consider the characteristics of a health savings account (HSA). What demographic of individuals would this type of coverage benefit the most?

2. Molly is three years old and has chronic ear infections. She sees her pediatrician at the neighborhood clinic often. She comes from a military family. Her grandfather is retired from the Air Force and is fighting COPD. Her parents both serve in the Army and have no chronic health issues, but they receive preventive services at the same clinic that Molly does. What type of health insurance does Molly have to treat her ear infections? What type of health insurance is provided to Molly's parents and grandfather? Explain your reasoning.

3. Compare and contrast the terms artificial intelligence and augmented intelligence within the context of healthcare delivery.

# References

Adams, L., E. Fontaine, S. Lin, T. Crowell, V. C. H. Chung, and A. A. Gonzalez. 2024. Artificial intelligence in health, health care, and biomedical science: An AI code of conduct principles and commitments discussion draft. *NAM Perspectives*. https://doi.org/10.31478/202403a.

AARC (American Association for Respiratory Care). n.d. "Understanding Credentials." https://www.aarc.org/your-rt-career/understanding-credentials/.

ABPTS (American Board of Physical Therapy Specialties). 2024. "ABPTS Specialty Councils." https://specialization.apta.org/about-abpts/specialty-councils.

AAMC (Association of American Medical Colleges). n.d. "About US." Accessed December 10, 2023. https://www.aamc.org/about/.

AANP (American Association of Nurse Practitioners). n.d. "What's a Nurse Practitioner (NP)? Discover Why

Americans Make More Than 1.06 billion Visits to NPs Each Year." https://www.aanp.org/about/all-about-nps/whats-a-nurse-practitioner.

AAPA (American Academy of Physician Associates). 2024. "What Is a PA?" https://www.aapa.org/about/what-is-a-pa/.

ACR (American College of Radiology). n.d. "What is a Radiologist?" https://www.acr.org/Practice-Management-Quality-Informatics/Practice-Toolkit/Patient-Resources/About-Radiology.

AHA (American Hospital Association). 2024a. "Fast Facts on US Hospitals." https://www.aha.org/statistics/fast-facts-us-hospitals.

AHA (American Hospital Association). 2024b. "Census Bureau Database to Provide Better Context on Retail Clinics Market." https://www.aha.org/aha-center-health-innovation-market-scan/2023-04-04-census-bureau-database-provide-better-context-retail-clinics-market.

AHA (American Hospital Association). 2022 (August). *Pandemic-Driven Deferred Care Has Led to Increased Patient Acuity in America's Hospitals*. https://www.aha.org/guidesreports/2022-08-15-pandemic-driven-deferred-care-has-led-increased-patient-acuity-americas.

AHA (American Hospital Association). 2019. *Fact Sheet: Post-Acute Care*. https://www.aha.org/system/files/media/file/2019/07/fact-sheet-post-acute-care-0719.pdf.

AHRQ (Agency for Healthcare Research and Quality). 2022. "Six Domains of Healthcare Quality." https://www.ahrq.gov/talkingquality/measures/six-domains.html.

AHRQ (Agency for Healthcare Research and Quality). 2020. "Understanding Quality Measurement." https://www.ahrq.gov/professionals/quality-patient-safety/quality-resources/tools/chtoolbx/understand/index.html.AAA (American Academy of Audiology). 2024. "Become an Audiologist". https://www.audiology.org/careers/become-an-audiologist/.

AMA (American Medical Association). n.d. "AMA History." Accessed December 10, 2023. https://www.ama-assn.org/about/ama-history/ama-history.

AMIA (American Medical Informatics Association). n.d. "AMIA's Role in CIS and History". https://amia.org/careers-certifications/clinical-informatics-subspecialty/amias-role-cis-and-history.

AOTA (American Occupational Therapy Association). n.d.a. "What Is Occupational Therapy?" Accessed July 25, 2024. https://www.aota.org/about/what-is-ot.

AOTA (American Occupational Therapy Association). n.d.b. "Become an Occupational Therapy Practitioner." Accessed July 25, 2024. https://www.aota.org/career/become-an-ot-ota.

APA (American Psychiatric Association). 2022. "The Psychiatric Bed Crisis in the US: Understanding the Problem and Moving towards Solutions." https://www.psychiatry.org/getmedia/81f685f1-036e-4311-8dfc-e13ac425380f/APA-Psychiatric-Bed-Crisis-Report-Full.pdf.

APTA (American Physical Therapy Association). n.d. "Licensure." Accessed July 25, 2024. https://www.apta.org/your-practice/licensure.

ARRT (American Registry of Radiologic Technologists). n.d. "Radiation Therapy." Accessed July 25, 2024. https://www.arrt.org/pages/earn-arrt-credentials/credential-options/radiation-therapy.

ASCLS (American Society for Clinical Laboratory Science). n.d. "Becoming a Clinical Laboratory Professional." Accessed July 25, 2024. https://ascls.org/how-do-i-become-a-laboratory-professional.

ASHA (American Speech-Language-Hearing Association). n.d. "One Discipline. Two Professions. Hearing and Speech." Accessed July 25, 2024. https://hearingandspeechcareers.org.

ASAHP (Association of Schools Advancing Health Professions). n.d. "What is Allied Health?" Accessed December 10, 2023. http://www.asahp.org/what-is/.

BLS (Bureau of Labor Statistics). 2024a. "Surgical Assistant and Technologist." https://www.bls.gov/ooh/healthcare/surgical-technologists.htm.

BLS (Bureau of Labor Statistics). 2024b. "Clinical Laboratory Technologists and Technicians." https://www.bls.gov/ooh/healthcare/clinical-laboratory-technologists-and-technicians.htm.

CFPB (Consumer Financial Protection Bureau). 2024 (May 1). "Issue Spotlight: Health Savings Accounts." https://www.consumerfinance.gov/data-research/research-reports/issue-spotlight-health-savings-accounts/.

Claxton, G., M. Rae, A. A. Winger, and E. Wager. 2023. *2023 Employer Health Benefits Survey*. KFF. https://www.kff.org/report-section/ehbs-2023-section-1-cost-of-health-insurance/.

CMS (Centers for Medicare and Medicaid Services). 2024a (January 24). "Historic 21.3 million People Choose ACA Marketplace Coverage" [press release]. https://www.cms.gov/newsroom/press-releases/historic-213-million-people-choose-aca-marketplace-coverage.

CMS (Centers for Medicare and Medicaid Services). 2024b (April 16). "Hospital Quality Initiative Public Reporting: Hospital Care Compare and Provider Data

Catalog." https://www.cms.gov/medicare/quality/initiatives/hospital-quality-initiative/hospital-compare.

CMS (Centers for Medicare and Medicaid Services). 2024c (February 20). "Accreditation of Medicare Certified Providers & Suppliers." https://www.cms.gov/medicare/health-safety-standards/accreditation-programs.

CMS (Centers for Medicare and Medicaid Services). 2024d. "The Data." https://data.cms.gov/provider-data/topics/long-term-care-hospitals/data.

CMS (Centers for Medicare and Medicaid Services). 2024e. "Participation Continues to Grow in CMS' Accountable Care Organization Initiatives in 2024." https://www.cms.gov/newsroom/press-releases/participation-continues-grow-cms-accountable-care-organization-initiatives-2024.

CMS (Centers for Medicare and Medicaid Services). 2024f (June 12). "NHE Fact Sheet." https://www.cms.gov/data-research/statistics-trends-and-reports/national-health-expenditure-data/nhe-fact-sheet.

CMS (Centers for Medicare and Medicaid Services). 2023a (December 27). "Hospital Inpatient Quality Reporting Program." https://www.cms.gov/medicare/quality/initiatives/hospital-quality-initiative/inpatient-reporting-program.

CMS (Centers for Medicare and Medicaid Services). 2023b. "Hospital Value-Based Purchasing Program." https://www.cms.gov/medicare/quality/initiatives/hospital-quality-initiative/hospital-value-based-purchasing.

CMS (Centers for Medicare and Medicaid Services). 2023c. "History." https://www.cms.gov/about-cms/who-we-are/history/.

CMS (Centers for Medicare and Medicaid Services). 2023d (November 22). "Nursing Home Quality Initiative." https://www.cms.gov/medicare/quality/nursing-home-improvement.

CMS (Centers for Medicare and Medicaid Services). 2023e. "HealthCare.gov Enrollment Exceeds 15 Million, Surpassing Previous Years' Milestones." https://www.cms.gov/newsroom/press-releases/healthcaregov-enrollment-exceeds-15-million-surpassing-previous-years-milestones.

CMS (Centers for Medicare and Medicaid Services) 2022. *What are Long-Term Care Hospitals?* https://www.medicare.gov/publications/11347-What-are-long-term-care-hospitals.pdf.

CMS (Centers for Medicare and Medicaid Services). 2021. *Medicare Benefit Policy Manual*. https://www.cms.gov/Regulations-and-Guidance/Guidance/Manuals/downloads/bp102c01.pdf.

CMS (Centers for Medicare and Medicaid Services). n.d.a. "What's Medicare." Accessed May 25, 2024. https://www.medicare.gov/what-medicare-covers/your-medicare-coverage-choices/whats-medicare.

CMS (Centers for Medicare and Medicaid Services). n.d.b. "Healthcare Reimbursement Account." Accessed May 25, 2024. https://www.healthcare.gov/glossary/health-reimbursement-account-hra/.

Cooke, M., D. Irby, W. Sullivan, and K. M. Ludmerer. 2006. American medical education 100 years after the Flexner report. *New England Journal of Medicine* 355:1339–1344. http://doi.org/10.1056/NEJMra055445.

Cures Act (21st Century Cures Act of 2016). Public Law 114-225. https://www.congress.gov/bill/114th-congress/house-bill/34.

Dayama, N., R. Pradhan, G. Davlyatov, and R. Weech-Maldonado. 2024. Electronic health record implementation enhances financial performance in high Medicaid nursing homes. *Journal of Multidisciplinary Healthcare* 17 (May):2577–89. doi:10.2147/JMDH.S457420.

DHA (Defence Health Agency). 2024. "Eligibility." https://tricare.mil/Plans/Eligibility.

Elwood, T. W. 2019. The changing nature of language. *Journal of Allied Health* 48(4):235.

Flexner, A. 1910. *Medical Education in the United States and Canada: A Report to the . Carnegie Foundation for the Advancement of Teaching.* http://archive.carnegiefoundation.org/publications/pdfs/elibrary/Carnegie_Flexner_Report.pdf.

Foley, D. J., R. W. Manderscheid, J. E. Atay, J. Maedke, J. Sussman, and S. Cribbs. 2004. "Highlights of Organized Mental Health Services in 2002 and Major National and State Trends." Edited by R. Manderscheid and J. Berry. Chapter 19 in *Mental Health, United States, 2004.* HHS Publication No. (SMA) 06-4195. http://www.yolocounty.org/home/showdocument?id=13935.

Freeman, W. J., A. J. Weiss, and K. C. Heslin. 2018. *Overview of U.W. Hospital Stays in 2016: Variation by Geographic Region.* Agency for Healthcare Research and Quality. https://www.hcup-us.ahrq.gov/reports/statbriefs/sb246-Geographic-Variation-Hospital-Stays.pdf.

Galan, N. 2023 (April 25). The Affordable Care Act: An update. *Medical News Today*. https://www.medicalnewstoday.com/articles/247287.

Goldberg, C. B., L. Adams, D. Blumenthal, P. F. Brennan, N. Brown, A. J. Butte, M. Cheatham, et al. 2024. To do no harm—and the most good—with AI in health care. *NEJM AI* 1(3). https://doi.org/10.1056/AIp2400036.

Grand View Research. 2022. *U.S. Home Healthcare Market Size, Share & Trends Analysis Report by Component (Equipment, Service), and Segment Forecasts, 2023–2030*. https://www.grandviewresearch.com/industry-analysis/us-home-healthcare-market-report.

Haseltine, W. 2018 (April 2). Aging populations will challenge healthcare systems all over the world. *Forbes*. https://www.forbes.com/sites/williamhaseltine/2018/04/02/aging-populations-will-challenge-healthcare-systems-all-over-the-world/#2549cf3a2cc3.

Hazelwood, A., E. Cook, and S. Hazelwood. 2005. The Joint Commission on healthcare oganization's sentinel events policy. *Academy of Healthcare Management Journal*. Annual.

Healthcare.gov. n.d. "Children's Health Insurance Program." Accessed October 31, 2024. https://www.healthcare.gov/medicaid-chip/childrens-health-insurance-program/.

HealthJob. 2024 (July 30). "How to Become a Patient Care Technician/Associate (PCT/A): A Step-by-Step Guide." https://www.healthjob.org/guide/how-to-become-a-patient-care-technician.

HHS (Department of Health and Human Services). 2024 (March 18). "About the Office of the Surgeon General." http://www.surgeongeneral.gov/about/index.html.

HHS (Department of Health and Human Services). 2022. "Strategic Plan FY 2022–2026." https://www.hhs.gov/about/strategic-plan/2022-2026/index.html.

HHS (Department of Health and Human Services). 1976. "200 years of American Medicine 1776–1976." https://www.nlm.nih.gov/hmd/pdf/200years.pdf.

HHS (Department of Health and Human Services). n.d. "About HHS." Accessed July 25, 2024. https://www.hhs.gov/about/index.html.

HPAC (Health Professions Accreditors Collaborative). 2024 (May 27). "Members." https://healthprofessionsaccreditors.org/members.

IHS (Indian Health Service). n.d. "About IHS." Accessed December 10, 2023. https://www.ihs.gov/aboutihs/.

Joint Commission. 2020. "The Joint Commission: Over a Century of Quality and Safety." https://www.jointcommission.org/-/media/tjc/documents/about-us/tjc-history-timeline-through-2020.pdf.

Joint Commission. n.d. "Federal Deemed Status Fact Sheet." Accessed July 25, 2024. https://www.jointcommission.org/resources/news-and-multimedia/fact-sheets/facts-about-federal-deemed-status/.

Kacik, A. 2018 (June 13). Healthcare costs increasing at unsustainable pace. *Modern Healthcare*. https://www.modernhealthcare.com/article/20180613/NEWS/180619961/healthcare-costs-increasing-at-unsustainable-pace.

Keisler-Starkey, K., L. N. Bunch, and R. A. Lindstrom. 2023. *Health Insurance Coverage in the United States*. US Census Bureau. https://www.census.gov/library/publications/2023/demo/p60-281.html.

Knickman, J. R., and B. B. Elbel. 2024. *Jonas and Kovner's Health Care Delivery in the United States*, 13th ed. New York: Springer Publishing Company.

Mark, T., E. Stranges, and K. Levit. 2010 (September 7). Using healthcare cost and utilization project state inpatient database and medicare cost reports data to determine the number of psychiatric discharges from psychiatric units of community hospitals. *Psychiatry Online* 61(6). https://ps.psychiatryonline.org/doi/full/10.1176/ps.2010.61.6.562.

MarkWideResearch. 2024. *Retail Clinics Market Analysis—Industry Size, Share, Research Report, Insights, COVID-19 Impact, Statistics, Trends, Growth and Forecast 2024–2032*. https://markwideresearch.com/retail-clinics-market/.

Mayo Clinic College of Medicine and Science. n.d. "Radiation Therapist." Accessed July 25, 2024. https://college.mayo.edu/academics/explore-health-care-careers/careers-a-z/radiation-therapist.

Merriam-Webster. n.d. "Biotechnology." Accessed December 10, 2023. https://www.merriam-webster.com/dictionary/biotechnology.

Mesko, B. 2024 (May 1). "10 Ways Technology is Changing Healthcare." *Medical Futurist*. https://medicalfuturist.com/ten-ways-technology-changing-healthcare.

Morris, G. 2023 (February 28). "What Is a Registered Nurse?" *NurseJournal*. https://nursejournal.org/registered-nursing.

Morris, G. 2024. "Types of Nursing Degrees and Levels." *NurseJournal*. https://nursejournal.org/degrees/types-of-nursing-degrees/.

Munday, R. 2022. "Certified Nursing Assistant (CNA) Career Overview." *NurseJournal*. https://nursejournal.org/cna.

NIH (National Institutes of Health). 2023 (January 10). "Decades in the Making: mRNA COVID-19 Vaccines." https://covid19.nih.gov/nih-strategic-response-covid-19/decades-making-mrna-covid-19-vaccines.

ONC (Office of the National Coordinator for Health Information Technology). 2018. "Percent of Hospitals by Type That Possess Health IT." https://www.healthit.gov/data/quickstats/percent-hospitals-type-possess-certified-health-it.

Orlousky, H. 2024. "The 21st Century Cures Act Effect on Patients, Physicians, and Interoperability." Rxnt.com. https://www.rxnt.com/21st-century-cures-act-effect-patients-physicians-interoperability

Penn Medicine. n.d. "History of Pennsylvania Hospital." Penn Medicine. Accessed December 10, 2023. http://www.uphs.upenn.edu/paharc/features/creation.html.

Peterson, E., M. T. Keehn, M. Hasnain, V. Gruss, M. Axelsson, E. Carlson, J. Jakobsson, and A. Kottorp. 2024. Exploring differences in and factors influencing self-efficacy for competence in interprofessional collaborative practice among health professions students. *Journal of Interprofessional Care* 38(1), 104–112.

Sahni, N. R., and B. Carrus. 2023. Artificial intelligence in US health care delivery. *New England Journal of Medicine* 389(4):348–358. https://doi.org/10.1056/NEJMra2204673.

Sand, J. 2021. Student perceptions of an undergraduate interprofessional capstone course including health information management. *Perspectives in Health Information Management* 18(3).

Schneider, E., A. Shah, P. Sah, S. M. Moghadas, T. Vilches, and A. P. Galvania. 2021. "The U.S. COVID-19 Vaccination Program at One Year: How Many Deaths and Hospitalizations Were Averted?" Commonwealth Fund. https://doi.org/10.26099/3542-5n54.

Starr, P. 1982. *The Social Transformation of American Medicine*. New York: Basic Books.

Steiner, C. A., Z. Karaca, B. Moore, M. Imshaug, and G. Pickens. 2020. "Surgeries in Hospital-Based Ambulatory Surgery and Hospital Inpatient Settings." https://www.hcup-us.ahrq.gov/reports/statbriefs/sb223-Ambulatory-Inpatient-Surgeries-2014.pdf.

Thomasson, M. 2003 (April 17). "Health Insurance in the United States." EH.Net Encyclopedia. Edited by Robert Whaples. http://eh.net/encyclopedia/health-insurance-in-the-united-states/.

Tichy, E. M., J. M. Hoffman, M. Tadrous, M. H. Rim, S. Cuellar, J. S. Clark, M. K. Newell and G. T. Schumock. 2024. National trends in prescription drug expenditures and projections for 2024. *American Journal of Health-System Pharmacy*. https://doi.org/10.1093/ajhp/zxae105.

Townsend, C. M. 2016. Franklin H. Martin and the American College of Surgeons. *BULLETIN American College of Surgeons* 101(12):12–21. https://www.facs.org/media/itwkgsfo/2016-townsend-16decbull.pdf.

Wager, E., I. Telesford, C. Cox, and K. Amin. 2023. "What Are the Recent and Forecasted Trends in Prescription Drug Spending?" Peterson-KFF Health System Tracker. https://www.healthsystemtracker.org/chart-collection/recent-forecasted-trends-prescription-drug-spending.

WHO (World Health Organization). 2010. *Framework for Action on Interprofessional Education and Collaborative Practice*. http://apps.who.int/iris/bitstream/10665/70185/1/WHO_HRH_HPN_10.3_eng.pdf.

WHO (World Health Organization). n.d. "Medical Devices." Accessed December 10, 2023. https://www.who.int/health-topics/medical-devices.

VA (Department of Veterans Affairs). 2024. "CHAMPVA benefits." https://www.va.gov/family-and-caregiver-benefits/health-and-disability/champva/.

VA (Department of Veterans Affairs). 2023. "Veterans Health Administration." https://www.va.gov/health/aboutVHA.asp.

29 CFR 825.118. "What Is a 'Health Care Provider'?" https://www.govinfo.gov/app/details/CFR-2002-title29-vol3/CFR-2002-title29-vol3-sec825-118.

# chapter 2

# Governing Data and Information Assets

*Joseph C. Brown, DHA, CHDA*

## Learning Objectives

- Distinguish between the functions of data governance and information governance
- Compare and contrast the data management domains
- Defend the importance of a business case for a data governance program
- Compare examples of prominent frameworks and organizational structure for data governance and information governance

## Key Terms

Accountability
Application programming interface (API)
Artifacts
Batch processing
Big data
Business case
Business intelligence (BI)
Cloud computing
Content management
Controls
Corporate governance
Cross-functional
Customer data platform
Data
Data, information, knowledge, and wisdom (DIKW) hierarchy
Data architecture
Data augmentation
Data capture
Data center
Data cleanroom
Data dashboard
Data democratization
Data dictionary
Data governance (DG)
Data governance office
Data governance steering committee
Data lake
Data life cycle
Data quality management
Data security
Data security management
Data stack
Data stakeholders
Data steward
Decision rights
Enterprise governance
Executive data governance council
Extract, transform, and load (ETL)
Health Level 7 Fast Healthcare Interoperability Resources (HL7 FHIR)
Framework
Governance
Information
Information governance (IG)
Information system
Interoperability
Machine learning
Master data management
Planning
Rules of engagement
Stakeholder analysis
Structured data
Terminology and classification management
Unstructured data

While the phrases **data governance (DG)** and **information governance (IG)** appear to define themselves, there are many definitions of each. The differences between DG and IG can be summarized by the following:

DG is the overall administration, through clearly defined procedures and plans, that assures the availability, integrity, security, and usability of the structured and unstructured data available to an organization.

IG uses policies, procedures, and multi-disciplinary arrangements to manage and optimize an organization's information for its immediate and future needs including regulatory, legal, risk, environmental, and operational requirements. (Foote 2016)

As healthcare struggles with the bombardment of digital data and regulatory reporting requirements, DG and IG have also received significant hype. Service companies, consultants, and vendors have latched onto the terms, but the divergence of thought on DG and IG sometimes makes the concepts and their implementation tough to pin down (Johns 2015, xxi). In many cases, the definitions are subjective. Many organizations are doing the same tasks but naming them differently, which makes it difficult for organizations to implement. Fortunately, several professional organizations and academic researchers are helping to create a roadmap for developing sound principles and practices for DG and IG in healthcare. The focus of this chapter is to help clarify the concepts of DG and IG, provide approaches for applying each in a cogent manner, and to suggest best practices for establishing DG and IG in a healthcare environment.

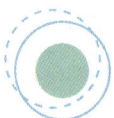

## Navigating Emerging Terms in Data and Information Governance

The topics of DG and IG are evolving and becoming more mainstream to those who might not even work in data management for any sector. It is important to be aware of key terms that are commonly used in the industry.

The starting point for all data is usually a **data lake** (Microsoft Azure n.d.). In short, the lake holds data in its raw format. A user may need to regularly obtain data from one interface and place it in another. This is common for systems such as price aggregators that compare prices for the same item from multiple websites. In the healthcare space, it is not uncommon to see web pages that display ongoing emergency department wait times from a variety of hospitals. If this is the case, an **application programming interface (API)**, the set of defined rules and protocols explaining how the applications talk to one another, is used (IBM 2024). Data can be loaded by following the **extract, transform, and load (ETL)** process, which collects and processes data from various sources into a single data store (IBM n.d.a). Many times, health data is categorized as being **big data**, meaning that the data sets are so large or complex that it is difficult to process using traditional methods (Tiao 2024). Once a system for using the data is established, automation is applied to increase efficiency. Not to be confused with automation, **batch processing** describes a high-volume of repetitive data jobs that run without manual intervention (AWS n.d.). An example of batch processing is loading a claims file, provider file, and member file all at once. Batch processing can be enhanced through **machine learning**, when a system uses artificial intelligence (AI) to identify trends and patterns for improvement (IBM n.d.b). From there, the data is consolidated in one external view that customers see known as the **customer data platform**.

Within these topics, it is very common for the word *data* to precede many descriptors that indicate how the data are being used. **Data capture** is simply collecting the data. In healthcare, it is the process of recording healthcare-related data in a health record or system or clinical database. In this context, an **information system** is an automated system that uses computer hardware and software to record, manipulate, store, recover, and disseminate data (that is, a system that receives and processes input and provides output). Captured data should be accompanied by a **data dictionary**, a descriptive list of the names, definitions, and attributes of data elements to be collected within an information system or database whose purpose is to standardize definitions and ensure consistent use. The data dictionary is a primary contributor to ensuring data **interoperability**, which is the ability of different information technology (IT) systems to exchange data accurately, effectively, and consistently so information can be used. Once collected, that data might be used for training; if so, it could be augmented. **Data augmentation** is when training data is artificially derived from existing data without collecting new data. A **data center** is where the hardware and software for the electronic information systems are held. It is a physical space where the servers, mainframes, and databases reside that house the data. The servers in a data center house the **data cleanroom,** which is a virtual environment to ensure personal identifiable information is anonymized (Kerner 2022). The cleanroom is part of a **data stack**, which is a complete suite of tools focused on loading, warehousing, transforming, and analyzing data (MongoDB n.d.). After anonymizing the data the owner might allow for **data democratization**, which is when data are made available without barriers, much like some government databases (Lefebvre et al. 2023). This allows many researchers to analyze the data from different angles for different reasons, enhancing the impact it will have on improving overall quality. Once analysis is in process or complete, the **data dashboard** provides a visual expression of the output (charts, graphs, and so on) (Tableau n.d.).

When discussing DG and IG as they relate to health specific data, it is imperative to understand **Health Level 7 Fast Healthcare Interoperability Resources (HL7 FHIR)**. This standard defines how healthcare information can be exchanged between computer systems regardless of how it is stored in those systems. In July 2021, the US Centers for Medicare and Medicaid Services mandated the use of FHIR for organizations it regulates (ONC 2024). These are just some of the many common terms that assist in aligning DG and IG professionals when discussing ways to improve standards and processes.

## Governance

The concept of governance has various meanings, and its characteristics and definition depend upon the desired end results to be achieved and the domain and the level to which governance is applied. A general definition of **governance** is the establishment of policies and the continual monitoring of their proper implementation for managing organization assets to enhance the prosperity and viability of the organization.

**Corporate governance** is the terminology most often used to describe the roles and responsibilities of boards of directors who protect shareholders' interests in publicly held companies. The Organisation for Economic Co-operation and Development expanded the meaning to indicate corporate governance "involves a set of relationships between a company's management, board, shareholders and stakeholders. Corporate governance also provides the structure and systems through which the company is directed and its objectives are set, and the means of attaining those objectives and monitoring performance are determined" (OECD 2023).

The top authority in an organization, such as the board of directors or executive officers, exercises governance by applying a conceptual structure, called a **framework**, for classifying, organizing, and showing interrelations among activities and is used as a guide for taking and coordinating action to achieve a goal. The framework is used as a guide for establishing policies, standards, rules, and decision rights and implementing these through the formal structure of assigned roles, responsibilities, and accountabilities. Good corporate governance helps to build the environment of trust, transparency, and accountability necessary for fostering long-term investment, financial stability and business integrity, thereby supporting stronger growth and more inclusive societies. This is achieved with well-designed corporate governance policies that do the following:

1. Help companies access financing, particularly from capital markets. By doing so, they promote innovation, productivity, and entrepreneurship, and foster economic dynamism more broadly. […]
2. Provide a framework to protect investors, which include households with invested savings. […]
3. Support the sustainability and resilience of corporations and in turn, may contribute to the sustainability and resilience of the broader economy. (OECD 2023)

**Enterprise governance**, in contrast to corporate governance, is a broader concept visible in every aspect of an organization through establishment, application, and monitoring of strategies, policies and procedures to all organizational entities and levels. Enterprise governance is typically applied, for example, in accounting and audit management, human resources management, financial reporting, record keeping, and risk management.

## Data Governance and Information Governance

The terms DG and IG are sometimes used interchangeably in popular literature and by vendors and consultants. However, they are not the same (Azhar 2022). Given the lack of consensus on the definition of DG or IG, it is understandable that lines between the two and what constitutes each are blurred. To improve quality and efficiency, agreed-upon definitions and accompanying standards provide benchmarks by which organizations can measure themselves and by which comparisons can be made among organizations. For example, if Health System A develops its IG program on the basis of a definition that emphasizes personal information, while Health System B develops and uses its own definition that emphasizes corporate information, comparing the outcomes between the IG programs at Health System A and Health System B is difficult because what is measured and how it is measured differ. A sample of formal definitions in figure 2.1 demonstrates the differing perspectives among organizations and experts in the governance field about the meaning of DG and IG.

Figure 2.2 depicts how DG is concerned with governing the input (data), whereas IG is concerned with governing the output (information) of an information system. The distinction between DG and IG begins with examining the difference between the assets that are being governed, namely data and information. A vital contribution of the National Health Service (NHS) of England is the distinction made between data and information:

- "**Data** is used to describe qualitative or quantitative statements or numbers that are assumed to be factual, and not the product of analysis or interpretation.
- **Information** is the output of some process that summarizes, interprets, or otherwise represents data to convey meaning" (Caldicott 2013, 24).

**Figure 2.1.** Health information technology vendor definitions of information and data governance

---

**Information Governance**

"The specification of decision rights and an accountability framework to ensure appropriate behavior in the valuation, creation, storage, use, archiving and deletion of information. It includes the processes, roles and policies, standards and metrics that ensure the effective and efficient use of information in enabling an organization to achieve its goals" (Gartner n.d.).

"Information Governance can be considered as a holistic approach that helps manage information by implementing controls, processes, metrics, and roles. It helps ensure that the information is treated as a valuable business asset in today's changing marketplace. The goal of Information Governance is to make the information available when needed, while reducing storage costs, ensuring compliance, and streamlining management" (Casepoint n.d.).

"Information governance is a broader category that includes data governance within its framework. It involves the principles, policies, and procedures around the lifecycle of all information, whether it is structured data, unstructured data, or paper documents. So, while data governance is about managing data, information governance is about managing all kinds of information in an organization" (Atlan 2023).

"It pertains to the framework used to manage information at an enterprise level, which includes ensuring regulatory compliance, mitigating risks, and aiding strategic decisions. Importantly, information governance is not limited to structured data; it also covers unstructured information like emails, documents, images, and more" (DataGalaxy 2023).

"Information governance provides a framework to help use information in a legal and ethical way, ensuring that data is safe and secure, available, current and accurate. It helps patients understand clearly and transparently what their data is used for, why it used, and how it is used" (NHS 2023).

**Data Governance**

"Data governance refers to the formal management of data to ensure its availability, usability, integrity, and security within an enterprise. It's a structured process that ensures that the data is trustworthy, reliable, and consistent, making it a critical part of any organization's data management strategy" (DataGalaxy 2023).

"Data governance provides a set of procedures and a plan to execute those procedures that ensures that important data assets are formally managed throughout the enterprise. It encompasses the people, processes, and IT required to create consistent and proper handling of an organization's data across the business enterprise. Key elements include data quality, data integration, data privacy, data strategy, and data operations" (Atlan 2023).

"Data governance refers to the set of roles, processes, policies and tools which ensure proper data quality throughout the data lifecycle and proper data usage across an organization. Data governance allows users to more easily find, prepare, use, and share trusted datasets on their own, without relying on IT" (Qlik n.d.).

The differences are best illustrated through the **data, information, knowledge, and wisdom (DIKW) hierarchy** that is an essential principle of computer information and library sciences. In the DIKW hierarchy, data are facts. For example, blood pressure readings of 140/90, 150/95, 138/95 have no meaning other than they are recorded as fact. When a fact is related to some other fact (data), the relationship produces a piece of information. For instance, if the blood pressure readings are associated with a specific patient, such as Mrs. Smith, the data that compose the relationship become information. Interpreting Mrs. Smith's blood pressure over time and recognizing a pattern suggestive of a prehypertensive stage transforms information into knowledge.

Each level in the DIKW hierarchy depends on the previous levels, as shown in figure 2.3. For instance, there can be no information without data. Likewise, there is no knowledge without information (Cato et al. 2020). In DG, the input (data) into an information system is the governed asset. The form of data may include text, video, and images, among others.

IG focuses on the control and use of the actual documents, reports, and records created from data (Smallwood 2020). Consequently, IG establishes policies and standards for governing how information is used, shared, and analyzed. These may include policies and standards that apply to information confidentiality, ethical use of information, record retention and disposal, and regulatory or legal compliance (Johns 2015). For example, policies about the maintenance of data models, development and maintenance of metadata schema, requirements for master and reference data, and processes for assessing and measuring data quality would fall under DG, while policies on legal holds for records, amendments and deletion of clinical notes, ethical use of statistical data, and release of information would fall under IG.

While the definitions and functions of DG and IG may vary, there are several core concepts associated with both: privacy and security, compliance, IT partnership, and quality (Azhar 2022). Based on these concepts, the following is a working definition of governance that is applied in this chapter to DG and

**Figure 2.2.** Comparison of data and information governance functions

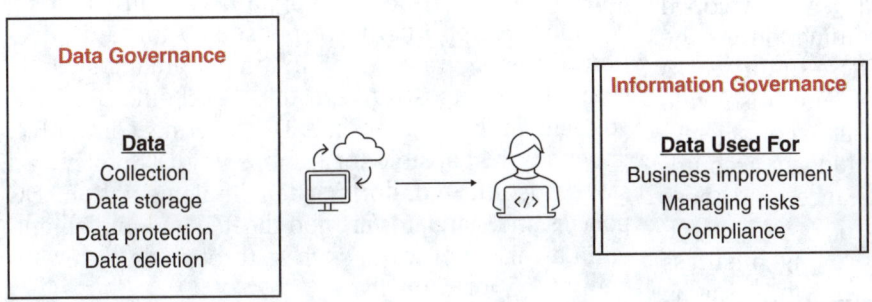

**Figure 2.3.** DIKW pyramid

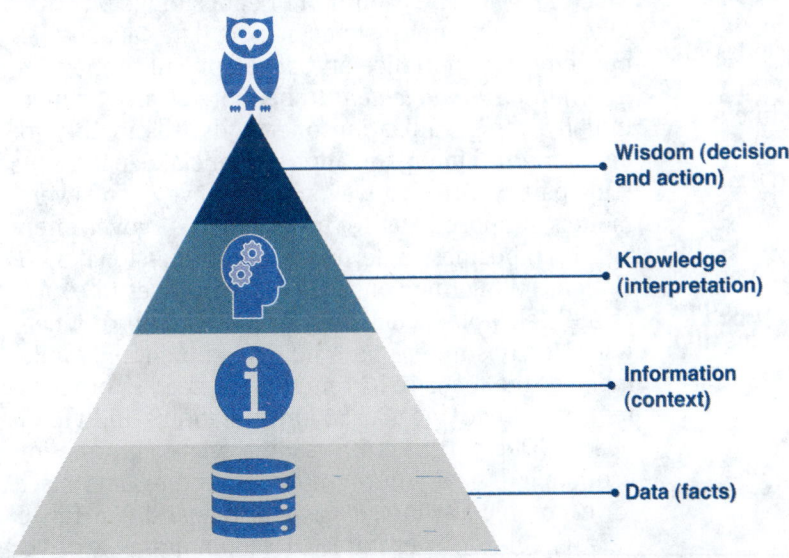

**IG:** *Data and information governance are defined as a subset of corporate governance. Top enterprise authority ensures risk management and accountability for enterprise data and information by establishing a framework of policies, standards, rules, and decision rights. This framework is implemented through a formal structure of assigned roles, responsibilities, and accountabilities for the management of data and information.*

Thus, the purpose of both DG and IG within an organization is to influence the behaviors of stakeholders toward the effective and efficient use of data and information to support the organization's strategy and meet its goals.

## Data Governance Background

While not officially called "data governance," related activities have occurred since the inception of information storage in any kind of computer hard drive. The concept of DG gained prominence in the early 2000s. Over time, technology became faster and more sophisticated. As a result, data could contribute to improved business. Due to ongoing breaches and privacy concerns, security has really ignited the DG boom (Hinkle 2020).

Academics and business enterprises developed various frameworks to serve as a foundation for the development of DG programs. These frameworks usually propose that DG consists of enterprise-wide policies, guidelines, and standards that encourage desirable behavior for data use and include an accountability structure that ensures compliance with these (Bento et al. 2022).

As it relates to healthcare, improving business includes improving patient outcomes while saving money, and privacy includes protecting patient data. DG piques the interest of patients, providers, and payers. It is essentially intertwined with any kind of patient information whether it is in paper or electronic format. All data needs to be regulated. DG includes any information-related processes; it is not limited to only certain kinds of data (Data Governance Institute n.d.).

Today, DG is accomplished through a formal organizational structure and applied to several data management functions. The areas are commonly called domains and referred to as data management domains (a term unique to healthcare) or data management knowledge areas (DAMA 2024). This chapter uses the following data management domains that fall within the purview of a DG program:

- Data life cycle management
- Data architecture management
- Metadata management
- Master data management
- Content management
- Data security management
- Business intelligence
- Data quality management

As shown in figure 2.4, these domains constitute a model of enterprise health information management (EHIM) for health information management (HIM) practice (Johns 2015).

The principal purpose of DG is to coordinate and synchronize all data management domains. The scope of the DG effort varies among organizations. For example, some organizations may take a focused approach and apply the DG effort to one or two data management domains, such as master data management and data security management. Others may take a broad scope and implement the DG effort in several or all data management domains. Effective DG will promote value and outcomes by focusing on transparency and ethics, risk and security, education and training, collaboration and culture, accountability and decision rights, and trust (Gartner 2021).

The organizational structure, discussed later in the chapter, depends on organization culture and size, and the scope of the DG program. Typically, DG is a collaborative effort with responsibility for authorization of the program vested in a high-ranking steering committee composed of executive level officials. A DG council, authorized by the DG steering committee, is usually responsible for establishing DG policy and standards and monitoring their implementation. DG policies and standards are coordinated and implemented in a variety of ways, such as through data steward committees or councils.

## Information Governance Background

Much like DG, the evolution of data storage on paper to within computer systems in a big data capacity has pushed the importance and development of the term *information management* to be more clearly defined. Initially, the organization of records was mainly for decisions within organizations' financial departments (Dogiparthi 2019). However, there have been several models proposed for IG by academics, government agencies, business enterprises, and professional associations. While the concept of IG continues to evolve as the stakeholders debate how IG should be defined, what it constitutes, and how it should be implemented, the focus of IG remains the need to organize information to meet each organization's individual needs (Dogiparthi 2019). Some view information economics—how information is bundled and used for economic advantage—as a principal driver for IG (CGOC 2017). An example of economics as a driver

**Figure 2.4.** EHIM model of HIM practice

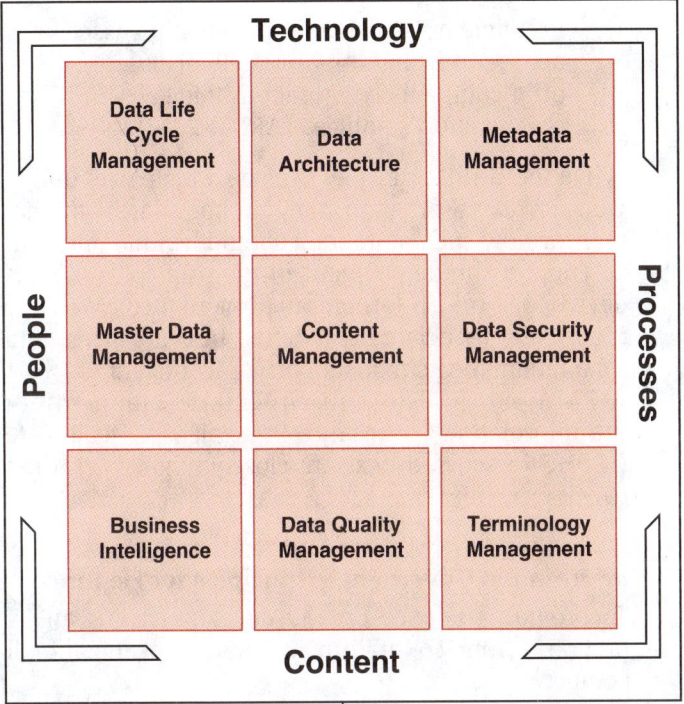

*Source:* Adapted from Johns 2015.

of IG would be collecting data on consumer online purchasing patterns and bundling the data as information for resale or reuse to increase the company's bottom line. On the other hand, some, such as the NHS, have seen IG from the perspective of information security and confidentiality (Caldicott 2013) and would not permit the resale or reuse of information derived from patient data.

Continued change is necessary to improve quality beyond financial endeavors. Electronic data security breaches have significantly increased in recent years and require attention. Tracking fatal bacteria and viruses has become more sophisticated, and that topic needs attention too. So, IG processes will not be static across all organizations, specifically healthcare ones. The number and variation among existing IG principles are too extensive to discuss within this chapter. However, three principles closely related to HIM will be described in the following sections.

### National Health Service Information Governance Principles

The term *information governance* was first used scientifically at the NHS in England as a framework for governing security and confidentiality for electronic health systems at multiple levels while addressing issues related to data protection, records management, and data quality (Kooper et al. 2011). The primary focus was on the requirements and standards that organizations and their suppliers needed to meet to ensure healthcare information was handled legally, securely, efficiently, effectively, and in a manner that maintained public trust. The NHS IG framework was implemented to ensure the necessary safeguards were in place to guide those working in the health and social care system in deciding when to share or not share patient information. A vital contribution of the NHS in defining IG is the distinction made between data and information:

- "**Data** is used to describe qualitative or quantitative statements or numbers that are assumed to be factual, and not the product of analysis or interpretation.
- **Information** is the output of some process that summarizes, interprets, or otherwise represents data to convey meaning" (Caldicott 2013, 24).

The NHS IG framework was developed in 1997, and at the time it consisted of six guiding principles organizations could use for access to patient data. As of 2020, there are eight principles, which are as follows:

1. Justify the purpose(s) for using confidential information.
2. Use confidential information only when it is necessary.
3. Use the minimum necessary confidential information.
4. Access to confidential information should be on a strict need-to-know basis.
5. Everyone with access to confidential information should be aware of their responsibilities.
6. Comply with the law.
7. The duty to share information before individual care is as important as the duty to protect patient confidentiality.
8. Inform patients and service users about how their confidential information is used (NDG 2020).

Edits to this list will be ongoing based on the needs of the industry in general (laws and regulations, employees, patients, and so forth).

## Generally Accepted Recordkeeping Principles

ARMA International (ARMA) was one of the first professional organizations to develop an IG framework. The framework, developed in 2008 and updated in 2017, is composed of eight principles with the intent of providing a consistent standard for recordkeeping across all industries, large or small. The principles, called Generally Accepted Recordkeeping Principles (GARP), serve as a high-level framework for an effective organizational IG program:

- Principle of Accountability: An IG program is overseen by a senior executive.
- Principle of Transparency: Business processes, activities, and IG program are documented openly and verifiable and available to all interested and appropriate parties.
- Principle of Integrity: An IG program ensures that information assets have authenticity and reliability.
- Principle of Protection: An IG program ensures an appropriate level of protection for information assets.
- Principle of Compliance: An IG program complies with applicable laws, binding authorities, and organization's policies.
- Principle of Availability: Information assets can be timely, efficiently, and accurately retrieved.
- Principle of Retention: Information assets are maintained for an appropriate time in accordance with legal, regulatory, fiscal, operational, and historical requirements.
- Principle of Disposition: Information assets are securely and appropriately disposed of in compliance with applicable laws and organization's policies (ARMA 2017).

While the GARP principles provide a high-level framework for an IG program, they do not address the details for how such a program should be implemented. To support the deployment of the principles, ARMA developed the Information Governance Maturity Model and associated standards, best practices, and legal requirements that support an IG program in 2011 (ARMA n.d.). The subsequent development of the Information Governance Principles for Healthcare (IGPHC) discussed next are closely aligned with the GARP principles.

## Information Governance Principles for Healthcare

To provide guidance on the development of an IG program, Iron Mountain maintains 10 organizational competencies:

- *IG* connects the organizational structure, programmatic structures, and supporting structures.
- *Strategic alignment* demonstrates valuation of information as a strategic asset and communicates that IG is an organizational imperative.
- *Enterprise information management* includes the policies and processes for managing information across the organization, throughout all phases of its life: creation/capture, processing, use, storing, preservation, and disposition.
- *DG* provides for the design and execution of data needs planning and data quality assurance in concert with the strategic information needs of the organization.
- *IT governance* establishes a construct for aligning IT strategy with the strategy of the business and a means of fostering success in achieving those strategies.
- *Analytics* is the ability to use data and information to achieve its strategy, goals, and mission, or, in short, to realize the value of its information is critical to success with IG.

- *Privacy and security* safeguards processes, policies, and technologies necessary to protect data and information across the organization from breach, corruption, and loss.
- *Regulatory and legal* focuses on the organization's ability to respond to regulatory audits, e-discovery, mandatory reporting, releases to patients upon requests, and compliance with information-related requirements of any and all regulatory and other bodies of authority.
- *Awareness and adherence* aims to ensure the workforce learns and understands IG program principles, processes, practices, and procedures consistent with respective roles.
- *IG performance* includes addressing capability for mandatory business, regulatory reporting, reliability of information, and measures for each of the areas of IG organizational competence (Iron Mountain 2021).

Iron Mountain views domains such as enterprise information management (EIM), DG, and IT governance as subdomains within IG as opposed to separate domains collaborating with IG.

## Check Your Understanding 2.1

**Answer the following questions in a separate document.**

1. There is no consistent definition for data governance nor information governance, based on the information provided in this chapter and other credible external sources. Write what you would consider a universal definition for each term. *Note this should not be a word-for-word copy of any of the definitions provided in the chapter.*

2. Describe one of your future desired healthcare-related jobs and indicate how its functions are affected by information governance and data governance.

3. Of the 10 Iron Mountain information governance competencies, rank the top five from your perspective. Justify your choices.

4. The data and information hierarchy (pyramid) is represented by an acronym. Following is a scrambled acronym for the terms: WKID. Put it in proper order from the bottom to the top of the pyramid, then define and describe what each letter means.

5. A healthcare system established an IG council and appointed a chief IG officer to facilitate the council's work. Which GARP principle is the organization meeting in designating the chief governance officer for this position? Explain why you chose this answer.

## Data Management Domains

Good IG depends on good data management. The principal domain that coordinates all other data management domains is DG. A model for describing what data management domains fall within the scope of DG is depicted in figure 2.4. Other models, such as the DAMA model, identify 11 data management domains (DAMA 2017). The Data Governance Institute (DGI), a vendor-neutral organization founded in 2003, consolidates these into fewer domains or includes variations of these domains. For the purposes of this chapter, the data management domains that support both DG and IG are based on the work of Johns that describe EHIM (figure 2.4) and are aligned with those included in the DAMA with the addition of terminology management (Johns 2015, 63–70). The descriptions of each of these data management domains are provided in the following sections.

### Data Life Cycle Management

Data management assumes all data have a life cycle that is "a series of successive stages: beginning, developmental, maturation, declining, and ending" (Johns 2015, 66). Each stage in the life cycle has a function and must be managed appropriately to fulfill its purpose. A life cycle is a component of a larger system. In addition to the functions performed within each life cycle stage, inputs from and outputs to a larger system are accommodated.

There are many models of the data life cycle, and while each portrays a slightly different view of life cycle stages, there are striking similarities among them. A typical data life cycle includes the stages of data planning, data inventory and evaluation, data capture, data transformation and processing, data access and distribution, data maintenance, data archival, and data destruction (Johns 2015, 67). Typical data life cycle functions requiring DG include:

- Establishing what data are to be collected and how they are to be captured
- Setting standards for data retention and storage
- Determining processes for data access and distribution
- Establishing standards for data archival and destruction (Johns 2015, 67)

In a professional setting, workers might not use the exact term "data life cycle." However, it is important to realize when the functions of this term are executed so the best practices can be implemented and the best decisions are made.

## Data Architecture Management

Data architecture is defined as "specifications used to describe existing state, define data requirements, guide data integration, and control data assets as put forth in a data strategy" (DAMA 2017, 98). The data architecture domain assumes data are essential components in complex systems, which require abstractions and models to describe data, and the relationships among data, and the processes they support (Johns 2015, 68). The artifacts developed through data architecture management—such as data models, use cases, data flow diagrams, and data dictionaries—are as important to data management as the blueprints prepared by an architect are to building design and maintenance. Typical functions of data architecture management requiring DG include the following:

- Establishing standards, policies, and procedures for the collection, storage, and integration of enterprise data and design of information systems
- Identifying and documenting data requirements that meet the needs and support the processes of the organization
- Developing and maintaining enterprise and conceptual data and process models that represent the organization's business rules (Johns 2015, 68)

Data architecture provides the underpinning of an organization's information system.

## Metadata Management

Metadata are often referred to as "data about data." Metadata are structured information used to increase the effective use of data. By describing data, metadata makes them easier to locate, retrieve, use, and manage (NISO 2017, 2). There are several types of metadata. For example, some metadata describe data for the purposes of locating data; search engines use this type of metadata. Other metadata describe when data were created or changed; this kind of metadata is used in computer audit trails. Another type of metadata describes who has access rights to create, review, update, and delete data. This metadata is used for access control and security purposes. One of the most familiar types of metadata is used to describe data in databases. Data element name, data type, and field length are examples of this kind of metadata. There are numerous metadata standards, many of which are industry sector-specific.

Metadata are used for discovery purposes to maintain, update, and retain data to meet regulatory and legal obligations. They may be embedded with the data they describe or maintained in large metadata repositories. Usual metadata management functions requiring DG include the following:

- Managing data dictionaries
- Establishing enterprise metadata strategy
- Developing policies, goals, and objectives for metadata management and use
- Adopting metadata standards
- Establishing and implementing metadata metrics
- Monitoring procedures to ensure metadata policy implementation (Johns 2015, 68)

Metadata play an important role in achieving interoperability among different computer systems and providing search and navigation capabilities.

## Master Data Management

Master data management refers to master data that an enterprise maintains about key business entities (such as customers, employees, or patients) and to reference data that is used to classify other data or identify allowable values for data such as codes for state abbreviations or products. A good healthcare example of master data is the master patient index that includes master data on the key entity—the patient—and usually includes patient medical record number; patient last, middle, and first names; birthdate; gender; and address. Typical functions associated with master data management include the following:

- Identifying reference data sources (such as databases and files)
- Maintaining authoritative reference data values lists and associated metadata
- Implementing change management processes for reference data

- Establishing organizational master data sets
- Defining and maintaining match rules for master data
- Identifying and reconciling duplicate master
- Establishing policies and procedures for applying data quality and matching rules, and incorporating data quality checks for master data
- Implementing change management processes for master data (Johns 2015, 68–69)

Since master and reference data are used across the organization, it is critical that they are consistent. Data quality issues are often attributable to poor management of one or both types of data. Inconsistencies or redundancies among either can have profound, negative effects on data quality and make it impossible to share data across computer applications both internal and external to the organization.

## Content Management

**Content management** encompasses managing both structured data (for example, data stored in databases) and unstructured data (such as data contained in text documents). **Structured data** commonly refers to data that are organized and easily retrievable and interpreted by traditional databases and data models. **Unstructured data** are data that do not have a predefined data model or are not stored in a traditional database structure. Unstructured data are typically found in documents, emails, and images. To manage data in both forms, policies and standards must be established for the creation, storage, and retrieval of documents and records and the cataloging and categorizing of information within these. Typically, content management functions requiring DG include the following:

- Developing and implementing policies and procedures for the organization and categorization of unstructured data (content) in electronic, paper, image, and audio files for their delivery, use, reuse, and preservation
- Developing and adopting taxonomic systems for the indexing, cataloging, and categorizing of data for purposes of information searching and retrieval
- Developing and maintaining an information architecture and metadata schema that identify links and relationships among documents and define the content within a document (Johns 2015, 69)

In addition to knowing the difference between structured and unstructured data, knowing the kind of data expected for an organization or specific department can be critical. If someone receives an unexpected file, there needs to be a process for ensuring the data stays secure and is rerouted to the correct intended recipient.

## Data Security Management

**Data security** is the process in which organizations implement protection measures and tools for safeguarding data and information from unauthorized, accidental, or intentional modification, destruction, or use. **Data security management** includes policies and procedures that address confidentiality and security concerns of organizational stakeholders (for example, patients, providers, and employees), protecting organizational proprietary interests, and compliance with government and regulatory requirements, while accommodating legitimate access needs. The typical functions of data security management that require DG include the following:

- Data security planning and organization
- Developing, implementing, and enforcing data security policies and procedures
- Establishing a data security risk management program
- Developing a business continuity plan
- Monitoring audit trails to identify potential and actual security violations
- Managing employee, contractor, and business partner security and confidentiality agreements
- Implementing employee security awareness training (Johns 2015, 69)

Training is one of the most important coinciding components of security. Not only must it occur once, but it must be scheduled regularly to ensure workers are aware of the latest scams and old concepts are not forgotten.

## Business Intelligence Management

**Business intelligence (BI)** is the end product or goal of knowledge management. BI can have varying definitions depending on the source and the environment in which the term is being used. However, no matter the industry, the most common and important theme is that BI is a unit that makes the business smarter. The source of guidance from BI comes from the data the organization maintains or has access to (currently and historically).

Usual functions associated with enterprise information intelligence that require DG include the following:

- Identifying enterprise intelligence needs
- Assessing current intelligence resources and use

- Determining scope and defining requirements and architecture for enterprise intelligence
- Developing and implementing policies and procedures for enterprise information intelligence
- Identifying, assessing, and resolving data quality issues
- Implementing data warehouses and data marts that store massive amounts of data
- Identifying and implementing appropriate business intelligence tools and interfaces (Johns 2015)

BI systems use structured data extracted from an organization's transactional databases that are stored in data warehouses. Since unstructured data—such as those found in word processed documents and emails—make up for a large percentage of an organization's data, it is becoming more common to analyze this type of data. However, unstructured data are difficult to define and categorize. Therefore, special text analysis tools are used to process, extract, and create clusters of text that are subsequently arranged in a data model and can be analyzed.

Because of increased internet speeds (both hard wired and wireless), the use of cloud computing has skyrocketed within the BI sector of many organizations. **Cloud computing** is defined as "on-demand access, via the internet, to computing resources—applications, servers (physical servers and virtual servers), data storage, development tools, networking capabilities, and more—hosted at a remote data center managed by a cloud services provider" (Susnjara and Smalley 2024). Large files located in the cloud (rather than on a personal computer's hard drive) allow for devices to run more smoothly. Additionally, cloud-based software is easier to update because it can be done without user intervention in most cases. The downstream impact has been the expedited development of more sophisticated tools such as predictive analytics and AI.

Predictive analytics does what its name indicates. A data analyst analyzes to predict what could occur next. For example, an analyst for a health plan might initiate a query to predict the health plan's next set of HEDIS rates, which is patient-focused quality data from the health plan (NCQA n.d.). Based on prior years' results that might be in the health plan's data warehouse or data lake, quality improvement focus areas can be identified from the predicted outcomes alone. The sibling of predictive analytics is AI. AI tools utilize advanced computing to simulate humans and problem solving (IBM n.d.c). The key to both predictive analytics and AI is "the more data the better." However, AI is usually more dynamic in the queries and algorithms used, and it utilizes machine learning to constantly update predictions.

To ensure AI is used effectively and responsibly, it is important to have a strong DG framework. This includes having a clear understanding of the data being used to train AI models, ensuring the data is of high quality and free from bias, and having processes in place to monitor and manage AI workflows. AI can also help organizations with DG by analyzing large amounts of data and automating tasks. AI has the potential to generate a lot of data. In many cases this data is stored in the cloud. Cloud computing has a plethora of resources that enhance IG and DG, which is critical for regulatory compliance, risk mitigation, and long-term profitability of data assets. Organizations would benefit from developing clear governance strategies and plans to obtain the most benefit from their predictive analytics, AI, and cloud initiatives. While the growth potential for predictive and AI tools are limitless, human intervention is still critical for development, security, trouble shooting and gauging things that cannot be measured, like someone's mood, possible pain tolerance, or a desired outcome that does not necessarily align with the status quo of historical data. When developing an IG and DG plan, think of the current issues and possible issues that do not exist yet.

## Data Quality Management

**Data quality management** is characterized as a continuous process "setting standards, building quality into the processes that create, transform, and store data, and measuring data against standards" (DAMA 2017, 454). Typical functions of a data quality management program that require DG include the following:

- Identifying data quality requirements and establishing data quality metrics
- Identifying and implementing data quality projects
- Profiling data and measuring conformance to established quality metrics and business rules
- Identifying data quality problems and assessing their root cause
- Managing data quality issues
- Implementing data quality improvement measures
- Providing training for ensuring data quality (Johns 2015)

All enterprise operations depend on accurate data. The purpose of data quality management is to ensure data meet quality characteristics such as accuracy, completeness, accessibility, precision, relevance, and timeliness.

## Terminology and Classification Management

**Terminology and classification management** consists of the processes for managing the breadth of healthcare terminologies, vocabularies, classification systems, and data sets an organization may use, and serves as a terminology authority for the enterprise. Typical functions assumed by this domain include assurance of appropriate adoption, maintenance, dissemination, and accessibility of vocabularies, terminologies, classification systems, and code sets for semantic interoperability and data integrity. Also, this domain includes developing algorithmic translations, concept representations, and mapping among clinical nomenclatures. The last important aspect of this domain is providing oversight for clinical and diagnostic coding to ensure compliance with established standards (Johns 2015).

### Check Your Understanding 2.2

**Answer the following questions in a separate document.**

1. The HIM director wants to ensure state regulations are followed with regard to retention of the health records of minors. Which of the following data management domains is responsible for ensuring these regulations are followed?
   a. Data architecture management
   b. Metadata management
   c. Data life cycle management
   d. Master data management

2. Community Hospital specifies that medical record numbers are 13 characters in length. Which of the following best describes this standard for medical record numbers?
   a. Master data
   b. Metadata
   c. Structured data
   d. Unstructured data

3. Describe at least two ways a small provider office could have a data breach. For each, provide steps the office could take to minimize that risk.

4. Describe how predictive analytics, artificial intelligence, and cloud computing relate to each other.

5. Why is data governance important in relation to the use of artificial intelligence?

## Governance Program Planning

It is imperative that organizations develop a comprehensive, enterprise-wide program for managing data and information as organizational assets. In some organizations, DG, IG, IT governance, and EIM may be considered separate and collaborating areas that constitute an organization's overall program for managing its data and information assets. In other organizations, IG is considered the overarching program. In still other organizations, different configurations may be employed depending upon an organization's strategy, goals, culture, and resources. Independent of these, general principles for developing a comprehensive program for governance of the development, maintenance, and use of an organization's data and information assets can be applied.

First, development of a comprehensive program plan should be incorporated with the organization's strategic IM planning efforts. A strategic IM plan is developed so all IM efforts are aligned with the organization's strategic plan and ensure IM goals and strategies support the organization's high-level initiatives. An IM plan usually includes a description of the business needs for IM. Business needs are identified from the organization's strategic plan and through conducting an external and internal environmental analysis of the current status and future projection of needs. An IM plan typically states the IM vision, mission, values, and high-level goals. The IM plan includes the key objectives, activities, and timeline for reaching each goal and establishes the metrics for evaluating the plan's success. To illustrate the connection between these planning processes, consider the process depicted in figure 2.5. An organization's strategic plan includes a goal of having an IM infrastructure in place that advances quality patient care, efficient operations, competitive advantage, and decision-making, and also ensures compliance with data regulations and mandates. To support the organization's strategic

**Figure 2.5.** Relationship among organizational planning efforts

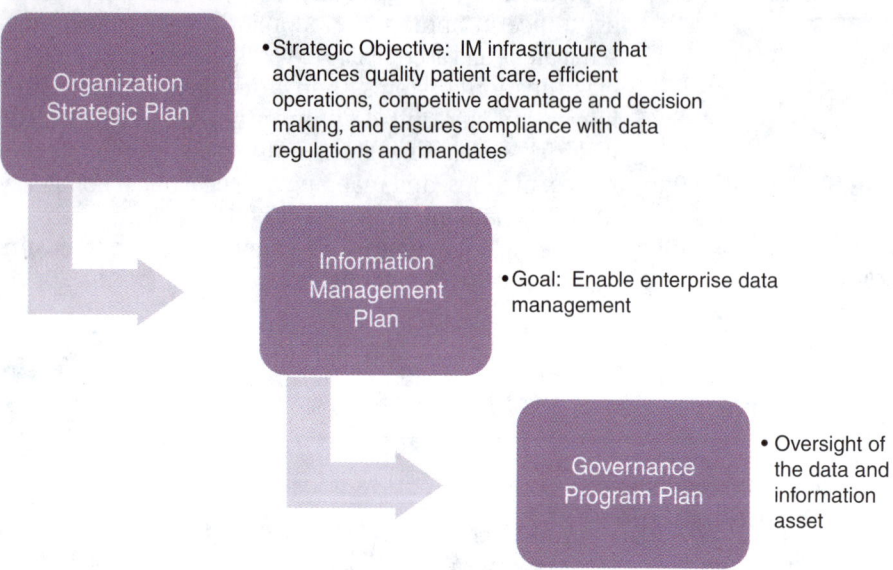

*Source:* ©Merida L. Johns, PhD. Reprinted with permission.

objective, the IM plan includes a goal for enabling enterprise data management. The IM plan identifies the development of a governance plan as one of the key activities for meeting the strategic objective.

Development of a governance program includes the typical management processes of planning, organizing, directing, and controlling. The DGI incorporates these processes for developing a DG program. DGI recommends the following seven steps, which are easily adapted for IG or IT governance:

1. Develop a value statement
2. Prepare a program roadmap
3. Plan and fund the program
4. Design the program
5. Deploy the program
6. Govern the data
7. Monitor the program, measure program effectiveness, report results (DGI n.d.b)

When launching any organizational effort, determining what must be done and why is called **planning**. In developing a governance program, identifying the purpose and value of the program should be the first step. Sometimes this is referred to as a **business case** or value proposal. The business case lays out the benefits and value for the organization that implementation of the DG program can obtain by anticipating a positive change from the current status. For instance, the current status may be framed by stating, business efficiency and effectiveness rests on timely access to accurate data. Inaccurate data leads to rework and reduces efficiency; incomplete data leads to wasted time and inefficiencies; late data leads to idle resources and increases costs. Based on this example, the business case or outcome of a DG program might be stated in the following way:

- If we reduce duplicate records in our MPI [master patient index], then we reduce clinical and administrative errors, which should lead to better patient care.
- If we improve the integration of our data, then we increase our efficiency, which should lead to lower costs and faster efficiency.
- If we establish an organization-wide data dictionary, then we have better interoperability among different information systems, which should lead to better and faster clinical and administrative decision-making. (Johns 2015, 88)

After a business case is established, executive support for the program is solicited, usually in the form of an executive sponsor. At this stage, a governance executive council (described later) is formed, and the planning process commences. Development of a governance mission statement, identification of program scope and priorities, and establishment of an organizational structure are the usual outcomes of the initial planning process.

Tackling all the data management domains requiring DG can be an overwhelming effort. Therefore, organizations usually start a DG program by focusing on a specific area or activity, such as master data management, content management, BI, or customer relationship management. It is best to start the DG program by completing small steps that bring immediate value to the organization.

After the mission, scope, and focus of the program is established, identifying and organizing resources for the program is typically the next step. This includes identifying which individuals and organizational bodies will be included or created, establishing lines of authority and responsibility, and determining how funding will be obtained. A DG office and DG steering committee (explained in the next section) may be established to begin the initial DG work. Once the appropriate organizational bodies and people are in place, DG goals are usually refined, tasks and timelines are developed, and controlling processes are put in place.

### Check Your Understanding 2.3

Answer the following questions in a separate document.

1. The CIO at Community Health System is presenting her business case for implementing an IG function to the C-suite leaders. Which of the following would be considered a business case?
   a. Turnaround time to information requests from third-party payers will be reduced, thus improving the timeliness of our revenue stream.
   b. Competitor health systems in our region are implementing an IG function.
   c. AHIMA recommends establishing an IG function.
   d. IG is the best way to manage information.

2. What should the first step be when developing an IG program? Explain your rationale.

3. Describe the correlation between a value statement and a business case when developing a governance program.

4. Describe why an organization may choose to not implement a full governance program.

5. Once the mission and scope of the program are established, what is included in the next step?

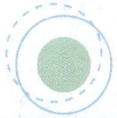

## Data and Information Governance Implementation and Stewardship

Governance is the overarching authority that ensures policies, standards, and accountabilities are in place and enforced for data management. Governance is implemented through a formal organizational structure with both authority and responsibility for managing an organization's data assets. Typical governance functions include the following:

- Advocating for the data or information assets
- Establishing data or information strategy
- Establishing data or information policies
- Approving data or information procedures and standards
- Communicating, monitoring, and enforcing data or information policy and standards
- Ensuring regulatory compliance
- Resolving data or information issues
- Approving data or IM projects
- Coordinating data management or information management organization (Johns 2015)

Note the governance structure varies among organizations but is normally headed by a high-level governance committee. Sometimes called a DG council, in the case of DG, or an IG council, in the case of an IG council, the committee is sponsored by the highest levels of organizational authority and supported by a network of data stewards.

### Data Governance Implementation Frameworks

Many frameworks are available for implementing DG. In the case of DG, a framework assists an organization in determining what constitutes the DG mission and scope, DG responsibilities, authority, organizational structure, and governance processes. Examples of DG frameworks include the Method for an Integrated Knowledge Environment (MIKE2.0), Data Governance Institute Framework, Data Management Association Framework, and Contingency Approach to Data Governance. While frameworks differ, they all assume the following:

- DG views data as a corporate asset requiring the same priority for management as other high-stake organizational assets.

- DG is an enterprise-wide program, linked to organizational strategy, and supported by a business case. The portfolio of DG initiatives is determined by organizational strategy.
- DG is a repetitive process. It initially prioritizes initiatives and focuses on small, select business imperatives that quickly deliver value and expand as the program matures.
- DG is a collaborative effort requiring participation from all organizational levels and stakeholders.
- DG specifies who has the authority and accountability for data decisions and who is responsible for carrying out the activities associated with these decisions. This requires identification and codification in written documents of the priorities, goals, main activities, roles, and responsibilities that are undertaken.
- The DG program includes an executive sponsor, a high-level and strategic oversight committee, and supporting committees or task forces composed of data stewards.
- The DG program is usually supported by a DG office, headed by the chief data steward, chief data officer, or other senior data management professional.

There is no one right way to structure the DG program. The structure and reporting lines of the DG program vary among organizations and are usually based on the mission and scope of the DG program and the customary way the organization operates.

The DGI framework encompasses many of the key characteristics of other DG frameworks and is closely associated with organizational management concepts and is an example of how a DG program can be implemented.

The DGI framework consists of four overarching parts that help classify, organize and communicate complex activities surrounding making decisions about enterprise data. There are four major parts of the framework:

- Why and for whom data governance programs exist
- What the program outputs are
- How the outputs are delivered
- Who participates in data governance programs

This framework establishes a pathway for increased value from data assets while managing risks and organizational clarity (Data Governance Institute n.d.a). Each of the framework components are illustrated in table 2.1 and explained in the following sections.

**Table 2.1.** 10 universal components of data governance

|  | Component | Description |
|---|---|---|
| Why and for whom? | Mission and value | Ways the data governance program can add value to the organization's end goals. |
|  | Beneficiaries of data governance | The stakeholders and their needs from data governance program. |
| What? | Data products | Usually, datasets from various sources used for analysis and intended as reusable assets. |
|  | Controls | Process, technical, automated, manual or technology-enabled manual processes that manage risks and increase data value. |
|  | Accountabilities | Who should complete tasks and when should they be completed. |
|  | Decision rights | Who makes decisions, when, and based on what criteria. |
|  | Policy and rules | Standards and requirements related to data sharing and usage of data. This ensures business, legal, and technical teams are aligned in their understanding of the policies. |
| How? | Data governance processes, tools, and communication | Working in conjunction, the governance process should be standardized, documented, and repeatable. To achieve this, the technical tools used must drive the mission, and there must be communication for all the moving parts. |
|  | DG work program | Individual workstreams for related tasks and ensuring all data governance participants are aware of what success is for each workflow along with how to measure it. |
| Who participates? | Participants | Decision bodies<br>Data governance office<br>Data stewards and custodians |

*Source:* Adapted from DGI n.d.a.

## Rules and Rules of Engagement

Operation of a DG program depends upon having rules in place. Rules are a set of principles and regulations; examples include policies, standards, controls, and accountabilities. Rules of engagement specify the way that policy makers, data owners, data stewards, and other stakeholders interact with each other. The following are considered essential rules of engagement in the DGI framework.

## Mission Statement

A mission statement identifies the fundamental purpose, scope, and high-level goals of the DG program so all stakeholders understand and agree on what is to be accomplished. A good mission statement helps to unify and motivate stakeholders, keeps the DG program on track, and holds the organization accountable for achieving the stated goals. The mission of a DG program will vary among organizations and depends upon overall organizational strategy as well as the scope of the program. One example mission statement may be, "To improve data search and retrieval and integration of transactional data for executive decision-making." In this case, the DG program scope may be narrowly focused on metadata management and developing a BI infrastructure. For another organization the DG mission statement may be, "To increase data integrity to improve operational performance." In this case, the DG program scope may be focused on data architecture and master data management. In some cases, the DG mission statement may be very broad, such as, "To increase data integrity, best practices in data management, reporting standards, and information consistency." Here, the DG scope would likely include governance of all the data management domains.

## Data Governance Beneficiaries

The value of the DG program is described in this category. It includes but is not limited to the data itself, data products (such as glossaries), policies, checkpoints, experts, and decision making. When considering the beneficiaries, the DGI warns against the following pitfalls: the perception that starting small equals failure, the perception that governance is too easy and forgetting governance was in the room.

## Data Products

The tools used for this category are considered to contain the source of truth for the organization. These might include datasets (dashboards, analytic models, data feeds, and such) used across multiple departments within the organization. With the rise of widely available high speed internet connections, data products are more widely available in a cloud setting allowing users to be aware of data updates in real time with little to limited software being downloaded.

## Controls

Controls are measures and functionality established for the purpose of preventing and mitigating risks (Johns 2015). Data are at risk for corruption, improper use, breach, and destruction at every point of the data life cycle. During the data capture life cycle stage, data is at risk for being incomplete or incorrect. To mitigate this risk, data capture controls might include forced field completion, use of drop-down lists of predefined terms, and automatic data type and format edit checks. When data are updated in a database, data concurrency controls are used to ensure data integrity. In addition to mitigating risks, the DG emphasizes that this category ensures data provides value.

## Accountabilities

Having accountabilities ensures the questions of who should be doing what and when can be answered. Accountabilities emphasizes the post-compliance paradigm (do it, control it, document it, and prove compliance). For example, patient billing information is maintained by the billing department; policies should be in place to ensure data remains in that department unless there is an organizational need for it to leave.

## Decision Rights

Assignment of decision rights is defined as appointing authority to specific individuals or categories of individuals to make data-related decisions and designating when and how those decisions are made. Assigning decision rights specifies commitments, is a precursor for establishing accountability for data decisions, and is a critical component of the rules of engagement. Decision rights must be clearly defined to avoid conflict and inconsistencies. For example, they must identify who has the decision rights for establishing data policies and standards for the master data model; who has the decision rights for developing data security policies and standards; and who has the decision rights for establishing standards for data element naming conventions, determining the length of a data field, or determining data access.

## Policy and Rules

At its basic level, DG entails policy development, implementation, and enforcement. Policies and rules double as translators between business teams, legal teams, and technical teams that must follow the rules. Typically, a DG program includes the following:

- Policies on data availability, access accountability, and ownership that clarify who is accountable for the quality and security of critical data
- Specific roles and responsibilities of data committees, data stewards, and data custodians
- Established data capture and validation standards and reference data rules
- Data access and usage rules
- Standards security, privacy rules, and master data, metadata, data definition, and data model standards (Johns 2015)

An organization could add more to this list, and components of each item will be unique from organization to organization. For example, a rural hospital might have completely different policies from a major metropolitan hospital.

## Data Governance Processes, Tools, and Communication

Processes are specific steps or actions taken to achieve a goal or outcome. DG processes are the steps required for governing data and ensuring compliance with DG policies and standards. The following 12 processes are considered DG best practices to be incorporated into any DG program:

- Aligning policies, requirements, and controls
- Establishing decision rights
- Establishing accountability
- Performing stewardship
- Managing change
- Defining data
- Resolving data issues
- Specifying data quality requirements
- Building governance into technology
- Providing stakeholder care
- Communications and program reporting
- Measuring and reporting value (DGI n.d.a, 16)

Processes can be proactive, reactive, or ongoing. Proactive processes are those that anticipate events and are associated with initiating change. Reactive processes, on the other hand, are those initiated as a response to an immediate and specific incident and usually do not continue beyond the event. Ongoing processes are those that maintain a steady state and stability within a system. Ideally, DG processes should be both proactive and ongoing, like those listed here.

## Data Governance Work Program

No matter the industry, the DG program's outputs will do one or more of the following: add value, reduce cost and complexity, and manage risks. The risks managed could include those related to data usage, strategy, product management, access, and such.

## Participants

There are many participants responsible for the operation of a DG program including decision bodies, a DG office, and data stewards. Decision bodies are responsible for appointing authority to specific individuals or categories of individuals to make data-related decisions and designating when and how those decisions are made. Assigning decision rights specifies commitments, is a precursor for establishing accountability for data decisions, and is a critical component of the rules of engagement. Typically, the DG program is led by a high-level committee, frequently referred to as the executive data governance council, committee, or board. This group of executives and senior-level managers is responsible for making the business case for the DG program, providing the authorization for the DG program, establishing the program's mission and scope, setting the program's strategic direction, securing funding and resources for the program, and evaluating and measuring the overall program success. It also has final responsibility and authority for approving DG policies and standards and resolving data-related issues that come to them.

The data governance steering committee is usually composed of representatives from various business or functional organizational units. This group serves as the coordinating body for the DG program. It develops the goals of the DG program, identifies and sequences project and task priorities, coordinates the data steward committees, monitors DG program outcomes, recommends policy and standards, and reports the status of the DG program to the executive data governance council.

A DG program should have an assigned staff that administratively supports efforts of the various DG committees, maintains DG documentation, and provides communication among all DG parties. Most DG efforts are supported by a data governance office that is led by an individual with the title of chief data officer or DG program director. The office's general responsibilities include the following:

- Providing centralized communication and archive for DG initiatives
- Working with stakeholders

- Coordinating DG initiatives
- Facilitating and coordinating data steward committees, task forces, and meetings
- Supporting the data governance council
- Collecting and analyzing DG metrics (Johns 2015)

The number of staff required for the DG program depends on the size of the organization and scope and structure of the DG program.

There are many definitions of a **data steward**, but the central concept includes an individual appointed with responsibility and accountability for data, usually in a specific domain. **Accountability** is the duty of an individual, group, or organization to be answerable for specific activities. Data stewardship is therefore a formalization of accountability for data across its life cycle. It involves a range of stewardship responsibilities from data capture through data disposition and is carried out by a network of data stewards. The way the stewardship function is operationalized varies among organizations. Some organizations arrange stewardship responsibilities in a hierarchy with different levels of accountabilities. Others organize the function based on DG initiatives, and some may have designated tactical teams by business unit throughout the organization. Some of the tasks that data stewards may perform include development of data definitions and data models, resolution of data issues, continuous data quality monitoring, and testing of data security procedures. Data stewards are typically designated within business units throughout the enterprise, including IT, and classified in the following way:

- Subject matter managers (domain stewards) within business areas who have a high level of accountability for the management of the data, but not necessarily the day-to-day hands-on responsibilities.
- Data definition stewards (domain coordinators) who function in a business, as opposed to a technical role; major responsibilities include identifying the specific data needed to operate business processes, recording business definitions and metadata, identifying and enforcing quality standards, communicating data issue concerns, and communicating new or changed business requirements.
- Data production stewards (operational stewards) who can be either in a business or technical role and are responsible for inserting, updating, and deleting business and technical data in IT systems; validating data that enters and exits business processes; coding and editing data quality standards such as format and content; and communicating data issue concerns and new or changed business requirements.
- Data usage stewards who are data users who access and use data for its intended purpose; access information about the data (metadata); ensure the quality, completeness, and accuracy of data usage; and communicate data issue concerns and new or changed business requirements (Seiner 2019).

Data stewards may be organized in program teams focused on specific initiatives that support the organization's DG mission and scope. Usually these teams are **cross-functional**, meaning they are composed of individuals who represent different business units, including IT. For example, an organization whose DG focus is on master data management may have a cross-functional stewardship team composed of representatives from HIM, human resources, finance and business, registration and admissions, medical staff services, procurement, compliance, and IT. These units have a vested interest in ensuring the quality of master data, such as master person data, master vendor data, and master provider data. A sample of the tasks this team may perform includes identifying deficiencies in the organization's master data and determining resolutions for them, developing a master data model, ensuring data from source systems are mapped to the master data model, recommending data quality metrics for monitoring master data quality, and drafting policies and standards for the management of master data and recommending these to the DG steering committee.

**Data stakeholders** are those who have an interest or stake in organizational data (Johns 2015). Among internal stakeholders are executive and senior management, front line management, healthcare providers, and business and service staff. Among external stakeholders are patients, public health and state and federal governmental agencies, other healthcare providers, and vendors (Johns 2015). Because an important DG purpose is to serve stakeholder interests, understanding stakeholder needs is pivotal to DG program success. For example, a top data priority of a senior executive may be to retrieve timely and aggregated operational data for strategic decision-making, whereas the human resource unit may need timely personnel and staffing data for daily staffing decisions. Determining stakeholder needs can be assessed by conducting a stakeholder analysis with key stakeholders. A **stakeholder analysis** is a process that identifies and analyzes the attitudes or opinions of stakeholders. It may be performed in different ways, such as a focus group or survey.

## Chapter 2 Governing Data and Information Assets

### Check Your Understanding 2.4

Answer the following questions in a separate document.

1. To initially present the concept of DG to the C-suite leaders, which of the following would the HIM director use to describe the functions, responsibilities, and expected outcomes of DG?
   a. A DG maturity model
   b. A DG framework
   c. An example of a DG mission statement
   d. An example of a DG vision statement

2. The executive data governance council at Community Health System is developing the organizational structure for the new DG function. Which of the following would the team assign responsibility for overall coordination of the DG program?
   a. DG officer
   b. Data steward committee
   c. DG steering committee
   d. Data steward

3. Community Health System is experiencing multiple data entry errors at the time of patient registration. Which of the following techniques would be the best first step in determining the potential causes of the errors?
   a. Develop a strategic plan.
   b. Conduct a stakeholder analysis.
   c. Develop a business case.
   d. Conduct an external environmental analysis.

4. Describe three similarities among data governance implementation frameworks that resonate with you as most critical.

5. Describe what is meant by the term *decision rights*.

## Information Governance Implementation Frameworks

As organizations identify the need for and expand their informative governance programs, key IG principles are considered best practices among varying IG implementation frameworks. Common principles of IG are:

1. Information as an asset—Organizations should be aware of what data they have and can get and know how that information adds value to the organization's mission and statement.
2. Stakeholder consultation—Communication regarding the unique impact of IG on each department and employee across the enterprise should occur regularly.
3. Information integrity—Data should be accurate so correct decisions can be made.
4. Information organization and classification—Information should be categorized and be accompanied with a map of where it can be found when needed. Also, this includes documentation on information layout.
5. Information security and policy—Safeguards must be put in place to limit security breaches, and disaster recovery plans should be established in case a security breach occurs on any level.
6. Information accessibility—This aligns with limiting security concerns. Access to all information should not be given to everyone.
7. Information control—This involves controlling the access, creation, and updating of any information within the organization.
8. Information governance monitoring and auditing—This utilizes metrics to make sure IG progress is measured, and employees are adhering to the IG program.
9. Executive sponsorship—The IG program needs to be implemented and overseen with executive support to reinforce its importance and ensure it is properly resourced.
10. Change management—IG will change the way users utilize systems to improve productivity as needs evolve.
11. Continuous improvement—An information governance program is not static. It should adapt with business needs, regulations, and security vulnerabilities. (Smallwood 2020)

This section covers some of the more notable frameworks: ARMA International Information Governance Maturity Model (ARMA n.d.), Cloudficient's Information Security Governance Framework: The Key Components (Bougnague 2023), and Iron Mountain's Enterprise Information Governance Framework (Iron Mountain 2023, 2).

### ARMA International Framework

The Information Governance Maturity Model was developed based on GARP and other standards and best practices and legal and regulatory requirements associated with IG. The model was designed for organizations to use to assess their level of IG implementation in meeting the GARP principles as a quality improvement tool. In the model, each GARP principle is described in relation to five different levels of deployment. Each level provides criteria to help an organization assess which level of implementation is currently functioning. The five levels include the following:

- Level 1 (Substandard): Principle is minimally addressed, not addressed, or sporadically addressed. Organization likely does not meet legal, regulatory, or business requirements.
- Level 2 (In Development): Recognition that the principle has an impact on the organization, but practices are ill-defined, incomplete, marginally effective, or insufficiently developed, leaving the organization vulnerable to legal or regulatory risks.
- Level 3 (Essential): There are defined policies and procedures and implementation processes that support the principle, but additional opportunities for streamlining business processes and controlling costs exist.
- Level 4 (Proactive): Supports the principle with a focus on continuous improvement with IG issues routinized and integrated into business decisions.
- Level 5 (Transformational): IG is embedded into the organization's infrastructure and business processes such that compliance with the organization's policies and legal and regulatory responsibilities is routine. (ARMA n.d.)

An organization determines the maturity of its IG program by evaluating its deployment level regarding each principle.

## Cloudficient's Information Security Governance Framework: The Key Components

Cloudficient's information security governance framework is important to mention as its overarching focus is security, which is important given the extreme uptick in health focused security breaches over the past 10 years. It is important to consider security no matter what tasks are in focus. Cloudficient's framework is made of six components, which are summarized with examples in table 2.2.

## Iron Mountain's Enterprise Information Governance Framework

Iron Mountain's enterprise IG framework includes four strategy categories to help an organization get to a state of operational effectiveness, regulatory compliance, cybersecurity, cost efficiency, and data quality and integrity:

- Information governance—how assets will be managed
- Information interoperability—two or more exchanging information
- Enterprise life cycle management—information assets, physical and electronic, across the enterprise including design, acquisition, processing, use and disposition
- Information and data quality—assessing and improving data quality and information

These efforts are geared toward helping improve client outcomes, delivering data-driven decision-making, mitigating compliance and security risks, leveraging operational and transactional information for analytics and insights, and improving productivity (Iron Mountain 2023).

Table 2.2. Example information security governance framework components

| Component | Description | Example(s) |
|---|---|---|
| Policies and procedures | Requirements and best practices for everyone in the organization | Password management |
| Risk management | Identifying and limiting possible threats | Requiring multi-factor authentication |
| Compliance | Staying up to date on and following regulations | HIPAA and NIST |
| Incident response | Having a plan to minimize impact in case a negative incident occurs and ensuring the plan can be executed | Creating an incident response team and establishing communication channels |
| Technology solutions | Ensuring the latest software updates are applied to the data stack and implementing tools to support security including automation | Encryption and firewalls |
| People and roles | Identifying and documenting responsibilities and accountabilities | Incident response team and chief information security officer |

*Source:* Adapted from Bougnague 2023.

### Check Your Understanding 2.5

Answer the following questions in a separate document.

1. One of the functions of the IG council at Community Health System is to grant decision rights. Which of the following would be directed to the council for a decision?
   a. Granting authority to HIM professionals to release health information
   b. Granting permission to registration personnel to access data
   c. Assigning responsibility for establishing standards for the enterprise data dictionary
   d. Granting physicians and nurses security clearances

2. Community Healthcare System has a DG council and an IG council. Which of the following responsibilities would *not* be assigned to the DG council?
   a. Developing policies for identifying master data management
   b. Enforcing data security policies
   c. Assessing the ethical use of statistical data
   d. Establishing policies for data model maintenance

3. Organize and describe the ARMA levels from 1 to 5: Essential, Development, Proactive, Substandard, Transformational

4. Give a specific password management example related to Cloudficient's IG Framework Policies and Procedures component.

5. Why is the common IG framework principle of Stakeholder Consultation important?

# References

ARMA (ARMA International). 2017. "Generally Accepted Recordkeeping Principles." https://cdn.ymaws.com/www.arma.org/resource/resmgr/files/Learn/2017_Generally_Accepted_Reco.pdf.

ARMA (ARMA International). n.d. "The Principles® Maturity Model." Accessed August 2, 2024. https://www.arma.org/page/PrinciplesMaturityModel.

Atlan. 2023. "Data Governance vs. Information Governance: What's Your Priority?" Accessed June 12, 2024. https://atlan.com/data-governance-vs-information-governance/.

AWS (Amazon Web Services). n.d. "What Is Batch Processing?" Accessed June 12, 2024. https://aws.amazon.com/what-is/batch-processing/.

Azhar, A. 2022 (September 12). "What Is the Difference between Data Governance and Information Governance?" https://www.techrepublic.com/article/data-governance-vs-information-governance/.

Bento, P., M. Neto, and N. Corte-Real. 2022 (June). "How Data Governance Frameworks Can Leverage Data-driven Decision Making: A Sustainable Approach for Data Governance in Organizations." Presented at the 17th Iberian Conference on Information Systems and Technologies (CISTI), Madrid, Spain. https://www.researchgate.net/publication/363101208.

Bougnague, S. 2023. "Information Security Governance Framework: The Key Components." https://www.cloudficient.com/blog/information-security-governance-framework-the-key-components.

Caldicott, F. 2013. "Information: To Share or Not to Share. Information Governance Review." https://assets.publishing.service.gov.uk/government/uploads/system/uploads/attachment_data/file/192572/2900774_InfoGovernance_accv2.pdf.

Casepoint. n.d. "Goals of Information Governance. Why Is It Important?" Accessed June 12, 2024. https://www.casepoint.com/resources/spotlight/goals-of-information-governance-why-is-it-important/.

Cato, K. D., K. McGrow, and S. C. Rossetti. 2020. Transforming clinical data into wisdom. *Nursing Management* 51(11):24–30. https://doi.org/10.1097/01.numa.0000719396.83518.d6.

CGOC (Compliance, Governance and Oversight Council). 2017. "Information Governance Process Maturity Model." https://community.ibm.com/community/user/dataops/viewdocument/updated-cgoc-information-governance?CommunityKey=73ce24ad-a006-4d3a-bc1e-7a509a0e2e7d&tab=librarydocuments#:~:text=The%20CGOC%20Information%20Governance%20Process.

DAMA (Data Administration Management Association). 2017. *The DAMA Guide to the Data Management Body of Knowledge,* 2nd ed. Basking Ridge, NJ: Technics Publications.

DAMA (Data Administration Management Association). 2024. *DAMA-DMBOK: Data Management Body of Knowledge,* 2nd ed. Revised. Basking Ridge, NJ: Technics Publications.

DataGalaxy. 2023. "Data Governance vs Information Governance." https://www.datagalaxy.com/en/blog/data-governance-vs-information-governance/.

Data Governance Institute (DGI). n.d.a. "DGI Data Governance Framework." Accessed June 4, 2024. https://datagovernance.com/the-dgi-data-governance-framework/.

DGI (Data Governance Institute). n.d.b. "Data Governance Program Phases." Accessed June 5, 2024. https://datagovernance.com/data-governance-program-phases/.

Dogiparthi, H. 2019 (February). *History of Information Governance* [research paper]. https://www.researchgate.net/publication/330844911_History_of_Information_Governance.

Foote, K. D. 2016 (September 13). "Data Governance and Information Governance: Contemporary Solutions." Dataversity. http://www.dataversity.net/data-governance-information-governance-contemporary-solutions/.

Gartner. 2021 (July 23). "7 Key Foundations for Modern Data and Analytics Governance." https://insider.govtech.com/california/sponsored/7-key-foundations-for-modern-data-and-analytics-governance.

Gartner. n.d. "Information Governance." Accessed June 12, 2024. https://www.gartner.com/en/information-technology/glossary/information-governance.

IBM. 2024 (April 8). "What Is an API (Application Programming Interface)?" Accessed June 12, 2024. https://www.ibm.com/topics/api.

IBM. n.d.a. "What Is ETL (Extract, Transform, Load)?" Accessed June 12, 2024. https://www.ibm.com/topics/etl.

IBM. n.d.b. "What Is Machine Learning?" Accessed June 12, 2024. https://www.ibm.com/topics/machine-learning.

IBM. n.d.c. "What Is Artificial Intelligence (AI)?" Accessed June 5, 2024. https://www.ibm.com/topics/artificial-intelligence.

Iron Mountain. 2023. *Measuring Enterprise Information Governance Maturity with IGHealthRate™*. https://edge.sitecorecloud.io/ironmountain-c8dd68e9/media/project/iron-mountain/iron-mountain/files/resources/whitepapers/m/measuring-enterprise-information-governance-maturity-with-ighealthrate.pdf?sc_lang=en-gb.

Johns, M. 2015. *Enterprise Health Information Management and Data Governance.* Chicago: AHIMA.

Kerner, S. M. 2022 (August). "Data Clean Room." https://www.techtarget.com/searchcustomerexperience/definition/data-clean-room.

Kooper, M. N., R. Maes, and R. Lindgreen. 2011. On the governance of information: Introducing a new concept of governance to support the management of information. *International Journal of Information Management* 31:195–200.

Lefebvre, H., C. Legner, and E. A. Teracino. 2023 (November 24). 5 pillars for democratizing data at your organization. *Harvard Business Review*. https://hbr.org/2023/11/5-pillars-for-democratizing-data-at-your-organization.

Microsoft Azure. n.d. "What Is a Data Lake?" Accessed June 12, 2024. https://azure.microsoft.com/en-us/resources/cloud-computing-dictionary/what-is-a-data-lake.

MongoDB. n.d. "What is a Modern Data Stack?" Accessed June 12, 2024. https://www.mongodb.com/resources/basics/data-stack.

NCQA (National Committee for Quality Assurance). n.d. "HEDIS and Performance Measurement." Accessed June 13, 2024. https://www.ncqa.org/hedis/.

NDG (National Data Guardian). 2020 (December). *The Eight Caldicott Principles*. https://assets.publishing.service.gov.uk/media/5fcf9b92d3bf7f5d0bb8bb13/Eight_Caldicott_Principles_08.12.20.pdf.

NHS (National Health Service England). 2023. "Information Governance and Data Protection." https://www.england.nhs.uk/long-read/information-governance-and-data-protection/.

NISO (National Information Standards Organization). 2017. *Understanding Metadata*. Bethesda: NISO Press. https://www.niso.org/publications/understanding-metadata.

OECD (Organisation for Economic Cooperation and Development). 2022. *G20/OECD Principles of Corporate Governance*. https://www.oecd-ilibrary.org/sites/ed750b30-en/1/1/3/index.html?itemId=/content/publication/ed750b30-en&_csp_=7a1eca165fad928a70a0300d1e07c36f&itemIGO=oecd&itemContentType=book.

ONC (Office of the National Coordinator). 2024 (March 19). "Health Level 7 (HL7) Fast Healthcare Interoperability Resources (FHIR)." https://www.healthit.gov/topic/standards-technology/standards/fhir.

Seiner, R. 2019 (May 1). Data governance roles and responsibilities. *The Data Administration Newsletter*. http://tdan.com/data-governance-roles-and-responsibilities/24774.

Smallwood, R. F. 2020. *Information Governance: Concepts, Strategies, and Best Practices,* 2nd ed. Hoboken, NJ: John Wiley and Sons.

Susnjara, S., and I. Smalley. 2024 (February 14). "What is Cloud Computing?" https://www.ibm.com/topics/cloud-computing?mhsrc = ibmsearch_a&mhq = cloud%20computing.

Tableau. n.d. "What Is a Dashboard? A Complete Overview." Accessed June 12, 2024. https://www.tableau.com/learn/articles/dashboards/what-is.

Tiao, S. 2024 (March 11). "What Is Big Data?" https://www.oracle.com/big-data/what-is-big-data/.

Qlik. 2024. "What Is Data Governance, Why It Matters and Best Practices." https://www.qlik.com/us/data-governance.

# chapter 3

# Health Record Content and Documentation

*Katie Kerr, EdD, RHIA*

## Learning Objectives

- Assess the factors that determine the content of the health records
- Compare the major content areas of the health record, including administrative and demographic data, clinical data, and specialized content
- Identify examples of general requirements for the primary documentation necessary in most health records
- Assess policies and procedures on health record creation, identification, storage, retrieval, retention, and destruction
- Examine issues related to identity management and assess the functions of the master patient index

## Key Terms

Bylaws
Closed record
Closed-record review
Concurrent analysis
Consultation
Delinquent health record
Discharge summary
Disposition
Duplicate
Durable power of attorney
Electronic signature

History
Joint Commission
Longitudinal health record
Master patient index (MPI)
Medication administration records
Notice of privacy practices
Open-record review
Overlap
Overlay
Patient portal
Personal health record (PHR)

Problem-oriented medical record (POMR)
Progress notes
Qualitative analysis
Quantitative analysis
Record retention
Scanning
Serial-unit numbering system
SOAP note
Unique identifier
Unit numbering system

The patient health record, once strictly maintained in a paper format, now primarily exists as an electronic health record (EHR). An EHR is an electronic record of health-related information on an individual that conforms to nationally recognized interoperability standards and that authorized clinicians and staff across more than one healthcare organization can create, manage, and consult. The accuracy of clinical documentation upon entry into the EHR is vital for all secondary uses of the data. The effectiveness of EHR systems relies heavily on the data collected during patient registration and continues throughout the patient's care journey. Standardized clinical documentation practices are essential in ensuring data accuracy and thorough data capture while respecting each patient's unique needs. Embedding these content standards in data capture tools, such as templates, within EHRs is crucial, as "documentation and data content within an EHR must be accurate, complete, concise, consistent, timely, and universally understood by data users" (Berry et al. 2019).

Establishing clinical documentation policies and guidelines, applicable to both electronic and paper formats, is essential to complying with governmental, regulatory, accreditation, and industry standards. These standards address accuracy, timeliness, copy functionality, and privacy and security protocols.

Today's health records include digital images and handwritten notes. Data are entered by electronic transfer from computerized laboratory or radiological testing systems, through direct voice entry into documentation systems, and from providers' wireless devices. However, the use of paper-based health records causes several problems in day-to-day operations. Paper-based records can only be maintained at one location at a time and accessed by one person at a time. This limits their use and effectiveness in contributing to patient care. Even with hybrid record formats, the paper aspect of the record must be scanned and indexed into an electronic system, which takes additional processing time and considerable employee effort. The organization must decide what to do with the original paper chart and how to control the printing of the chart, which creates even more paper. While the momentum to move away from paper has dramatically increased, a fully operational EHR for all types of healthcare providers and facilities remains a goal.

The widespread implementation of EHRs is due to the many positive solutions they bring to the challenge of collecting, maintaining, and utilizing patient information. Fully electronic health record systems make patient information available to any practitioner at any time or location based on the practitioner's level of approved access to the system. Multiple providers may access the record simultaneously and there is no delay for information processing. Abstracting data and comparing it across patients and over time is done quickly and without accessing individual records. The system can automatically track which users reviewed each piece of information and for how long. EHRs can even provide decision support by alerting providers to medication interaction issues, health status changes, and so forth. EHRs can be key to enhancing coordination of care, driving cost savings, and improving patient outcomes.

This chapter provides a historical overview of the health record and describes the kinds of information it contains, the formats in which it is kept, the documentation standards for health record management, and the health information technology systems used to manage health information. The chapter also focuses on the health information management (HIM) professional's role in managing patient information through the record life cycle, from the creation and storage of information to its long-term retention and eventual destruction, and in ensuring its accuracy, completeness, and security. Finally, this chapter describes the functions of the master or enterprise patient index, which is critical for proper patient identification and record linkage.

## Evolution of the Health Record

The patient health record has evolved as medical and health information technology have evolved. Once simply the notation of the patient's name and a brief description of his or her illness or injury, the health record has grown into a detailed collection of documentation templates, electronic data, digital images, and pathology reports reflecting the contributions of numerous healthcare providers.

### Historical Overview

Health records have existed for as long as there has been a need to communicate information about patient treatment. Archeological evidence indicates that maintaining information on patient care and treatment techniques is an ancient art.

Health records are maintained by all organizations that deliver healthcare services, including physician and provider offices, long-term care facilities, emergency clinics, rehabilitation facilities, home health agencies, behavioral health facilities, correctional institutions, and various delivery systems and organizations. Health records are also generated by patients with the increasing use of personal heath monitoring devices and individuals' ability to record and transmit data to providers.

Records vary by facility type. Healthcare records in acute-care hospitals, for example, require rapid documentation by many providers. Patients are often in the hospital for life-threatening injuries or conditions, and various healthcare practitioners may access and record information in their patients' EHRs. Records in non-acute-care hospital settings have much of the same content found in acute-care settings. The records also contain specialized content to meet requirements related to those settings. Although format and content of the EHR may differ among healthcare settings, all providers of care must maintain information to meet patient care needs and to comply with relevant laws, standards, and regulations.

Today's HIM professional is responsible for records that may still contain paper and are maintained in a variety of formats other than paper. There is an increasing demand to share information among providers to improve continuity of care. Today's records come in multiple formats and are a challenge to the goal of uniform information sharing. HIM professionals' skills are in great demand to ensure the quality and integrity of shared health information.

## Factors Influencing the Content of the Health Record

A variety of factors influence what is included in the health record and how it is formatted. In the physician office, for example, provider preference may influence what and how much data are collected about the patient. The process of providing healthcare is another factor. The healthcare provider must gather enough information to determine a diagnosis and to direct treatment. The data must then be structured in a way that is useful for all record users. For many settings, such as acute care, long-term care, and home health, data sets were developed to indicate what data elements should be found in records for that type of facility. Finally, there are accrediting and certifying bodies' external standards and regulations and state licensure standards, in addition to internal standards such as medical staff bylaws that outline requirements for content of the health record. Federal programs promoting interoperability and patient data exchange also drive the content and format of the health record as providers are required to collect and transmit certain data elements electronically.

## Documentation and Maintenance Standards for the Health Record

Health records provide proof of what has been done for the patient. As the complexity of care has evolved, so has the need for improved documentation. Standards for record documentation and maintenance have been established and are constantly refined and revised. These standards and regulations have a major impact on what is documented in the health record. The following includes an overview of the common sources of documentation and maintenance standards for the health record.

### The Joint Commission

The Joint Commission is the successor organization to the American College of Surgeons (ACS) regarding standardization. It assumed responsibility for the accreditation process in 1952, as a collaborative effort of the ACS, the American College of Physicians, the American Medical Association, and the American Hospital Association. Initially responsible for the accreditation of hospitals, the Joint Commission has since expanded its accreditation process to home health, long-term care, and other types of healthcare facilities.

The Joint Commission offers resources and benchmark standards to uphold and enhance the quality and safety of care, treatment, and services rendered. The Joint Commission provides information management standards to address the planning of information management systems, and it provides record of care, treatment, and service standards for compiling and maintaining a complete health record.

### Medicare Conditions of Participation

In 1965, the federal government passed legislation creating the Medicare program, which provides healthcare insurance coverage to Americans aged 65 or older. Since then, the legislation has been expanded to cover persons disabled for two years and persons with chronic kidney disease or ALS (also called Lou Gehrig's disease). The Centers for Medicare and Medicaid Services (CMS) is the division of the federal Department of Health and Human Services responsible for developing and enforcing regulations regarding the participation of healthcare providers in the Medicare program.

The regulations for health record content and documentation were originally established in the Conditions of Participation—guidelines and regulations established by CMS under which facilities are allowed to participate in Medicare and Medicaid programs. As health record documentation became increasingly important, CMS focused on reviewing it for medical necessity and compliance with the decision-making rules established by the federal government. In addition, CMS publishes guidelines for documentation to support physician evaluation and management coding.

### State Licensure

Every state has licensure regulations that healthcare facilities must meet to operate. Licensure regulations may include very specific requirements for the content, format, retention, and use of patient records. These regulations are established by state governments, usually under the direction of state departments of health.

### Internal Standards

Bylaws, rules, and regulations are developed by the medical staff and approved by the board of trustees or governing bodies in healthcare facilities. In addition to describing the organization's manner of operation, bylaws outline the content of patient health records, identify the exact personnel who can enter information in health records, and may restate applicable Joint Commission and CMS requirements. In addition, bylaws describe the time limits for completing patient health records. External surveyors review the bylaws to ensure healthcare facilities abide by their own established rules and regulations and that the bylaws agree with current standards and regulations. All medical staff personnel are required to abide by the approved bylaws. The HIM professional must be able to work effectively with the medical staff to ensure they follow the medical staff bylaws and regulations and adhere to the many laws and regulations that specify the need for proper documentation.

Of great importance to the HIM professional is individual medical staff members' adherence to bylaws related to completion of health records and compliance with documentation guidelines and requirements. The HIM professional supports the patient care process by ensuring quality and timely documentation in the patient record. This also supports the facility's patient safety and quality efforts. The typical medical staff bylaws contain provisions for timely and proper completion of health records, including the requirements to write legibly or use the EHR to record patient notes; for communicating and coordinating the care of the patient with other members of the staff; and for creating reports of history and physical examinations, operative notes, and other required documents based on best practices and facility policies. Failure to comply with any of the provisions of health record documentation may result in progressive discipline up to and including suspension of medical staff membership. One common process is suspending admission privileges until the delinquent health records are completed. Suspension limits the ability of the practitioner to schedule time in the operating room or admit patients. Suspension regulations should be set forth in the facility's bylaws.

Generally, a medical staff committee is responsible for HIM and patient record issues including EHRs. Information about incomplete and delinquent health records is typically reported by the director of the HIM department during committee meetings. Because of this, it is important that HIM professionals know the medical staff bylaws, Joint Commission standards, the CMS Conditions of Participation, any state statutes, and other facility licensure requirements regarding the timely completion of health records.

## Today's Health Record

The patient health record is the foundation for most decisions made in any healthcare facility. Decisions relative to patient care and financial reimbursement depend on the quality of documentation in the health record. The health record is the communication tool among the members of the patient's healthcare team. It is evidence of what was done for the patient, and the information it contains is used to evaluate the quality of care and to provide important information for research and public health needs. The information in the health record protects the legal interests of both the patient and the facility. The traditional saying in healthcare, "if it wasn't documented, it wasn't done," is a reminder of how important the record is for the patient, the facility, and the numerous other users of the record and the information it contains.

Today's health record includes the contributions of numerous healthcare providers. In addition, it includes information provided by the patient or a person acting on his or her behalf describing the reasons for the patient's visit to the healthcare provider and other pertinent background facts. The modern health record is patient-centered, meaning that the patient is the focus of all documentation of the activities that revolve around the patient while under the provider's care.

The health record must outline and justify the patient's treatment, support the diagnosis of the patient's condition, describe the patient's progress and response to medications and services, and explain the outcomes of the care provided. The health record promotes continuity of care among all the providers who treat the patient by documenting all activities revolving around the patient.

### Functions of Health Records and Health Information

The most important use of the health record is patient care, and the person to whom the record is of most value is the patient. To providers, the health record is valuable as the principal source of information in determining care for the patient. To the healthcare facility, it is valuable as a primary source of information in determining the reimbursement for care. In addition, payment models emphasizing the quality of care provided strengthen the need for health records to be accessible and to grant a timely, accurate, and complete picture of patient care.

The primary functions of the health record are as follows:

- Facilitate the ongoing care and treatment of individual patients
- Support clinical decision-making and communication among providers
- Document the services provided to patients in support of reimbursement
- Provide information for the evaluation of the quality and efficacy of the care provided
- Provide information in support of medical research and education
- Help facilitate the operational management of the facility
- Provide information as required by local and national laws and regulations

***Ongoing Care and Treatment of Individual Patients*** When physicians were the only caregivers, they knew the patient and family and decided how detailed the patient's records needed to be. Often, a small card or a ledger listing the patient's problem at a particular time was all the recordkeeping physicians needed. As healthcare has come to depend on technology and the skilled personnel to use it, health records have become more complex. Patients often have multiple caregivers. Providers cannot remember all the patient information provided by the available technology, and fast access to past information about the patient's care is vital to the continuity of care.

***Clinical Decision-Making and Communication*** Health information serves the vital function of allowing all the patient's providers to enter and analyze information and to make decisions. Each member of the healthcare team must have access to the information to review what others are doing and communicate with them through the record. Thus, the health record is the healthcare team's primary reference and communication tool. Because of EHRs, this is extending outside of the healthcare organization as the amount of data sharing and reporting increases with promotion of interoperability requirements and health information exchange efforts.

***Reimbursement*** Information in the health record is used to document the services provided to the patient so that coding and payment for the care provided can be made by those responsible for creating the bill. Insurance companies, managed care organizations, and CMS require that specific information be submitted to support the services billed to the patient and to demonstrate the care provided was medically necessary and effective.

***Evaluation of the Quality and Efficacy of Care*** The health record is used to assess the quality of care rendered by the healthcare provider and serves as the organization's legal business record. Accurate and complete documentation in the EHR allows healthcare providers to provide the best care, improve their ability to diagnose diseases, and improve patient outcomes. The documentation in the record provides information for accrediting and licensing activities. Joint Commission surveyors routinely review the health records of current patients to obtain knowledge about the facility's performance and process of care. The content of the health record also provides evidence of compliance with evidence-based medicine guidelines.

***Medical Research and Education*** Data from many health records may be aggregated and analyzed for research studies and can provide statistical information on medical conditions and treatment modalities. As an example, public health agencies need data on certain diseases and conditions to develop prevention and control procedures as well as to monitor disease trends. Moreover, the information in health records serves to provide continuing education for students in a variety of health professions.

***Operational Management*** Information gathered from health records helps facilities plan ahead based on the types of patients and diagnoses treated. Aggregate statistical information provides data on the use of services, provider patterns, and other important issues. Management often uses the information to make comparisons with other facilities. Finally, the quality of information in the health record aids managerial decision-making in terms of improving the quality of patient care.

***Legal Purposes*** The health record serves the legal interests of the patient, the provider, and the facility. It serves as evidence in legal cases addressing the treatment received by the patient or the extent of injuries. It serves to prove the patient's allegations in a malpractice case and is used by the clinical provider and the facility to defend the care they provided the patient. The record is admissible as evidence in court under the business records provision because the documentation occurs routinely as part of the healthcare facility's daily operation. This is one of the HIM professional's roles, serving as the custodian of the health record.

The health record itself belongs to the owner of the healthcare facility where the health record was created. However, patients have the right to be informed about the use of their protected health information (PHI). The federal Health Insurance Portability and Accountability Act (HIPAA) Privacy Rule allows patients to request an accounting of disclosures of their PHI, amend their record, and inspect and obtain a copy of their PHI (45 CFR 164). The Office of the National Coordinator (ONC) established the 21st Century Cures Act in 2016, which allows patients to electronically access all of their electronic health information at no cost and prohibits information blocking (interfering with access, exchange, or use or electronic information) (45 CFR 171).

## The Longitudinal Health Record

The longitudinal health record is a record compiled about an individual containing health records from various encounters and numerous healthcare delivery settings. This is not a new concept, and it is commonly accomplished through health information exchange projects in the US. The Cures Act "encourages partnerships between health information exchange organizations and networks and healthcare organizations to promote patient access to their electronic health information in a 'single, longitudinal format that is easy to understand, secure, and updated automatically'" (Lye et al. 2018, 1219). The longitudinal health record serves as a reference of medical history and helps the provider avoid repeating details and duplicating tests for the same conditions. Moreover, the longitudinal health record helps prevent medical errors because information on allergies, drug interactions, surgeries, and past medical problems is available before treatment decisions are made.

## Responsibility for Quality Documentation

Ensuring data accuracy of health record content is one of the HIM professional's primary responsibilities. HIM professionals must have a thorough understanding of the organization's EHR and lead the effort in healthcare organizations to ensure the availability of quality health information. Integrity of health information is one of the biggest challenges to health record quality.

One EHR documentation issue is copy and paste functionality, which is also called copy and paste, cloning, or copy forward. This occurs when a provider copies a note from a previous patient encounter either into the same health record or another patient's health record. Copying and pasting health information can lead to what is called "note bloat," inaccurate information being entered in the health record, patient safety concerns, unnecessary tests and procedures being performed, and misdiagnosis. Organizational policies should be established to address copy and paste functionality in the electronic health record.

Modifications, corrections, additions, and deletions—also known as amendments—to health information, will need to be made in an electronic health record. To ensure health information integrity, the HIM professional must understand the functionality of the organization's EHR system, implement best practices, and ensure policies address who may amend a record, when, and how (Berry et al. 2019). Policies should also address how to process patient amendment requests according to the HIPAA Privacy Rule (45 CFR 164). Legacy systems, which are older systems that are being phased out, and standalone source systems in ancillary areas, like radiology and other diagnostic areas, can create issues for the HIM professional in records management. Before these systems are discontinued or data is migrated to the current EHR, the legacy system must be analyzed. A testing environment should be established, the data stored in the legacy system should be evaluated, and the creation of a plan for data mapping to transfer the necessary data from the legacy system to the current EHR must take place before any data is migrated over to the current EHR. Record retention policies should also be considered. If the entirety of the legacy system data is transferred to the current EHR or another storage solution, such as an archival system, the legacy system could be discontinued and adherence to retention guidelines for the new storage method would apply (Berry et al. 2019).

Patient identity management is a huge issue in today's environment. Ensuring that the right patient connects with the right information relies on accurate patient identity management. To that end, implementing access controls that limit the ability to update or change key demographic data is imperative.

The provider of care is responsible for ensuring that entries made in the record are of high quality. Although the facility's medical staff bylaws establish the rules and regulations for record content, the individual care providers are ultimately responsible for the quality of entries they make and authenticate (sign). Healthcare organizations may transition from paper health records to EHRs in stages due to cost and the substantial impact EHR implementation can have on an organization. This transition can lead to inconsistent documentation methods, requiring some documentation to be stored in the EHR and some to remain on paper. HIM professionals should develop a record matrix, such as the one in table 3.1, to track the transition of documentation from paper to electronic formats, when data is interfaced with the EHR, and is migrated to a new system.

**Table 3.1.** Sample record matrix

| Type of Record or Document | Media Type: (P)Paper, (E)Electronic, (S)Scanned, (T)Transcribed | Primary Source System (If not paper based) | Electronic Storage Start Date | Stop Printing Start Date | Part of (LHR) Legal Health Record, (DRS) Designated Record Set, or (B) Both |
|---|---|---|---|---|---|
| Facesheet | | | | | B |
| Advance Directive | | | | | DRS [NOTE: if the advance directive is used to make decisions regarding providing health care services to a patient, it may also be considered part of the LHR] |
| H&Ps: Dictated Hospital Report | | | | | B |
| Short Form | | | | | B |
| Clinic Notes | | | | | B |
| ACOG Forms | | | | | B |
| OB Outpatient Record | | | | | B |
| Newborn Physical Examination Sheet | | | | | B |
| Fetal strips | | | | | B |
| Inpatient ER Dr./Nurse Reports | | | | | B |
| Inpatient ER Orders, Vitals, Etc. | | | | | B |
| Inpatient Ambulance Reports | | | | | B |
| Inpatient Code Blue Forms | | | | | B |
| Outpatient ER Orders, Vitals, Etc. | | | | | B |
| Outpatient ER Ambulance Report | | | | | B |
| Outpatient ER Code Blue Forms | | | | | B |
| Discharge Summary | | | | | B |

*Source:* NLC 2013, 10.

### Check Your Understanding 3.1

**Answer the following questions in a separate document.**

1. Examine the evolution of the patient health record from simply noting the patient's name and illness to an EHR. Why do you think this evolution was necessary, and what benefits and challenges do we now face with the EHR?

2. The medical staff is upset by the number of admitting privilege suspensions. The HIM director is asked to attend a meeting of the medical staff to address this issue. What information should the director present?

3. Patient health records hold a plethora of information. What are three ways patient health record data can be used aside from direct patient care?

4. What is the role of each of the following in the development of standards for health information: Joint Commission, CMS, state licensure, and medical staff bylaws?

5. Explain the significance of the health record for healthcare providers.

6. The care provider is ultimately responsible for ensuring the quality of health record documentation. What is the HIM professional's role regarding quality documentation?

# Content and Format of the Health Record

All health records contain information that can be classified into two broad categories: administrative and demographic data, or clinical data. All health record entries must be legible, complete, dated, and authenticated according to the healthcare organization's policies. Because the hospital record contains the most complex content, it will be the basis for describing health record content.

## Administrative Information

Administrative and demographic information is generally found through a login screen or dashboard in an EHR. The information entered provides data that identify the patient and data related to payment, reimbursement, and other operational needs of the healthcare facility. This information is entered into the system by administrative staff when the patient presents for care or may be entered electronically by the patient or staff from a physician's office. Facility patient portals may allow patients to enter this information prior to an elective admission or edit it after discharge from the facility. Other types of administrative documentation, including consent for treatment forms, advanced directives, patient rights statements, and valuables lists, are listed in the administrative section of an EHR.

### Demographic Data

Demographic data represent one type of administrative information. Demographic information includes facts such as the patient's name, address, telephone number, date of birth, social security number, health insurance number, next of kin, and other specific identifying information.

A unique identifier is a combination of numbers or alphanumeric characters assigned to each patient of a specific healthcare organization, which is often called the health record number. More information about health record number assignment is covered later in this chapter. Facilities use the unique identifier to ensure all information about the patient is entered in the correct record and the correct record is accessed when a query is entered into the computer system. Demographic information helps to specifically identify the patient and can be aggregated from many patients to provide statistical information that is vital for planning, research, statistics, and other needs.

### Consent to Treatment

Through the consent process, the patient agrees to undergo the treatments and procedures to be performed by practitioners and acknowledges the receipt of patient rights. A general consent form is often part of the admission or intake process into the healthcare facility and allows the facility to provide routine care. The general consent to treatment form including the statement that patient rights have been explained, must be signed by the patient and made part of the health record. The general consent to treatment form does not replace the individual informed consent forms the patient must complete and sign for each operation or special procedure to indicate he or she is fully informed about the care to be provided.

Written consent forms signed by the patient for experimental drugs and treatment and for participation in research also must be included in the health record. Refusal of treatment or procedures likewise must be written to ensure the consequences of the decision to refuse treatment have been explained and the patient is aware of them.

### Acknowledgement of Receipt of Patient's Rights Statement

The consent to treatment form typically includes patient's rights statements that are required by state laws and regulations and CMS. State laws and regulations determine which rights must be explained to patients regardless of their insurance. At the national level, CMS requires Medicare patients to be informed of their rights, including the right to know who is treating them, the right to confidentiality, the right to refuse treatment, to participate in care planning, and to be safe from abuse.

### Consent to Use or Disclose Protected Health Record Information

Under HIPAA, at the time of admission to the facility or prior to treatment by the provider, patients must be informed about the use of individually identifiable health information. This notice of privacy practices must explain and give examples of the uses of the patient's health information for treatment, payment, and healthcare operations, as well as other disclosures for purposes established in the regulations. If a particular use of information is not covered in the notice of privacy practices, the patient must sign an authorization form specific to the additional disclosure before his or her information can be released.

### Advance Directives

An advance directive is a written document, such as a living will, that states the patient's preferences for care if the patient's condition prevents him or her from making care decisions. It also can be in the form of a durable power of attorney for healthcare in which the patient names another person to make medical decisions on his or her behalf in the event he or she is incapacitated. The advance directive goes into effect when the physician determines the patient is no longer able to communicate about healthcare decisions.

When the patient has a written advance directive, its existence must be noted in the health record. Patients or family members may bring the document to the facility to show the patient's wishes in case of terminal disease, traumatic injury, or cardiac arrest. The advance directive can be included as a part of the health record, although its inclusion may not be required. Rather than a formal written document, there may be documentation by the physician outlining the discussion with the patient or the family about the patient's wishes. Patients must be informed that they have the right to have an advance directive. Further, they must be notified of the provider's policies regarding its refusal to comply with advance directives. Caring Connections is a program of the National Hospice and Palliative Care Organization and provides links to information about advance directives in each state. This information is helpful for HIM professionals since legal processes and procedures are primarily dictated by state law.

## Property and Valuables List

Although facilities encourage patients to leave jewelry and other valuables at home, patients often will have clothing, dentures, eyeglasses, hearing aids, and other personal articles. Patients may be asked to list these items and sign a release of responsibility form to absolve the facility of responsibility for loss or damage to their personal property. This form then becomes part of the patient health record.

# Clinical Data

Clinical data include information related to the patient's condition, course of treatment, and progress. The patient health record includes mainly clinical data.

## History and Physical

The history and physical form (also referred to as H&P) includes information about what has led up to the current medical issue and the practitioner's investigation into its cause. The history is a summary of the illness or injury from the patient's point of view. Its purpose is to allow the patient or the patient's authorized representative to give the practitioner as much background information about the patient's illness as possible.

The physical examination is a comprehensive assessment of the patient's physical condition through examination and inspection of the patient's body by the practitioner. The practitioner usually tailors the physical examination to symptoms described in the patient's history and begins an assessment. The end of the physical examination should include the impression, which is a list of the patient's problems based on the information obtained. Thus, the history and physical provides a base on which the practitioner can develop an initial plan of care. Appropriate treatment can then begin.

*Components of the Medical History* It is important that the person recording the patient's medical history documents whether the information was given by the patient or by another person (in cases where the patient is unable to communicate). Table 3.2 lists the information usually included in a complete medical history.

*Components of the Physical Examination* The physical examination is conducted by observing the patient, palpating or touching the patient, tapping the thoracic and abdominal cavities, listening to the patient's breath and heart sounds, and taking the patient's blood pressure. In a comprehensive physical examination, each of the patient's body systems is examined thoroughly. If the patient is admitted for a particular procedure, a more focused physical examination may take place. Table 3.3 shows the components of a comprehensive physical examination.

*Time Frame of the History and Physical Examination* The facility must have a policy that establishes a time frame for completing the history and physical. Most facilities set the time frame as within the first 24 hours following admission and require that the history and physical be completed by the practitioner who is admitting the patient. CMS Conditions of Participation requires that the history and physical examination be completed no more than 30 days before or 24 hours after admission, and the report must be placed in the record within 24 hours after admission (42 CFR 482.24(4)(i)(A)). If the history and physical have been completed within the 30 days prior to admission, there must be an updated entry in the health record that documents an examination for any changes in the patient's condition since the original history and physical examination, and this entry must be included in the record within the first 24 hours of admission (42 CFR 482.24(4)(i)(B)). CMS

**Table 3.2.** Information usually included in a complete medical history

| Components of the history | Complaints and symptoms |
|---|---|
| Chief complaint (CC) | Nature and duration of the symptoms that caused the patient to seek medical attention as stated in his or her own words |
| History of present illness/present illness (HPI) | Detailed chronological description of the development of the patient's illness, from the appearance of the first symptom to the present situation |
| Past medical history | Summary of childhood and adult illnesses and conditions, such as infectious diseases, pregnancies, allergies and drug sensitivities, accidents, operations, hospitalizations, and current medications |
| Social and personal history | Marital status; dietary, sleep, and exercise patterns; use of coffee, tobacco, alcohol, and other drugs; occupation; home environment; daily routine; and so on |
| Family medical history | Diseases among relatives in which heredity or contact might play a role, such as allergies, cancer, and infectious, psychiatric, metabolic, endocrine, cardiovascular, and renal diseases; health status or cause of and age at death for immediate relatives |
| Review of systems (ROS) | Systemic inventory designed to uncover current or past subjective symptoms that includes the following types of data:<br>• *General:* Usual weight, recent weight changes, fever, weakness, fatigue<br>• *Skin:* Rashes, eruptions, dryness, cyanosis, jaundice; changes in skin, hair, or nails<br>• *Head:* Headache (duration, severity, character, location)<br>• *Eyes:* Glasses or contact lenses, last eye examination, glaucoma, cataracts, eyestrain, pain, diplopia, redness, lacrimation, inflammation, blurring<br>• *Ears:* Hearing, discharge, tinnitus, dizziness, pain<br>• *Nose:* Head colds, epistaxis, discharges, obstruction, postnasal drip, sinus pain<br>• *Mouth and throat:* Condition of teeth and gums, last dental examination, soreness, redness, hoarseness, difficulty in swallowing<br>• *Respiratory system:* Chest pain, wheezing, cough, dyspnea, sputum (color and quantity), hemoptysis, asthma, bronchitis, emphysema, pneumonia, tuberculosis, pleurisy, last chest x-ray<br>• *Neurological system:* Fainting, blackouts, seizures, paralysis, tingling, tremors, memory loss<br>• *Musculoskeletal system:* Joint pain or stiffness, arthritis, gout, backache, muscle pain, cramps, swelling, redness, limitation in motor activity<br>• *Cardiovascular system:* Chest pain, rheumatic fever, tachycardia, palpitation, high blood pressure, edema, vertigo, faintness, varicose veins, thrombophlebitis<br>• *Gastrointestinal system:* Appetite, thirst, nausea, vomiting, hematemesis, rectal bleeding, change in bowel habits, diarrhea, constipation, indigestion, food intolerance, flatus, hemorrhoids, jaundice<br>• *Urinary system:* Frequent or painful urination, nocturia, pyuria, hematuria, incontinence, urinary infections<br>• *Genitoreproductive system:* Male—venereal disease, sores, discharge from penis, hernias, testicular pain, or masses; Female—age at menarche, frequency and duration of menstruation, dysmenorrhea, menorrhagia, symptoms of menopause, contraception, pregnancies, deliveries, abortions, last Pap smear<br>• *Endocrine system:* Thyroid disease; heat or cold intolerance; excessive sweating, thirst, hunger, or urination<br>• *Hematologic system:* Anemia, easy bruising or bleeding, past transfusions<br>• *Psychiatric disorders:* Insomnia, headache, nightmares, personality disorders, anxiety disorders, mood disorders |

rules specify the history and physical examination must be completed by the physician or another qualified individual who has medical staff privileges in accordance with state law and hospital policy. State licensure laws vary on the acceptable time frame for completion of the history and physical. The Joint Commission requires the history and physical examination be recorded and made part of the patient health record prior to any operative procedure (Joint Commission 2023, RC.02.01.03).

The HIM professional is responsible for ensuring the most stringent time requirements are followed so that the facility complies with state and federal laws and regulations, licensure standards, CMS Conditions of Participation, and accreditation requirements for the specific type of facility.

## Diagnostic and Therapeutic Orders

Physicians or other credentialed practitioners generate orders that direct the healthcare team. Orders may be for treatments, ancillary medical services, laboratory tests, radiological procedures, medications, devices, related materials, restraint, or seclusion. Orders change according to the patient's needs and responses to previous treatment. In the case of medications, the

**Table 3.3.** Information usually documented in the report of a physical examination

| Report components | Content |
|---|---|
| General condition | Apparent state of health, signs of distress, posture, weight, height, skin color, dress and personal hygiene, facial expression, manner, mood, state of awareness, speech |
| Vital signs | Pulse, respiration, blood pressure, temperature |
| Skin | Color, vascularity, lesions, edema, moisture, temperature, texture, thickness, mobility and turgor, nails |
| Head | Hair, scalp, skull, face |
| Eyes | Visual acuity and fields; position and alignment of the eyes, eyebrows, eyelids; lacrimal apparatus; conjunctivae; sclerae; corneas; irises; size, shape, equality, reaction to light, and accommodation of pupils; extraocular movements; ophthalmoscopic exam |
| Ears | Auricles, canals, tympanic membranes, hearing, discharge |
| Nose and sinuses | Airways, mucosa, septum, sinus tenderness, discharge, bleeding, smell |
| Mouth | Breath, lips, teeth, gums, tongue, salivary ducts |
| Throat | Tonsils, pharynx, palate, uvula, postnasal drip |
| Neck | Stiffness, thyroid, trachea, vessels, lymph nodes, salivary glands |
| Thorax, anterior | Shape, symmetry, respiration and posterior |
| Breasts | Masses, tenderness, discharge from nipples |
| Lungs | Fremitus, breath sounds, adventitious sounds, friction, spoken voice, whispered voice |
| Heart | Location and quality of apical impulse, trill, pulsation, rhythm, sounds, murmurs, friction rub, jugular venous pressure and pulse, carotid artery pulse |
| Abdomen | Contour, peristalsis, scars, rigidity, tenderness, spasm, masses, fluid, hernia, bowel sounds and bruits, palpable organs |
| Male genitourinary | Scars, lesions, discharge, penis, scrotum, epididymis, varicocele, hydrocele |
| Female reproductive | External genitalia, Skene's glands and organs, Bartholin's glands, vagina, cervix, uterus, adnexa |
| Rectum | Fissure, fistula, hemorrhoids, sphincter tone, masses, prostate, seminal vesicles, feces |
| Musculoskeletal | Spine and extremities, deformities, swelling, system redness, tenderness, range of motion |
| Lymphatics | Palpable cervical, axillary, inguinal nodes; location; size; consistency; mobility and tenderness |
| Blood vessels | Pulses, color, temperature, vessel walls, veins |
| Neurological system | Cranial nerves, coordination, reflexes, biceps, triceps, patellar, Achilles, abdominal, cremasteric, Babinski, Romberg, gait, sensory, vibratory |
| Diagnosis(es) | |

physician orders a specific drug in a particular dosage stating how often the drug is to be given, by what means (orally, intravenously, or by other method), and for how long.

Orders for tests and services must demonstrate the medical necessity and explain the reason for the order. This explanation is required because payers may not reimburse the facility if the reason for the test or treatment is not properly entered in the Computerized Provider Order Entry application.

**Clinicians Authorized to Give and Receive Orders** Orders must be written or entered directly into the EHR by the physician or other credentialed practitioner or verbally communicated to persons qualified and authorized to receive and record verbal orders either in person or by telephone. For verbal orders, the person accepting the order should record the order, read it back to the ordering physician, and authenticate it as appropriate. State licensure regulations vary, and each organization should be familiar with any relevant state-specific laws and regulations regarding who is allowed to give verbal orders and who is allowed to record them.

Medical staff policies and procedures must specifically state the categories of personnel authorized to accept and record orders. Verbal orders for medication are usually required to be given to, and to be accepted only by, nursing or pharmacy personnel. Some categories of personnel that may accept verbal orders for services within the specific area of practice include physical therapists, registered nurse anesthetists, dietitians, and medical technologists. The Joint Commission requires that the hospital identifies, in writing, staff who are authorized to receive and record verbal orders. This is typically included in the medical staff bylaws (Joint Commission 2023, RC.02.03.07).

The time the order was given should be recorded in the health record. Some facilities do not allow verbal orders for treatments or procedures that might put the patient at risk. The Joint Commission requires the documentation of verbal orders to include the date and names of individuals who gave, received, and implemented the orders (Joint Commission 2023, RC.02.03.07).

**Signatures on Orders** Orders must be dated and authenticated manually or electronically by the treating practitioner responsible for the patient's care who gave the orders. CMS requires orders to be authenticated promptly. The Joint Commission does not have a standard for the timeframe in which orders must be authenticated and directs healthcare organizations to follow state or local laws or regulations.

Standing orders are "written protocols that authorize designated members of the healthcare team (e.g., nurses or medical assistants) to complete certain clinical tasks without having to first obtain a physician order" (Leubner and Wild, 2018, 13). CMS requires standing orders to be based on evidence-based guidelines and recommendations, and they must be documented as an order in the patient's health record and authenticated by the provider responsible for the care of the patient (42 CFR 482.24(3)(c)(3)). A responsible provider must sign the standing orders while the order is being carried out or soon after the order is carried out.

**Special Types of Orders** Certain categories of medications, such as narcotics and sedatives, have an automatic time limit or stop order. This means these medications will be discontinued unless the practitioner gives a specific order to continue the medication. This method prevents patients from receiving drugs for a longer period than is necessary.

Do not resuscitate (DNR) orders must contain documentation that the decision to withhold resuscitative services was discussed, when the decision was made, and who participated in the decision. This discussion is often documented in the progress notes. Generally, patients are presumed to have consented to CPR unless a DNR order is present in the record. DNR orders may be part of the advance directives in the record. The Joint Commission offers guidance through standards about end-of-life care and patient decision-making regarding withdrawing life-sustaining treatment and withholding resuscitative services (Joint Commission 2023, RI.01.05.01).

Orders for seclusion and restraint, including drugs used for restraint, must comply with facility policies and CMS regulations, state laws, and Joint Commission standards. The most restrictive guidance should be followed. These should never be standing or as-needed orders. Instead, such treatments must be ordered only when necessary to protect the patient or others from injury or harm. These orders must follow specific time limits, and there must be continuous oversight of the patient under restraint or seclusion. The Joint Commission has a standard on documentation of the use of restraint and seclusion in patient care (Joint Commission 2023, PC.03.05.05).

**Discharge Orders** Discharge orders for hospital patients must be documented in the health record and can only be issued by a physician. When a patient leaves against medical advice, this fact should be noted in lieu of a discharge order because the patient was not actually discharged. In the case of death, some facilities require a discharge to the morgue order.

## Clinical Observations

In addition to orders, clinical observations of the patient are documented in the health record in several areas, including areas of medical services, nursing services, ancillary services, surgical services, autopsy reporting, organ transplantation, and obstetrical services. These observations are usually documented in two primary areas: progress notes and consultation reports.

**Progress notes** are chronological statements about the patient's response to treatment during their stay in the facility. Facility procedures and policies must state exactly what categories of personnel are allowed to write or enter information into progress notes. Generally, these personnel include physicians, nurse practitioners, physician assistants, nurses, physical therapists, occupational therapists, respiratory therapists, social workers, case managers, registered dietitians, nurse anesthetists, pharmacists, radiologic technologists, speech therapists, and others providing direct treatment or consultation to the patient. Each person authorized to enter documentation into the progress notes must write or enter their own note, authenticate, and date it. In some facilities, various practitioners record progress notes on a common form or within one electronic section (integrated progress notes) while in other record formats, there may be separate sections for physician, nursing, and therapy progress notes.

Each progress note should include changes in the patient's condition, findings based on the facts of the case, test results, and response to treatment, as well as an analysis of the findings. The final part of the note contains the decisions or actions planned for future care. The **SOAP (subjective, objective, assessment, plan) note** format, detailed in table 3.4, is a

**Table 3.4.** SOAP documentation format

| Letter in acronym | Letter stands for | Definition |
|---|---|---|
| S | Subjective findings | Includes patient statements including symptoms |
| O | Objective findings | Laboratory and other test results |
| A | Assessment | Based on findings and observations from clinicians |
| P | Plan | Methods and actions to address the identified problems |

common method for recording progress notes. SOAP is an easy acronym that helps providers remember the specific and systematic decision-making process being documented. Many providers routinely use the SOAP method, or an adaptation of it, to document progress notes.

The patient's condition dictates how often progress notes are recorded, and the frequency is generally established by the healthcare facility or payers. In a hospital, the physician primarily responsible for the patient's care is often required to document a progress note daily. Doing so shows the physician's involvement and that he or she is aware of changes in the patient's condition.

A **consultation** is the opinion of a physician with specialty training beyond general board certification such as an oncologist, cardiologist, or dermatologist. If the attending physician requests that a specialist see the patient, the specialist prepares a consultation report, which is included in the health record. Each consultant is responsible for writing, dictating, or entering his or her own report. The report should show evidence of the consultant's review of the record; examination of the patient; and any pertinent findings, opinions, and recommendations. Moreover, the documentation should show that the physician requesting the consultation reviewed the report. Not all patients receive consultations, so a consultation report is not found in every health record.

***Nursing Services*** Nursing personnel have the most frequent contact with patients, and their documentation provides a complete record of the patient's progress and condition and demonstrates the continuity of care. Licensed registered nurses, licensed practical nurses (sometimes called licensed vocational nurses), and nursing assistants record the patient's vital signs and facts of the physician's orders being carried out; observe the patient's response to treatment interventions and nursing interventions; and describe the patient's condition and complaints and the outcome of care as reflected in the patient's status at discharge or termination of treatment. Nursing documentation is predominantly made by entering discrete data into flowsheets and responding to assessment checklist questions.

Nursing personnel begin recording information in the health record when the patient is admitted to the facility. They coordinate the patient's care to ensure that orders are carried out. The initial nursing assessment must summarize the date, time, and method of admission; the patient's condition, symptoms, and vital signs; and other information. Nurses may use a variation of the SOAP notes from the **problem-oriented medical record (POMR)** format when recording notes. The POMR is a patient record in which clinical problems are defined and documented individually. All nursing notes must be signed, using full names and titles, by the individuals who provided the service or observed the patient's condition.

**Medication administration records** are maintained by nursing staff for all patients and include medications given, time, form of administration, and dosage and strength. Medication administration records are the "source of truth" confirming the administration of a medication because they document the time medication is given. Orders document the medication prescribed. This is especially important when reviewing medications prescribed "as needed" or "prn" in the providers' orders. The records are updated each time the patient is given medication. The health record must reflect when a medication is given in error, indicating what was done about it and the patient's response. Adverse drug reactions must be fully documented and reported to the provider and to the performance improvement or risk management program according to the facility's guidelines.

Flow sheets are often used in addition to narrative notes for intake and output records showing how much fluid the patient consumed and how much they release from their body through urine or other means. In addition, blood glucose records are often charted on flow sheets for ease of comparison.

***Ancillary Services*** Laboratory and radiology reports and reports from other ancillary services, such as electrocardiographs (EKGs) and electroencephalographs (EEGs), must be signed by the physician responsible for the interpretations. A pathologist is responsible for the work of the pathology laboratory; a radiologist is responsible for the work of the radiology department. The final interpretations of the radiology or other reports become part of the health record and are kept however long the health records are kept.

Healthcare facility policies and procedures must state that the practitioner approved by the medical staff to interpret diagnostic procedures, such as nuclear medicine procedures, MRIs, EEGs, and EKGs, should sign and date their interpretations. It is important that all tests or procedures ordered have corresponding reports in the health record.

Orders and records of services rendered to patients from rehabilitation, physical therapy, occupational therapy, audiology, or speech pathology should be included in the record, as appropriate to the patient's condition. These reports must contain evaluations, recommendations, goals, course of treatment, and response to treatment. Nutritional care plans must be developed in compliance with a physician's order, and information on nutrition and diet should be included in the discharge plan and transfer orders.

**Surgical Services**  The operative section of the health record includes the anesthesia record, the intraoperative record, and the recovery record. The history and physical examination, informed consent signed by the patient or his or her authorized representative, and the postoperative progress note also are part of the documentation about the operative procedure. Every patient's record must include a complete history and physical examination prior to any surgery or invasive procedure unless there is an emergency. The Joint Commission's standards require that prior to high-risk procedures and those involving the use of anesthesia of deep sedation, a provisional diagnosis is recorded by the licensed independent practitioner involved in the patient's care (Joint Commission 2023, RC.02.01.03).

Moreover, the anesthesiologist or the certified registered nurse anesthetist must document a preanesthesia evaluation or an updated evaluation prior to surgery. This evaluation must cover information on the anesthesia to be used, risk factors, allergy and drug history, potential problems, and a general assessment of the patient's condition. An intraoperative anesthesia record of all events during surgery, including complete information on the anesthesia administration, blood pressure, pulse, respiration, and other monitors of the patient's condition must be maintained. Finally, after surgery, the appropriate anesthesia personnel must document a postoperative anesthesia follow-up report including any anesthetic complications. The Joint Commission requires that the health record contain postoperative information, including the patient's vital signs, level of consciousness, medications including fluids, and any dispensed blood or blood products; and any unforeseen incidents or complications and the handling of those occurrences (Joint Commission 2023, RC.02.01.03).

The operative report must be completed by the surgeon immediately after surgery and must include the names of the surgeon and assistants, the name of the procedures performed, a description of the procedures, findings of the procedures, any specimens removed, any estimated blood loss, and the postoperative diagnosis. The surgeon must enter a brief operative progress note in the record immediately after surgery before the patient is transferred to the next level of care. The postoperative progress notes and completion of the operative reports must be carefully monitored to ensure this documentation is promptly entered in the health record.

Pathology reports are required for cases in which a surgical specimen is removed or expelled during a procedure. The medical staff and a pathologist must decide which specimens require both a microscopic and macroscopic (gross or with the naked eye) evaluation of the tissue and which require a gross examination only. These reports are part of the operative section of the health record and must be authenticated by the pathologist. (Authentication validates content and proves authorship.) The preoperative diagnosis and pathological diagnosis can then be compared for quality-of-care purposes.

Information on the patient's discharge from the postoperative or post-anesthesia care unit must be documented as part of the recovery record and authenticated by the licensed independent practitioner responsible for the discharge or by the provider verifying that the patient is ready for discharge according to specific discharge criteria.

The operative section also contains data on implants, including product numbers, and additional information for follow-up.

**Autopsy Reporting**  If a patient dies under questionable circumstances or if a patient's family requests it, an autopsy may be performed on a deceased patient. The autopsy report includes exam details provided by the medical examiner or pathologist that leads to a determination of a cause of death. It will contain a summary of a disease process or trauma along with related treatments (if known), gross and microscopic findings, and a clinical diagnosis. An autopsy may be conducted on the whole body, trunk only, or head only. A provisional diagnosis should be documented in the chart within three days, and the final report should be made part of the chart within 60 days of the examination.

**Organ Transplantation**  The Federal Conditions of Participation and the Joint Commission require hospitals to establish an agreement with an Organ Procurement

Organization (OPO) and to develop and implement a protocol to notify the OPO of patients who have died and of patients whose death is imminent (42 CFR 482.45; Joint Commission 2023, TS.01.01.01). CMS and the Joint Commission require hospitals to inform families of the opportunity to donate organs, tissues, or eyes. The hospital, in collaboration with the medical staff, must institute policies and procedures for the donation and procurement of organs and tissues (Joint Commission 2023, TS.01.01.01). The hospital must work with the OPO to develop and implement policies and procedures for notifying the family of each potential donor about the option to donate or decline the donation of organs, tissues, or eyes. An individual at the hospital is designated as the person responsible for notifying the family and then must document that the patient or family accepts or declines the organ, tissue, or eye donation (Joint Commission 2023, TS.01.01.01). Sample forms and other information are available on the United Network for Organ Sharing website.

***Obstetrical Services*** For obstetrical cases, the health record includes the antepartum record, the labor and delivery record, and the postpartum record. The antepartum or prenatal record is information usually collected in the physician's office before the birth event and made available to the hospital by the 36th week of pregnancy. It summarizes the patient's current health issues, menstrual history, past pregnancy details, drug sensitivities, blood transfusions, blood group and Rh type, and gynecologic abnormalities. It also includes any family history of disease, abnormalities, and multiple births along with a risk assessment indicating past cesarean sections or surgeries, diagnoses such as diabetes or hypertension, history of premature onset of labor or prolonged labor, multiple births or abortions, syphilis screening, and use of alcohol, tobacco, or drugs.

The labor and delivery record includes information collected from the time the patient is admitted to the hospital through to the delivery. It includes an updated history and physical detailing the frequency and severity of contractions, the status of membranes, abnormal bleeding, leaking of amniotic fluid, fetal position and presentation and heart rate, type of delivery, instruments used, amount of blood loss, description of placenta and cord, need for episiotomy, and whether medications or anesthesia were used. Infant data, such as APGAR score (Activity, Pulse, Grimace, Appearance, Respiration scoring system), gender, weight, length, and abnormalities, are also documented.

The postpartum record provides details about the patient after delivery through the recovery process. It provides details on the status of the breasts, fundus, and perineum after the birthing process and discusses any medications or treatments given during this time. If a cesarean section was required, surgical and anesthesia information will also be included.

In the case of a live birth, a new record with a separate health record number will be created for each child. This record will include a history and physical assessment summarizing the pregnancy and delivery details, along with date and time of birth, sex, length, weight, circumference of head and chest, temperature, and exam details or abnormalities. Vital signs will be documented along with input and output of fluids and the condition of the umbilical stump.

## Conclusions at Termination of Care

At the time of discharge, the physician must summarize the patient's condition at the beginning of treatment and basic information about tests, examinations, procedures, and results occurring during treatment. This conclusion at the termination of care is called the discharge summary.

### Discharge Summary

The discharge summary provides details about the patient's stay while in the facility and is the foundation for future treatment. It is prepared when the patient is discharged or transferred to another facility or when the patient dies. The summary states the patient's reason for hospitalization and gives a brief history explaining why he or she needed to be hospitalized. Pertinent laboratory, x-ray, consultation, and other significant findings, as well as the patient's response to treatment or procedures, are included. In addition to a description of the patient's condition at discharge, the discharge summary delineates specific instructions given to the patient or family for future care, including information on medications, referrals to other providers, diet, activities, follow-up visits to the physician, and the patient's final diagnoses. The discharge summary must be authenticated and dated by the physician.

When a patient dies in the hospital, the facility often requires the physician who pronounced death to write a note that gives the time and date of death. This documentation, in addition to the discharge summary, is required in all cases when a patient dies no matter how long the patient was in the facility. In some cases, nurses are allowed to declare a patient dead and subsequently complete the necessary documentation.

A discharge summary is not typically required for patients who are in the hospital for 48 hours or less. Such patients usually have a short-stay or short-service record, which can be used to record the history and physical examination, the operative report, the discharge summary, and discharge instructions. A final discharge progress note may also suffice in these cases to provide a summary of the hospitalization at the patient's discharge. When the patient dies 48 hours or less after admission, the short-stay record is insufficient, and a complete discharge summary must be prepared. Also, most facilities do not require a discharge summary for normal newborns, no abnormal medical conditions or need for special care, and obstetrical cases without complications, if there is a final progress note.

Typically, the discharge summary must be completed within 30 days after discharge; however, facility policy may require a quicker completion date Joint Commission 2023, RC.01.03.01). When a patient is transferred, the physician should complete the discharge summary within 24 hours. The Joint Commission allows for a transfer summary when the patient is transferred to another level of care in the facility or the patient's care is transferred to another provider (Joint Commission 2023, RC.02.04.01).

### Discharge Plan

Discharge planning information regarding further treatment of the patient after discharge should be part of the acute-care health record. The discharge planning process begins at admission and must include information on the patient's ability to perform self-care as well as other services the patient needs. The case manager, the social worker, utilization review personnel, or nursing personnel may write this plan.

## External Records Filed with the Health Record

In the past, there was much debate about whether patient records received from other facilities should be made part of the receiving facility's health record. HIPAA regulations require that all information, including information from other facilities, is included as part of the health record when the information is used in treating the patient (45 CFR 164.524). Unsolicited health information can come from many sources, such as the patient, the patient's family, and other healthcare facilities. Healthcare facilities must develop policies to determine the types of unsolicited information that will be incorporated into the EHR. Working with the medical staff to establish protocols to determine the types of health information that will be retained routinely and sent to a provider for review, the process for handling information falling outside the protocol, and how health information falling outside of the protocol will not be retained. Administrative policies should also define the legal health record, guidelines for the use of a patient's personal health record, and how health information in different types of media formats will be managed (Kadlec 2016).

### The Personal Health Record, Patient Portal, and Electronic Communication

Healthcare facilities work to improve healthcare quality though many means, including patient engagement. One way for patients to become engaged in managing their healthcare is through a **personal health record (PHR)**. PHRs are tools that individuals can use to collect, track, and share past and current information about their health or the health of someone in their care. These records may be in paper or electronic format and consist information from providers, insurance companies, pharmacies, and hospitals; immunization records; allergy information; and information from wellness trackers and mobile devices.

A PHR offered by the patient's healthcare provider is referred to as a **patient portal**. It allows patients to pay their bills online and to securely view all or portions of their provider-based EHR. The ONC Cures Act Final Rule prohibits information blocking, meaning it requires the timely release of electronic health information (EHI) upon request and without delay (45 CFR 171). To comply, many healthcare organizations have chosen to immediately release EHI through a patient portal rather than wait for provider review.

HIPAA allows providers and patients to communicate by email; however, access controls, audit controls, integrity controls, ID authentication, and transmission security measures must be in place before emails containing PHI are sent. The email communication must also become part of the patient's health record. Today's patient portal systems allow for secure messaging between the provider, the care team, and the patient. The communication is automatically captured and documented in the EHR (Alder 2023).

## Specialized Health Record Content

The content of the health record varies according to the type of care provided. When specialized services are provided to the patient, additional documentation is required, which may require special templates and custom forms. Joint Commission standards and regulations for the type of facility often specify content to include in the record, as do data sets specific to each setting.

### Emergency Care

The health records used in the emergency department (ED) may be handwritten, dictated or transcribed, templated on paper or documented in an EHR, or dictated to a scribe who then transcribes the information into the EHR (ACEP 2022). The content of the emergency health record should include the following items:

- Identification data
- Time of arrival
- Means of arrival (by ambulance, private automobile, or police vehicle)
- Name of person or organization transporting patient to the ED
- Pertinent history, including chief complaint and onset of injury or illness
- Significant physical findings
- Laboratory, x-ray, and EKG findings
- Treatment rendered
- Conclusions at termination of treatment
- Disposition of patient, including whether sent home, transferred, or admitted
- Condition of the patient upon discharge or transfer
- Diagnosis upon discharge
- Instructions given to the patient or the family regarding further care and follow-up
- Signatures and titles of the patient's caregivers

When the patient leaves the ED before being seen or against medical advice, this fact should be noted on the ED form. Consent forms for treatment also must be included in the record.

## Ambulatory or Outpatient Care

Ambulatory or outpatient care means that patients move from location to location and do not stay overnight. Ambulatory or outpatient care may be given in a freestanding clinic (which is not owned or operated by a hospital) a hospital-based clinic, private physician practice, public health department, a federally qualified health center, rural health clinic, urgent care center, or ambulatory surgery center (ASC).

Contents of the ambulatory care record vary depending on the type of facility and the treatment received. Ambulatory facilities that only perform surgery are called ASCs. The ASC record must include the following:

- Patient identification
- Significant medical history and results of physical examination (as applicable)
- Pre-operative diagnostic studies (entered before surgery), if performed
- Findings and techniques of the operation, including a pathologist's report on all tissues removed during surgery, except those exempted by the governing body
- Any allergies and abnormal drug reactions
- Entries related to anesthesia administration
- Documentation of properly executed informed patient consent
- Discharge diagnosis (42 CFR 416.47)

## Behavioral Healthcare

Treatment and healthcare for behavioral health or mental health-related issues are provided in a variety of care settings, including community mental health centers, traditional inpatient psychiatric hospitals, short-term psychiatric crisis facilities, residential treatment facilities, alcohol and drug rehabilitation facilities, partial hospitalization program (also called day programs), intensive outpatient programs, private practitioners, and telemental health services. Behavioral health records, also known as mental health records or psychiatric records, must include diagnostic, assessment, and treatment information related to both the patient's mental condition and their physical health. The Medicare Conditions of Participation require that the health records of inpatients within a psychiatric hospital include the development of an assessment and diagnostic data, psychiatric evaluation, treatment plan, progress notes, and discharge planning and discharge summary (42 CFR 482.61).

In general, the HIPAA privacy rule does not provide special protection for mental health records; however, it does provide special protection for psychotherapy notes. Psychotherapy notes are defined as "notes recorded (in any medium) by a healthcare provider who is a mental health professional documenting or analyzing the contents of conversation during a private counseling session or a group, joint, or family counseling session and that are separated from the rest of the individual's medical record" (45 CFR 164.501). Psychotherapy notes must be kept separate from the health record and are treated differently because they contain highly sensitive information and are the therapist's personal notes.

## Home Healthcare Services

According to the National Association for Home Care and Hospice, home healthcare is prescribed by a provider and comprises a wide range of health and social services delivered in the "home to recovering, disabled, chronically or terminally ill persons in need of medical, nursing, social, or therapeutic treatment and/or assistance with the essential activities of daily living" (NAHC n.d.). Home healthcare services include professional nursing; home care aides; physical, occupational, respiratory, and speech therapies; social work, nutritional care, and medical equipment and supply services (NAHC n.d.). The home healthcare health record is comprised of an initial assessment, a comprehensive assessment, the Outcome and Assessment Information Set (OASIS), and updated comprehensive assessments. After a physician orders home healthcare, a registered nurse must conduct an initial assessment visit to determine the patient's immediate care and support needs within 48 hours of referral, within 48 hours of the patient's return home, or on the physician or allowed practitioner-ordered start of care date (42 CFR 484.55). When the provider orders only rehabilitation therapy service, an appropriate rehabilitation skilled professional may complete the initial assessment visit (42 CFR 484.55). Before physicians or non-physician practitioners certify a Medicare beneficiary (the patient) for home healthcare services, they are required to have a face-to-face encounter with the patient and document a clinical note or discharge summary in the health record (CMS 2018). A home healthcare comprehensive assessment must include the following:

- The patient's current health, psychosocial, functional, and cognitive status
- The patient's strengths, goals, and care preferences, including information that may be used to demonstrate the patient's progress toward achievement of the goals identified by the patient and the measurable outcomes identified by the home health agency
- The patient's continuing need for home care
- The patient's medical, nursing, rehabilitative, social, and discharge planning needs
- A review of all medications the patient is currently using in order to identify any potential adverse effects and drug reactions, including ineffective drug therapy, significant side effects, significant drug interactions, duplicate drug therapy, and noncompliance with drug therapy
- The patient's primary caregiver(s), if any, and other available supports, including their willingness and ability to provide care, and availability and schedules
- The patient's representative (if any)
- Incorporation of the current version of the OASIS items (42 CFR 484.55 (c))

The comprehensive assessment must be updated and revised as often as the patient's condition warrants due to a major decline or improvement in the patient's health status. See 42 CFR 484.55 for further details about the comprehensive assessment update requirements.

### Hospice Care Services

Hospice care is "a model of care that focuses on relieving symptoms and supporting patients with a life expectancy of six months or less. Hospice involves an interdisciplinary approach in the provision of medical care, pain management, and emotional and spiritual support" (NAHC n.d.). Hospice services are provided in numerous types of settings, including homes, hospitals, and long-term care facilities. Special documentation for the election of hospice care is required for CMS to reimburse for services. This includes certification by the patient's attending physician and the hospice organization that the patient has a terminal illness. The Medicare Conditions of Participation require that hospice patients' health records include the following:

- The initial plan of care, updated plans of care, initial assessment, comprehensive assessment, updated comprehensive assessments, and clinical notes
- Signed copies of the notice of patient rights and hospice election statement
- Responses to medications, symptom management, treatments, and services.
- Outcome measure data elements, as described in § 418.54(e) of this subpart.
- Physician certification and recertification of terminal illness
- Any advance directives
- Physician orders (42 CFR 418.104)

Bereavement counseling may also be provided to the patient's family and significant other up to one year after the patient's death. Bereavement counseling "means emotional, psychosocial, and spiritual support and services provided before and after the death of a patient to assist with issues related to grief, loss, and adjustment" (42 CFR 418.3). When bereavement services are provided, an initial bereavement assessment needs to be performed and then incorporated into the plan of care and documented in the health record.

### Rehabilitation Services

Rehabilitation covers a wide range of services provided to build or rebuild the patient's abilities to perform the usual activities of daily living. Rehabilitation services include physical therapy, occupational therapy, and speech pathology. Oftentimes, rehabilitation is a continuum of care that begins in the inpatient, acute-care hospital setting, through the post-acute hospital phase, and to the outpatient setting. The Medicare Conditions of Participation outlines the health record documentation requirements for outpatient physical therapy and speech pathology services. The following must be documented in these outpatient health records:

- Medical history and prior treatment
    - The patient's significant past history.
    - Current medical findings, if any.
    - Diagnosis(es), if established.

- Physician's orders, if any.
- Rehabilitation goals, if determined.
- Contraindications, if any.
- The extent to which the patient is aware of the diagnosis(es) and prognosis.
- If appropriate, the summary of treatment furnished and results achieved during previous periods of rehabilitation services or institutionalization.

• Plan of care
- A written plan of care established by the physician or by the physical therapist or speech language pathologist who furnishes the services.
- Indicates anticipated goals and specifies for those services the type, amount, frequency, and duration.
- The results of treatment are reviewed by the physician or by the individual who established the plan at least as often as the patient's condition requires, and the indicated action is taken.
- Changes in the plan of care are noted in the clinical record. (42 CFR 485.711)

In the rehabilitation setting, the history and physical must include a functional history covering the patient's functional status before and after injury or onset of illness. Additionally, the history should describe the equipment the patient uses at home, including orthotics and prosthetics. It is important that the physician outline the goals for the patient's care to coordinate the interdisciplinary team involved in the care.

### Long-Term Care and Skilled Nursing Facilities

There are several settings where long-term care is provided. Long-term care (LTC) is healthcare rendered in a non-acute-care facility to patients who require inpatient nursing and related services for more than 30 consecutive days. Skilled nursing facilities (SNFs) are a type of nursing facility with the necessary staff and equipment to treat, manage, and observe a person's condition, and evaluate their care (CMS 2024). SNF patients receive the same level of nursing care as they would receive in a hospital. According to CMS, a SNF must maintain clinical records for each resident that are complete, accurately documented, readily accessible, and systematically organized (42 CFR 483.70). The SNF clinical records must encompass a complete representation of the resident's experience in the facility. It should include "sufficient information to identify the resident, a record of the resident's assessments, plan of care and services provided, the results of any preadmission screening conducted by the state, and progress notes" (Larkey n.d.). Additionally, the SNF record should demonstrate the facility's awareness of the resident's health status, to include comprehensive care plans and substantial evidence of the care's impact. SNFs must use a federally mandated Resident Assessment Instrument that includes the Minimum Data Set (MDS) 3.0 and Care Area Assessment (CAA). The MDS is a standardized assessment tool that is used to measure the health status of skilled nursing facility residents. The assessment is completed every three months or more frequently as the resident's health status changes and they drive reimbursement for the long-term care facility. The CAA is an assessment that allows care providers to assess the resident in specific areas and to identify areas where residents may require assistance, such as activities of daily living, cognition, mobility, and continence. These assessments serve as the foundation for documentation standards and determine the reimbursement rates from Medicare (Larkey n.d.).

## Check Your Understanding 3.2

**In a separate document, match the scenario with the part of the record needed or referred to.**

1. _____ A physician called the unit coordinator to specify the medications needed for her patient.

2. _____ As a surgeon prepares for surgery, she looks to the patient record for a comprehensive assessment of the patient.

3. _____ A physical therapist documented which exercises his patient did today including the level of improvement.

4. _____ A patient explained how difficult it was for her to see her mother develop dementia at only age 42.

5. _____ A 70-year-old patient arrived unconscious in the emergency department following a heart attack with no family by her side; the physician on duty needs direction in providing her care.

6. _____ An attending physician reviewed the health record to determine if the patient's blood pressure was coming down.

7. _____ A patient's family practitioner needs direction in following up on her condition after a recent brief hospitalization.

8. _____ A patient's family practitioner stopped by the hospital to review what the cardiologist recommends.
    a. Care path
    b. History
    c. History and physical
    d. Orders
    e. Consultations
    f. Nursing notes
    g. Advance directives
    h. Emergency record
    i. Discharge summary
    j. Ancillary notes

**Answer the following questions in a separate document.**

9. Explain the significance of the Minimum Data Set (MDS) 3.0 and Care Area Assessment (CAA) in SNFs, and analyze how these tools impact both the quality of care provided to residents and the reimbursement process from Medicare.

10. Dr. Z's patient is feeling light-headed and has a hemoglobin of 7.8. Dr. Z determines that the patient is anemic and needs a transfusion. How will Dr. Z document his progress note using the SOAP format?

11. What documentation is required for CMS to reimburse for hospice care services?

12. What is included in a home healthcare comprehensive assessment?

## Management of Health Record Content

The HIM professional manages health record content through oversight responsibilities. The health record is also used for abstracting patient data and reporting information both internally and externally. The HIM responsibilities for incomplete records include analyzing and monitoring incomplete records to ensure they are properly completed to meet facility standards and patient healthcare needs, and controlling the design and production of forms and electronic templates to ensure all health records are in a standardized format.

### Document Creation

Completion of the health record and managing paper records in an electronic environment is greatly enhanced by the sophisticated technology in use today. Physicians and other providers have various methods for documenting the care they provide, such as speech recognition applications with and without transcription support, electronic templates and free text in the EHR, a scribe documenting health information in the EHR, and different forms of these methods continue to evolve as technology advances, such as artificial intelligence (AI).

### Transcription

Transcription is still used by providers to create healthcare reports, such as, history and physical examinations, operative reports, discharge summaries, consultation reports, progress notes, clinic notes, pathology reports, and radiology reports. The provider dictates the report, which is transcribed to produce the final output in the EHR, to become a part of the legal health record. Personnel who type—that is, transcribe—the dictation are traditionally called medical transcriptionists. Medical scribes can also transcribe medical information, as they provide real-time documentation in the EHR while sitting with the patient and the provider during a visit or exam.

### Speech Recognition Technology

Speech recognition technology is a software trained to recognize generic speech and speech patterns. It can identify speech without needing to be trained for each person, letting them talk without pauses. Providers create reports using front-end or back-end speech recognition by dictating their reports into a microphone, and the spoken words are converted to text by the speech recognition software. Front-end speech recognition software is used to create a report in real-time that is edited immediately by the provider. Speech recognition software can learn a provider's speech patterns through editing the document. In back-end speech recognition, the provider's dictation is stored as a digital voice file which is then processed and converted by the speech recognition software to a draft document. A transcriptionist will then listen to the voice file while proofreading and editing the draft document (AHDI n.d.).

## Templates

Standardized electronic forms and templates are also used in document creation. EHR templates are customizable and allow for the collection of detailed, standardized, and structured health information at the point of care. Templates can be designed to capture clinical documentation at a level necessary for ICD-10 code assignment and reporting and patient safety and quality outcomes can be better achieved using EHR templates. EHR templates also offer features such as smart text or text expanders or macros. A text expander or macro is a tool that removes the need to type the same information repeatedly and allows for the insertion of common phrases and sentences. Typically, these are inserted into the template through keyboard shortcuts and dot phrases.

## Managing Paper Records in an Electronic Environment

Imaging involves preparing the documents before the records are scanned. Staples must be removed, papers repaired, and each page checked to ensure the presence of a barcode on both the front and back of every form in the record. The barcode identifies the type of form being scanned and contains patient information that allows the record to be identified automatically after being scanned. The scanning process involves inserting the paper into the optical scanner so that both the front and back of the forms are scanned at the same time.

Indexing—a critical activity—involves identifying each individual page according to the type of form, such as discharge summary. If the image is not indexed to the appropriate patient and the correct form for that admission, the information cannot be retrieved. A scanner is the device that scans a human-readable document and uses software to create a picture of the document. After being scanned and indexed, records must be verified and generally are not submitted to the final stored archive until the physician completes them. Verifying that the image is clear and the indexing is correct is important to make sure the image can be retrieved and used in the future. Facilities assign personnel to handle the tasks of preparation and scanning. Emergency department reports, outpatient reports, and reports submitted from physicians often do not have the correct patient numbers or encounter numbers, and all this information must be entered so that each form in the record can be appropriately indexed and retrieved. A concern for HIM professionals is that scanning equipment from one vendor may not work with equipment from another vendor. The long-term storage capability of optical disk has not been evaluated for long-term quality because the technology is still evolving.

## Artificial Intelligence

AI continues to advance, and the ways it can be used to support document creation in healthcare are evolving. Rather than depending on manual inputting of data, using AI in medical documentation can enhance note-taking through instantaneous comprehension and processing of language. Additionally, organizations can incorporate AI into current systems and databases, allowing documentation systems to integrate information from various sources. Using systems that combine natural language processing and speech recognition technology provider conversations with patients are captured automatically and AI-enabled devices can extract and synthesize key points to create a transcribed report. Ambient clinical intelligence, a form of augmented intelligence, is technology that autonomously records vital medical details from interactions between patients and providers. This technology supports providers by utilizing natural language processing and generative AI models to evaluate discussions in healthcare applications and telehealth devices to produce a succinct clinical summary (Bas 2023).

# Incomplete Record Control

Health records must be complete to provide all the information necessary for patient care, billing, and reimbursement. Incomplete health records include but are not limited to unauthenticated progress notes and reports and missing documentation for the intent to order services, such as unauthenticated orders, and missing reports such as a discharge summary (MLN 2023).

The business office notifies the HIM department of bills that are waiting for information from the physician so that the record can be coded and the bill prepared. The administrative team places a great deal of pressure on the HIM department to process bills in a timely manner so revenue can be generated for the facility. In turn, the HIM professional must motivate physicians to provide the information the department needs to do its work. Incomplete records are less of a problem in most healthcare facilities with EHRs. However, monitoring incomplete health records is a constant challenge for the HIM professional.

## Quantitative Analysis

Quantitative analysis, often called discharge analysis, is a review of the health record for completeness and accuracy. It is generally conducted retrospectively—

after the patient's discharge from the facility or at the conclusion of treatment. Quantitative analysis may also be done while the patient is in the facility, in which case it is referred to as concurrent review or **concurrent analysis**. The concurrent analysis and discharge analysis review typically analyze the health records for the same documentation.

EHR systems facilitate the record completion process with workflows that notify providers when record entries require authentication or further documentation. These systems are also used to automate the division of work to the HIM personnel by routing specific record types to designated personnel for analysis, coding, and other HIM operations. These workflows can reduce the manpower requirements and shorten the record completion time.

Any corrections or amendments to the record must be entered properly. In paper records, the provider should draw a single line through the error, add a note explaining the error, initial and date the error with the date it was discovered, and enter the correct information in chronological order. For electronic entries, a procedure should be followed that explains how to correct errors and enter addenda to the health record including the current date and reason for the information being added to the record. In cases of medical identity theft, when someone presents using another's identity, the record must be identified as such so the appropriate health information is entered into the correct health record. This is a growing area of concern for the HIM professional, and procedures and guidance will continue to evolve until a standard of practice is established.

## Qualitative Analysis

In **qualitative analysis**, HIM personnel carefully review the quality and adequacy of record documentation and ensure that it is in accordance with the policies, rules, and regulations established by the facility; the standards of licensing and accrediting bodies; and government requirements. Like quantitative analysis, qualitative analysis may be done concurrently or retrospectively.

Qualitative analysis is a more in-depth review of health records than quantitative analysis, although the processes may overlap somewhat, depending on the facility. When qualitative analysis is done while the patient is in the facility or under active treatment, it is called **open-record review**, ongoing records review, point-of-care review, or continuous record review. Joint Commission requires an open-record review to ensure that its documentation standards are met at the point of care delivery (Joint Commission 2023, RC.01.04.01). HIM personnel as well as case management personnel, nurses, physicians, and other providers should participate in the open-record review process.

This review process looks at requirements such as presence of the history and physical examination prior to surgery and whether it thoroughly describes the condition of the patient upon admission, completion of the postoperative note with all requirements documented, and many other aspects of the care process as documented in the health record. Open-record review should be done on a continuous basis.

Qualitative review also is performed on **closed records**, which are records of discharged patients. **Closed-record review** means that the qualitative review is done retrospectively following discharge or termination of treatment. The benefit of open-record review is that problems in the care process that are revealed through the review can be corrected immediately. Closed-record review is an important way to obtain information about trends and patterns of documentation.

## Criteria for Adequacy of Documentation

Documentation must reflect the care rendered to the patient and the patient's response to care. It must be timely and legible and authenticated by the person who wrote it. The health record is considered a legal document and a business record because it records events at or around the time they happen. Personnel in the HIM department analyze the health record for timeliness, accuracy, and completeness of entries in the health record. There are many patient safety concerns. However, one that relies on proper documentation is the use of abbreviations in the health record. The health record must be analyzed to ensure that symbols and abbreviations used in documentation have been approved by the medical staff and have only one clear meaning. The HIM department staff often analyze the health record for adequacy of documentation during (concurrent analysis) and after (discharge analysis) the patient's stay in the hospital.

## Authentication of Health Record Entries

Authentication means to prove authorship and can be done in several ways. Signatures handwritten in ink are the most common method for signing paper-based health records. An **electronic signature** or e-signature is "a computer data compilation of any symbol or series of symbols executed, adopted, or authorized by an individual to be the legally binding equivalent of the individual's handwritten signature" (21 CFR 11.3 (b)(7)). Methods of electronically signing documentation include a digital signature, a digitized image of a signature, a biometric identifier such as fingerprint or retinal scan, or a code or password. If a password or code is used, a statement ensuring that the password or code is controlled and used only by the responsible provider should be required to protect patient confidentiality and to ensure others do not use it. Password security is critical. In today's health record, electronic signatures are used more frequently as more documents in the record are produced by, and remain in, the system rather than becoming part of the paper record.

Authentication of record entries in teaching hospitals is especially important to show the attending physician responsible for the patient is actively involved in the patient's care. Signatures by attending physicians are generally required on all reports completed by medical residents and students. In electronic signature programs, the attending physician's co-signature should be entered after the resident has reviewed and signed the report to confirm the attending physician's participation.

### Record Completion Policies and Procedures

The health record is not complete until all its parts are assembled, organized, and authenticated or until all documentation and reports are entered into the EHR system and authenticated. The HIM professional, the administration, and the medical staff must develop record completion policies and procedures and include them in the medical staff bylaws. Although the facility's governing body has overall responsibility for patient care, responsibility for the delivery and documentation of patient care is delegated to the medical staff. The medical staff and the individual physician have primary responsibility for completing the health record to document the process of care that was rendered.

The health record committee chair may communicate directly with physicians or other medical staff members to solve problems related to record completion. The committee can be a valuable resource to the HIM professional because it has representation from every area that enters documents into the patient record. Committee members can often assist the HIM department in acquiring equipment and personnel needed to properly perform its responsibilities. The committee generally reports to the executive committee of the medical staff and makes recommendations for executive staff action to improve patient record services.

### Management of Incomplete Records

The HIM professional is responsible for ensuring health records, whether manual or electronic, are readily accessible and adequate equipment and personnel are available to facilitate record completion. No matter how well-staffed and well-organized the HIM department is, it can only facilitate the process. Providers are responsible for the documentation and must authenticate and complete the patient health record.

*Storage, Retrieval, and Tracking of Incomplete Records* With the hybrid health record system, the paper-based portion of the record may be scanned into the EHR at the time of the patient's discharge, and providers are allowed to electronically authenticate incomplete records. This method is convenient for the providers as deficient health records may be simultaneously routed to multiple providers via workflow software. It is more efficient than the paper-based routing of health records as it requires fewer HIM personnel to locate, transport, and refile the paper-based health record. It is also more efficient for the providers who may access, authenticate, and complete the hybrid or fully electronic health record remotely. Hybrid and EHR systems have decreased the health record delinquency rates in many facilities.

*Policies and Procedures on Record Completion* CMS, accrediting bodies, and state licensure standards require that the health record be completed in a timely manner. The completion time clock begins running when the patient is discharged, the patient dies, or treatment is terminated. Records are considered deficient or incomplete immediately at discharge. Some facilities choose to begin the time clock after the records are reviewed quantitatively by the HIM staff and made available to the providers; however, regulations and standards do not allow for extra time for analysis or transcription delays, computer system downtime, or physician unavailability. Healthcare facility policies and medical staff bylaws must define when incomplete or deficient records become delinquent.

A delinquent health record is a record that is not completed within the specified time frame, for example, within 14 days of discharge. The definition of a delinquent health record varies according to the facility, but most facilities require records be completed within 30 days of discharge as mandated by CMS regulations and Joint Commission standards. Some facilities require a shorter time frame for completing records because of concerns about timely billing.

Numerous methods may be used to encourage the timely completion of records. Concurrent analysis by HIM or other facility personnel can speed up completion time. HIM professionals rely on medical staff committees, such as the health record committee, chiefs of medical services, and medical staff leaders, to motivate providers to complete records. As previously discussed, hybrid and EHRs alleviate some of the past issues with completion of the health record.

### Role of Health Information Management Professionals in Health Record Management

The Conditions of Participation require hospitals to have a health record service (42 CFR 482.24). Additionally, some states require hospitals to assign the responsibility of health record management to a trained health information professional. This requirement includes having the staff, equipment, and policies and procedures to ensure records are current and accurate, and that information is accessible.

The HIM department works closely with the business department regarding record completion. The business department and the entire organization depend on the HIM staff to work with physicians and other healthcare professionals to provide the necessary information so that bills can be finalized in a timely manner, usually within two to three days after discharge. The health information manager receives daily notification of accounts that need information, and procedures must be established to expedite the flow of information for payment purposes.

The HIM department must work closely with the medical staff. Medical staff members are responsible for developing bylaws governing their operations. The medical staff bylaws include the requirements for documentation and completion of health records and penalties for not adhering to these rules. Each member of the medical staff signs a statement that he or she will abide by the bylaws, and each is responsible for documentation. The HIM department ensures the medical staff bylaws related to documentation and record completion are upheld.

## Template (Forms) Design and Management

The management and design of forms used in the healthcare environment is a concern of all providers because well-designed forms and electronic screens can facilitate the documentation of care. Forms within the paper record must be developed and approved in a careful, systematic process to ensure they meet facility standards, are compatible with scanning systems, and do not duplicate information on existing forms. HIM department personnel must be constantly vigilant to ensure only approved forms become part of the permanent health record.

This vigilance is especially important as healthcare facilities encounter planned and unplanned EHR downtime. This is an increasingly complex issue as system downtimes may be caused by cyberattacks or other outside threats to the healthcare organization and require business continuity planning for documenting patient care. Many EHR systems maintain view-only backup systems that provide access to documentation from the most recent period before the downtime, typically the last 30 minutes to two hours of care. The organization should determine whether providers and staff will resort to paper documentation during downtime. If paper documentation forms are utilized during downtime, decisions must be made regarding which data can be electronically recovered once the system is restored and what data must be scanned into the EHR, based on the duration of the downtime (AHIMA 2019). The HIM department should maintain a forms management policy, design standards, and a forms inventory to manage the paper forms used during downtime, for information that cannot be captured in electronic format, and in situations where there is a hybrid health record.

With fully electronic health records, the forms design process becomes the process of designing computer views and templates for data entry, but the principles of control still apply. Facilities with hybrid health records must transition existing forms into templates for the EHR. This transition requires extensive input and expertise from the HIM professional. A well-designed form or template improves the reliability of the data entered on it. A form or template should be designed to collect information in a consistent way and to remind providers of information that must be included. Considerations include the number of clicks required to enter patient information into an electronic form or computer view. (Examples of commonly used health record forms are provided in appendix B of this book.)

### Check Your Understanding 3.3

**Answer the following questions in a separate document.**

1. Are the following examples of quantitative or qualitative analysis? Please explain your reasoning.
    a. Whether a surgeon signed the operative report or not
    b. Whether a history and physical report was dictated and present in the patient's health record or not
    c. Whether all the required elements were present on the history and physical report or not
    d. Reference to the same patient as a "he" in some reports and a "she" in other reports
    e. Whether all ordered labs have corresponding lab reports present in the health record or not

2. How does concurrent analysis facilitate record completion?

3. Why is the finance department concerned about the timely completion of records?

4. The medical staff bylaws state that discharge summaries must be complete and a part of the patient's health record within 14 days. Dr. Jones has three records flagged for completion; one is 10 days post-discharge, one is 13 days post-discharge, and one is 16 days post-discharge. Does Dr. Jones have any delinquent or incomplete records?

5. How do health information management professionals ensure detailed review of the content and documentation of the health record documentation through qualitative analysis?

6. What measures are taken to ensure the authentication of health record entries, and why is this important?

7. Explain the difference between front-end and back-end speech recognition technology in the context of health record documentation.

8. What is the importance of templates in EHRs, and how do they contribute to documentation quality?

# Health Record Life Cycle

Healthcare organizations need policies covering the access and storage of health records to ensure the records can be accessed by healthcare providers and staff when required. EHR management "requires planning and decision making for the entire life cycle of the information contained in EHR systems—from creation or capture, review, modification, and sharing through searching, tracking, preserving, retention, and, ultimately, destruction of the information that has been designated as health records of the organization or entity" (Glondys and Kadlec 2016). Management of health records includes three processes: creation and identification, storage and retrieval, and retention and disposition.

## Health Record Creation and Identification

As discussed earlier, the health record is created when the patient is first admitted to or treated in a healthcare facility. Every patient is assigned a unique identifier, and the health record is initiated with the collection of admission or registration information.

### Health Record Identification Systems

For the correct health record to be quickly retrieved when it is needed, each record must be assigned a unique identifier. The choice of record identification system is tied to the organization's EHR system.

Prior to EHR systems, health record identification systems were tied to the organization's paper health record filing system. Small healthcare facilities, such as physician offices, often used a simple alphabetical identifier: the patient's last and first names. Larger facilities used a unit numbering system.

In a unit numbering system, the patient was assigned a number during the first encounter for care and kept it for all subsequent encounters. In a serial-unit numbering system, the patient was issued a different number for each admission or encounter for care and the records of past episodes of care were brought forward to be filed under the last number issued. This created a unit record that contained information from all the patient's encounters.

### Paper Health Record Filing Systems

Paper health records can be filed in different ways. In a straight numeric filing system, paper records are filed in numerical order according to the number assigned. In a terminal-digit filing system, paper records are filed according to a three-part number made up of two-digit pairs. The basic terminal-digit filing system contains 10,000 divisions, made up of 100 sections ranging from 00 to 99 with 100 divisions within each section ranging from 00 to 99.

### Patient Identity Management

As healthcare delivery becomes more connected, correctly identifying patients and linking patient records is more important and has elevated the role of the HIM professional in patient identity management. HIM professionals have long been charged with the correct assignment of the health record or health record number, which is used to assimilate, store, and access patient health records.

The master patient index (MPI) is a permanent database including patient-identifiable data for every patient ever admitted to or treated by the facility. Even though patient health records may be destroyed after legal retention periods have been met, the information contained in the MPI must be kept permanently. The MPI is also referred to as the master person index, master name file, enterprise master patient index (EMPI), regional master patient index (RMPI), and master patient database. Whatever it is called, the MPI is an important key to the health record because it contains the patient's identifying information including the patient's name and health record number.

Each facility has an MPI, which includes information for all patients who have been registered or treated at any location in the facility. The MPI associates the patient with the number under which patient treatment information can be located.

The challenges in maintaining the MPI are many. For example, patients may not remember previous admissions or may have been admitted under a different name. A person other than the patient may have provided incorrect information, resulting in a new number being assigned when the patient returns for an appointment or is readmitted to the hospital. Sometimes patients use different middle initials or a nickname rather than a given name, or their names may have many possible spellings or may be hyphenated. Babies may have names changed, first and last names can be reversed, and outside laboratories may use different data. Basic demographic information such as addresses can be abbreviated incorrectly. In some cases, patients do not speak the same language as the clerk entering the information, resulting in miscommunication and incorrect data. Facilities that have either merged or separated must keep information on patients treated and often have problems combining information from two computer systems into one MPI.

The challenge for facilities is to maintain a correct and current MPI so each patient has a unique identifier number. Duplication, overlays, and overlaps are major problems. A **duplicate** occurs "when two or more medical record numbers are created for the same person, causing them to have two or more records" (AHIMA 2020). An **overlap** occurs when a patient has more than one health record number assigned across more than one database. An **overlay** occurs when one patient record is overwritten with data from another patient's record. The goal is to have a true longitudinal record from birth to death, and the MPI serves as the link to information and certainty of identification that are critical to the quality and safety of patient care. Healthcare facilities have hired HIM professionals as EMPI coordinators or have hired consultants to clean and maintain EMPI systems to ensure the correct information on the correct patient is available to the provider and others who need it. This has become even more important with the growth of EHRs and the implementation of health information exchange. With an EMPI, patient information is included from all entities within the enterprise and shared as needed. The sharing of data is a worthy goal, but incorrect information can adversely affect the quality and safety of care; thus, accuracy of the MPI is a critical issue. There has been some interest in a uniform patient identifier that would be used nationwide, but action toward creating such a universal identifier has not progressed.

The MPI usually includes the following information, though some variation occurs:

- Patient's full name and any other names the patient uses
- Patient's date of birth
- Patient's complete address
- Patient's phone numbers including cellular phone number
- Patient's health record number
- Patient's social security number
- Patient's billing or account number
- Name of the attending physician
- Dates of the patient's admission and discharge or the date of the visit or encounter
- Patient's disposition at discharge or the conclusion of treatment
- Patient's marital status
- Patient's legal sex
- Patient's race
- Patient's ethnicity
- Name of the patient's emergency contact

Healthcare facilities should also consider that the discrete data the MPI captures may not match what is captured in the health record where the patient's preferred pronouns, name, gender identity, and so on are documented. Developing standardized collection tools to accurately capture sexual orientation and gender identity demographic data is essential to providing quality care to a diverse patient population (AHIMA Work Group 2017). The initial misidentification of a patient upon registration or admission can lead to repeat testing, patient safety concerns, delays in treatment, compliance risks, financial costs, and many other issues.

The first step in maintaining an accurate index is to obtain the correct information at admission or registration and identify the correct patient information contained in the registration system. Staff must be trained to understand the importance of accurate patient data collection and patient matching during registration. Many facilities develop an algorithm using a group of common fields, such as a patient's name, legal sex, date of birth, and social security number, to search for each new entry in the MPI and to review the MPI database for potential duplicate entries. A data integrity team that includes HIM professionals can work together to identify, review, and correct duplicates, overlays, and overlaps in patient health records. Obtaining patient photos at the time of registration, checking photo ID or driver's license, and address verification through the United States Postal Service are also ways for registration staff to verify patient identity. In addition to these patient identity matching practices, several tools have been developed to further assist facilities in addressing patient identification issues, including, biometric authentication tools like palm vein scans, retinal scans or iris identification, facial recognition, and speaker or voice recognition (AHIMA Work Group 2016).

## Health Record Storage and Retrieval

While the healthcare industry has transitioned to EHRs, the HIM department is still responsible for the management, storage, and retrieval of paper health records. Health record retention guidelines must be followed, and until that retention period expires the HIM department must ensure the record is available for patient care and other patient needs, such as litigation, workers compensation, continuity of care, ROI requests, and so forth.

### Health Record Storage

Storage is the application of efficient procedures for the use of physical filing equipment and storage media to keep records secure and available to those providers and other healthcare personnel authorized to access them.

Health record storage is a responsibility for the HIM professional. He or she must maintain a leadership role in ensuring that sufficient, conveniently accessible space is available for the storage of paper records. A sufficient filing room for paper records must be maintained by purging and destroying records according to an approved retention schedule. EHR storage will depend on the type of EHR the facility has implemented. The data is either stored in the cloud or on-premises locally hosted servers. Archival systems are used when migrating from one EHR to another and not all the information will be migrated but still must be retained.

Because physical storage space is expensive, administrators and facilities management personnel are always looking for ways to better use available space. However, HIM professionals must make sure all storage spaces are easy to locate and their environmental conditions protect paper health records from damage by flooding, fire, pests, mold, and dust.

With increased use of EHRs and the volume of electronic data to be retained, electronic storage services and media are a less expensive option. For example, cloud-based storage solutions, storage area networks, and Software as a Service (SaaS) services provided by EHR vendors can be utilized for a fraction of the cost. HIM professionals must firmly assert the need to protect the original records for the duration of the legally required period. The potential need for health records should be considered when deciding to send records to an off-site storage facility. Many companies specialize in the storage of vital records and provide the proper conditions for the protection of records as well as access to records.

HIM professionals have had to deal with the restoration of paper records damaged by water resulting from hurricanes, earthquakes, and tornadoes. There are companies that specialize in the restoration of records and handle disaster recovery.

### Health Record Retrieval

Retrieval is concerned with locating requested records and information. With a paper health record, it involves signing out or checking out records from the filing area and tracking their location. In an EHR system, HIM professionals must have a broader understanding of all the data sources that feed into the EHR's data warehouse, where the data resides, and understand the data attributes.

HIM professionals are charged with safeguarding patient information by ensuring the person accessing the record has a need to know and an appropriate reason to access the patient record. In both paper and electronic retrievals, the HIM professional is responsible for ensuring that access is appropriate.

HIM personnel must be able to quickly determine the exact location of a specific paper health record at any time. Physical security safeguards should be put in place for the paper record storage area, and chart location should be tracked and out guides should be used when a paper record is pulled from the shelf or box. In the case of EHRs, HIPAA privacy and security standards support role-based security, where the needs of groups of end-users are evaluated to determine the level of access, they will have within the EHR and other systems that store PHI. Each EHR system has its own access control capabilities that can be very granular, such as controlling the access to a specific document type or data field.

The facility or provider is responsible for maintaining the health record. When the facility or provider cannot produce a record, it must be able to prove that the loss was unintentional. In a paper record filing system, periodic audits can take place to ensure files are in the correct order. In the case of an EHR, access audits are typically part of a comprehensive security program.

## Health Record Retention and Disposition

HIM professionals must ensure records in all formats are securely stored and promptly retrievable, and determine how long health records are retained. Record retention involves determining the schedule to be followed to protect and preserve active and inactive records. Disposition involves the process of destroying the records once the end of the retention period has been reached. Establishing policies that incorporate state and federal laws and maintaining a disaster plan are part of the disposition process.

### Accreditation and Legal Health Record Retention Requirements

Health record retention is the responsibility of the HIM professional. Record retention policies and procedures must be established along with a retention schedule. Federal and state laws, statutes of limitations, accreditation standards, AHIMA recommendations, and operational needs should all be considered when developing facility retention policies and procedures (Brodnik et al. 2023). The Joint Commission asserts that the length of health record retention depends on laws, regulations, and the use of health records (Joint Commission 2023, RC.01.05.01).

The HIM professional must adhere to the strictest time limit if the recommended retention period varies among different laws and regulations. In addition to the length of time for maintaining health records, the HIM professional must consider the required length of retention for other documentation such as immunization records, mammography records, x-rays, and radiographs. It is important to realize that the retention periods are different for the records of minors and incompetent patients.

CMS requires health records to be maintained for at least five years (42 CFR 482.24(b)(1)). This requirement includes committee reports, physician certification and recertification reports, radiologist records (printouts, films, scans, and other images), home health agency records, long-term care records, laboratory records, and any other records that document information about claims. The Occupational Safety and Health Administration (29 CFR 1910.1020) requires records of employees with occupational exposure to be maintained for the duration of employment plus 30 years (29 CFR 1910.1020). The statutes of limitation (deadline for filing a lawsuit) in various types of legal actions are important considerations in developing a retention schedule.

Other departments rely on the expertise of the HIM professional to assist them in developing record retention procedures. A retention plan for the facility must be carefully written and included in the departmental policy and procedure manual to ensure that record destruction is part of the normal course of business and that no one health record or group of health records is singled out for destruction.

### Retention Requirements for Ancillary Materials

Email messages and faxes are used for instructions, information about appointments, and the reporting of information. These must be scanned, indexed, and included in the EHR.

Whenever possible, standalone devices and systems should be incorporated into the EHR through an interface. If the system output is not able to be incorporated into the EHR, the information should be scanned into the EHR. The original interpretations of the results must be part of the patient health record. State laws should be reviewed to determine the retention requirement of other images.

Fetal monitoring strips should also be incorporated into the EHR through an interface or scanning. These strips are part of the mother's record, but because the strips relate to the newborn, they should be maintained according to the length of time stipulated for a minor's records.

Magnetic tapes containing the digital versions of MRI and CT studies are not considered permanent health records if a hard copy of the final images (radiographic film) is in the patient's health record. The signed interpretation of the studies must be maintained in the record for the full retention period required by law. Per Federal regulation, mammograms must be maintained for 5 to 10 years, depending on whether additional mammograms are performed (21 CFR 900.12(c)(4)). State laws may require a retention period for mammograms of 20 to 30 years. This is another example of the HIM professional having to ensure that the longer period is followed when retention schedules are determined.

### Destruction and Transfer of Health Records

After time limits for retention have been reached, the HIM professional must decide on the destruction process for paper health records, which must ensure that health records are burned, shredded, or destroyed in such a way that PHI is not revealed. Physical destruction of electronic media which makes it unusable is the most secure method. Depending on the type of storage media, pulverizing, shredding, degaussing, or demagnetizing may also be appropriate (Brodnik et al. 2023).

When the facility is closed or sold, its health records are transferred to the successor provider, meaning the entity or individual that purchases the facility. In ambulatory care settings or physician offices, patients are informed of their options to transfer their records to another provider of choice before their health records are transferred to the successor provider. When a physician leaves a group practice, patients should be given the choice to transfer their health records, to have the health records and the responsibility for care transferred to another provider in the group, or to receive copies of their health record (AMA n.d.).

## Development of a Record Retention Program

The record retention program must ensure current health records are retained; that inactive records are maintained; that retention is cost-effective in terms of storage space, equipment, and personnel; that a formal health record destruction process is in place; and that retention periods are established. A task force or committee might be established with representation from administration, medical staff, health information services, risk management, and legal counsel to consider the needs of all groups who use patient health information. The steps in developing a record retention program are as follows: conduct an inventory of the facility's records; determine the format and location of record storage; assign each record a retention period; and purge, destroy, or archive records that are no longer needed.

***Conduct an Inventory of Records*** The first step in establishing a record retention program is to carefully and completely inventory the records or categories of records maintained. In this phase, it is important to determine all the locations and formats of patient information, including images, video files, emails, tracings, electronic records, and other formats. The inventory also must include the records and registries maintained by all departments. Both primary and secondary records must be identified. A comprehensive list of all software and versions used should be maintained so that health records, documents, and images can be retrieved in the future. Specialized computer systems used by individual departments should be included.

***Determine Storage Format and Location*** Determining the method of storage is the second step in retention program development. For electronic information, an organization must consider the type of media on which to store the data as well as how quickly the data will need to be accessed. For paper records, the facility will need to decide whether the records will be scanned or stored in hard copy. If the records are retained in hard copy, will they be stored on-site or in off-site contract storage? Off-site contract storage should be located at a distance far enough away from the facility to ensure that a disaster affecting the facility will not affect the storage location. Records maintained electronically are dependent on the hardware and software used by the provider.

***Assign a Retention Period*** After all departments have been inventoried, the third step is to assign a retention period for each type of record. The retention period should be defined as time in active files, time in inactive storage, and total time before destruction. In practice, the reference column of the retention schedule would be populated with the statutes and regulations applicable to the state where the facility is located.

As discussed previously, state and federal laws and regulations must be reviewed to ensure records are maintained for the longest length of time required. Many states recommend that patient health records be retained for 10 years following patient discharge or death. There are usually special requirements for patients who are minors. For example, the state of Minnesota requires that the records of minor patients be maintained for seven years following the age of majority. Therefore, the record of a newborn in Minnesota would be maintained until the patient reaches the age of majority, which is 18 years, plus seven years or a total of 25 years (Office of the Revisor of Statutes 2023).

The retention period should reflect the scope and needs of the facility, along with the preliminary costs associated with scanning, archiving, and other methods of maintaining and storing records. Storage mechanisms that protect records and provide ease of access and employee safety should be selected.

Protection of paper-based, hybrid, and electronic health records during the legally required retention period is extremely important and needs to be considered before a disaster occurs or a situation occurs where a health record in storage cannot be located or available.

***Destroy Unnecessary Records*** Destroying unneeded records is the fourth step in developing a record retention program. PHI stored in paper or electronic formats should be destroyed at the end of the retention period. Shredding, pulverization, and incineration are acceptable methods of destruction. A permanent destruction log, such as the one shown in figure 3.1, should be developed and maintained to identify and track the records and PHI destroyed. The destruction log should include the date of destruction, name(s) of the individual(s) responsible for destroying the records, name of the individual witnessing the destruction, the method of destruction, and patient information including their full name, health record number, date of admission, and date of discharge. If a third-party destruction company is hired, a business associate agreement must be in place, and they must provide the health information manager with a certificate attesting to the destruction of the records.

When paper records are scanned and no longer considered the legal record, they should be destroyed as per the organizational policy. The destruction of electronic and digital records should follow security guidelines to ensure information is permanently destroyed. Facilities must maintain basic information about the patient in the MPI, which is maintained permanently even though the corresponding health record is destroyed.

***Dealing with Outdated Media*** Patient health information may be stored on the hard drives of workstations, laptops, servers, copiers, and other hardware. When this hardware is no longer used by the facility, the facility must determine if there was patient health information stored on its hard drive. The files containing patient health information cannot simply be deleted as the data is not erased. The following guidelines should be followed for the destruction of hard drives:

1. To ensure any patient's health information has been removed, utility software that overwrites the entire disk drive must be used, which may be accomplished by overwriting the data with a series of characters. Total data destruction does not occur until the backup tapes have been overwritten. Magnetic neutralization will leave the domain in random patterns with no preference to orientation, rendering previous data unrecoverable.

2. If the computer is being redeployed internally or disposed of owing to obsolescence, the aforementioned utility must be run against the computer's hard drive, after which the hard drive may be reformatted, and a standard software image loaded on the reformatted drive.

3. If the computer is being disposed of owing to damage and it is not possible to run the utility to overwrite the data, then the hard drive must be removed from the computer and physically destroyed. Alternatively, the drive can be erased by use of a magnetic bulk eraser. This requirement applies to PC workstations, laptops, and servers. (Glondys and Kadlec 2016)

**Figure 3.1.** Health record destruction log

| Patient Name (First and Last) | Health Record Number | Admission Date | Discharge Date | General Description of Records | Media Type (paper, CD, microfiche, etc.) |
|---|---|---|---|---|---|
|  |  |  |  |  |  |
|  |  |  |  |  |  |
|  |  |  |  |  |  |
|  |  |  |  |  |  |
|  |  |  |  |  |  |

Date of Destruction: _____  Method of Destruction: _____
Destroyed By: _____  Witness: _____
**Retain log permanently.**

## Check Your Understanding 3.4

**Answer the following questions in a separate document.**

**For questions 1 through 4, refer to the following scenario.**

John Smith, a 50-year-old man from Atlanta, GA, was recently admitted to Seaside Hospital. During the admissions process, the registration clerk found that there are 20 John Smiths already in the MPI system with three of them having similar but not the same dates of birth. The clerk chose to add the John Smith being admitted as a "new" patient in the MPI system and he was assigned a new health record number. After he was discharged, it was discovered that he was one of the three John Smiths in the system with a similar birth date.

1. Why is this a problem?
2. How could this mistake have occurred?
3. What are the consequences of this mistake for John Smith, and how will it impact his care?
4. How would you approach cleaning up the MPI after discovering that John Smith, who was recently admitted to Seaside Hospital, was already in the system under a different health record number?
5. Discuss the various rules, regulations, and standards that must be taken into consideration when determining how long health records are maintained.
6. Sue Shelley, RHIA, the HIM manager at St. Mary's hospital, has noticed that the duplicate health record number rate has increased significantly over the past six months. The CFO has asked Shelly to work with the admissions manager to address the issue and create a policy or procedure for correctly identifying patients in the admissions process. What information or best practices should be included in an admissions policy or procedure to reduce duplicate health record numbers?
7. John Richardson, RHIA, is the new HIM director at Nearby Hospital. This hospital has kept all health records since it opened in 1950 in two rented warehouses located two miles from the main hospital. The warehouse property is being sold, and the records must be moved to the hospital location. Before that happens, the CFO would like John to determine whether any of the records should be purged and destroyed. Determine how John should proceed with this request and how he would establish an effective record retention program.
8. Create a draft policy for destruction of health records.
9. What are the key considerations for health record storage to ensure their security and availability?
10. In the age of electronic health record systems; why would it be important for HIM professionals to understand paper record filing systems?

# References

ACEP (American College of Emergency Physicians). 2022. "Patient Medical Records in the Emergency Department." https://www.acep.org/patient-care/policy-statements/patient-medical-records-in-the-emergency-department.

AHDI (Association for Healthcare Documentation Integrity). n.d. "Speech Recognition Technology." Accessed March 14, 2024. https://www.ahdionline.org/page/srt.

AHIMA (American Health Information Management Association). 2020. White Paper. "A Realistic Approach to Achieving a 1% Duplicate Record Error Rate." https://ahima.org/media/m1pldevh/ahima-pim-whitepaper.pdf.

AHIMA (American Health Information Management Association). 2011. Retention and Destruction of Health Information. http://library.ahima.org/xpedio/groups/public/documents/ahima/bok1_049252.hcsp?dDocName&#xF03D;bok1_049252 (page discontinued).

AHIMA (American Health Information Management Association). 2010. Role of the Personal Health Record in the EHR (Updated). http://library.ahima.org/xpedio/groups/public/documents/ahima/bok1_048517.hcsp?dDocName&#xF03D;bok1_048517 (page discontinued).

Alder, S. 2023. HIPAA compliance for email. *The HIPAA Journal*. https://www.hipaajournal.com/hipaa-compliance-for-email/.

American Health Information Management Association Work Group. 2017. Improved patient engagement for LGBT populations: Addressing factors related to sexual orientation/gender identity for effective health information management. *Journal of AHIMA* 88(3).

AMA (American Medical Association). n.d. "AMA Code of Medical Ethics, Chapter 3, Opinion 3.3.1: Management of Medical Records." Accessed March 24, 2024. https://code-medical-ethics.ama-assn.org/sites/amacoedb/files/2022-08/3.3.1.pdf.

Bas, A. 2023 (December 14). "How AI Improves Healthcare Documentation." https://www.uptech.team/blog/ai-medical-documentation.

Berry, S., A. Campbell, J. Flanigan, D. Paulson, B. Ryznar, and J. Woebkenberg. 2019. Ensuring the integrity of the EHR. *Journal of AHIMA* 90(1):34–37.

Brodnik, M. S., L. A. Rinehart-Thompson, and R. B. Reynolds. 2023. *Fundamentals of Law for Health Informatics and Information Management*. Chicago: AHIMA.

CMS (Centers for Medicare and Medicaid Services). 2024. *Medicare & Skilled Nursing Facility Care: Skilled Care When You Need It*. https://www.medicare.gov/publications/11359-getting-started-medicare-and-skilled-nursing-facility-care.pdf.

CMS (Centers for Medicare and Medicaid Services). 2018. "Home Health Care: Proper Certification

Required." https://www.cms.gov/outreach-and-education/medicare-learning-network-mln/mlnproducts/fast-facts/home-health-care.

Glondys, B. and L. Kadlec. 2016. EHRs serving as the business and legal records of healthcare organizations. *Journal of AHIMA* 87(5). https://bok.ahima.org/topics/healthcare-data-lifecycle/ehrs-serving-as-the-business-and-legal-records-of-healthcare-organizations-2016-update/.

Joint Commission. 2023. *Comprehensive Accreditation Manual for Hospitals*. Oak Brook Terrace, IL: Joint Commission.

Kadlec, L. 2016. Practice Brief: Managing unsolicited health information in the electronic health record. https://bok.ahima.org/topics/privacy-and-security/managing-unsolicited-health-information-in-the-electronic-health-record-2016-update/.

Larkey, K. n.d. "Medicare Documentation Guidelines for Skilled Nursing Facilities." Accessed March 24, 2024. https://www.intelycare.com/facilities/resources/medicare-documentation-guidelines-for-skilled-nursing-facilities/.

Leubner, J., and S. Wild. 2018. Developing standing orders to help your team work to the highest level. *Family Practice Management*. 25(3):13–16.

Lye, C. T., H. P. Forman, J. G. Daniel, and H. M. Krumholz. 2018. The 21st Century Cures Act and electronic health records one year later: will patients see the benefits? *Journal of the American Medical Informatics Association: JAMIA* 25(9):1218–1220. https://doi.org/10.1093/jamia/ocy065.

MLN (Medicare Learning Network). 2023. *Complying with Medical Record Documentation Requirements*. https://www.cms.gov/outreach-and-education/medicare-learning-network-mln/mlnproducts/downloads/certmedrecdoc-factsheet-icn909160.pdf.

NAHC (National Association for Home Care and Hospice). n.d. "NAHC FAQ." Accessed March 13, 2024. https://www.nahc.org/about/faq/#111.

NHPCO (National Hospice and Palliative Care Organization). 2019. "The Hospice Team." https://www.nhpco.org/patients-and-caregivers/about-hospice-care/the-hospice-team/.

NLC (National Learning Consortium). 2013. Legal health record policy template [Microsoft Word document]. https://www.healthit.gov/sites/default/files/legal_health_policy_template.docx.

Office of the Revisor of Statutes. 2023. 2023 Minnesota statutes. https://www.revisor.mn.gov/statutes/?id=145.32.

UNOS (United Network for Organ Sharing). Accessed June 30, 2024. https://unos.org/.

21 CFR 11.3: Definitions. 1997 (March 20).

21 CFR 900.12: Mammography quality standards. 2000 (July 14).

29 CFR 1910.1020: Access to employee medical records. 2011 (June 8).

42 CFR 482.24: Conditions of participation: Medical record services. 2012 (May 16).

42 CFR 482.45: Conditions of participation: Organ, tissue, and eye procurement program. 2017

42 CFR 482.61: Condition of participation. 2007 (October 26).

42 CFR 483.70: Administration. 2016 (October 4).

42 CFR 484.55: Condition of participation: Comprehensive assessment of patients. 2021 (November 9).

45 CFR 164.524: Access of individuals to protected health information. 2014 (February 6).

45 CFR 171: Information blocking. 2020 (May 1).

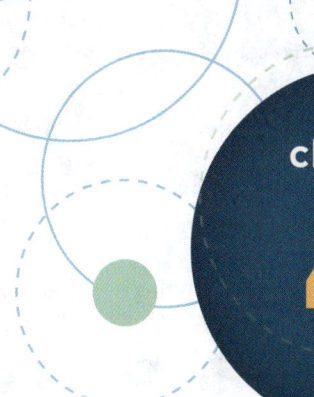

# Clinical Classifications, Vocabularies, Terminologies, and Standards

*Brooke Palkie, EdD, RHIA, CPHIMS, FAHIMA*

## Learning Objectives

- Differentiate among and identify the correct uses of classifications, vocabularies, terminologies, and standards
- Describe the characteristics of ICD-10-CM and ICD-10-PCS
- Apply clinical classifications and code sets appropriately
- Select a terminology most likely to meet clinical data representation and data retrieval needs
- Explain the need for a terminology in an electronic health record (EHR) system
- Discuss the role of mapping and conduct mapping among clinical terminologies, vocabularies, and classifications
- Explain electronic applications and systems for clinical classifications
- Explain healthcare data sets and describe their purpose
- Describe organizations that are key players in current efforts to develop standards for EHRs
- Demonstrate knowledge of and explain healthcare informatics standards
- Describe data standard development, testing, coordination, and harmonization
- Examine how ICD-10-CM and ICD-10-PCS codes are connected to health information systems, machine learning and artificial intelligence

## Key Terms

Artificial intelligence (AI)
Basic interoperability
Clinical Care Classification (CCC)
Clinical classification
Clinical Document Architecture (CDA)
Clinical terminology
Clinical vocabulary
Concept
Continuity of Care Document (CCD)
Current Dental Terminology (CDT)
Current Procedural Terminology (CPT)
*Diagnostic and Statistical Manual of Mental Disorders, Fifth Edition, Text Revision* (DSM-5-TR)
Functional interoperability
Healthcare Common Procedure Coding System (HCPCS)
Interface terminology
*International Classification of Diseases* (ICD)
*International Classification of Diseases, Eleventh Revision* (ICD-11)
*International Classification of Diseases, Tenth Revision, Clinical Modification* (ICD-10-CM)
*International Classification of Diseases, Tenth Revision, Procedure Coding System* (ICD-10-PCS)
*International Classification of Diseases for Oncology*, Third Edition (ICD-O-3)

*International Classification of Primary Care* (ICPC-3)
*International Classification on Functioning, Disability, and Health* (ICF)
International Health Terminology Standards Development Organization (IHTSDO)
Interoperability
Lexicon
Logical Observation Identifiers Names and Codes (LOINC)
Machine Learning
Mapping
MEDCIN
Medical Subject Headings database (MeSH)
Morphology
National Drug Codes (NDCs) directory
National Library of Medicine (NLM)
Nomenclature
Patient medical record information (PMRI)
Reference terminology
RxNorm
Semantic interoperability
Systematized Nomenclature of Medicine Clinical Terminology (SNOMED CT)
Terminology
Topography
Transitions of care (ToC) initiative
Unified Medical Language System (UMLS)

Healthcare is faced with many challenges, including an aging population, the need to conserve resources, medical data that are increasing exponentially, and a technologically savvy consumer population. To meet these challenges, healthcare organizations must have the ability to operate effectively and efficiently using current medical data and knowledge. Although moving closer to standardization, the US healthcare industry has yet to fully agree on common terminologies that would allow healthcare facilities and providers throughout the country to exchange and use information reliably.

The quest to establish common terminologies to classify morbidity and mortality is quite old. London parishes first began to keep death records in 1532. In the 1600s, Sir William Petty was able to extrapolate from mortality rates an estimate of community economic loss caused by deaths (Encyclopedia Britannica n.d.). Two hundred years later, in *Notes on a Hospital*, Florence Nightingale wrote,

In attempting to arrive at the truth, I have applied everywhere for information, but in scarcely an instance have I been able to obtain hospital records fit for any purposes of comparison. If they could be obtained ... they would show subscribers how their money was being spent, what amount of good was really being done with it, or whether the money was not doing mischief rather than good. (Barnett et al. 1993, 1046)

Many of the issues with availability of information remain in healthcare today. It is vitally important to be able to compare data for outcomes measurement, quality improvement, resource utilization, best practices, medical research, public health, and reimbursement purposes. These tasks can be accomplished only when healthcare has fully standardized terminology that is easily integrated into the EHR. This chapter examines the history, current practices, and desired characteristics of classifications, terminologies, vocabularies, and standards in the healthcare industry.

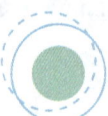

## Development of Classification Systems, Vocabularies, and Terminologies for Healthcare Data

As the discussion of classification systems, terminologies, and vocabularies for healthcare data begins, it is important to understand several terms related to clinical content representation. It is difficult to get standards developers to completely agree on definitions for even basic concepts; however, there are some commonly accepted definitions. Table 4.1 provides definitions and examples of classification system terms. A clinical classification is a clinical vocabulary, terminology, or nomenclature that lists words or phrases with their meanings; provides for the proper use of clinical words as names or symbols; and facilitates mapping of standardized terms to broader classifications for administrative, regulatory, oversight, and fiscal requirements. A classification system provides easy storage, retrieval, and analysis of data for the purposes of transmitting and comparing data. A nomenclature is a recognized system of terms used in a science or an art that follows preestablished naming conventions. The terms *classification* and *nomenclature* are often used interchangeably. However, the two can be distinguished: "classifications and nomenclatures can be more helpfully regarded as lying along a continuum, where the first categorizes and aggregates while the second supports detailed descriptions" (Chute 2000, 298). The *International Classification of Diseases, Tenth Revision* (ICD-10) is a classification system that organizes

Table 4.1. Definitions and examples of classification system terms

| Terms | Definition | Example |
|---|---|---|
| Clinical classification | A clinical vocabulary, terminology, or nomenclature that "arranges together similar diseases and procedures and organizes related entities for easy retrieval" (AMIA and AHIMA Terminology and Classification Policy Task Force 2007, 32). | ICD-10-CM |
| Nomenclature | A recognized system of terms that follows preestablished naming conventions. | DSM-5-TR |
| Clinical terminology | "A set of standardized terms and their synonyms that record patient findings, circumstances, events, and interventions with sufficient detail to support clinical care, decision support, outcomes research, and quality improvement" (AMIA and AHIMA Terminology and Classification Policy Task Force 2007, 35). | SNOMED CT |
| Clinical vocabulary | A formally recognized list of preferred medical terms; also called medical vocabulary. | HL7 (in terms of structural vocabulary) |

(categorizes) many of its disease entries by body system or etiology. For example, disorders related to the circulatory system are organized and classified within a single chapter. The Diagnostic Statistical Manual (DSM) is an example of a nomenclature that provides a listing of the terms and definitions (criteria) used to describe mental health disorders.

A **terminology** is a set of terms representing a system of concepts of a particular subject or field. Another generic term often used when discussing terminologies is **lexicon**, which refers to the listings of words or expressions in a language (terminology) and information about the language such as definitions, related principles, and description of (grammatical) structure (NLM 2016a).

It is important to recognize that the problem of multiple definitions and names is endemic in the field of healthcare terminology. A **clinical terminology** is "a set of standardized terms and their synonyms that record patient findings, circumstances, events, and interventions with sufficient detail to support clinical care, decision support, outcomes research, and quality improvement" (AMIA and AHIMA Terminology and Classification Policy Task Force 2007, 41). A **clinical vocabulary** is a formally recognized list of preferred medical terms. The definition for the vocabulary is like that of terminology except that it includes the meanings or definitions of words. Because of their very similar meanings, the terms *clinical terminology* and *clinical vocabulary* are often used interchangeably. To further complicate the issue, many working within the field also often use *terminology* to refer to the entire spectrum of issues related to clinical data representation from classifications and nomenclatures to clinical terminologies (Chute 2000, 299). The pyramid in figure 4.1 illustrates how these terms are all related. A nomenclature can be less specific than a terminology, which is less specific than a language. So, while a classification or nomenclature categorizes and aggregates, a terminology represents the whole of

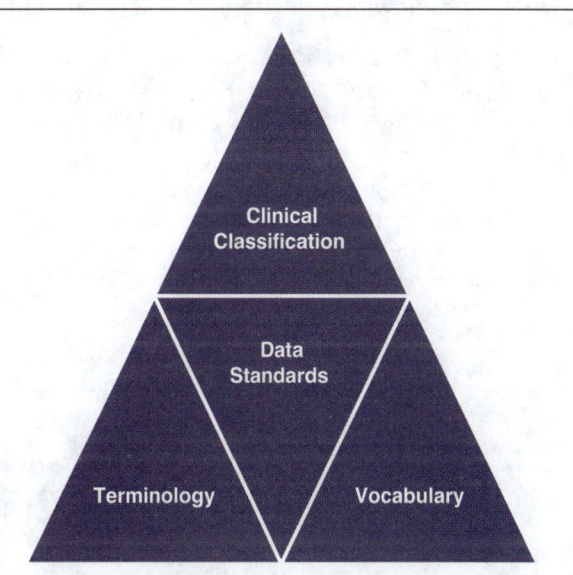

Figure 4.1. Comparative level of detail in classifications, terminologies, vocabularies, and data standards

a subject field. Each plays a specific yet interdependent role in data standardization.

Clinical classifications and terminologies do serve different functions. For example, the classification systems *International Classification of Diseases, Tenth Revision, Clinical Modification* (ICD-10-CM), *International Classification of Diseases, Tenth Revision, Procedure Coding System* (ICD-10-PCS), and Current Procedural Terminology (CPT) represent similar procedures and diagnoses with single codes. This broad categorization of information is useful for functions such as billing and monitoring resource utilization. In contrast, terminologies support the capture and representation of information collected within an EHR at the time of documentation (SNOMED International 2020). Terminologies exist to represent topics ranging from nursing documentation and laboratory data to medical devices. This detailed level of data capture is useful to support functions such as clinical decision support and clinical alerts.

Depending on the purpose of a given classification or terminology, differences are also seen at the level of granularity (detail) used to represent content. For example, the CPT classification system has a single code (86003 Allergen specific IgE: quantitative or semiquantitative, allergen extract, each) to report a laboratory test to detect a specific allergen. The same code is used regardless of the allergen (for example, food, weeds, dust). On the other hand, Logical Observation Identifiers Names and Codes (LOINC), a clinical terminology, provides a common language for clinical and laboratory observations (LOINC n.d.a). LOINC provides many different codes (for example, 11195-5 (rapeseed), 11196-3 (orange roughy Ige Ab), 11197-1 (sardine (pilchard)) to represent the test for each unique allergen (NLM 2012). In this case, the LOINC representation of the allergen tests is more granular; that is, more specific. Granularity is important because it represents the degree to which a term specifies the concept it is representing.

### Check Your Understanding 4.1

**Answer the following questions in a separate document.**

1. Articulate why it is important to incorporate classification, vocabularies, and terminologies. Interpret the similarities and differences. Explain why only one would not suffice within an EHR.
2. How is the use of clinical terminologies important for the accurate capture and representation of health information within EHRs? Provide an example for each of the following SNOMED CT, LOINC, and ICD-10-CM in terms of use within an EHR:
3. Which clinical terminology is used to represent common language for a clinical laboratory observation?
4. What was the initial purpose of collecting healthcare data for mortality, and how does this data collection compare to the current-day capture of both mortality and morbidity data?
5. Why is it important to standardize data and information for healthcare purposes?

## Common Healthcare Classifications and Code Sets

Systems for classifying diseases have progressed through various stages since the first classification system was developed in the late 19th century. The following section describes past, current, and near-future developments for a variety of classification systems.

### International Classification of Diseases

The *International Classification of Diseases* (ICD) began as the Bertillon Classification of Diseases in 1893. In 1900, the French government convened an international meeting to update the Bertillon classification to the International List of Causes of Death (WHO n.d.a). The goal was to develop a common system for describing the causes of mortality. The World Health Organization (WHO) became responsible for maintaining ICD in 1948. Currently, ICD is used by more than 100 countries worldwide to classify diseases and other health issues (WHO n.d.a). The *International Classification of Diseases* (ICD) facilitates the storage and retrieval of diagnostic information and serves as the basis for compiling mortality and morbidity statistics reported by WHO members. The US transitioned to the clinical modification of ICD-10 (meaning capturing diseases or causes of illness—morbidity) in 2015. ICD-10 is no longer updated by WHO since its replacement by ICD-11 on January 1, 2022. The development of an 11th edition of ICD integrates updated medical data discovered since ICD-10 was published. *International Classification of Diseases, Eleventh Revision* (ICD-11) still needs to be clinically modified for use in the US. A significant difference in ICD-11 is that it is designed to include linkages to standardized healthcare terminologies to facilitate processing and use of the data for a variety of purposes such as research (WHO n.d.b). The US transition from ICD-10 to ICD-11 is pending for both cause of death coding for mortality reporting to WHO and for its use to capture morbidity coding based upon the needs of the US healthcare system (NCVHS 2023).

## International Classification of Diseases, Tenth Revision, Clinical Modification

CMS and NCHS modified the *International Classification of Diseases, Tenth Revision, Clinical Modification* (ICD-10-CM) for the reporting of morbidity data and reimbursement in the US. In 2008, the Department of Health and Human Services (HHS) published a notice of proposed rulemaking that identified the replacement of ICD-9-CM with ICD-10-CM for diagnosis coding and ICD-10-PCS for inpatient procedure coding. However, the implementation was delayed twice and the effective date for ICD-10-CM and ICD-10-PCS implementation became October 1, 2015.

The Centers for Medicare and Medicaid Services (CMS) identifies ICD-10-CM as the US clinical modification of WHO's ICD-10 and is maintained by the National Center for Health Statistics (NCHS). "It is a morbidity classification system that classifies diagnoses and other reasons for healthcare encounters" (CMS 2023d). The code structure is alphanumeric, with codes comprised of three to seven characters.

ICD-10-CM content and format components are as follows:

- Information relevant to ambulatory care
- Cause of injury codes
- Combination diagnosis and symptom codes to reduce the number of codes needed to fully describe a condition and reduce coding errors
- Specificity in code assignment
- Laterality information (right and left)
- Achievement of the benefits of an EHR
- Ability to meet the Health Insurance Portability and Accountability Act (HIPAA) electronic transaction/code set requirements
- Value in the US investment in Systematized Nomenclature of Medicine Clinical Terminology (SNOMED CT)
- Use of seven-character alphanumeric format, which facilitates expansion and further revision of classification (space to accommodate future expansion) (CMS 2023b)

Figure 4.2 provides an example of an entry in the Tabular List of Diseases, ICD-10-CM. In the figure, the category level is flush with the left-hand margin (T40) and subcategory level is indented once and bold (T40.0). This code itself is not a valid ICD-10-CM code. In this case, the coding note identifies that code T40.0 must include a seventh character; meaning, it will be seven-character code (for example, T40.0X6A).

## International Classification of Diseases, Eleventh Revision

The WHO released the International Classification of Diseases 2018 Revision for Mortality and Morbidity Statistics (ICD-11-MMS) in June 2018, 18 years after the launch of ICD-10. It became effective on January 1, 2022. ICD-11-MMS is the replacement for WHO's ICD-10. Commonly referred to as ICD-11, it has been released in a completely electronic format and includes additional details such as anatomy, substances, infectious agents, and place of injury. ICD-11 intends for users to combine several codes to describe the level of detail of clinical conditions. Its electronic format allows for unique identifiers to be assigned to conditions listed independently. While the format remains consistent, this revision includes updates of known issues from ICD-10 in addition to scientific groups with a clinical perspective, field-testing, and member state input. The new features are further defined in table 4.2.

**Figure 4.2.** Example of an ICD-10-CM entry

| | | |
|---|---|---|
| **T40 Poisoning by, adverse effect of and underdosing of narcotics and psychodysleptics [hallucinogens]** | | |
| Excludes2: drug dependence and related mental and behavioral disorders due to psychoactive substance use (F10.-F19.-) | | |
| The appropriate seventh character is to be added to each code from category T40 | | |
| A | initial encounter | |
| D | subsequent encounter | |
| S | sequela | |
| **T40.0** | **Poisoning by, adverse effect of and underdosing of opium** | |
| | T40.0X | Poisoning by, adverse effect of and underdosing of opium |
| | T40.0X1 | Poisoning by opium, accidental (unintentional) |
| | | Poisoning by opium NOS |
| | T40.0X2 | Poisoning by opium, intentional self-harm |
| | T40.0X3 | Poisoning by opium, assault |
| | T40.0X4 | Poisoning by opium, undetermined |
| | T40.0X5 | Adverse effect of opium |
| | T40.0X6 | Underdosing of opium |

*Source:* CMS 2023b.

Table 4.2. New features of ICD-11

| ICD-11 Term | Explanation |
|---|---|
| Foundation Component | Multidimensional collection of ICD entities (diseases, disorders, injuries, external causes, signs, and symptoms), serving as an underlying structure. |
| Stem Code | Codes that can used alone and can be entities or groupings of clinical conditions that should always be described as one single category. |
| Extension Code | Codes designed to add detail to a stem code. |
| Precoordination | When a stem code contains all pertinent information about a clinical concept in a pre-combined fashion. |
| Postcoordination | Linking (through cluster coding) two or more stem codes or stem codes with one or more extension codes to fully describe a clinical concept. |
| Cluster Coding | A convention used to show more than one code used together to describe a clinical concept. I.e. slash (/) or ampersand (&) |
| Primary and Secondary Parents | Entity classified in two different places, e.g. by site or by etiology; similar format to ICD-10. |

*Source:* WHO n.d.c.

The US modifications will be subject to the same international process as all other prior changes to ICD to date. One significant difference between ICD-10 and ICD-11 is the Foundation Component. The Foundation Component represents the knowledge base, a large collection of concepts that includes all ICD concepts and the relationships needed to build tabular lists (WHO 2019). Specifically, the tabular list ICD-11 for Mortality and Morbidity Statistics (ICD-11 MMS) is the classification that replaces WHO's ICD-10 (WHO 2023).

The WHO provides online access to ICD-11 (WHO n.d.c). It can also be accessed through user-specific software. For this route, ICD-11 provides an IT guide for compatibility requirements.

## International Classification of Diseases, Tenth Revision, Procedure Coding System

In the mid-1990s, CMS awarded a contract to the 3M Health Information Systems group to develop a new procedure coding system, the *International Classification of Diseases, Tenth Revision, Procedure Coding System* (ICD-10-PCS). It includes the use of standardized definitions, ease of expandability, ease of use, and comprehensiveness. ICD-10-PCS uses very precise definitions. For example, a percutaneous approach is defined as "entry, by puncture or minor incision, of instrumentation through the skin or mucous membrane and any other body layers necessary to reach the site of the procedure" (CMS 2023c).

ICD-10-PCS is composed of seven-character alphanumeric codes. Each character can be one of 34 values (numbers 0 through 9 and the letters of the alphabet, excluding I and O). The classification is divided into 16 sections, each of which covers a specific diagnostic area (for example, medical and surgical, radiation oncology, and mental health). Depending on the requirements

Figure 4.3. ICD-10-PCS code structure

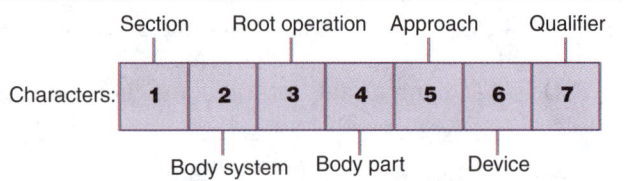

*Source:* Butler et al. 2016.

of each section, the seven characters are assigned different meanings. For example, in the medical and surgical section, the fourth character represents the body part or region involved in the procedure; in the placement section, it represents the body region or orifice; and in the chiropractic section, it represents the body region (CMS 2023c). It is important to note that ICD-10-PCS is separate from ICD-10 and ICD-11 and will not be replaced with ICD-11 when the ICD-11 clinical modification is complete for use in the US.

Figure 4.3 illustrates the meanings of each character of ICD-10-PCS codes in the medical surgical section of the classification. Table 4.3 is an excerpt from a table used for code assignment in the medical and surgical section of ICD-10-PCS. All codes represented in the table begin with the three characters identified in the header and are completed with characters selected from each of the four columns depending upon the nature of the procedure being coded.

## International Classification of Diseases for Oncology, Third Edition, Second Revision

The *International Classification of Diseases for Oncology, Third Edition* (ICD-O-3) is currently in its third edition via the WHO. This classification is used in the US and abroad for coding diagnoses of neoplasms in

## Table 4.3. ICD-10-PCS table

Within a PCS table, valid codes include all combinations of choices in characters 4 through 7 contained in the same row of the table. In the following example, 0JHT3VZ is a valid code, and 0JHW3VZ is not a valid code.
**Section: 0** Medical and Surgical
**Body System: J** Subcutaneous Tissue and Fascia
**Operation: H** Insertion: Putting in a nonbiological appliance that monitors, assists, performs, or prevents a physiological function but does not physically take the place of a body part

| Body part | Approach | Device | Qualifier |
|---|---|---|---|
| 0 Subcutaneous Tissue and Fascia, Scalp<br>1 Subcutaneous Tissue and Fascia, Face<br>4 Subcutaneous Tissue and Fascia, Right Neck<br>5 Subcutaneous Tissue and Fascia, Left Neck<br>9 Subcutaneous Tissue and Fascia, Buttock<br>B Subcutaneous Tissue and Fascia, Perineum<br>C Subcutaneous Tissue and Fascia, Pelvic Region<br>J Subcutaneous Tissue and Fascia, Right Hand<br>K Subcutaneous Tissue and Fascia, Left Hand<br>Q Subcutaneous Tissue and Fascia, Right Foot<br>R Subcutaneous Tissue and Fascia, Left Foot | 0 Open<br>3 Percutaneous | N Tissue Expander | Z No Qualifier |
| 6 Subcutaneous Tissue and Fascia, Chest Pectoral fascia | 0 Open<br>3 Percutaneous | 0 Monitoring Device, Hemodynamic<br>2 Monitoring Device<br>4 Pacemaker, Single Chamber<br>5 Pacemaker, Single Chamber Rate Responsive<br>6 Pacemaker, Dual Chamber<br>7 Cardiac Resynchronization Pacemaker Pulse Generator<br>8 Defibrillator Generator<br>9 Cardiac Resynchronization Defibrillator Pulse Generator<br>A Contractility Modulation Device<br>B Stimulator Generator, Single Array<br>C Stimulator Generator, Single Array Rechargeable<br>D Stimulator Generator, Multiple Array<br>E Stimulator Generator, Multiple Array Rechargeable<br>F Subcutaneous Defibrillator Lead<br>H Contraceptive Device<br>M Stimulator Generator<br>N Tissue Expander<br>P Cardiac Rhythm Related Device<br>V Infusion Device, Pump<br>W Vascular Access Device, Totally Implantable<br>X Vascular Access Device, Tunneled<br>Y Other Device | Z No Qualifier |
| 7 Subcutaneous Tissue and Fascia, Back | 0 Open<br>3 Percutaneous | B Stimulator Generator, Single Array<br>C Stimulator Generator, Single Array Rechargeable<br>D Stimulator Generator, Multiple Array<br>E Stimulator Generator, Multiple Array Rechargeable<br>M Stimulator Generator<br>N Tissue Expander<br>V Infusion Device, Pump<br>Y Other Device | Z No Qualifier |

*Continued*

**Table 4.3.** ICD-10-PCS table (continued)

| Body part | Approach | Device | Qualifier |
|---|---|---|---|
| 8 Subcutaneous Tissue and Fascia, Abdomen | 0 Open<br>3 Percutaneous | 0 Monitoring Device, Hemodynamic<br>2 Monitoring Device<br>4 Pacemaker, Single Chamber<br>5 Pacemaker, Single Chamber Rate Responsive<br>6 Pacemaker, Dual Chamber<br>7 Cardiac Resynchronization Pacemaker Pulse Generator<br>8 Defibrillator Generator<br>9 Cardiac Resynchronization Defibrillator Pulse Generator<br>A Contractility Modulation Device<br>B Stimulator Generator, Single Array<br>C Stimulator Generator, Single Array Rechargeable<br>D Stimulator Generator, Multiple Array<br>E Stimulator Generator, Multiple Array Rechargeable<br>H Contraceptive Device<br>M Stimulator Generator<br>N Tissue Expander<br>P Cardiac Rhythm Related Device<br>V Infusion Device, Pump<br>W Vascular Access Device, Totally Implantable<br>X Vascular Access Device, Tunneled<br>Y Other Device | Z No Qualifier |
| D Subcutaneous Tissue and Fascia, Right Upper Arm<br>F Subcutaneous Tissue and Fascia, Left Upper Arm<br>G Subcutaneous Tissue and Fascia, Right Lower Arm<br>H Subcutaneous Tissue and Fascia, Left Lower Arm<br>L Subcutaneous Tissue and Fascia, Right Upper Leg<br>M Subcutaneous Tissue and Fascia, Left Upper Leg<br>N Subcutaneous Tissue and Fascia, Right Lower Leg<br>P Subcutaneous Tissue and Fascia, Left Lower Leg | 0 Open<br>3 Percutaneous | H Contraceptive Device<br>N Tissue Expander<br>V Infusion Device, Pump<br>W Vascular Access Device, Totally Implantable<br>X Vascular Access Device, Tunneled | Z No Qualifier |
| S Subcutaneous Tissue and Fascia, Head and Neck<br>V Subcutaneous Tissue and Fascia, Upper Extremity<br>W Subcutaneous Tissue and Fascia, Lower Extremity | 0 Open<br>3 Percutaneous | 1 Radioactive Element<br>3 Infusion Device<br>Y Other Device | Z No Qualifier |
| T Subcutaneous Tissue and Fascia, Trunk | 0 Open<br>3 Percutaneous | 1 Radioactive Element<br>3 Infusion Device<br>V Infusion Device, Pump<br>Y Other Device | Z No Qualifier |

*Source:* Adapted from CMS 2023c.

tumor and cancer registries. It is also used in pathology laboratories. The **topography** code describes the site of origin of the neoplasm and uses the same three-character categories as in the neoplasm section of the second chapter of ICD-10. The morphology, grading and anatomy content identified in ICD-O is reflected within the histopathology part of ICD-11. The **morphology** code describes the characteristics of the tumor itself, including cell type and biologic activity (Fritz et al. 2019). The topography codes remain the same as in the previous edition, but the morphology codes have been thoroughly revised where necessary in the third edition, second revision. ICD-O is accessible on the ICD-11 maintenance platform. ICD-O-4 is expected in spring 2025 with the addition of a fifth digit due to the lack of available codes for new morphology diagnoses. To the greatest extent possible, ICD-O uses the nomenclature published in the WHO series, International Histological Classification of Tumors. ICD-O is under the purview of WHO Collaborating Centres for Classification of Disease (WHO 2019).

## International Classification on Functioning, Disability, and Health

The *International Classification on Functioning, Disability, and Health* **(ICF)** is a classification developed by the WHO of health and health-related domains that describe body functions and structures, activities, and participation and is used within the US. Three lists exist within ICF:

- Body functions and structure
- Domains of activity and participation
- Environmental factors that interact with all these components

ICD-11, ICD-10, and ICF are complementary, and users are encouraged to use them together to create a broader and more meaningful picture of the experience of health of individuals and populations (WHO n.d.d). Table 4.4 provides examples of ICF self-care codes (WHO n.d.e).

## Healthcare Common Procedure Coding System

Healthcare Common Procedure Coding System (HCPCS) is used to report services and supplies primarily for reimbursement purposes in the outpatient or ambulatory setting. The system is divided into two sections referred to as levels. Level I of HCPCS is composed of the CPT codes as published by the American Medical Association (AMA) and represents medical services and procedures performed by physicians and other healthcare providers. Level II of HCPCS contains codes that represent products, supplies, and services not included in the CPT codes. The Level I (CPT) codes are primarily five-digit numeric codes; however, there are CPT codes that have letters in the fifth character. Level II codes are five-character alphanumeric codes. HCPCS codes may also be reported with two-character modifiers which provide further detail about the service or procedure.

HCPCS codes are updated every year on January 1. The HCPCS Level II codes are updated quarterly and can be downloaded from the HCPCS website. Table 4.5 contains examples of various types of HCPCS Level II codes (CMS 2023a).

## Current Procedural Terminology

The AMA publishes the Current Procedural Terminology (CPT). The "CPT codes offer doctors and health care professionals a uniform language for coding medical services and procedures to streamline reporting, increase accuracy and efficiency" (AMA n.d.). CPT was first developed and published by the AMA in 1966. In 1983, the system was adopted by CMS as Level I of the HCPCS. HCPCS has two identified subsections, Level I CPT and Level II, and is a standardized coding system to identify products, supplies, and services not included in CPT (CMS 2023a). Since that time, CPT has become widely used as a standard for outpatient and ambulatory care procedural coding in contexts related to reimbursement.

CPT is updated annually on January 1. However, certain components of CPT category codes are updated more frequently. The American Medical Association (AMA) should be followed for all code updates. The codebook is organized into chapters by specialty, body system, and service provided. The codes themselves consist of five digits, and the descriptions of the codes are often accompanied by inclusion and exclusion notes (for example, 90630 Influenza virus vaccine). Modifiers to the five-digit codes also are

**Table 4.4.** Examples of ICF self-care codes 2018 version

| Chapter | Description | Categories | Category description | Subcategories |
|---|---|---|---|---|
| Self-Care | This chapter is about caring for oneself, washing and drying oneself, caring for one's body and body parts, dressing, eating, and drinking; and looking after one's health | d530 Toileting | Planning and carrying out the elimination of human waste (menstruation, urination, and defecation) and clean oneself afterwards. | d5300 Regulating urination<br>d5301 Regulating defecation<br>d5302 Menstrual care<br>d5308 Other specified toileting<br>d5309 Toileting, unspecified |
| | | d540 Dressing | Carrying out the coordinated actions and tasks of putting on and taking off clothes and footwear in sequence and in keeping with climatic and social conditions, such as by putting on, adjusting, and removing shirts, skirts, blouses, pants, undergarments, saris, kimono, tights, hats, gloves, coats, shoes, boots, sandals, and slippers. | d5400 Putting on clothes<br>d5401 Taking off clothes<br>d5402 Putting on footwear<br>d5403 Taking off footwear<br>d5404 Choosing appropriate clothing<br>d5408 Other specified dressing<br>d5409 Dressing, unspecified |

*Source:* WHO n.d.d. ©WHO. Used with permission.

**Table 4.5.** Examples of HCPCS Level II codes

| HCPCS Level II code | Code title |
|---|---|
| A0130 | Nonemergency transportation: wheelchair van |
| A4918 | Venous pressure clamp, for hemodialysis, each |
| B4036 | Enteral feeding supply kit: gravity fed, per day, includes but not limited to feeding/flushing syringe, administration set tubing, dressings, tape |
| E0619 | Apnea monitor, with recording feature |
| J3370 | Injection, vancomycin hcl, 500 mg |
| Q0480 | Driver for use with pneumatic ventricular assist device, replacement only |
| S0274 | Nurse practitioner visit at member's home, outside of a capitation arrangement |

*Source:* CMS 2023a.

used extensively to offer additional information (for example, 19120-LT Biopsy or Excision Procedures on the breast—left). CPT also contains two supplemental sections. The first, Category II codes, contains optional codes used for performance measurement reporting purposes. The second, CPT Category III codes, are temporary codes assigned to facilitate data collection for emerging technologies.

CPT is maintained by the CPT Editorial Panel, which is authorized to revise, update, and modify CPT. Many on the panel are physicians, with the rest coming from industry and government. Supporting the work of the CPT Editorial Panel is the CPT Health Care Professionals Advisory Committee (HCPAC). The HCPAC includes participation in the CPT process from organizations representing licensed independent practitioners and allied health professionals.

The AMA is responsible for developing and publishing the official guidelines for CPT. The association provides support in several ways. It publishes *CPT Assistant*, a monthly newsletter, and offers CPT Information Services, detailed descriptions, coding tips and articles that provides users with expert advice on code use. The association also conducts an annual CPT coding symposium (AMA n.d.).

## Diagnostic and Statistical Manual of Mental Disorders

The *Diagnostic and Statistical Manual of Mental Disorders, Fifth Edition, Text Revision* (DSM-5-TR) is the handbook used by healthcare professionals as a guide to diagnose mental disorders and was first published by the American Psychiatric Association (APA) in 1952. The fifth and most recent complete revision was developed in 2019 and published in 2022 to replace the DSM-IV-TR (APA n.d.a).

Historically, the DSM used a multiaxial (five-axis) coding system to document diagnoses. In this context, multiaxial is a method of evaluation that considers factors from multiple mental health diagnosis axes. The DSM-5-TR has transitioned away from the multiaxial coding system, combining the former Axes I clinical disorders, II personality disorders, and III general medical conditions and has created a separate notation for psychosocial and contextual factors (formerly Axis IV), and for disability (formerly Axis V) (APA n.d.b). The psychosocial and environmental elements are now captured with ICD-10-CM Z-codes. The Global Assessment of Functioning (GAF) (scale for level of functioning and formerly Axis V) was replaced with the WHO Disability Assessment Schedule (WHODAS), which is a scale developed by the WHO as the recommended best global measure of disability. The DSM-5-TR chapters have been restructured based on disorders' apparent relatedness to one another (similarities in disorders' underlying symptom characteristics) that now align with ICD-11.

The APA states two general uses for DSM: as a source of diagnostic information that enhances clinical practice, research, and education, and as a tool for collecting and communicating accurate public health statistics. The APA updates DSM information to correspond to the ICD (APA n.d.b). However, there are several differences between DSM-5-TR and ICD-10-CM. DSM-5-TR diagnoses are reclassified, criteria are clarified, not otherwise specified (NOS) designation is removed, and there is no longer the axis system. In comparison to ICD-10, at certain times different disorders or subtypes share the same diagnostic code. Behavioral health professionals must be fluent in both systems, focusing on the diagnostics sets that have the greatest differences. There has been an alignment of the mental and behavioral disorders in ICD-11 and DSM-5-TR from the ICD-DSM Harmonization Coordination Group formed by WHO for this harmonization effort.

## International Classification of Primary Care

The *International Classification of Primary Care* (ICPC-3) is a coding terminology for the classification of primary care developed by the World Organization of Family Doctors (WONCA) International Classification Committee (WICC) (ICPC-3 n.d.). ICPC-3 has been developed as a tool for general practitioners and family doctors throughout the world. It has been mapped to classifications of WHO, ICD-11, ICD-10, ICF, and the International Classification of Health Interventions (ICHI) so that conversion systems can be used (Della Mea et al. 2023). ICPC-3 is a concise, person-centered health issues classification that provides more granularity for visits related to primary care (WONCA 2020). Table 4.6 depicts code examples from the ICPC-3.

## Current Dental Terminology

The Current Dental Terminology (CDT) is a reference manual maintained and updated annually by the American Dental Association (ADA). Included in the manual is the Code on Dental Procedures and Nomenclature (the Code), which is a classification system for dental treatment procedures and services. The Code has been designated as the national standard for reporting dental services by the federal government under HIPAA and is recognized by third-party payers nationwide. The CDT code is a five-character alphanumeric code beginning with the letter *D* followed by four numbers (ADCA 2010). The code set is organized into 12 categories of service, each with its own series of five-digit alphanumeric codes. Each category of service is divided into subcategories of generally recognized related procedures (ADA n.d.).

## National Drug Codes

The Food and Drug Administration (FDA) developed the National Drug Codes (NDCs) directory to serve as a universal product identifier for human drugs. It identifies the labeler or vendor, product, and trade package size. It is an approved HIPAA billing and financial transaction code set for reporting drugs and biologicals. In 2004, the NDCs were adopted as a federal healthcare information interoperability standard to enable the federal healthcare sector to share information regarding drug products (HHS 2018, 25).

Each drug product is assigned a unique 10-digit or 11-digit, 3-segment number. The three segments of an NDC represent the following:

- First segment—labeler code, assigned by the FDA. A labeler is a firm that manufactures, repacks, or distributes a drug product.

- Second segment—product code, identifies a specific strength, dose form, and formulation for a particular firm.

- Third segment—package code, identifies package sizes; both the product and package codes are assigned by the firm. (FDA 2024)

The 10-digit NDCs will be in one of the following current configurations of digits in each segment: 4-4-2, 5-3-2, or 5-4-1 (see table 4.7). However, in a proposed rule, the FDA will move to a 6-digit labeler code, with a new 11-digit native NDC configuration (4-4-2 with a leading zero) for the purposes of equaling the number of digits required by HIPAA standards (21 CFR Parts 201 and 207).

Table 4.6. ICPC-3: Example diagnosis codes in primary care

| Code | |
|---|---|
| DD72 | Appendicitis |
| KD73 | Hypertension, uncomplicated |
| DD78 | Irritable bowel syndrome |
| AS04 | General weakness or tiredness (example inclusion: fatigue) |

*Source:* ICPC-3 n.d. ©WHO. Reprinted with permission.

Table 4.7. Examples of NDC codes

| Drug | NDC Product Code |
|---|---|
| Fluoxetine | 63739-493 |
| Prenatal Plus | 42291-686 |
| Glycolax Osmotic Laxative | 62175-190 |
| Flonase Allergy Relief Nasal Spray 20 Spray metered | 0135-0576 |
| Amoxicillin 500 mg Capsule | 10544-007 |

*Source:* FDA 2024.

### Check Your Understanding 4.2

**Answer the following questions in a separate document.**

1. Using figure 4.2, determine the correct code for a subsequent visit for underdosing of opium.

2. Using figure 4.3, ICD-10-PCS code structure, determine the appropriate character for each of the following:
   a. Endoscopic
   b. Pacemaker
   c. Excision

3. Do HCPCS and CPT codes apply within the inpatient or outpatient setting? What level within HCPCS defines CPT? In your own words, describe the primary function of CPT. What classification system provides the diagnostic codes that tie to the HCPCS and CPT codes? Finally, identify example settings where HCPCS and CPT codes are used.

4. Based on your reading, explain the major differences between DSM-5-TR and ICD-10. Explain what impact you expect using the two companion systems has had on behavioral health services?

5. What purpose does the NDCs directory serve in healthcare? Which of the segment would the following **bold** part of the NDC code example fall in and what information does this specific section contain?

   NDC for a 100-count bottle of Prozac 20 mg is 0777 – **3105** – 02

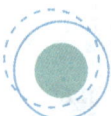

## Other Healthcare Terminologies, Vocabularies, and Classification Systems

Healthcare terminologies facilitate health information exchange by standardizing the data collected. Through this standard representation of data, terminologies provide shared meaning and a sense of context for the information being used. In simple terms, this ability to exchange information between computer systems is referred to as **interoperability**, the capability of different information systems (ISs) and software applications to communicate and exchange data. A more detailed definition for interoperability is the ability of different information technology systems and software applications to communicate; to exchange data accurately, effectively, and consistently; and to use the information that has been changed. Many experts have identified a lack of interoperability as a major obstacle to realizing the full potential of EHR systems and the exchange of health information (Turbow et al. 2021).

The National Committee on Vital and Health Statistics (NCVHS) has identified three levels of interoperability: basic, functional, and semantic. **Basic interoperability** relates to the ability to successfully transmit and receive data from one computer to another. The ability to understand or interpret the information being transmitted is not essential to basic interoperability. **Functional interoperability** refers to sending messages between computers with a shared understanding of the structure and format of the message. With functional interoperability, the receiving computer can store information in a similar data field because the nature (context) of the data being sent is understood. For example, the receiving computer could recognize that the information being sent is a lab result and store it accordingly. The NCVHS definition of **semantic interoperability** is like that of the Health Level Seven (HL7) EHR Interoperability Work Group, in which the information being transmitted is understood (NCVHS 2018). Building on the previous example, the receiving system would not only recognize that what was being sent is a lab value but would also understand the method used to calculate the value and the reference ranges for a normal result. The use of clinical terminologies in EHRs to provide standardized data is essential to achieving semantic interoperability. Progress is being made in the incorporation of clinical terminologies into EHR systems.

There are different types of clinical terminologies, each of which serves unique purposes. A **reference terminology** for clinical data is defined as a set of concepts and relationships that provide a common consultation point for comparison and aggregation of data about the entire healthcare process, recorded by multiple individuals, systems, or institutions. A reference terminology provides a common source to which data captured through other terminologies and classifications can be mapped. This linkage back to a common source facilitates aggregation and comparison of data. SNOMED CT, a widely used reference terminology, is discussed later in this chapter. An **interface terminology** is concerned with facilitating clinician documentation within the standardized structure (for example, menus, drop-down boxes) needed for an EHR. An interface terminology provides a limited set of words and phrases in a manner that is consistent with a clinician's thought process used while documenting. Information represented by an interface terminology is often mapped to similar concepts in a comprehensive reference terminology. In this sense, the interface terminology serves as a conduit between the natural language expression of the healthcare provider and the data as they are represented by the reference terminology (Bronnert et al. 2012). Some of the common terminologies in EHRs and their uses are described in the sections that follow.

## Systematized Nomenclature of Medicine Clinical Terminology

Systematized Nomenclature of Medicine Clinical Terminology (SNOMED CT) is a comprehensive, multilingual, multi-hierarchical, concept-oriented clinical terminology owned, maintained, and distributed by the International Health Terminology Standards Development Organization (IHTSDO), an international nonprofit organization based in Denmark. Figure 4.4 lists the top-level hierarchies into which SNOMED CT is organized.

The size of the terminology conveys how extensive it is. SNOMED CT is updated and released every six months. SNOMED CT includes more than 360,000 active concepts, 1,000,000 active descriptions, and 957,000 defining relationships (SNOMED International n.d.b). A concept is the most granular unit within a terminology. In SNOMED CT, it represents a "unique clinical meaning, which is referenced using a unique, numeric and machine readable SNOMED CT identifier" (SNOMED 2023). Multiple descriptions are often assigned to a single concept. For example, the descriptions *heart attack*, *myocardial infarction*, and *cardiac infarction* are all linked to a single concept (myocardial infarction 22298006). Relationships describe how the concepts within SNOMED CT are linked to one another. An example of a relationship is that the concept *diabetes mellitus* is an *endocrine disorder*, another concept with a broader meaning (SNOMED International n.d.b).

The HHS recommended SNOMED CT as part of a core set of patient medical record information (PMRI) terminology in 2003, for the adoption of uniform data standards for PMRI and electronic information exchange (NCVHS 2003) and currently still supported for use. Then in 2004, SNOMED CT was adopted as a federal information technology interoperability standard to do the following:

- Describe specific nonlaboratory interventions and procedures performed or delivered
- Exchange results of laboratory tests between facilities
- Describe anatomical locations for clinical, surgical, pathological, and research purposes
- Define diagnosis and problem lists
- Define terminology of the delivery of nursing care (SNOMED International n.d.c)

Tables 4.8 and 4.9 illustrate level of detail comparisons between SNOMED CT concepts and codes to ICD-10-CM and CPT, respectively.

SNOMED CT is currently being used in EHR systems as a clinical reference terminology to capture data for problem lists and patient assessments at the point of care. It also supports alerts, warnings, or reminders used

**Figure 4.4.** Example of SNOMED CT hierarchies

| | |
|---|---|
| Clinical finding | Qualifier value *(Right)* |
| • Finding *(Acute skin disorder)* | Record artifact *(Death certificate)* |
| • Disorder *(Acute eczema)* | Physical object *(Suture needle)* |
| | Physical force *(Friction)* |
| Procedure *(Biopsy of lung)* | Environments/geographical locations *(Intensive care unit)* |
| Observable entity *(Tumor stage)* | Social context *(Organ donor)* |
| Body structure *(Structure of thyroid)* | Situation with explicit content *(No nausea)* |
| • Morphologically abnormal structure *(Granuloma)* | Staging and scales *(Barthel index)* |
| | Linkage concept |
| Substance *(Gastric acid)* | • Link assertion *(Has etiology)* |
| Pharmaceutical/biologic product *(Tamoxifen)* | • Attributes *(Finding site)* |
| Specimen *(Urine specimen)* | Special concept *(Inactive concept)* |

**Source:** SNOMED International n.d.a.

**Table 4.8.** SNOMED CT ICD clinical detail comparison

| SNOMED CT | Description | ICD-10 |
|---|---|---|
| 49455004 | Diabetic polyneuropathy (disorder) | E08.42 |
| | | E09.42 |
| | | E10.42 |
| | | E11.42 |
| | One to many | E13.42 |
| 190502001 | Pituitary-dependent Cushing's Disease (disorder) Exact Match | E24.0 |
| 26237000 | Ankle edema (finding) Inexact Match | R60.0 |

*Source:* NLM n.d.

**Table 4.9.** SNOMED CT CPT clinical detail comparison: Procedures

| SNOMED CT | Description | CPT |
|---|---|---|
| | Total abdominal hysterectomy with or without removal of tubes, with or without removal of ovaries | 58150 |
| 116144002 | –with bilateral salpingo-oophorectomy | |

*Source:* Adapted from UMLS 2017.

for decision support. The US Department of Veterans Affairs (VA) is using SNOMED CT for standardization of problem list entries, allergic reactions, and anatomy coding in autopsy reports. A subset of SNOMED CT terms that can be used to represent problem list entries documented within an EHR is available for download at the website of the Unified Medical Language System (UMLS). The list is being provided without any licensing or intellectual property restrictions to facilitate use of the SNOMED CT terms for problem list data representation (NLM 2012). The incorporation of SNOMED CT into EHR applications is increasing (SNOMED International n.d.b).

## Logical Observation Identifiers Names and Codes

Development of the Logical Observation Identifiers Names and Codes (LOINC), the exchange standard for laboratory results, began in February 1994. The Regenstrief Institute maintains the LOINC database and its supporting documentation. Most healthcare facilities and reference laboratories use their own protocols for storing lab test and result information. The goal for LOINC is not to replace the laboratory fields in facility databases but, rather, to provide a mapping mechanism. The LOINC committee hoped that laboratories would create fields in their master files for storing LOINC codes and names as attributes of their own data elements (Regenstrief Institute n.d.). Each LOINC name identifies a distinct laboratory observation and is structured to contain up to six parts, including the following:

- Analyte or component (for example, potassium, hemoglobin)
- Kind of property measured or observed (for example, mass, mass concentration, enzyme concentration)
- Time aspect of the measurement or observation (a point in time versus an observation integrated over time)
- System and sample type (for example, urine, blood, serum)
- Type of measurement or observation scale (quantitative [a number] versus qualitative [a trait such as cloudy])
- Type of measurement or observation method used (for example, clean catch or catheter)

Table 4.10 provides an example of a LOINC code and the characteristics with its corresponding attributes.

The primary disadvantage to LOINC is that it may require significant modifications to work with a current laboratory information system that has been previously using its own protocols for lab data representation. A distinct advantage to using LOINC is that it enables the standardized communication of laboratory results. Large integrated delivery systems that have very diverse laboratory processing systems (the machines that perform the tests) will find it easier to maintain and use an EHR with LOINC-identified laboratory results.

LOINC is divided into two major sections: Lab LOINC and Clinical LOINC. Lab LOINC was established by the Regenstrief Institute to identify observations in HL7 messages as a universal standard for laboratory test names. Clinical LOINC includes entries for vital signs,

**Table 4.10.** Example of a LOINC code and its attributes

| LOINC number | 10968-6 |
|---|---|
| Component/Analyte | Glucose^4.5H post 75 g glucose PO |
| Property | PrThr (presence or threshold) |
| Time aspect | Pt (point in time) |
| System (sample type) | Urine |
| Scale type | Ord (ordinal) |
| Method type | Test strip |

*Source:* This material contains content from LOINC® (http://loinc.org). LOINC is copyright © 1995–2023, Regenstrief Institute, Inc. and the Logical Observation Identifiers Names and Codes (LOINC) Committee and is available at no cost under the license at http://loinc.org/terms-of-use.

intake and output, EKG, obstetric ultrasound, cardiac echo, urologic imaging, gastroendoscopic procedures, and other clinical observations (LOINC n.d.b).

In 2003, LOINC was adopted as a federal health information interoperability standard for the electronic exchange of laboratory test orders and drug label section headers using Structured Product Labeling (SPL) (Regenstrief Institute n.d.). LOINC has been implemented in several different healthcare settings. Many large commercial laboratories have adopted LOINC as an alternate format for reporting lab data. The current LOINC content server uses the terminology services defined by HL7's Fast Healthcare Interoperability Resources (FHIR) standard in a beta status. FHIR is a standard for healthcare data exchange published by HL7 and is discussed further later in the chapter.

## Clinical Care Classification

The Clinical Care Classification (CCC) system is a free empirically developed system consisting of (a) standardized coded nursing terminology and (b) an information model designed for documenting the essence of care in EHR systems (CCC n.d.). This system increases the opportunities for health information and interoperability in the important area of nursing.

The CCC system can be used for many purposes. Primarily, it facilitates capturing standardized data with the electronic documentation of patient care at the point of care. It can be used to track nursing activities in patient care, clinical pathways, decision support, and the effect of nursing care on patient outcomes. Furthermore, it can be used to predict workload, assess resource needs, and determine costs of nursing care. This is difficult to capture without a standardized method for codifying nursing data.

The CCC also has applications in nursing education. It can be used to teach students how to electronically document patient care and the characteristics of a nursing terminology for documentation purposes.

Another important functionality the CCC provides is in nursing research and informatics. It supports analysis and evaluation of patient outcomes, facilitates the design of expert systems, and advances nursing practice knowledge. The CCC's standardized terminology allows much higher quality data for the research. It also allows the data to be captured and reviewed more quickly than paper documentation. Thus, the knowledge gained can be utilized to improve measurement and evaluation of outcomes and better the nursing care provided to patients at the point of care (Moss et al. 2005). Nursing informatics is the "specialty that integrates nursing science with multiple information and analytical sciences to identify, define, manage and communicate data, information, knowledge and wisdom in nursing practice" (HIMSS n.d.). At its core, nursing informatics promotes innovation while driving enhanced clinical workflows and improved outcomes.

## RxNorm

RxNorm is a standardized nomenclature for clinical drugs that provides information on a drug's ingredients, strengths, and form in which it is to be administered or used. It is produced by the National Library of Medicine (NLM) and allows various systems using different drug nomenclatures to share data efficiently at the appropriate level of detail (NLM 2024a). RxNorm's standard names for clinical drugs are connected to the names of drugs present in many other controlled vocabularies, including those available in drug information sources today. These connections facilitate interoperability among the EHR systems that record or process data dealing with clinical drugs (NLM 2017). Examples of the linkages provided through RxNorm include from brand-named and generic-named clinical drugs to their active ingredients, drug components, and related brand names. They can also be connected to the FDA's NDCs (refer to table 4.7) for specific drug products and many of the drug vocabularies commonly used in pharmacy management and drug interaction (NIST 2021). This nomenclature provides a detailed level of codified data that facilitates interoperability between pharmacy systems. It allows these systems to check for drug–drug or drug–allergy interactions so that providers can avoid prescribing certain drugs and to give them other prescription choices with no adverse effects. This functionality is available today on a limited basis for patients who are treated in both the VA and Department of Defense (DoD) medical treatment facilities. It has already been shown to significantly decrease medication errors, reduce duplicate prescriptions, and most importantly, improve patient safety.

## MEDCIN

MEDCIN is a proprietary clinical terminology owned and maintained by Medicomp Systems. The system was initially developed by Peter Goltra in 1978 and has been updated regularly (NLM 2023b). MEDCIN contains approximately 400,000 clinical concepts created with a strong focus on facilitating documentation by providing clinically relevant choices in a format that is consistent with the provider's clinical thought processes. Because of this feature, the system is considered an interface terminology (Medicomp n.d.). MEDCIN is licensed by EHR developers that incorporate the terminology into their EHR systems. For example, MEDCIN is the clinical terminology used by the DoD in its Armed Forces Health Longitudinal Technology Application system. MEDCIN also identifies relationships through multiple hierarchies for each of its clinical elements. These linkages support other functionalities of the system such as clinical alerts, compliance tracking with clinical quality measures, automated note generation, and computer-assisted coding for CPT evaluation and management codes (Medicomp 2023).

## Specialty Healthcare Terminologies, Vocabularies, and Classifications

No single terminology, vocabulary, or classification has the depth and breadth to represent the broad spectrum of medical knowledge; thus, a core group of well-integrated, nonredundant methods will be needed to serve as the backbone of clinical information (Roy and Auld 2018).

Table 4.11 provides a reference to many of the specialized terminologies, vocabularies, and classifications available for use in healthcare. Tables 4.12 through 4.16 provide examples of the coding methodologies for several of these systems.

**Table 4.11.** Other healthcare terminologies, vocabularies, and classifications

| Name | Description |
|---|---|
| The National Cancer Institute (NCI) Thesaurus (table 4.12) | Contains the working vocabulary used in NCI data systems. It covers clinical, translational, and basic research as well as administrative terminology. In May 2004, the NCI Thesaurus was adopted as a federal healthcare information interoperability standard to describe anatomical locations for clinical, surgical, pathological, and research purposes (NCI 2024). |
| The Human Gene Nomenclature Committee (HGNC) (table 4.13) | Approves a gene name and symbol (short-form abbreviation) for each known human gene. It is managed by the Human Genome Organisation (HUGO) Gene Nomenclature Committee (HGNC) as a confidential database containing over 16,000 records and 43,000 approved symbols. Web data are integrated with other human gene databases, and approved gene symbols are carefully coordinated with the Mouse Genome Database (MGD). HUGO was adopted as a federal health information interoperability standard for exchanging information regarding the role of genes in biomedical research and healthcare (HGNC 2024). |
| The Global Medical Device Nomenclature (GMDN) FDA Device Classification Panels (table 4.14) | Consists of medical devices such as home blood pressure monitors, blood glucose devices, and ventilators. A standard is needed to inventory devices, document their use by healthcare providers, and regulate the devices as well as ensuring the safety and effectiveness of these products. GMDN is a collection of internationally recognized terms used to describe and catalog medical devices and supplies. GMDN is currently divided into 12 categories that encompass all of these products. It is strongly supported by the FDA for communicating these data (table 4.14 FDA Device Classification Panels). The agency also recommends that the GMDN eventually replace the FDA terminology for devices. The nomenclature is used extensively outside the US and is recognized by the European Committee for Standardization (CEN) and other international bodies.<br><br>The FDA and Emergency Care Research Institute (ECRI) are currently producing a map of UMDNS to GMDN to coordinate their practices leading to a merger between them. This should result in a terminology that enables the US federal system to utilize one set of medical device names, definitions, and codes. These identifiers may also be used to communicate with foreign entities (GMDN 2024; FDA 2018). |
| The Universal Medical Device Nomenclature System (UMDNS) | Is a standard international nomenclature and computer coding system for medical devices. It facilitates identifying, processing, filing, storing, retrieving, transferring, and communicating data about medical devices. It is primarily used by healthcare institutions. It has been adopted by many nations, including the entire European Union (EU). It is used in applications ranging from hospital inventory and work-order controls to national agency medical device regulatory systems. It is incorporated into the UMLS. UMDNS has been merged with the GMDN (WHO n.d.f). |

Continued

**Table 4.11.** Other healthcare terminologies, vocabularies, and classifications (continued)

| Name | Description |
|---|---|
| The Environmental Protection Agency (EPA) Substance Registry System (SRS) (table 4.15) | Provides information on substances and how they are represented in the EPA's regulations and information systems. It provides a common basis for identification of chemicals, biological organisms, and other substances listed in EPA regulations and data systems, as well as substances of interest from other sources, such as publications. The EPA SRS was adopted as the federal health information interoperability standard for chemicals in May 2004 (EPA SRS 2023). |
| The Breast Imaging Reporting and Data System Atlas (BI-RADS) (table 4.16) | Is designed to serve as a comprehensive guide providing standardized breast imaging terminology, a report organization, an assessment structure, and a classification system for mammography, ultrasound, and MRI of the breast (ACS 2022). BI-RADS assessment categories are listed in table 4.17.<br><br>BI-RADS is the product of a collaboration effort among members of various committees of the American College of Radiology with cooperation from the National Cancer Institute, the Centers for Disease Control and Prevention, the FDA, and the College of American Pathologists. Results are compiled in a standardized manner that permits the maintenance and collection analysis of demographic, mammographic, and outcome data (ACR 2023, 123). |
| The Medical Dictionary for Regulatory Activities (MedDRA) | Is a medically valid terminology that has an emphasis on ease of use for data entry, retrieval, analysis, and display. It was developed by the International Conference on Harmonisation (ICH) to provide a single standardized international medical terminology.<br>MedDRA terminology applies to all phases of drug development and also applies to the health effects and malfunction of devices. |
|  | Those who should subscribe to MedDRA include the following:<br>• Pharmaceutical companies<br>• Biotechnology companies<br>• Device manufacturers<br>• Regulatory authorities<br>• Contract research organizations<br>• Systems developers<br>• Other support service organizations<br>The Maintenance and Support Services Organization (MSSO) serves as the repository, maintainer, and distributor of MedDRA (ICH n.d.). |
| The Systematized Nomenclature of Dentistry (SNODENT) | Is a clinical vocabulary developed by the American Dental Association (ADA) for data representation of clinical dentistry content. The need for interoperable dental information is increasing as the field of dentistry is moving more into the medical management of oral diseases. For example, dentists now sometimes perform saliva testing for the purpose of substance abuse and disease monitoring. This type of information may need to be shared with other healthcare providers (ADA n.d.). |

**Table 4.12.** NCI Thesaurus taxonomy concept details

| Identifiers: | |
|---|---|
| Name | Pancreas |
| Code | C12393 |
| **Relationships to other concepts:** | |
| Anatomic_Structure_Has_Location | Epigastric Region |
| Anatomic_Structure_is_Physical_Part_of | Pancreatobiliary System |
| **Information about this concept:** | |
| Display_Name | Pancreas |
| Preferred_Name | Pancreas |
| Semantic_Type | Body Part, Organ, or Organ Component |
| Subsource | ICDO |
| Unified Medical Language System | C0030274 |

*Source:* NCI 2024.

**Table 4.13.** Human genes with approved symbols: Single-letter amino acid codes

| Amino Acid | Approved Symbol |
|---|---|
| Alanine – glyoxylate aminotransferase | AGXT |
| Arginine vasopressin | AVP |
| Cysteine rich protein 1 | CRIP1 |
| Glutamine rich 2 | GRICH2 |

*Source:* HGNC 2023.

**Table 4.14.** FDA classification panels

Most medical devices can be classified by finding the matching description of the device in Title 21 of the Code of Federal Regulations (CFR), Parts 862-892. FDA has classified and described over 1,700 distinct types of devices and organized them in the CFR into 16 medical specialty panels:

| Medical Specialty | | Regulation Citation (21 CFR) |
|---|---|---|
| 73 | Anesthesiology | Part 868 |
| 74 | Cardiovascular | Part 870 |
| 75 | Chemistry | Part 862 |
| 76 | Dental | Part 872 |
| 77 | Ear, Nose, and Throat | Part 874 |
| 78 | Gastroenterology and Urology | Part 876 |
| 79 | General and Plastic Surgery | Part 878 |
| 80 | General Hospital | Part 880 |
| 81 | Hematology | Part 864 |
| 82 | Immunology | Part 866 |
| 83 | Microbiology | Part 866 |
| 84 | Neurology | Part 882 |
| 85 | Obstetrical and Gynecological | Part 884 |
| 86 | Ophthalmic | Part 886 |
| 87 | Orthopedic | Part 888 |
| 88 | Pathology | Part 864 |
| 89 | Physical Medicine | Part 890 |
| 90 | Radiology | Part 892 |
| 91 | Toxicology | Part 862 |

*Source:* FDA 2018.

**Table 4.15.** Example of an EPA SRS substance list

| Name | Liquid Nitrogen (Containing) |
|---|---|
| Molecular Formula | N2 |
| Substance Type | Chemical Substance |
| Classification | All |
| Display Option | Substance Name |
| Sort Option | Name |
| Systematic Name | Nitrogen |
| EPA Registry Name | Nitrogen |
| IUPAC Name | Nitrogen |
| Classification | Chemical |
| CAS number | 7727-37-9 |
| EPA ID | 153122 |

*Source:* EPA SRS 2023.

### Table 4.16. BI-RADS mammography assessment categories

| Assessment | Category |
|---|---|
| a. Mammographic Assessment is Incomplete | 0: Incomplete<br>Additional imaging evaluation and/or comparison to prior mammograms (or other imaging tests) is needed. |
| b. Mammographic Assessment is Complete–Final Categories | 1: Negative<br>This is a normal test result. In this case, negative means nothing new or abnormal was found. Continue routine screening. |
| | 2: Benign (non-cancerous) finding<br>This is also a negative test result, but the radiologist chooses to describe a finding that is not cancer, such as benign calcifications, masses, or lymph nodes in the breast. This can also be used to describe changes from prior procedures. Ensures that others who look at the mammogram in the future will not misinterpret the benign finding as suspicious. Continue routine screening. |
| | 3: Probably Benign Finding—Follow-up in a short timeframe is suggested<br>Short-term follow-up mammogram at 6 months, then every 6 to 12 months for 1 to 2 years. A finding in this category has a very low (no more than 2%) chance of being cancer. Monitoring to see if the area in question does change over time. |
| | 4: Suspicious Abnormality—Biopsy should be considered<br>These findings do not definitively look like cancer but could be cancer and can have a wide range of suspicion levels. Perform biopsy, preferably needle biopsy (4A Low suspicion, 4B Moderate suspicion, 4C High suspicion). |
| | 5: Highly Suggestive of Malignancy—Appropriate action should be taken<br>Findings look like cancer and have a high chance of being cancer. Biopsy and treatment, as necessary. |
| | 6: Known Biopsy–Proven Malignancy—Appropriate action should be taken<br>This category is only used for findings on a mammogram (or ultrasound or MRI) that have already been shown to be cancer by a previous biopsy, treatment pending (ensure that treatment is completed) and imaging to monitor how well the cancer is responding to treatment. |

*Source:* Adapted from ACR 2023, 134–138.

## Check Your Understanding 4.3

**Answer the following questions in a separate document.**

1. In your own words, explain interoperability and describe how terminologies play a role in interoperability.
2. Identify two data standards for each class of the following data-sharing interoperability standards and describe the data set's purpose. Explain the relationship to a classification or clinical terminologies utilized and identify the associated Standards Development Organization(s) (SDO[s]).
3. Identify an appropriate classification, terminology, vocabulary, or standard that is a good candidate to represent: (a) laboratory data, (b) nursing documentation, and (c) problem list documentation.
4. Based on your reading, provide an example where SNOMED-CT is being used within the EHR as clinical reference terminology and explain how it is used.
5. Distinguish the two major sections for LOINC.

| Class of Standards | Example Standards | Standards Development Organization(s) | Purpose of Data Set |
|---|---|---|---|
| Data Interchange | | | |
| EHR | | | |

## Data Standardization

Data standardization exists to support different healthcare functions. Classifications are used to aggregate data for functions such as data analysis and reimbursement. Clinical terminologies play an essential role in capturing and sharing data in a manner that meets the requirements of semantic interoperability, which is essential for reliable health information exchange. **Mapping** is the process of associating concepts from one coding system and defining their equivalence in accordance with a documented rationale and a given purpose. Maps that link related content in classifications and terminologies allow data collected for one purpose to be used for another. For example, a laboratory system that manages data using the LOINC terminology can map the LOINC terms to CPT codes to be used for billing purposes. The NLM, within the framework of the UMLS, contains many sets of mapping among terminologies including LOINC to CPT mapping and SNOMED CT to ICD-10-CM mapping (UMLS 2016a). Many maps are created to support a specific use case. For example, the map created for a reimbursement use case might be very different from that for a public health use case. This is even true if the two use cases were mapping between the same two systems. Therefore, successful mapping requires a thorough understanding of the intended use of the map (use case), the structure and purpose of the source, and target terminologies (UMLS 2016b).

To reach the full potential of health information exchange, health information management (HIM) professionals must participate in the development, implementation, and maintenance of information systems that use standards for collecting and reporting data. As HIM professionals search for ways to formalize the myriad types of data contained in EHRs, it helps to evaluate the different classifications and terminologies. Certain characteristics are desirable. Several organizations are actively involved in developing standards for healthcare. See table 4.17 for examples of standards development organizations. Both private organizations and government agencies such as the Office of the National Coordinator for Health Information Technology (ONC), CMS, FDA, the Agency for Health Care Policy and Research, the Office of the Assistant Secretary for Planning and Evaluation, and the Centers for Disease Control and Prevention (CDC) work collaboratively in the development and maintenance of these standards.

The critical importance of healthcare information standards has been recognized in federal initiatives, including the legislatively mandated ONC and the establishment of two official HHS advisory committees as the initial result of the Health Information Technology for Economic and Clinical Health (HITECH) Act, part of the American Recovery and Reinvestment Act of 2009 (ARRA). Since then, CMS has transitioned, and the current program's objectives and measures can be found on the CMS Medicare Promoting Interoperability Program Objectives & Measures fact sheet (CMS 2023e).

The government used one of its health outcomes policy priorities, improving care coordination, to create the framework for meaningful use of EHRs. A key component of this framework is to achieve interoperability, which is the ability of different information technology systems and software applications to communicate; to exchange data accurately, effectively, and consistently; and to use changed information. To achieve interoperability, electronic information exchange requires having a defined core data sets such as from the American Society for Testing and Materials International (ASTM). ASTM International was instrumental in identifying a core data set for a patient's clinical summary with the of Standard Specification for Continuity of Care Record (CCR). Another organization, HL7, developed the **Clinical Document Architecture (CDA)**. The CDA provides an exchange model for clinical documents (such as discharge summaries and progress notes). ASTM International and HL7 combined their work to create the **Continuity of Care Document (CCD)**. The CCD is an implementation guide for sharing CCR patient summary data using the CDA. The CCD was recognized as part of the first set of interoperability standards.

Continuing the work toward interoperability is the **transitions of care (ToC) initiative**, one of the projects of the ONC Standards and Interoperability (S&I) Framework. The S&I Framework empowers healthcare stakeholders to establish standards, specifications, and other implementation guidance that facilitate effective healthcare information exchange. Another ONC initiative includes the Interoperability Standards Advisory (ISA). The ISA process "represents the model by which the Office of the National Coordinator for Health Information Technology (ONC) will coordinate the identification, assessment, and determination of 'recognized' interoperability standards and implementation specifications for industry use to fulfill specific clinical health IT interoperability needs" (ONC n.d.a).

Standards in the healthcare industry evolve over time. While the CCD remains relevant, the development

**Table 4.17.** Standards development organizations

| Resource | Description | Source |
|---|---|---|
| AIIM | AIIM is a standards development organization accredited by the American National Standards Institute (ANSI). AIIM also holds the Secretariat for the ISO (International Organization for Standardization) committee focused on information management compliance issues, TC171. | https://www.aiim.org |
| Accredited Standards Committee (ASC) X12 | ASC X12 is a designated committee under the Designated Standard Maintenance Organization (DSMO), which develops uniform standards for cross-industry exchange of business transactions through electronic data interchange (EDI) standards. ASC X12 is an ANSI-accredited standards development organization. | https://www.x12.org |
| American Dental Association (ADA) | The ADA is an ANSI-accredited standards developing organization that develops dental standards that promote safe and effective oral healthcare. | https://www.ada.org/resources/practice/dental-standards |
| ASTM International | Formerly the American Society for Testing and Materials, ASTM International is an ANSI-accredited standards development organization that develops standards for healthcare data security, standard record content, and protocols for exchange of laboratory data (ASTM 2023). | https://www.astm.org |
| European Committee for Standardization (CEN) | CEN contributes to the objectives of the European Union and European Economic Area with voluntary technical standards that promote free trade, the safety of workers and consumers, interoperability of networks, environmental protection, exploitation of research and development programs, and public procurement. | Sustainability Reporting - CEN-CENELEC https://www.cencenelec.eu |
| Clinical and Laboratory Standards Institute (CLSI) | CLSI is a global, nonprofit, standards development organization that promotes the development and use of voluntary consensus standards and guidelines within the healthcare community. Its core business is the development of globally applicable voluntary consensus documents for healthcare testing. | https://www.clsi.org |
| Clinical Data Interchange Standards Consortium (CDISC) | CDISC is an open, multidisciplinary, nonprofit organization that has established worldwide industry standards to support the electronic acquisition, exchange, submission, and archiving of clinical trials data and metadata for medical and biopharmaceutical product development. | https://www.cdisc.org |
| Designated Standard Maintenance Organization (DSMO) | A category of organizations established under HIPAA to maintain the electronic transaction standards | (45 CFR 162.910 2013) |
| Health Industry Business Communications Council (HIBCC) | HIBCC is an industry-sponsored and supported nonprofit organization. As an ANSI-accredited organization, its primary function is to facilitate electronic communications by developing standards for information exchange among healthcare trading partners. | https://www.hibcc.org |
| Health Level 7 (HL7) | HL7 is an ANSI-accredited standards development organization that develops messaging, data content, and document standards to support the exchange of clinical information. | https://www.hl7.org |
| Institute of Electrical and Electronic Engineers (IEEE) | IEEE is a national organization that develops standards for hospital system interface transactions, including links between critical care bedside instruments and clinical information systems. | https://standards.ieee.org/ |
| International Organization for Standardization (ISO) | ISO is a nongovernmental organization and network of national standards institutes from 157 countries. | https://www.iso.org/about-us.html |
| National Council for Prescription Drug Programs (NCPDP) | NCPDP is a designated committee under the DSMO that specializes in developing standards for exchanging prescription and payment information. | https://www.ncpdp.org/Who-We-Are.aspx |
| National Information Standards Organization (NISO) | NISO is an ANSI-accredited, nonprofit association that identifies, develops, maintains, and publishes technical standards to manage information. NISO standards address areas of retrieval, repurposing, storage, metadata, and preservation. | https://www.niso.org |
| National Uniform Billing Committee (NUBC) | NUBC is a designated committee under the DSMO that is responsible for identifying data elements and designing the UB-04. | https://www.nubc.org |
| National Uniform Claim Committee (NUCC) | NUCC is the national group that replaced the Uniform Claim Form Task Force in 1995 and developed a standard data set to be used in the transmission of noninstitutional provider CMS-1500 claims to and from third-party payers. | https://www.nucc.org |
| The United States Core Data for Interoperability (USCDI) | The USCDI is a set of standards that define the minimum health data elements for interoperability. It is an aggregation of data elements by a common theme. The USCDI data element is a piece of data defined in USCDI for access, exchange or use for electronic health information. | https://www.healthit.gov/isa/united-states-core-data-interoperability-uscdi |

and adoption of United States Core Data for Interoperability (USCDI) standards reflect the healthcare industry's commitment to continually improving and standardizing health data exchange for better patient care and outcomes. The 21st Century Cures Act delivers the next phase in standardization (45 CFR 170; 45 CFR 171). The USCDI standard will replace the Common Clinical Data Set. Certified health IT must be updated to support the USCDI for all certification criteria.

The Cures Act requires the Secretary of HHS to establish Conditions and Maintenance of Certification requirements for the ONC Health IT Certification Program (ONC n.d.b). There are seven Conditions of Certification with accompanying Maintenance of Certification Requirements (HHS 2023). As of June 2023, the HHS Office of the National Coordinator for Health Information Technology (ONC) released proposals to implement provisions of the Cures Act to make enhancements to the ONC Health IT Certification Program, including updating standards and implementation specifications to advance interoperability (HHS 2023).

## Interoperability

FHIR plays a pivotal role in advancing health information interoperability and exchange. FHIR is a standard developed by HL7 to facilitate the bi-directional exchange of healthcare information electronically (ONC n.d.c). It serves as a framework for integrating various terminologies including ICD-10-CM and ICD-10-PCS, SNOMED CT, LOINC, and RxNorm (HL7 2023). FHIR plays a critical role in promoting health information interoperability by using modern web standards such as HTTP and RESTful APIs (Representational State Transfer) to enable communication and interoperability between different healthcare systems and applications (ONC n.d.c). FHIR is designed with a modular approach using resources, discrete units of healthcare information such as medication and observation. Using resources enhances flexibility and adaptability, which reduces the need to transfer large datasets and improves efficiency. FHIR defines interoperability standards, which supports a harmonized approach to data exchange and promotes a standardized understanding of how specific data elements, such as coded clinical data, should be represented (ONC n.d.c). For example, a coding professional can use FHIR resources to encode and represent clinical information to share and exchange coded data across different healthcare systems. FHIR includes resources for representing various types of coded clinical data such as conditions, procedures, medications, and observations. These resources leverage standardized code systems, including ICD-10, SNOMED-CT, and LOINC for example to ensure consistency (HL7 2023). FHIR serves as a common framework for representing coded clinical data, aligning with established coding systems and standards. Coding professionals can leverage FHIR to encode and exchange coded information.

## National Library of Medicine's Role in Healthcare Terminologies

The National Library of Medicine (NLM) is the world's largest medical library. It collects materials in all aspects of biomedicine and healthcare, as well as works on biomedical aspects of technology, the humanities, and the physical, life, and social sciences (NLM 2023b). It is a standards-supporting and promoting organization that explores the uses of computer and communication technologies to improve organizations and the use of biomedical information.

### Medical Subject Headings

The Medical Subject Headings database (MeSH) is the NLM's controlled vocabulary thesaurus. It consists of terms naming descriptors in a hierarchical structure that permits searching at various levels of specificity (NLM 2021). The descriptors exist in both alphabetic and hierarchical structures. It contains very broad headings, such as "Mental Disorders," and more specific levels, such as "Conduct Disorder." There are more than 30,000 descriptors in MeSH and more than 139,000 headings, called Supplementary Concept Records, within a separate thesaurus (UMLS 2022). Thousands of cross-references also exist. MeSH is used by the NLM for indexing articles from 4,600 of the world's leading biomedical journals for the MEDLINE/PubMed database. Each bibliographic reference is associated with a set of MeSH terms that describe the content of the item (UMLS 2022). Staff subject specialists are responsible for revising and updating the vocabulary on a continuous basis. MeSH is available in electronic format at no charge at the NLM website and a hard copy version is published each January (UMLS 2022).

### Unified Medical Language System

The Unified Medical Language System (UMLS) is a government-funded project from the NLM that has been in development since 1986. The purpose of the UMLS is "to facilitate the development of computer systems that behave as if they 'understand' the meaning of the language of biomedicine and health. The UMLS provides data for system developers as well as search and report functions for less technical users"

(NLM 2021). This goal is achieved through the three knowledge sources found in the UMLS:

- UMLS Metathesaurus: A list containing information on biomedical concepts and terms
- SPECIALIST Lexicon: An English-language vocabulary containing many biomedical terms
- UMLS Semantic Network: A consistent categorization of all concepts represented in the UMLS Metathesaurus

More information on the UMLS can be obtained from the NLM website. When looking in-depth at the UMLS, it is important to keep in mind that it has been designed for computer use; its layouts and other structures are meant to be read by machines. It is not structured to be readable by humans.

The VA has used the UMLS Metathesaurus as a lookup tool for finding concepts, synonyms, and linkages to other terminologies in the allergy data standardization. The VA also uses the UMLS RxNorm for standardizing pharmacy data and shares those data with the DoD. It has also been proposed to use UMLS as the mediation terminology for VA drug classes.

## Artificial Intelligence

Artificial intelligence (AI) is defined as high-level information technologies used in developing machines that imitate human qualities such as learning and reasoning. AI systems enhance the medical coding role as well as clinical documentation integrity (CDI) by automating routine tasks, providing real-time suggestions, improving accuracy, and facilitating continuous learning and adaptation to evolving healthcare standards.

AI, particularly with the use of natural language processing (NLP) and machine learning models, can analyze unstructured clinical notes, provider documentation, and other free text data. Machine learning is "a process by which machines can be given the capability to learn about a given dataset without being explicitly programmed on what to learn" (NIH 2023). This is invaluable for coding professionals as a significant portion of patient information in an EHR is stored in an unstructured format. AI systems integrate with EHRs to provide real-time coding assistance within an existing workflow. See figure 4.5 as an example. AI can help analyze clinical documentation for missing or incomplete information that is necessary for accurate code assignment and can learn from historical coding patterns, updates in guidelines, and feedback directly from coding professionals (Gallegos 2023). NLP helps AI identify and extract pertinent information from the unstructured narratives. This assists in CDI efforts by identifying areas that require queries for clarification or specificity. AI systems can also be trained to automatically assign appropriate codes based on clinical documentation. AI can analyze large datasets to identify specific coding trends, patterns and areas of concern (Pluard 2023). Machine learning is an area of computer science that studies algorithms and computer programs that improve employee performance on some tasks by exposure to a training or learning experience. Machine learning models can analyze historical coding data to identify trends. The models can then apply predictive analytics to help anticipate documentation needs for specific conditions or procedures, allowing for proactive measures with quality documentation. The models also assist in speeding up the coding process while reducing the risk of human error. By suggesting the codes in real-time, AI systems guide both providers and coding professionals toward more accurate and specific documentation, which improves the overall documentation quality of patient health records. The collaboration and interaction between AI systems, coding professionals, and CDI specialists contribute to efficient and accurate health documentation, compliance in coding processes, and ultimately contribute to better patient care and financial outcomes for healthcare organizations (Smith 2023).

Figure 4.5. AI system integration with coding assistance workflow

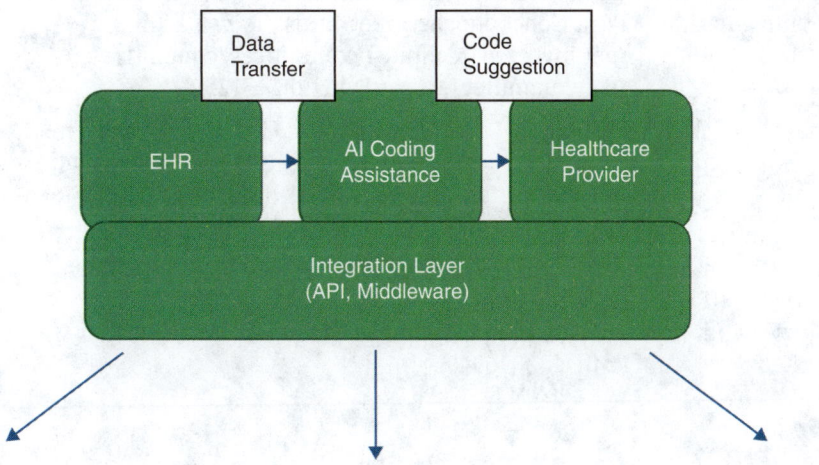

### Check Your Understanding 4.4

**Answer the following questions in a separate document.**

1. Examine the reasons data standardization is important in healthcare today.
2. Identify the five desirable characteristics of terminologies and classifications for data standardization.
3. Describe how AI is incorporated into the ICD-10-CM coding workflow within the EHR.
4. Explain why mapping is needed.
5. Healthcare informatics standards are frameworks and guidelines designed to ensure healthcare information is accurately captured, securely stored, and effectively exchanged among different systems and stakeholders within healthcare. Identify the key components of the example healthcare informatics standards provided in the following table:

| Healthcare Informatics Standard | Key Components |
|---|---|
| Health Level Seven (HL7) | |
| Clinical Documentation Architecture (CDA) | |
| ASTM E2369 Continuity of Care Record (CCR) | |
| LOINC | |
| ISO/IEC 27000 Series | |
| SNOMED-CT | |
| ICD | |

# References

ACS (American Cancer Society). 2022. "BI-RADS." https://www.cancer.org/cancer/types/breast-cancer/screening-tests-and-early-detection/mammograms/understanding-your-mammogram-report.html.

ACR (American College of Radiology). 2013 *BI-RADS Atlas*, 5th ed. https://www.acr.org/-/media/ACR/Files/RADS/BI-RADS/Mammography-Reporting.pdf.

ADA (American Dental Association). n.d. "Code on Dental Procedures and Nomenclature (CDT Code)." Accessed December 2023. http://www.ada.org/en/publications/cdt/.

ADCA (American Dental Coders Association). "Dental Billing and Coding 101 for 2024." Accessed July 15, 2024. https://www.adcaonline.org/dental-billing-and-coding-101/.

AMA (American Medical Association). n.d. "CPT Overview and code approval." Accessed May 20, 2024. https://www.ama-assn.org/practice-management/cpt/cpt-overview-and-code-approval.

AMIA (American Medical Informatics Association) and AHIMA (American Health Information Management Association) Terminology and Classification Policy Task Force. 2007 (June 27). Healthcare terminologies and classifications: An action agenda for the United States. *Perspectives in Health Information Management*. https://library.ahima.org/PdfView?oid=71880.

APA (American Psychiatric Association). n.d.a. "History of DSM-5 -TR." Accessed May 20, 2024. https://www.psychiatry.org/psychiatrists/practice/dsm/about-dsm/history-of-the-dsm.

APA (American Psychiatric Association). n.d.b. "Diagnostic and Statistical Manual." Accessed May 20, 2024. https://www.psychiatry.org/psychiatrists/practice/dsm/updates-to-dsm/updates-to-dsm-5-tr-criteria-text.

ASTM. 2023. "Standard Guide for Quality Indicators for Health Classifications." ASTM International. West Conshohocken, PA: https://www.astm.org/get-involved/technical-committees/committee-e31/subcommittee-e31/jurisdiction-e3125.

Barnett, O. G., R. Jenders, and H. Chueh. 1993. The computer-based clinical record: Where do we stand? *Annals of Internal Medicine* 119(10):1046–1048.

Bronnert, J., C. Masarie, F. Naeymi-Rad, E. Rose, G. Aldin. 2012. Problem-centered care delivery: how interface terminology makes standardized health information possible. *Journal of AHIMA* 83(7):30–35. PMID: 22896949.

Butler, R. R., R. L. Mullin, T. M. Grant, R. F. Averill, and B. A. Steinbeck. 2016 *ICD-10-PCS Reference Manual*. https://www.cms.gov/files/document/icd-10-pcs-reference-manual-2016.pdf.

CMS (Centers for Medicare and Medicaid Services). 2023a. "HCPCS General Information." https://www.cms.gov/Medicare/Coding/MedHCPCSGenInfo/index.html.

CMS (Centers for Medicare and Medicaid Services). 2023b. *2024 ICD-10-CM Code Tables and Index*. https://www.cms.gov/files/zip/2024-code-tables-tabular-and-index-updated-02/01/2024.zip.

CMS (Centers for Medicare and Medicaid Services). 2023c. "2024 ICD-10-PCS." https://www.cms.gov/medicare/coding-billing/icd-10-codes/2024-icd-10-pcs.

CMS (Centers for Medicare and Medicaid Services). 2023d. *2024 ICD-10-PCS Official Coding Guidelines*. https://www.cms.gov/files/document/2024-official-icd-10-pcs-coding-guidelines-updated-12/19/2023.pdf.

CMS (Centers for Medicare and Medicaid Services). 2023e. *Medicare Promoting Interoperability Program Objectives and Measures*. https://www.cms.gov/files/document/pi-program-objective-overview-05-2023.pdf.

Chute, C. G. 2000. Clinical classification and terminology: Some history and current observations. *Journal of the American Medical Informatics Association* 70(3):298–303.

Della Mea, V., A. H. Almborg, M. Martinuzzi, S. W. Tu, and A. Martinuzzi. 2023. Harmonization of ICF Body Structures and ICD-11 Anatomic Detail: One foundation for multiple classifications. *PloS one 18*(7), e0280106. https://doi.org/10.1371/journal.pone.0280106.

Encyclopedia Britannica. n.d. "Sir William Petty." Accessed May 29, 2024. http://www.britannica.com/EBchecked/topic/454631/Sir-William-Petty.

EPA SRS (Environmental Protection Agency Substance Registry Services). 2023. "Find Chemicals or Substances." http://iaspub.epa.gov/sor_internet/registry/substreg/searchandretrieve/substancesearch/search.do?details=displayDetails.

FDA (Food and Drug Administration). 2023. "National Drug Code Directory." https://www.accessdata.fda.gov/scripts/cder/ndc/index.cfm.

FDA (Food and Drug Administration). 2018. "Device Classification Panels." https://www.fda.gov/medical-devices/classify-your-medical-device/device-classification-panels.

Fritz, A. C. Percy, A. Jack, K. Shanmugarathan, L. Sobin, D. M. Parkin, and S. Whelan. 2019. *International Classification of Diseases for Oncology (ICD-O)*, 3rd ed. World Health Organization.

Gallegos, A. 2023. Keeping up with artificial intelligence: The role of HI professionals. *Journal of AHIMA*. https://journal.ahima.org/page/keeping-up-with-artificial-intelligence-the-role-of-hi-professionals.

GMDN (The Global Medical Device Nomenclature). 2024. https://www.gmdnagency.org/.

HHS (U.S. Department of Health and Human Services). 2023. "HHS Proposes New Rule to Further Implement the 21st Century Cures Act." https://www.hhs.gov/about/news/2023/04/11/hhs-propose-new-rule-to-further-implement-the-21st-century-cures-act.html.

HHS (U.S. Department of Health and Human Services). 2018. Health Terminologies and Vocabularies Environmental Scan. https://ncvhs.hhs.gov/wp-content/uploads/2018/10/Report-Health-Terminologies-and-Vocabularies-Environmental-Scan.pdf.

HIMSS (Healthcare Information and Management Systems Society). n.d. "What Is Nursing Informatics?" Accessed January 2, 2024. https://www.himss.org/resources/what-nursing-informatics.

HL7 FHIR. 2023. "Terminology Code Systems." https://www.hl7.org/fhir/terminologies-systems.html.

HGNC (HUGO Gene Nomenclature Committee). 2024. http://www.genenames.org.

ICH (International Council for Harmonisation of Technical Requirements for Pharmaceuticals for Human Use). n.d. "Welcome to MedDRA." Accessed May 29, 2024. https://www.meddra.org/.

ICPC-3 (International Classification of Primary Care). n.d. "Introduction to ICPD-3." Accessed January 1, 2024. https://www.icpc-3.info/.

ICPC-3 (International Classification of Primary Care). 2024. "ICPC-3 Browser." https://browser.icpc-3.info/.

LOINC (Logical Observation Identifiers Names and Codes). n.d.a. "About LOINC." Accessed May 29, 2024. https://loinc.org/about/.

LOINC (Logical Observation Identifiers Names and Codes). n.d.b. "Scope of LOINC." Accessed May 20, 2024. https://loinc.org/get-started/.

Medicomp Systems. n.d. "The Medicomp MEDCIN Engine." Accessed May 2024. https://medicomp.com/medcin-details/.

Moss, J. A., M. Damrongsak, and K. Gallichio. 2005. Representing critical care data using the clinical care classification. *AMIA Annual Symposium Proceedings. AMIA Symposium, 2005*, 545–549.

NCI (National Cancer Institute). 2024. "NCI Thesaurus (NCIT)." http://ncit.nci.nih.gov/ncitbrowser/ConceptReport.jsp?dictionary=NCI%20Thesaurus&code=C12393.

NCVHS (National Committee on Vital and Health Statistics). 2018. "NCVHS Subcommittee on Standards and Security." https://ncvhs.hhs.gov/subcommittees-work-groups/subcommittee-on-standards/.

NCVHS (National Committee on Vital and Health Statistics). 2003. Recommendations for PMRI Terminology Standards. http://www.ncvhs.hhs.gov/wp-content/uploads/2014/05/031105lt3.pdf.

NIH (National Institutes of Health). 2023. "Artificial Intelligence, Machine Learning and Genomics Fact Sheet." https://www.genome.gov/about-genomics/educational-resources/fact-sheets/artificial-intelligence-machine-learning-and-genomics.

NIST (National Institute of Standards and Technology). 2021. "HIT Implementation Support and Testing." http://healthcare.nist.gov/testing_infrastructure/index.html.

NLM (National Library of Medicine). 2023a. "RxNorm Overview." http://www.nlm.nih.gov/research/umls/rxnorm/overview.html.

NLM (National Library of Medicine). 2023b. "Collection Development Guidelines of the National Library of Medicine." https://www.ncbi.nlm.nih.gov/books/NBK518702/?report = reader.

NLM (National Library of Medicine). 2023c. "SNOMED CT Browser." https://browser.ihtsdotools.org/?perspective = full&conceptId1 = 404684003&edition = MAIN/SNOMEDCT-US/2023-09-01&release = &languages = en.

NLM (National Library of Medicine). 2021. "UMLS Metathesaurus Browser." https://uts.nlm.nih.gov/uts/umls/home.

NLM (National Library of Medicine). 2017 (January 27). "UMLS Knowledge Source Server Mappings: Draft LNC215 to CPT2005 Mapping." http://www.nlm.nih.gov/research/umls/mapping_projects/loinc_to_cpt_map.html.

NLM (National Library of Medicine). 2016a (July 29). "Unified Medical Language System Glossary." http://www.nlm.nih.gov/research/umls/new_users/glossary.html.

NLM (National Library of Medicine). 2016b (March 32). "Basic Mapping Project Assumptions." http://www.nlm.nih.gov/research/umls/mapping_projects/mapping_assumptions.html.

NLM (National Library of Medicine). 2012 (April 2). "UMLS enhanced VA/KP problem list subset of SNOMED CT." http://www.nlm.nih.gov/research/umls/licensedcontent/vakpproblemlist.html.

NLM (National Library of Medicine). n.d. "I-MAGIC SNOMED-CT to ICD-10-CM Map." Accessed May 20, 2024. https://imagic.nlm.nih.gov/imagic/code/map.

ONC (Office of the National Coordinator for Health Information Technology). n.d.a. "Interoperability Standards Advisory (ISA)." Accessed January 1, 2024. https://www.healthit.gov/isa/.

ONC (Office of the National Coordinator for Health Information Technology). n.d.b. *United States Core Data for Interoperability*. Accessed January 1, 2024. https://www.healthit.gov/sites/default/files/page2/2020-03/USCDI.pdf.

ONC (Office of the National Coordinator for Health Information Technology). n.d.c. ONC Fact Sheet. "What Is FHIR." Accessed May 29, 2024. https://www.healthit.gov/sites/default/files/2019-08/ONCFHIRFSWhatIsFHIR.pdf.

Pluard, D. 2023 (January 31). "AI in Healthcare: How Can It Be Applied to Medical Records & Interoperability?" *Intely* (blog). https://www.intely.io/blog/ai-in-healthcare-how-can-it-be-applied-to-medical-records-interoperability/.

Regenstrief Institute, Inc. n.d. "Logical Observation Identifiers Names and Codes." Accessed January 1, 2024. http://loinc.org.

Roy, S. L., and V. A. Auld. 2018. *Health Terminologies and Vocabularies Environmental Scan*. https://ncvhs.hhs.gov/wp-content/uploads/2018/10/Report-Health-Terminologies-and-Vocabularies-Environmental-Scan.pdf.

Smith, G. 2023 (November 1). "AI and Coding: Can It Reduce Cognitive Overload?" *Coder's Corner* (blog). https://libmaneducation.com/ai-and-coding-can-it-reduce-cognitive-overload.

SNOMED International. n.d.a. "SNOMED CT Browser". Accessed May 29, 2024. http://browser.ihtsdotools.org/?.

SNOMED International. n.d.b. "What Is SNOMED CT." Accessed May 29, 2024. https://www.snomed.org/five-step-briefing.

SNOMED International. n.d.c. "Why SNOMED CT?" Accessed May 29, 2024. https://www.snomed.org/news/why-snomed-ct%3F-new-platform-presents-a-refreshed-case-for-investing-in-the-comprehensive-clinical-terminology.

SNOMED International. 2020. "What Is the Difference Between a Classification Such as ICD-10 or ICPC and a Terminology like SNOMED CT?" https://ihtsdo.freshdesk.com/support/solutions/articles/4000144252-what-is-the-difference-between-a-classification-such-as-icd-10-or-icpc-and-a-terminology-like-snomed-.

Turbow S., J. R. Hollberg, and M. K. Ali. 2021. Electronic health record interoperability: How did we get here and how do we move forward? *JAMA Health*

*Forum* 2(3):e210253. https://jamanetwork.com/journals/jama-health-forum/fullarticle/2777782.

UMLS (Unified Medical Language System). 2022. "RxNorm." http://www.nlm.nih.gov/research/umls/rxnorm/.

UMLS (Unified Medical Language System). 2017 (January 27). "SNOMED CT Browsers." https://www.nlm.nih.gov/research/umls/Snomed/snomed_browsers.html.

UMLS (Unified Medical Language System). 2016a. "UMLS Metathesaurus–Mapping Projects." https://www.nlm.nih.gov/research/umls/knowledge_sources/metathesaurus/mapping_projects/index.html.

UMLS (Unified Medical Language System). 2016b. "UMLS Basic Mapping Project Assumptions." https://www.nlm.nih.gov/research/umls/mapping_projects/mapping_assumptions.html

WHO (World Health Organization). 2022. *2023 ICD-11 Reference Guide*. https://icdcdn.who.int/icd11referenceguide/en/html/index.html.

WHO (World Health Organization). 2019 (May 27). "The 72nd World Health Assembly Resolution for ICD-11 Adoption." https://www.who.int/publications/m/item/eleventh-revision-of-the-international-classification-of-diseases-adoption-wha72.

WHO (World Health Organization). n.d.a. "History of ICD." Accessed May 29, 2024. https://www.who.int/news-room/spotlight/international-classification-of-diseases#:~:text=In%20the%201940s%2C%20the%20World,Causes%20of%20Death%20(ICD).

WHO (World Health Organization). n.d.b. "ICD-11 Fact Sheet." Accessed January 1, 2024. https://icd.who.int/en/docs/icd11factsheet_en.pdf.

WHO (World Health Organization). n.d.c. "*International Classification of Diseases*, 11th Revision." Accessed January 1, 2024. https://icdcdn.who.int/icd11referenceguide/en/html/index.html#general-features-of-icd11/.

WHO (World Health Organization). n.d.d. "*International Classification of Primary Care*, 2nd Edition (ICPC-2)." Accessed May 29, 2024. https://www.who.int/standards/classifications/other-classifications/international-classification-of-primary-care.

WHO (World Health Organization). n.d.e. "International Classification of Functioning, Disability and Health (ICF)." Accessed May 29, 2024. https://icd.who.int/dev11/l-icf/en.

WHO (World Health Organization). n.d.f. "Nomenclature of medical devices." May 29, 2024. https://www.who.int/teams/health-product-policy-and-standards/assistive-and-medical-technology/medical-devices/nomenclature.

WONCA (World Organization of National Colleges, Academies and Academic Associations of General Practitioners/Family Physicians). 2020. "ICPC-3 field test invitation." https://www.globalfamilydoctor.com/News/ICPC-3fieldtestinvitation.aspx.

21 CFR Parts 201 and 207. Food and Drug Administration. 2022. https://www.govinfo.gov/content/pkg/FR-2022-07-25/pdf/2022-15414.pdf.

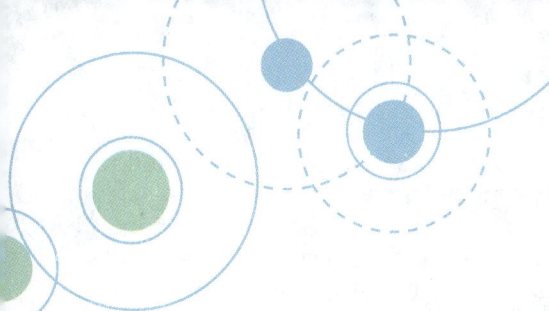

# chapter 5

# Data Management

*Marcia Y. Sharp, EdD, MBA, RHIA, FAHIMA*
*Charisse Madlock-Brown, PhD, MLS*

## Learning Objectives

- Explain the difference among data categories
- Compare the indices commonly found in hospitals
- Differentiate among the registries used in hospitals according to purpose, methods of case definition and case finding, data collection methods, reporting and follow-up, and pertinent laws and regulations affecting registry operations
- Propose methods for database design, development, and use
- Evaluate elements of AHIMA's data quality model
- Discuss the role of the health information management professional in creating, using, and maintaining databases, data standards, and data warehouses

## Key Terms

Abbreviated injury scale (AIS)
Accession number
Accession registry
Agency for Healthcare Research and Quality (AHRQ)
Aggregate data
Attributes
Cancer staging
Case definition
Case finding
Data dictionary
Data modeling
Database management system (DBMS)
Disease index
Entity
Entity relationship diagram (ERD)
Facility-based registry
Foreign keys
Healthcare Cost and Utilization Project (HCUP)
Index
Information system
Injury severity score (ISS)
Medical Literature, Analysis, and Retrieval System Online (MEDLINE)
Medicare Provider Analysis and Review (MEDPAR)
National Center for Health Statistics (NCHS)
National Health Care Survey (NHCS)
Normalization
Operation index
Patient-identifiable data
Physician index
Population-based registry
Primary data source
Primary keys
Public health
Registry
Relational databases
Relationships
Schema mapping
Secondary data source
Staging system
Structured Query Language (SQL)
Traumatic injury
Unified Medical Language System (UMLS)
Vital statistics

As a rich source of data about an individual patient, the health record fulfills the uses of patient care and reimbursement for individual encounters. However, it is not easy to see trends in a population of patients by looking at individual records. For this purpose, data must be extracted from individual records and entered in specialized databases that support analysis across individual records. A database is an organized collection of data typically stored in a structured format in a computer system. These data may be used in a facility-specific or population-based registry for research and improvement in patient care. Also, data may be reported to the state and become part of state- and federal-level databases used to set health policy and improve healthcare.

The health information management (HIM) professional plays various roles in managing secondary records, data, and databases, with a key responsibility in assisting with database set-up. This task includes determining the content of the database or registry and ensuring compliance with the laws, regulations, and accrediting standards that affect the content and use of the registry or database. All data elements included in the database or registry must be defined in a data dictionary. In this role, the HIM professional may oversee the completeness and accuracy of the data abstracted for inclusion in the database or registry.

This chapter explains the difference between primary and secondary data and offers an in-depth look at various types of secondary databases and how they are processed and maintained, in addition to indices and registries and their functions. The chapter also examines relational database management systems (RDBMSs) and data warehouses and explores data quality standards, models, and requirements.

## Data and Data Sources

The health record is considered a **primary data source** because it is a "record that was developed by healthcare professionals in the process of providing care or services to a patient" (White 2023, 3). A **secondary data source** is created using the data from a primary data source. Registries, indices, and reports are considered secondary data sources because the data are derived from the health record or a primary source.

Data are also categorized as either patient-identifiable data or aggregate data. The health record consists entirely of **patient-identifiable data**. In other words, every fact recorded in the record relates to a particular patient. Secondary data also may be patient identifiable. In some instances, data—including the patient's name—are entered into a database and maintained in an identifiable form. Registries are an example of patient-identifiable data on groups of patients.

More often, however, secondary data are considered aggregate data. **Aggregate data** include data on groups of people or patients without identifying any patient individually. Examples of aggregate data are statistics on the average length of stay (ALOS) for patients discharged within a particular diagnosis-related group (DRG).

Secondary data sources consist of facility-specific indices; registries, either facility or population-based; and other healthcare databases. Healthcare organizations maintain the data sources relevant to their specific operations. States and the federal government also maintain databases to assess the health and wellness of their populations.

Secondary data sources provide information that is not easily available by looking at individual health records. For example, with a diagnosis index, one could review the list of diagnoses in numerical order and select those with the appropriate diagnosis code for myocardial infarction for inclusion in a study.

Data extracted from health records and entered in disease-oriented databases can, for example, help researchers determine the effectiveness of alternate treatment methods. They can quickly demonstrate survival rates at different stages of disease as well.

### Check Your Understanding 5.1

Answer the following questions in a separate document.

1. Is an operative report a primary or secondary data source? Explain why.
2. Is an operative report patient-identifiable or aggregate data? Explain why.
3. Explain how secondary data sources are used in research.
4. A 10-percent increase in the prevalence of influenza is reported to the Centers for Disease Control (CDC). Are these data patient-identifiable or aggregate? Is the CDC an internal or external user of secondary data? Explain your rationale.
5. Why are secondary data sources developed?

# Indices

The secondary data sources that have been in existence the longest are the indices that have been developed within facilities to meet their individual needs. An **index** is simply a report from a database that enables health records to be located by diagnosis, procedure, or physician, indices are computerized reports available from data included in databases routinely maintained in the healthcare facility. Most acute-care facilities maintain indices described in the following sections.

## Master Patient Index

The master patient index (MPI), which is sometimes called the master person index, contains patient-identifiable data such as name, address, date of birth, dates of hospitalizations or encounters, name of attending physician, and health record number. The MPI is an important source of patient health record numbers. These numbers enable the facility to retrieve health information for specific patients quickly. Most of the information in the MPI is entered into the facility database during the admission, preadmission, or registration process. Thus, it is imperative that all departments in the facility work collaboratively to avoid unnecessary issues in the workflow process.

## Disease and Operation Indices

The **disease index** is a list of diagnosis codes in numerical order for patients discharged from the facility during a particular period. Each patient's diagnoses are converted from a verbal description to a numerical code, usually using a coding system such as the International Classification of Diseases (ICD). In most cases, patient diagnosis codes are entered into the facility's health information system (HIS) as part of the discharge processing of the patient health record.

The index always includes the patient's health record number and the diagnosis codes so records can be retrieved by diagnosis. Because each patient is listed with the health record number, the disease index is considered patient-identifiable data. The disease index also may include the attending physician's name or the date of discharge. In an acute-care setting, the list is of patients discharged from the facility during a particular period. In nonacute settings, the disease index might be generated to reflect patients currently receiving services in the facility. In essence, the disease index is a comprehensive tool for healthcare providers to manage information effectively and efficiently.

The **operation index** is similar to the disease index except that it is arranged in numerical order by the patients' procedure code(s), usually using ICD or Current Procedural Terminology (CPT) codes. The other information listed in the operation index is generally the same as that listed in the disease index except that the surgeon may be listed in addition to, or instead of, the attending physician. In many cases, facilities no longer have an actual list for the diagnosis and operation indices. Instead, a query from the HIS utilizing the diagnosis or procedure code generates the index.

## Physician Index

The **physician index** is a list of cases in order by physician name or physician identification number. It also includes the patient's health record number and may include other data, such as the date of discharge. The physician index enables users to retrieve information about a particular physician, including the number of cases seen during a particular period. As with the disease and operation indices, facilities generally query the HIS to obtain physician data.

## Check Your Understanding 5.2

**Answer the following questions in a separate document.**

1. How do HIM departments use indices?
2. Summarize the purpose of the master patient index and its significance to the broader context of healthcare. Explain the elements found in an MPI.
3. If the chief of staff wants to know which patients had sepsis last year for a quality improvement study, what index would he use? Explain why.
4. Choose the type of index to use if the quality improvement analyst wants to find out what patients had a total hip replacement in the first six months of last year.
5. Recommend the type of index the medical staff executive committee would use if it wanted to know what types of patients Dr. Smith treated in January.

## Registries

A **registry** is a collection of care information related to a specific disease, condition, or procedure that makes health record information available for analysis and comparison. Registries often require more extensive data from the patient record. Each registry must determine the cases that are to be included, a process called **case definition**. In a trauma registry, for example, the case definition might be *all patients admitted with a diagnosis falling into ICD-10 code numbers S00 through S99*, the trauma diagnosis codes.

After the cases to be included have been determined through the case definition process, the next step in collecting data is usually case finding. **Case finding** includes the methods used to identify the patients who have been seen and treated in the facility for the disease or condition of interest to the registry. After cases have been identified, extensive data are abstracted from the patient record into the registry database or fed from other databases and entered in the registry database.

Registries are crucial for improving public health and patient care. The sole purpose of some registries is to collect data from the patient's health record and make them available to users. Other registries take further steps to enter additional information in the registry database, such as routine follow-up of patients at specified intervals. Follow-up can include tracking the rate of survival and monitoring quality-of-life issues over time. Common types of registries include those for cancer, diabetes, trauma, immunizations, and more, all of which contribute to understanding disease patterns, improving health outcomes, and shaping public health strategies.

### Cancer Registries

The cancer registries aggregate clinical information to improve the diagnosis and treatment of cancer. The first hospital cancer registry was founded in 1926 at Yale-New Haven Hospital (NCRA n.d.b). The registry may be a **facility-based registry** (located within a facility such as a hospital or a clinic) or a **population-based registry** (gathering data from multiple facilities within a geographic area such as a state or region).

The data from facility-based registries are used to provide information for the improved understanding of cancer, including its causes and methods of diagnosis and treatment. The data collected also may provide comparisons in survival rates and quality of life for patients with different treatments and at different stages of cancer at the time of diagnosis. In population-based registries, the emphasis is on identifying trends and changes in the incidence (new cases) of cancer within the area covered by the registry.

The Cancer Registries Amendment Act of 1992 funded the National Program of Cancer Registries (NPCR) with population-based registries in each state. This law authorized the CDC to provide funding and technical assistance to statewide, population-based cancer registries and established CDCs national cancer surveillance system (CDC 2024a).

#### Case Definition and Case Finding in the Cancer Registry

In a cancer registry all cancer cases except certain skin cancers might meet the definition for the cases to be included. Skin cancers such as basal cell carcinomas might be excluded because they do not metastasize and do not require the follow-up necessary for other cancers included in the registry. Data on benign and borderline brain or central nervous system tumors must be collected according to the NPCR (CDC 2024b).

In the facility-based cancer registry, the first step is case finding. One way to find cases is through the discharge process in the HIM department. During the discharge process, coding or HIM professionals can easily identify cases of patients with cancer for inclusion in the registry. Another case-finding method is to use the facility-specific disease indices or the HIS to identify patients with diagnoses of cancer. Additional methods may include reviews of pathology reports and lists of patients receiving radiation therapy or other cancer treatments to determine cases that have not been found by other methods.

Population-based registries usually depend on hospitals, physician offices, radiation facilities, ambulatory surgery centers (ASCs), and pathology laboratories to identify and report cases to the central registry. The population-based registry has a responsibility to ensure that all cases of cancer in the target area have been identified and reported to the central registry. All cancer registry data are formally reported to the state central registry and the CDC (CDC 2024c).

#### Data Collection for the Cancer Registry

When a case is first entered in the registry, an **accession number** is assigned; this number is used to identify the patient. The accession number consists of the first digits of the year the patient was first seen at the facility, with the remaining digits assigned sequentially throughout the year. The first case in 2017, for example, might be 17-0001. An **accession registry** of all cases can be obtained by the database software. This list of patients in accession number order provides a way to monitor that all cases have been entered into the registry.

Data collection methods vary between facility-based registries and population-based registries. In a facility-based registry, data are initially obtained by reviewing and collecting them from the patient's health record. In addition to demographic data (such as name, health record number, address), patient data in a cancer registry include the following:

- Type and site of the cancer
- Diagnostic methodologies
- Treatment methodologies
- Stage at the time of diagnosis

Cancer staging is the process of determining the size and extent of spread of the tumor throughout the body. Historically, several different staging systems have been used. A staging system is a classification system that describes the extent of cancer within a patient (NCI 2022). Frequently, the population-based registry only collects information when the patient is diagnosed. Sometimes, however, it receives follow-up information from its reporting entities, healthcare providers, clinics, or other organizations. These entities usually submit the information to the central registry electronically.

### Reporting and Follow-up for Cancer Registry Data

Formal reporting of cancer registry data is done through an annual report that goes to the state central cancer registry and the CDC (CDC 2024b). The annual report includes aggregate data on the number of cases in the past year by site and type of cancer. It also may include information on patients by sex, age, and ethnic group. Often, a particular site or type of cancer is featured with more in-depth data provided.

Other reports are provided as needed. Data from the cancer registry are frequently used in the quality assessment process for a facility as well as in research. Data on survival rates by site of cancer and methods of treatment, for example, would be helpful in researching the most effective treatment for a type of cancer.

Another activity of the cancer registry is patient follow-up. On an annual basis, the registry attempts to obtain information about each patient in the registry, including whether he or she is still alive, the status of the cancer, and treatment received during the period. Various methods are used to obtain this information. For a facility-based registry, the facility's patient health records may be checked for return hospitalizations or visits for treatment. The patient's physician also may be contacted to determine whether the patient is still living and to obtain information about the cancer.

When patient status cannot be determined through these methods, an attempt may be made to contact the patient using information in the registry, such as address and telephone number of the patient and other contacts. Also, contact information from the patient's health record may be used to request information from the patient's relatives. Other methods used include using the internet to locate patients through sites such as the Social Security Death Index and online directories. The information obtained through follow-up is important to allow the registry to develop statistics on survival rates for specific cancers and different treatment methodologies.

Population-based registries do not always include follow-up information on the patients in their databases. They may, however, receive information from the reporting entities such as hospitals, physician offices, and other organizations providing follow-up care.

### Standards and Approval Agencies for Cancer Registries

Several organizations have developed standards or approval processes for cancer programs (see table 5.1). The American College of Surgeons (ACS) Commission on Cancer has an approval process for cancer programs. One of the requirements of this process is the existence of a cancer registry as part of the program. The ACS standards are published in the Cancer Program Standards (ACS 2023a). When the ACS surveys the cancer program, part of the survey process is a review of cancer registry activities.

The North American Association of Central Cancer Registries (NAACCR) has a certification program for state population-based registries. Certification is based on the quality of data collected and reported by the state registry. The NAACCR has developed standards for data quality and format, and it works with other cancer organizations to align their various standards sets (NAACCR n.d).

The CDC also has national standards regarding completeness, timeliness, and quality of cancer registry data from state registries through the NPCR (CDC 2024a). The NPCR was developed because of the Cancer Registries Amendment Act of 1992. The CDC collects data from the NPCR state registries.

### Education and Certification for Cancer Registrars

Traditionally, cancer registrars have been trained through on-the-job training and professional workshops and seminars. The NCRA has worked with colleges to develop formal educational programs for cancer registrars

**Table 5.1.** Standard-setting or approval agencies for cancer registries

| Agency | Type of registry |
|---|---|
| American College of Surgeons (ACS) | Facility-based |
| North American Association of Central Cancer Registries (NAACCR) | Population-based |
| Centers for Disease Control and Prevention (CDC) | Population-based |

either through a certificate or an associate's degree program. A cancer registrar may become certified as an Oncology Data Specialist by passing an examination provided by the NCRA's certification board. Eligibility requirements for the certification examination include a combination of experience and education (NCRA n.d.a).

## Trauma Registries

Trauma registries maintain databases on patients with severe traumatic injuries. A traumatic injury is a wound or another injury caused by an external physical force such as an automobile accident, a shooting, a stabbing, or a fall. Examples of such injuries would include fractures, burns, and lacerations. Information collected by the trauma registry may be used for performance improvement and research in trauma care. Trauma registries are usually facility-based, but in some cases may include data for a region or state.

### Case Definition and Case Finding for Trauma Registries

The case definition for the trauma registry varies from registry to registry. To find cases with trauma diagnoses, the trauma registrar may query the facility's HIS looking for cases with codes in the trauma section of ICD-10-CM. Also, the registrar may look at deaths in services with frequent trauma diagnoses such as trauma, neurosurgery, orthopedics, and plastic surgery to find additional cases.

### Data Collection for Trauma Registries

After the cases have been identified, data are abstracted from the health records of the injured patients and entered in the trauma registry database. The data elements collected in the abstracting process vary from registry to registry but usually include the following:

- Demographic data on the patient
- Information on the injury
- Care the patient received before hospitalization (such as care at another transferring hospital or care from an emergency medical technician (EMT) who provided care at the scene of the accident or in transport from the accident site to the hospital)
- Status of the patient at the time of admission
- Patient's course in the hospital
- ICD diagnosis and procedure codes
- Abbreviated injury scale
- Injury severity score

The abbreviated injury scale (AIS) reflects the nature and severity (threat to life) of the injury by body system. It may be assigned manually by the registrar or generated as part of the database from data the registrar enters. The injury severity score (ISS) is an overall severity measurement calculated from the AIS scores for the patient's three most severe injuries (ACI n.d.). The AIS and ISS classify and describe the severity of injuries and can be used for reporting registry activity.

### Reporting and Follow-up for Trauma Registries

Reporting varies among trauma registries. An annual report is often developed to show the activity of the trauma registry. Other reports may be generated as part of the performance improvement process, such as self-extubation (patients removing their own tubes) and delays in abdominal surgery or patient complications.

Trauma registries may or may not follow-up on patients in the registry. When follow-up is done, the emphasis is frequently on the patient's quality of life after a period. Unlike cancer, where physician follow-up is crucial to detect recurrence, many traumatic injuries do not require continued patient care over time. Thus, follow-up on trauma registry patients is less common than follow-up on cancer registry patients.

### Standards and Agencies for Approval of Trauma Registries

The ACS certifies levels I, II, III, and IV trauma centers. As part of its certification requirements, the ACS states that the level I trauma center, the type of center receiving the most serious cases and providing the highest level of trauma service, must have a trauma registry (ACS n.d.b). Refer to table 5.2 for a description of each trauma center level.

### Education and Certification of Trauma Registrars

Trauma registrars may be registered health information technicians (RHITs), registered health information administrators (RHIAs), registered nurses (RNs), licensed practical nurses (LPNs), EMTs, or other health

**Table 5.2.** Trauma center levels and definitions

| Trauma center level | Description |
|---|---|
| Level I | Able to provide total care for every aspect of injury from prevention through rehabilitation |
| Level II | Able to initiate definitive care for all injured patients |
| Level III | Able to provide prompt assessment, resuscitation, surgery, intensive care, and stabilization of injured patients and emergency operations |
| Level IV | Able to provide advanced trauma life support (ATLS) before the transfer of patients to a higher-level trauma center; provides evaluation, stabilization, and diagnostic capabilities for injured patients |
| Level V | Able to provide initial evaluation, stabilization, and diagnostic capabilities and prepares patients for transfer to higher levels of care |

*Source*: ATS n.d.

professionals. Training for trauma registrars is accomplished through workshops and on-the-job training. The American Trauma Society (ATS), for example, provides core and advanced workshops for trauma registrars and a certification examination for trauma registrars through its Registrar Certification Board. Certified trauma registrars have earned the certified specialist in trauma registry (CSTR) credential (ATS n.d.).

## Diabetes Registries

Diabetes registries collect data about patients with diabetes to assist with care management and to support research. Patients whose diabetes is not well managed frequently have numerous complications. The diabetes registry can document whether the patient has been seen by a physician to prevent complications.

### Case Definition and Case Finding for Diabetes Registries

There are two types of diabetes mellitus, type 1 and type 2. Type 1 diabetes, previously known as juvenile diabetes, is insulin-dependent diabetes (Mayo Clinic n.d.a). Type 2 diabetes, previously known as adult-onset diabetes, is non-insulin-dependent (Mayo Clinic n.d.b). Registries sometimes limit their cases by type of diabetes. In some instances, there may be further definition by age; for example, some diabetes registries only include children with diabetes.

Case finding includes the review of health records of patients with diabetes. Other case-finding methods include the reviews of ICD diagnostic codes, billing data, medication lists, physician identification, and health plans.

Although facility-based registries for cancer and trauma are usually hospital-based, facility-based diabetes registries are often maintained by physician offices and clinics because they are the main location for diabetes care. Thus, the data about the patient to be entered into the registry are available at these sites rather than at the hospital. Patient health records of diabetes patients in the physician practice may be identified through ICD-10 code numbers for diabetes, billing data for diabetes-related services, medication lists for patients on diabetic medications, or identification of patients at the patient visit.

### Data Collection for Diabetes Registries

In addition to demographic data about the cases, other data collected may include laboratory values such as HbA1c. This test is used to determine the average patient's blood glucose level for a period of approximately 60 days before the time of the test. Moreover, facility registries may track patient visits to follow-up with patients who have not been seen in the past year.

### Reporting and Follow-up for Diabetes Registries

A variety of reports may be developed from the diabetes registry. For facility-based registries, one report may keep up with laboratory monitoring of the patient's diabetes to allow intensive intervention with patients whose diabetes is not well controlled. Another report might be of patients who have not been tested within a year or who have not had a primary care provider visit within a year.

Population-based diabetes registries might provide reporting on the incidence of diabetes for the geographic area covered by the registry. Registry data also may be used to investigate risk factors for diabetes. Follow-up is aimed primarily at ensuring the diabetic is seen by the physician at appropriate intervals to prevent complications.

## Transplant Registries

Transplant registries have varied purposes. Some organ transplant registries maintain databases of patients who need organs. When an organ becomes available, an equitable way may be used to allocate the organ to the patient with the highest priority. In other cases, the purpose of the registry is to provide a database of potential donors for transplants using live donors, such as bone marrow transplants. Posttransplant information on organ recipients and donors also is kept. Data collected in the transplant registry may be used for research, policy analysis, and quality control projects. Because transplant registries are used to match donor organs with recipients, they are often national or even international in scope. Examples of national registries include the UNet of the United Network for Organ Sharing and the registry of the National Marrow Donor Program.

### Case Definition and Case Finding for Transplant Registries

Physicians identify patients who need transplants and provide information about the patient to the registry. When an organ becomes available, information about it is matched with potential donors. For donor registries, donors are often solicited through community outreach efforts like those carried out by blood banks to encourage blood donations.

### Data Collection for Transplant Registries

Data collection is an integral component of transplant registries. The type of data collected varies according to the type of registry. Pretransplant data about the recipient include the following:

- Demographics
- Patient's diagnosis
- Patient's status codes regarding medical urgency
- Patient's functional status
- Whether the patient is on life support
- Previous transplantations

Information on donors varies according to whether the donor is living. For organs harvested from patients who have died, information is collected on the following:

- Cause and circumstances of the death
- Organ procurement and consent process
- Medications the donor was taking
- Other donor history

For a living donor, the information includes the relationship of the donor to the recipient (if any), clinical information, and information on organ recovery.

### Reporting and Follow-up for Transplant Registries

Reporting includes information on donors and recipients as well as survival rates, length of time on the waiting list for an organ, and death rates. Follow-up information is collected for recipients as well as living donors. For living donors, the information collected might include procedure complications and length of stay (LOS) in the hospital. Follow-up information about recipients includes information on status at the time of follow-up (for example, living, dead, lost to follow-up), functional status, graft status, and treatment, such as immunosuppressive drugs. Follow-up is carried out at intervals throughout the first year after the transplant and then annually after that.

## Immunization Registries

Children are encouraged to receive a large number of immunizations during the first six years of life and several more, at lower frequency, thereafter. These immunizations are so important that the federal government has set several objectives related to immunizations in Healthy People 2030, a set of health goals for the nation (HHS n.d.). These include increasing the proportion of children and adolescents who are fully immunized and increasing the proportion of children in population-based immunization registries.

Immunization registries usually have the purpose of increasing the number of infants and children who receive proper immunizations at the proper intervals. To accomplish this goal, each state is required to collect information within its geographic area about children and their immunization status. The state's immunization registry is a central source of information for a particular child's immunization history, even when the child has received immunizations from a variety of providers. By having this central location for immunization information, parents are relieved of the responsibility of maintaining immunization records for their children.

### Case Definition and Case Finding for Immunization Registries

All children in the population area served by the registry should be included in the registry. Some registries limit their inclusion of patients to those seen at public clinics, excluding those seen exclusively by private practitioners. Although children are usually targeted in immunization registries, some registries do include information on adults for influenza, COVID-19, and pneumonia vaccines.

Children are often entered in the registry at birth, in some cases electronically through a connection with an electronic birth record system. Registry personnel may review birth and death certificates and adoption records to determine what children to include and what children to exclude because they died after birth. Accuracy and completeness of the data in the registry are dependent on the thoroughness of the submitters reporting immunizations.

### Data Collection for Immunization Registries

The CDC has worked with the National Vaccine Advisory Committee to develop a set of core immunization data elements to be included in all immunization registries. The required data elements include the following, but are not limited to:

- Patient's name (first, middle, and last)
- Patient's birth date
- Patient's sex
- Patient's birth state and country
- Mother's name (first, middle, last, and maiden)
- Responsible person (first, middle, last, relationship to patient)
- Vaccine type
- Vaccine manufacturer
- Vaccination date
- Vaccine lot number
- Vaccine ordering provider (person)
- Vaccine administering provider suffix
- Vaccine administering provider (person) (CDC 2018)

Other items may be included, as needed, by the individual registry.

### Reporting and Follow-up for Immunization Registries

Because the purpose of immunization registries is to increase the number of children who receive immunizations promptly, reporting should emphasize immunization rates, especially rate changes target areas. Immunization registries also can automatically report children's immunization to schools or allow schools to check their students' immunization status.

Follow-up is directed toward reminding parents that it is time for immunizations as well as monitoring whether or not parents bring the child in for the immunization after a reminder. Moreover, the entity managing the registries must decide how frequently to follow up with parents who do not bring their children for immunization. Parents may be allowed to opt out of the registry if they prefer not to be reminded.

### Standards and Agencies for Approval of Immunization Registries

The CDC, through its National Immunization Program, provides funding for some population-based immunization registries. The Immunization Information System Functional Standards Version 4.1 Resource Guide is available on the CDC website (CDC 2022). The guide includes information on regulatory elements, essential infrastructure related to data security, and data quality standards, all of which are crucial for health information professionals.

## Other Registries

Registries may be developed for any disease or condition. Examples of other types of registries that are commonly kept include implant, birth defects, and long COVID. An implant is a material or substance inserted in the body, such as breast implants, heart valves, and pacemakers. Implant registries, such as the American Joint Replacement Registry, have been developed to track the performance of implants, including complications, deaths, and defects resulting from implants, as well as longevity.

Birth defect registries collect data on newborns diagnosed with birth defects. This type of registry is used to track the prevalence of birth defects and identify other factors that may increase or decrease the risk of birth defects.

Researchers worldwide are actively establishing long COVID registries to track symptoms that last for weeks or months after the acute phase of the COVID-19 virus. In New Zealand, the University of Auckland is spearheading a research project aimed at gathering data on the prevalence of long COVID (Ang 2022). Similarly, the Australian Institute of Health and Welfare is engaged in a linked data project. Through the AIHW national-linked data platform, COVID-19 data from various states and territories is integrated with additional datasets covering areas like aged care, deaths, and hospitalizations. This initiative is designed to enhance our understanding of the correlation between COVID-19 and other potential risk factors (Ang 2023). The CDC, in partnership with the Census Bureau, added questions about long-COVID on the Household Pulse Survey. Questions about long COVID are also included in the National Health Interview Survey (CDC 2024d).

Registries may be developed for administrative purposes also. The National Provider Identifier (NPI) Registry is an example of an administrative registry. The NPI Registry enables users to search for a provider's national plan and provider enumeration system information, including the national provider identification number. The NPI number is a 10-digit unique identification number assigned to healthcare providers in the US. There is no charge to use the registry, and it is updated daily. Data collected for healthcare administrative purposes are also discussed later in the chapter.

> **Check Your Understanding 5.3**
>
> Answer questions 1 through 6 for each of the following registries by creating a comparison table: cancer, trauma, diabetes, transplant, and immunization.
>
> 1. Is it facility-based, population-based, or both?
> 2. What methods are used for case definition and case finding?
> 3. What methods of follow-up are used?
> 4. What standards are applicable, and what agencies approve or accredit the registry?
> 5. What education is required for registrars?
> 6. What certification is available for registrars?
>
> Answer the following question in a separate document.
>
> 7. You are the trauma registrar for a large healthcare system responsible for maintaining the accuracy of the trauma registry. A new trauma case has been assigned to you. Which of the following tasks are you responsible for in this situation? *(Select all that apply.)*
>    a. Abstracting information from the HIS for trauma cases
>    b. Assigning Abbreviated Injury Scale scores
>    c. Training new staff on how to use the trauma registry
>    d. Ensuring all data elements are included

## Database Management and Design

Information retrieval and storage are at the heart of medical activities. Databases contain patient demographics, financial, and health-related data. They store information about supplies, staff, and system use. A **database management system (DBMS)** is software used to store, analyze, modify, and access data.

### Relational Databases

There are several types of database systems, and DBMSs can be characterized by the way they model data. **Relational databases** are the most widely used in numerous industries, including healthcare. This model consists of a database with a set of formally described tables, related (linked) to each other by a shared reference (Hernandez 2020). It is widely used because it offers a simple, yet powerful view of stored information. Developers can easily understand how information is organized, and users can create their own interactive queries. It is flexible enough that databases can be simple or complex, and yet each part has an easy-to-understand representation. There are three steps to database design: conceptual, logical, and physical design. Figure 5.1 details the processes for each design phase.

### Entity Relationship Modeling

**Data modeling**, a fundamental aspect of database design, involves formalizing data requirements and structuring data to meet specific needs. One widely used form of data modeling is entity-relationship modeling, which visually represents and defines the relationships between data entities (Bagui and Earp 2022, 71–72). An **entity relationship diagram (ERD)** has three basic graphical symbols. First, there are entities, which are data objects represented as rectangles. An **entity** can be considered a class of objects that exist in the real world and have related properties. Entities can be a type of person, place, or thing. Second, there are **attributes**, which describe characteristics and are represented as circles. Third, there are **relationships**, which describe associations between entities and are represented with diamonds.

Entity-relationship modeling is a type of conceptual modeling. Conceptual models are abstract and encourage high-level problem structuring. They help establish a common ground for communication between users and developers. They also help developers understand how an existing model can be modified. ERDs are used often in conceptual design; an example of an entity relationship is displayed in figure 5.2.

ERDs are converted into tables by a process called **schema mapping** (Bagui and Earp 2022, 94–98). There are a few simple rules used for mapping. The main rule used to determine table structure is based on the **cardinality** of the relationship (the maximum number of occurrences of each entity that occurrences of other entities can link to). For example, if a patient can have only one doctor, the mapping would differ from a model where the patient can have multiple doctors. The example in figure 5.3 shows that each doctor can have one associated clinic, but each clinic

**Figure 5.1.** Database design process

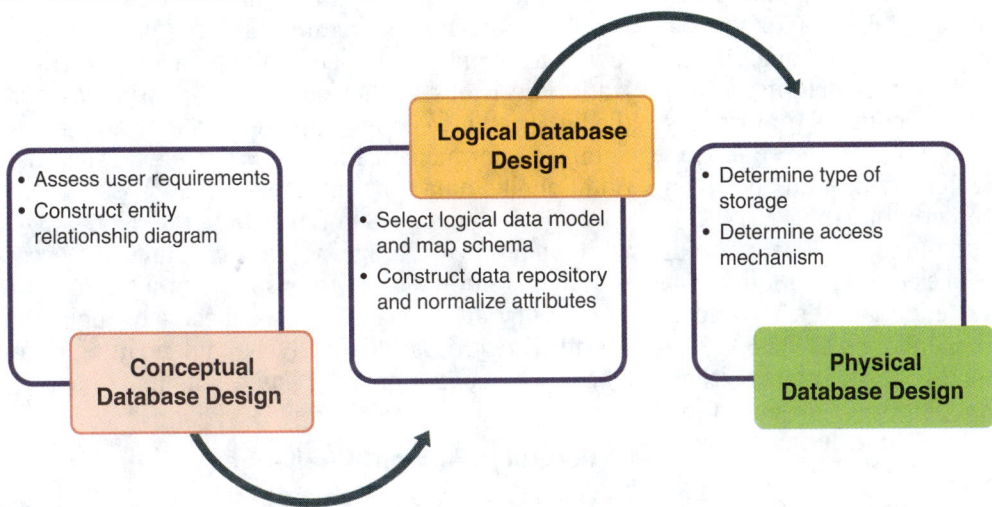

**Figure 5.2.** Example of an entity relationship

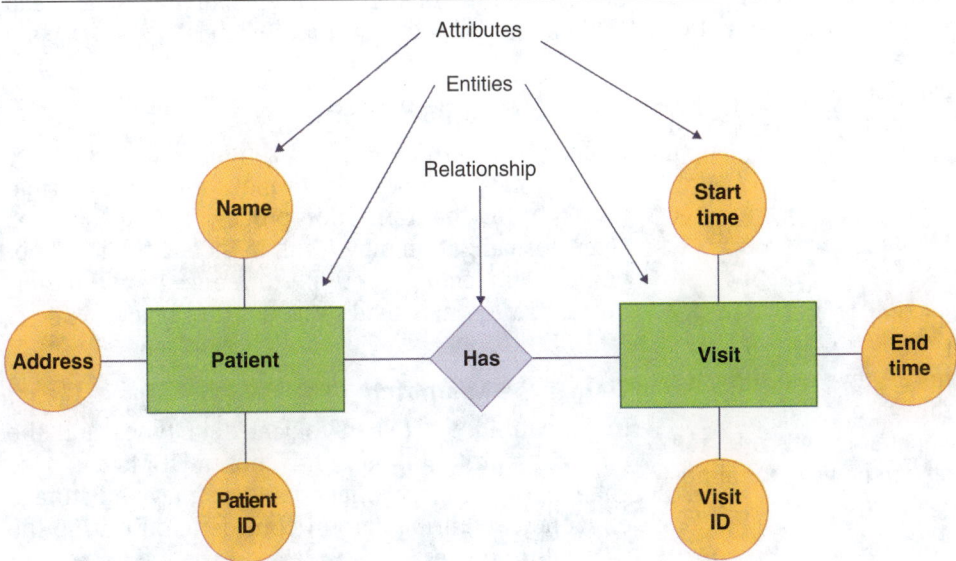

**Figure 5.3.** ERD notation and example

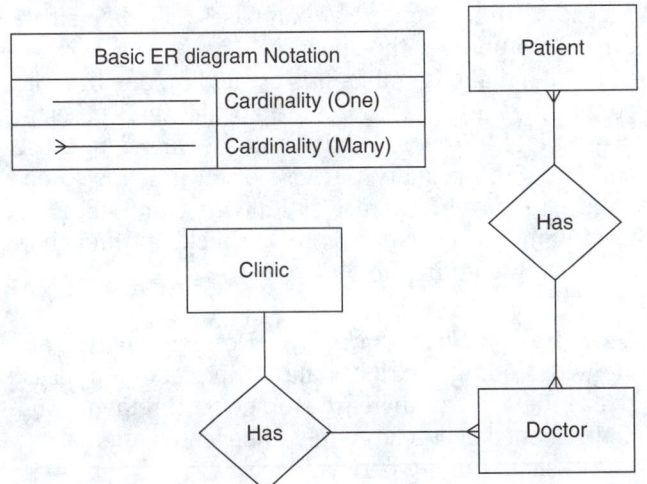

can have many associated doctors. In addition, each patient can have many doctors, and each doctor can have many patients. The type of relationship and the unique identifier (for example, patient ID and visit ID in figure 5.2) for each entity further determine how tables will be linked as unique identifiers (or **primary keys**) for one table are represented as **foreign keys** (which are fields in a table that create a link between the data in two tables) in other tables.

Entity relationship diagramming is a very useful process because it helps reduce errors. **Normalization** is intrinsic to the process. It eliminates errors associated with updates, deletions, and data insertions into the database. This process reduces redundancy and improves data quality. Mapping and normalization are performed in the logical database design phase.

## Structured Query Language

**Structured Query Language (SQL)** is the formal language used to retrieve information stored in relational databases. SQL defines some operations, or activities, which can be used to access data across tables based on a set of conditions (Friedrichsen et al. 2021, 83–95). The following example shows a query to select patient names from a patient table where the gender is female (indicated by F):

    SELECT patient_name FROM patients WHERE gender = 'F';

In this simple example, the operator "select" indicates what data to get. The keyword "from" specifies the table or tables to access. The "where" keyword indicates the criteria for selection, in this case, gender = 'F'. F. SQL's syntax consists of many operators and conditionals. It is a flexible language that can be used for almost any information need.

## Database Implementation

Implementing the database using a specific DBMS is the goal of the physical design phase. In this phase, designers select a storage system, translate the data model from the logical design phase into a physical representation, create indices for ease of access, and grant user access rights (Friedrichsen et al. 2021, 207–235). Designers must make decisions based on the specific type of DBMS used. The most popular type of DBMS is the relational database management system (RDBMS). RDBMSs follow a set of integrity rules that ensure accuracy and accessibility.

### Issues with Translating into Physical Representation

Translating database schemas into their physical representation presents several challenges. One primary issue is structural alignment, where the logical structure of the schema must be accurately mapped to the physical storage architecture, often requiring adjustments to maintain efficiency and integrity. Normalization decisions further complicate this process, as the balance between reducing redundancy and maintaining performance can lead to complex trade-offs. Additionally, data type mismatches can arise, where the logical schema's data types do not perfectly align with the physical storage system's capabilities, necessitating careful handling to ensure data integrity and consistency. These challenges collectively highlight the intricate process of effectively implementing a database schema in a physical environment.

### Structural Alignment Challenges

Designers may face difficulties in structurally aligning the logical data model with the physical representation. This involves defining tables, relationships, and other structural elements, and misalignment can lead to data inconsistency and inefficiency.

### Normalization Decisions

Decisions regarding normalization levels (such as first normal form, second normal form, third normal form) during the translation process can be complex. Over-normalization may result in increased "join" operations, impacting query performance, while under-normalization may lead to data redundancy.

### Data Type Mismatch

Incompatibility between logical data types and the physical representation in the chosen DBMS can pose challenges. This may affect data accuracy and storage efficiency, requiring careful consideration during the translation process.

### Issues with Creating Indices

An index, in the context of databases, is a data structure that improves the speed of data retrieval operations on a database table. It is created on one or more columns of a table to provide a quick and efficient way to look up records based on the values in those columns. The primary purpose of an index is to enhance query performance by allowing the DBMS to locate and retrieve specific rows quickly, rather than scanning the entire table.

***Over- Versus Under-Indexing*** Designers may grapple with finding the right balance in creating indices. Over-indexing can increase storage requirements and maintenance overhead, while under-indexing may result in slower query performance.

***Dynamic Data Characteristics*** Dynamic changes in data characteristics over time can pose challenges in maintaining effective indices. Designers need to anticipate changes in query patterns and adjust indices accordingly to ensure ongoing optimal performance.

## Issues with User Access Rights

Granting user access rights in healthcare settings demands a careful balance between security, compliance, and operational efficiency. Navigating regulatory requirements to protect sensitive patient information, defining roles and permissions in large organizations, and implementing robust audit trails are critical components of this process. Ensuring access rights are properly managed is essential for maintaining both security and functionality within healthcare systems.

***Security and Compliance Concerns*** Granting user access rights involves navigating security and compliance considerations, particularly in healthcare. Designers must ensure access rights align with regulatory requirements to safeguard sensitive patient information.

***Role Definition Complexity*** Defining roles and permissions can be complex, especially in large healthcare organizations. Striking a balance between providing access for necessary tasks and preventing unauthorized access requires thorough role definition and management.

***Audit Trail Implementation*** Establishing an effective audit trail to monitor user access and activities adds another layer of complexity. Ensuring traceability of actions and adherence to privacy regulations requires careful implementation and ongoing management. By addressing these issues during the physical design phase, designers can enhance the effectiveness and efficiency of the database implementation process in the context of the chosen DBMS, such as an RDBMS.

## Database Implementation and HIM

Database implementation is a critical aspect of HIM, particularly within the context of EHR systems. Choosing an appropriate DBMS is crucial for developing functional EHR systems. EHR platforms often have specific requirements and recommendations for compatible DBMS. The selection process involves evaluating the scalability, performance, and security features of the DBMS to ensure it aligns with the demands of healthcare data storage. Granting user access rights is a critical aspect of database implementation, especially in the context of healthcare where data confidentiality is paramount. Designers must carefully define and manage user roles and permissions within the EHR system to ensure only authorized personnel can access sensitive patient information.

Both systems include graphical user interfaces (GUIs) that allow users to query the database without requiring an in-depth knowledge of SQL. These interfaces are designed to provide healthcare professionals with user-friendly tools for accessing and analyzing patient data. Some EHR systems have tools that enable users to create and run reports without directly using SQL. Some key features include a user-friendly interface, pre-built templates, data visualization and role-based access. Some systems offer tools without querying capabilities involving SQL but have graphical tools available for users. GUIs play a crucial role in making the querying process accessible to a broader range of users, including clinicians and healthcare administrators who may not be SQL experts. These tools enhance efficiency, reduce the learning curve, and empower users to extract meaningful insights from the vast data stored in EHR systems.

## Common Data Models for EHR Data Warehouses

In the rapidly evolving healthcare landscape, digitizing patient records has become paramount. EHRs not only streamline patient information management but also offer an invaluable resource for clinical research and healthcare analytics. HIM professionals rely on robust data models that standardize and organize diverse and complex healthcare information to harness the full potential of these vast datasets.

Two prominent data models frequently employed in EHR data warehouses are the National Patient-Centered Clinical Research Network (PCORnet) (PCORnet Steering Committee n.d.) and the Observational Medical Outcomes Partnership (OMOP) (Observational Health Data Sciences and Informatics n.d.). These models are pivotal in ensuring interoperability, facilitating data exchange, and supporting meaningful analysis across diverse healthcare settings.

PCORnet is a collaborative effort that aims to transform the landscape of clinical research through a patient-centric approach (Forrest et al. 2020). The PCORnet Common Data Model (CDM) is designed to harmonize data from various electronic health record systems, claims databases, and other healthcare sources. Its core focus is capturing patient-reported outcomes and incorporating patient-generated health data, making it valuable for studies emphasizing patient perspectives. PCORnet is ideal for studies focused on understanding and evaluating patient-reported outcomes (PROs). For instance, research examining the impact of chronic diseases on patients' daily lives and well-being can leverage PCORnet's emphasis on capturing patient experiences. Additionally, PCORnet is well-suited for research that incorporates patient-generated data found in activity trackers, wearable devices, and patient diaries. Research that uses patient-generated data could include investigating the correlation between lifestyle factors (tracked by patients themselves) and health outcomes. The OMOP takes a different but equally vital approach to standardizing healthcare data (Voss et al. 2015). OMOP's CDM is designed to support observational research by standardizing disparate data sources into a consistent format. This model enables data integration from diverse healthcare systems, allowing researchers to conduct large-scale studies and generate real-world evidence. For instance, a study comparing the long-term effectiveness and safety of various medications in real-world clinical practice, using data from different healthcare systems, could benefit from OMOP's ability to harmonize diverse sources.

### Check Your Understanding 5.4

Answer the following questions in a separate document.

1. Compare and contrast the three different phases of database design. Assess the separation of tasks into phases for potential benefits.
2. Draw a simple entity relationship diagram that represents a staff member entity (with the attribute staff_id as the primary key) in a many-to-many relationship with a patient visit entity (with the attributes visit_id as primary key, patient id, and visit date). Then, describe a many-to-many relationship. *(EditPlus is a free online tool that can be used to answer this question.)*
3. Describe a one-to-one entity relationship.
4. Write an SQL query to list the names of all male patients. Consider what information is needed and what tables in which it might be found. Tables include the patients table and the visits table.
5. Compare and contrast PCORnet and OMOP based on the information provided. Discuss each data model's key features, strengths, and potential limitations in standardizing healthcare information for research. Consider their focus areas, treatment of patient-generated data, and suitability for different studies. Highlight any commonalities they share in terms of goals and functionalities. This comparison should provide insights into the unique characteristics that make each model valuable in the context of healthcare data management and research.
6. Explain the crucial steps in the physical design phase of implementing a database, specifically in the context of electronic health record systems like EPIC and Cerner. Consider the impact of choosing a Relational Database Management System (RDBMS). Ensure your answer covers the following aspects: storage system selection, translation to logical design, creation of indices, user access rights, considerations of the specific requirements of RDBMS, GUIs, and querying without SQL knowledge.

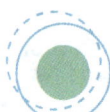

## Healthcare Databases

Databases may be developed for a variety of purposes. The federal government, for example, has developed a wide variety of databases that enable it to carry out surveillance, improvement, and prevention duties. Health information managers may provide information for these databases through data abstraction or from data reported by a facility to state and local entities. They also may use these data to do research or work with other researchers on issues related to reimbursement and health status.

### National and State Administrative Databases

Some databases are established for administrative rather than disease-oriented reasons. Data banks are developed, for example, to collect claims data submitted on Medicare claims. Other administrative databases assist in the credentialing and privileging of health practitioners.

### Medicare Provider Analysis and Review File

The **Medicare Provider Analysis and Review (MEDPAR)** file is made up of acute-care hospital and skilled nursing facility (SNF) claims data for all Medicare claims. It consists of the following types of data:

- Demographic data on the patient
- Data on the provider
- Information on Medicare coverage for the claim
- Total charges

- Charges broken down by specific types of services, such as operating room, physical therapy, and pharmacy charges
- ICD-10-CM diagnosis and ICD-10-PCS procedure codes
- DRGs

The MEDPAR file is frequently used for research on topics such as charges for different types of care and analysis by DRG. The limitation of the MEDPAR data for research purposes is that it only contains data about Medicare patients.

### National Practitioner Data Bank

The US Congress created the National Practitioner Data Bank (NPDB), a confidential information distribution system, to improve healthcare quality, protect the public from professionals with a history of malpractice, and reduce healthcare fraud and abuse in the US (NPDB 2018). Federal legislation and regulations are the foundation of the NPDB, which was mandated under the Health Care Quality Improvement Act of 1986 to provide a database of medical malpractice payments, adverse licensure actions, and certain professional review actions (such as denial of medical staff privileges) taken by healthcare entities such as hospitals against physicians, dentists, and other healthcare providers (NPDB 2018). The NPDB was developed to address the lack of information on malpractice decisions, denial of medical staff privileges, or loss of medical license. Because these data were not widely available, physicians could move to another state or another facility and begin practicing again with the current state or facility unaware of the previous actions against the physician. This workforce tool helps protect the public and healthcare entities from such occurrences. The law requires healthcare facilities to query the NPDB as part of the credentialing process when a physician initially applies for medical staff privileges and every two years thereafter (NPDB 2018). A query result may include no reports, one report or more, notification if there are future updates to the report, and notifications if there are new reports for enrolled subjects. Physicians and providers may search the NPDB for their own information and may submit a subject statement explaining the circumstances which will become part of the report.

### State Administrative Data Banks

States also frequently have health-related administrative databases. Many states, for example, collect either Uniform Hospital Discharge Data Set (UHDDS) or UB-04 data on patients discharged from hospitals located within their area. The goal of UHDDS is to obtain uniform comparable discharge data on all inpatients. These datasets contain four categories of data elements: patient identification, provider information, clinical information about the patient visit, and financial information. The Statewide Planning and Research Cooperative System (SPARCS) in New York is an example of this type of administrative database. It is an all-payer data reporting system, combining UB-04 data with data required by the state of New York. SPARCS includes both hospital inpatient stays and outpatient (ambulatory surgery, emergency department, and outpatient services) visit data (NYSDH 2024).

## National, State, and County Public Health Databases

Public health is the area of healthcare dealing with the health of populations in geographic areas such as states or counties. Publicly reported healthcare data vary from quality and patient safety measurement data to patient satisfaction results. The aggregated data range from a local to a national perspective, such as state-specific public health conditions to national morbidity and mortality statistics. Also, consumers are becoming more actively involved in their healthcare. Publicly reported data might be presented for consumer use through various ratings on different quality measures via organizations such as the Leapfrog Group, HealthGrades, or Hospital Compare. These companies provide patients with hospital ratings concerning patient safety, errors, accidents, infections, and more. One of the duties of public health agencies is the surveillance of health status within their jurisdiction.

Databases developed by public health departments provide information on the incidence and prevalence of diseases, possible high-risk populations, survival statistics, and trends over time. Data for these databases may be collected using a variety of methods including interviews, physical examination of individuals, and review of health records. At the national level, the National Center for Health Statistics (NCHS) has responsibility for these databases. NCHS provides a database of statistical health information to guide public health actions and policymaking. Their website provides information on population health status and trends in health status and care delivery (CDC 2024).

### National Health Care Survey

One of the major public health surveys is the National Health Care Survey (NHCS). This collection of surveys covers a broad spectrum of healthcare settings (CDC 2023a). Largely, it relies on data from surveys. This dataset includes the following:

- National Ambulatory Medical Care Survey
- National Hospital Ambulatory Medical Care Surgery
- National Hospital Care Survey
- National Study of Long-Term Care Providers (CDC 2024e)

Table 5.3 lists the component databases of the NHCS along with their corresponding data sources.

The NHCSs are designed to answer questions of interest to healthcare policy makers, public health professionals, and researchers. Data from these surveys encompass a wide range of healthcare settings, are provider-based, and are designed to be nationally representative. Samples of patient (or discharge) encounters gathered from a sample of care-providing organizations represent entities such as home healthcare agencies, inpatient hospital units, and physician offices (CDC 2023a). Other national public health databases include the National Health Interview Survey, which is used to monitor the health status of the population of the US, and the National Health and Nutrition Examination Survey, which collects data on the health and nutritional status of adults and children in the US.

State and local public health departments also develop databases as needed to perform their duties of health surveillance, disease prevention, and research. An example of a state database is the infectious and notifiable disease database. Each state has a list of diseases that must be reported to the state—such as AIDS, measles, and syphilis—so that containment and prevention measures may be taken to avoid large outbreaks. These state and local reporting systems are connected to the CDC through the National Electronic Disease Surveillance System (NEDSS) to evaluate trends in disease outbreaks. Statewide databases and registries also may collect extensive information on specific diseases and conditions.

## Vital Statistics

Vital statistics include data on births, deaths, fetal deaths, marriages, and divorces. Responsibility for the collection of vital statistics rests with the states; vital statistics are collected at the local level and shared with NCHS. For example, birth certificates are completed at the facility where the birth occurred and are then sent to the state level vital records, health statistics, and information systems agencies. An information system (IS) is "an automated system that uses computer hardware and software to record, manipulate, store, recover, and disseminate data (that is, a system that receives and processes input and provides output)" (Sayles and Kavanaugh-Burke 2021, 1). From the vital statistics collected, states and the national government develop a variety of databases and statistics about vital events in the state or country. Various

**Table 5.3.** Components of the National Health Care Survey Registry

| Database | Type of setting | Content | Data source | Method of data collection |
|---|---|---|---|---|
| National Ambulatory Medical Care Survey (NAMCS) | Ambulatory care setting | Data on the facility and patients | Physician | Abstract |
| National Hospital Ambulatory Medical Care Survey (NHAMCS) | Hospital-based emergency and outpatient departments and freestanding ambulatory surgery centers | Data on the facility and patients | Facility response to survey and patient records | Survey and abstract |
| National Hospital Care Survey (NHCS) | Inpatient, Emergency, Outpatient departments | Uniform Hospital Discharge Data Set and data on the patient and the visit | Discharged patient records | Electronic submission and completion of online Annual Hospital Interview Abstract |
| National Study of Long-Term Care Providers (now called National Post-acute and Long-Term Care Study (NPALS) | Adult day services center, assisted living and similar residential care communities, home health agencies, hospices, inpatient rehabilitation facilities, long-term care hospitals and nursing homes. | Facility data and patient data | Administrator; owner, operators, or designated staff | Provider and services user questionnaires |

*Source:* CDC 2021a; CDC 2023b; CDC 2024f; CDC 2024g.

vital statistics datasets can be found on the National Vital Statistics Systems website (CDC 2024h).

## Clinical Trials Databases

A clinical trial is a research project in which new treatments and tests are investigated to determine whether they are safe and effective. The trial proceeds according to a protocol, which is the list of rules and procedures to be followed. Clinical trials databases have been developed to allow physicians and patients to find clinical trials. For example, a patient with cancer or high blood pressure might be interested in participating in a clinical trial but not know how to locate one applicable to his or her type of disease. Clinical trials databases provide the data to enable patients and practitioners to determine what clinical trials are available and applicable to the patient. The Food and Drug Administration Modernization Act of 1997 mandated that a clinical trials database be developed. The National Institute of Health and the FDA worked together to create the modernized ClinicalTrials.gov website, which is maintained by the National Library of Medicine (NLM 2024). These databases contain information like that found on ClinicalTrials.gov. Although ClinicalTrials.gov has been set up for use by both patients and health practitioners, some databases are more oriented to practitioners.

## Health Services Research Databases

Health services research concerns healthcare delivery systems, including organization, delivery, care effectiveness, and efficiency. Within the federal government, the organization most involved in health services research is the **Agency for Healthcare Research and Quality (AHRQ)**. AHRQ looks at issues related to the efficiency and effectiveness of the healthcare delivery system, disease protocols, and guidelines for improved disease outcomes. AHRQ also provides access to different types of data that are primarily used for quality and utilization management purposes.

A major initiative for AHRQ has been the **Healthcare Cost and Utilization Project (HCUP)**. HCUP uses data collected from nationwide databases and state-specific databases at the state level from either claims data from the UB-04 or discharge-abstracted data, including UHDDS items reported by individual hospitals and, in some cases, by freestanding ambulatory care centers. Data selected for reporting depends on the individual state. Data may be reported by the facilities to a state agency or to the state hospital association, depending on state regulations. The data are then reported from the state to AHRQ, where they become part of the HCUP databases (AHRQ 2022). HCUP consists of the following set of databases:

- National (Nationwide) Inpatient Sample consists of inpatient discharge data from all hospitals participating in HCUP
- Kids' Inpatient Database is made up of inpatient discharge data on children younger than 19 years
- Nationwide Ambulatory Surgery Sample is the largest all-payer ambulatory surgery database in the US
- Nationwide Emergency Department Sample consists of national estimates about emergency department visits across the country
- Nationwide Readmissions Database includes discharges for patients with and without repeat hospital visits in a year and those who have died in the hospital
- State Inpatient Database includes data collected by states on hospital discharges
- State Ambulatory Surgery Databases include information from a sample of states on hospital-affiliated ASCs and, from some states, data from freestanding surgery centers
- State Emergency Department Databases include data from hospital-affiliated EDs

These databases are unique because they include data on inpatients whose care is paid for by all types of payers including Medicare, Medicaid, and private insurance, as well as self-paying and uninsured patients. Data elements include demographic information, information on diagnoses and procedures, admission and discharge status, payment sources, total charges, LOS, and information on the hospital or freestanding ASC. Researchers may use these databases to look at issues such as those related to the costs of treating diseases, the extent to which treatments are used, and differences in outcomes and cost for alternative treatments.

## National Library of Medicine

The National Library of Medicine produces two databases of special interest to the HIM professional: MEDLINE and UMLS. **Medical Literature, Analysis, and Retrieval System Online (MEDLINE)** is the best-known database from the National Library of Medicine. It includes bibliographic lists for publications in medicine, dentistry, nursing, pharmacy, allied health, and veterinary medicine. and HIM professionals use MEDLINE to locate articles on HIM issues and articles on medical topics necessary to carry out quality improvement and medical research activities. The **Unified**

Medical Language System (UMLS) integrates biomedical concepts from various sources to show their relationships. This process supports linking ISs using standardized vocabularies for purposes like connecting patient records from different EHR systems. The vocabularies provide standardized language to describe drugs, procedures, diagnoses, and the like.

The UMLS system provides a crosswalk between the vocabularies so an IS using one can link to an IS using another. UMLS is of particular interest to HIM professionals because medical classifications such as ICD-10-CM, CPT, and the Healthcare Common Procedure Coding System (HCPCS) are among the items included.

### Check Your Understanding 5.5

Answer the following questions in a separate document.

1. Discuss how HIM professionals use databases like MEDLINE and systems like the Unified Medical Language System (UMLS) in their work. How do these tools support their efforts in quality improvement, medical research, and integrating information systems?

2. How do national and state administrative healthcare databases, such as the Medicare Provider Analysis and Review (MEDPAR) file, the National Practitioner Data Bank (NPDB), and state-level databases like the Statewide Planning and Research Cooperative System (SPARCS), support healthcare research, quality improvement, and public health initiatives?

3. What type of information is collected via HCUP? Provide an example of a report or study you could do using HCUP data. Are there any limitations to these data?

4. How might UMLS be used to integrate information from one research database to the other when the databases use different medical vocabularies to describe health conditions? What data might UMLS not be able to link?

5. How does the NPDB affect physician hiring practices? How does this system promote patient safety?

## Processing and Maintenance of Secondary Databases

Several issues surround the processing and maintenance of secondary databases. HIM professionals are often involved in decisions concerning these issues.

### Automated versus Manual Methods of Data Collection

Although registries and databases are computerized, data collection is sometimes done manually. The most frequent method is abstracting, the process of reviewing the patient health record and entering the required data elements into the database. In some cases, the abstracting may initially be done on an abstract form. The data then would be entered into the database from the form. In many cases, it is done directly from the primary patient health record into a data collection screen in the computerized database system.

In some cases, data can be downloaded directly from other electronic systems. Birth defects registries, for example, often download information on births and birth defects from the vital records system. In some cases, providers such as hospitals and physicians send information in electronic format to the registry or database. As the EHR develops further, less data will need to be manually abstracted since it will be available electronically through the EHR.

### Vendor Systems Versus Facility-Specific Systems

Each registry must determine what information technology solution best meets its needs. In some cases that will be a vendor-created product specifically for registries. In other cases, the registry system may be part of an overall facility HIS. It is important that either type of product can incorporate demographic and other pertinent information from the facility HIS. In this way, time is saved and data integrity between the registry information and the HIS is maintained. If registries use registry applications as part of a facility-wide HIS, it is important that the registry manager is included in the decision of which HIS to purchase for the facility as well as in pertinent training and implementation decisions.

## Data Security and Confidentiality Issues

Concerns exist about collecting healthcare data in an environment without clear guidance about ownership of secondary data, unauthorized reuse of data, and spotty confidentiality and security regulations. Patients have concerns that secondary data collected about them may adversely affect their employment or ability to obtain health insurance. It is much more difficult for patients to determine what information about them is maintained in secondary databases than it is to view their primary health records.

For HIPAA-covered entities, the data collection registries are considered part of healthcare operations. The patient does not, therefore, authorize release of protected health information (PHI) to be included in the registry. Reporting of notifiable diseases to the state falls under "required reporting" and does not require patient authorization for release (Brodnik 2023, 301–302). Release of information to requestors other than the state will depend on the requestor. Data may be released to internal users, such as physicians for research, without the patient's consent because research is part of healthcare operations. External users, such as the ACS, collect aggregate data from facilities so individual patient authorization is not required. At the initial encounter with a healthcare facility, patients are notified about how their information may be included in registries or other secondary data sources and reported to outside entities through receipt of the facility's Notice of Privacy Practices.

HIPAA security regulations, which require policies in administrative, technical, and physical security, also apply to data in registries and indices. However, registries that are not part of a HIPAA-covered entity, such as a healthcare provider organization, or as a business associate, may not be covered under HIPAA (Brodnik 2023, 302). Central registries would be an example of a registry that is not covered under HIPAA. In such cases, the general norms for data security and confidentiality should be followed.

### Data Security

Registries and secondary databases must ensure the security of the information that they maintain. Some methods, such as passwords and role-based access, may be used to ensure that only authorized people have access to patient data in the facility's computer system. Loss of data is another important consideration in data security that could severely affect registries and secondary data sources. Data stored onsite are sometimes lost because of unauthorized access, hardware failure, or computer viruses. An alternative is a cloud-based service providing a single platform to store data within a cloud provider's infrastructure. These systems offer access controls, data monitoring, encryption capabilities and robust data backup mechanisms to prevent data loss (Nafea and Amin Almaiah 2021).

### Data Privacy and Confidentiality

When considering methods to protect secondary records, patient-specific information requires more control than secondary databases that include only aggregate data because individual patients cannot be identified in aggregate data. Policies on who may access the data provide the basic protection for confidentiality.

The type of data maintained also may affect policies on confidentiality. Many of the government databases discussed previously, such as those related to public health, include aggregate data that are readily available to any interested user.

All employees who work with patient data, including those working with data in indices, registries, and databases, should receive confidentiality training. Further, the NCHS requires staff to complete yearly training to ensure employees understand the implications of failure to maintain data confidentiality (CDC 2021b).

## Trends in Collecting Secondary Data

The most significant trend in collecting secondary data is the increased use of automated data entry. Registries and databases most commonly use data already available in electronic form rather than manually abstracting all data. EHR systems eliminate the need for separate databases for various diseases and conditions such as cancer, diabetes, and trauma. The patient health record itself is shifting into a database that can be queried for information currently obtained from specialized registries. Since not all data can currently be entered through automated means, other facilities are using existing technologies such as point-of-care data collection at the patient's bedside using wireless technology (Pérez-Martí et al. 2022).

Secondary data collection is becoming more common, and more secondary data are being collected about patients. Because of this, national stakeholders such as the American Medical Informatics Association and the National Center for Vital and Health Statistics are becoming more involved in setting national policy related to secondary data. One of the concerns is secondary data ownership. "'Who can do what to which data and under which circumstances' is the central question that must be asked in determining the rights and responsibilities of each stakeholder"

(Burrington-Brown and Hjort 2007). As the collection of secondary patient data expands, HIM professionals play an increasingly vital role in managing, protecting, and utilizing this information. Their expertise in EHRs, clinical documentation, coding, and legal compliance makes them essential when it comes to data governance and stewardship. Additionally, the increased use of this data necessitates a comprehensive understanding of information systems and technology, as well as familiarity with data analytics, for HIM professionals to fully leverage their expertise (Sherifi et al. 2021).

> ### Check Your Understanding 5.6
>
> **Answer the following questions in a separate document.**
>
> 1. Give an example of data that should be incorporated electronically into a registry, if possible. Explain why.
> 2. How does an HIM professional function as a data steward in regard to creating and maintaining secondary records?
> 3. What trends are evident in the collection of secondary data? What impact do these trends have on the HIM professional?
> 4. How might a registry manager assist in the implementation and maintenance of a registry that is part of a facility-wide HIS?
> 5. How might an HIM professional champion privacy of secondary data in their organization?

## Data Quality

Healthcare delivery systems use quality metrics to benchmark and assess the quality of care and inform improvement initiatives. Effectively, data management requires attention to data quality. Otherwise, data comparison and aggregation are impossible, and effective measurement cannot take place. To address this issue, data quality standards, requirements, and data dictionaries are used, providing a framework for maintaining the accuracy and consistency needed for meaningful data analysis and reporting.

### Data Quality Standards

For quality measurements to be constructive, data must conform to recognized standards. However, there are no universally accepted sets of healthcare quality guidelines, which hinders health information managers from ensuring data quality. This lack of guidelines is partially because the intended use of the data determines the quality of data needed. For example, a larger margin of error is more acceptable in census counts than for a critical lab test in a patient care setting. In the latter example, the margin of error must be near zero to ensure patient safety. Therefore, data quality standards must be specific to the intended use of the data or resulting information.

Two organizations have published guidance that can help healthcare organizations establish their own data quality standards. The Centers for Medicare and Medicaid Services (CMS) provides a "Documentation Matters Toolkit," which underscores the necessity of complete, accurate, and timely documentation to ensure high-quality patient care and adherence to federal regulations (CMS n.d.), and the American Health Information Management Association (AHIMA) has published the data quality management model (Davoudi et al. 2015).

### CMS Documentation Matters Toolkit

The "Documentation Matters Toolkit" is a comprehensive resource to enhance documentation practices in healthcare settings. This toolkit underscores the significance of complete, accurate, and timely documentation to improve patient care quality and ensure compliance with federal regulations. It includes several key components: the Documentation Matters Fact Sheet for Medical Professionals, providing guidelines for documenting patient encounters; the Documentation Matters Fact Sheet for Behavioral Health Practitioners, addressing the specific needs of behavioral health documentation; and the Documentation Matters Fact Sheet for Medical Office Staff, offering practical advice for office staff. The Medicaid Medical Records Resource Guide also serves as a quick reference of resources for Medicaid documentation and billing rules. At the same time, the Documentation Matters Educational Video and its accompanying Handout and Case Study provide in-depth educational content. The toolkit also includes the Electronic Health Records Fact Sheet and the Electronic Health Records Resource Guide, which discuss the effective use of

EHR systems. These resources collectively aim to improve documentation quality, promote self-auditing, reduce errors, and ensure regulatory compliance.

### AHIMA Data Quality Model

AHIMA Data Quality Management Task Force has published a data quality model and an accompanying set of general data characteristics (Davoudi et al. 2015). The model is used as a framework for the design and management process of database systems and warehouses using data quality measures. There are some similarities between the AHIMA characteristics and the CMS "Documentation Matters Toolkit." However, unlike the CMS "Documentation Matters Toolkit," which provides guidelines for very specific needs, AHIMA's model provides a comprehensive framework instead of specific instructions. Figure 5.4 illustrates AHIMA's data quality model.

**Figure 5.4.** AHIMA characteristics of data quality

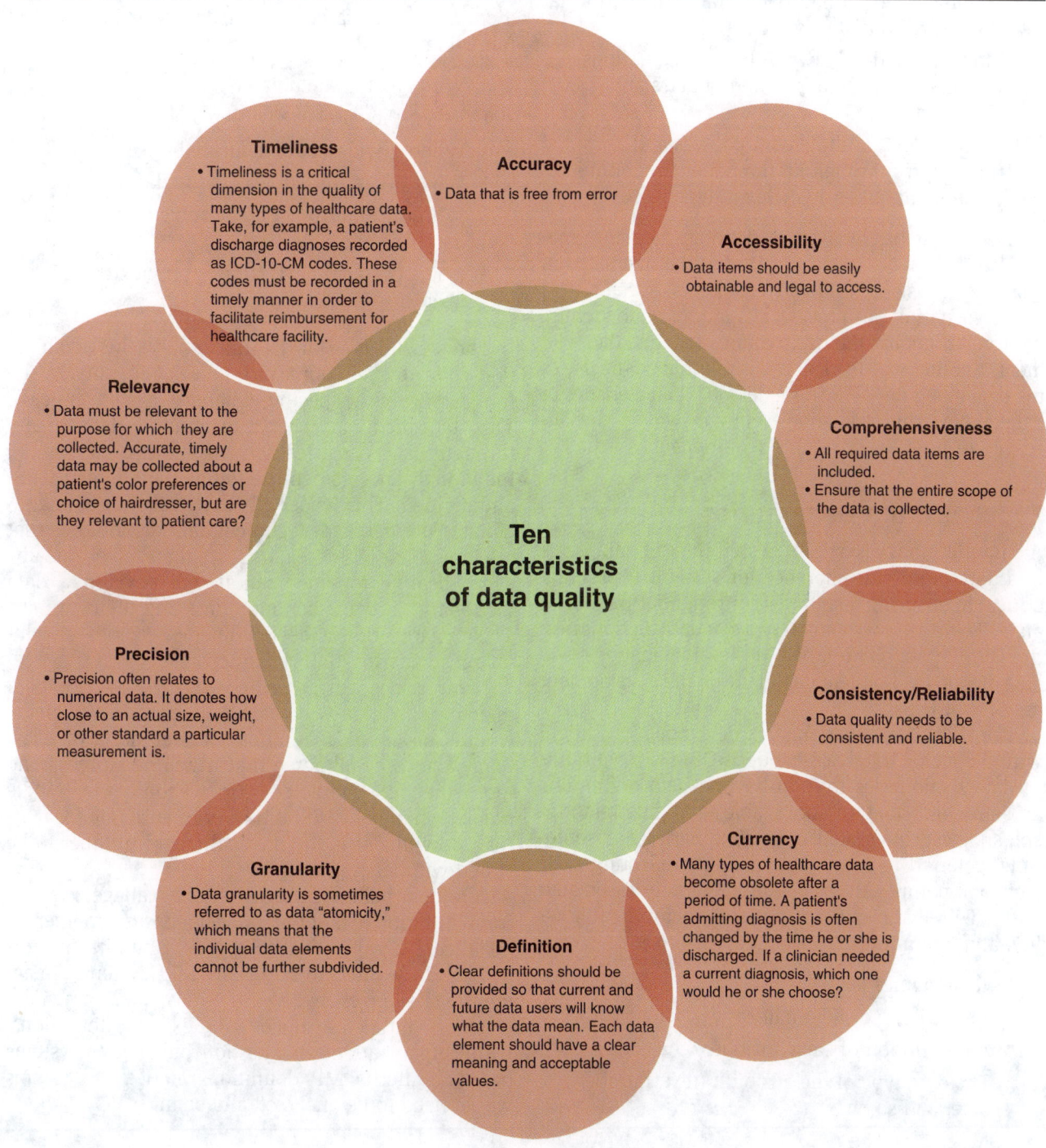

*Source:* AHIMA Data Quality Management Task Force 2012.

## Data Quality Requirements for Information Systems

In addition to the 10 characteristics of data quality, AHIMA has published data quality best practices:

- Access permissions: Define and enforce access to data.
- Data dictionary: A data dictionary exists and each data element is defined. The definitions are communicated to all staff.
- Standardized format: Use a standardized format to ensure consistency.
- State and federal laws: All laws, regulations, accreditation standards, and policies are followed.
- Data integrity: Implement policies and procedures throughout the patient encounter to ensure data integrity. (Davoudi et al. 2015)

Users must be involved in defining their information needs and designing ISs. One of the first steps in systems analysis is to identify the users' specific data needs. As part of this process, it is important to identify the level of quality the user requires for each data element. Another way to view this is to evaluate the use of the data along the AHIMA model's 10 characteristics of data quality. This evaluation eventually will be translated into technical performance requirements for the IS.

## Types of Data Dictionaries

A data dictionary is a set of descriptions of data items in a data model for reference for systems users. It is critical to ensuring data quality throughout the use of an IS. There are two general types of data dictionaries: the DBMS data dictionary and the organization-wide data dictionary. Both are important for the development and use of HISs.

The DBMS data dictionary is developed in tandem with a specific database. Modern DBMSs have built-in data dictionaries that go beyond data definitions and store information about tables and data relationships. These integrated data dictionaries are sometimes referred to as system catalogs, reflecting their technical nature. A typical data dictionary associated with a DBMS allows for documentation of the following, at a minimum:

- Table names
- All attribute or field names
- A description of each attribute
- The data type of the attribute (text, number, date, and so on)
- The format of each attribute, such as DD_MM_YYYY
- The size of each attribute, such as 12 characters in a phone number with dashes
- An appropriate range of values, such as integers 100000–999999 for the health record number
- Whether the attribute is required
- Relationships among attributes

Other descriptions that might be stored in the data dictionary associated with a database include the following:

- Who created the database
- When the database was created
- Where the database is located
- What programs can access the database
- Who the end users and administrators of the database are
- How access authorization is provided to all users

The second type of data dictionary, the organization-wide data dictionary, is developed outside the framework of a specific database design process. This data dictionary serves to promote data quality through data consistency across the organization. Individual data element definitions are agreed upon and defined. This leads to better quality data and facilitates the detailed, technical data dictionaries that are integrated with the databases themselves. Ideally, every healthcare organization will develop a data dictionary to define common data and their formats. This organization-wide document becomes a valuable resource for IS development.

Many issues can be settled with the development of an organization-wide data dictionary. Although everyone may think they know the definition of a last name, can they all agree that it will be stored as no more than 25 characters? How should the middle name be handled? Will it be a prior surname for married individuals? Is the medical record number to be stored with leading zeros?

Another challenge for healthcare managers results from interorganizational projects or the merger of healthcare organizations. Suppose a multifacility organization wanted to merge its MPI systems. Imagine the challenges involved not only in defining data elements but also in uncovering existing definitions. If the organizations in question built other systems based on internal MPI definitions, all of these systems would need to be analyzed and changed.

## Development of Data Dictionaries

The health information manager should be a key member of any data dictionary project team. Developing a data dictionary can be an overwhelming task considering the diversity of data users and the size and scope of some healthcare organizations.

To assist with data dictionary development, AHIMA has published recommended guidelines:

- Design a plan: Preplan the development, implementation, and maintenance of the data dictionary.
- Develop an enterprise data dictionary: Integrate common data elements across the entire institution to ensure consistency.
- Ensure collaborative involvement: Make sure there is support from all key stakeholders.
- Develop an approvals process: Ensure a documentation trail for all decisions, updates, and maintenance.
- Identify and retain details of data versions: Version control is important.
- Design for flexibility and growth.
- Design room for expansion of field values.
- Follow established International Organization for Standards (ISO)/International Electrotechnical Commission (IEC) 11179 guidelines for metadata registry: To promote interoperability, follow standards.
- Adopt nationally recognized standards.
- Beware of differing standards for the same concepts.
- Use geographic codes and conform to the National Spatial Data Infrastructure and the Federal Geographic Data Committee. This committee provides standards on acquiring, accessing, storing, and distributing geospatial data.
- Test the IS: Develop a test plan to ensure the system supports the data dictionary.
- Provide ongoing education and training.
- Assess the extent to which the data elements maintain consistency and avoid duplication. (AHIMA e-HIM Workgroup on EHR Data Content 2006; Davoudi et al. 2016)

Data dictionaries support medical professionals in exchanging accurate information linked across various clinical systems through data standardization. Standardized clinical data supports interoperability and ensures consistent use. Health information managers are increasingly inundated with complex information requests and data standardization can help provide the structure to enable decision support, reporting, and information retrieval.

### Check Your Understanding 5.7

**Answer the following questions in a separate document.**

1. What is the major difference between AHIMA's data quality model and the CMS "Documentation Matters Toolkit?" Are they compatible with one another? Explain your rationale.
2. Choose 3 of the 10 AHIMA data quality model characteristics and explain why each of these 3 stand out to you in ensuring data quality in healthcare. This can be from your own personal experience, experiences you have heard from others, or experiences you have read about (either positive or negative).
3. Name three characteristics that you may find in a DBMS type of data dictionary for the "patient first name" field. How will these characteristics impact data quality?
4. Why is it important to maintain an organization-wide or enterprise-wide data dictionary? What problems might an organization face without one?
5. What are AHIMA's recommended guidelines for the development of data dictionaries?

# References

ACI (Agency for Clinical Innovation). n.d. "Institute of Trauma and Injury Management." Accessed December 7, 2023. https://aci.health.nsw.gov.au/networks/trauma/data/injury-scoring.

AHIMA Data Quality Management Task Force. 2012. Practice brief: Data quality management model. *Journal of AHIMA* 83(7).

AHIMA e-HIM Workgroup on EHR Data Content. 2006. Practice Brief: Guidelines for developing a data dictionary. *Journal of AHIMA* 77(2):64A–D.

AHRQ (Agency for Healthcare Research and Quality). 2022 (April 21). "Healthcare Cost and Utilization Project (HCUP)." https://hcup-us.ahrq.gov/databases.jsp.

ACS (American College of Surgeons). n.d.a. "Commission on Cancer." Accessed December 4, 2023. https://www.facs.org/quality-programs/cancer-programs/commission-on-cancer/standards-and-resources/.

ACS (American College of Surgeons). n.d.b. "Trauma Programs." Accessed December 7, 2023. https://www.facs.org/quality-programs/trauma/quality/national-trauma-data-bank/about-ntdb/.

Ang, A. 2022 (August 30). Australian Institute of Health and Welfare gets $2M for COVID-19 linked data project. Healthcare IT News. https://www.healthcareitnews.com/news/anz/australian-institute-health-and-welfare-gets-2m-covid-19-linked-data-project.

Ang, A. 2023 (July 13). New Zealand researchers building long-COVID Registry. Healthcare IT News. https://www.healthcareitnews.com/news/anz/new-zealand-researchers-building-long-covid-registry.

ATS (American Trauma Society). n.d. "Trauma Center Levels Explained." Accessed December 7, 2023. https://www.amtrauma.org/page/TraumaLevels?&hhsearchterms=%22trauma+and+center+and+levels+and+explained%22.

Bagui, S. S., and R. W. Earp. 2022. *Database Design Using Entity-Relationship Diagrams*, 3rd ed. Auerbach Publications.

Brodnik, M. 2023. "Required Reporting and Mandatory Disclosure Laws." Chapter 12 in *Fundamentals of Law for Health Informatics and Information Management*, 4th ed., edited by M. S. Brodnik, L. A. Rinehart-Thompson, and R. B. Reynolds. Chicago: AHIMA.

Burrington-Brown, J. and B. Hjort. 2007. Health data access, use and control. *Journal of AHIMA* 78(5): 63–66.

CDC (Centers for Disease Control and Prevention). 2024a. "National Data Quality Standard." http://www.cdc.gov/cancer/npcr/standards.htm.

CDC (Centers for Disease Control and Prevention). 2024b. "How Cancer Registries Work." https://www.cdc.gov/national-program-cancer-registries/about/how-cancer-registries-work.html.

CDC (Centers for Disease Control and Prevention). 2024c. "About the National Program of Cancer Registries." https://www.cdc.gov/national-program-cancer-registries/about/index.html.

CDC (Centers for Disease Control and Prevention). 2024d. "Long COVID: Household Pulse Survey." https://www.cdc.gov/nchs/covid19/pulse/long-covid.htm.

CDC (Centers for Disease Control and Prevention). 2024e. "National Health Care Surveys." https://www.cdc.gov/nchs/dhcs/nhcs_registry_landing.htm.

CDC (Centers for Disease Control and Prevention). 2024f. "Hospital Health Care Data." https://www.cdc.gov/nchs/ahcd/index.htm.

CDC (Centers for Disease Control and Prevention). 2024g. "National Hospital Care Survey." https://www.cdc.gov/nchs/nhcs/index.htm.

CDC (Centers for Disease Control and Prevention). 2024h. "National Center for Health Statistics." https://www.cdc.gov/nchs/index.htm.

CDC (Centers for Disease Control and Prevention). 2023a. "DHCS—National Health Care Surveys." https://www.cdc.gov/nchs/dhcs/index.htm.

CDC (Centers for Disease Control and Prevention). 2023b. "NPALS Adult Day Services Survey." https://www.cdc.gov/nchs/npals-adsc/.

CDC (Centers for Disease and Prevention). 2022. *IIS Functional Standards Version 4.1 Resource Guide*. https://www.cdc.gov/vaccines/programs/iis/functional-standards/func-stds-v4-1-resource-guide.pdf.

CDC (Centers for Disease Control and Prevention). 2021a (December 30). "Ambulatory Health Care Surveys." https://www.cdc.gov/nchs/ahcd/about_ahcd.htm.

CDC (Centers for Disease Control and Prevention). 2021b (June 15). "National Hospital Care Survey—Confidentiality." https://www.cdc.gov/nchs/nhcs/confidentiality.htm.

CDC (Centers for Disease Control and Prevention). 2018. "National Immunization Program." https://www.cdc.gov/vaccines/programs/iis/core-data-elements/iis-func-stds.html.

CMS (Centers for Medicare and Medicaid Services). n.d. "Documentation Matters Toolkit CMS." Accessed May 29, 2024. https://www.cms.gov/medicare/medicaid-coordination/states/dcoumentation-matters-toolkit.

Davoudi, S., J. Flanigan, S. Houser, L. Kadlec, A. Kirby, D. VanSlyke, and A. Wendicke. 2016. Practice Brief: Managing a data dictionary (2016 update). https://bok.ahima.org/topics/healthcare-data-lifecycle/managing-a-data-dictionary-2016-update/.

Davoudi, S., J. A. Dooling, B. Glondys, T. D. Jones, L. Kadlec, S. M. Overgaard, K. Ruben, and A. Wendicke. 2015. Practice Brief: Data quality management model (2015 update). https://bok.ahima.org/topics/healthcare-data-lifecycle/data-quality-management-model-2015-update/.

Forrest, C. B., K. M. McTigue, A. F. Hernandez, L. W. Cohen, H. Cruz, K. Haynes, R. Kaushal, A. N. Kho, K. A. Marsolo, V. P. Nair, et al. 2020. PCORnet® 2020:

Current state, accomplishments, and future directions. *Journal of Clinical Epidemiology*, 129:60–67. https://doi.org/10.1016/j.jclinepi.2020.09.036.

Friedrichsen, L., L. Ruffolo, E. Monk, J. L. Starks, and P. J. Pratt. 2021. *Concepts of Database Management*, 10th edition. Cengage Learning.

Hernandez, M. J. 2020. The relational database. In *Database design for mere mortals: 25th anniversary edition* (4th ed.). Addison-Wesley Professional.

HHS (Department of Health and Human Services). n.d. "Healthy People 2030." Accessed May 29, 2024. http://www.healthypeople.gov/.

Nafea, R. A., and M. Amin Almaiah. 2021. Cyber security threats in cloud: Literature review. Paper presented at the 2021 International Conference on Information Technology (ICIT), Amman, Jordan, July 2021. IEEE. https://doi.org/10.1109/ICIT52682.2021.9491638.

NCI (National Cancer Institute). 2022 (October 14). "Cancer Staging." https://www.cancer.gov/about-cancer/diagnosis-staging/staging.

NCRA (National Cancer Registrars Association). n.d.a. "Education." Accessed December 5, 2023. http://www.ncra-usa.org/Education.

NCRA (National Cancer Registrars Association). n.d.b. "History of Cancer Registries." Accessed December 5, 2023. https://www.ncra-usa.org/About/History.

NLM (National Library of Medicine (NLM). n.d. "NCBI Insights." Accessed July 26, 2024. https://ncbiinsights.ncbi.nlm.nih.gov/2024/06/25/modern-clinicaltrials-gov-website/.

NPDB (National Practitioner Data Bank). 2018. *NPDB Guidebook*. Rockville, MD: US Department of Health and Human Services. https://www.npdb.hrsa.gov/resources/aboutGuidebooks.jsp.

NYSDH (New York State Department of Health). 2024. "Statewide Planning and Research Cooperative System (SPARCS)." https://www.health.ny.gov/statistics/sparcs/.

NAACCR (North American Association of Central Cancer Registries). n.d. "About NAACCR." Accessed December 5, 2023. https://www.naaccr.org/about-naaccr/.

Mayo Clinic. n.d.a. "Diseases and Conditions: Type diabetes" Accessed July 26, 2024. https://www.mayoclinic.org/diseases-conditions/type-1-diabetes/symptoms-causes/syc-20353011.

Mayo Clinic. n.d.b. "Diseases and Conditions: Type 2 diabetes" Accessed July 26, 2024. https://www.mayoclinic.org/diseases-conditions/type-2-diabetes/symptoms-causes/syc-20351193.

Observational Health Data Sciences and Informatics. n.d. "Data Standardization: The OMOP Common Data Model." Accessed May 28, 2024. https://www.ohdsi.org/data-standardization/.

PCORnet Steering Committee. n.d. *The National Patient Centered Clinical Research Network*. The National Patient-Centered Clinical Research Network. Accessed July 29, 2024. https://pcornet.org/.

Pérez-Martí, M., L. Casadó-Marín, and A. Guillén-Villar. 2022. Electronic records with tablets at the point of care in an internal medicine unit: Before-after time motion study. *JMIR Human Factors* 9(1):e30512. https://doi.org/10.2196/30512.

Sayles, N., and L. Kavanaugh-Burke. 2021. *Introduction to Information Systems for Health Information Technology*, 4th ed. Chicago: AHIMA.

Sherifi, D., M. Ndanga, T. J. Hunt, and S. Srinivasan. 2021. The symbiotic relationship between health information management and health informatics: Opportunities for growth and collaboration. *Perspectives in Health Information Management* 18(4):1c. https://pmc.ncbi.nlm.nih.gov/articles/PMC8649705/.

UNOS (United Network for Organ Sharing). n.d. "UNet." Accessed July 26, 2024. https://unos.org/technology/unet/.

Voss, E. A., R. Makadia, A. Matcho, Q. Ma, C. Knoll, M. Schuemie, F. J. DeFalco, A. Londhe, V. Zhu, and P. B. Ryan. 2015. Feasibility and utility of applications of the common data model to multiple, disparate observational health databases. *Journal of the American Medical Informatics Association* 22(3): 553–564. https://doi.org/10.1093/jamia/ocu023.

White, S. 2023. *Calculating and Reporting Healthcare Statistics*, 7th ed. Chicago: AHIMA.

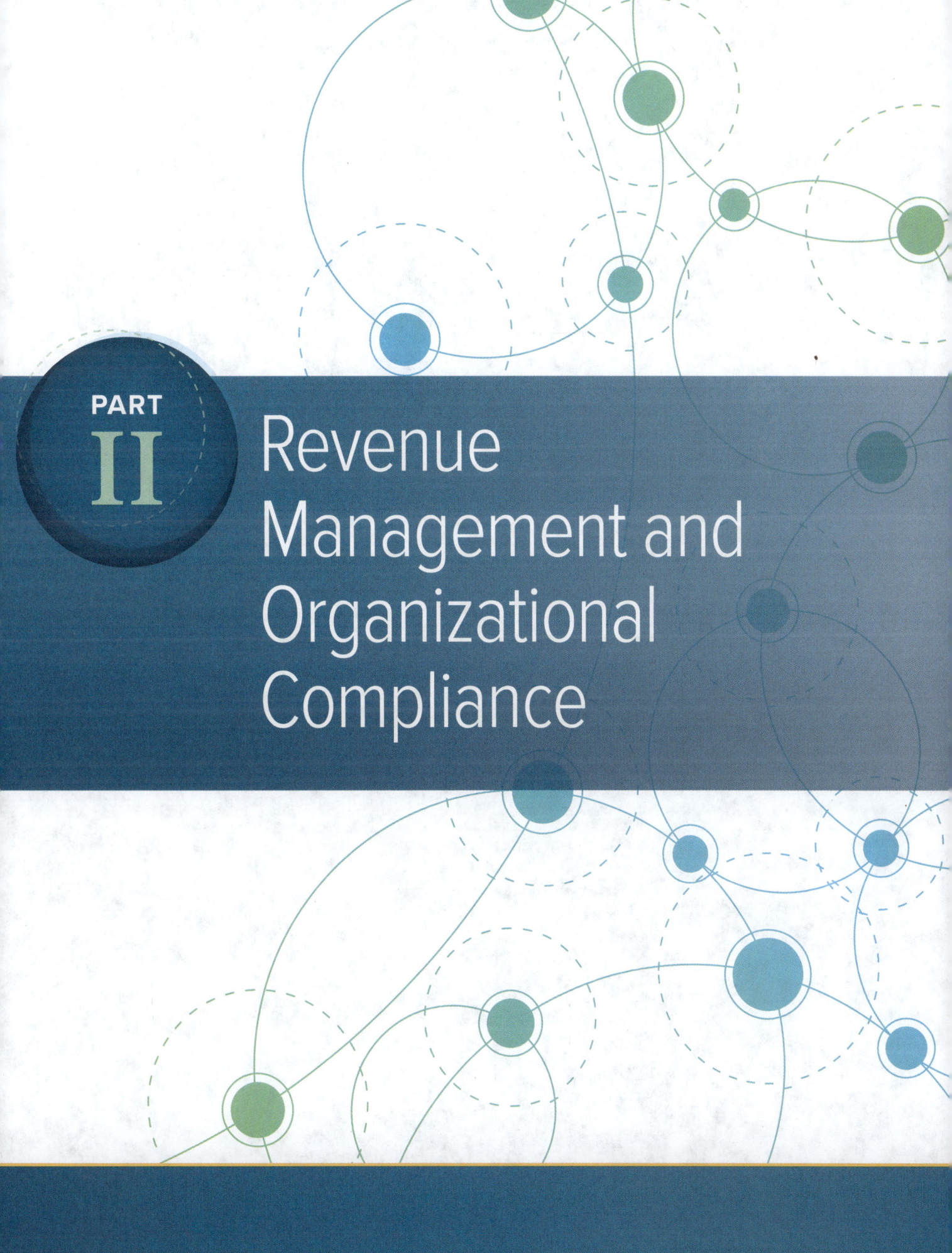

# PART II

# Revenue Management and Organizational Compliance

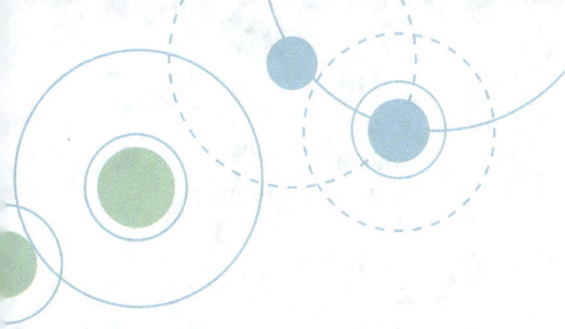

# Reimbursement Methodologies

*Anita C. Hazelwood, EdD, RHIA, FAHIMA*

## Learning Objectives

- Assess current reimbursement processes and support practices for healthcare reimbursement
- Explain the difference between private health insurance plans and employer self-insurance plans
- Outline the purpose and basic benefits of the following government-sponsored health programs: Medicare Part A through D, Medicaid, Veterans Administration, TRICARE, IHS, PACE, CHIP, and workers' compensation
- Compare the different types of managed care organizations
- Compare the different types of healthcare reimbursement methodologies
- Discuss the changes in telehealth reimbursement that were made due to COVID-19.
- Analyze prospective payment systems for various types of healthcare facilities and services

## Key Terms

Accountable Care Organization (ACO)
Acute-care prospective payment system
Administrative services only (ASO) contract
Ambulatory surgery center (ASC)
Balanced Budget Refinement Act (BBRA) of 1999
Capitation
Care area assessment (CAA)
Case-mix group (CMG) relative weight
Case-mix groups (CMGs)
Case-mix index (CMI)
Children's Health Insurance Program (CHIP)
Civilian Health and Medical Program–of the Department of Veterans Affairs (CHAMPVA)
Claim
Comorbidity
Complication
Cost outlier
Diagnosis-related group (DRG)
Discounting
Employer-based self-insurance
Episode-of-care (EOC) reimbursement
Exclusive provider organization (EPO)
Fee-for-service (FFS) reimbursement
Flexible spending account (FSA)
Geographic practice cost index (GPCI)
Global payment
Global surgery payment
Group model HMO
Health reimbursement account (HRA)
Health savings account (HSA)
Healthcare Effectiveness Data and Information Set (HEDIS)
Hierarchical Condition Category (HCC)
Home health agency (HHA)
Home health resource groups (HHRGs)
Hospital-acquired conditions (HAC)
Independent practice association (IPA)

Indian Health Service (IHS)
Long-term care hospital (LTCH)
Major diagnostic category (MDC)
Medically needy option
Medicare Advantage plan
Medicare fee schedule (MFS)
Medicare severity diagnosis-related groups (MS-DRGs)
Medigap
Minimum Data Set 3.0 (MDS)
National conversion factor (CF)
Network model HMO
Network provider
Omnibus Budget Reconciliation Act (OBRA)
Outcome and Assessment Information Set D (OASIS-D)
Outpatient prospective payment system (OPPS)
Packaging
Patient-Driven Payment Model (PDPM)
Payment status indicator (PSI)
Premium
Present on admission (POA)
Primary care physician (PCP)
Principal diagnosis
Programs of All-Inclusive Care for the Elderly (PACE)
Prospective payment system (PPS)
Relative value unit (RVU)
Resident assessment instrument (RAI)
Resource-based relative value scale (RBRVS)
Respite care
Retrospective payment system
Risk adjustment
Skilled nursing facility prospective payment system (SNF PPS)
Staff model HMO
Tax Equity and Fiscal Responsibility Act of 1982 (TEFRA)
Telehealth
TRICARE

In the US, complex systems are used to pay healthcare entities and individual healthcare providers for their services. This complexity is due in part to the variety of reimbursement methods in use and the strict requirements for detailed documentation to support medical claims. The government and other third-party payers are also concerned about potential fraud and abuse in claims processing. Therefore, ensuring bills and claims are accurate and correctly presented is an important focus of healthcare compliance.

A reimbursement **claim** is a statement of services submitted by a healthcare provider to a third-party payer (for example, an insurance company or Medicare). The claim documents the medical and surgical services provided to a specific patient during a specific period of care. Accurate reimbursement is critical to the operational and financial health of healthcare organizations. In most healthcare organizations, health insurance specialists process reimbursement claims. Health information management (HIM) professionals also play an important role in healthcare reimbursement by doing the following:

- Ensuring health record documentation supports services billed
- Assigning diagnosis and procedural codes according to patient record documentation
- Applying coding guidelines and edits when assigning codes or auditing for coding quality and accuracy
- Appealing insurance claims denials

This chapter explains the different reimbursement systems commonly used since the adoption of various types of prospective payment systems (PPSs). It then discusses a variety of healthcare reimbursement methodologies with a focus on Medicare PPSs.

## Healthcare Reimbursement Systems

Before the widespread availability of health insurance coverage, individuals were assured access to healthcare only when they could pay for the services themselves. They paid cash for services on a retrospective fee-for-service (FFS) basis in which the patient was expected to pay the healthcare provider the amount of the billed charges after a service was rendered. Until the advent of managed care, capitation, and other PPSs, private insurance plans and government-sponsored programs also reimbursed providers on a retrospective FFS basis.

FFS reimbursement is now rare for most types of medical services. Today, many Americans are covered by some form of health insurance, and most health insurance plans compensate providers according to predetermined discounted rates rather than FFS charges. However, some types of care are not covered by most health insurance plans and are still paid for directly by patients on an FFS basis. Cosmetic surgery is one example of a medical service that is not considered medically necessary and so is not covered by most insurance plans. Third-party-payors fall into one of a few categories, which are discussed in the sections that follow.

### Commercial Insurance

Many Americans are covered by private group insurance plans tied to their employment. Typically, employers and employees share the cost of such plans. Two types of commercial insurance are commonly available, private insurance and employer-based self-insurance.

### Private Health Insurance Plans

Private commercial insurance plans are financed through the payment of premiums. Each covered individual or family pays a preestablished amount (usually monthly) called a premium, and the insurance company sets aside the premiums from all the people covered by the plan in a special fund. When a claim for medical care is submitted to the insurance company, the claim is paid out of the fund's reserves. The amount of premiums that individuals pay depends on the size of the risk pool they are in. When the risk pool or number of individuals in a plan is large, premiums tend to be lower, while individuals in small risk pools pay higher premiums. In a large risk pool, the higher costs of the unhealthy are offset by the lower cost of the healthy.

Before payment is made, the insurance company reviews every claim to determine whether the services described on the claim are covered by the patient's policy. The company also reviews the claim to ensure services provided were medically necessary. Payment is made to either the provider or the policyholder.

An insurance policy represents a legal contract for services between the insured and the insurance company. Most insurance policies include the following information:

- What medical services the company will cover
- When the company will pay for medical services
- How much and for how long the company will pay for covered services
- What process is to be followed to ensure that covered medical expenses are paid

### Employer-Based Self-Insurance Plans

During the 1970s, several large companies discovered they could save money by self-insuring their employee health plans (employer-based self-insurance) rather than purchasing coverage from private insurers. Large companies have large workforces, and so aggregate (total) employee medical experiences and associated expenses vary only slightly from one year to the next. The companies understood that it was in their best interest to self-insure their health plans because yearly expenses could be predicted with relative accuracy.

The cost of self-insurance funding is lower than the cost of paying premiums to private insurers because the premiums reflect more than the actual cost of the services provided to beneficiaries. Private insurers build additional fees into premiums to compensate them for assuming the risk of providing insurance coverage. In self-insured plans, the employer assumes the risk. By budgeting a certain amount to pay its employees' medical claims, the employer retains control over the funds until the time when group medical claims need to be paid.

Employer-based self-insurance has become a common form of group health insurance coverage. Many employers enter administrative services only contracts with private insurers and fund the plans themselves. An administrative services only (ASO) contract is an agreement between an employer and an insurance organization to administer the employer's self-insurance health plan. The private insurers administer self-insurance plans on behalf of the employers.

### Not-for-Profit Insurance Companies

As with other types of health insurance, not-for-profit or nonprofit health insurance provides coverage for hospital and other medical expenses. The difference is that not-for-profit companies do not exist to make a profit for shareholders; any profits are put back into the company. The best known of the not-for-profits are the Blue Cross and Blue Shield (BCBS) companies. Currently, BCBS supplies coverage to more than 115 million members in all 50 states, the District of Columbia, and Puerto Rico. Across the nation, more than 95 percent of providers contract with BCBS (BCBS n.d.). Consumers may elect to adopt a type of healthcare savings account to assist in paying the high cost of medical expenses.

### Types of Healthcare Savings Accounts

A health savings account (HSA) is like a personal savings account, but the money deposited into it can be used only for healthcare expenses. The individual decides how much money is placed into the account and, in the case of employer-sponsored accounts, the employer may contribute as well. Any unused money at the end of the year can roll over to the next year; copays or deductibles, qualifying prescriptions, and certain medical equipment can be paid from the HSA.

A flexible spending account (FSA) is similar to an HSA, but unused money from one year cannot be rolled over to the next year. Money not used is forfeited. In both cases, funds are deposited into the account on a pretax basis, so employees reduce their tax liability. There are three types of flexible spending accounts: the healthcare FSA, the limited expense healthcare FSA, and the dependent care FSA.

A health reimbursement account (HRA), which is also called a health reimbursement arrangement, is an employer-funded health plan that helps employees pay for their qualified medical expenses. One advantage of a HRA is that unused amounts may roll or carry over from one year to another. Only the employer can put money into the HRA (UHC n.d.).

## Government-Sponsored Healthcare Programs

The federal government administers several healthcare programs. The best known are Medicare and Medicaid. The Medicare program pays for the healthcare services provided to Social Security beneficiaries aged 65 and older, individuals with permanent disabilities, people with end-stage renal disease, and other groups of individuals. State governments work with the federal Medicaid program to provide healthcare coverage to individuals and families with low-income status.

In addition, the federal government offers the Veterans Health Administration (VHA) and TRICARE health programs to address the military personnel and their dependents' needs, and the Indian Health Service (IHS) to provide federal health services to Native Americans of federally recognized tribes.

### Medicare

For Americans receiving Social Security benefits, Medicare automatically provides hospitalization insurance (Medicare Part A). It also offers voluntary supplemental medical insurance (SMI) (Medicare Part B) to help pay for physicians' services, medical services, and medical-surgical supplies not covered by the hospitalization plan. Enrollees pay extra for Part B benefits. To fill gaps in Medicare coverage, most Medicare enrollees also supplement their benefits with private insurance policies. These private policies are referred to as **Medigap** or supplemental insurance. The **Medicare Advantage plan** (a type of supplemental plan) was established by the Balanced Budget Act (BBA) of 1997 to expand the options for participation in private healthcare plans. Established in 2003, Medicare Part D covers prescription drugs.

***Medicare Part A*** Medicare Part A is generally provided free of charge to individuals aged 65 and over who are eligible for Social Security or Railroad Retirement benefits. In addition, workers (and their spouses) who have been employed in federal, state, or local government for a sufficient period qualify for Medicare coverage beginning at age 65. Requirements for receiving Medicare Part A before the age of 65 are disability, a diagnosis of end-stage renal disease, and receipt of either Social Security or Railroad Retirement disability benefits for a minimum of 24 months.

The following healthcare services are covered under Medicare Part A: inpatient hospital care, skilled nursing facility (SNF) care, home healthcare, hospice care, and inpatient care in a religious nonmedical healthcare institution. (See table 6.1.) Medicare Part A

**Table 6.1.** Medicare Part A benefit period, beneficiary deductibles and copayments, and Medicare payment responsibilities according to healthcare setting

| Healthcare setting | Benefit period | Patient's responsibility | Medicare payments |
|---|---|---|---|
| Hospital (inpatient) | • First 60 days<br>• Days 61–90<br>• Days 91–150 (these reserve days can be used only once in the patient's lifetime)<br>• Beyond 150 days | • $1,632 annual deductible<br>• $408 per day<br>• $816 per day<br>• All costs | • All but $1,632<br>• All but $408/day<br>• All but $816/day<br>• Nothing |
| Skilled nursing facility | • First 20 days<br>• Days 21–100<br>• Beyond 100 days | • Nothing<br>• $204.00 per day<br>• All costs | • 100% approved amount<br>• All but $204.00 per day<br>• Nothing |
| Home healthcare | For as long as patient meets Medicare medical necessity criteria | Nothing for services, but 20% of approved amount for durable medical equipment (DME) | 100% of the approved amount, and 80% of the approved amount for DME |
| Hospice care | For as long as physician certifies need for care | Limited costs for outpatient drugs and inpatient respite care ($5 per outpatient prescription and 5% for respite care) | All but limited costs for outpatient drugs and inpatient respite care |
| Blood banks | Unlimited if medical necessity criteria are met | First three pints unless patient or someone else donates blood to replace what patient uses | All but first three pints per calendar year |

***Source:*** Adapted from CMS 2024a, 25–29.

pays for inpatient hospital care and skilled nursing care when such care is medically necessary. An initial deductible payment is required for each hospital admission. Copayments are required after 60 days of care in each benefit period.

Each benefit period begins the day the Medicare beneficiary is admitted to the hospital and ends when the beneficiary has not been hospitalized for a period of 60 consecutive days. Inpatient hospital care is usually limited to 90 days during each benefit period. There is no limit to the number of benefit periods covered by Medicare hospital insurance during a beneficiary's lifetime. However, copayment requirements apply to days 61 through 90. When a beneficiary exhausts the 90 days of inpatient hospital care available during a benefit period, a nonrenewable lifetime reserve of up to a total of 60 additional days of inpatient hospital care can be used. Copayments are required for such additional days.

SNF care is covered when it occurs within 30 days of a three-day-long or longer hospitalization and is certified as medically necessary. Medicare will pay up to 100 days in a skilled nursing facility per benefit period. There is a copayment required for days 21–100. Medicare Part A will only pay for care in an SNF when it is determined skilled nursing care or skilled rehabilitation is needed (CMS 2024a, 28–29).

Care provided by a **home health agency (HHA)**, a program or organization that provides a blend of home-based medical and social services to homebound patients and their families, may be provided part-time in a homebound beneficiary's home when intermittent or part-time skilled nursing or certain other therapy or rehabilitation care is needed. Certain medical supplies and durable medical equipment (DME) also may be paid for under the Medicare home health benefit.

The Medicare program requires the HHA to develop a treatment plan periodically reviewed by a physician. Home healthcare under Medicare Part A has no limitations on duration, no copayments, and no deductibles. For DME, beneficiaries must pay 20 percent coinsurance, as required under Medicare Part B.

Terminally ill persons whose life expectancies are six months or less may elect to receive hospice services. Hospice is an interdisciplinary program of palliative care and supportive services that addresses the physical, spiritual, social, and economic needs of terminally ill patients and their families. To qualify for Medicare reimbursement for hospice care, patients must elect to forgo standard Medicare benefits for treatment of their illnesses and agree to receive only hospice care. When a hospice patient requires treatment for a condition unrelated to his or her terminal illness, however, Medicare does pay for all covered services necessary for that condition. The Medicare beneficiary pays no deductible for hospice coverage but does pay coinsurance amounts for drugs and inpatient respite care. **Respite care** is any inpatient care provided to the hospice patient for the purpose of giving primary caregivers a break from their caregiving responsibilities.

***Medicare Part B*** Medicare Part B covers medically necessary services as well as preventive services. Medically necessary services are those performed to diagnose or treat a medical condition. Preventive services are those that help prevent illness or detect illness at an early stage. Part B covers services such as doctor's services, outpatient or home healthcare, durable medical equipment, mental health services and other medical services (CMS 2024a). Part B services are generally subject to deductibles and coinsurance payments. (See table 6.2.)

Note that some healthcare services are usually not covered by Medicare Part A or B and are only covered by private health plans, for example, long-term nursing care, cosmetic surgery, dentures and dental care, acupuncture, and hearing aids and exams for fitting hearing aids. Beneficiaries pay a monthly premium starting at $174.70.

***Medicare Advantage*** Medicare Advantage, also called Medicare Part C, provides expanded coverage of many healthcare services. Although any Medicare beneficiary may receive benefits through the original FFS program (Parts A and B), some beneficiaries choose to participate in a Medicare Advantage plan instead.

Primary Medicare Advantage products include the following types of plans:

- *Health maintenance organization (HMO) plans*: In most HMOs, the patient pays a monthly membership premium and then can only go to doctors, other healthcare providers, or hospitals in network, except in an emergency. Patients may also need to get a referral from their primary care doctor.

- *Preferred provider organization (PPO) plans*: In a PPO plan, patients use doctors, specialists, and hospitals in the plan's network and can go to doctors and hospitals not on the list, usually at an additional cost. Patients do not need referrals to see doctors or go to hospitals that are not part of the plan's network and may pay lower copayments and receive extra benefits.

- *Private FFS plans*: A private FFS plan is similar to original Medicare in that the patient can generally go to any doctor, other healthcare provider, or hospital as long as they agree to

**Table 6.2.** Medicare Part B benefit deductibles and copayments and Medicare payment responsibilities according to type of service

| Type of service | Benefit | Deductible and copayment | Medicare payment |
|---|---|---|---|
| Medical expense | • Physicians' services, inpatient and outpatient medical and surgical services and supplies, and durable medical equipment (DME)<br>• Behavioral healthcare | • $240 annual deductible, plus 20% of approved amount after deductible has been met, except in outpatient setting<br>• 20% of most outpatient care | • 80% of approved amount (after patient has paid $240 deductible)<br>• 80% of most outpatient care |
| Clinical laboratory services | Blood tests, urinalysis, etc. | Nothing | 100% of approved amount |
| Home healthcare | Intermittent skilled care, home health aide services, DME and supplies, and other services | Nothing for home care service, 20% of approved amount for DME | 100% of approved amount 80% of approved amount for DME |
| Outpatient hospital services | Services for diagnosis and treatment of an illness or injury | A coinsurance (for doctors' services) or a copayment amount for most outpatient hospital services; the copayment for a single service cannot be more than the amount of the inpatient hospital deductible Charges for items or services that Medicare does not cover | All but deductible and copayment/coinsurance |
| Blood | Unlimited if medical necessity criteria are met | First three pints or have blood donated by someone else (if met under Part B, does not have to be met again under Part A) | All but first three pints |

*Source:* Adapted from CMS 2024a, 29–55.

treat the patient. This plan determines how much it will pay doctors, other healthcare providers, and hospitals and how much the patient must pay when receiving care.

- *Special needs plans*: Special needs plans provide focused and specialized healthcare for specific groups of people, such as those who have both Medicare and Medicaid, who live in a nursing home, or who have certain chronic medical conditions.
- *HMO point-of-service (HMO POS) plans*: These are HMO plans that may allow the patient to get some services out-of-network for a higher copayment or coinsurance. (CMS 2024a, 66–69)

**Medicare Prescription Drug Improvement and Modernization Act of 2003** The Medicare Prescription Drug Improvement and Modernization Act of 2003, provides older individuals and individuals with disabilities with a prescription drug benefit, more choices, and better benefits under Medicare. Medicare drug plans are run by insurance companies and other private companies approved by Medicare. Each plan can vary in cost and drugs covered, and beneficiaries select their preferred plan.

**Medigap Insurance** Medigap, or supplemental insurance, is private health insurance that pays, within limits, most of the healthcare service charges not covered by Medicare Parts A or B. These policies must meet federal and state laws. Medigap insurance, which generally covers copayments, coinsurance, and deductibles, is sold by private companies. Some Medigap policies also cover care outside the US (CMS 2024a).

## Medicaid

Title XIX of the Social Security Act enacted Medicaid in 1965. The Medicaid program pays for medical assistance provided to individuals and families with low incomes and limited financial resources. Individual states must meet broad national guidelines established by federal statutes, regulations, and policies to qualify for federal matching grants under the Medicaid program. Individual state medical assistance agencies, however, establish the Medicaid eligibility standards for residents of their states. The states also determine the type, amount, duration, and scope of covered services, calculate the rate of payment for covered services, and administer local programs.

Medicaid policies on eligibility, services, and payment are complex and vary considerably among states, even among states of similar size or geographic proximity. Therefore, an individual who is eligible for Medicaid in one state may not be eligible in another. In addition, the amount, duration, and scope of care provided vary considerably from state to state.

Moreover, Medicaid eligibility and services within a state can change from year to year.

***Medicaid Eligibility Criteria*** Low income is only one measure for Medicaid eligibility. Other financial resources are compared against eligibility standards. The Patient Protection and Affordable Care Act of 2010 established a new methodology for determining income eligibility for Medicaid, which is based on Modified Adjusted Gross Income. It is the basis for determining the Medicaid income eligibility for most children, pregnant women, parents, and adults. This methodology considers taxable income and tax filing relationships to determine financial eligibility.

States also have the option of providing Medicaid coverage to other categorically related groups. Categorically related groups share the characteristics of the eligible groups (that is, they fall within defined categories), but the eligibility criteria are somewhat more liberally defined. Some examples include individuals who are institutionalized or living with tuberculosis. Individuals with disabilities or who are blind and do not meet income eligibility and the medically needy are also covered. A medically needy option also allows states to extend Medicaid eligibility to persons who would be eligible for Medicaid under one of the mandatory or optional groups except that their income and resources are above the eligibility level set by their state (CMS n.d.a).

Federal welfare reform legislation established the Temporary Assistance for Needy Families program, which provides states with grant money to be used for time-limited cash assistance. A family's lifetime cash welfare benefits are generally limited to a maximum of five years. Individual states are allowed to impose other eligibility restrictions and provisions for childcare assistance or job preparation.

***Medicaid Services*** To be eligible for federal matching funds, each state's Medicaid program must offer medical assistance for the following basic services:

- Inpatient hospital services
- Outpatient hospital services
- Tobacco cessation counseling and prescription drugs for pregnant women
- Freestanding birth centers
- Medical transportation
- Physicians' services
- Skilled nursing facility (SNF) services for persons aged 21 or older
- Family planning services and supplies
- Rural health clinic services
- Home healthcare
- Laboratory and x-ray services
- Pediatric and family nurse practitioner services
- Nurse-midwife services
- Federally qualified health center (FQHC) services and ambulatory services performed at the FQHC that would be available in other settings
- Early and periodic screening and diagnostic and therapeutic services (CMS n.d.b)

States also may receive federal matching funds to provide optional services such as eyeglasses, dental care, personal care services, prosthetic devices, prescription drugs, and intermediate care facilities.

***Medicaid-Medicare Relationship*** Assistance from the Medicaid program may be available to individuals with low-income status who receive Medicare benefits. Medicaid benefits available may include, nursing facility care for longer than the usual Medicare benefit (100 days), prescription drugs, hearing aids, or eyeglasses. For individuals enrolled in both Medicare and Medicaid, any services covered by Medicare are paid for by the Medicare program before any payments are made by the Medicaid program because Medicaid is always the payer of last resort (Medicare Interactive n.d.)

### Programs of All-Inclusive Care for the Elderly

The BBA also called for implementation of a state option called Programs of All-Inclusive Care for the Elderly (PACE). PACE is a joint Medicare-Medicaid venture that provides an alternative to institutional care for individuals aged 55 or older who require a level of care usually provided at nursing facilities. It offers and manages all the health, medical, and social services needed by a beneficiary and mobilizes other services, as needed, to provide preventive, rehabilitative, curative, and supportive care. A state may or may not elect to offer PACE services to its citizens.

PACE services can be provided in day healthcare centers, homes, hospitals, and nursing homes. States that offer PACE services must provide at least one facility in a geographic service area. The program helps its beneficiaries maintain their independence, dignity, and quality of life. Individuals enrolled in PACE receive benefits solely through the PACE program and are not eligible for other government healthcare benefits (CMS n.d.c).

### Children's Health Insurance Program

The Children's Health Insurance Program (CHIP) (Title XXI of the Social Security Act) is a program initiated by the BBA. CHIP became available in 1997 and is jointly funded by the federal government and the states. Following broad federal guidelines, states establish eligibility and coverage guidelines and have flexibility in the way they provide services. CHIP allows states to expand existing insurance programs to cover children up to age 19. It provides additional federal funds to states so that Medicaid eligibility can be expanded to include a greater number of children.

States may design their CHIP programs in one of three ways:

- As a separate CHIP program under which the federal government provides the funding for qualified children
- As a Medicaid expansion CHIP where states receive funding to expand the Medicaid program
- As a combination CHIP where a state receives funding to implement both a Medicaid expansion and a separate CHIP (CMS n.d.d)

Benefits provided differ by state, but all states must provide comprehensive coverage including well-baby and well-child care, dental benefits, vaccines, and behavioral healthcare (CMS n.d.e).

## TRICARE

**TRICARE** is a federal healthcare program for active-duty members of the military and qualified family members. Eligible retirees and their family members, as well as eligible survivors of members of the uniformed services, are also eligible for TRICARE. The Department of Defense operates many military clinics and hospitals, but civilian health providers are also used. TRICARE offers a variety of plans. The most widely used are TRICARE Prime and TRICARE Select, which will be covered in the following sections.

***TRICARE Prime*** TRICARE Prime is the managed care option for active duty and retired service members and their families, activated National Guard or Reserve members and their families, retired National Guard or Reserve members, survivors, Medal of Honor recipients and their families, and qualified former spouses. Primary care managers provide most of the healthcare, but they can refer individuals to specialists for care when needed.

Additional Prime options include Prime Remote, for individuals living in remote areas of the US; Prime Overseas, for individuals in overseas areas near military hospitals and clinics; and Prime Remote Overseas, for individuals located in remote overseas locations in Eurasia-Africa, Latin America, Canada, and the Pacific. TRICARE Prime offers fewer out-of-pocket costs but less freedom to choose providers.

***TRICARE Select*** TRICARE Select is a self-managed, PPO plan available in the United States. TRICARE Select allows eligible beneficiaries to choose any physician or healthcare provider. It pays a set percentage of the providers' fees, and the enrollee pays the rest. This option permits flexibility but may be the most expensive for the beneficiary, particularly when the provider's charges are higher than the amounts allowed by the program. There is also an annual outpatient deductible. TRICARE Select Overseas provides coverage in overseas areas. TRICARE Reserve Select is a premium-based option for Select Reserve National Guard members and their families. TRICARE Retired Reserve is similar but has higher premiums and higher coinsurance and copayment amounts. Additional TRICARE options are TRICARE for Life and TRICARE Young Adult. TRICARE for Life is available to individuals who have both Part A and Part B of Medicare. TRICARE Young Adult is available for unmarried, adult children ages 21 to 26 who aged out of their parents' TRICARE coverage (DHA 2023).

### Veterans Health Administration

The VHA is the largest integrated healthcare delivery system, with more than 1,321 care sites available to serve more than 9 million veterans each year (VA 2024). Enrollment is based on priority groups (PGs); there are eight PGs, which are based on individual service and circumstances of discharge (VA 2023a). PG 1, for example, includes veterans who have service-related disabilities rated by the US Department of Veterans Affairs (VA) as 50 percent or more disabling or veterans deemed to be unemployable due to a service-connected condition. Veterans who have been awarded the Medal of Honor are also included in PG 1. The VA also offers healthcare services for a veteran's family members and dependents who meet eligibility requirements:

- The **Civilian Health and Medical Program–Veterans Administration (CHAMPVA)** is a healthcare program for dependents and survivors of permanently and totally disabled veterans, survivors of veterans who died from service-related conditions, and survivors of military personnel who died in the line of duty. CHAMPVA is a voluntary program that allows beneficiaries to be treated for free at participating VA healthcare facilities, with the VA sharing the cost of covered healthcare services and supplies.
- The Camp Lejeune Family Member program is for family members of veterans that lived or served at the US Marine Corps Base Camp

Lejeune and were exposed to contaminated water (VA 2023a).
- The Children of Women Vietnam Veterans Health Care Benefits Program provides benefits to individuals who have certain birth defects and were born to female Vietnam veterans.
- The Spina Bifida Health Care Benefits program provides training and rehabilitation for children diagnosed with spina bifida born to Korea and Vietnam veterans (VA 2022).

These programs provide care and services for approximately 700,000 spouses and dependents.

## Indian Health Service

The Indian Health Service (IHS) is an agency within the HHS. It is responsible for providing healthcare services to American Indians and Indigenous People of Alaska. This group comprises approximately 2.6 million people and 574 federally recognized nations. These individuals receive preventive healthcare services, primary medical services (hospital and ambulatory care), community health services, substance abuse treatment services, and rehabilitative services. Secondary medical care, highly specialized medical services, and other rehabilitative care are provided by private healthcare providers working under contract with the IHS.

A system of acute- and ambulatory-care facilities operates on American Indian reservations and in communities where American Indians and Indigenous People of Alaska reside. In locations where the IHS does not have its own facilities or is not equipped to provide a needed service, it contracts with local hospitals, state and local healthcare agencies, reservation-run health institutions, and individual healthcare providers (IHS n.d.).

## Workers' Compensation

Most employees are eligible for some type of workers' compensation insurance. Workers' compensation programs cover healthcare costs and lost income associated with work-related injuries and illnesses. Federal government employees are covered by the Federal Employees' Compensation Act. Individual states pass legislation that addresses workers' compensation coverage for nonfederal government employees. Some states exclude certain workers, for example, business owners, independent contractors, farm workers, and so on.

***Federal Workers' Compensation Funds*** Four disability compensation programs are offered by the US Department of Labor's Office of Workers' Compensation Programs (OWCP) for federal workers and their dependents. These programs provide rehabilitation services, medical care, and wage replacement benefits. In addition to the Federal Employees' Compensation Program, the OWCP administers the Longshore and Harbor Workers' Compensation Program, the Federal Black Lung Program, and the Energy Employees Occupational Illness Compensation Program. The need for these programs stemmed from the industrial revolution. As industrial activities flourished, the number of work injuries increased (DOL n.d.).

***State Workers' Compensation Funds*** State workers' compensation insurance was developed in response to employers' concerns of going out of business when insurance companies refused to provide coverage or charged excessive premiums (AASCIF n.d.). Legislators in most states have addressed these concerns by establishing state workers' compensation insurance funds that provide a stable source of insurance coverage and serve to protect employers from uncertainties about the continuing availability of coverage. Because state funds are provided on a nonprofit basis, the premiums can be kept low. In addition, the funds provide only one type of insurance: workers' compensation. This specialization allows the funds to concentrate resources, knowledge, and expertise in a single field of insurance.

State workers' compensation insurance funds do not operate at taxpayer expense because, by law, the funds support themselves through income derived from premiums and investments. As nonprofit departments of the state or as independent nonprofit companies, they return surplus assets to policyholders as dividends or safety refunds. This system reduces the overall cost of state-level workers' compensation insurance. Numerous court decisions have determined that the assets, reserves, and surplus of the funds are not public funds but, instead, the property of the employers insured by the funds. In states where state funds have not been mandated, employers purchase workers' compensation coverage from private carriers or provide self-insurance coverage.

## Managed Care

Healthcare costs in the US rose dramatically during the 1970s and 1980s. As a result, the federal government, employers, and other third-party payers began investigating more cost-effective healthcare delivery systems. While the federal government decided to move toward PPSs for the Medicare program in the mid-1980s, commercial insurance providers looked to managed care.

Managed care is the generic term for prepaid health plans that integrate the financial and delivery aspects of healthcare services. In other words, managed care organizations work to control the cost of, and access to, healthcare services while they strive to meet high quality standards. They manage healthcare costs by negotiating discounted providers' fees and controlling patients' access to expensive healthcare services. In managed care plans, a primary care provider coordinates services to ensure they are medically appropriate and necessary. The cost of providing appropriate services is also monitored continuously to determine whether services are being delivered in the most efficient and cost-effective way possible.

Since 1973, several pieces of federal legislation have been passed with the goal of encouraging the development of managed healthcare systems. (See table 6.3.) The Health Maintenance Organization Assistance Act of 1973 authorized federal grants and loans to private organizations that wished to develop HMOs. Another important advancement in managed care was development of the **Healthcare Effectiveness Data and Information Set (HEDIS)** by the National Committee for Quality Assurance (NCQA) (NCQA n.d.).

The NCQA is a private, not-for-profit organization that accredits, assesses, and reports on the quality of managed care plans in the US. In 1989, NCQA worked with public and private healthcare purchasers, health plans, researchers, and consumer advocates to develop HEDIS. HEDIS (formerly known as the Health Plan

**Table 6.3.** Federal legislation relevant to managed care

| Year | Legislative title | Legislative summary |
|---|---|---|
| 1973 | Federal Health Maintenance Organization Assistance Act of 1973 (HMO Act of 1973) | • Authorized grants and loans to develop HMOs under private sponsorship<br>• Defined a federally qualified HMO (certified to provide healthcare services to Medicare and Medicaid enrollees) as one that has applied for and met federal standards established in the HMO Act of 1973<br>• Required most employers with more than 25 employees to offer HMO coverage when local plans were available |
| 1974 | Employee Retirement Income Security Act of 1974 (ERISA) | • Mandated reporting and disclosure requirements for group life and health plans (including managed care plans)<br>• Permitted large employers to self-insure employee healthcare benefits<br>• Exempted large employers from taxes on health insurance premiums |
| 1981 | Omnibus Budget Reconciliation Act of 1981 (OBRA) | • Provided states with flexibility to establish HMOs for Medicare and Medicaid programs<br>• Resulted in increased enrollment |
| 1982 | Tax Equity and Fiscal Responsibility Act of 1982 (TEFRA) | • Modified the HMO Act of 1973<br>• Created Medicare risk programs, which allowed federally qualified HMOs and competitive medical plans that met specified Medicare requirements to provide Medicare-covered services under a risk contract<br>• Defined risk contract as an arrangement among providers to provide capitated (fixed, prepaid basis) healthcare services to Medicare beneficiaries<br>• Defined competitive medical plan (CMP) as an HMO that meets federal eligibility requirements for a Medicare risk contract but is not licensed as a federally qualified plan |
| 1985 | Preferred Provider Health Care Act of 1985 | • Eased restrictions on preferred provider organizations<br>• Allowed subscribers to seek healthcare from providers outside the PPO |
| 1985 | Consolidated Omnibus Budget Reconciliation Act of 1985 (COBRA) | • Established an employee's right to continue healthcare coverage beyond scheduled benefit termination date (including HMO coverage) |
| 1988 | Amendment to the HMO Act of 1973 | • Allowed federally qualified HMOs to permit members to occasionally use non-HMO physicians and be partially reimbursed |
| 1989 | Healthcare Effectiveness Data and Information Set (HEDIS)—developed by National Committee for Quality Assurance (NCQA) | • Created standards to assess managed care systems in terms of membership, utilization of services, quality, access, health plan management and activities, and financial indicators |
| 1994 | Health Care Financing Administration's Office of Managed Care established | • Facilitated innovation and competition among Medicare HMOs |
| 2010 | Patient Protection and Affordable Care Act of 2010 | • Individual mandate requirements; expansion of public programs; health insurance exchanges; changes to private insurance; employer requirements; and cost and coverage estimates |

Employer Data and Information Set) is a set of standardized measures used to compare managed care plans in terms of the quality of services they provide. HEDIS, one of the most prevalent performance improvement tools in healthcare, includes more than 90 measures across six domains of care: effectiveness of care, access to and availability of care, experience of care, utilization and risk-adjusted utilization, health plan descriptive information, and measures collected using electronic clinical data systems (NCQA 2023).

## Health Maintenance Organizations

An HMO is a prepaid voluntary health plan that provides healthcare services in return for the payment of a monthly membership premium. HMO premiums are based on a projection of the costs likely to be involved in treating the plan's average enrollee over a specified period. If the actual cost per enrollee exceeded the projected cost, the HMO would experience a financial loss. If the actual cost per enrollee turned out to be lower than the projection, the HMO would show a profit. Because most HMOs are for-profit organizations, they emphasize cost control and preventive medicine.

The benefit to third-party payers and enrollees alike is cost savings. Most HMO enrollees have significantly lower out-of-pocket expenses than enrollees of traditional FFS and other types of managed care plans. The HMO premiums shared by employers and enrollees also are lower than the premiums for other types of healthcare plans.

HMOs often use a primary care primary care physician (PCP) to coordinate care for the patient. Patients under this care plan receive their preventive and primary care from the PCP who refers the patient to a specialist as needed.

HMOs can be organized in several ways, including the group model HMO, the independent practice association (IPA), the network model HMO, and the staff model HMO. A combination of the staff, group, and network models is called a mixed model.

***Group Model HMOs*** In the **group model HMO**, the HMO contracts with an independent multispecialty physician group to provide medical services to plan members. The providers usually agree to devote a fixed percentage of their practice time to the HMO. Alternatively, the HMO may own or directly manage the physician group, in which case the physicians and their support staff would be considered its employees.

Group model HMOs are closed-panel arrangements, meaning the physicians are not allowed to treat patients from other managed care plans. Enrollees of group model HMOs are required to seek services from the designated physician group.

***Network Model HMOs*** **Network model HMOs** are like group model HMOs except that the HMO contracts for services with two or more multispecialty group practices instead of just one practice. Members of network model HMOs receive a list of all the physicians on the approved panel and are required to select providers from the list.

***Independent Practice Associations*** In an **independent practice association (IPA)** model, the HMO contracts with an organized group of physicians who join for purposes of fulfilling the HMO contract but retain their individual practices. The IPA serves as an intermediary during contract negotiations. It also manages the premiums from the HMO and pays individual physicians as appropriate. The physicians are not considered employees of the HMO. They work from their own private offices and continue to see other patients. The HMO usually pays the IPA according to a pre-negotiated list of discounted fees. Alternatively, physicians may agree to provide services to HMO members for a set prepaid capitated payment for a specified period. The IPA is an open-panel HMO, which means the physicians are free to treat patients from other plans. Enrollees of such HMOs are required to seek services from the designated physician group.

***Staff Model HMOs*** **Staff model HMOs** directly employ physicians and other healthcare professionals to provide medical services to members. Members of the salaried medical staff are considered employees of the HMO rather than independent practitioners. Premiums are paid directly to the HMO, and ambulatory care services are usually provided within the HMO's corporate facilities. The staff model HMO is a closed-panel arrangement and the most rigid model (Falkson and Srinivasan 2023).

## Preferred Provider Organizations

Preferred provider organizations (PPOs) involve agreements between healthcare providers and a self-insured employer or a health insurance carrier. Beneficiaries of PPOs are able to select providers from a list of participating providers who have agreed to furnish healthcare services to the beneficiaries. Non-participating physicians or facilities can be used but beneficiaries must pay a greater portion of the total cost. Providers are usually reimbursed on a discounted FFS basis. Patients do not have to get referrals from a primary care doctor to see a specialist.

## Point-of-Service Plans

Point-of-service (POS) plans are like HMOs in that subscribers must select a **primary care physician (PCP)** from a network of participating physicians. The PCP is usually a family or general practice physician or an internal medicine specialist. The PCP acts as a service gatekeeper to control the patient's access to specialty, surgical, and hospital care as well as expensive diagnostic services.

POS plans are different from HMOs in that subscribers are allowed to seek care from providers outside the network. However, the subscribers must pay a greater share of the charges for out-of-network services. POS plans were created to increase the flexibility of managed care plans and to allow patients more choice in providers.

### Exclusive Provider Organizations

Exclusive provider organizations (EPOs) are like PPOs except that EPOs provide benefits to enrollees only when the enrollees receive healthcare services from network providers, healthcare professionals who are members of a managed care network. In other words, EPO beneficiaries do not receive reimbursement for services furnished by nonparticipating providers.

### Integrated Delivery Systems and Integrated Delivery Networks

Integrated delivery systems (IDSs) and integrated delivery integrated delivery networks (IDNs) are both terms used in the healthcare industry to describe organizational structures that provide a coordinated and comprehensive approach to healthcare delivery. While the terms are sometimes used interchangeably, they can have slightly different meanings in different contexts. An IDS typically refers to a healthcare organization or entity that seeks to integrate various components of healthcare services within its own system. These components can include hospitals, primary care clinics, specialty care clinics, long-term care facilities, and sometimes health insurance. The primary focus of an IDS is on consolidating the delivery of care and services under a single organizational umbrella. The goal is to achieve better coordination of care, improved quality, and potentially cost savings through the elimination of duplication and inefficiencies.

An IDN is a broader concept that encompasses multiple healthcare organizations working together to deliver a coordinated and comprehensive approach to healthcare delivery within a specific geographic area or community. IDNs can include multiple hospitals, clinics, physician practices, long-term care facilities, and other healthcare providers that may not all be owned or operated by a single entity. Instead, they collaborate through partnerships, affiliations, or contractual agreements. The primary focus of an IDN is on creating a network of care providers who share patient information and collaborate to ensure a patient's healthcare needs are met across the network, even if the individual components of the network are not all owned by the same organization. IDNs often involve shared electronic health records and other health information exchange mechanisms to facilitate coordination among different healthcare entities.

### Check Your Understanding 6.1

Answer the following questions in a separate document.

1. Summarize the services provided in Medicare Parts A and B. Create an infographic to visually present the differences in the two parts.

2. Differentiate between TRICARE Prime and TRICARE Select. Evaluate the best option for a military member stationed in Iraq.

3. Explain the difference between an IDS and an IDN.

4. Which HMO model directly employs physicians and other healthcare professionals to provide medical services to members? How does this model work? Visually describe the differences between this type of HMO model and the network model using Microsoft PowerPoint, infographic, or another creative method.

5. Distinguish between private health insurance plans and employer-based self-insurance plans. Based on the differences in these plans, which one would generally be more cost-effective for the employer?

6. How do EPOs differ from PPOs? A potential patient lives in one state and has college-age students in other states. Send a memo to the prospective client summarizing her potential financial responsibilities if her children need medical care out of state.

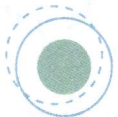

# Healthcare Reimbursement Methodologies, Accountable Care Organizations, and Risk Adjustment

Most healthcare expenses in the US are reimbursed through third-party payers rather than by the actual recipients of the services. The recipients can be considered the first parties and the providers the second parties. Third-party payers include commercial for-profit insurance companies, nonprofit BCBS organizations, self-insured employers, federal programs (Medicare, Medicaid, CHIP, TRICARE, VHA, and IHS), and workers' compensation programs.

Providers determine their own charges for services rendered. However, providers are rarely reimbursed this full amount because third-party payers likely have a unique reimbursement methodology. For example, commercial insurance plans usually reimburse healthcare providers under some type of retrospective payment system. In retrospective payment systems, the exact amount of the payment is determined after the service has been delivered. In a prospective payment system (PPS), the exact amount of the payment is determined before the service is delivered. The federal Medicare program uses several unique PPSs.

An Accountable Care Organization (ACO), while not strictly a reimbursement methodology, supports shared responsibility for the coordination of care, the quality of care, and the cost of care using metrics and incentives for excellent care and cost-savings. A risk adjustment model is used to predict patient costs based on previous diagnoses. This method allows organizations to forecast future costs to develop capitation models and provide higher reimbursement for providers seeing patients with complex medical conditions or multiple chronic conditions (AAFB 2024). Fee-for-service and episode-of-care reimbursement will be described in the sections that follow.

## Fee-for-Service Reimbursement Methodologies

Fee-for-service (FFS) reimbursement methodologies issue payments to healthcare providers based on the charges assigned to each separate service performed for the patient. The total bill for an episode of care represents the sum of all itemized charges for every element of care provided. Independent clinical professionals such as physicians and psychologists who are not employees of the facility issue separate itemized bills to cover their services after the services are completed or monthly when the services are ongoing.

Before prepaid insurance plans became common in the 1950s and the Medicare and Medicaid programs were developed in the 1960s, healthcare providers sent itemized bills directly to their patients, who were responsible for payment. When prepaid health plans and the Medicare and Medicaid programs were originally developed, the FFS method was used. A similar type of reimbursement methodology is the traditional fee-for-service type.

### Traditional Fee-for-Service Reimbursement

In traditional FFS reimbursement systems, third-party payers or patients issue payments to healthcare providers after healthcare services have been provided (for example, after the patient has been discharged from the hospital). Payments are based on the specific services delivered. The fees charged for services vary considerably by the type of services provided, the resources required, and the type and number of healthcare professionals involved. Payments can be calculated based on actual billed charges, discounted charges, pre-negotiated rate schedules, or the usual or customary charges in a specific community.

For example, some third-party payers pay only the maximum allowable charges as determined by the plan. Maximum allowable charges may be significantly lower than the provider's billed charges. Some payers issue payments based on usual, customary, and reasonable charges. Commercial insurance and BCBS plans often issue payments based on pre-negotiated discount rates and contractual cost-sharing arrangements with the patient.

For many plans, the health plan and the patient share costs on an 80/20 percent arrangement. The portion of the claim covered by the patient's insurance plan would be 80 percent of allowable charges. After the third-party payer transmits its payment to the provider, the provider's billing department issues a final statement to the patient. The statement shows the amount for which the patient is responsible (in this example, 20 percent of allowable charges). The traditional FFS reimbursement methodology is still used by many commercial insurance companies for visits to physicians' offices.

### Managed Fee-for-Service Reimbursement

Managed FFS reimbursement is similar to traditional FFS reimbursement except that managed care plans control costs primarily by managing their members' use of healthcare services. Most managed care plans also negotiate with providers to develop discounted fee schedules. Managed FFS reimbursement is common for inpatient hospital care. In some areas of the country, however, it also is applied to outpatient and ambulatory services, surgical procedures, high-cost diagnostic procedures, and physicians' services.

Utilization controls include the prospective and retrospective review of the healthcare services planned for, or provided to, patients. For example, a prospective review of a plan to hospitalize a patient for minor surgery might determine that the surgery could be safely performed less expensively in an outpatient setting. Prospective utilization review is sometimes called precertification.

In a retrospective utilization review, the plan might determine that part or all of the services provided to a patient were not medically necessary or were not covered by the plan. In such cases, the plan would disallow part or all of the provider's charges and the patient would be responsible for paying the provider's outstanding charges.

Discharge planning can be considered a type of utilization control. The managed care plan may be able to move the patient to a less intensive, and therefore less expensive, care setting as soon as possible by coordinating his or her discharge from inpatient care. The episode of care reimbursement methodology is used by many healthcare providers.

## Episode-of-Care Reimbursement Methodologies

Plans that use case rate or **episode-of-care (EOC) reimbursement** methods issue lump-sum payments to providers to compensate them for all the healthcare services delivered to a patient for a specific illness or over a specific period. EOC payments also are called bundled payments. Bundled payments cover multiple services and may involve multiple providers of care. EOC reimbursement methods include capitated payments, global payments, global surgery payments, Medicare ASC rates, and Medicare PPSs.

### Capitation

**Capitation** is based on per-person premiums or membership fees rather than on itemized per-procedure or per-service charges. The capitated managed care plan negotiates a contract with an employer or a government agency representing a specific group of individuals. According to the contract, the managed care organization agrees to provide all the contracted healthcare services that covered individuals need over a specified period (usually one year). In exchange, the individual enrollee or third-party payer agrees to pay a fixed premium for the covered group. Like other insurance plans, a capitated insurance contract stipulates as part of the contract which healthcare services are covered and which ones are not.

Capitated premiums are calculated on the projected cost of providing covered services per patient per month (PPPM) or per member per month (PMPM). The premium for an individual member of a plan includes all the services covered by the plan, regardless of the number of services provided during the period or their cost. If the average member of the plan used more services than originally assumed in the PPPM calculation, the provider (who contracts with the managed care plan) would show a loss for the period. If the average member used fewer services, the provider would show a profit. An advantage to the provider is that they have a guaranteed monthly income.

The purchasers of capitated coverage (usually the member's employer) pay monthly premiums to the managed care plan. The individual enrollees usually pay part of the premium as well. The plan then compensates the providers who furnished the services. In some arrangements, the managed care plan accepts all the risk involved in the contract. In others, some of the risk is passed on to the PCPs who agreed to act as gatekeepers for the plan.

The capitated managed care organization may own or operate some of or all the healthcare facilities that provide care to members and directly employ clinical professionals. Staff model HMOs operate in this way. Alternatively, the capitated managed care organization may purchase services from independent physicians and facilities, as do group model HMOs.

### Global Payment

Global payment methodology is sometimes applied to radiological and similar types of procedures that involve professional and technical components. **Global payments** are lump-sum payments distributed among the physicians who performed the procedure or interpreted its results and the healthcare facility that provided the equipment, supplies, and technical support required. The procedure's professional component is supplied by physicians (for example, radiologists), and its technical component (for example, radiological supplies, equipment, and support services) is supplied by a hospital or freestanding diagnostic or surgical center. Consider the following example:

> Larry Timber underwent a scheduled carotid angiogram as a hospital outpatient. He had complained of ringing in his ears and dizziness, and his physician scheduled the procedure to determine whether there was a blockage in one of Larry's carotid arteries. The procedure

required a surgeon (not the radiologist) to inject radiopaque contrast material through a catheter into Larry's left carotid artery. A radiological technician then took an x-ray of Larry's neck. The technician was supervised by a radiologist, and both were employees of the hospital.

*Professional component*: Injection of radiopaque contrast material by the surgeon
*Technical component*: X-ray of the neck region (the technician and radiologist are employees of the hospital and are paid by the hospital)
*Global payment*: The facility received a lump-sum payment for the procedure and paid for the services of the surgeon from that payment.

A single **global surgery payment** covers all healthcare services entailed in planning and completing a specific surgical procedure. In other words, every element of the procedure from the treatment decision through normal postoperative patient care is covered by a single bundled payment. This is exemplified in the following scenario:

Dr. Michaels provided Tammy Murdock with all the prenatal, perinatal, and postnatal care involved in the birth of her daughter. She received one bill from the Dr. Michaels for a total of $2,200. The bill represented the total charges for the obstetrical services associated with her pregnancy. However, the two-day inpatient hospital stay for the normal delivery was not included in the global payment, nor were the laboratory services she received during her hospital stay. Tammy received a separate bill for these services. In addition, if she had suffered a postdelivery complication (for example, a wound infection) or an unrelated medical problem, the physician and hospital services required to treat the complication would not have been covered by the global payment.

## Reimbursement for Telehealth

**Telehealth** refers to the use of electronic information and telecommunications technologies to support long-distance clinical healthcare, patient and professional health-related education, public health, and health administration. Telehealth can include various services such as virtual consultations, remote monitoring of patients, and the transmission of medical images and data for diagnostic purposes.

Telehealth has become increasingly popular due to its ability to provide convenient and accessible healthcare, especially in remote or underserved areas. It can also facilitate timely access to medical services, reduce the need for in-person visits, and lower healthcare costs. Telehealth can encompass a range of healthcare services, including primary care, specialty care, mental health services, and follow-up care.

Telehealth gained significant attention and adoption, particularly during the COVID-19 pandemic and the Medicare rules for reimbursement were changed to accommodate the increase in telehealth visits. Many of the changes made to the Medicare reimbursement policies were extended beyond the end of the COVID-19 pandemic, and some changes were made permanent. For example, there are no geographic restrictions for the originating site for behavioral or mental telehealth services. Medicare continues to refine telehealth policies.

## Accountable Care Organizations

Signed into law in 2010, the Affordable Care Act (ACA) aimed to improve the quality and affordability of healthcare in the United States. One of the key provisions of the ACA was the establishment of Accountable Care Organizations. ACOs are designed to encourage coordination and cooperation among various healthcare providers to improve the quality of care for patients, while also reducing unnecessary costs. ACOs are groups of providers such as doctors, hospitals and laboratories that come together to coordinate the care given to Medicare beneficiaries. The ACA also introduced the Medicare Shared Savings Program, which incentivizes ACOs to meet certain quality and savings requirements (Mayo Clinic n.d.). ACOs that met these requirements are eligible to receive a share of the savings they help generate in the Medicare program. Those ACOs that do not meet quality and savings requirements share the losses with the Medicare program. Specific quality measures and performance standards must be met by the ACO to be eligible for shared savings. These measures ensure that ACOs provide high-quality care to patients and improve overall health outcomes. A primary goal of the ACO models is to help reduce healthcare costs by promoting efficiency and eliminating unnecessary procedures and services. By focusing on preventative care and managing chronic conditions, ACOs aim to improve health outcomes while reducing the overall cost of care. Overall, the ACA's establishment of ACOs was intended to shift the healthcare system toward a more integrated and value-based model, with a greater emphasis on delivering high-quality, cost-effective care to patients. The success of ACOs has been mixed, with some demonstrating improved quality and reduced costs, while others have faced challenges in meeting their targets and achieving desired outcomes (CMS n.d.f).

## Risk Adjustment Models

In an ACO, risk adjustment refers to the process of adjusting financial benchmarks or performance measures to account for the health status and demographic characteristics of the patient population. This ensures that providers are fairly evaluated, recognizing that patients with more complex health needs may require more resources and care. Risk adjustment considers the underlying health issues and health spending of patients when examining their healthcare outcomes and healthcare costs (HealthCare.gov n.d.). The basis of risk adjustment is to be able to predict which patients will be more expensive to treat and to adjust payment rates for those patients. The Department of Health and Human Services has developed several risk adjustment models including CMS' Hierarchical Condition Categories (HCCs). HCCs categorize diseases and health conditions for the purpose of risk adjustment in healthcare. HCCs are hierarchical in nature, meaning they are organized to reflect the complexity of diseases and the costs associated with those diseases. These categories consider the severity of illnesses and the expected healthcare costs associated with managing these conditions. They allow for a more accurate prediction of the healthcare costs for a specific individual or population group. The HCCs are used in Medicare's managed care plans under Medicare Advantage.

The HCC coding system considers age, sex, and the presence of certain chronic conditions in classifying conditions. By using this system, healthcare providers and insurers can adjust their payments based on the relative risk of the patient population they are serving. Proper documentation and coding of HCCs are crucial for healthcare entities and providers participating in risk-adjustment programs. This ensures they receive appropriate payments for the care provided to patients with complex health needs (IMO n.d.).

### Check Your Understanding 6.2

Answer the following questions in a separate document.

1. Differentiate between a traditional FFS reimbursement methodology and a managed FFS reimbursement methodology. Which system would be more successful in keeping healthcare costs down?
2. How did the reimbursement for telehealth services change due to the COVID-19 pandemic?
3. A patient is scheduled for x-ray images to evaluate the shape and structure of the uterine cavity and the patency of the fallopian tubes. The OB-GYN injects a contrast material into the uterus through the cervix. Once the contrast material is injected, the patient is positioned, and the facility-employed radiology technician captures a series of x-ray images. These images are then assessed by the facility-employed radiologist to determine the distribution of the contrast material within the uterus and fallopian tubes to identify any abnormalities such as blockages or structural issues. Assess how each of the three principal players (OB-GYN, radiologist, and technician) are paid under a global payment methodology?
4. Assess EOC payments. How do they relate to bundled payments? Using the knowledge of EOC payments and bundled payments, prepare a memo for your OB-GYN physicians summarizing the payment methodologies for their obstetric patients' prenatal, delivery, and post-natal care.
5. Justify the value of a capitated managed care plan to a group of physicians.
6. What is the link between Accountable Care Organizations and Medicare's Shared Savings Program?

## Medicare's Prospective Payment Systems

Congress enacted the first Medicare PPS in 1983 as a cost-cutting measure. Implementation of the acute-care prospective payment system, which is the reimbursement system for inpatient hospital services provided to Medicare and Medicaid beneficiaries that is based on the use of diagnosis-related groups (DRGs) as a classification tool, resulted in a shift of clinical services and expenditures away from the inpatient hospital setting to outpatient settings. As a result of the cost containment efforts in the acute-care setting, spending on nonacute care exploded. Congress responded by passing the Omnibus Budget Reconciliation Act (OBRA) of 1986, which mandated that CMS develop a prospective system for hospital-based outpatient services provided to Medicare beneficiaries. In subsequent years, Congress mandated the development of PPSs for other healthcare providers.

## Medicare's Acute-Care Prospective Payment System

Prior to 1983, Medicare Part A payments to hospitals were determined on a traditional FFS reimbursement methodology. Payment was based on the cost of services provided, and reasonable cost or per diem costs were used to determine payment.

During the late 1960s, Congress authorized a group at Yale University to develop a system for monitoring quality of care and utilization of services. This system was known as **diagnosis-related groups (DRGs)**. A DRG is a unit of case-mix classification adopted by the federal government and some other payers as a prospective payment mechanism for hospital inpatients in which diseases are placed into groups because related diseases and treatments tend to consume similar amounts of healthcare resources and incur similar costs. DRGs were implemented on an experimental basis by the New Jersey Department of Health in the late 1970s to predetermine reimbursement for hospital inpatient stays.

At the conclusion of the New Jersey DRG experiment, Congress passed the **Tax Equity and Fiscal Responsibility Act of 1982 (TEFRA)**. TEFRA modified Medicare's retrospective reimbursement system for inpatient hospital stays by requiring implementation of the DRG PPS in 1983. Under DRGs, Medicare paid most hospitals for inpatient hospital services according to a predetermined rate for each discharge. Very simply, the DRG system was a way of classifying patients based on diagnosis. Patients within each DRG were said to be "medically meaningful"—that is, patients within a group were expected to evoke a set of clinical responses that statistically would result in an approximately equal use of hospital resources. On October 1, 2007, the DRG system became known as the **Medicare severity diagnosis-related groups (MS-DRGs)**, which better accounts for severity of illness and resource consumption.

To determine the appropriate MS-DRG, a claim for a healthcare encounter is first classified into one of 25 **major diagnostic categories (MDCs)**. Most MDCs are based on body systems and include diseases and disorders relating to a particular system. However, some MDCs include disorders and diseases involving multiple organ systems (for example, burns). The number of MS-DRGs within a particular MDC varies.

The **principal diagnosis** is defined as the condition that, after study, is determined to have caused the patient's admission to the hospital for care, and it determines the MDC assignment. Within each MDC, decision trees are used to determine the correct MS-DRG. Within most MDCs, cases are divided into surgical MS-DRGs (based on a surgical hierarchy that orders individual procedures or groups of procedures by resource intensity) and medical MS-DRGs. Medical MS-DRGs generally are differentiated based on diagnosis and age. Some surgical and medical MS-DRGs are further differentiated according to the presence or absence of complications or comorbidities (CCs).

A **complication** is a secondary condition that arises during hospitalization and is thought to increase the length of stay (LOS) by at least one day for approximately 75 percent of patients. A **comorbidity** is a condition that existed at admission and is thought to increase the LOS at least one day for approximately 75 percent of patients. During the initial years of DRGs, there was a standard list of diagnoses that were considered CCs. Each year new CCs are added, and others deleted from the CC list.

Each base MS-DRG can be subdivided in one of three possible alternatives:

- MS-DRGs with three subgroups (Major Complication/Comorbidity [MCC, CC, and non-CC; referred to as: with MCC, with CC, and w/o CC/MCC])
    - MS-DRG 682 Renal Failure with MCC
    - MS-DRG 683 Renal Failure with CC
    - MS-DRG 684 Renal Failure w/o CC/MCC
- MS-DRGs with two subgroups (MCC and CC/non-CC; referred to as: with MCC and w/o MCC)
    - MS-DRG 725 Benign Prostatic Hypertrophy with MCC
    - MS-DRG 726 Benign Prostatic Hypertrophy w/o MCC
- MS-DRGs with two subgroups (non-CC and CC/MCC; referred to as: with CC/MCC and w/o CC/MCC)
    - MS-DRG 294 Deep Vein Thrombophlebitis with CC/MCC
    - MS-DRG 295 Deep Vein Thrombophlebitis w/o CC/MCC (CMS, 2024b)

The increased number of classifications is intended to differentiate between the levels of resource consumption within a base MS-DRG group.

Under the acute-care prospective payment system, a predetermined rate based on the MS-DRG assigned to each case (only one is assigned per case) is used to reimburse hospitals for inpatient care provided to Medicare and TRICARE beneficiaries. CMS adjusts the Medicare MS-DRG list and reimbursement rates every fiscal year (October 1 through September 30). There are currently 767 MS-DRGs (CMS 2024b).

Hospitals determine MS-DRGs by assigning ICD-10-CM or ICD-10-PCS codes to each patient's principal diagnosis, comorbidities, complications, major complications, principal procedure, and secondary procedures. These code numbers and other information on the patient (age, sex, and discharge status) are entered into a grouper. An MS-DRG grouper is a computer software program that assigns appropriate MS-DRGs according to the information provided for each episode of care.

Reimbursement for each episode of care is based on the MS-DRG assigned. Different diagnoses require different levels of care and expenditures of resources. Therefore, each MS-DRG is assigned a different weight that reflects the average amount of resources required to treat a patient assigned to that MS-DRG. Each MS-DRG is associated with a description, a relative weight, a geometric mean LOS, and an arithmetic mean LOS. The relative weight represents the average resources required to care for cases in a given MS-DRG relative to the national average of resources used to treat all Medicare patients. An MS-DRG with a relative weight of 2.000, on average, requires twice as many resources as an MS-DRG with a relative weight of 1.000. The geometric mean LOS is defined as the total days of service, excluding any outliers or transfers, divided by the total number of patients; the arithmetic mean LOS is defined as the total days of service divided by the total number of patients.

For example, MS-DRG 1, organized within MDC 01, is described as heart transplant or implant of a heart assist system with MCC, and has a relative weight of 25.3518, a geometric mean LOS of 28.3, and an arithmetic mean LOS of 35.9.

In some cases, the MS-DRG payment the hospital receives may be lower than the actual cost of providing Medicare Part A inpatient services. In such cases, the hospital must absorb the loss. In other cases, the cost of providing care is lower than the MS-DRG payment; that is, the hospital may receive a payment for more than its actual cost and, therefore, make a profit.

Special circumstances can also apply to inpatient cases and result in an outlier payment to the hospital. An outlier case results in exceptionally high costs when compared with other cases in the same MS-DRG. To qualify for a **cost outlier**, a hospital's charges for a case (adjusted to cost) must exceed the payment rate for the MS-DRG by a fixed dollar amount, which changes each year. The additional payment amount is equal to 80 percent of the difference between the hospital's entire cost for the stay and the threshold amount. The fixed-loss threshold amount is the sum of the MS-DRG payment amount, and the annual outlier threshold set by CMS.

There can be further hospital-specific adjustments resulting in add-on payments:

- *Disproportionate share hospital (DSH)*: If the hospital treats a high percentage of low-income patients, it receives a percentage add-on payment applied to the MS-DRG-adjusted base payment rate.
- *Indirect medical education (IME)*: If the hospital is an approved teaching hospital, it receives a percentage add-on payment for each case paid under MS-DRGs. This percentage varies depending on the ratio of residents to beds.
- *New technologies*: If the hospital demonstrates the use of a new technology that is a substantial clinical improvement over available existing technologies and the new technology is approved, additional payments are made. Hospitals must submit a formal request to CMS with a significant sample of data to demonstrate the technology meets the high-cost threshold.

The MS-DRG system bases a hospital's **case-mix index (CMI)**—types or categories of patients treated by the hospital—on the relative weights of the MS-DRG. The sum of all total weights divided by the sum of total patient discharges equals the CMI. A hospital may relate its CMI to the costs incurred for inpatient care. This information allows the hospital to make administrative decisions about services to be offered to its patient population. For example, if a hospital's case-mix report indicates that a small population of patients receives obstetrical services, but the costs associated with providing such services are disproportionately high, this report along with other data might result in the hospital's administrative decision to discontinue its obstetrical services department.

## Hospital-Acquired Conditions and Present on Admission Indicator Reporting

The Deficit Reduction Act of 2005 (DRA) mandated a quality adjustment in the MS-DRG payments for certain hospital-acquired conditions (HACs). CMS titled the program "Hospital-Acquired Conditions and Present on Admission Indicator Reporting." **Present on admission (POA)** is defined as a condition present at the time the order for inpatient admission occurs—conditions that develop during an outpatient encounter, including in the emergency department, observation, or outpatient surgery, are considered as POA. A POA indicator is assigned to principal and secondary diagnoses and the external cause of injury codes. The reporting options that are available are as follows:

- Y = Yes, diagnosis was present at the time of inpatient admission.
- N = No, diagnosis was not present at the time of inpatient admission.
- U = Unknown, documentation is insufficient to determine if condition was present at the time of inpatient admission.
- W = Clinically undetermined, the provider is unable to clinically determine whether the condition was present at the time of admission.
- 1 = Unreported/not used = Exempt from POA reporting.

The following hospitals are exempt from the POA indicator requirement: critical access hospitals (CAHs), long-term care hospitals (LTCHs), Maryland waiver hospitals, cancer hospitals, children's inpatient facilities, inpatient rehabilitation facilities (IRFs), and psychiatric hospitals.

CMS identified eight **hospital-acquired conditions (HACs)** (not POA) as reasonably preventable, and hospitals will not receive additional payment for cases in which one of the eight selected conditions was not POA. This is termed the HAC payment provision. Conditions identified have been added or dropped over time. There are currently 14 HACs:

- Foreign object retained after surgery
- Air embolism
- Blood incompatibility
- Stage III and IV pressure ulcers
- Falls and trauma
- Catheter-associated urinary tract infection
- Vascular catheter-associated infection
- Surgical site infection—mediastinitis after coronary artery bypass graft
- Surgical site infections following certain orthopedic procedures of the spine, shoulder and elbow
- Surgical site infections following bariatric surgery for obesity
- Manifestations of poor glycemic control
- Deep vein thrombosis (DVT) and pulmonary embolism (PE) following certain orthopedic procedures
- Iatrogenic pneumothorax with venous catheterization
- Surgical site infection following cardiac implantable electronic devices procedure (CMS n.d.g)

## Inpatient Psychiatric Facilities Prospective Payment System

The Balanced Budget Refinement Act of 1999 mandated the development of a per diem PPS for inpatient psychiatric services furnished in hospitals and exempt units. The PPS became effective on January 1, 2005, establishing a standardized per diem rate to inpatient psychiatric facilities (IPFs) based on the national average of operating, ancillary, and capital costs for each patient day of care in the IPF.

Patient-level or case-level adjustments are provided for age, specified MS-DRGs, and certain comorbidity categories. Payment adjustments are made for eight age categories beginning with age 45 at which point, statistically, costs increase as the patient ages.

The IPF receives an MS-DRG payment adjustment for a principal diagnosis that groups to 1 of 17 psychiatric MS-DRGs (shown in table 6.4). Certain comorbidity categories that require comparatively more costly treatment during an inpatient stay also generate a payment adjustment.

In addition, there is a variable per diem adjustment to recognize higher costs in the early days of a psychiatric stay.

The IPF PPS also includes an outlier policy for those patients who require more expensive care than expected to minimize the financial risk to the IPF. Although the basis of the system is a per diem rate, outlier payments are made on a per case basis rather than on the per diem basis. Payment is also adjusted for patients who are given electroconvulsive therapy.

The PPS also includes regulations on payments when there is an interrupted stay, meaning the patient is discharged from an IPF and returns to the same or another facility before midnight on the third consecutive day. The intent of the policy is to prevent a facility from prematurely discharging a patient after the maximum payment is received and subsequently readmitting the patient.

Facility adjustments include a wage-index adjustment, a rural location adjustment, a teaching status adjustment, a cost-of-living adjustment for Alaska and Hawaii, and a qualifying emergency department adjustment. Payment is made based on a per diem basis adjusted for geographic areas. The 2024 IPF per diem rate was $895.63 (CMS 2023a, 1).

**Table 6.4.** Psychiatric DRGs

| MS-DRG | MS-DRG description |
|---|---|
| 056 | Degenerative nervous system disorders with MCC |
| 057 | Degenerative nervous system disorders w/o MCC |
| 080 | Nontraumatic stupor and coma with MCC |
| 081 | Nontraumatic stupor and coma w/o MCC |
| 876 | OR procedure with principal diagnoses of mental illness |
| 880 | Acute adjustment reaction and psychosocial dysfunction |
| 881 | Depressive neuroses |
| 882 | Neuroses except depressive |
| 883 | Disorders of personality and impulse control |
| 884 | Organic disturbances and intellectual disabilities |
| 885 | Psychoses |
| 886 | Behavioral and developmental disorders |
| 887 | Other mental disorder diagnoses |
| 894 | Alcohol/drug abuse or dependence, left Against Medical Advice (AMA) |
| 895 | Alcohol/drug abuse or dependence with rehabilitation therapy |
| 896 | Alcohol/drug abuse or dependence w/o rehabilitation therapy with MCC |
| 897 | Alcohol/drug abuse or dependence w/o rehabilitation therapy w/o MCC |

*Source:* CMS 2023a, 30.

## Resource-Based Relative Value Scale System

In 1992, CMS implemented the resource-based relative value scale (RBRVS) system for physicians' services such as office visits covered under Medicare Part B. The system reimburses physicians according to a fee schedule based on predetermined values assigned to specific services.

The Medicare fee schedule (MFS) is the listing of allowed charges that are reimbursable to physicians under Medicare. Each year's MFS is published by CMS in the *Federal Register*.

To calculate fee schedule amounts, Medicare uses a formula that incorporates the following relative value units (RVUs):

- Physician work (RVUw)
- Practice expenses (RVUpe)
- Malpractice costs (RVUm)

RVUs are a measurement that represents the value of the work involved in providing a specific professional medical service in relation to the value of the work involved in providing other medical services. Sample RVUs for selected Healthcare Common Procedure Coding System (HCPCS) codes are shown in table 6.5.

Payment localities are adjusted according to three geographic practice cost indices (GPCIs):

- Physician work (GPCIw)
- Practice expenses (GPCIpe)
- Malpractice costs (GPCIm)

A geographic practice cost index (GPCI) is a number used to multiply each RVU so that it better reflects a geographical area's relative costs. For example, costs of office rental prices, local taxes, average salaries, and malpractice costs are all affected by geography. Sample GPCIs for selected US cities are shown in table 6.6.

A national conversion factor (CF) converts the RVUs into payments. The conversion factor changes annually.

The RBRVS fee schedule uses the following formula:

$$[(RVUw \times GPCIw) + (RVUpe \times GPCIpe) + (RVUm \times GPCIm)] \times CF = Payment$$

As an example, payment for performing a repair of a nail bed (code 11760) in Birmingham, AL, can be calculated. RVU values include the following:

- RVUw = 1.63
- RVUpe = 1.91
- RVUm = 0.22

**Table 6.5.** Sample 2023 RVUs for selected HCPCS codes

| HCPCS Code | Description | Work RVU | Facility practice expense RVU | Malpractice expense RVU |
|---|---|---|---|---|
| 99203 | Office visit | 1.60 | 0.68 | 0.17 |
| 99204 | Office visit | 2.60 | 1.11 | 0.23 |
| 11010 | Debridement skin at fracture site | 4.19 | 3.30 | 0.74 |
| 45380 | Colonoscopy with biopsy | 3.56 | 1.89 | 0.44 |
| 52601 | TURP, complete | 13.16 | 6.74 | 1.56 |

*Source*: CMS 2023b.

**Table 6.6.** Sample GPCIs for selected US cities

| City | Work GPCI | Practice expense GPCI | Malpractice expense GPCI |
|---|---|---|---|
| Baltimore | 1.024 | 1.087 | 1.311 |
| Dallas | 1.017 | 1.017 | 0.711 |
| Miami | 1.000 | 1.025 | 2.564 |
| New Orleans | 1.000 | 0.931 | 1.342 |

*Source*: CMS 2023b.

GPCI values include the following:

- $GPCI_w = 1.00$
- $GPCI_{pe} = 0.850$
- $GPCI_m = 0.617$
- National CF for 202X = $32.75 (changes annually)

The calculation is as follows:

$(1.63 \times 1.00) + (1.91 \times 0.850) + (0.22 \times 0.617) \times CF$
$1.63 + 1.6235 + 0.13574 = 3.38924 \times \$32.75$

There is a fee schedule payment of $110.99.

## Medicare and Medicaid Outpatient Prospective Payment System

The **outpatient prospective payment system (OPPS)** was first implemented for services furnished on or after August 1, 2000. OPPS is the Medicare PPS used for hospital-based outpatient services and procedures. Services included under OPPS follow:

- Surgical procedures
- Radiology including radiation therapy
- Clinic visits (evaluation and management or E/M)
- Emergency department visits
- Partial hospitalization services for the mentally ill
- Chemotherapy
- Preventive services and screening exams
- Dialysis for other than end-stage renal disease
- Vaccines, splints, casts, and antigens
- Certain implantable items

The OPPS does not apply to CAHs, hospitals in Maryland that are excluded, IHS hospitals, or hospitals outside the 50 states, the District of Columbia, and Puerto Rico. CAH is a designation given by CMS to rural hospitals that meet eligibility guidelines. The CAH designation was created by the BBA after numerous rural hospitals closed in the 1980s and 1990s. The ACA and American Recovery and Reinvestment Act (ARRA) both included provisions for strengthening these rural hospitals. The purpose of the CAH is to reduce financial vulnerability often plaguing rural communities. CAHs receive benefits including cost-based reimbursement from Medicare.

CMS uses three separate reimbursement methods to reimburse hospital outpatient services. These include fee schedule payment, prospective payment using ambulatory payment classification (APC), and reasonable cost basis. Examples of services paid using a fee schedule include DME, physical therapy (PT), and diagnostic lab services. Influenza and pneumococcal immunizations, and acquisition of corneal tissue are examples of services paid on a reasonable cost basis.

The calculation of most payment for most services under the OPPS is based on the categorization of outpatient services into APC groups according to Current Procedural Terminology (CPT) and HCPCS codes. ICD-10-CM and ICD-10-PCS coding is not used in the selection of APCs. The APCs are categorized into significant procedure APCs, radiology and other diagnostic APCs, medical visit APCs, and partial hospitalization APCs. Services within an APC are similar, both clinically and regarding resource consumption, and each APC is assigned a fixed payment rate for the facility fee or technical component of the outpatient visit. Payment rates are also adjusted according to the hospital's wage index. Multiple APCs may be appropriate for a single episode of care as the patient may receive various types of services such as radiology or surgical procedures.

The OPPS **payment status indicators (PSIs)** that are assigned to each HCPCS code and APCs play an important role in determining payment for services under the OPPS. PSIs indicate whether a service is payable under the OPPS or one of the other reimbursement systems mentioned above. For example, status indicator "C" is used to show that a procedure is performed on an inpatient basis only. This inpatient-only list is updated each year. Other notable PSIs include the following:

- A   Fee schedule payment
- F   Reasonable cost payment
- G   APC pass-through payment
- K   APC payment
- S   APC payment
- T   APC payment (Noridian 2023)

Services that are packaged into APC rates are indicated with the status indicator "N." **Packaging** means that payment for that service is packaged into payment for other services and, therefore, there is no separate APC payment. Packaged services might include minor ancillary services, inexpensive drugs, medical supplies, and implantable devices (Noridian 2023).

**Discounting** applies to multiple surgical procedures furnished during the same operative session. For discounted procedures, the full APC rate is paid for the surgical procedure with the highest rate, and other surgical procedures performed at the same time are reimbursed at 50 percent of the APC rate. When a surgical procedure is terminated after a patient is prepared for surgery but before induction of anesthesia, the facility is reimbursed at 50 percent of the APC rate. Modifier 73 should be appended to the procedure code indicating that the procedure was discontinued. Modifier 74 is appended to the procedure code when a procedure is interrupted after its initiation or the administration of anesthesia. The facility receives the full APC payment.

The OPPS does pay outlier payments on a service-by-service basis when the cost of furnishing a service or procedure by a hospital exceeds 1.75 times the APC payment amount and exceeds the APC payment rate plus a fixed-dollar threshold. If a provider meets both conditions, the outlier payment is calculated as 50 percent of the amount by which the cost of furnishing the service exceeds 1.75 times the APC payment rate. The fixed-dollar threshold changes each year.

Special payments are also made for new technology in one of two ways. Transitional pass-through payments are temporary additional payments that are made when certain drugs, biological agents, brachytherapy devices, and other expensive medical devices new to medicine are used. These new technology APCs were created to allow new procedures and services to enter the OPPS quickly even though their complete costs and payment information are not known. New technology APCs house modern procedures and services until enough data are collected to properly place the new procedure in an existing APC or to create a new APC for the service or procedure. Coding for E/M medical visits is different under the APC system than it is for physician billing. CMS states that each facility should develop a system for mapping the provided services furnished to the different levels of effort represented by E/M codes. If services furnished are documented and medically necessary and the facility is following its own system, which reasonably relates the intensity of hospital resources to the different levels of codes, CMS assumes the hospital is in compliance with its reporting requirements.

## Ambulatory Surgery Center Prospective Payment System

For Medicare purposes, an **ambulatory surgery center (ASC)** is a distinct entity that operates exclusively for the purpose of furnishing outpatient surgical services to patients. An ASC is either independent or operated by a hospital. If it is operated by a hospital, it has the option of being covered under Medicare as an ASC, or it can continue to be covered as an outpatient surgery department. To be considered an ASC of a hospital it must be a separately identifiable entity physically, administratively, and financially.

The Medicare Modernization Act (MMA) of 2003 extensively revised the ASC payment system with changes going into effect on January 1, 2008. The system is called the ambulatory surgery center prospective payment system (ASC PPS).

ASCs must accept assignment as payment in full. Eighty percent of the payment comes from the government and 20 percent from the beneficiary. Under the ASC payment system, Medicare will make payments to ASCs only for services on the ASC list of covered procedures. The surgical procedures included in the list are those determined to pose no significant risk to beneficiaries when furnished in an ASC. The ASC payment includes services such as medical and surgical supplies, nursing services, surgical dressings, implanted prosthetic devices not on a pass-through list, and splints and casts. Examples of services not included in the ASC payment are brachytherapy, procurement of corneal tissue, and certain drugs and biologicals.

The payment rates for most covered ASC procedures and covered ancillary services are established prospectively based on a percentage of the OPPS payment rates while a small number of services are contractor based, such as the pass-through items.

The HCPCS code is used as the basis for payment. Each HCPCS code falls into one of more than 1,500 ASC groups, with each group having a unique payment. Medicare pays 80 percent of the wage-adjusted rate, and the beneficiary is responsible for the other 20 percent. Like the OPPS, each HCPCS code has a payment indicator that determines whether the surgical procedure is on the ASC list (A2); device-intensive procedure paid at adjusted rate (J8); or packaged service or item for which no separate payment is made (N1). These are just a few examples of some of the payment indicators.

Again, like the OPPS, there are guidelines for payment of terminated procedures. The following rules apply:

- Zero percent payment for procedures terminated for unforeseen circumstances before the ASC has expended substantial resources
- Fifty percent payment for procedures that are terminated due to medical complications prior to anesthesia
- One hundred percent payment for procedures that have started but are terminated after anesthesia is induced

## Ambulance Fee Schedule

A Medicare payment system for medically necessary transports effective for services provided on or after April 1, 2002, was included as part of the BBA. The payment system applies to all ambulance services including volunteer, municipal, private, independent, and institutional providers (hospitals, CAHs, SNFs, and home health agencies [HHAs]).

Ambulance services are reported on claims using HCPCS codes that reflect the seven categories of ground service and two categories of air service. Mandatory assignment is required for all ambulance service providers. There are seven categories of ground (which includes land and water) services for ambulance use. These are basic life support, advanced life support (level 1), advanced life support (level 2), specialty care transport, paramedic intercept, fixed wing air ambulance, and rotary wing air ambulance (42 CFR 414.605).

## Medicare Skilled Nursing Facility Prospective Payment System

The BBA mandated implementation of a skilled nursing facility prospective payment system (SNF PPS). An SNF PPS is defined as a per diem reimbursement system for all costs (routine, ancillary, and capital) associated with covered SNF services furnished to Medicare Part A beneficiaries. The SNF PPS was implemented on July 1, 1998. Under the PPS, SNFs are no longer paid under a system based on reasonable costs. Instead, they are paid according to a per diem PPS based on case mix–adjusted payment rates.

Medicare Part A covers post-acute SNF services, and all items and services paid under Medicare Part B before July 1, 1998 (other than physician and certain other services specifically excluded under the BBA). Major elements of the SNF PPS include rates, coverage, transition, and consolidated billing. OBRA required CMS to develop an assessment instrument to standardize the collection of SNF patient data. The Resident Assessment Instrument (RAI) has three components: the Minimum Data Set 3.0 (MDS), the Care Area Assessment (CAA) process, and the RAI utilization guidelines. The CAA process involves a comprehensive assessment of a resident's needs in specific areas or care domains, such as medical, functional, cognitive, psychosocial, and behavioral. These assessments help care providers identify the resident's strengths, weaknesses, preferences, and potential areas for improvement. The MDS is the minimum core of defined and categorized patient assessment data that serves as the basis for documentation and reimbursement in an SNF. The MDS form contains a face sheet for documentation of resident identification information, demographic information, and the patient's customary routine. The PPS for SNF changed as described in the section that follows. Consolidated billing remains an important component of the PPS for SNFs.

### Patient Driven Payment Model

Prior to October 1, 2019, the PPS used for SNFs was based on the Resource Utilization Groups, Version IV, also called RUG-IV. Payment under RUGs was based primarily on the amount of therapy provided to a patient, regardless of the patient's characteristics, needs, or goals.

In 2019, the **patient driven payment model (PDPM)** was developed to improve payment accuracy and appropriateness by focusing on the patient and their characteristics, rather than on the volume of services provided, to reduce administrative burden on providers, and to improve SNF payments to underserved beneficiaries.

Under PDPM, payment is determined using six separate payment components. Five of these are case-mix adjusted and include the PT component, the OT component, the speech-language pathology (SLP) component, the non-therapy ancillary (NTA) services component, and the nursing component. The sixth is a non-case-mix-adjusted component meaning that it does not vary according to patient characteristics and is used to cover utilization of SNF resources.

The per diem payment under PDPM is determined by the base rates that correspond to the five payment components and the standard sixth component amount and the CMI values that correspond to each classification group within the case-mix adjusted payment components. The PDPM also adjusts the per diem rate over the course of the stay. An additional payment adjustment is applied for residents with HIV/AIDS.

The PT and OT components are based on the patient's functional score and an appropriate clinical category. There are 10 clinical categories into which diagnosis codes are mapped. Surgeries prior to admission may affect the clinical category assigned. The score for the PT and OT components is arrived at by scoring the following items: two bed mobility items (for example, lying on the bed to sitting up), three transfer items (for example, moving from the chair to the bed), one eating item, one toileting item, one oral hygiene item, and two walking items.

The SLP component group is determined by the patient's clinical category, cognitive function, possible SLP-related comorbidity, and the presence of a swallowing disorder or an altered diet. The nursing component is based on the patient's clinical conditions, use of services, presence of depression, restorative nursing services provided, and the resident's functional score to assign a patient to a nursing case-mix group (CMG). The NTA component uses a comorbidity score as well as number of extensive services to group to a CMG. The non-case-mix payment is determined by a base rate. Adding the reimbursement determined for each of the six components results in the final SNF payment.

The PDPM has an interrupted stay policy. If a patient is discharged from an SNF and readmitted to the same SNF no more than three consecutive calendar days after discharge, then the subsequent stay is considered a continuation of the previous stay. Another important component of the SNF PPS is consolidated billing (Acumen 2018; CMS 2019).

## Consolidated Billing Provision

The BBA includes a billing provision that requires an SNF to submit consolidated Medicare bills for its residents for services covered under either Part A or Part B except for a limited number of specifically excluded services. For example, when a physician provides a diagnostic radiology service to an SNF patient, the SNF must bill for the technical component of the radiology service because this is included in the SNF consolidated billing payment. The rendering physician must develop a business relationship with the SNF to receive payment from the SNF for the services he or she rendered. The professional component of the physicians' services is excluded from SNF consolidated billing and must be billed separately to the Medicare administrative contractor. There are, of course, other exclusions to this provision, including physician assistant services, nurse practitioner services, and clinical nurse specialist services when these individuals are working under the supervision of, or in collaboration with, a physician, certified midwife services, qualified psychologist services, and certified registered nurse anesthetist services. Other exclusions include hospice care, maintenance dialysis, selected services furnished on an outpatient basis such as cardiac catheterization services, CT scans and MRIs, radiation therapy, and ambulance services. In addition, SNFs report HCPCS codes on all Part B bills.

# Home Health Prospective Payment System

The BBA called for the development and implementation of a home health prospective payment system (HHPPS) for reimbursement of services provided to Medicare beneficiaries. The PPS for HHAs was implemented on October 1, 2000. Medicare pays a predetermined payment rate for each 30-day period of home healthcare. Payment is expected to cover all costs that providers are expected to incur while furnishing, physical, occupational, and speech therapy, skilled nursing care, medical social work services and aide services.

Payments to home health agencies are determined using a base payment adjusted for the geographical area where the services are provided. CMS uses a home health case-mix system, the Patient Driven Groupings Model (PDGM) to adjust payment for differences in patient characteristics. Cost outliers can also affect payment. The OASIS-D data set is used to collect the data needed to properly bill (MedPAC 2021).

## Patient Driven Groupings Model (PDGM)

During each 30-day period, the PDGM is used to categorizes each patient into one of 432 home health resource groups (HHRGs). The HHRGs are based on the source of admission, comorbidities that are present, the level of the patient's function (low, medium, or high), payment period timing (early or late), and the clinical category based on diagnoses or treatments provided. There are 12 clinical categories for which a patient is admitted to home health, for example, musculoskeletal or stroke rehabilitation, wound care, behavioral healthcare, or surgical aftercare. An early episode is the first 30-day payment period, and a late episode is any subsequent 30-day payment period. Each HHRG has a national relative weight that reflects the average costliness of patients in the group compared with the average Medicare home health patient (MedPAC 2021). Reimbursement can be increased by identifying high-cost outliers.

## High-cost Outliers

Outlier payments are used to mitigate the financial risk of care given to extremely high-cost cases. If a patient requires a high number of visits, the HHA may receive an outlier payment. To be eligible, actual costs must exceed the payment rate by an amount determined annually by CMS. If estimated costs exceed the outlier threshold, the HHA will receive an additional payment equal to 80 percent of the difference between the period payment with the threshold and the period's estimated costs.

## Outcome and Assessment Information Set

HHAs conduct all patient assessments using the Outcome and Assessment Information Set D (OASIS-D) data set. It was developed by CMS and consists of data elements that represent core items for the comprehensive assessment of an adult home care patient and form the basis for measuring patient outcomes for the purpose of outcome-based quality improvement (OBQI). OASIS-D is a key component of Medicare's partnership with the home care industry to foster and monitor improved home healthcare outcomes.

## Consolidated Billing

Home health agencies are subject to consolidated billing, which means that the agency provides and bills for all services offered to the patient. CMS established this mechanism to prevent double billing for services. For example, if a patient needs speech and language pathology therapy and does not have a professional on staff, the agency bills CMS for the services and contracts with a speech and language professional to provide the services. The agency pays the speech and language therapist; the therapist does not bill CMS for the services provided.

# Inpatient Rehabilitation Facility Prospective Payment System

The BBA (as amended by the Balanced Budget Refinement Act of 1999 [BBRA]) authorized implementation of a per-discharge PPS for care provided to Medicare beneficiaries by inpatient rehabilitation hospitals and rehabilitation units, referred to as IRFs. The PPS for IRFs became effective on January 1, 2002.

IRFs must meet the regulatory requirements to be classified as a rehabilitation hospital or rehabilitation unit excluded from the PPS for inpatient acute-care services. To meet the criteria, an IRF must operate as a hospital. Requirements state that during the most recent, consecutive, and appropriate 12-month time period, the hospital will have treated an inpatient population of whom at least 60 percent required intensive rehabilitative services for treatment of conditions such as stroke, spinal cord injury, congenital deformity, amputation, major multiple trauma, hip fracture, brain injuries, neurological disorders, burns, rheumatoid arthritis, osteoarthritis, polyarthritis, systemic vasculitides, or knee or hip replacement (CMS 2024c).

## Patient Assessment Instrument

IRFs are required by CMS to complete a patient assessment instrument (PAI) upon each patient's admission *and* discharge from the facility. These data are used in assessing clinical characteristics of patients in rehabilitation settings. Ultimately, they can be used to provide survey agencies with a means to objectively measure and compare facility performance and quality and allow researchers to develop improved standards of care. The Functional Independence Assessment is a major element of the PAI and includes data on 18 items which reflect the characteristics of the patient. Data on the cognitive and motor skills of the patient are collected.

The IRF PPS uses information from the IRF-PAI to classify patients into distinct groups based on clinical characteristics and expected resource needs. Data used to construct these groups, called case-mix groups (CMGs), include rehabilitation impairment categories (RICs), functional status (both motor and cognitive), age, comorbidities, and other factors deemed appropriate to improve the explanatory power of the groups.

### Case-Mix Group Relative Weight

An appropriate weight, called the case-mix group (CMG) relative weight, is assigned to each CMG and measures the relative difference in facility resource intensity among the various groups. A standard payment conversion factor is used to convert the CMG relative weight into payment. Comorbidity codes will impact final payment as well. Additional payments are calculated for each group, including the application of case- and facility-level adjustments. Facility-level adjustments include wage-index adjustments, low-income patient adjustments, and rural facility adjustments. Case-level adjustments include transfer adjustments, interrupted-stay adjustments, and high-cost outlier adjustments (CMS 2024c).

## Long-Term Care Hospital Prospective Payment System

The Balanced Budget Refinement Act (BBRA) of 1999 amended by the Benefits Improvement Act of 2000 mandated the establishment of a per-discharge, DRG-based PPS for longer-term care hospitals beginning October 1, 2002.

Long-term care hospitals (LTCHs) are defined as having an average inpatient LOS greater than 25 days (CMS 2024d). Typically, patients with the following conditions are treated in LTCHs:

- Chronic cardiac disorders
- Neuromuscular and neurovascular diseases such as after-effects of strokes or Parkinson's disease
- Infectious conditions requiring long-term care such as methicillin-resistant *staphylococcus aureus*
- Complex orthopedic conditions such as pelvic fractures or complicated hip fractures
- Wound care complications
- Multisystem organ failure
- Immunosuppressed conditions
- Respiratory failure and ventilation management and weaning
- Dysphagia management
- Postoperative complications
- Multiple intravenous therapies
- Chemotherapy
- Pre- and postoperative organ transplant care
- Chronic nutritional problems and total parenteral nutrition issues
- Spinal cord injuries
- Burns
- Head injuries

As with all PPSs, there are CMGs and adjustments.

### MS-LTC-DRGs

Patients are classified into distinct diagnosis groups based on clinical characteristics and expected resource use. These groups are based on the current inpatient MS-DRGs. The payment system includes the following three primary elements: patient classification into a MS-LTC-DRG weight; relative weight of the MS-LTC-DRG, as the weights reflect the variation in cost per discharge as they consider the utilization for each diagnosis; and federal payment rate. Payment is made at a predetermined per-discharge amount for each MS-LTC-DRG.

### Adjustments

The PPS provides for adjustments at the case (patient) level such as short-stay outliers, interrupted stays, and high-cost outliers. Facility-wide adjustments include area wage index and cost of living adjustments.

A short-stay outlier is an adjustment to the payment rate for stays that are considerably shorter than the average length of stay (ALOS) for a particular MS-LTC-DRG. A case would qualify for short-stay outlier status when the LOS is between one day and up to and including five-sixths of the ALOS for the MS-LTC-DRG. Both the ALOS and the five-sixths of the ALOS periods are published in the *Federal Register*. Payment under the short-stay outlier is made using different payment methodologies. (See table 6.7 for examples of MS-LTC-DRGs and the ALOS for each.)

An interrupted stay occurs when a patient is discharged from the LTCH and then is readmitted to the same facility for further treatment after a specific number of days away from the facility. There are different policies if the patient is readmitted to the facility within three days (called three-day or less interrupted-stay policy) or if the patient is away from the facility more than three days (called the greater than three-day interrupted-stay policy).

A high-cost outlier is an adjustment to the payment rate for a patient when the costs are unusually high and exceed the typical costs associated with a MS-LTC-DRG. High-cost outlier payments reduce the facility's potential financial losses that can result from treating patients who require more costly care than is normal. A case qualifies for a high-cost outlier payment when the estimated cost of care exceeds the high-cost outlier threshold, which is updated each year.

**Table 6.7.** Examples of MS-LTC-DRGs, relative weights, and geometric ALOS

| MS-LTC-DRG | Description | Relative weight | Geometric ALOS |
|---|---|---|---|
| 28 | Spinal procedures with MCC | .6366 | 19.3 |
| 114 | Orbital procedures w/o CC/MCC | .7813 | 21.1 |
| 150 | Epistaxis with MCC | 1.0424 | 26.9 |
| 163 | Major chest procedure with MCC | 2.9476 | 39.9 |
| 181 | Respiratory neoplasm with CC | .4545 | 15.7 |
| 194 | Simple pneumonia and pleurisy with MCC | .5534 | 16.42 |

*Source:* CMS 2024d.

## Check Your Understanding 6.3

**Answer the following questions in a separate document.**

1. What are the consequences of shifts in the CMI?
2. Summarize the major components of the RBRVS. Justify the difference between values for facility versus non-facility practice expenses.
3. Critique the appropriateness of the high-cost outlier threshold.
4. Evaluate the impact of POA on hospital reimbursement. Consider what policies would need to be addressed to receive appropriate reimbursement.
5. Compare the acute inpatient prospective payment system to the long-term care hospitals prospective payment system. Summarize the similarities and differences.
6. Summarize the similarities and differences between the Home Health Prospective Payment System and the Skilled Nursing Facility Prospective Payment System.

# References

AAFB (American Academy of Family Physicians). 2024. "Hierarchical Condition Category Coding." https://www.aafp.org/family-physician/practice-and-career/getting-paid/coding/hierarchical-condition-category.html.

AASCIF (American Association of State Compensation Insurance Funds). n.d. "About Us." Accessed July 18, 2024. https://www.aascif.org/.

Acumen. 2018. *Skilled Nursing Facilities Patient-Driven Payment Model Technical Report.* https://www.cms.gov/Medicare/Medicare-Fee-for-Service-Payment/SNFPPS/Downloads/PDPM_Technical_Report_508.pdf.

BCBS (Blue Cross Blue Shield). n.d. "The Blue Cross and Blue Shield System." Accessed October 31, 2023. https://www.bcbs.com/about-us/blue-cross-blue-shield-system.

CMS (Centers for Medicare and Medicaid Services). 2024a. "Medicare and You 2025." https://www.medicare.gov/Pubs/pdf/10050-medicare-and-you.pdf.

CMS (Centers for Medicare and Medicaid Services). 2024b. "FY 2024 IPPS Final Rule Home Page." https://www.cms.gov/medicare/payment/prospective-payment-systems/acute-inpatient-pps/fy-2024-ipps-final-rule-home-page#Tables.

CMS (Centers for Medicare and Medicaid Services). 2024c. "Inpatient Rehabilitation Facility PPS." https://www.cms.gov/medicare/payment/prospective-payment-systems/inpatient-rehabilitation.

CMS (Centers for Medicare and Medicaid Services). 2024d. "LTC-DRG Files." https://www.cms.gov/medicare/payment/prospective-payment-systems/long-term-care-hospital/drg-files.

CMS (Centers for Medicare and Medicaid Services). 2023a. "Inpatient Psychiatric Facility PPS." https://www.cms.gov/medicare/payment/prospective-payment-systems/inpatient-psychiatric-facility.

CMS (Centers for Medicare and Medicaid Services). 2023b. "RVU23A." https://www.cms.gov/medicare/medicare-fee-service-payment/physicianfeesched/pfs-relative-value-files/rvu23a.

CMS (Centers for Medicare and Medicaid Services). 2019. *Fact Sheet: PDPM Patient Classification.* https://www.cms.gov/medicare/medicare-fee-for

-service-payment/snfpps/downloads/pdpm_fact_sheet_template_payment-overview_v5.zip.

CMS (Centers for Medicare and Medicaid Services). n.d.a. "Medicaid Eligibility." Accessed October 31, 2023. https://www.medicaid.gov/medicaid/eligibility/index.html.

CMS (Centers for Medicare and Medicaid Services). n.d.b. "Medicaid." Accessed October 31, 2023. https://www.medicaid.gov/medicaid/benefits/mandatory-optional-medicaid-benefits/index.html.

CMS (Centers for Medicare and Medicaid Services). n.d.c. "Program of All-Inclusive Care for the Elderly." Accessed October 31, 2023. https://www.medicaid.gov/medicaid/long-term-services-supports/program-all-inclusive-care-elderly/index.html.

CMS (Centers for Medicare and Medicaid Services). n.d.d. "Children's Health Insurance Program." Accessed October 31, 2023. https://www.medicaid.gov/chip/index.html.

CMS (Centers for Medicare and Medicaid Services). n.d.e. "Children's Health Insurance Program. Benefits." Accessed October 31, 2023. https://www.medicaid.gov/chip/benefits/index.html.

CMS (Centers for Medicare and Medicaid Services). n.d.f. "Accountable Care and Accountable Care Organizations." Accessed October 31, 2023. https://www.cms.gov/priorities/innovation/key-concepts/accountable-care-and-accountable-care-organizations.

CMS (Centers for Medicare and Medicaid Services). n.d.g. "Hospital-acquired Conditions." Accessed May 22, 2024. https://www.cms.gov/medicare/payment/fee-for-service-providers/hospital-aquired-conditions-hac.

DHA (Defence Health Agency). 2023. "Tricare 101." https://tricare.mil/Plans/New.

DOL (US Department of Labor). n.d. "Workers' Compensation." Accessed May 21, 2024. https://www.dol.gov/general/topic/workcomp.

Falkson, S., and V. Srinivasan. 2023. "Health Maintenance Organization." National Library of Medicine. https://www.ncbi.nlm.nih.gov/books/NBK554454/.

HealthCare.gov. n.d. "Risk Adjustment. Glossary." Accessed October 31, 2023. https://www.healthcare.gov/glossary/risk-adjustment/.

IHS (Indian Health Service). n.d. "About IHS." Accessed October 31, 2023. https://www.ihs.gov/aboutihs/.

IMO (Intelligent Medical Objects). n.d. "HCC 101: What You Need to Know about Hierarchical Condition Categories." Accessed May 22, 2024. https://www.imohealth.com/ideas/article/hcc-101-what-you-need-to-know-about-hierarchical-condition-categories/.

Mayo Clinic. n.d. "Medicare Accountable Care Organization (ACO) Frequently Asked Questions." Accessed July 19, 2024. https://www.mayoclinic.org/about-mayo-clinic/aco/frequently-asked-questions.

Medicare Interactive. n.d. "How Medicare works with Medicaid." Accessed July 20, 2024. https://www.medicareinteractive.org/get-answers/cost-saving-programs-for-people-with-medicare/medicare-and-medicaid/how-medicaid-works-with-medicare.

MedPAC (Medicare Payment Advisory Commission). 2021. "Home Health Care Services Payment System." https://www.medpac.gov/wp-content/uploads/2021/11/medpac_payment_basics_21_hha_final_sec.pdf.

NCQA (National Committee for Quality Assurance). n.d. Accessed October 31, 2023. https://www.ncqa.org/.

Noridian Healthcare Solutions. 2023. "OPPS Payment Status Indicators." https://med.noridianmedicare.com/web/jea/provider-types/opps/opps-payment-status-indicators.

UHC (United Healthcare). n.d. "What Is a Health Reimbursement Account." Accessed May 21, 2024. https://www.uhc.com/understanding-health-insurance/understanding-health-insurance-costs/health-reimbursement-accounts.

VA (Veterans Health Administration). 2024. "Veterans Health Administration." https://www.va.gov/health/.

VA (Veterans Health Administration). 2023a. "About VA Health Benefits." https://www.va.gov/health-care/about-va-health-benefits/.

VA (Veterans Health Administration). 2023b. "Camp Lejeune Water Contamination Health Issues." https://www.va.gov/disability/eligibility/hazardous-materials-exposure/camp-lejeune-water-contamination/.

VA (US Department of Veterans Affairs). 2022. "Health Care for Spouses, Dependents, and Family Caregivers." https://www.va.gov/health-care/family-caregiver-benefits/.

42 CFR 414.605. 2019. Definitions. https://www.ecfr.gov/current/title-42/chapter-IV/subchapter-B/part-414/subpart-H.

# chapter 7

# Revenue Cycle Management

*Lauree Handlon, MHA, RHIA, CCS, CHCRS, CRCR, CSAF, FAHIMA, FHFMA*

## Learning Objectives

- Evaluate the key processes in each phase of the revenue life cycle from patient access to claims adjudication
- Evaluate the impact of case management and utilization management on the revenue cycle
- Build a successful denial management program
- Evaluate the purpose of revenue cycle support services
- Utilize key performance indicators to measure operations
- Assess various opportunities for integration of artificial intelligence on each revenue cycle process

## Key Terms

Accounts receivable (A/R) days
Advance beneficiary notice of noncoverage (ABN)
Adverse determination
Artificial intelligence (AI)
Bill hold period
Case management
Charge capture
Charge description master (CDM)
Charity care
Claims adjudication
Claims scrubber software
Clean claims
Denial
Discharged, not final billed (DNFB)
Electronic remittance advice (ERA)
Explanation of benefits (EOB)
Financial counselor
Hospital-issued notice of noncoverage (HINN)
Insurance verification
Integrated Outpatient Code Editor (IOCE)
Key performance indicators (KPIs)
Local coverage determinations (LCDs)
MAP Keys
Medical necessity
Medically unlikely edits (MUEs)
Medicare administrative contractor (MAC)
Medicare code editor (MCE)
National Correct Coding Initiative (NCCI)
National coverage determinations (NCDs)
No Surprises Act (NSA) of 2022
Physician credentialing
Point-of-service (POS) collection
Preauthorization
Precertification
Remittance advice (RA)
Revenue cycle
Revenue cycle management (RCM)
Utilization management (UM)

Financial viability is critical for healthcare organizations to provide the services necessary to treat patients. For an organization to fund its purpose, many key financial activities are required to flow efficiently. Without efficient and effective processes to manage the entire life of a patient account, healthcare organizations will struggle to achieve successfully functioning revenue cycle operations.

The **revenue cycle** refers to the sequence of processes to progress a patient account from creation to closing. Healthcare **revenue cycle management (RCM)** refers to the strategy implemented to direct administrative and clinical functions associated with capturing, monitoring, and collecting patient service revenue. In practice, RCM involves balancing people, tools, methodologies, technology, and the environment in which the processes occur. For many years, organizations approached the revenue cycle as a segmented process and operated as independent, nonrelated departments, creating significant communication and organizational effectiveness challenges. However, for healthcare organizations to succeed, all revenue cycle contributors must understand the big picture, collaborate, regularly and promptly communicate, and work cohesively to ensure revenue moves efficiently. Today's RCM needs industry-wide collaboration to place patient interactions and quality care at the center of the RCM processes (HFMA 2018). The revenue life cycle can be broken down into three general phases: the front end, middle, and back end (see figure 7.1).

The term *revenue cycle* suggests the patient account flow is cyclical. While the life of an individual patient account flows through specific stages from beginning to end, successful operations require that patient accounts continuously progress through the cycle. The patient account process involves numerous steps, moving from scheduling or registration through payment adjudication (determination of payment from the payer) and account closure, affected by interrelated operations along the way. Figure 7.2 illustrates the flow of an individual patient account through the healthcare revenue cycle. The typical account flow shown applies to both inpatient and outpatient settings.

**Figure 7.1.** Revenue management life cycle

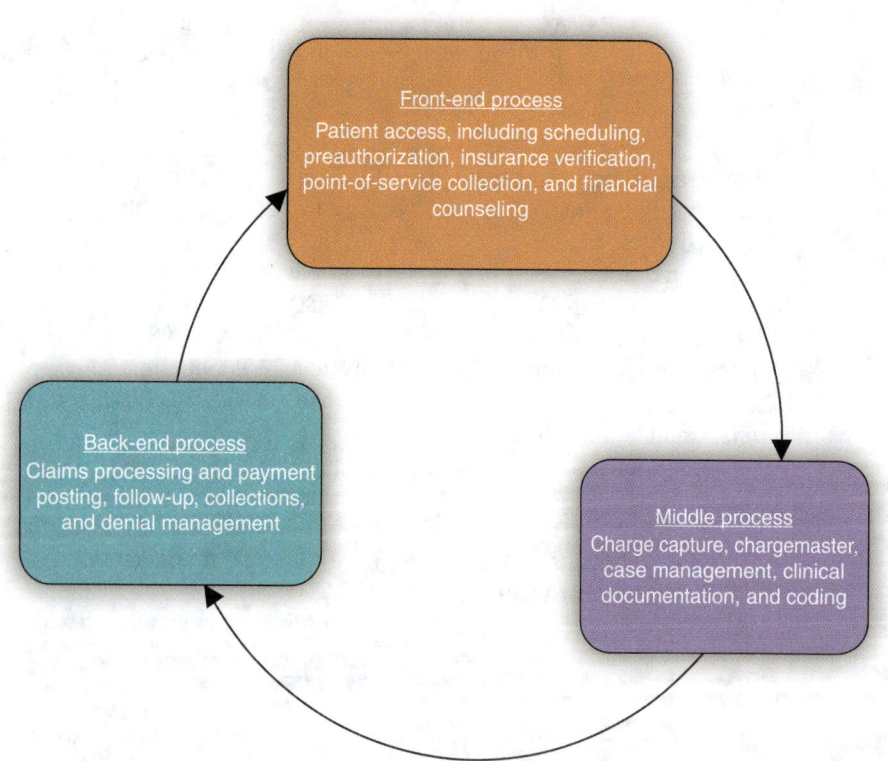

**Figure 7.2.** Healthcare revenue cycle for an individual account

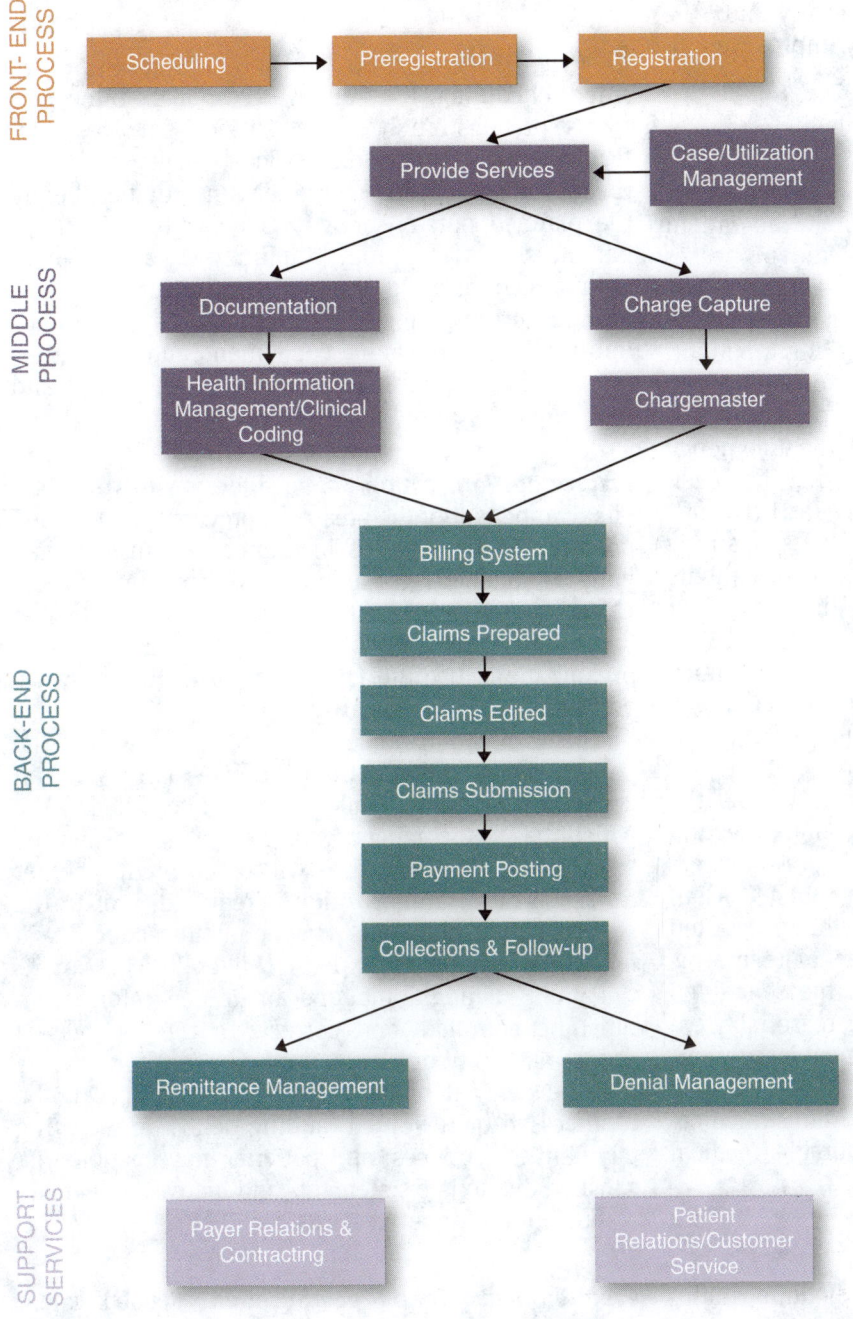

## Revenue Cycle Front-End Process

The front end of the healthcare revenue cycle starts at the point of scheduling a patient for healthcare services or when the patient presents for nonscheduled services. During this phase, healthcare organizations must establish the payment source for services rendered, follow requirements specified by the payer, accurately collect the patient's demographic information, and ensure a positive patient experience. The best opportunity to improve the overall revenue cycle process occurs during the patient access stage with accurately identifying, scheduling, and registering patients (LaPointe 2021). Many organizations are enhancing the front-end process operations through automation efforts and applying artificial intelligence (AI) techniques. AI integrates seamlessly into the healthcare revenue cycle processes by improving efficiencies and supporting quality of care (Montroy and Rakes 2022).

## Patient Access Components

Patient access represents the stage where the patient encounter is initiated and involves the processes of scheduling, preregistration, and registration. The flow of the patient account through the revenue cycle begins with scheduling and registering a patient, except in emergency visit situations. For emergency situations, depending on their severity, patients could be registered at different points during the emergency department (ED) encounter. Scheduling, however, is excluded from the cycle completely for ED visits. Initiating the registration function during scheduling saves time and is often more convenient for patients when they arrive for services. Each time a patient presents for clinical services, the data collected during previous encounters must be verified for accuracy and updated to address any changes to prevent registration errors. The accuracy of information captured in the patient access stage is vital to many of the processes occurring later in the revenue cycle, and the goal is to continuously improve the data collection and accuracy. During this stage, healthcare providers are required under the **No Surprises Act (NSA) of 2022** to prepare good faith estimates when requested for uninsured patients. The good faith estimate informs the patient of the charges related to the scheduled care, describing the items and services reasonably expected to be delivered. The estimate must be presented in a single, comprehensive format and the items or services may include charges for procedures, medical tests, supplies, prescription drugs, durable medical equipment, or encounter fees (CMS 2022a).

### Scheduling

Patient access staff responsible for scheduling functions must have significant knowledge regarding data collection requirements, including insurance carrier conditions and provider preferences. The scheduling function involves setting the patient's appointment and creating an account to prepare for the clinical visit and subsequent billing for the visit. The scheduler tells the patient what information to bring to the visit, the expected copayment or deductible at the time of the visit, what time to arrive for the visit, and any additional administrative information to be completed at the time of registration. Accurate communication is essential to beginning the visit efficiently, enhancing patient satisfaction, and initiating appropriate revenue-generating processes.

### Preregistration

After scheduling, the patient access team often performs preregistration. Preregistration involves confirming eligibility and insurance benefits, including preauthorization and precertification activities, before the planned date-of-service visit. During this stage, patient access staff may remind the patient about the planned visit. Other administrative functions performed during preregistration are updating insurance information, confirming copayment and deductible information, screening for medical necessity, and ensuring all required referrals are on file.

*Insurance Verification* **Insurance verification** is a vital component of the prearrival process for scheduled patients. Verification of insurance for unscheduled patients, such as those patients presenting to the ED or urgent care, occurs at the time of registration for clinical services or shortly thereafter. Many organizations institute a policy requiring ED insurance verification after medical screening.

The verification process entails validating that the patient is a member of the insurance plan given and is covered for the scheduled service date, whether the patient has forthcoming coverage changes, whether the scheduled service expenses will be covered, whether a referral or an authorization is required prior to the service being rendered and whether the patient will incur an out-of-pocket expense (Miller 2023).

Patient demographic and insurance information must be complete and correct. In the absence of proper eligibility determination, payment for services may be delayed or denied; claims may need to be reprocessed or reworked, adding delays in receiving payment for services; and patients may become dissatisfied due to late statements and increased financial responsibility for services (Reiner 2018).

*Preauthorization and Precertification* Reimbursement for services without preauthorization and precertification are frequent reasons for denial by insurers (Optum 2023). **Preauthorization**, or prior authorization, occurs when the provider obtains permission to provide the service from the insurance carrier, usually to ensure the patient has the benefits available. **Precertification** is when the insurance carrier must review the proposed service or procedure and approve it as medically necessary before payment will be granted to the provider.

Insurers have established more stringent approval guidelines to address increases in high-technology and high-cost procedures and tests. For example, if a physician orders a fluorodeoxyglucose (FDG) positron emission tomography (PET) for a Medicare patient, the Centers for Medicare and Medicaid Services (CMS) provides a list of oncological conditions that must be present to receive payment for the FDG-PET service (CMS 2014). This example reflects the precertification action to verify specific requirements for payment coverage.

Patient access teams must understand medical procedures and tests, initial diagnoses, and scheduled treatments to obtain the necessary preauthorization or precertification by the insurance company. Complex rules and regulations surround preauthorization requirements and criteria may vary widely among payers (Ingrao 2019). Therefore, it is important for healthcare providers to have current lists of procedures and tests requiring prior authorization from all health insurers and have processes in place to obtain the authorization prior to services being rendered.

***Medical Necessity Coverage Issues*** During the preregistration process, patients are screened for medical necessity. Health insurance companies provide coverage only for health-related services they define or establish to be medically necessary. The American Medical Association (AMA) defines medical necessity as

> Health care services or products that a prudent physician would provide to a patient for the purpose of preventing, diagnosing or treating an illness, injury, disease or its symptoms in a manner that is: (a) in accordance with generally accepted standards of medical practice; (b) clinically appropriate in terms of type, frequency, extent, site, and duration; and (c) not primarily for the economic benefit of the health plans and purchasers or for the convenience of the patient, treating physician, or other health care provider. (AMA 2023)

The AMA has developed application of its definition of medical necessity into a medical review policy. The principles of the AMA's explanation and its recommended use are shown in figure 7.3.

Medicare defines **medical necessity** as a determination that a service is reasonable and necessary for the related diagnosis or treatment of illness or injury (CMS n.d.a). Therefore, Medicare coverage is limited to items and services considered reasonable and necessary for the diagnosis or treatment of the patient's condition. Medicare's national coverage policies are known as **national coverage determinations (NCDs)**, and local **Medicare Administrative Contractor (MAC)** policies are known as **local coverage determinations (LCDs)**. A MAC is a private healthcare insurer awarded by Medicare for a geographic jurisdiction for multistate or regional contractor responsibilities to process Medicare Part A and Part B (A/B) medical claims. NCD or LCD policies are not available for every type of procedure or service that could be provided for a patient. Therefore, healthcare organizations must maintain knowledge of current regulatory requirements and revisions to reduce billing denials and ensure payment is received for the services rendered. Without an NCD, or if an NCD requires further clarification, MACs may develop an LCD to cover an item or service.

Providers are required to issue an **advance beneficiary notice of noncoverage (ABN)** to Medicare patients when Medicare is not likely to provide coverage. An ABN is a written notice to inform patients when an outpatient item or service is not considered reasonable and necessary or may not be covered. By signing the ABN, the patient is accepting financial responsibility if the insurer denies payment. The patient may not be held financially liable if the patient does not receive written notice represented by

**Figure 7.3.** Definition and application of medical necessity

1. Practice of the term "medical necessity" must be consistent between the medical profession and the insurance industry.
2. Payer denials for non-covered services should clearly state so and not confuse this with a determination of lack of medical necessity.
3. Providers are encouraged to carefully review their health plan medical services agreements to ensure that they do not contain definitions of medical necessity that emphasize cost and resource utilization above quality and clinical effectiveness.
4. Private sector health care accreditation organizations are encouraged to develop and incorporate standards that prohibit the use of definitions of medical necessity that emphasize cost and resource utilization above quality and clinical effectiveness.
5. Determinations of medical necessity shall be based only on information that is available at the time that health care products or services are provided.

*Source:* Adapted from AMA 2023.

the ABN when required (CMS 2022b). A **hospital-issued notice of noncoverage (HINN)** may be provided to patients when an inpatient service has been deemed noncovered due to medical necessity (CMS 2023a). HINNs can be issued at any point prior to or during a hospital admission. Since inpatient medical necessity determination may not always occur during the front-end process, the discussion of HINNs is continued later in this chapter. Resources to support specific requirements include payer billing manuals, Medicare billing manuals, and local MAC policies.

## Registration

The registration stage, also referred to as admissions, begins when the patient arrives for the visit. The patient access team should confirm the patient's demographic information, make copies of the patient's insurance card and driver's license or other government-issued ID to verify identity, initiate financial counseling if applicable, collect copayment or deductible amounts, and obtain the patient's signature for insurance payment, patient consent, and often for release of medical information. Another important registration function is avoiding duplicating the health record number, account number, or patient identification when the patient encounter file is originated. Key fields gathered during the patient access stage to assist in uniquely identifying an individual include full name (first, middle, last), former names, date of birth, Social Security number, residence, gender, marital status, race and ethnicity, employer, insurance carrier, and guarantor (person considered responsible for the patient's bill). Collecting complete patient information enhances registration accuracy. When registration accuracy improves, organizations experience an improved revenue cycle overall (Cohen et al. 2019). The most common registration errors are:

- Punctuation errors with hyphens or apostrophes
- Use of maiden or marital names
- Name changes
- Misspelled name
- Incorrect address/phone number
- Incorrect or missing date of birth
- Policy number/health insurance number missing or invalid
- Physician orders incomplete or missing
- Transcription errors (for example, language barriers during the registration process)
- Multiple medical record numbers per patient (Cohen et al. 2019)

When registration errors arise, the organization should focus on detecting the root cause, correcting the actions that create errors, and implementing prevention techniques.

*Financial Counseling* A healthcare organization must ensure the patient understands the financial aspects of his or her care encounter and the process for resolving any fiscal responsibility. **Financial counselors** are staff dedicated to helping patients and physicians determine sources of reimbursement for healthcare services. The counselors are responsible for identifying and verifying the method of payment and debt resolution for services rendered to patients. Counselors must understand a patient's financial assets and discuss payment alternatives with patients. Some patients are eligible for **charity care**, which is defined as healthcare services that have been or will be provided but are never expected to result in cash inflows. Charity care results from a provider's policy to provide healthcare services free or at a discount to individuals who meet the criteria each organization establishes (Levinson et al. 2022). The counselors can establish payment options such as credit card payments, bank loans, and interest-bearing, hospital-funded payment arrangements as necessary.

Strategies for financial counselors can include the ability to provide discounts on hospital bills for patients who do not have health insurance and who meet certain eligibility criteria. The discount amount is determined after an assessment of the patient's or a family's financial need and is typically based on current federal poverty guidelines. Incentives for prompt-payment discounts can also be offered to patients. Healthcare facilities must follow consistent procedures and steps to obtain appropriate payment and to enhance revenue cycle processes (Stewart 2017).

*Point-of-Service Collection* Patients have taken on greater financial responsibility for their healthcare costs. The patient financial portion represents approximately 30 percent of total net patient revenue (Sanborn 2018). **Point-of-service (POS) collection** is the collection of the portion of the bill that is the patient's responsibility to pay prior to the provision of service being rendered. The patient's responsibility is the cost-sharing portion, which could involve a deductible amount in addition to a copayment or coinsurance amount. All payment collection amounts are determined based on the service to be provided and the insurance coverage of the patient's plan.

POS collection works well with scheduled and non-emergent patient visits. Access to billing data from both payers and the healthcare's own system is necessary to estimate what a patient owes at the point of service. Patient access teams must communicate with the patient to set expectations regarding the cost of the services, insurance coverage, and the expected payment at the time of service. ED POS collections tend to be more challenging in some situations due to the nature of the visit and the patient's diminished ability to interact. While the patient is informed about financial responsibility after the medical screening, the request for payment for ED visits often does not occur until services are complete and the patient is to be discharged.

### Pre-encounter Services

Many healthcare facilities have combined patient access team resources related to the revenue cycle front-end process and developed comprehensive pre-encounter service centers for specific outpatient services. The centers handle scheduling, preregistration, insurance eligibility and benefit verification, payer authorizations, and POS collections for all scheduled diagnostic testing and surgery patients. Healthcare organizations that have developed goals to streamline workflows and performance characteristics are set to support front-end processes such as the following:

- All areas performing registration functions will follow standardized policies and procedures
- Approved services require preregistration of the patient
- All patients will be contacted by phone at a minimum of five days prior to the appointment

- Estimation of patient out-of-pocket responsibilities will be determined using real-time tools
- Payment plan options will be personalized to each patient's ability to pay
- Uninsured patients will be connected with available financial assistance programs when appropriate (Barton and Shelton 2018)

Combining the front-end processes can eliminate last-minute cancellations of scheduled services, improve patient flow, and increase patient satisfaction. An additional front-end approach producing significant advances in front-end processes is incorporating **artificial intelligence (AI)**. AI is high-level information technologies used in developing machines that imitate human qualities such as learning and reasoning. Front-end processes benefit primarily from using AI in prior authorization, registration, eligibility, and medical necessity through data validation and scrubbing techniques (LaPointe 2023). Even encounter-level payment estimations are being generated by AI. Through access to numerous data sources, AI can rapidly identify errors and opportunities for complete health information, ultimately saving time and resources on downstream issues that stem from front-end process challenges. In addition, AI enriches front-end staff training and provides necessary answers to complex issues in a fraction of the typical resource time (LaPointe 2023).

### Check Your Understanding 7.1

**Answer the following questions in a separate document.**

1. Compare the revenue cycle and revenue cycle management (RCM). What is the key differentiator between them? What would you suggest as a best practice approach to RCM success?

2. A newly hired registration professional notices that registration processes produce incorrect patient information. What are some strategies to reduce the occurrence of duplicate patient record registration errors?

3. The financial counselor is meeting with a patient struggling to pay for an emergency appendectomy last month. How can strategies be prioritized for the counselor in considering how to obtain appropriate payment for services provided to the patient?

4. Evaluate common registration errors and provide rationales for why such errors may occur. Suggest at least three solutions to prevent them from happening. Consider your own healthcare experiences to help formulate your answer.

5. The patient access staff is scheduling a patient for bariatric surgery. What actions should the staff take before completing registration for the patient for this procedure to be performed? Why are those actions important to the provider? Evaluate the choices to be made if the bariatric procedure was not a benefit under the patient's insurance plan.

6. The director of the patient access department has requested your assistance with creating the provider's pre-encounter service center for outpatient same-day surgeries. She specifically tasked you with point-of-service (POS) collections. What are at least two performance characteristics you would recommend to the director to support the integration of this front-end process? Suggest additional performance characteristics for POS collection and explain why these selections would benefit the organization in this type of environment.

# Revenue Cycle Middle Process

The middle process of the healthcare revenue cycle represents the intersection of clinical practice, documentation, and coding with charge capture to bill for services provided. The middle process also includes case and utilization management. The key objective of this phase is to ensure that captured clinical and charge information is accurate, complete, compliant, and timely.

## Clinical Services

As the clinical team and the patient interact while services are delivered, information is documented about the encounter. The patient's visit with the clinical team becomes the basis of the remaining processes within the revenue cycle. The clinical documentation recorded in the patient's health record establishes a means of communication about the services rendered and this communication is an essential foundation of reimbursement to the provider.

## Clinical Documentation

Clinical documentation is the foundation for communication—clinically, legally, and financially. Complete, accurate, and timely documentation of patient encounters are important aspects of the revenue cycle. Clinicians must document the services performed and the medical necessity of the services, and staff must verify the charges match the services being performed prior to bill submission. CMS regulations require adequate documentation to support payment for reported care provided to the patient (CMS 2023b). To comply with these regulations, hospitals have placed an increased focus on clinical documentation management and coding practices due to their direct impact on the healthcare facility's revenue.

Healthcare providers have invested in clinical documentation integrity (CDI) programs to ensure the health record accurately reflects the patient's actual condition. A focus on appropriate clinical documentation reduces the risk of incomplete and unclear documentation, resulting in lost revenue for the healthcare facility. Accurate and thorough clinical documentation that is properly coded and billed to payers results in benefits such as increased third-party payer billing compliance, improved quality reporting to external parties, and increased revenues by applying the most appropriate clinical codes and minimizing denials. Physician documentation enhancements can be gained through AI-assisted speech recognition and formatting support. Using AI with documentation ultimately creates efficiencies in coding as accurate information reduces the need for queries (Montroy and Rakes 2022).

## Case Management and Utilization Management

As focus shifts to value in the healthcare industry, case management and utilization management (UM) have significantly progressed. Delivering the appropriate care at the appropriate time in the appropriate patient setting while reflecting the appropriate cost is key to the concept of successful case and utilization management (Mehrabian 2018).

The Case Management Society of America (CMSA) defines **case management** as "a means for achieving client wellness and autonomy through advocacy, communication, education, identification of service resources and service facilitation" (CMSA n.d.). The American Case Management Association (ACMA) and the Commission for Case Manager Certification (CCMC) defines case management as follows:

> A dynamic process that assesses, plans, implements, coordinates, monitors, and evaluates to improve outcomes, experiences, and value. The practice of case management is professional and collaborative, occurring in a variety of settings where medical care, mental health care, and social supports are delivered. Services are facilitated by diverse disciplines in conjunction with the care recipient and their support system. In pursuit of health equity, priorities include identifying needs, ensuring appropriate access to resources/services, addressing social determinants of health and facilitating safe care transitions. Professional case managers help navigate complex systems to achieve mutual goals, advocate for those they serve, and recognize personal dignity, autonomy, and the right to self-determination. (ACMA n.d.)

The CMSA, ACMA, and CCMC support professionals, called case managers, who evaluate the appropriateness of hospital admissions according to preestablished criteria, are assigned to a patient during their stay, remain with the patient during their care to ensure their medical and psychosocial needs are appropriately being met, and assist in facilitation of ongoing needs after discharge.

Case managers' responsibilities were initially to manage and ensure the appropriate utilization of acute-care resources, focusing on improving quality and reducing costs. The case manager assumes many roles, including patient advocate, assessor, and educator, and the role has evolved to include the following:

- Supporting continuity of care by providing individualized care coordination through identified cost-effective pathways
- Performing as an intra-interprofessional intermediary by communicating disease management programs, outcomes assessment, and complex health management
- Championing as a care manager by representing the patient and their families with the care team (De Luca et al. 2022)

These responsibilities allow the case managers to quickly identify barriers that may impede the efficient progression of the patient through the healthcare service process. Case and utilization management assessments could occur at various stages in the revenue cycle process as assessments involve prospective, concurrent, and retrospective reviews. A prospective review occurs prior to services being performed and some aspects of case and utilization management, such as the preauthorization and prior authorization activities, are integrated into the registration process. Concurrent reviews occur during the care episode. Retrospective reviews occur after services have been rendered and generally are focused on the setting and timing of the services provided (LaPointe 2018). Therefore, case management and utilization management activities may occur in all revenue cycle processes. However, most often, the actions of case and utilization management assessments support the middle-process at the time the patient is being treated.

**Utilization management (UM)** is a collection of systems and processes to ensure that facilities and resources, both human and nonhuman, are used maximally and are consistent with patient care needs. UM works in conjunction with case management and the terms and responsibilities sometimes are used interchangeably. Healthcare UM is a planned, systematic review of patients receiving healthcare services against criteria for appropriateness of services being provided as well as admission, continued stay, and discharge planning. Evidence-based, decision support criteria from Milliman, InterQual, and similar clinical intelligence support are essential to any UM program. These decision support solutions provide objective criteria to assist the UM staff in determining appropriate care. UM ensures that benefits a payer provides are effectively used. The UM staff is responsible for the day-to-day provisions of the hospital's utilization plan, which is also a requirement of the Medicare Conditions of Participation.

The UM staff works with external quality improvement organizations who are under the direction of CMS to support the quality of patient care and services. UM also collaborates with third-party reviewers to manage the provision of requested clinical information, facilitate access to health records, supervise external insurance reviewers, and ensure effective communication to patients and their families based on direction from the external review organizations.

According to CMS, hospitals have the responsibility to issue HINNs to Medicare beneficiaries prior to admission, at admission, or at any point during an inpatient stay if the hospital determines that the care the beneficiary is receiving, or is about to receive, is not covered for one of the following reasons:

- Is not medically necessary
- Is not delivered in the most appropriate setting
- Is custodial in nature (CMS 2023a)

Medicaid requirements for notification of denial of care or termination of benefits vary from state to state. Additionally, many commercial payers also establish specific guidelines, and many commercial payers publish UM guideline workbooks for providers as a general educational tool to assist with compliance and formulation of a utilization program. The healthcare facility's UM program should include federal, state, and commercial payer specific requirements. Commercial payers are responsible for providing written documentation to the patient or the patient's family, attending physician, and facility of an **adverse determination**. Adverse determinations represent when a healthcare insurer denies payment for proposed or already rendered healthcare service. Payers work with the hospital department responsible for UM to communicate the decision. Case and utilization management programs assist providers with delivering high-quality, cost-efficient care and are a critical element to successful revenue cycle operations.

## Health Information Management and Clinical Coding

The health information management (HIM) professional performs a variety of functions, but the primary one related to the revenue cycle involves code assignment. HIM professionals are responsible for reviewing clinical documentation and assigning clinical codes. Table 7.1 illustrates the categories of HIPAA-approved code sets used in clinical coding by provider type, setting, and patient type to be reported to both public and private payers.

The process of human interaction with assessing clinical documentation and selecting code assignment

**Table 7.1.** Code set by provider, by setting, by patient type

| Provider | Inpatient | | Outpatient | |
| --- | --- | --- | --- | --- |
| | Diagnosis | Procedure | Diagnosis | Procedure |
| Physician/Professional | ICD-10-CM | HCPCS (Level I = CPT & Level II) | ICD-10-CM | HCPCS (Level I = CPT & Level II) |
| Facility/Hospital | ICD-10-CM | ICD-10-PCS | ICD-10-CM | HCPCS (Level I = CPT & Level II) |

is often referred to as "soft coding" as opposed to "hard coding." Experienced, well-trained coding professionals ensure accurate and complete code assignment and optimum reimbursement. Coding professionals must be skilled at reading through documentation in a variety of different forms and formats and interpreting that documentation to arrive at the correct code assignment. When documentation is vague or ambiguous, querying the provider for clarification is necessary. The provider query process (often referred to as the physician query process) can create significant delays in the revenue cycle when the coder must wait for the physician's response to complete coding.

Third-party payers generally will not reimburse a claim that does not include the clinical diagnostic and procedural codes. This is true whether the reimbursement is based on a prospective payment system (PPS), actual charges, or some other method. For this reason, the patient accounts department cannot drop a bill until the patient record has been coded. Therefore, timely, accurate coding is critical to the reimbursement process and directly affects the facility's cash flow.

A bill cannot be generated until the coding is complete, so organizations routinely monitor the **discharged, not final billed (DNFB)** days. Generally, this is done by reviewing the DNFB report that includes all patients who have been discharged from the facility, but for whom the billing process is not complete. The goal for an efficient revenue cycle is to eliminate any backlog of uncoded charts and to complete the coding process within the number of bill hold days the organization has established.

Clinical documentation completeness and code assignment accuracy can influence a facility's case-mix index (CMI). By missing diagnoses or procedures that should be coded, or failing to assign the most specific code possible, the coding professionals can cause the CMI to be lower than it should be. The CMI allows an organization to compare the cost of providing care with the mix of patients in relation to other hospitals. While computer-assisted coding (CAC) has been available for some time, AI further enriches the coding process by applying coding guidelines in conjunction with documentation review, producing codes readily available by each encounter for a professional to review for accuracy instead of generating all the codes manually. As with the other revenue cycle processes, AI enhances middle-process staff training and supports learning by delivering critical responses to questions in minimal time (LaPointe 2023).

## Charge Capture

**Charge capture** is a method of recording services and supplies or items delivered to the patient and directing them to be billed on a claim form. It is the process of documenting, posting, and reconciling the charges for services rendered to patients. For example, consider a patient who is seen in the ED. The patient is assessed, appropriate services (such as laboratory tests and x-rays) are determined, and medications are provided. The time spent with the patient during the assessment corresponds to an evaluation and management charge, and the radiology charge for x-ray, laboratory charges depending on the tests provided, and then pharmacy charges for medications administered during the visit. The recording of charges is used for a variety of purposes including reimbursement, tracking utilization, and monitoring inventory. While clinical staff may not view charge capture as a priority, it is important to recognize and ensure clinical staff and charge capture efforts work toward the same purpose, which is to sustain the organization's mission of caring for patients (NAHRI 2018). Organizational success directly depends on accurately documenting and reporting charges in a timely manner; and the aim is to have policies, procedures, and resources in place to ensure quality charge capture that enhances revenue and adheres to compliance and other standards.

Quality charge capture is critical for the following reasons:

- Payments are often related to charges; reimbursement for outpatient services is often driven by the specific charges along with Current Procedural Terminology (CPT) and Healthcare Common Procedure Coding System (HCPCS) codes listed on the claim.

- Charges drive prices and rates for reimbursement; payment rates established for diagnosis-related groups (DRGs) and ambulatory patient classifications (APCs) are determined by analyzing historical cost data; if true costs are not being reflected, reimbursement rates are set too low.
- Charges reflect resource utilization; this allows analysis and comparison of the resources used for patients with similar diagnoses treated in similar service lines or receiving similar treatments.
- Charges help with measuring labor cost and productivity; this assists the organization in monitoring the cost of doing business and determining staffing needs.
- Errors in charge capture create significant rework and billing delays; errors may also go undetected and result in loss of revenue or put the organization at risk by not meeting regulatory requirements.

A variety of charge capture mechanisms may be in place to enter charges in the billing system. Charges are captured electronically or manually, but generally the electronic health record (EHR) integrates charges directly from the documented services. Additional interfaces from source systems used in areas such as a lab or pharmacy that submit large volumes of charges contribute to the complete charge capture of the services provided to patients. EHR systems may also be configured to apply charges to patient accounts, and HIM coding staff often has responsibility for some charge entry based on clinical documentation. A common situation where HIM coding staff could be accountable for some charge entry is with surgical procedures in the ED. Some providers may place the responsibility of procedure service, such as a wound repair or fracture repair, on the HIM department to not only code the service but also select the corresponding charge for that service based on the provider charge criteria. Regardless of the mechanism for charge entry, it is important to verify the accuracy of the charge codes being entered and ensure they are posted to the correct patient accounts for the correct dates of service.

The primary responsibility for charge capture is assigned to staff in the departments providing the services. However, complex regulatory requirements surround compliant charge capture, so ongoing charge capture education with well-documented policies and procedures is vital. Many organizations refer to the department or program responsible for overseeing charge capture processes as revenue integrity. Revenue integrity is an approach in which organizations prioritize efforts to maximize warranted reimbursement operationally through a legally and contractually compliant business strategy. Revenue integrity success depends on the strategy implemented involving process, teams, and technology. Related departments such as HIM, CDI, quality improvement, and RCM, must commit to transparency with activities associated with charge capture and collaborate with the revenue integrity program team. Proven success involves evaluating and managing coding and billing accuracy issues early in the revenue cycle.

One of the most prominent examples of common challenges with revenue integrity involves pharmaceuticals. Medication dosage versus billing descriptions often differ requiring approaches to ensure the coding in the chargemaster is representative of the medications provided. Many pharmaceutical items are crucial reimbursement risk areas where the code description is different than the common dosage and requires a conversion factor to be billed and paid appropriately. For example, Keytruda, a common medication used to treat melanoma, is reported with HCPCS code J9271. The code description is for an injection of 1 milligram. The recommended dosage is 200 milligrams. Consider if a hospital has the charge set up for this medication based on the vial of 100 milligram/4 milliliter. Initially the hospital may show two units for this service. A conversion of the units to be reported on the claim form is necessary to be paid correctly if payment is on a per unit basis, which is common for drugs and biologicals. In this situation, if a dosage of 200 milligram of Keytruda was provided but anything less than 200 units of J9271 is charged, the provider will not be paid accurately. Incorporating software to assist in detecting miscoding items or pharmacy conversion issues will assist in increasing the organization's revenue integrity efforts.

Timely submission of charges is also critical for revenue cycle success. Each facility has a defined number of days during the **bill hold period**. These are the number of days in which accounts will be held from billing so charges can be entered after the patient is discharged. Bill hold assumes there will be a delay in accumulating the charges incurred by a patient. By incorporating this predicted delay into normal operations, the facility creates a preventive control to avoid under billing or having to submit late charges to the payer. Charges added after this bill hold (typically two to five days) are considered late charges.

An additional responsibility in RCM is determining which items or services are separately chargeable and which items or services are separately billable. An area of confusion involves supplies. Medicare provides minimal guidance for hospitals to determine if a supply item is routine, nonroutine, separately billable or separately chargeable and much is left to the preference of the facility and the payer. However, some payers publish policies related to supplies. An example is Blue Cross Blue Shield of Texas (BCBSTX). BCBSTX has published an inpatient and outpatient unbundling policy that addresses routine services, equipment, and supplies by providing payer-specific guidance on items that should not be billed separately (BCBSTX 2022). A few questions providers can address to determine whether a supply item can be separately billed are as follows:

- Is the supply medically necessary and furnished at the direction of a physician (i.e., not personal convenience items such as slippers, powders, lotions, etc.)?
- Is the supply used for a specific patient (excluding gowns, gloves, and masks used by staff)?
- Is the supply not ordinarily used for or on most patients (excluding blood pressure cuffs, thermometers and patient gowns)?
- Is the supply not basically a stock (bulk) supply (excluding drapes, pads, cotton balls, urinals, bedpans, bed linen and gauze)? (BCBSTX 2022)

If the answer to all these questions is yes, the item may be separately billable. However, best practice for providers is to create their own internal policies surrounding billing decisions and apply across all charging practices.

Medicare provides more direction for outpatient services under the hospital Outpatient Prospective Payment System (OPPS). Even if Medicare does not separately pay for a service or item (including supplies), CMS instructs hospitals when a service has a corresponding HCPCS code to charge for the service. The Medicare Claims Processing Manual states, "it is extremely important that hospitals report all HCPCS codes consistent with their descriptors; CPT and/or CMS instructions and correct coding principles, and all charges for all services they furnish, whether payment for the services is made separately or is packaged" (CMS 2024a). After review of governmental and commercial payer charging guidelines applicable in each patient type setting, whether inpatient or outpatient, providers need to develop and execute charge capture policies and procedures meeting organization-approved compliant practices.

## Charge Description Master

The **charge description master (CDM)**, commonly referred to as a chargemaster, is an electronic file that represents a master list of all services, supplies, devices, and medications charged for inpatient or outpatient services. A sample CDM is shown in table 7.2. The CDM contains the basic elements for identifying, coding, and billing items and services provided to patients, and it is the mechanism for representing captured charges on the billing claim.

Each billable service or supply is set up in the CDM and assigned an internal charge code number, which links it to the various data elements necessary for billing and for tracking charge activity within the

**Table 7.2.** Sample charge description master

| Charge code | Charge code description | CPT/HCPCS code | Modifier | Revenue code | Price |
|---|---|---|---|---|---|
| 2721159 | CATHETER, DRAINAGE | C1729 | | 0272 | 79.00 |
| 2786337 | CATHETER, HEMODIALYSIS LONG TERM | C1750 | | 0278 | 438.00 |
| 3008423 | DRUG TEST PRESUMPTIVE, ANY NUMBER | 80305 | | 0300 | 41.00 |
| 3007215 | CBC COMPLETE, WITH DIFFERENTIAL | 85025 | | 0300 | 123.00 |
| 3207721 | VENOGRAM EXTREMITY BILATERAL | 75822 | | 0320 | 1,320.00 |
| 3406973 | PARATHYROID SCAN | 78070 | | 0340 | 798.00 |
| 3600223 | O.R. MINOR SERVICE, 1ST 30 MIN | | | 0360 | 816.00 |
| 3600224 | O.R. MINOR SERVICE, EACH ADDL 15 MIN | | | 0360 | 276.00 |
| 3618306 | DRAINAGE OF HEMATOMA/SEROMA | 10140 | | 0361 | 1,517.00 |
| 3612905 | INJECTION SACROILIAC JOINT | G0259 | | 0361 | 786.00 |
| 4245986 | PT EVAL, HIGH COMPLEX 45 MIN | 97163 | GP | 0424 | 196.00 |
| 4302398 | OT RE-EVAL EST PLAN CARE | 97168 | GO | 0430 | 134.00 |
| 4802563 | ECHO TRANSTHORACIC, CONGENITAL W/ CONTRAST | 93303 | | 0480 | 1,232.00 |

organization. The CDM contains the following general data elements:

- Charge code—a unique identifier to distinguish and represent each billable service or supply. The number is meaningful only to the organization and does not appear on the billing claim.
- Charge code description—a narrative description of the service or supply. It does not appear on the billing claim but would be available on an itemized patient statement.
- CPT or HCPCS code—a nationally recognized five-character alphanumeric code. Not all CDM line items have a CPT or HCPCS code because there are services and supplies for which no code has been developed. These charges are represented on the claim using only the revenue code. Charges for operating room time are an example of a CDM line item often without a CPT or HCPCS. Most hospitals charge operating room services on a time or level basis. A time or level charge structure initiates the intersection of the chargemaster with HIM and coding of outpatient accounts. The trained coding professional will assign the most appropriate code(s). This process, as discussed prior, is often referred to as "soft coding" or dynamic coding. When a CPT or HCPCS code exists to represent a chargemaster line item and is directly placed in the chargemaster file this is referred to as "hard" coding or static coding. Many services, supplies, and pharmacy items can be accurately described and coded without requiring review of documentation to select the most appropriate code; therefore, they can be directly coded in the chargemaster.
- Modifiers—two-character numeric or alphanumeric extensions added to the CPT or HCPCS codes to provide further information about the code. The electronic claim form allows for up to four modifiers to be attached to a CPT or HCPCS code. Therefore, organizations may consider including multiple modifier fields in the chargemaster build.
- Revenue code—a nationally recognized and standardized four-digit code that identifies what the line-item charge represents. More than 500 revenue codes are available to represent categories like room and board, lab services, radiology services, pharmacy items, therapy services, supply items, and surgical procedures. The revenue code and its description are required on each line item of a billing claim for both inpatients and outpatients.
- Price—the per unit charge amount for the line-item service, item, or supply. Factors influencing the price the organization establishes include the following:
  - Medicare and Medicaid reimbursement rates (set by federal and state government agencies)
  - Reimbursement provided by other third-party payers (set by contract negotiations with the payers)
  - Cost information that is calculated by the accounting or finance area (the cost to the organization to provide that service, such as supplies, equipment, and labor)
  - Standard markup rates for services or supplies (to factor in indirect costs to the organization or discount rates that are negotiated with the third-party payers)
  - Benchmark data on pricing in comparable organizations
  - Market competitive services

Medicare "charges refer to the regular rates established by the provider for services rendered to both beneficiaries and to other paying patients. Charges should be related consistently to the cost of the services and uniformly applied to all patients whether inpatient or outpatient" (CMS n.d.b). However, organizations may establish different prices when multiple hospitals are involved, and cost difference by location is determined. All established prices should be reviewed and updated at least annually.

Additional CDM data elements may include the date the charge code was created or activated; the date the charge code was deactivated; a code that uniquely identifies the department cost center that uses the code; and payer-specific requirements for reporting the charge; for example, a different CPT, HCPCS, modifier, or revenue code that needs to be reported to the payer for the charge submitted. These additional data elements allow the CDM to be used as a tool to collect data to evaluate costs related to resources, to prepare departmental budgets, and provide information necessary in contract negotiations with managed care payers.

The chargemaster must continually be updated to ensure it represents all billable services and supplies and to keep up with changes in CPT or HCPCS codes, revenue code assignment, and payer-specific requirements. Any number of events may trigger a need for CDM modifications. Examples include the following:

- Regulatory changes such as CPT or HCPCS code changes, including new, revised, or deleted codes
- Changes in CMS reimbursement guideline
- Changes in other public and private payer-specific policies

- New service area offered by clinical staff
- Changes in department codes to represent where charge item is charged
- Increase in claim errors or denials due to chargemaster elements (Emery and Smith 2019)

Other scenarios that require modification to the chargemaster include identification of an existing item code description and CPT or HCPCS code descriptions that do not match or that do not correspond to the service being provided, encountering recurring claim scrubber or outpatient code editor (OCE) edits indicating inappropriate chargemaster setup, or duplicate line items potentially causing charging confusion.

A variety of resources may be used to support the maintenance of the CDM and are listed in figure 7.4. Additional resources are coding and reporting guidelines as set by the CPT coding manual, CPT Assistant, and Optum's Uniform Billing Editor.

Many larger organizations use a software system to assist with maintenance of the CDM and to view items that are set up in a department or cost center's chargemaster. The software is primarily designed to continuously apply edits that point out compliance issues, the validity of elements such as CPT codes and revenue codes, and identification of items priced below national reimbursement levels.

Maintaining the CDM is a multidisciplinary activity. Proper chargemaster maintenance requires expertise in coding, clinical procedures, health record or clinical documentation, and billing regulations. For example, the HIM department is knowledgeable of the codes, the patient accounts department knows the general ledger codes, the pharmacy department is familiar with the drugs and their costs, and the finance or revenue integrity department knows the associated charge formulas. The staff in the pharmacy department cannot reliably update the radiology department chargemaster data, just as the finance staff cannot update charges without knowledge of underlying costs and input from the specific department (Casto 2023, 181).

During creation of a CDM committee, involving representatives from various areas that impact the revenue life cycle is critical to the success of the CDM team. It is equally beneficial to include representatives from those departments that capture and generate charges; additional representatives may be included depending on the facility structure. Department representation typically includes the following individuals and departments: chargemaster coordinator; patient access, including admitting, registration, and scheduling; compliance; revenue integrity; patient financial services (PFS), also known as the billing department; contracting; finance; information services; HIM; ancillary departments such as radiology, laboratory, surgery, or pharmacy; and physicians as needed.

Responsibilities of the CDM committee include oversight of the following chargemaster maintenance actions:

- Creating policies and procedures for the chargemaster review process
- Reviewing the CDM at least annually and when new CPT and HCPCS codes are available, or changes are made throughout the year
- Attending to key elements of the annual chargemaster review, including reviewing the following:
  - All CPT and HCPCS codes for accuracy, validity, and relationship to charge description number
  - All charge descriptions for accuracy and clinical appropriateness
  - All revenue codes for accuracy and linkage to charge description numbers
- Ensuring that the usage of all CPT, HCPCS, and revenue codes follow Medicare guidelines or other existing payer contracts
- Assessing all charge dollar amounts for appropriateness by payer
- Evaluating all charge codes for uniqueness and validity
- Reviewing all department code numbers for uniqueness and validity
- Performing ongoing chargemaster maintenance as the facility adds or deletes new procedures, updates technology, or changes services provided
- Ensuring that all necessary maintenance to systems affected by changes to the chargemaster (such as order entry feeder systems, charge tickets, and interfaces) is performed when chargemaster maintenance is performed
- Performing tests to make sure that changes to the chargemaster result in the desired outcome
- Educating all clinical department directors on the chargemaster and the effect of the chargemaster on corporate compliance
- Establishing a procedure to allow clinical department directors to submit chargemaster change requests for new, deleted, or revised procedures or services
- Ensuring there is no duplication of code assignment by coders and chargemaster-assigned codes in any department (for

example, interventional radiology or cardiology catheterization laboratory)
- Reviewing all charge ticket and order entry screens for accuracy against the chargemaster and appropriate mapping to CPT or HCPCS codes when required
- Assessing and fulfilling directives in Medicare transmittals, Medicare manual updates, and official coding guidelines
- Complying with guidelines in the National Correct Coding Initiative (NCCI), Outpatient Code Editor edits, and any other coding or bundling edits
- Carefully considering any application that involves one charge description number that expands into more than one CPT or HCPCS code to prevent inadvertent unbundling and unearned reimbursement for services
- Reviewing and taking action on all remittance advice denials involving HCPCS or CPT coding rules and guidelines or CMS rules and regulations
- Educating all staff affected by changes to the chargemaster in a timely fashion (Kadlec et al. 2023)

The CDM staff must also communicate with staff that negotiates commercial and managed care contracts for a hospital or healthcare organization to ensure data elements meet specific payer requirements. Chargemaster maintenance also involves communicating with the billing staff about payment denials related to an incorrect revenue code or CPT or HCPCS code so that necessary changes are made to the chargemaster.

Consequences of an improperly maintained or inaccurate chargemaster are the following:

- Services are provided, but associated charges are not set up in the CDM, so the organization is unable to bill and is providing free service.
- If a charge is not set up in the CDM until after the service is provided, the charge might not get posted to the patient's account during the bill hold time.
- When all services are not set up in the CDM, the department is only capturing part of its charges, and the result is reduced revenue.
- If charges are not set up in the CDM or if there are errors in the way they are set up, billing edits and OCE edits may be generated, holding up processing of the claim. All billing delays result in increased accounts receivable (A/R) days.
- OCE and billing edits result in multiple individuals investigating the issues and making necessary changes, which results in increased cost to the organization.

An up-to-date, complete, and well-maintained chargemaster is a significant financial, operational, and compliance asset to a healthcare organization.

**Figure 7.4.** CDM resources

- Medicare contractor bulletins and advisories
- Medicare manuals
  - Claims Processing Manual (combination of the old hospital, intermediary, and carrier manuals)
  - Benefit Policy Manual
  - Provider Reimbursement Manual
  - National Coverage Determinations Manual
- Transmittals related to:
  - Hospital OPPS
  - Fraud and abuse
- Coverage determinations
- Durable medical equipment regional carriers (DMERCs)
- Orthotics, prosthetics, and supplies
- Ambulance billing
- HIPAA
- Clarifications of previous transmittals
- Office of Inspector General
- National Correct Coding Initiative (NCCI) edits
- Medicare Addendum B

*Source:* Shuler 2011.

## Check Your Understanding 7.2

**Answer the following questions in a separate document.**

1. What negative effects could poor charge capture processes have on the reimbursement received for services?

2. To ensure appropriate and effective resource coordination, what roles should be performed by the case managers or utilization management staff? How does this coordination impact the revenue cycle?

3. Understanding hard coding and soft coding are essential to a complete and accurate outpatient claim. Using the two examples below, describe the necessary collaboration of the HIM department and the chargemaster and explain how these two departments could work together on soft coding and hard coding.

**Example 1**

| Charge code | Charge code description | CPT/HCPCS code | Modifier | Revenue code | Price |
|---|---|---|---|---|---|
| 3600223 | O.R. MINOR SERVICE, 1st 30 min | | | 0360 | $816.00 |

**Example 2**

| Charge code | Charge code description | CPT/HCPCS code | Modifier | Revenue code | Price |
|---|---|---|---|---|---|
| 4245986 | PT EVAL | 97001 | GP | 0424 | $196.00 |

4. The charge description master (CDM) has been neglected since the previous manager retired, which has caused billing issues. Robert has been asked to take on the role of coordinating the CDM. What areas should he investigate first to start making improvements?

5. What areas of clinical documentation integrity programs and coding activities benefit from artificial intelligence applications? What opportunities are created for CDI specialists and coders?

# Revenue Cycle Back-End Process

The back end of the revenue cycle—often referred to as the business office—involves all aspects of claims processing to prepare and submit a claim for payment. The information from the front-end and middle processes are combined during the billing system stage to create meaningful communication with the payer to represent the patient encounter. Claims processing involves synchronizing charges for all services, submitting claims for reimbursement, and ensuring claims are satisfied. In nonhospital ambulatory care, claims processing is often outsourced because physician offices and other small facilities generally do not have the resources to perform this complex activity effectively.

The PFS area is responsible for collecting revenue for the patient encounter. PFS is also typically responsible for merging the clinical and financial data through all associated back-end processes, which include managing the billing system, claims preparation, claims editing, claims submission, payment posting, collections and account follow-up, and remittance management, including revenue audit and revenue recovery. The business office is also responsible for ensuring effective communication about the patient's responsibility for the healthcare claim by following specific regulations centered around the services rendered due to the NSA. Once a patient has ended their encounter, the goal is to generate a complete and accurate claim and submit for payment as quickly as possible.

The revenue cycle back-end process may experience the largest impact with the application of AI practices. Prominent areas of AI use involve denials management, including appeal letter generation, payer contract management, and claim auditing (Montroy and Rakes 2022). The time efficiency alone provides significant cost benefits. As with the other revenue cycle processes, AI supports back-end process staff training and enhances knowledge gains by providing timely answers to essential questions (LaPointe 2023).

## Billing System

At the billing system stage, administrative and clinical information including charges and all applicable clinical coding from a variety of information systems are merged through a software module to reflect the patient encounter. Figure 7.2 reflects the billing system action of combining information from such separate systems, representing the first stage in the back-end process of the revenue cycle for an account. This action begins with creating the bill or claim that will eventually be submitted to the payer. Typically, healthcare organizations have a waiting period before the claim moves on through the cycle. As described earlier during the charge capture process, this is the bill hold period. The account cannot progress through the cycle until all applicable administrative and clinical systems provide the necessary information to unite the account in the billing system.

## Claims Preparation

The billing system merges the account information, but the claims preparation stage involves placing the pieces of information accumulated into the respective fields on the claim. Two different methods are used to prepare and deliver healthcare claims to payers, including public and private insurers. Providers must submit Medicare claims electronically unless the provider qualifies for a waiver or exception. Many private and other public payers follow Medicare guidance.

The 837i is the HIPAA-approved electronic format for healthcare institutions, also referred to as facilities, and the 837p is the electronic version for professional reporting. The manual format, or paper-claim form, for healthcare facilities is UB-04, also known as CMS-1450. The paper-claim format for professional claims (used primarily by physicians, allied health professionals, and suppliers) is known as CMS-1500. However, most claims in today's healthcare environment are electronically submitted to the payer. Yet, in conversation, it is common to hear the claims referred to as the "UB" and the "1500." The paper and electronic forms healthcare facilities in current use were developed and are maintained by the National Uniform Billing Committee (NUBC). The NUBC was formed to create and adopt a standard set of data to be used nationally by institutional, private, and public providers and payers for handling healthcare claims (NUBC n.d.). The payer and electronic forms in current use for professional reporting were developed and are maintained by the National Uniform Claim Committee (NUCC). The NUCC was formed to develop a standard set of data to be used by noninstitutional providers to communicate claim and encounter information to and from all third-party payers (NUCC n.d.). Data elements in the electronic format are consistent with the paper copy (CMS 2023c). The claims are then transmitted to a data clearinghouse, where the data are held for the claims editing process.

## Claims Editing

Healthcare organizations often use internal billing system edits designed to detect and correct errors before submitting claims to the payer. Prior to claims submission, the claim is scrubbed for data accuracy. To "scrub" a claim is to conduct an elaborate review just prior to submission to the payer. **Claims scrubber software** contains a series of edits to determine if the claim is ready to be submitted. The scrubber software usually includes standard edits, but it is also customizable to accommodate payer issues the healthcare organization may have experienced in past claim submissions. AI is becoming increasingly integrated into the claims editing process by searching available payer policies with speed and identifying updates and guidelines affecting accurate code reporting during the editing process (AIHC 2024).

Standard edits are uniform edits developed by CMS. Depending on the patient type—inpatient or outpatient—a series of edits are publicly available to incorporate into claims scrubber software. For example, the **Medicare Code Editor (MCE)** is the inpatient code editor used to detect various claim errors. Some MCE edits include invalid diagnosis or procedure code, unacceptable principal diagnosis, age conflict, questionable admission, noncovered procedure, and procedure inconsistent with length of stay (CMS 2023d).

The **Integrated Outpatient Code Editor (IOCE)** validates complete and accurate outpatient claims. Part of the IOCE is the **National Correct Coding Initiative (NCCI)**. CMS developed the NCCI to promote correct coding methodologies and to control improper coding leading to inappropriate payment. Some of the IOCE edits include the following:

- Invalid diagnosis code
- Diagnosis and age conflict
- Invalid procedure code
- Questionable covered service
- Inpatient procedure
- Invalid revenue code
- Service is not separately payable
- Revenue center requires HCPCS
- Add-on code reported without required primary procedure code (CMS 2023e, 14–22)

Another outpatient-specific edit enacted by the CMS is **medically unlikely edits (MUEs)**. An MUE identifies CPT and HCPCS codes reported with units greater than what has been deemed appropriate. MUEs are maximum units of services a provider would report under most circumstances for a single beneficiary on a single date of service (CMS 2024b).

Custom edits are written specifically to ensure claims comply with certain payer rules or to identify common issues experienced in previous claims. Common custom edits include reporting charges for a blood product transfused but there is no indication a blood transfusion was performed (opposite of standard edit IOCE 43), a pharmaceutical item requiring injection or infusion is present without the administration procedure, or a fracture diagnosis code is present on an ED claim without a fracture treatment procedure.

As errors are detected, reports or electronic record work queues should be generated to be reviewed by the appropriate staff. Charge or coding corrections can then be made, if supported by the health record documentation. Trending the errors can assist in identifying sources of inaccuracies and provide data for meaningful staff education. Integrating AI into initial claims preparation before submission to predict denials by payer is an effective method to potentially reduce known denial trends prospectively. AI-generated line-specific predictions allow providers to develop the most appropriate edits to ensure a clean claim before submission (Pal et al. 2022). The overall objectives of the claims editing process are to ensure accurate claims for maximum payment for the services provided and shorten the amount of time from claim submission to payment posting.

## Claims Submission

The activity of submitting a claim is often called dropping a bill. Reimbursement for clinical services provided is the healthcare facility's largest source of revenue, so timely and accurate claims submission is necessary. Most billing systems are programmed to automatically submit claims to payers after the bill hold time frame if the account is not being held for any type of edit resolution. These are often referred to as clean claims. CMS indicates providers play a vital role in protecting the integrity of the Medicare program by submitting accurate claims. Many complex rules and edits apply, so many claims require manual intervention. However, the goal is to continually increase the percentage of clean claims that can be billed with no intervention. The sophistication level of an organization's billing system determines how much can be programmed into the system versus how much the billing staff must handle manually. Through machine learning and a robotic process, AI assists in ensuring claims are as clean as possible (Williams 2024).

Timely filing is an important consideration for all payers. Medicare claims must be filed to the appropriate contractor no later than 12 months, or one calendar year, after the service date. In general, the 12-month timely filing period begins based on the account's "from" date on the claim. If the claim arrives to Medicare after the deadline date, the claim in most cases will be denied and not subject to appeal (CMS 2023c). Commercial payers may follow Medicare's timely filing rules, but many commercial payers require a much shorter period. The provider must recognize individual payer requirements on timely filing for claims submission.

## Payment Posting

After claim submission, the payer processes the claim for payment. Payment is received from third-party payers and patients in various ways, and the payments must be posted to the correct individual patient accounts. The payer will pay, adjust and pay, suspend, reject, or deny either in full or in part (Casto 2023, 214). The payer will provide an explanation of benefits (EOB) or explanation of payment (EOP) to describe the payment made on the claim. Since multiple claim payments may be sent to the provider as a single submission, the EOB or EOP is essential for claims reconciliation. Internally, some revenue must be allocated to the various areas that provided services. The organization's financial accounting area establishes this process, and the allocation methods may vary. Since payment received usually does not equal the amount billed, it is a complex process to determine the correct allocations and to post the necessary payments, adjustments, and discounts to the correct accounts.

Ultimately, the patient's account should have a zero balance, but how and why the balance reaches that goal produces important insight (HFMA 2021). There are instances when too many payments are posted to the accounts because there can be multiple payments from one or more insurance companies and copayment, or coinsurance payments received from the patient. In these cases, the account has a negative balance, and it must be determined where the overpayments occurred so refunds can be made to the correct payer or to the patient.

Organizations routinely measure **accounts receivable (A/R) days**—the average number of days between the discharge date and the receipt of payment for services rendered as a measure of revenue cycle success. A low A/R value is favorable. The median days for not-for-profit healthcare facilities in A/R for the US were 52.6 in 2022 (Pickett and Zagar 2023) An efficient revenue cycle helps the organization lower the A/R days, which in turn improves cash flow. Key performance indicators (KPIs) and high performer benchmarking measures are discussed later in this chapter.

## Collections and Account Follow-Up

Once payment is received from third-party payers and the discounts and adjustments are applied to the balance on the account, there may still be a portion that the patient owes (related to deductibles, coinsurance, and copayments). This process is called claims adjudication. After claims are adjudicated, any remaining balance on a patient account should be sent to collections at the point determined by the organization's established formal, board-approved collection action policy. The PFS staff works to collect this portion from the patient and to appropriately refer patients to medical assistance or other programs or apply charge discounts as appropriate. Patient collections can be a major challenge for providers because the patient is contacted directly to pay for the patient responsible portion. Taking at least a month to receive payments from patients is not uncommon. Offering electronic payment options through patient portals is one increasingly popular method to improve patient collections and enhance the consumer experience.

The appropriate resolution of the patient balance of an account has been addressed through a best practices report based on the partnership of the Healthcare Financial Management Association (HFMA), the Association of Credit and Collection Professionals (ACA International), and stakeholders of providers, consumer advocates, collection agencies, and credit bureaus. This partnership formed a task force to communicate a standardized process for resolving the patient portion of bills and provide a framework for educating patients about the process of resolving patient balance situations (HFMA and ACA 2020). Aligning with the HFMA's Patient Friendly Billing principles and federal requirements, the initiative provides the process for best practices of account resolution. The area still recognized as needing improved framework is assigning average time to the various steps in the process, including when an account should go to collections. However, the current framework also offers flexibility for organizations to manage those timeframes in accordance with the individual organization's operations and board-approved policy (HFMA and ACA 2020).

Organizations may also use third-party collection agencies to assist with collection of payment on problem accounts. These engagements may also necessitate a relationship with a third-party collection attorney and an internal legal review team that reviews all accounts prior to legal collection. The patient account is then closed if the account has been collected to the level expected to be received.

## No Surprises Act

Unforeseen and substantial out-of-pocket financial requirements continue to emerge when out-of-network providers treat unknowing private insurance patients.

Authorized into law as part of the Consolidated Appropriations Act (CAA) of 2021 on December 27, 2020, and effective January 1, 2022, the NSA created change at the federal level to protect patients from being subject to healthcare costs beyond their control when receiving out-of-network care (Hoadley and Lucia 2022). Patients are federally protected by limiting out-of-network cost-sharing, and the NSA prohibits patients from being billed for any higher amounts resulting from a variance between the provider's billed charge and the amount collected from the payer in addition to the patient's initial cost-sharing requirement (Requirements Related to Surprise Billing 2022). The provisions of the act apply to certain types of private health insurers and specific provider types. Comprehensive individual and group health plans, self-funded plans, and fully insured plans purchased through individual and group markets are included in the provisions of the act (AHA 2021a, 3).

The NSA also protects against most surprise bills for specified settings and defined types of services, essentially categorized into two areas. First, emergency services involving screening and stabilizing treatment provided in hospital EDs, freestanding EDs, and urgent care centers qualified to deliver emergency care are included in the NSA. Post-emergency stabilization services are also included in the act and cover the care provided to a patient until a physician establishes the patient can be transported safely to another in-network provider. In addition, air ambulance transportation suppliers are included in the NSA for initial emergency treatment. However, it is important to note that ground ambulance transportation suppliers are not included in the Act (Pollitz 2021).

The second defined type of service in the NSA involves non-emergency services delivered at in-network facilities. However, a portion of the treatment is supplied by out-of-network medical staff. Additional aspects are stipulated for the non-emergency service coverage. These include services provided in hospitals, hospital outpatient service areas, and ambulatory surgery centers, delivering care involving direct medical treatment, radiology, laboratory, pre- and post-operative care, telemedicine, and equipment or devices (Pollitz 2021). The policy scope defines the provider types, services, and insurance payers.

The law limits the patient responsibility amount while dictating a process for resolving provider-payer payment responsibility disputes. Since the NSA is recent, it may be too soon to understand its effects. The NSA must be closely monitored, evaluated, and modified to meet the goal of patient access, quality of care, and lowering healthcare costs while ensuring the implementation and policy outcomes are reasonable to stakeholders involved.

## Denial Management

**Denials** may simply be defined as a payer's refusal to provide partial or full payment. A study by Change Healthcare using facility inpatient and outpatient claims showed that for a typical health system in 2020, as much as 12 percent of claims on average across the US were at risk due to denials, with the Pacific region topping at 17 percent. Change Healthcare also reported 82 percent of denied claims are avoidable on average (Change Healthcare 2022). The front-end processes continue to cause the largest percent of denials, with registration or eligibility as the most significant reason. The most common causes for denials include the following:

- Registration or eligibility
- Missing or invalid claim data
- Authorization or precertification

- Medical documentation requested
- Service not covered
- Medical coding
- Medical necessity
- Provider eligibility
- Untimely filing
- Avoidable care (Change Healthcare 2022)

A denial management program requires facilities to seek both prevention and recovery. Denial management requires a cross-functional team to evaluate reasons for the denials and to facilitate changes in work processes to prevent additional denials. Denial team stakeholders often include staff or managers from departments such as PFS or billing; HIM; compliance; revenue integrity or chargemaster; patient access, including registration, admissions, and surgery scheduling; utilization or case management; contracting; finance; and various ancillary services and clinics where the denials may be occurring. With new systems and technologies available, a successful denial management program must be based in core analytics—which means using tools to assist in understanding available data and detail—to inform and educate (Poland and Harihara 2022). A successful denial management program includes the following best practices:

- Create a team of experts to manage the denials
- Organize data, analyze statistics, and identify trends in claims denials
- Meet deadlines by payer policy
- Collaborate with payers
- Validate patient information
- Master claim formats for the most efficient identification and resolution
- Leverage knowledge from previous rejections
- Target quality over quantity through regular follow-up instead of higher number of low dollar claims
- Conduct performance audits of write-off adjustments, zero payment claims, and remittance advice reviews
- Monitor progress for system efficiency and improvement efforts
- Use technology to assist with processes (Poland and Harihara 2022)

A successful denial management program requires consistent focus and evaluation of denial trends. Denials should be addressed within one week of receipt from the insurer. Identifying the root cause of the denial and then analyzing to determine significance of impact allows for a strategic approach to prevent and manage denials (Poland and Harihara 2022). Findings from trends or patterns identified must be shared on a routine basis with denial management stakeholders. Allowing the organization's denial data to drive the organization's denial management program is an efficient strategy. The organization's denial management team can develop action plans based on the initial denial data. Focusing efforts on the denials with greatest impact provides the best opportunity to improve overall revenue cycle performance.

## Remittance Management

After payers process claims, **remittance advice (RA)** files are provided with final individual claim adjudication and payment information. The payment information can then be used to determine revenue audit and recovery efforts. Government and most commercial payers use electronic remittances. The electronic file format adopted as the national HIPAA **electronic remittance advice (ERA)** standard is the X12 835 version 5010, more commonly known as the 835 (CMS 2020). RAs provide explanation through itemized claims processing decision information about any adjustments made regarding payments, deductibles and copayments, adjustments, denials, missing or incorrect data, refunds, and claims withholding due to Medicare Secondary Payer (MSP) or penalty situations (CMS 2020).

### Revenue Audit

For healthcare plans, after the payment is received, the organization should audit against the contract terms to determine whether the organization has received the correct reimbursement. Even while Medicare payment is prospectively determined, auditing the payment is still necessary to determine whether payment is as expected. To achieve optimum benefit, audits should occur for all payment relationships that can be modeled. Since the terms of payer contracts are usually complex, the revenue audit and recovery function is enhanced by the use of software systems that model the contracts and produce reports of accounts with variation from the expected reimbursement.

Payments are examined against the EOB to determine if specific items were paid, considered bundled services, denied, or returned to the provider for correction. Payment audits may detect errors in the applied modeling or in insurance assignment at the time of registration. This provides an opportunity to offer feedback and further educate staff. Audits can detect patterns of underpayments or overpayments, so the organization can initiate a focus on accounts with similar charges. It may reveal the need to revise the chargemaster setup, or to prices established in the fee schedules. Payment audits may also identify the need to evaluate the quality of documentation and coding, or to implement or enforce compliance standards. Revenue audit and recovery processes are extremely important to ensure reimbursement follows the agreed-upon contracted amounts from all possible sources.

### Revenue Recovery

In organizations that use modeling software, the information about expected reimbursement is calculated after all charges are posted to the account and the bill is submitted to the payer. The level of detail specified in negotiated contracts requires the software modeling programs to create a hierarchy when multiple types of services are provided to the patient. Once payment is received and the reimbursement amounts are posted to the account, the software system generates a weekly or monthly report of all accounts with payment variation. A threshold is usually established for the percentage of variation that must exist for an account to be included in the variation report. The number of accounts may be too high to enable a 100 percent review, so guidelines should be established to determine which accounts will be reviewed for revenue recovery efforts. Reports are generated to allow review of accounts by a specific payer, a payer plan, inpatients versus outpatients, accounts with high dollar amounts, and others.

---

**Check Your Understanding 7.3**

Answer the following questions in a separate document.

1. How are an organization's accounts receivable (A/R) days impacted by their bill hold days and their percentage of clean claim submission? How do A/R days impact cash flow?

2. Why would a patient account balance display a negative amount? What action would you recommend resolving the negative balance?

3. How does the No Surprises Act influence the amount that a patient can be charged for an out-of-network provider at an in-network hospital?

4. Cooper has been asked to develop a denial management program. Where should he begin?

5. What criteria are used to select claims that should be audited to determine whether proper reimbursement has been received? How would you prioritize the focus of a claim audit for reimbursement? Why?

---

## Revenue Cycle Support Services

While payer relations and patient relations activities are not directly involved in the day-to-day flow of a patient account, they are essential to the success of the revenue cycle processes. Building collaborative relationships with data sharing and transparency for both payers and patients advances the organization through trust and higher-quality care.

### Payer Relations and Health Plan Contracts

The management of payer contracts is an essential function of the revenue cycle, although it is not directly involved with an account moving through the cycle. Healthcare facilities negotiate contract terms with third-party insurers for payment of services rendered to patients. Health plan contracts include two specific components. The first is the basis of payment. This section includes contract language indicating the administration of the contract. Allowable costs, chargeable services, hierarchy of payment, and supplies provided by a hospital or physician that qualify as covered expenses are defined. Second, the contract includes the payment terms or schedules (Cleverley and Cleverley 2018, 164). The contract terms need to benefit and be cost-effective for the facility, its patients, and the insurer.

Contract management has its own life cycle, and contract managers need to understand competitor and local market rates to negotiate reasonable reimbursement rates that cover the healthcare organization's expenses while remaining competitive. As discussed in the Remittance Management section of this chapter, tracking variances from contract terms and understanding the root cause and responsible party of the variances is extremely important. A variance may be caused by the healthcare organization's internal processes, a payer's contract term modeling in their software system, or a payer's or provider's lack of understanding of the contract terms negotiated.

Payment variance may be alleviated by the organization negotiating proactively through establishing several payment terms with the payers to allow specific actions. Several recommended proactive contract terms include the following:

- Prompt payment and penalties for lack of compliance
- Eliminate retroactive denials
- Address precluding language of reducing inpatient stays from higher to lower paying service categories
- Establish a reasonable appeal process
- Define clean claims
- Remove most favored nation clauses (meaning the provider must give the payer the lowest rate given to any other payer)
- Prohibit silent PPO arrangements
- Include terms for outliers or technology-driven cost increases
- Establish ability to recover payment after termination
- Remove unclear language
- Preserve the ability to be paid for service when patient consent is granted (Cleverley and Cleverley 2018, 163)

Assessing payer performance and payment accuracy can help organizations negotiate better reimbursement rates and improve medical billing compliance. However, ideally, the payer and provider should work collaboratively with a shared vision for improvement and prevention of variance. A collaborative approach creates a greater opportunity for an efficient system environment (Poland and Harihara 2022).

## Payer Relations and Physician Credentialing

**Credentialing** is a screening process to evaluate and validate a healthcare provider's qualifications for medical staff membership, allowing them to provide care to patients within the facility. This process is also used by third-party payers before allowing healthcare providers to deliver services to patients covered by their plans. The activity is critical to ensure healthcare providers meet certain standards of education, training, and licensure (Murphy 2020). While specific requirements may vary depending on the healthcare institution, payer, and the type of practice, the general process typically includes the following steps:

1. Application submission: Physicians or representatives typically submit a credentialing application to the third-party payer, including detailed information about the physician's education, training, work experience, and professional references.
2. Verification of credentials: The payer reviews the application and verifies the physician's credentials, which may include checking medical school diplomas, residency training, board certifications, and any additional training or specialization.
3. Licensure verification: The payer confirms that the physician holds a valid and current medical license to practice in the state where the services will be provided. This step often involves contacting the relevant state medical board.
4. Malpractice history check: The payer may review the physician's malpractice history, including any past claims or lawsuits, to assess the risk associated with the physician's practice.
5. Privileges verification: If the physician is practicing in a hospital or other healthcare facility, the payer may also verify the physician's clinical privileges at that facility.
6. Background screening: Some payers may conduct a background check to ensure the physician has no criminal history or other red flags that could raise concerns about the physician's ability to provide safe and effective care.
7. Peer review: Sometimes, the payer may request peer reviews or references from other healthcare professionals who have worked with the physician to assess their clinical competence and professionalism.
8. Contracting: After completing the credentialing process, the physician may enter a contract with the third-party payer, outlining the reimbursement terms and other relevant details (Bell and Katz 2021; Medaket n.d.; Murphy 2020)

Credentialing is important in ensuring patients receive high-quality and reliable healthcare services from qualified providers. Regardless of the number of hospitals a physician has served, how many states in which the physician holds appropriate licensure, or the number of payer plans the physician has successfully been enrolled in, each hospital and payer must independently perform the credentialing process (Bell and Katz 2021). Generally, providers are required to repeat the credentialing process every one to three years (Medaket n.d.).

## Patient Relations and Customer Service

The patient experience is of increasingly high importance for healthcare organizations as the healthcare industry moves toward value-based care. Maintaining patient satisfaction even after healthcare services are provided is a primary goal. Treating patients with respect and dignity regardless of their account status assists in building patient loyalty. Managing patient perceptions is challenging, but not impossible. To build customer service in the healthcare revenue cycle process, providers should consider the following approaches:

- Patient engagement: represents a shared decision approach and giving patients choice along with establishing a connection and exchanging ideas
- Transparency: providing financial information in a user-friendly format along with all relevant past and current patient obligations
- Consumer-centric: allowing for easy access to financial information for the patient represents the organization understands the patient situation and has taken steps to anticipate needs. Also permitting creation of payment plans specific to their needs shows desire for organization-to-patient collaboration. (Considine 2018)

The organization's relationship with the patient impacts its revenue flow. As more financial responsibility shifts to the patient, providers must focus on communicating with them about care and financial obligations. Usually, the last experience regarding the patient encounter involves the bill. The organization should desire to create a positive last experience (AHA 2021b, 1). Creating a positive patient experience is essential to healthy revenue and a healthy future for the organization. Understanding coverage, patient financial responsibility, availability of payment plans, and alternate financing options may influence a patient's place of care decision. Communicating with patients and making them feel they are more important to providers than their financial obligation improves the patient experience and results in better financial outcomes (HFMA 2023a).

## Performance Measures for Improvement

Measuring and monitoring performance frequently, along with setting appropriate goals, is key for performance improvement. Increasing revenue cycle performance can positively impact a healthcare organization's financial bottom line (see table 7.3). To determine how successful healthcare organizations are at achieving set performance goals, **key performance indicators (KPIs)** must be selected. KPIs allow healthcare facilities to measure and benchmark their data against best practice. Measuring the various processes of the revenue cycle against established benchmarks provides an opportunity for organizations to focus on areas to improve.

Organizations select different measures for claims management and may change their KPIs over time. Success depends on selecting relevant indicators that align with the organization's goals. Leaders must continuously pursue appropriate indicators for each revenue cycle process at the operational level, not just at the overall system level (Dazley and Halpin 2020). Common front-end revenue cycle KPIs include pre-registration rate, insurance verification rate, POS with cash collections, and service authorization rate. Middle process measures may consist of KPIs such as accuracy and timeliness of department charge capture and late charges as a percentage of total charges. The back-end process may include KPIs related to DNFB, A/R, clean claim rate, bad debt, and initial denial rate (HFMA 2023b).

The HFMA directed industry leaders to develop indicators to consistently measure the KPIs. These strategic KPIs set the new standard for revenue cycle excellence and are known as **MAP Keys**, which stands for measure, apply, perform. MAP represents "the comprehensive revenue cycle strategy to *measure* performance, *apply* evidence-based improvement strategies, and *perform* to the highest standards to improve financial results and patient satisfaction" (HFMA n.d.). The industry-standard metrics classify revenue cycle performance in a reliable, distinct, and neutral manner. MAP Keys are comprised of 29 KPIs for revenue cycle benchmarking separated into five major groups: patient access, pre-billing, claims, account resolution, and financial management (HFMA n.d.).

Each MAP Key measures a specific revenue cycle function and details the purpose for the measurement, the value of the measure, the specific equation (numerator and denominator), and inclusions and exclusions to consistently calculate the measure. Examples of MAP Keys are found in table 7.4.

RCM success depends on multiple processes, people, and technology. Effective management requires identification of trends and then adjustment to processes and procedures and, at times, software technology

**Table 7.3.** Benchmarking against MAP award for high performance in revenue cycle winners for 2023

| Use of benchmarking can drive significant improvements | | | |
|---|---|---|---|
| Key performance indicator | 90th Percentile | Median | Difference |
| Net Days in A/R | 26.1 | 38.6 | 12.5 |
| Point-of-service cash collection | 40.7% | 27.8% | 12.9% |

*Source*: HFMA 2024.

**Table 7.4.** Examples of MAP Keys

| Group | Measure | Purpose | Value | Equation* |
|---|---|---|---|---|
| Patient Access | Point-of-service cash collections | Trending indicator of point-of-service collection efforts | Accelerates cash collections and may reduce collection costs | N: Patient POS payments<br>D: Total self-pay cash collected |
| Patient Access | Preregistration rate | Trending indicator for timely and efficient patient access processes | Indicates revenue cycle efficiency and effectiveness | N: Number of patient encounters preregistered<br>D: Number of scheduled patient encounters |
| Patient Access | Insurance verification rate | Trending indicator for timely and efficient patient access functions | Indicates revenue cycle process efficiency and effectiveness | N: Number of verified encounters<br>D: Number of registered encounters |
| Pre-Billing | Days in total discharged, not final bill (DNFB) | Trending indicator of claims generation process | Indicates revenue cycle performance and can identify performance issues impacting cash flow | N: Gross dollars in discharged not final billed (DNFB)<br>D: Average daily gross patient service revenue |
| Pre-Billing | Days in total discharged, not submitted to payer (DNSP) | Trending indicator of total claims generation and submission process | Indicates revenue cycle performance and can identify performance issues impacting cash flow | N: gross dollars in DNFB + gross dollars in FBNS<br>D: Average daily gross patient service revenue |
| Claims | Clean Claim Rate | Trending indicator of claims data as it impacts revenue cycle performance | Indicates quality of data collected and reported | N: Number of claims that pass edits requiring no manual intervention<br>D: Number of claims accepted into claims processing tool for billing |
| Claims | Late charges as percentage of total charges | Measure of revenue capture efficiency | Helps identify opportunities to improve revenue capture, reduce unnecessary cost, and accelerate cash flow. | N: Gross charges with postdate greater than three days from last service date<br>D: Total gross charges |
| Account Resolution | Net days in credit balance | Trending indicator to accurately report account values, ensure compliance with regulatory requirements, and monitor overall payment system effectiveness | Indicates process failure in timely cash posting, incorrect posting or incorrect payment | N: Dollars in credit balance<br>D: Average daily net patient service revenue |
| Financial Management | Net days in accounts receivable (A/R) | Trending indicator of overall A/R performance | Indicates revenue cycle (RC) efficiency | N: Net A/R<br>D: Average daily net patient service revenue |

*N = Numerator, D = Denominator.
*Source*: HFMA n.d.

updates. The revenue cycle could be considered the heart of the organization as it impacts patients and their families; physicians and other providers of care; ancillary departments, such as radiology and laboratory; support departments, such as scheduling and registration; finance; HIM; clinical documentation; PFS; and information technology. Combining efforts across departments and staff members to improve the revenue cycle processes and establishing performance expectations will lead to a successful revenue cycle program.

### Check Your Understanding 7.4

**Answer the following questions in a separate document.**

1. What are three areas providers should focus on when building patient relations and customer service in the revenue cycle? Why is building patient relations important to the revenue cycle?

2. Why do healthcare institutions and third-party payers credential physicians?

3. Payment variance has been detected with the organization's current major payer contract. T. J., the new director of managed care, examines the contract and notices the contract includes payment language that could be interpreted various ways. Which component is lacking in this contract and what should T. J. do to improve payer performance?

4. How do payer relations support the various revenue cycle processes? Why is a good relationship with the payers important?

5. If C. Lewis Medical Center's last fiscal year's value for POS cash collections was 25.3 percent and the current fiscal year has a value of 28.1 percent, is this considered favorable or unfavorable? Explain why.

# References

ACMA (American Case Management Association). n.d. "Definition of Case Management." Accessed December 16, 2023. http://acmaweb.org/section.aspx?mn=mn1&sn=sn1&wpg=mh.&sid=4.

AHA (American Hospital Association). 2021a. Legislative advisory: Detailed summary of No Surprises Act. Comprehensive legislation to address surprise medical billing at the federal level. https://www.aha.org/system/files/media/file/2021/01/detailed-summary-of-no-surprises-act-advisory-1-14-21.pdf.

AHA (American Hospital Association). 2021b. Improving the patient billing experience: A strategic imperative for hospitals and health systems. https://www.aha.org/system/files/media/file/2021/10/Improving-Patient-Billing-Experience_IB_Final_10-22-21.pdf.

AIHC (American Institute of Healthcare Compliance). 2024. "AI and Algorithms: The Other Side of Medical Claims Processing." https://aihc-assn.org/ai-and-algorithms-the-other-side-of-medical-claims-processing/.

AMA (American Medical Association). 2023. "Definitions of 'Screening' and 'Medical Necessity' H-320.953." https://policysearch.ama-assn.org/policyfinder/detail/H-320.953?uri=%2FAMADoc%2FHOD.xml-0-2625.xml.

Barton, J., and D. Shelton. 2018. "Transforming Patient Access and Engagement. Revenue Cycle Strategist." https://www.hfma.org/revenue-cycle/patient-access/62346/.

Bell, D. L., and M. H, Katz. 2021. Modernize medical licensing, and credentialing, too—lessons from the COVID-19 pandemic. *JAMA Internal Medicine* 181(3), 312–315. https://doi.org/10.1001/jamainternmed.2020.8705.

BCBSTX (Blue Cross Blue Shield of Texas). 2022. "Clinical Payment and Coding Policy." https://www.bcbstx.com/docs/provider/tx/standards/clinical-pay-coding/2022/cpcp002-in-op-unbundling-01142022.pdf.

Casto, A. B., and S. White 2023. *Principles of Healthcare Reimbursement,* 8th ed. Chicago: AHIMA.

Change Healthcare. 2022. The Change Healthcare 2022 Revenue Cycle Denials Index. https://media.bitpipe.com/io_16x/io_164605/item_2612841/2022-revenue-cycle-denials-index.pdf.

Cleverley, W., and J. Cleverley. 2018. "Revenue Determination." Chapter 6 in *Essentials of Healthcare Finance,* 8th ed. Burlington, MA: Jones and Bartlett Learning.

CMS (Centers for Medicare and Medicaid Services). 2024a. *Medicare Claims Processing Manual:*

*Chapter 4—Part B Hospital*. https://www.cms.gov/Regulations-and-Guidance/Guidance/Manuals/Downloads/clm104c04.pdf.

CMS (Centers for Medicare and Medicaid Services). 2024b. "Medicare NCCI Medically Unlikely Edits (MUEs)." https://www.cms.gov/Medicare/Coding/NationalCorrectCodInitEd/MUE.html.

CMS (Centers for Medicare and Medicaid Services). 2023a. "HINNs." http://www.cms.gov/Medicare/Medicare-General-Information/BNI/HINNs.html.

CMS (Centers for Medicare and Medicaid Services). 2023b. *Complying with Medical Record Documentation Requirements*. https://www.cms.gov/Outreach-and-Education/Medicare-Learning-Network-MLN/MLNProducts/Downloads/CERTMedRecDoc-FactSheet-ICN909160.pdf.

CMS (Centers for Medicare and Medicaid Services). 2023c. *Medicare Billing: 837I and Form CMS-1450*. https://www.cms.gov/Outreach-and-Education/Medicare-Learning-Network-MLN/MLNProducts/Downloads/837I-FormCMS-1450-ICN006926.pdf.

CMS (Centers for Medicare and Medicaid Services). 2023d. Definitions of Medicare Code Edits_v41. Medicare Severity Diagnosis Related Group (MS-DRG) Grouper Software and Medicare Code Editor (MCE) Version 41, ICD-10 Software. https://www.cms.gov/files/zip/ms-drg-mce-pc-software-v41.zip.

CMS (Centers for Medicare and Medicaid Services). 2023e. Integrated OCE (IOCE) CMS Specifications V24.3. https://www.cms.gov/apps/aha/license.asp?file=/files/zip/i/oce-quarterly-data-files-v243r0.zip.

CMS (Centers for Medicare and Medicaid Services). 2022a. "The No Surprises Act's Good Faith Estimate and Patient-Provider Dispute Resolution Requirements." https://www.cms.gov/files/document/gfe-and-ppdr-requirements-slides.pdf.

CMS (Centers for Medicare and Medicaid Services). 2022b. *Medicare Advance Written Notices of Noncoverage*. https://www.cms.gov/Outreach-and-Education/Medicare-Learning-Network-MLN/MLNProducts/downloads/abn_booklet_icn006266.pdf.

CMS (Centers for Medicare and Medicaid Services). 2020. *Understanding Your Remittance Advice Reports*. https://www.hhs.gov/guidance/sites/default/files/hhs-guidance-documents/ICNMLN8788099-final_0.pdf.

CMS (Centers for Medicare and Medicaid Services). 2014. "CMS Manual System, Transmittal 168." https://www.cms.gov/Regulations-and-Guidance/Guidance/Transmittals/Downloads/R168NCD.pdf.

CMS (Centers for Medicare and Medicaid Services). n.d.a. "Glossary M, Medically Necessary." Accessed December 16, 2023. https://www.healthcare.gov/glossary/medically-necessary/.

CMS (Centers for Medicare and Medicaid Services). n.d.b. *The Provider Reimbursement Manual–Part 1*. Chapter 22. Accessed October 14, 2024. https://www.cms.gov/regulations-and-guidance/guidance/manuals/downloads/p151_22.zip.

CMSA (Case Management Society of America). n.d. "What Is a Case Manager?" Accessed December 16, 2023. http://www.cmsa.org/who-we-are/what-is-a-case-manager/.

Cohen, R., S. Ning, M. T. Yan, and J. Callum. 2019. Transfusion safety: The nature and outcomes of errors in patient registration. *Transfusion Medicine Reviews* 33(2):78–83. https://doi.org/10.1016/j.tmrv.2018.11.004.

Considine, J. 2018. Better patient experience hinges on improving financial journey. *Health Management Technology*. https://www.hcinnovationgroup.com/home/article/13010171/better-patient-experience-hinges-on-improving-financial-journey.

Davenport, T. and R. Kalakota. 2019. The potential for artificial intelligence in healthcare. *Future Healthcare Journal* 6(2):94–98. https://doi.org/10.7861/futurehosp.6-2-94.

Dazley, M., and T. Halpin. 2020. "Healthcare Revenue Cycle: Five Keys to Financial Sustainability." Health Catalyst. https://www.healthcatalyst.com/insights/healthcare-revenue-cycle-5-keys-success.

De Luca, E., C. Cosentino, S. Cedretto, A. L. Maviglia, J. Bucci, J. Dotto, G. Artioli, and A. Bonacaro. 2022. Multidisciplinary team perceptions of the Case/Care Managers' role implementation: a qualitative study. *Acta bio-medica: Atenei Parmensis* 93(3), e2022259. https://doi.org/10.23750/abm.v93i3.13371.

Emery, D. and D. Smith. 2019. *Chargemaster Maintenance Ensures Financial Viability of Hospitals* [White paper]. Optum360. https://www.optum.com/content/dam/optum3/optum/en/resources/white-papers/WF1476481_SPRJ6133_Enterprise%20ChargemasterExpert%20maintenance%20white%20paper_HR.pdf.

HFMA (Healthcare Financial Management Association). 2024. *MAP Award Winner Statistical Data*. https://www.hfma.org/wp-content/uploads/2024/07/MAP_230608_Winner-Resources_Stats-2024.pdf.

HFMA (Healthcare Financial Management Association). 2023a (April 28). "How the Patient Financial

Experience Impacts Loyalty." https://www.hfma.org/revenue-cycle/patient-financial-communications/how-the-patient-financial-experience-impacts-loyalty/.

HFMA (Healthcare Financial Management Association). 2023b (April 6). "7 KPIs Providers Should Be Tracking." https://www.hfma.org/revenue-cycle/kpis/7-kpis-providers-should-be-tracking/.

HFMA (Healthcare Financial Management Association). 2021 (January 6). "Managing Self-pay with a Patient Satisfaction Mindset: 4 Tips for Success." https://www.hfma.org/revenue-cycle/self-payment-collection/managing-self-pay-with-a-patient-satisfaction-mindset-4-tips-fo/.

HFMA (Healthcare Financial Management Association). 2018 (November 18). "The Path to a Patient-centric Revenue Cycle." HFMA. https://www.hfma.org/revenue-cycle/patient-financial-communications/62489/.

HFMA (Healthcare Financial Management Association). n.d. "MapKeys." Accessed December 17, 2023. http://www.hfma.org/MAP/MapKeys/.

HFMA (Healthcare Financial Management Association) and ACA International. 2020. *Best Practices for Resolution of Medical Accounts: A Report from the Medical Debt Collection Task Force.* https://www.hfma.org/wp-content/uploads/2022/10/best-practices-medical-resolution-medical-accounts.pdf.

Hoadley, J., and K. Lucia. 2022. The no surprises act: A bipartisan achievement to protect consumers from unexpected medical bills. *Journal of Health Politics, Policy and Law* 47(1):93–109. https://doi.org/10.1215/03616878-9417470.

Ingrao, C. 2019. Addressing prior authorization with blockchain, the first step in revenue cycle transformation. HIMSS. https://www.himss.org/news/addressing-prior-authorization-blockchain-first-step-revenue-cycle-transformation.

Kadlec, L., T. Selmon, S. L. Goodman, J. Krush, and T. Ortiz. 2023. *Care and Maintenance of Chargemasters 2023 Update.* https://bok.ahima.org/topics/coding-compliance-and-revenue-cycle/care-and-maintenance-of-chargemasters-2023-update/.

LaPointe, J. 2023 (October 19). "Generative AI's potential shines on revenue cycle management." TechTarget. https://www.techtarget.com/revcyclemanagement/answer/Generative-AIs-Potential-Shines-on-Revenue-Cycle-Management.

LaPointe, J. 2021 (May 6). "Why Patient Access Is Key to Revenue Cycle Management Success." TechTarget. https://www.techtarget.com/revcyclemanagement/answer/Why-Patient-Access-is-Key-to-Revenue-Cycle-Management-Success.

LaPointe, J. 2018 (March 23). "Hospital Utilization Management Care Reduce Denials, Improve Care." TechTarget. https://www.techtarget.com/revcyclemanagement/feature/Hospital-Utilization-Management-Can-Reduce-Denials-Improve-Care.

Levinson, K., S. Hulver, and T. Neuman. 2022 (November 3). "Hospital Charity Care: How It Works and Why It Matters." Kaiser Family Foundation (KFF). https://www.kff.org/health-costs/issue-brief/hospital-charity-care-how-it-works-and-why-it-matters/.

Medaket. n.d. "The Definitive Guide to Provider Credentialing and Payer Enrollment." Accessed October 14, 2024. https://www.madakethealth.com/definitive-guides/the-definitive-guide-to-provider-credentialing-and-payer-enrollment.

Mehrabian, N. 2018 (February 22). Reinventing utilization management to bring value to the point of care. *Healthcare Innovation.* https://www.hcinnovationgroup.com/policy-value-based-care/accountable-care-organizations-acos/article/13029840/reinventing-utilization-management-to-bring-value-to-the-point-of-care.

Miller, M. 2023 (April 7). "Best Practices in Patient Eligibility and Benefits Verification." American Institute of Healthcare Compliance. https://aihc-assn.org/best-practices-in-patient-eligibility-and-benefits-verification/.

Montroy, T., and G. Rakes. 2022 (October 17). What is AI, and how can it benefit the healthcare revenue cycle? *Journal of AHIMA.* https://journal.ahima.org/page/what-is-ai-and-how-can-it-benefit-the-healthcare-revenue-cycle.

Murphy, B. 2020 (October 14). "Credentialing 101: What Medical Residents Need to Know." American Medical Association. https://www.ama-assn.org/medical-residents/transition-resident-attending/credentialing-101-what-medical-residents-need-know.

NAHRI (National Association of Healthcare Revenue Integrity). 2018 (April 4). Build bridges to solve charge capture and reconciliation issues before they hit denials. *Revenue Integrity Insider.* https://nahri.org/articles/build-bridges-solve-charge-capture-and-reconciliation-issues-they-hit-denials.

NUBC (National Uniform Billing Committee). n.d. "About the NUBC." Accessed December 17, 2023. https://www.nubc.org/about-nubc.

NUCC (National Uniform Claim Committee). n.d. Accessed December 17, 2023. http://www.nucc.org/.

Optum. 2023. *The Optum 2022 Revenue Cycle Denials Index.* https://www.changehealthcare.com/content/dam/change-healthcare/sales—marketing-content/revenue-cycle-management-provider-engagement

/rcm-general/ebook/change-healthcare-2022-denials-index-report/optum-denials-index-2022-ebook.pdf.

Pal, S., M. Gaur, R. Chaudhuri, R. Kalaivanan, K. V. Chetan, B. H. Praneeth, and U. Ramamurthy. 2022. Driving impact in claims denial management using artificial intelligence. *Communications in Computer and Information Science*, 1613:107–120. https://doi.org/10.1007/978-3-031-12638-3_10.

Pickett, C. A., and P. Zagar. 2023. US Not-for-profit health care stand-along hospital median financial ratios—2022. S&P Global. https://www.spglobal.com/ratings/en/research/articles/230807-u-s-not-for-profit-health-care-stand-alone-hospital-median-financial-ratios-2022-12811732.

Poland, L., and S. Harihara. 2022 (April 25). Claims denials: A step-by-step approach to resolution. *Journal of AHIMA*. https://journal.ahima.org/page/claims-denials-a-step-by-step-approach-to-resolution.

Pollitz, K. 2021 (December 10). No surprises act implementation: What to expect in 2022. KFF. https://www.kff.org/health-reform/issue-brief/no-surprises-act-implementation-what-to-expect-in-2022/.

Reiner, G. 2018. "Success in Proactive Denials Management and Prevention." HFMA. https://www.hfma.org/revenue-cycle/denials-management/61778/.

Sanborn, B. J. 2018 (February 6). Revenue cycle expert: The patient is the new payer. Healthcare Finance News. https://www.healthcarefinancenews.com/news/revenue-cycle-expert-patient-new-payer.

Shuler, G. 2011. "Chargemaster 101—Let's Start at the Beginning." Paper provided at the Minnesota Hospital Association Education Program, St. Paul, MN, August 2011.

Stewart, J. K. 2017. Patient discounts the fine line between leniency and liability. Medical Economics. https://www.medicaleconomics.com/view/patient-discounts-fine-line-between-leniency-and-liability.

Williams, J. 2024 (March 28). Battle of the bots: As payers use AI to drive denials higher, providers fight back. HFMA. https://www.hfma.org/revenue-cycle/denials-management/health-systems-start-to-fight-back-against-ai-powered-robots-driving-denial-rates-higher/.

# chapter 8

# Clinical Documentation Integrity and Coding Compliance

*T. J. Hunt, PhD, RHIA, CHDA, FAHIMA*
*Megan Tober, MBA, RHIA*

## Learning Objectives

- Determine processes for compliance with laws and standards related to coding and revenue cycle
- Develop methods to ensure the accuracy of coded data based on established guidelines
- Determine processes to monitor healthcare fraud and abuse
- Develop methods to manage elements of the clinical documentation integrity process functions of a healthcare corporate compliance program
- Interpret the importance of the Office of the Inspector General workplan to organize compliance
- Differentiate the elements of the Federal Sentencing Guidelines, False Claims Act, Anti-Kickback Statute, Emergency Medical Treatment and Labor Act, and Stark Law that relate to the healthcare industry
- Distinguish between identity theft and medical identity theft

## Key Terms

Abuse
Anti-Kickback Statute (AKS)
Benchmarks
Case mix
Civil Monetary Penalties Law
Clinical
Clinical documentation integrity (CDI)
Coding optimization
Compliance
Computer-assisted coding (CAC)
Concurrent review
Corporate integrity agreements (CIAs)
Exclusion Provisions
Extrapolation method
Federal False Claims Act of 1863
Identity theft
Maximization
Medical identity theft
Office of the Inspector General (OIG)
OIG workplan
Physician champion
Query
Qui tam relators
Red Flags Rule
Retrospective review
Stark Law
Unbundling
Upcoding
Waste
Whistleblowing

For as long as the patient health record has existed, it has been a central hub for communication between healthcare providers. The first widely known reference regarding health records, *Manual for Medical Records Librarians*, was authored in 1941 by health information management (HIM) pioneer Edna Huffman. It was in print as the recognized authority on the profession for over 50 years. She defines the complete health record as consisting of "sufficient data written in sequence of events to justify the diagnosis and warrant the treatment and end results" (Huffman 1941, 21).

The format of patient records has evolved in the last century. Whether the record storage medium is paper, microfilm, microfiche, or electronic, the purpose remains the same. Today the information justifying the diagnosis, warranting the treatment, and detailing the progress and result for the patient is used for patient care, quality improvement, research, provider payment, decision-making, and more. It is the legal business record of the care provider (Rinehart-Thompson 2023, 140).

In many ways, the record can be compared to an itemized receipt for services. It communicates what was done and why it was necessary.

> Clinical documentation is the cornerstone of medical data and the foundation of patient care. It provides a lasting record of the patient's history, diagnoses, tests, and treatments. An accurate and complete health record is beneficial not only to ensure that the severity and risk of illness of the patient is accurately reflected, but it also benefits the patient-provider relationship and aids in population health management and research. (AHIMA and ACDIS 2021, 1)

The term **clinical** refers to work done with real patients, about or relating to the medical treatment given to patients in facilities such as hospitals and clinics. Documentation regarding the clinical evaluation and treatment of the patient is the core of the health record in paper, scanned, or electronic form. Other functions of the patient health record are facilitating the care and treatment of patients, serving as a communication method among caregivers and healthcare organizations, being a resource for clinical and organizational decision-making, and providing information for research and quality improvement.

Information found in the patient health record is the foundation on which decision-making is based. The many functions and uses of the record, including communication, reimbursement, compliance, and more, drive the need for accuracy. Accurate clinical documentation is an important organizational asset in the healthcare industry. Incomplete, inaccurate, or nonspecific information in the record has negative consequences on all the record functions listed here. This is why many healthcare organizations have formalized processes and compliance programs to support the integrity of clinical documentation.

## Clinical Documentation Integrity

There are many examples in healthcare where improved documentation will benefit both patients and providers. **Clinical documentation integrity (CDI)**—previously referred to as clinical documentation improvement—is a "process an organization undertakes that will improve clinical specificity and documentation that will allow coding professionals to assign more concise disease classification codes" (AHIMA 2017, 45). Information is collected from the patient health record and recorded as codes representing the diagnoses and procedures performed. This information is then used for many purposes in healthcare. CDI programs initiate reviews of health records for conflicting, incomplete, or nonspecific provider documentation with end goal of a precise representation of the patient's clinical status (AHIMA 2021, 5).

The primary reason for excellent documentation is improved patient care through clear communication between providers and an accurate picture of the patient's medical situation and course of treatment. Additional examples are more accurate reimbursement and data reporting through programs dependent on diagnosis and procedure codes such as the following:

- Medicare severity diagnosis-related groups (MS-DRG)
- Value-based purchasing (VBP)
- Quality of care measures including inpatient quality reporting (IQR)
- Severity of illness (SOI)
- Expected risk of mortality (ROM)
- Present on admission (POA) or hospital-acquired condition (HAC) reporting
- Patient safety measures
- Utilization of resource measures such as case-mix and medical necessity
- Protection from liability

- Reduction of claim denials
- Public health monitoring (AHIMA 2018a, 17; AHIMA 2021, 9)

In addition, measures such as these may also be used as a comparison with peers for both physicians and facilities. The benefit of better documentation has been apparent for over 100 years, articulated in one example in the foreword of *Manual for Medical Records Librarians*:

> Meagre information other than nurses' notes was to be found in the medical records of most hospitals when the American College of Surgeons initiated its program of Hospital Standardization in 1918... Many a surgeon, wishing to become a Fellow of the College, could not qualify because acceptable records of the operations he had performed were not obtainable... Better medical records have had a share in, and will continue to affect, medical progress. (Huffman 1941, VII, IX)

While HIM professionals had been reviewing documentation even before the *Manual for Medical Record Librarians* was published, the increased need for information about the care provided to the patient from these programs and functions made the existence of CDI programs shift from a program for improvement used by some providers to a standard function in many healthcare organizations, throughout many care settings (Casto and White 2024, 241). The *International Classification of Diseases, Tenth Revision, Clinical Modification* (ICD-10-CM) and *International Classification of Diseases, Tenth Revision, Procedure Coding System* (ICD-10-PCS) require a higher level of specificity than the *International Classification of Diseases, Ninth Revision, Clinical Modification* (ICD-9-CM) system and has been a major factor in the growth of CDI programs. CDI professionals seek to ensure clinical documentation is accurate, timely, complete, and specific to fully describe the patient's condition and course of treatment (Casto and White 2024, 241). They are "translators and validators of the health record, working to ensure complete and accurate information" (AHIMA and ACDIS 2021, 1) for the coding process. The result of improving clinical documentation is not to amass *more*, but to produce *better* documentation that easily communicates what patient care was delivered and the reason for the treatment.

## Documentation for Coded Data

Many of the reporting and communication needs of healthcare that are dependent on documentation are accomplished using coded data. On October 1, 2015, the US transitioned to the ICD-10-CM and ICD-10-PCS coding system from ICD-9-CM, which had been in effect since 1979. The new system has greater capability to capture specific detail about the care provided; this includes ensuring higher quality information to make decisions about patient care, offering more accurate reimbursement to providers, and benefiting from improved data for information needs. The challenge continues to be ensuring that detailed clinical documentation matches the detailed capability of ICD-10-CM (and future ICD-11-CM) coding system.

The need for a CDI process in these cases not only impacts the accuracy and detail of diagnosis and procedure codes, but perhaps even the ability to assign a code at all. For example, laterality of a disease or procedure was not a detail captured in ICD-9-CM. However, in ICD-10-CM and ICD-10-PCS, knowing if the condition or procedure affects the right or left eye is essential to assigning a code. Without the necessary documentation, complete coding for the care encounter will take longer. A longer coding timeframe causes delayed action on all processes in which coded information is needed, including financial functions.

## Clinical Documentation Integrity Goals

The purpose of a CDI program is to "facilitate the precise representation of a patient's clinical status. This is accomplished by reviewing health records to assure they meet high-quality clinical documentation standards that will translate into the appropriate coded data" (AHIMA 2021, 5). Concurrent and retrospective reviews are completed to reduce the amount of conflicting, incomplete, or nonspecific documentation (AHIMA 2016). **Concurrent review** of the record occurs while the patient care is ongoing, and often the reviewers are alongside the healthcare providers in the patient care service areas to facilitate communication. **Retrospective review** occurs later after that patient has been discharged.

The goals of the reviews should be clearly defined by the organization embarking on the CDI process. Key stakeholders must be involved in the goal-setting process and throughout the program to achieve success (ACDIS 2017, 9; CHIMA 2021). Examples of key stakeholders in an acute-care or integrated organization are displayed in figure 8.1.

The range of stakeholders is wide because the information from a patient record is used for multiple functions throughout a healthcare organization. Clinical documentation is generated by healthcare providers, which then has a domino effect on many other functions related to patient care such as communication

**Figure 8.1.** List of key CDI stakeholders

- Executive leadership
- Health information management/coding
- Risk management
- Utilization management
- Case management
- Patient financial services/billing
- Medical staff and provider leadership
- Compliance
- Finance/revenue cycle
- Nursing
- Quality improvement
- Ethics committee

*Source:* AHIMA 2021; AHIMA 2016a; CHIMA 2021.

between caregivers. Some examples of CDI program goals include the following:

- Obtain clinical documentation that captures the patient severity of illness (SOI) and risk of mortality (ROM)
- Identify and clarify missing, conflicting, or nonspecific physician documentation related to diagnoses and procedures
- Support accurate diagnostic and procedural coding and MS-DRG assignment, leading to appropriate reimbursement and fewer claim denials
- Promote health record completion during the patient's course of care, which promotes patient safety
- Improve communication between physicians and other members of the healthcare team
- Provide awareness and education
- Improve documentation to reflect quality and outcome scores
- Improve coding professionals' clinical knowledge (AHIMA 2018a,17; AHIMA 2021, 5)

Overarching themes in a CDI program are identifying areas of documentation deficiencies, improving documentation to be more specific or clear, and providing ongoing education for future excellence. An initial gap assessment indicating a need for CDI and the service areas in which it is required is an important benchmark at the beginning of a CDI process.

## Operational Considerations

The following decisions must be made before implementing a CDI program to ensure the right people, processes, and technology are in place:

- Who will comprise the CDI staff
- How the CDI program will be aligned
- What types of records will be reviewed
- How many health records will be reviewed and at what frequency
- Amount budgeted for CDI activities
- What training is needed
- Who will do the training
- Where the training will take place
- The scope of CDI practice
- How activities will be reported and performance monitored (AHIMA 2016a, 16)

Each facility or organization can use this list as a starting point in creating their CDI process. It is a roadmap including topics of discussion and investigation for planning a successful CDI implementation.

### Composition of the CDI Staff

The many uses and users of information derived from clinical documentation support the need for an individualized approach to CDI. Each facility, provider, or organization's CDI program will or should be uniquely comprised to meet their specific needs (Casto and White 2024, 241). While there are multiple stakeholders involved in creating goals for the CDI process, the team performing review functions should include physicians, other healthcare providers, and coding professionals. Formal CDI programs using concurrent review teams can use a single discipline model (teams consisting of all nurses, HIM professionals, or physicians) or a hybrid (interdisciplinary) staffing model utilizing the skills from a combination of disciplines, often HIM and nursing (Butler 2019, 11). Employers report hiring CDI specialists from a mix of educational backgrounds (Combs 2019, 20). This suggests that organizations have evolved to the point of using an interdisciplinary approach.

As previously mentioned, the HIM staff has been performing retrospective quantitative and qualitative analysis for many years. Utilization management (UM) is a planned, systematic review of patients in a healthcare facility against care criteria for admission, continued stay, and discharge. UM professionals review documentation concurrently for specific indicators and criteria related to appropriate and resource-efficient patient care. When developing the process, CDI teams have sometimes incorporated existing HIM and UM functions instead of creating a completely new process.

One approach to CDI involves using only physician reviewers to communicate findings peer-to-peer with other physicians. While this provides advantages in relationship building between CDI programs and physicians, not all organizations can devote full-time physician resources to the process. Even when the CDI team is comprised of other healthcare professionals, a physician champion is often included to assist in communicating with their peers. The **physician champion**, also known in some organizations as the physician advisor, is an individual who assists in communicating with and educating medical staff in areas such as documentation procedures for accurate billing and electronic health record (EHR) procedures. Another approach to clinical review is to use only clinical staff, such as nursing professionals, who are familiar with the patient care unit and working with clinicians to treat patients. This has the benefit of communication and strong relationships. However, if the team lacks knowledge of documentation requirements for coding compliance, reimbursement, and other uses of coded data, the CDI program still struggles. Many CDI teams have incorporated the best of these approaches, with one or more physician champions and a mix of reviewers, some with a clinical background and others with an HIM or coding background (Butler 2019). This interdisciplinary approach makes the documentation review, communication of findings, and education more effective by including talent from clinical documentation users.

Regardless of professional background, those performing CDI must be able to work with a wide variety of team members. Treating each discipline, department, and individual with respect is important in the support and success of a CDI process. Cultural compatibility with the organization, leadership, and communication skills, and the ability to succeed in the complex healthcare environment, are all important aspects to consider (AHIMA 2013, 59). Reviewers must have a mix of knowledge regarding the uses of documentation and coded data internally for the organization and externally for government, regulatory, and quality purposes. The preferred and required qualifications of CDI professionals vary and can include physicians, physician assistants, nurses and nurse practitioners, as well as those with AHIMA, American Academy of Professional Coders (AAPC), and Association of Clinical Documentation Integrity Specialists (ACDIS) credentials. The minimum threshold for most CDI roles is an associate's degree, and a bachelor's degree is preferred (Combs 2019, 20). Recruitment for people who can fit this dynamic role often starts with professionals working in HIM and coding, quality improvement, UM, nursing, or case management departments. AHIMA's Commission on Certification for Health Informatics and Information Management (CCHIIM) developed the Clinical Documentation Integrity Practitioner (CDIP®) credential to help individuals signal their CDI qualifications. The CDIP exam covers content including knowledge of clinical coding practice, education and leadership development, record review and document clarification, CDI metrics and statistics, and compliance (AHIMA n.d.b). Healthcare organizations seeking CDI staff may want to target candidates who have passed the exam, which indicates credential holders have the following qualifications:

- Distinguished as knowledgeable and competent in clinical documentation in patient health records,
- Ready for leadership roles in the health informatics and information management community,
- Able to demonstrate competency in capturing documentation necessary to fully communicate patients' health status and conditions and provide a strong base of CDI expertise in the industry (AHIMA n.d.b).

ACDIS also has certifications; the Certified Clinical Documentation Specialist (CCDS) and Certified Clinical Documentation Specialist-Outpatient (CCDS-O) exams (ACDIS n.d.), and the American Academy of Professional Coders (AAPC) offers the Certified Documentation Expert Inpatient (CDEI) and Certified Documentation Expert Outpatient (CDEO) exams (AAPC n.d.). Certification can offer employers seeking CDI staff some evidence of the applicant's baseline knowledge and can be a component of the organizational or departmental compliance plan in hiring qualified CDI professionals.

The entire CDI team must carry out its duties in an ethical manner following industry-recognized best practices and facility policies and procedures. AHIMA has also developed the Ethical Standards for Clinical Documentation Integrity (CDI) Professionals to guide CDI planning, decision-making, and creation of procedures. According to these standards, CDI professionals will do the following:

1. Facilitate accurate, complete, and consistent clinical documentation within the health record to demonstrate quality care, support coding and reporting of high-quality healthcare data used for both individual patients and aggregate reporting.

2. Support the reporting of healthcare data elements (e.g. diagnoses and procedure codes, hospital acquired conditions, patient safety indicators) required for external reporting purposes (e.g. reimbursement, value based purchasing initiatives and other administrative uses, population health, quality and patient safety measurement, and research) completely and accurately, in accordance with regulatory and documentation standards and requirements, as well as all applicable official coding conventions, rules, and guidelines.

3. Query the provider (physician or other qualified healthcare practitioner), whether verbal or written, for clarification and/or additional documentation when there is conflicting, incomplete, or ambiguous information in the health record regarding a significant reportable condition or procedure or other reportable data element dependent on health record documentation (e.g. present on admission indicators). Query the provider if the documentation describes or is associated with clinical indicators without a definitive relationship to an underlying diagnosis, or provides a diagnosis without underlying clinical validation.

4. Never participate in or support documentation practices intended to inappropriately increase payment, to qualify for insurance policy coverage, to avoid quality reporting issues, or to skew data by means that do not comply with federal and state statutes, regulations and official rules and guidelines.

5. Facilitate interdisciplinary education and collaboration in situations supporting proper documentation, reporting and data collection practices throughout the facility.

6. Advance professional knowledge and practice through continuing education.

7. Never participate in or conceal unethical reporting practices or support documentation practices intended to inappropriately increase payment, qualify for insurance policy coverage, or distort data by means that do not comply with federal and state statutes, regulations and official coding rules and guidelines.

8. Protect the confidentiality of the health record at all times and refuse to access protected health information not required for job-related activities.

9. Demonstrate behavior that reflects integrity, shows a commitment to ethical and legal reporting practices, and fosters trust in professional activities.

10. Collaborate in a team environment with the coding, quality, and other professionals in the organization.

11. Report unethical, noncompliant, or unlawful activity to the organization's compliance officer or similar official responsible for monitoring such activities. (AHIMA 2020)

Certification for CDI professionals supports a healthcare organization's CDI process. In the hiring process, certification can be helpful in assessing what knowledge the applicants bring in addition to any potential skill-based assessments during the hiring process. It is a development goal requiring continued education and growth to achieve the certification for professionals working in the CDI process who are not certified and gives job seekers an advantage in obtaining a CDI position.

## Alignment

A CDI program may be housed in various areas of the organization such as corporate compliance, HIM, or quality improvement; however, each organization must evaluate where it fits best. Many organizations have a dedicated CDI manager and staff structure. An inclusive CDI oversight committee working with the CDI manager is a beneficial to bringing together the multiple stakeholders identified in the previous section. Executive administration and medical staff leadership are essential pieces of the committee.

The organization's administrators and medical staff need to support documentation improvement efforts. Top-level administration support is required, as it would be for any organizational change, and documentation processes and practices affect the organization in every area of patient care.

Support of the medical staff leadership is a key driver of success. Depending on the medical staff model used, physicians and physician leaders are not necessarily employees of the healthcare organization, although they work in tandem with healthcare professionals to provide care regardless of the model. This can be described as the dual-pyramid organization of healthcare facilities (Liebler and McConnell 2021, 42). The responsibility and authority structure of the medical staff functions alongside the administrative functions of executives, directors, and managers in hospitals and health systems. Depending on size and type of facility and the medical staff bylaws, a chief of staff, medical director, or corresponding position is responsible as a counterpart to the hospital chief executive officer.

Physicians who are not employees of a facility can apply for clinical privileges to practice there. They would report to the chief of staff or to a departmental physician lead or chairperson who ultimately reports to the chief of staff or medical director. CDI teams need to know what type of physician model and reporting structure is used when seeking the support of medical staff. Even though the CDI process may not be initiated by a particular physician, service, or office, the support of the medical staff and leadership is just as important as support from hospital administration. Physician leadership and involvement is an essential component in a successful and sustainable CDI program (ACDIS 2020b, 5). Physician leaders must be able to connect with peers and communicate the benefits of improved documentation to both the facility and physicians.

The physician champion has a responsibility to communicate, educate, and build or maintain respectful relationships with peers in improving documentation practices. The physician champion is involved with CDI and HIM staff on a routine basis as the medical expert regarding clinical documentation. CDI teams without physician champions are missing a valuable resource. The physician champion must be actively influential for a CDI program to succeed and is tasked with devoting time to the following:

- Educating providers on the importance of documentation
- Planning education for different medical departments
- Communicating with the medical staff regarding CDI (through newsletters, website, presentations, and such)
- Participating in investigating admission denials, DRG changes, Medicare core measures documentation
- Assisting in formulating clinically appropriate and compliant queries for physicians to clarify documentation (AHIMA 2016a)

Physician CDI champions should be selected based on their medical experience, work well with their peers, and communicate requirements of a successful CDI process (Hess 2018, 250). Even in programs where all or most of the documentation review is performed by nonphysician CDI professionals, the physician component for reviewer support and peer-to-peer communication and education is essential.

## Record Review

In many cases, reviewing every record concurrently is not a feasible undertaking for the CDI team. Selecting the priority areas of service, patient care units, type of insurance, or other criteria that is high impact is often needed to direct the process. A retrospective review of documentation on accounts already billed in the past may help identify areas of need or significant impact to begin with (AHIMA 2016a). It is important to remember that more accurate reimbursement is a benefit of a successful CDI program as opposed to maximizing payments from third-party payers (ACDIS 2019, 5; AHIMA House of Delegates 2016). The goal is to obtain the most accurate clinical documentation that represents the patient's medical status and treatment received, not to target or exploit reimbursement programs. While many CDI programs started by looking at inpatient encounters, they are now reviewing documentation in all care settings. This indicates CDI programs are evolving to focus on more than reimbursement metrics and are aiming at a whole spectrum of outcomes, including quality measures and patient safety. A growing number of organizations have adopted outpatient CDI programs (AHIMA 2018b, 5; Combs 2019, 19). (Most of the information in this chapter refers to inpatient CDI, yet the concepts apply to both settings.) One challenge in outpatient CDI programs is concurrent documentation review, as the timeframe for visits is much shorter than for inpatient stays. Even so, accurate documentation is important to patient care regardless of setting (AHIMA 2018b, 15).

Seven items a CDI professional often needs to obtain more specific documentation about in order to achieve accurate coding are as follows:

- Disease type
  - The inclusion of descriptors is needed for the most accurate code and often needed before any code can be assigned. Is a fracture traumatic or pathological, or a tumor malignant or benign?
- Disease acuity
  - Is the disease chronic, acute, or subacute?
- Site specificity
  - Does the most accurate code require location such as a specific lobe, or distal, proximal, superior, or inferior location?
- Disease stage
  - How severe or advanced is the disease?
- Laterality
  - Specifying the left or right eye, ear, or limb
- Details needed to assign a combination code
  - Many diseases and conditions are related and could be communicated with one code instead of multiple if specified as related

in the documentation such as diabetic complications, while others can be assumed related unless specified otherwise like hypertension and kidney disease
- Documentation missing completely (Hinkle-Azzara and Carr 2014, 37)

Specificity in clinical documentation for medical coding has been and continues to be a challenge (AHIMA 2018b, 5). Conditions such as respiratory failure, sepsis, pressure ulcer, coma, and pregnancy that have detailed coding requirements are areas in which CDI had the potential to make the most difference regardless of the coding system. Diagnoses and procedures that posed documentation challenges in the past continue to be potential focus areas due to their complex nature and many clinical factors that need to be considered and documented (AHIMA 2016b).

In addition to potential code-system documentation gaps, record review can also begin with diagnoses that may impact the organization's case mix under MS-DRG. **Case mix** is a description of a patient population based on characteristics including age, gender, type of insurance, diagnosis, risk factors, treatment received, and resources used. Healthcare facilities review the case-mix index (CMI) by averaging the MS-DRG relative weights of each inpatient treated, which reflects the resource intensity and clinical severity of that group of patients. When looking at the MS-DRG, the focus is not to aggressively maximize payment from insurers but to work toward the most accurate payment the provider is justly and legally entitled to receive (AHIMA House of Delegates 2016).

**Upcoding** is the practice of assigning diagnostic or procedural codes that represent higher payment rates than the services that were provided. The resulting legal action for fraud has proved a lesson and guide for CDI programs to focus on accurate, quality data as opposed to only payment, and it is one reason both AHIMA and the Association of Clinical Documentation Integrity Specialists (ACDIS) have developed the Ethical Standards for Clinical Documentation Improvement (CDI) Professionals (AHIMA 2020) and the ACDIS Code of Ethics (ACDIS 2020a) (Refer to online appendix C to review these ethical standards.) In addition, the case mix is used for myriad patient severity measures. The multiple comorbidities and complications (CC) and major comorbidities and complications (MCC) that impact the organization the most regarding differences in MS-DRG assignment are good targets for record review.

Each organization may need to focus on a specific set of records. Past results of external reviews—such as Recovery Audit Contractor (RAC) audits, and Program for Evaluating Payment Patterns Electronic Report (PEPPER)—or types of services that have had claims denials or rejections are good indicators of where to begin reviewing.

In many cases, missing a small detail can delay the coding process as clarification is sought. In the example of the ICD-10-PCS system, missing information to determine just one of the seven characters representing different aspects of the procedure will prevent code assignment. This is one reason concurrent review is preferred, both to obtain more accurate documentation in a timely manner, and to facilitate communication with providers during the care episode. Working for improved documentation during the episode of care benefits patient care safety and quality. However, once the patient is discharged, the opportunity to improve the care provided has passed. Retrospective reviews *are* valuable and useful for identifying trends and gathering data for decisions; however, their ability to improve documentation for communication is limited.

Determining where to start when planning a CDI process can be difficult. One strategy is to identify the top 5 to 10 MS-DRGs and surgeries occurring in the organization. From there, CDI specialists can define the documentation requirements needed for ICD-10-CM and ICD-10-PCS coding, identify the current weaknesses through record review, and develop a plan for documentation improvement starting with these areas (AHIMA 2016a).

### Frequency and Number of Record Reviews

Each organization must determine how many records are reasonable to review depending on the size of the CDI team and the complexity and types of records to be reviewed in the target areas. As previously mentioned, 100 percent review is not possible in most cases. The frequency of record review is also a consideration and depends on the individual organization. In concurrent review, the records continue to grow as the patient stay progresses; one record may need to be reviewed multiple times throughout the stay, whether daily or every other day. Another option is to review upon admission and day of expected discharge, then an alternating schedule in between.

### Budget

The CDI team requires adequate resources to accomplish the organization's goals. The budget is a tool to be used both for the planning and controlling management functions (Liebler and McConnell 2021, 172). Budgetary needs for hiring staff; providing education; utilizing communication tools; and measuring, tracking, and reporting should be considered by the organization when planning the CDI process. The composition of the CDI team, number and type of records to be reviewed, methods of education, communication needs, and information and results tracking will vary among organizations. The number and types of records requiring review and frequency of desired review also impacts the budget for personnel and hours. Regardless of the final dollar amount, the budget should provide enough resources to complete essential CDI functions.

### CDI Staff Training

Both physicians and the CDI team need continuous education to stay current in regulatory, legal, coding and external reporting requirements. Because CDI professionals come from a variety of healthcare backgrounds and have strengths in different areas (clinical, coding, quality, legal, and others), it may also be beneficial to have a common orientation program for new team members to ensure everyone has the same understanding of documentation issues and considerations. Specific education may be required for CDI staff who are very strong in some areas but lack experience in others. For example, a CDI team member with a clinical background may need further knowledge in coding guidelines, or a professional with a coding background may need more orientation on completing concurrent reviews.

### CDI Physician and Healthcare Provider Training

The education component for physicians and healthcare providers, such as physician assistants, nurse practitioners, and therapists, should increase awareness of documentation issues. This includes the many uses and impacts of documentation and coded data, where areas of improvement are to be found, and feedback on the quality of documentation and what improvements and benefits have been discovered. One benefit of having a physician champion for CDI is peer-to-peer insight in planning and facilitating training sessions. While everyone on the CDI team should be comfortable speaking with physicians and building respectful working relationships, the physician champion(s) can be a great asset in both group sessions and individual meetings with physicians about specific documentation issues. Education before and after the CDI program begins reduces misunderstandings and grows physician engagement in the CDI process (ACDIS 2021, 4).

While many physicians are not experts in the method of determining facility reimbursement or the acuity and severity of the patients the hospital serves, documentation and the resulting coded data are used for much more than hospital reimbursement. Data collected are used for multiple purposes, including many that reflect upon the physician's medical practices such as physician profiling and public reporting; quality assessment, including mortality and surgical complications; credentialing and reappointment; peer review; and performance improvement. Physician reimbursement is also aided by better documentation, upon which coded data for third-party reimbursement systems are based.

Providing short education sessions incrementally over time to change documentation practices is more effective than attempting to schedule and conduct one or a few exhaustive sessions (AHIMA 2016b). Short sessions, even by department or specialty, could give an opportunity to tailor the message to different groups of physicians. The following methods may be used to facilitate effective training sessions:

- Utilize real, practical examples of actual documentation from the facility or physician in CDI review
- Communicate the specific documentation needs of the ICD-10-CM/PCS system
- Create templates for diagnoses, procedures, or services needing improvement in documentation
- Distribute handouts as communication tools
- Leverage newsletters
- Display posters or signage to increase awareness
- Utilize "pocket cards" for quick reference (AHIMA 2016b)

Multiple methods can be used to communicate, educate, and remind those who document in the health record of the CDI process. As with any change, more communication, even in a small or short message, is better than less.

### Scope of Practice

The duties of each participant in the CDI process should be planned, defined, communicated, and understood by all involved. The CDI process includes creating job descriptions, determining department-level responsibilities, and establishing the reporting structure for roles such as the physician champion, CDI manager, and CDI staff. A process flowchart may help in planning and to clearly communicate CDI responsibilities and procedures (AHIMA and ACDIS 2021, 13). The scope of each role can differ by healthcare organization depending on unique organizational factors. The key stakeholders can help set the scope based on what resources and goals the organization has.

## Administrative Reports and Performance Monitoring Metrics

Metrics and statistics are about decision-making (White 2023, 2). Data regarding the success of the CDI program are essential components not only to support the decision to continue CDI, but to identify areas in which documentation still needs to improve. Metrics are important for knowing what is working and how well, and what is not working. Measuring performance and using that feedback for either correction or further improvement is part of the management function of controlling (Liebler and McConnell 2021, 292). Multiple sources indicate the need for some essential measurements to assist in the development and continuing improvement of the CDI process. Metrics are identified in figure 8.2.

Organizations may have differing data reporting needs. For example, an outpatient CDI process would not use CC and MCC capture rates, as they are specific to inpatient data. The outpatient metric may be related to ambulatory payment classification (APC) or include the number of claim denials related to documentation (AHIMA 2018b, 6). Additionally, some facilities may have data points needed for state-level programs or for specific action plans in which improvement is captured in the medical documentation. The end goal of metrics is not simply to collect data, but to use the data to evaluate and improve the organization and CDI process. It may be useful to use a dashboard or scorecard as in figure 8.3 to assist stakeholders in keeping aware of progress and making decisions regarding strategy, policy, and processes (AHIMA 2016a).

## CDI Benchmarks

Benchmarks for measures and performance statistics are a comparison of one's own results with the results of other individuals, departments, or organizations (Liebler and McConnell 2021, 297). Organizations can also benchmark against their own previous performance and results. The purpose is to identify and compare best practices of organizations with similar characteristics to assist in improving performance. Because each organization is different, national industry benchmarks are not always the best measure. However, some examples of benchmarks for CDI metrics (ACDIS, 2019, 3; AHIMA 2016a) are found in figure 8.4.

Benchmarks are tools for performance improvement. Measurements provide important feedback regarding the outcomes of the CDI program and

**Figure 8.2.** Basic metrics for CDI program evaluation

| Metric | Description |
|---|---|
| Record Review Rate | Number of discharges reviewed divided by the number of discharges available for review |
| Query Review Rate | Number of records queried divided by the number of records reviewed |
| Query Response Rate | Number of responses divided by the number of records queried |
| Query Agreement Rate | Number of queries in which the physicians agree with the CDI staff divided by the number of responses |
| Co-morbidity and Complication (CC) and Major Co-morbidity and Complication Capture Rates | Number of MS-DRGs with diagnosis codes for CC/MCC divided by number of total MS-DRGs |
| Physician Clarification Impact Percentage | Number of queries initiated by a CDI that had an impact on the DRG divided by the total number of queries |
| Severity Clarification Percentage | Number of queries that resulted in a severity change divided by the total number of queries |
| CDI Productivity | Each CDI professional's individual results in the given metrics |
| Physician-specific Query Rate | Each physician's individual results in the given metrics |
| Physician Response Turnaround Time | Amount of turnaround time between the initiation of the query and the physician response |
| CDI/Coding Agreement | Number of queries where the CDI team anticipated DRG matches the final coding assignment DRG divided by total number of queries (a learning tool for both) |
| Baseline Medical/Surgical Case Mix Index (CMI) | Set at time of initial program assessment |
| Actual CMI | Medical and surgical—based on population CDI program reviews, such as Medicare only or all inpatient discharges, etc. May want to exclude OB, newborn, psychiatry, rehabilitation, etc. |
| Trending actual CMI to goal CMI | Can break the trend into medical and surgical CMI, physician specialty/service line CMI. Most healthcare facilities review CMI over time, both overall and by specialty |
| DRG Proportions/Pairs | Review low/high DRGs and opportunities for DRG movement, such as from DRG 193–195, Simple Pneumonia, to DRG 177–179, Respiratory Infections & Inflammations |

*Source:* AHIMA 2022; AHIMA 2016a; ACDIS 2020b; ACDIS 2019.

**Figure 8.3.** Example of a CDI dashboard

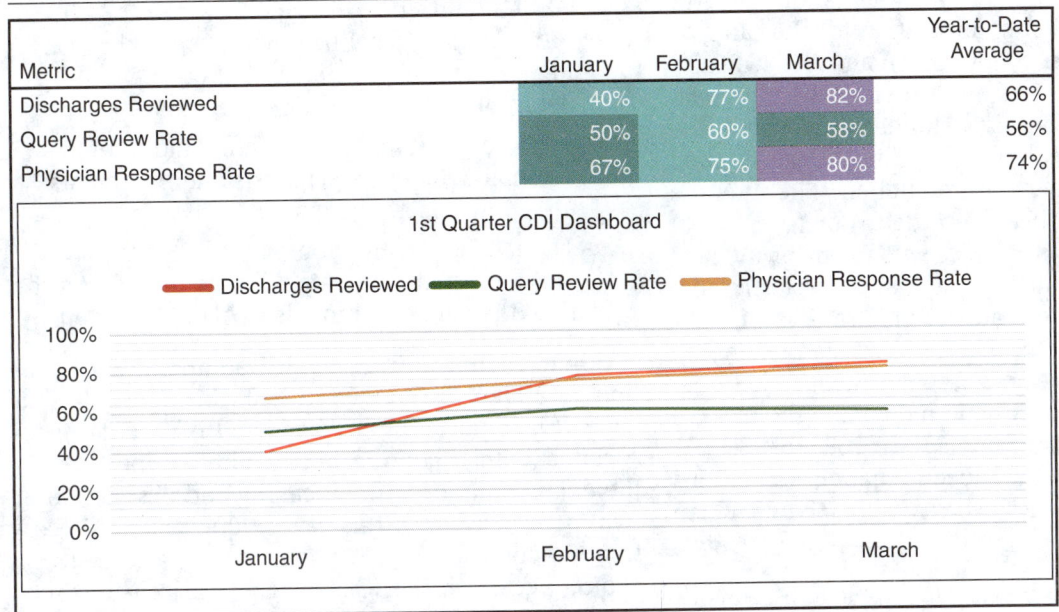

**Figure 8.4.** Sample CDI benchmarks

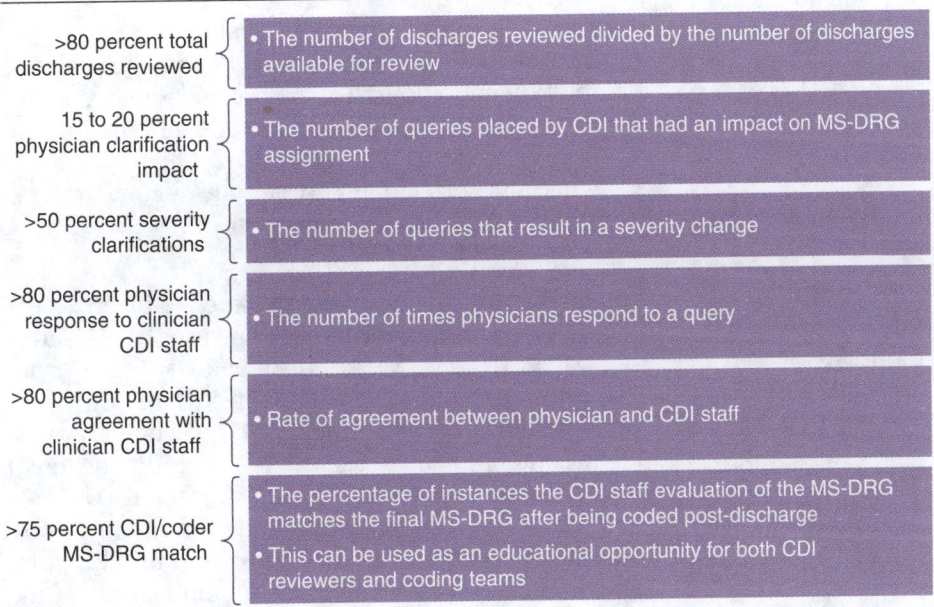

identify successes and areas for improvement. Achieving a certain score or number is not the most important consideration—the overall goal of these metrics is the accuracy of information, ultimately leading to better patient care.

## Query Process

Successful communication between the CDI team and the healthcare providers who are documenting care is identified as a key element to success (AHIMA 2021, 10). One form of communication is the process of asking providers for clarification on documentation. While methods of communication vary widely, there are some essential components. A sender must initiate and transmit the message, and a recipient must understand the message and acknowledge its receipt for both parties to be successful in the process. Both CDI professionals and physicians in the documentation improvement process must be senders and receivers to be successful. In cases where a CDI specialist or coder needs to ask a physician a question regarding documentation, it is referred to as a query (or, sometimes, a clarification). A **query** is a routine communication and education tool used to advocate for complete and compliant documentation (AHIMA 2016). This includes communication for the purpose of correct code assignment (AHIMA and ACDIS 2022). As a result of the variation in providers' documentation methods, querying is a standard practice and a common communication and educational method to advocate for proper documentation. The intent is to clarify what has been recorded, not to call into question the provider's clinical judgment or medical expertise. Both the query process and physician feedback about the process are essential pieces of communication. One role of the CDI physician champion is to assist and advocate for engagement when queries are lacking responses and help guide the process if misunderstandings occur (CHIMA 2023, 6).

As CDI staff review documentation, situations where a query may be necessary to include when documentation:

- is conflicting, imprecise, incomplete, illegible, ambiguous, or inconsistent;
- describes clinical indicators without a definitive relationship to an underlying diagnosis;
- includes clinical indicators, diagnostic evaluation, or treatment not related to a specific condition or procedure;
- provides a diagnosis without supporting clinical validation;
- is unclear for present on admission indicator assignment;
- leaves uncertainty of a cause-and-effect relationship between two conditions or organisms; or
- offers clinical evidence for a higher degree of specificity or severity (AHIMA and ACDIS 2022, 4; AHIMA 2018c, 3).

Queries may also be appropriate for documentation that is not legible, complete, clear, consistent, precise, reliable, or timely (AHIMA 2018c, 3). Definitions of these components of high-quality documentation are as follows:

- Legible: Documentation that is clear enough for the reader to easily interpret
- Complete: Documentation that is detailed and has maximum content fully addressing all concerns in the patient record
- Clear: Thoroughly describing what is occurring with the patient. Inpatient settings seek a definitive diagnosis while outpatient settings may be all that is known at the time
- Consistent: Documentation that does not contradict itself
- Precise: Clearly defined by including the highest level of specificity that can be determined from the clinical evidence
- Reliable: Trustworthy documentation, for example where the diagnosis and treatments are appropriately matched
- Timely: Documentation that is prepared, authenticated, and dated, by the provider at the time the care was provided (AHIMA 2018b, 15)

Some circumstances require additional information to assign the proper ICD-10-CM or ICD-10-PCS code. It is important to understand the exact term associated with a code is not required to be used in the documentation if the meaning and description of treatment is clear. In this case, a query is not necessary simply to have the matching term recorded. For coding accuracy, the ICD-10-PCS Official Guidelines for Coding and Reporting indicates that

> Many of the terms used to construct PCS codes are defined within the system. It is the coder's responsibility to determine what the documentation in the medical record equates to in the PCS definitions. The physician is not expected to use the terms used in PCS code descriptions, nor is the coder required to query the physician when the correlation between the documentation and the defined PCS terms is clear. (CMS 2024a, A11)

Coding professionals are not qualified to diagnose patients or perform procedures; however, the Centers for Medicare and Medicaid Services (CMS) do not expect physicians to be experts in ICD-10-PCS terminology and language either. CDI and coding professionals do not need to ask the physician to document using the exact phrasing contained in the ICD-10-PCS coding system if the documentation in the health record supports the code assigned based on PCS guidance. This CMS determination should be part of the education and training of both CDI staff and physicians as well as in policy for guidance to CDI and coding professionals. This will avoid needless queries to physicians.

### Developing a Query

When formulating a question about the specificity or clarity of information in the record, multiple factors should be considered. Just as the goal of CDI is accurate, specific, and clear documentation in the record, the query to the provider should also be easily understood and the reason for the question should be apparent. Including clinical indicators, focusing on accuracy, and, in most cases, creating open-ended questions that allow the results to be driven by physician medical expertise are some methods to employ.

It is important to include support from the documentation in the query. Including the reasoning for the query communicates to the clinician why they are being asked to clarify and what pieces of information are or are not already specified in the record.

The goal of querying is to achieve the greatest amount of specificity and accuracy (AHIMA 2018c). Reimbursement impact should not be the focus of the query, nor should the goal be to document the highest severity condition to obtain increased reimbursement. Inclusion of the reimbursement impact in the query confuses the motive of better communication and patient care with a monetary goal. It can also be viewed as a leading question to provide clinical indicators directing the response to a specific diagnosis or procedure that carries higher reimbursement.

It is wise to determine if open- or closed-ended questions are most appropriate. Some situations are acceptable for closed-ended, yes or no questions, such as clarifying a cause-and-effect relationship between diagnoses, seeking agreement or clarification between clinicians or reports, confirming details regarding established diagnosis, and determining if a diagnosis was POA. Looking at potential new diagnoses that are not already specified in the record could be viewed as attempting to lead a clinician to a particular diagnosis when presenting clinical support for only one diagnosis followed by only yes or no options. A better format in this case is an open-ended question asking if further detail can be provided or multiple-choice structure to allow for the most accurate response. Regardless of format, the query should not be formulated to lead the physician's response (AHIMA and ACDIS 2022, 11).

AHIMA and ACDIS's *Inpatient Query Toolkit* (2022, 6) suggests the following steps for a query process:

1. Queries may be either verbal or written and may be generated at any of the following times:
   - Concurrently (while the patient is still an inpatient)
   - Prebill (prior to the claim submission)
   - Retrospectively (post billing)
2. Written, electronically submitted, and email queries should be made utilizing compliant query templates and should follow all HIPAA [Health Insurance Portability and Accountability Act of 1996] security regulations.
3. The query templates provided in this toolkit may only be edited as follows:
   - Deletion of any part of the query form not pertinent to the query
   - Please delete any diagnosis listed in the multiple-choice query template that is not relevant to the patient's clinical picture
   - Add any pertinent clinical findings/diagnosis as documented in the health record
4. Verbal and telephonic queries should follow the same format as written queries.
5. All queries should:
   - Be clear, concise, and non-leading (if a title is included on a query, it should not be leading, and the query should include both supporting as well as conflicting documentation)
   - Be simple and direct. A query includes a synopsis of the encounter up to the time the query is being written that will support the intent of the query
   - Itemize the clinical indicators or clues (example: documentation found in nursing documentation, but not mentioned in the primary provider's documentation, lab findings, radiological findings) from the health record
6. The query should contain all the patient's identifying information such as name, date of admission or service, discharge date (if applicable), unit, etc. The query should also include a clear concise itemization of the clinical findings, with supporting documentation, that results in a specific question for the provider.
7. Queries are to be initiated by professionals trained and educated in the compliant query process, such as, but not limited to, coding and CDI professionals.
8. All queries should be logged for follow-up, to track responses and to trend for any documentation issues.

   Any issues identified may provide documentation improvement educational opportunities for providers as well as detecting the overuse of queries by CDI or coding professionals.
9. The highly specific nature of procedure coding systems (ICD-10-PCS, CPT/HCPCS) may

also require a query to obtain more detailed information. A compliant query can be directed to professionals who perform a procedure, as long as their documentation can be used for coding purposes. It is at times appropriate to query the surgeon or other providers, but the health record documentation is still ultimately the responsibility of the attending physician. (AHIMA 2018c, 5)

Queries are an important piece of both the concurrent CDI and coding process after patient discharge. They ensure the most accurate and specific documentation is recorded for multiple reasons, including patient care, coding, reimbursement, compliance, and more. Positive communication through queries helps lead to success in recording the best documentation possible.

### Documentation of Queries

Any documentation resulting from the query should be included in the patient record to communicate to other providers and support the patient's course of treatment. This is often recorded in the progress notes, discharge summary, or addendum to the documentation. Each organization must determine if the actual query is part of the permanent patient record or retained in other administrative records. Queries maintained as a part of the health record require more patient information than those recorded and stored elsewhere. A policy and procedure should be created to indicate if the query is a part of the patient health record, where is it located, and how long it is retained. Involvement of compliance and legal departments aid in determining the policy for each institution (AHIMA 2021, 9). Any information affecting the billed services obtained after the physician's documentation was completed must be included in accordance with accepted standards for amending the health record. During concurrent review, CDI professionals may have the opportunity to verbally communicate with physicians to clarify documentation. These queries and interactions should also be recorded to capture the impact of the CDI process. While not every verbal communication between CDI staff and physicians is an official query for clarification, instances where information that would have been communicated through a paper or electronic communication but has been discussed face-to-face should be recorded as a query.

### Format of Queries

Although the content of the question is more important than the format, some uniform format guidelines have been suggested:

- Patient name
- Admission date and time
- Account number
- Health record number
- Date the query is initiated
- CDI reviewer's contact information
- Individualized diagnosis-specific information relevant to the patient (AHIMA and ACDIS 2022)

In addition to the format or template of the query, other operational considerations must be determined, such as the following:

- Where in the record queries are placed
- The process for notifying a physician there is a query
- Standard procedures for how long a query is left open or unanswered before following up
- What happens to an open query after the patient is discharged
- Who will monitor the unanswered queries
- Feedback or corrective action to be taken and who will undertake it (AHIMA and ACDIS 2022)

Figures 8.5 and 8.6 provide examples of physician queries. Each situation requires different documentation considerations depending on the method of communication—paper, electronic, or verbal. Open-ended questions are also an effective method of querying physicians, as noted in the situations of figure 8.6.

## Technology Considerations in CDI

The meaningful use of technology has expanded in healthcare to provide many advances in treating patients and making recordkeeping and administrative functions more efficient. While technology such as the EHR, with its ability to integrate clinical pathways and provide real-time reminders to clinicians, is helpful, it is not an automatic fix to documentation deficiencies. In some cases, facilities have developed or used documentation templates specific to particular

**Figure 8.5.** Examples of closed-ended queries

**Compliant Example 1**

**Clinical scenario:** In the impression of the pathology report, ovarian cancer is documented; however, only ovarian mass is documented in the final discharge statement by the provider.

**Query:** Do you agree with the pathology report specifying the "ovarian mass" as an "ovarian cancer?" Please document your response in the health record or below.

Yes _____

No _____

Other _____

Clinically Undetermined _____

Name: _____ Date: _____

**Rationale:** This yes or no query involves confirming a diagnosis that is already present as an interpretation of a pathology specimen in the health record.

**Compliant Example 2**

**Clinical scenario:** Consulting pulmonologist documents pneumonia as an impression based on the chest x-ray. However, the attending physician documents bronchitis throughout the record, including in the discharge summary.

**Query:** Do you agree with the pulmonologist's impression that the patient has pneumonia? Please document your response in the health record or below.

Yes _____

No _____

Other _____

Clinically Undetermined _____

Name: _____ Date: _____

**Rationale:** This is an example of a yes or no query resolving conflicting practitioner documentation.

*Source:* AHIMA 2019.

**Figure 8.6.** Example of an open-ended query

A patient is admitted with pneumonia. The admitting H&P examination reveals WBC of 14,000; a respiratory rate of 24; a temperature of 102 degrees; heart rate of 120; hypotension; and altered mental status. The patient is administered an IV antibiotic and IV fluid resuscitation.

**Leading:** The patient has elevated WBCs, tachycardia, and is given an IV antibiotic for Pseudomonas cultured from the blood. Are you treating for sepsis?

**Nonleading:** Based on your clinical judgment, can you provide a diagnosis that represents the below-listed clinical indicators?

In this patient admitted with pneumonia, the admitting history and physical examination reveals the following:

- WBC 14,000
- Respiratory rate 24
- Temperature 102°F
- Heart rate 120
- Hypotension
- Altered mental status
- IV antibiotic administration
- IV fluid resuscitation

Please document the condition and the causative organism (if known) in the medical record.

*Source:* AHIMA 2019.

diagnoses, procedures, or services and can be very useful to help capture relevant and required details for ICD-10-CM and ICD-10-PCS coding, core measures, and other quality indicators. Reviews of the templates should be conducted each year as changes in coding and quality reporting occur (AHIMA 2016b). The AHIMA *Query Toolkit* (2019) provides specific examples of templates for different types of diagnoses that may be built into an electronic system; however, a generic template can be used as shown in figure 8.7. Templates, edits, and prompts are useful tools to encourage quality documentation but should not be relied upon as a sole solution for improving documentation.

**Computer-assisted coding (CAC)**, a tool intended for improved efficiency of the coding and claims submission process, is an emerging technology used in the coding process. While CAC can be useful in settings where documentation is structured and has a limited vocabulary, remember that specific and accurate documentation is the underlying resource for technologic advances relating to patient records, medical coding, and quality improvement. As healthcare continues to advance technologically, the content—including documentation of patient treatment—inside the software and hardware utilized provides the real benefit to patient care and the processes that support it.

**Figure 8.7.** Generic query template

| Dear | (add provider(s) name) |
|------|------------------------|
| Identify the opportunity | was documented within the Reference document location(s) |
| Clinical Indicators: Signs and Symptoms: | Signs and Symptoms: | Additional Indicators: | Risk Factors: |
| Additional Risk Factors: | Treatment: | Treatment: | Additional Treatment |

Based on the clinical indicators and your professional judgment Questions:
Please complete by selecting one of the options below.

- Click here to enter text:
- Click here to enter text:
- Findings of no clinical significance (optional)
- Other explanation of clinical findings  Click here to enter text:
- Unable to determine
- No further clarification needed (optional)

*Source:* AHIMA 2018c, 12.

HIM professionals are beginning to explore how artificial intelligence (AI) and machine learning (ML) affect HIM processes. AI is high-level information technologies used in developing machines that imitate human qualities such as learning and reasoning. ML is an area of computer science that studies algorithms and computer programs that improve employee performance on some task by exposure to a training or learning experience. As we see greater advances in AI and ML, HIM professionals must consider how to incorporate them in HIM job functions to maximize the benefits. HIM can celebrate and embrace working in partnership with AI, especially in the areas of CDI and compliance. Taking an objective look to see where AI and ML can improve human performance will prove to be challenging and rewarding as we see efficiency and accuracy improve without increasing staff.

A mutually beneficial integration of AI into HIM roles would start by identifying what AI can meaningfully contribute to each HIM job function including CDI, considering what a person can do that a computer cannot and vice versa. "To reap the benefits of all that AI has made possible while still valuing human intelligence and emotions, we need to approach it with excitement and an open mind. We must recognize our collective abilities and realize that the choice is not between people and AI, but rather how to create a future in which human intelligence and AI coexist and work together" (Muthukumaraswamy 2023).

Coding professionals can focus on things like upgrading their soft skills, such as communication, to interact with the many members of the healthcare team regarding documentation while using AI and ML software for other CDI tasks (Muthukumaraswamy 2023). This "technology is an important tool to support clinical documentation but does not eliminate the need for CDSs (clinical documentation specialists) whose clinical and critical thinking skills are paramount to CDI success" (AHIMA 2022). The overarching goal of AI and ML in the CDI process would be to improve coder and CDS productivity and accuracy for the organization while increasing job satisfaction for the professional. Determining which tasks are best suited for technology and which are best suited for human interaction will be the place to start in planning integration of AI and ML.

### Check Your Understanding 8.1

**Answer the following questions in a separate document.**

1. How would you present and defend the purpose and importance of a clinical documentation integrity (CDI) program to a healthcare provider?
2. Recommend a CDI process workflow design, and justify your choice.
3. How would you advocate for the importance of a CDI program to potential stakeholders? How will the CDI program benefit and impact each stakeholder?
4. Justify the importance of a CDI physician champion.
5. What factors need to be considered when proposing to implement a CDI process? Why is each factor important to the plan and what possible issues might be associated with each?
6. Compare and contrast the advantages and disadvantages of obtaining and keeping a CDI credential.

7. Review the AHIMA Ethical Standards for Clinical Documentation Integrity Professional. Create a scenario where an employee violates the ethical standards. Then recommend a path to avoiding the scenario in the future.
8. Articulate the need for CDI program goals and who should be involved in goal setting.
9. Examine why CDI is essential to an accurate case mix. Determine if CDI can have a negative impact on CMI. If so, why?
10. Explain what a benchmark is and why they are useful. Review the sample CDI benchmarks in figure 8.4. Using the categories provided in the figure, analyze each category. Then develop a new minimum threshold for each category with an explanation of why the change is needed.

## Corporate Compliance

Corporate compliance is intended to help detect and prevent the violations of fraud, waste, and abuse. Coding compliance is a part of an overall corporate compliance plan. Along with ensuring that employees adhere to ethical conduct, corporate compliance programs conform to the goals of the **Office of the Inspector General (OIG)**. The mission of the OIG is to protect the integrity of US Department of Health and Human Services (HHS) programs and operations, and the health and well-being of the people served. The OIG's strategic plan includes the following four goals:

- fight fraud, waste, and abuse;
- promote quality and safety;
- secure the future; and
- advance innovation (OIG n.d.a)

The OIG's work consists of a multidisciplinary and collaborative approach that includes auditing and evaluating its annual workplan and combating fraud, waste, and abuse by providing government oversight and resources to improve the efficiency of HHS programs. The **OIG workplan** "sets forth various projects to be addressed during the fiscal year by the Office of Audit Services, Office of Evaluation and Inspections, Office of Investigations, and Office of Counsel" to the Inspector General, including projects planned by CMS (OIG n.d.b). In addition to the workplan, the OIG makes legal and investigative efforts to help facilitate compliance in the healthcare industry.

Like the OIG, CMS develops compliance program guidance specific to Medicare fee-for-service contractors to promote adherence to all Medicare statutory and regulatory requirements (CMS 2005, 3). According to both CMS and the OIG, effective healthcare compliance programs are based on seven fundamental elements:

- Enforcing policies, procedures, and standards of conduct
- Establishing a formalized compliance committee and designating a compliance officer
- Regularly conducting, reviewing, and updating trainings
- Maintaining open lines of communication
- Continuously measuring effectiveness through ongoing internal monitoring and audits
- Enforcing standards though established guidelines
- Providing a swift response to all compliance issues (CMS 2005, 4; OIG n.d.f).

In the US, noncompliance in healthcare can lead to civil or criminal penalties. It is important to understand the minimum general corporate compliance program elements to help establish a culture that promotes prevention, detection, and appropriate resolution of conduct that does not conform to federal and state laws and healthcare program requirements.

Standards of conduct should exist as written organizational policy. Compliance officers are ultimately responsible for making sure employees adhere to the code of conduct and timely reporting of compliance violations. Although a distinction exists between unintentional mistakes and fraud, sound prevention and detection processes should be incorporated into compliance plans. The compliance officer is responsible for identifying and locating primary law sources to assist in this process. Primary sources such as the OIG, DOJ, and CMS should always be sought for review and cited to validate recommendations. The federal False Claims Act, Deficit Reduction Acts of 2005, and HIPAA are addressed with coding compliance in the following section. Additional topics which are not specifically for coding compliance but included in an overall corporate compliance plan include identify theft, kickbacks, the Stark Law, and the Emergency Medical Treatment and Labor Act (EMTALA).

## Coding Compliance

Compliance means abiding by rules, laws, standards, or regulations. Following the required rules and expected practices in regard to coding is of particular interest since coded data are used for many purposes, including the basis of most payment and reimbursement decisions made in the US healthcare system. This includes the federal Medicare and state Medicaid programs for which the discrepancy between submitted coded data and the actual service provided is an area often reviewed for fraud (CMS 2021, 6). Government investigators have the authority to examine claims for payment from any organization or provider who delivers services or treatments to Medicare beneficiaries as the Federal fraud and abuse laws apply (OIG n.d.c). Professional ethics and accepted practice are to comply with the rules of programs in which the healthcare provider participates; this is because accurate and complete coded data "is then translated into quality reporting, physician report cards, reimbursement, public health data, disease tracking and trending, and medical research" (AHIMA n.d.a.). In addition to the inherent benefits of ensuring accurately coded data, the risk of negative consequences is also a driver for coding compliance plans.

Numerous factors could result in organizational harm due to incorrectly coded data on claims for reimbursement. *Fraud* and *abuse* are two terms often used to describe actions of a provider or organization collecting undeserved payments. Fraud is an intentional deception or misrepresentation an individual makes with the knowledge that the deception could result in unauthorized benefit to self or others, and abuse describes practices or incidents that are inconsistent with sound fiscal, business, or medical practices and result in improper payments from Medicare (CMS 2021, 7).

Fraudulent activities misrepresent the care that took place. Billing for services that were not provided or providing a lesser service than what is reported is an example of fraud. Other examples are billing for new equipment while providing the patient with used or old equipment, reporting that services were completed at a different site than they were, or misrepresenting which practitioner provided the service. There are many more ways fraudulent requests for payment using coded data could occur, all of them involving a misrepresentation.

Abuse is defined as healthcare providers or suppliers performing actions that directly or indirectly result in unnecessary costs to any healthcare benefit programs (CMS 2021). Excessive or improper use of services or actions inconsistent with acceptable business practices is considered abuse. It does not have to be intentional; however, the idea that the person or organization "knows or should know better" applies when determining the difference between fraud and abuse (CMS 2021, 8). No proof of intent is required if a person or organization acts in deliberate ignorance of the truth or acts in reckless disregard; their actions can still be seen as fraud (Bowman 2023, 339). Examples of abuse include unintentional unbundling of codes or mistakenly reporting the wrong place of service or discharge status. By submitting a claim for payment, the provider is certifying they have earned the requested payment and complied with all requirements to receive it. If the provider or organization knew or should have known the claim for payment was false, they are in violation (CMS 2021). Penalties apply under federal and state law for both fraud and abuse, intentional or unintentional, which is why compliance programs are essential.

Although waste is not a legally defined term, CMS identifies waste as "overutilization, underutilization, or misuse of resources" (CMS 2019, 4). An example of overutilization is repeat lab tests. An example of underutilization is bypassing preventative screenings. An example of misuse is using a CT scan for routine mammography instead of x-ray when not warranted. Waste is typically not intentional or criminal in nature; however, waste does have a financial impact on services.

## Regulation

Many laws apply to healthcare fraud and abuse. For example, the federal False Claims Act, Civil Monetary Penalties Law, HIPAA, Balanced Budget Act of 1997, Tax Relief and Health Care Act of 2006, and others have aspects or outline programs specifically dealing with coded healthcare data used for financial purposes. The Deficit Reduction Act of 2005 necessitated that compliance programs by healthcare providers shift from voluntary to a mandatory practice (Bowman 2023, 346). Continuing awareness of new and changing legislation and regulation is important for HIM professionals.

### Federal False Claims Act of 1863

The federal False Claims Act of 1863 is a federal law that seeks to protect governmental programs from fraud by individuals and companies. It outlines how both deliberate ignorance and reckless disregard to the "truth or falsity" of a claim are included with having knowledge of the false information (CMS 2021). Even without intent to defraud the government, a provider, organization, or individual can be found in violation. A coding compliance plan will work to eliminate the ignorance or indifference throughout the organization regarding inaccurate data on claims. The civil False Claims Act was originally enacted during the American Civil War to prevent government contractors from collecting money for services or goods not actually provided or misrepresenting what was provided in the claim to the government. In 1986, the act was amended and one of the most significant updates included the provision to allow involvement of **qui tam relators**, or those acting on behalf of the government. This is sometimes referred to as **whistleblowing**, where anyone—including employees, patients, and competitors—can bring lawsuits based on their knowledge of fraud (DOJ 2024). Qui tam relators receive a minimum of 15 percent of the fraudulent monies recovered by the government.

### Deficit Reduction Act of 2005

The Deficit Reduction Act of 2005 is a multifaceted law concerning the nation's budget. One section specifically aims at fighting Medicaid fraud and abuse. The act requires any program that receives or makes payments of over $5,000,000 annually to provide education to employees regarding the False Claims Act (CMS n.d.a, 5). The act requires written policies for anyone working with claims, including contractors, to communicate details of the False Claims Act to employees, including the organizational process for reporting and correcting inaccuracies; whistleblower protections; the prevention and detection of waste, fraud, and abuse; as well as related laws (Bowman 2023, 346). It also allocated additional resources to identifying Medicare fraud and abuse.

### Health Insurance Portability and Accountability Act of 1996

HIPAA, enacted in 1996, is a law regarding many aspects of the healthcare system. Considerable attention has been paid to the patient privacy and information security aspects in the administrative simplification section, although there are pieces that relate to coding compliance as well. Preventing healthcare fraud and abuse is a major focus of the legislation. Providing medically unnecessary services, billing for services that were not provided, and misrepresentations in coding practices are examples that HIPAA outlines as fraud and abuse (OIG n.d.c, 10). Unbundling and upcoding are types of coding misrepresentations that lead to inaccurate and undeserved reimbursement. Both are practices investigated by the OIG.

### Governmental Audit Programs

There are many audit programs concerning the accuracy of coded data submitted to federal agencies. The reviews typically include reviewing the documentation in the patient record and comparing it to the codes submitted on a claim for payment. Some examples are listed in figure 8.8

In addition to the examples of governmental programs related to fraud, private insurers also administer audits and reviews. This ensures both quality and efficient care by providers and that appropriate payment by the insurer is provided for the privately insured population.

### Exclusion from Federal Programs

Providers and healthcare entities found to be fraudulent or abusive in receiving payments from the government are subject to penalties and exclusion from participating in federal programs. The **Exclusion Provisions**, a component of the Social Security Act, indicates that the OIG has the authority to "exclude individuals from participating in federal healthcare programs and will not pay for items or services furnished by an excluded individual or entity" (Social Security Act 1996). The **Civil Monetary Penalties Law** provides punitive fines imposed by a civil court to organizations that profit from illegal or unethical activities (OIG n.d.b). Depending upon the extent and intent of the fraudulent activity, one or both of these sanctions can be applied. An example would be billing for services that were not medically necessary, which is classified as healthcare abuse. Exclusion is significant as the government is the largest purchaser and provider of healthcare services in the country. Any provider or supplier convicted of Medicare fraud or other healthcare fraud, theft, or financial misconduct is required to be excluded from any federal healthcare program (CMS 2021).

Advances in technology are making the need for compliance plans apparent. More sophisticated tools and data analysis allow government entities and private insurers to identify trends in provider claims and more easily benchmark and compare data among similar providers to detect fraud, waste, and abuse. HIM professionals need to engage in continuing education throughout their career to remain aware of new and changing programs and agencies both governmental and nongovernmental.

### Auditing

When an auditor of a governmental agency or third-party payer is preparing to review records on-site or through remote access, a notification of what records

**Figure 8.8.** Governmental agencies and programs

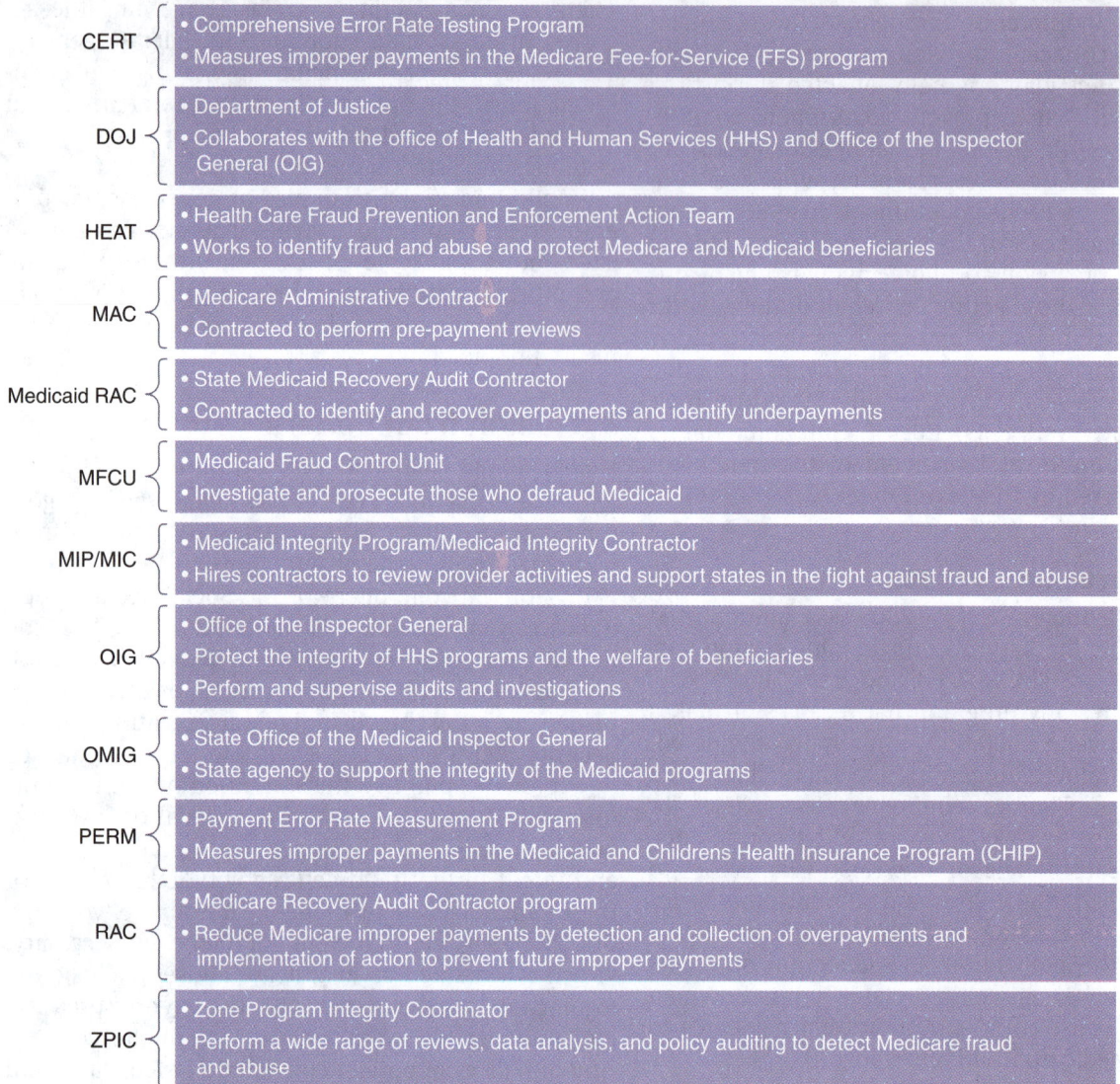

are needed and the method of review is provided. Auditors will select many records for review in some cases and a smaller sample in others. Audits may be performed for many reasons: reviewing quality indicators, compliance with regulations, reimbursement for services, and more. When the audit is for reimbursement purposes, any over- or underpayments might be corrected on only the accounts reviewed. Another method of adjustment is referred to as the extrapolation method. The extrapolation method of auditing claims looks at a small sample of records and applies the correction in reimbursement across many claims in a period or service area. One strategy for healthcare providers in preparation for the audit is to review the selected records beforehand, once the sample has been selected by the auditing agency or team (AHIMA 2013, 60). The purpose is not to make changes or alter ahead of time, but to be able to estimate any potential change in retroactive reimbursement and begin to prepare financially for any anticipated adjustments.

## Office of the Inspector General Compliance Guidance

The OIG was created in 1976 with the mission to "protect the integrity of the Health and Human Services (HHS) programs as well as the health and welfare of program beneficiaries" (OIG n.d.d). Different departments of the government have their own investigative agencies, although the HHS OIG is larger than any other governmental OIG. The OIG publishes guidelines organizations are strongly urged to follow; however, they are not mandates because every provider is different and specific guidelines may not apply to every organization (Bowman 2023, 346). Guidance to hospitals, nursing facilities, researchers, ambulance suppliers, pharmaceutical manufacturers, physicians, clinical laboratories, third-party billing agencies, Medicare + Choice programs, and durable equipment companies can be found on the OIG website. Some foundational guidelines provided by the OIG are as follows:

- The development and distribution of written standards of conduct, as well as written policies and procedures that promote the hospital's commitment to compliance (e.g., by including adherence to compliance as an element in evaluating managers and employees)...;
- The designation of a chief compliance officer and other appropriate bodies, e.g., a corporate compliance committee charged with the responsibility of operating and monitoring the compliance program and who report directly to the CEO and the governing body;
- The development and implementation of regular, effective education and training programs for all affected employees;
- The maintenance of a process, such as a hotline, to receive complaints, and the adoption of procedures to protect the anonymity of complainants and to protect whistleblowers from retaliation;
- The development of a system to respond to allegations of improper/illegal activities and the enforcement of appropriate disciplinary action against employees who have violated internal compliance policies, applicable statutes, regulations or Federal health care program requirements;
- The use of audits and/or other evaluation techniques to monitor compliance and assist in the reduction of identified problem areas; and
- The investigation and remediation of identified systemic problems and the development of policies addressing the non-employment or retention of sanctioned individuals. (OIG 2023, 32)

Benchmarking, longitudinal studies, and regular reporting are elements supported by the OIG as the essential components of an overall compliance plan. A compliance plan can include both internal self-audits as well as external reviewers with the aim to identify weaknesses and improve practices on a voluntary basis. The best practice for internal audits is to avoid having the same people review records who are initially responsible for the coding. Many healthcare organizations have a coding compliance reviewer separate from the HIM coding department. External reviewers are often consultants or agencies also designed to give outside, unbiased advice based on results of record review, coded data, and claims reviews. The goal is to prevent any practices that may not meet the standards of federal and state laws, as well as other accreditation or regulatory practices. While prevention is the best outcome, identification and correction of issues also fall within the realm of compliance.

### Target Areas and OIG Workplan

Each year the HHS OIG publishes planned projects and areas identified for review. These published workplans cover CMS and the Administrations for Children and Families and Administration on Aging. The workplan can be found on the HHS OIG website. It is advisable to include the OIG workplan items that may apply to an organization in the compliance plan, as well as address other high-risk areas for review including billing for noncovered services, inaccurate claim forms, duplicate billing, correction of overpayments, unbundling, overcoding, or upcoding (Bowman 2023, 358).

During the process of reviewing the health record for code assignment, fraud and abuse practices called unbundling and upcoding may be identified. **Unbundling** is the reporting of multiple codes to describe a service or procedure when, according to coding conventions, one code would accurately describe the procedure. Unbundling often results in additional reimbursement, as if the provider performed various smaller procedures separately although the procedure is intended to include all the essential components bundled together. Upcoding describes using diagnosis or procedure codes selected specifically because they result in higher payment from third-party payers. Unbundling and upcoding are examples of attempts to maximize reimbursement to the highest possible amount through coded data, or **maximization**. This practice puts an organization or provider at risk of violating the previously mentioned federal and state laws. A better focus is the intent of coding optimization. **Coding optimization** seeks the most accurate documentation, coded data, and resulting payment in the amount the provider is rightly and legally entitled to receive (AHIMA 2016). CDI and coding compliance programs support coding optimization.

### Developing a Coding Compliance Plan

While compliance in general refers to meeting the requirements of laws and regulations, a specific compliance plan related to coding is beneficial to healthcare organizations because of the relationship of coded data to financial reimbursement for services. Formal policies and procedures must be in place to provide instruction in the entire process from the provision of care through to the submission of claims (AHIMA 2010). The coding compliance plan should include the following components:

- Policy statement regarding the commitment of the organization to correctly assign and report codes
- The source of official coding guidelines used to direct code selection
- Identification of who is responsible for code selection
- The procedure to follow when clinical information is not clear or specific enough to assign the correct code
- Specification of policies and procedures by care setting (ER, OP, IP)
- Applicable reporting requirements mandated by specific agencies, including where payer-specific instructions can be found
- Procedures for correction of inaccurate code assignments
- Areas of risk that have been identified through audits and monitoring, a defined plan for audit and review, and corrective actions outlined for identified problems
- Identification of essential coding resources available to and used by coding professionals
- A process for coding new procedures or unusual diagnoses
- A procedure to identify any optional codes gathered for statistical purposes by the facility and clarification of the appropriate use of external cause codes
- Appropriate methods for resolving coding or documentation disputes with physicians
- A procedure for processing claim rejections
- A statement regarding "codes will not be assigned, modified, or excluded solely for the purpose of maximizing reimbursement or avoiding reduced payment. Clinical codes will not be changed or amended merely because of either physician or patient request to have the service in question covered by insurance. If the initial code assignment did not reflect actual services, codes may be revised on the basis of documentation" (AHIMA 2010, 3)
- Statement on the use and reliance on encoding software; coding staff will be skilled in the review of records and proper assignment of diagnostic and procedural codes, not dependent or relying solely on coding software
- Medical records are analyzed and codes selected only with complete and appropriate physician documentation available; official coding guidelines state codes are not assigned without supporting documentation from the provider and the entire record should be reviewed (AHIMA 2010)

In addition to policies and procedures, the individuals completing the coding function should have guidance as to the correct and ethical method of medical coding. All coding compliance plans should reference AHIMA's Standards of Ethical Coding (DeVault and Stanfill, 2019, 50–52). (Refer to online appendix C.) The guides used to determine coding process should be American Hospital Association (AHA) *Coding Clinic*, AHA *HCPCS Clinic*, American Medical Association (AMA) *CPT Assistant*, and additional guidance from CMS.

## Fraud Surveillance

Fraud, abuse, and waste divert significant resources away from healthcare services. Both state and federal initiatives have implemented steps against healthcare fraud. One important example of an anti-fraud effort is CMS's Center for Program Integrity (CPI). CPI serves as the central point for CMS's program integrity mission (CMS 2021, 19). In addition to CMS, the OIG issues annual guidelines for compliance to healthcare providers. The OIG protects the integrity of HHS programs, including CMS.

Increased attention on investigating, preventing, and prosecuting fraud and abuse in healthcare was apparent in 1996 with passage of HIPAA. HIPAA expanded the role of the OIG to include private insurance programs in addition to federally funded programs.

The OIG negotiates **corporate integrity agreements (CIAs)** with healthcare providers and other entities. "As part of the settlement of federal healthcare program investigations, providers or entities agree to the obligations in exchange for the OIG to not seek their exclusion from participation in federal healthcare programs" (OIG n.d.a). CIAs may last for many years and are imposed when serious misconduct (fraud and abuse) is discovered through an audit or self-disclosure. Remediation initiatives, such as training or designation of a compliance officer, are part of the CIA. Remediation activities are intended to offer providers another chance to prove they are worthy of participating in federal healthcare programs

(OIG n.d.a). CIAs generally do not result from unintentional errors and are imposed where there is evidence of intentional fraud.

As a preventative measure, the US Sentencing Commission has developed key criteria for establishing an effective compliance and ethics program, which includes the following:

- Standards and procedures to prevent and detect criminal conduct
- Oversight by high-level personnel
- Due care in delegating substantial discretionary authority
- Effective communication to all levels of employees
- Reasonable steps to achieve compliance, which include systems for monitoring, auditing, and reporting suspected wrongdoing without fear of reprisal
- Consistent enforcement of compliance standards including disciplinary mechanisms
- Reasonable steps to respond to and prevent further similar offenses upon detection of a violation (US Sentencing Commission 2018, 8B2.1)

These initiatives are designed to ensure fraudulent activities do not occur. Prevention approaches can be driven by both external and internal factors.

### External and Internal Fraud Prevention Drivers

External fraud surveillance approaches include whistleblower incentives, data mining and data validation, working with RACs, and other audits, such as those for complaints. Many of the commonly known government auditors in healthcare are listed in figure 8.8. Building fraud and abuse controls and cost-effective performance monitoring in all organization functional areas support a process of continuous improvement and eliminate waste. To operate an effective compliance program, it is important to have internal monitoring measures. These measures include the following:

- Continually reviewing fraud and abuse surveillance plans;
- Maintaining system hardware and software upgrades;
- Conducting risk assessments;
- Monitoring marketing practices;
- Enforcing policies and procedures; and
- Providing prompt response to compliance issues such as reporting and findings from compliance reviews and audits (OIG 2017, 1).

Another internal driver of compliance is the proactive review of coding, contracts, repayment, and post-payment, and the monitoring of third-party transactions.

### Key Clinical Documents

The official coding guidelines for ICD-10-CM and ICD-10-PCS indicate complete and appropriate documentation must be reviewed when assigning diagnostic and procedural codes. No external rule or regulation exists that outlines or defines specific documents required to be complete or appropriate for coding, only that the documentation must be from the patient's provider, a physician or other qualified healthcare practitioner legally accountable for establishing the patient's diagnosis (CMS 2024b, 15). As part of the compliance plan the organization should define what key clinical documents are required based on the care setting and type of record (Cassidy 2012). A policy should identify what documents the organization requires to be available and reviewed before assigning diagnostic or procedural codes. This can reduce the pressure to code an encounter without complete documentation to expedite the claims submission process. The required set also gives new and experienced coding professionals a facility- and service-specific guide as to what documentation to review. The documents listed in figure 8.9 are suggestions for defining the core designated clinical documentation set for coding compliance (Cassidy 2012).

Identifying these documents can also support successful implementation of electronic processes, including accurate CAC. Requiring any CAC process to include a specific and complete set of information allows the process to stay on track with the compliance plan to prevent errors (Cassidy 2012).

### Coding Compliance Education

Coding compliance education for everyone from providers to claims submission staff is integral to prevention. Formal policies and job descriptions typically specify that those hired to coding positions must have the appropriate training, experience, and credentials to successfully perform the job. It is also common for employers to require coding applicants to pass an assessment even if the candidate possesses coding credentials or certifications. Coding compliance training beyond the general orientation is recommended for any new employees responsible for assigning codes, as well as ongoing, regular education after hire (Bowman 2023, 366). Training content should ensure employees understand the organization's compliance plan and compliance laws and regulations.

Ongoing training needs to be a requirement of employment, and testing is encouraged to measure the

**Figure 8.9.** Core clinical documents for coding

| Inpatient Coding | Outpatient/Ambulatory Surgery Coding | Observation Coding | Emergency Department Coding | Outpatient/Ancillary Coding |
|---|---|---|---|---|
| • Face sheet (or similar document organization-specific)<br>• Progress notes<br>• History and physical<br>• Discharge summary<br>• Consultation report<br>• Operative reports<br>• Pathology reports<br>• Laboratory<br>• Radiology<br>• Physician's orders<br>• Nutritional assessments | • History and physical<br>• Results of previous diagnostics tests related to the encounter<br>• Operative/procedure report<br>• Pathology report<br>• Medication list | • History and physical<br>• Progress notes<br>• Physician orders (both for admission to observation and for treatment)<br>• Clinical observations<br>• Final progress note/summary | • Emergency department report<br>• Initial encounter<br>• Diagnostic interventions<br>• Treatment interventions<br>• Nursing notes<br>• Physician's orders<br>• Progress notes with principal diagnosis | • Authenticated physician order for services<br>• Clinician visit notes<br>• Diagnosis/reason the service was ordered<br>• Test results<br>• Therapies if applicable to the service<br>• Problem list if applicable to the service<br>• Medication list if applicable to the service |

success of the training (OIG 2023, 46). Referring to the definitions of fraud and abuse, the idea of what providers and organizations know or should know about coded data and billing practices should be the aim of ongoing education. Prevention, detection, and correction are the goals of a successful coding compliance program.

Some compliance training can be conducted in conjunction with CDI training sessions to foster communication and collaboration between clinicians, CDI professionals, and coding professionals. Other sessions can be role-specific depending on the topic, job responsibility, and intended audience. Topics for ongoing coding compliance education include the following:

- Yearly updates to ICD, CPT, and HCPCS coding systems
- New guidance from the AHA ICD-10 *Coding Clinic*, AHA *HCPCS Clinic*, and AMA *CPT Assistant*
- OIG workplan
- Review of ICD-10-CM/PCS Official Guidelines for Coding and Reporting
- POA reporting
- Complicated areas of coding depending on setting, such as modifiers, global surgery package, add-on codes, evaluation and management (E&M) codes
- Changes in reimbursement systems
- Uses of coded data—SOI, mortality, and CMI
- Organizational processes for reporting and resolving potential compliance violations (OIG 2023, 48)

The education sessions should be documented with attendance recorded.

## Medical Identity Theft

**Identity theft** is "a fraud attempted or committed using identifying information of another person without authority" (FTC 2021). When identity theft occurs in the context of medical care, it is known as medical identity theft. **Medical identity theft** is the inappropriate or unauthorized use of a person's identity to obtain medical goods or services or to falsify claims to fraudulently bill insurance companies. According to the Federal Trade Commission (FTC), medical identity theft "occurs when someone uses another person's name or insurance information to get medical treatment, prescription drugs, surgery, or even healthcare organizations using another person's information to submit false bills to insurance companies" (FTC 2021). To fight identity theft, the FTC enforces the Red Flags Rule requirements.

The **Red Flags Rule** is a set of Federal Trade Commission regulations that requires certain entities to develop and implement identity theft prevention programs. The intent is to deter identity theft and have a plan in place for quick detection if suspicious activity arises. The Red Flags Rule requires organizations to implement four basic identity theft prevention elements:

1. Include reasonable policies and procedures to identify the red flags of identity theft
2. Design the program to be able to detect red flags that have been identified in step 1
3. Detail appropriate actions when red flags are detected
4. Detail how to keep the plan current and to reflect new and emerging threats (FTC 2009)

Although policy is a very important approach to identity theft, the most important component of prevention is an organization's plan to incorporate these elements in day-to-day activities by alerting staff to watch for red flags, such as suspicious personal identifying information. An example of suspicious activity is inconsistencies, such as patient providing a Social Security number listed on the Social Security Administration's death list (FTC 2018). Finally, conducting risk assessments is an important activity to proactively determine potential risks.

## Anti-Kickback Statute

The Anti-Kickback Statute (AKS) makes knowingly offering, paying, soliciting, or receiving any remuneration that rewards referrals for services reimbursable by a federal program a criminal offense (CMS 2023). The only exception to the statute is the Safe Harbor Regulations that describe various payment and business practices that shall not be treated as a criminal offense under the AKSs and serve as an exclusion, such as an investment interest (42 CFR 1001.952). In these cases, AKS will not treat the arrangements as offenses.

## Stark Law

The Stark Law (or Physician Self-Referral Law) prohibits a physician from referring certain health services to "an entity in which the physician (or member of immediate family) has an ownership or investment or with which the physician has a compensation arrangement, unless an exception applies" (CMS 2021, 9). Financial relationships can meet the terms and conditions of an applicable exception; however, these need to be closely evaluated with the current CMS list. When an exception is not valid, CMS allows an additional avenue for physician self-referral reporting for noncompliance with the law through the Medicare self-referral disclosure protocol. The protocol is a tool intended to facilitate a resolution to the actual or potential violation of the Stark Law.

## Emergency Medical Treatment and Labor Act

EMTALA, otherwise known as the patient anti-dumping statute, was enacted by Congress in 1986 as part of the Consolidated Omnibus Budget Reconciliation Act (COBRA) (CMS n.d.b, 11). EMTALA is a component of the Social Security Act that assigns obligations to hospitals (including critical access hospitals) that offer emergency department (ED) services. "The obligations concern individuals who come to a hospital emergency department and request examination or treatment for medical conditions, and apply to all individuals, regardless of whether or not they are beneficiaries of any program under the Act" (CMS n.d.b, 10). EMTALA requires Medicare-participating hospitals with EDs to screen and treat the emergency medical conditions of patients in a nondiscriminatory manner to anyone, regardless of their ability to pay, insurance status, national origin, race, creed, or color. Its components include medical screening examinations, stabilization treatment, and transferring patients (to another organization or released from the ED). Under the EMTALA statute, "all participating hospitals with an emergency department would be required to provide an appropriate medical screening examination to determine whether an emergency medical condition exists or if the patient is in active labor" (CMS n.d.b, 10). Stabilization treatment for emergency medical conditions includes stabilizing the medical condition or transferring the patient to another medical facility only when the transfer is appropriate and when medical benefits outweigh the risks. The enforcement of EMTALA is initiated by a complaint. If a hospital's staff violates EMTALA, it may be subject to a civil monetary penalty or termination from a participation agreement with CMS.

### Check Your Understanding 8.2

**Answer the following questions in a separate document.**

1. How would you rationalize implementing a coding compliance plan?
2. How would you assess whether a healthcare provider is involved in fraud or abuse?
3. What is the difference between optimization versus maximization regarding coding and reimbursement? How do these differences align and potentially conflict with each other?
4. Recommend the resources and organizations that should be consulted for coding compliance guidance. Include a rationale of why they are the best sources.
5. What factors would you use to justify the significance of inclusion in or exclusion from Medicare and other federal programs?
6. CMS and OIG agree there are seven fundamental elements for effective compliance programs. Analyze each of the seven elements and examine the consequences of noncompliance.

7. Draft a memo to staff for the annual education on medical identity theft that includes the four basic identity theft prevention elements required by the red flag rule. In the memo, cover why they are key to helping eliminate medical identity theft.

8. Examine why the following regulations were necessary for compliance: Federal False Claims Act, Deficit Reduction Act of 2005, and HIPAA.

9. What are the external and internal drivers of fraud surveillance?

10. Choose one of the following topics, and then develop a departmental training outline for that topic: OIG workplan, uses of coded data- SOI, mortality, and CMI, or organizational processes for reporting and resolving potential compliance violations (OIG).

# References

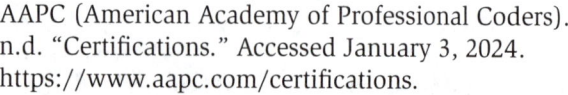

AAPC (American Academy of Professional Coders). n.d. "Certifications." Accessed January 3, 2024. https://www.aapc.com/certifications.

ACDIS (Association of Clinical Documentation Integrity Specialists). 2021. *Aligning CDI with Organizational Mission: What Matters?* [Position paper]. HCPro. https://acdis.org/sites/acdis/files/resources/CR-5372_ACDIS%20Risk%20Adjusted%20CDI-2_PP_Final.pdf.

ACDIS (Association of Clinical Documentation Integrity Specialists). 2020a. *Code of Ethics* [Position paper]. HCPro. https://acdis.org/system/files/resources/CR-727%20ACDIS%20Code%20of%20Ethics_position_paper_final_0.pdf.

ACDIS (Association of Clinical Documentation Integrity Specialists). 2020b. *Defining and Measuring an Engaged Provider Base* [Position paper]. HCPro. https://acdis.org/system/files/resources/CR-3179_ACDIS%20Provider%20Engagement-Measurement_PP_Final.pdf.

ACDIS (Association of Clinical Documentation Integrity Specialists). 2019. *CDI Yesterday, Today, and Tomorrow: Staying Relevant in Changing Times* [Position paper]. HCPro. https://acdis.org/sites/acdis/files/resources/CR-1913%20ACDIS%20White%20Paper%20CDI%20Yesterday.pdf.

ACDIS (Association of Clinical Documentation Integrity Specialists). 2017. *Developing Effective CDI Leadership: A Matter of Effort and Attitude* [Position paper]. HCPro. https://acdis.org/system/files/resources/37865_ACDIS%20Leadership_position_paper_final.pdf.

ACDIS (Association of Clinical Documentation Integrity Specialists). n.d. "About ACDIS' Certifications and Certificates." Accessed January 3, 2024. https://acdis.org/certification.

AHIMA (American Health Information Management Association). 2022. Practice Brief: Clinical documentation integrity key performance indicators. https://bok.ahima.org/topics/clinical-documentation-integrity/clinical-documentation-integrity-key-performance-indicators/.

AHIMA and Artifact (American Health Information Management Association and Artifact Health). 2022. *CDI: Compliant Technology Adoption and the Role of Clinical Documentation Specialists* [White Paper]. AHIMA. https://www.ahima.org/landing-pages/whitepapers/cdi-compliant-technology-adoption-and-the-role-of-clinical-documentation-specialists/.

AHIMA (American Health Information Management Association). 2021. *AHIMA Clinical Documentation Integrity (CDI) Toolkit Beginner's Guide*. Chicago: AHIMA.

AHIMA (American Health Information Management Association). 2020. *Ethical Standards for Clinical Documentation Improvement (CDI) Professionals*. AHIMA. https://www.ahima.org/media/r2gmhlop/ethical-standards-for-clinical-documentation-integrity-cdi-professionals-2020.pdf?oid=301868.

AHIMA (American Health Information Management Association). 2018a. *AHIMA CDI and Coding Collaboration in Denials Management Toolkit*. Chicago: AHIMA.

AHIMA (American Health Information Management Association). 2018b. *AHIMA Outpatient Clinical Documentation Toolkit*. Chicago: AHIMA.

AHIMA (American Health Information Management Association). 2018c. *AHIMA Inpatient Query Toolkit*. Chicago: AHIMA.

AHIMA (American Health Information Management Association). 2016a. *AHIMA Clinical Documentation Improvement (CDI) Toolkit*. Chicago: AHIMA.

AHIMA (American Health Information Management Association). 2016b. Practice Brief: Using CDI programs to improve acute care documentation in preparation for ICD-10-CM/PCS. AHIMA. https://pubmed.ncbi.nlm.nih.gov/23844546/.

AHIMA (American Health Information Management Association). 2013. Recruitment, selection, and orientation for CDI specialists. *Journal of AHIMA* 84(7):58–62.

AHIMA (American Health Information Management Association). 2010. Developing a coding compliance policy document (updated). *Journal of AHIMA* 81(3).

AHIMA (American Health Information Management Association). n.d.a. "Clinical Documentation Integrity." https://www.ahima.org/education-events/education-by-topic/.

AHIMA (American Health Information Management Association). n.d.b. "Certified Documentation Integrity Practitioner (CDIP®)." Accessed December 16, 2023. http://www.ahima.org/certification/cdip.

AHIMA and ACDIS (American Health Information Management Association and Association of Clinical Documentation Integrity Specialists). 2021. *AHIMA/ACDIS Compliant Clinical Documentation Integrity Technology Standards* [Position paper]. https://acdis.org/resources/acdisahima-compliant-clinical-documentation-integrity-technology-standards.

AHIMA and ACDIS (American Health Information Management Association and Association of Clinical Documentation Integrity Specialists). 2022. "Guidelines for Achieving a Compliant Query Practice (2022 update)." https://www.ahima.org/landing-pages/ahima-acdis-guidelines-for-achieving-a-compliant-query-practice/.

AHIMA House of Delegates. 2016. "American Health Information Management Association Standards for Ethical Coding." Chicago: AHIMA. https://bok.ahima.org/topics/coding-compliance-and-revenue-cycle/american-health-information-management-association-standards-of-ethical-coding-2016-version/.

Bowman, S. 2023. "Corporate Compliance". Chapter 14 in *Fundamentals of Law for Health Informatics and Information Management*, 4th ed. Edited by M. S. Brodnik, A. Rinehart-Thompson, and R. B. Reynolds. Chicago: AHIMA.

Butler, M. 2019. Coders or nurses for CDI teams: Why hiring both to collaborate works best. *Journal of AHIMA* 90(7): 10–13.

Cassidy, B. 2012. *AHIMA Thought Leadership Series: Defining the Core Clinical Documentation Set for Coding Compliance*. http://library.ahima.org/xpedio/groups/public/documents/ahima/bok1_049822.pdf (page for this edition discontinued).

CHIMA (Canadian Health Information Management Association). 2023. *A Physician's Guide to Clinical Documentation Improvement*. https://cchim.ca/wp-content/uploads/2023/03/A-Physicians-Guide-to-Clinical-Documentation-Improvement.pdf.

CHIMA (Canadian Health Information Management Association). 2021 (December 7). "CDI Community Meets to Discuss Engagement with Leadership Teams and Physicians." https://www.echima.ca/cdi-community-meets-to-discuss-engagement-with-leadership-teams-and-physicians/.

CMS (Centers for Medicare and Medicaid Services). 2024. Official ICD-10-PCS Guidelines. https://www.cms.gov/files/document/2025-official-icd-10-pcs-coding-guidelines.pdf.

CMS (Centers for Medicare and Medicaid Services). 2023. "Physician Self-Referral." https://www.cms.gov/medicare/regulations-guidance/physician-self-referral.

Centers for Medicare and Medicaid Services (CMS). 2024b. "2023 Official ICD-10-CM Guidelines." https://stacks.cdc.gov/view/cdc/158747.

CMS (Centers for Medicare and Medicaid Services). 2021 (January). *Medicare Fraud & Abuse: Prevent, Detect, Report*. https://www.cms.gov/Outreach-and-Education/Medicare-Learning-Network-MLN/MLNProducts/Downloads/Fraud-Abuse-MLN4649244.pdf.

CMS (Centers for Medicare and Medicaid Services). 2019. *Combating Medicare Parts C and D Fraud, Waste, and Abuse Web-Based Training Course*. https://www.cms.gov/Outreach-and-Education/Medicare-Learning-Network-MLN/MLNProducts/Downloads/CombMedCandDFWAdownload.pdf.

CMS (Centers for Medicare and Medicaid Services). 2017. Laws against Health Care Fraud. https://www.cms.gov/files/document/overviewfwalawsagainstfactsheet072616.pdf.

CMS (Centers for Medicare and Medicaid Services). 2005. Compliance Program Guidance for Medicare Fee-For-Service Contractors. https://www.cms.gov/Medicare/Medicare-Contracting/Medicare-Administrative-Contractors/Downloads/compliance.pdf.

CMS (Centers for Medicare and Medicaid Services). n.d.a. The Deficit Reduction Act: Important Facts for State Government Officials. Accessed January 3, 2024. https://www.cms.gov/regulations-and-guidance/legislation/deficitreductionact/downloads/guide.pdf.

CMS (Centers for Medicare and Medicaid Services). n.d.b. Guidance on 42 CFR Parts 413, 482, and 489. Accessed January 3, 2024. https://www.cms.gov/Regulations-and-Guidance/Legislation/EMTALA/downloads/cms-1063-f.pdf.

Combs, T. 2019. The state of CDI. *Journal of AHIMA* 90(4):18–21.

DOJ (Department of Justice). 2024. The False Claims Act. https://www.justice.gov/civil/false-claims-act.

DeVault, K, and M. H. and Stanfill. 2019. Components of an effective inpatient coding compliance program. *Journal of AHIMA* 7 (Jul–Aug):50–52.

FTC (Federal Trade Commission). 2021. "What to Know About Medical Identity Theft." https://consumer.ftc.gov/articles/what-know-about-medical-identity-theft.

Hess, P. C. 2023. Clinical Documentation Integrity in a virtual world. *Journal of AHIMA*. https://journal.ahima.org/page/clinical-documentation-integrity-in-a-virtual-world.

Hess, P. C. 2018. *Clinical Documentation Improvement for Outpatient Care*. Chicago: AHIMA.

Hinkle-Azzara, B., and K. J. Carr. 2014. Bird's eye view of ICD-10 documentation gaps. *Journal of AHIMA* 85(6):34–38.

Huffman, E. K. 1941. *Manual for Medical Record Librarians*. Chicago: Physicians' Record Company.

Liebler, J. G., and C. R. McConnell. 2021. *Management Principles for Health Professionals*, 8th ed. Sudbury, MA: Jones and Bartlett.

Muthukumaraswamy, V. 2023. Reinventing the Role of the Medical Coder in the Artificial Intelligence Era. *Journal of AHIMA*. Accessed October 16, 2023; https://journal.ahima.org/page/reinventing-the-role-of-medical-coders-in-the-artificial-intelligence-era.

OIG (Office of the Inspector General). 2023. "General Compliance Program Guidance." https://oig.hhs.gov/documents/compliance-guidance/1135/HHS-OIG-GCPG-2023.pdf.

OIG (Office of the Inspector General). 2017. "Measuring Compliance Program Effectiveness: A Resource Guide." https://oig.hhs.gov/compliance/compliance-resource-portal/files/HCCA-OIG-Resource-Guide.pdf.

Office of the Inspector General (OIG). n.d.a. "Corporate Integrity Agreements." Accessed January 3, 2024. https://oig.hhs.gov/compliance/corporate-integrity-agreements/.

Office of the Inspector General (OIG). n.d.b. "Civil Monetary Penalties and Affirmative Exclusions." Accessed January 3, 2024. https://oig.hhs.gov/fraud/enforcement/types-of-civil-monetary-penalties-and-affirmative-exclusions/.

OIG (Office of the Inspector General). n.d.c. "A Roadmap for New Physicians: Avoiding Medicare and Medicaid Fraud and Abuse." Accessed January 3, 2024. https://oig.hhs.gov/documents/compliance/981/roadmap_web_version_.pdf.

OIG (Office of the Inspector General. n.d.d. "About OIG." Accessed January 3, 2024. https://oig.hhs.gov/about-oig/about-us/index.asp.

Rinehart-Thompson, L. A. 2023. "Requirements for Legally Defensible Health Records." Chapter 7 in *Fundamentals of Law for Health Informatics and Information Management*, 4th ed. Edited by M. S. Brodnik, A. Rinehart-Thompson, and R. B. Reynolds. Chicago: AHIMA.

Social Security Act of 1996. 1128: Exclusion of Certain Individuals and Entities from Participation in Medicare and State Health Care Programs.

US Sentencing Commission. 2018. "Effective Compliance and Ethics Program." https://www.ussc.gov/guidelines/2018-guidelines-manual/2018-chapter-8.

White, S. 2023. *Calculating and Reporting Healthcare Statistics*, 7th ed. Chicago: AHIMA.

42 CFR 1001.952 Safe Harbor Regulations. 2018.

chapter 9

# Legal Issues in Health Information Management

*Laurie A. Rinehart-Thompson, JD, RHIA, CHP, FAHIMA*

## Learning Objectives

- Identify the three branches of government, sources and types of law, and the state and federal court systems
- Articulate the process for civil litigation and criminal proceedings
- Differentiate healthcare causes of action as they relate to tort liability and breach of contract
- Identify the purpose of and challenges associated with creation and maintenance of the health record and demonstrate how it can be used as evidence in legal proceedings, including e-discovery
- Examine release of information principles for proper disclosure of health information, including highly sensitive information
- Identify types and consequences of medical identity theft
- Identify types of quality improvement activities and examine likelihood of quality improvement documents being subject to discovery

## Key Terms

Acceptance
Acquittal
Actual causation
Adhesion contract
Adjudicated
Administrative law
Administrative branch
Advance directive
Answer
Apology statutes
Appellate court
Arbitration
Arraignment
Assault

Assumption of risk
Authentication
Authenticity
Battery
Bench trial
Beyond a reasonable doubt
Binding authority
Breach of confidentiality
Breach of warranty
Burden of proof
Business record
Business records exception
Charitable immunity
Circuit

Circuit courts
Civil law
Code of Federal Regulations (CFR)
Common law
Comparative negligence
Complaint
Confidentiality of Substance Use Disorder Patient Records
Consent
Consideration
Constitutional law
Contract
Contract law

Contributory negligence
Conviction
Corporate negligence
Counterclaim
Courts of appeals
Crimes
Criminal law
Criminal negligence
Cross-claim
Damages
Deemed status
Defamation of character
Default judgment
Defendant
Depositions
Discovery
District courts
Diversity jurisdiction
Do-not-resuscitate order (DNR)
Durable power of attorney for healthcare decisions
Economic compensatory (special) damages
E-discovery
Electronic health information (EHI)
Emergency Medical Treatment and Labor Act (EMTALA)
Evidence
Express warranty
False imprisonment
Fault
Federal question jurisdiction
*Federal Register*
Felony
Fiduciary duty
Fraud
Freedom of Information Act of 1967 (FOIA)
General consent
General jurisdiction
Good Samaritan Statutes
Governmental (sovereign) immunity
Grand jury
Gross negligence
Health Insurance Portability and Accountability Act of 1996 (HIPAA)
Hearsay
Holding
Hung jury
Implied warranty
Incident
Incident report
Indictment
Infliction of emotional distress
Informed consent
Injunction
Intent
Interrogatories
Invasion of privacy
Joinder
Judicial branch
Jurisdiction
Legal hold
Legal system
Legislative branch
Libel
Licensure
Limited jurisdiction
Litigation
Living will
Malfeasance
Mediation
Medical identity theft
Metadata
Misdemeanor
Misfeasance
Motions for summary judgment
Negligence
Non-economic compensatory (general) damages
Nonfeasance
Offer
Ordinary negligence
Original jurisdiction
Patient Self-Determination Act
Persuasive authority
Petition for writ of certiorari
Physician-patient privilege
Plaintiff
Potentially compensable event (PCE)
Preemption
Preponderance of the evidence
Privacy Act of 1974
Private law
Privilege
Product liability
Proximate causation
Prosecutor
Public law
Punitive damages
Regulations
Requests for production
*Res ipsa loquitur*
*Res judicata*
*Respondeat superior*
Restitution
Right to privacy
Settlements
Slander
Specific performance
Spoliation
Standard of care
Standard of proof
*Stare decisis*
Statute of limitations
Statutes
Statutory (legislative) law
Strict liability
Subject matter jurisdiction
Subpoenas
Summons
Supreme court
Tort
Tort law
Trial court
Trier of fact

To understand the health information management (HIM) professional's role in the legal system and in protecting confidential health information, one must first understand basic legal concepts and principles of appropriate access and disclosure. Because health records are often central to litigation, which is the resolution of legal disputes in the court system, the HIM professional should be comfortable with the legal process. The following sections present basic yet crucial information about the American legal system, including healthcare causes of action and legal considerations that must accompany the management of health information.

# Legal Foundations and Proceedings

To understand how law functions, it is important to know the branches of government, both at the federal and state levels, and the sources (types) of law that comprise our legal system. Further, one must be aware of branches of government that create each source of law. Finally, recognizing the ways law can be categorized, public versus private and civil versus criminal, provides a fundamental background toward understanding the US court system.

## Branches of Government

The legal system in the US consists of three related branches, or subsystems, that exist at varying levels of government (federal, state, and local): a judicial branch, a legislative branch, and an administrative branch. As each government branch or source of law is discussed, all three levels of government must be considered.

The judicial branch, which is the court system, provides an avenue to enforce rights and obligations through the resolution of disputes. Through the courts, a person or entity may bring a civil action against another person or entity believed to have caused harm. A wide variety of civil actions can be brought against an alleged wrongdoer, who likewise prepares a defense. The judicial system also provides a mechanism for a government to charge a person or entity with a crime. The system allows the charged person or entity the opportunity to defend against the charge or charges.

The legislative branch enacts laws. It controls many activities related to industry, including the healthcare industry, via statutes. Statutes, which often set forth required actions, are laws created by legislative bodies.

The administrative branch, which controls governmental administrative operations, operates through administrative agencies that enact regulations. Regulations are rules developed by administrative agencies after the passage of statutes. Regulations establish how statutes are to be carried out and have the same legal force or authority as statutes.

Understanding the US judicial, legislative, and administrative branches within a governmental organization at any level (federal, state, or local) gives the HIM professional an appreciation for the health record as a legal document and its role in each of these branches.

## Sources of Law

The laws that rule all Americans come from many sources, resulting in a rather complex legal system. Overall, there is a federal legal system, 50 individual state legal systems, and myriad local legal systems. US territories generally have their own court systems and federal territorial courts. Regardless of the source, the legal system is the mechanism through which members of society settle disputes. These disputes may occur between private individuals and organizations or between either of these entities and the government, whether state, federal, local, or a combination.

### Constitutional Law

Many of the rights and obligations of government, which subsequently affect the rights and obligations of individuals and entities, are set out in federal and state constitutions, establishing constitutional law. The Constitution of the United States is the highest law in the land. It takes precedence over constitutions and laws in the individual states and local jurisdictions (Rinehart-Thompson 2023a, 47). The US Constitution defines the federal government's general organization and grants powers to it. It also places limits on what federal and state governments may do. State constitutions have the same effect within each state. State constitutions can address many areas, including state lotteries and public sector employee retirement plans.

### Common Law

English common law is the primary source of many legal rules and principles and was based initially on tradition and custom. Common law also known as judicial law, judge-make law, or case law) is created by courts in the resolution of disputes. A court's decision is referred to as a holding. Courts are significant decision makers. Their dispute resolution authority includes interpreting statutes, regulations, and constitutions; resolving conflicting statutes and regulations; determining the constitutionality of statutes and regulations; using prior binding decisions to make determinations; and creating law where a void exists (Rinehart-Thompson 2023a, 46).

Federal courts create and make changes to federal common law. States add to their own bodies of common law through state court decisions. A common-law principle established in one state has no effect in another state unless the second state adopts the same principle. Even then, it may be applied differently. After a court establishes a new common-law principle, that principle becomes binding authority, which sets a precedent for future cases that address the same issues in that court system. The body of common law continually evolves as court decisions are created, modified, overturned or repealed. Although a precedent in one court system does not bind courts in other court systems, courts may use each other's precedents as persuasive authority, or guidance, in analyzing a specific legal problem (Rinehart-Thompson 2023a, 46). Lower courts must look to higher courts in the same court system for precedent; however, higher courts are not bound by the holdings of lower courts in the same court system. Courts at the same level within a court system are not obligated to follow the decisions of one another (Rinehart-Thompson 2023a, 46).

A legal principle related to precedent is *stare decisis*, which means "let the decision stand." It states that in lower court cases involving a fact pattern like that in a higher court within the same court system, the lower court is bound to apply the decision of the higher court (Rinehart-Thompson 2023a, 46).

### Statutory Law

Statutory (legislative) law is written law established by federal and state legislatures, or municipalities (where the law is frequently called an ordinance). It may be amended, repealed, or expanded by the legislature. Statutory law may be upheld or found by a court to violate or conflict with the state or federal constitution. Further, it may be found to conflict with a different state law or a federal law.

Courts also interpret laws in terms of how they apply to a given situation. Thus, statutory law may be revised by a court ruling in terms of its constitutionality and applicability. However, if the legislature disagrees with the court's interpretation, it can revise the statute.

### Administrative Law

When a matter is technical or complex, legislatures often delegate their authority to regulate to appropriate administrative agencies. These agencies are empowered to enact rules (also referred to as regulations) that have the same force of law as statutory law and that carry out the intent of the legislature. Rules can impose civil and criminal penalties for noncompliance. Accordingly, administrative law is the branch of law that controls a government's agency, or administrative, operations. Administrative agencies include licensing bodies (at all levels of government) and the Centers for Medicare and Medicaid Services at the federal level. Regulatory agencies can function in a legislative, adjudicative, and enforcement role regarding their own regulations (Pozgar 2021, 25). Federal administrative agencies must follow the Administrative Procedure Act (5 USC 500–576 (Law. Co-op. (1989)) One of their roles is to create agency rules (also referred to as regulations) and revisions to existing rules. Proposed and final administrative rules are published in the *Federal Register*, a daily publication issued by the Office of the Federal Register, an office within the National Archives and Records Administration. Proposed rules are published for a comment period, where the public is invited to provide feedback on the applicability and impact of the proposed rules. After the comment period, the administrative agency responsible for the proposed rule may or may not finalize the rules. If rules are finalized, notices and final rules are then published. Final rules are also codified and published in the appropriate code section of the Code of Federal Regulations (CFR), which is the compilation of federal administrative regulations. The Medicare Conditions of Participation (CoP) and the Health Insurance Portability and Accountability Act of 1996 (HIPAA) Privacy and Security Rules are examples of healthcare regulations published in the *Federal Register*.

Courts can review regulations and administrative decisions if there is a question as to whether an agency has overstepped its bounds or misinterpreted a law. Most states have procedural laws in place to govern the functions of state agencies.

## Public Law versus Private Law

Public law involves the relationship between the government (at any level) and individuals or organizations. The purposes of public law are defining, regulating, and enforcing rights where the government is a party. Criminal law, discussed later, is public law because it is the government that brings criminal action (prosecution) against individuals or entities. Public law also encompasses statutory and administrative law because it involves the carrying out of statutes and regulations created by a governmental body. Public statutory and administrative law can be civil or criminal, depending on how the statute or regulation is written.

Private law involves the relationship between private individuals or entities; the government is not a party. Private law often includes torts, contracts, and property issues. Because torts are civil (noncriminal) wrongs that result in injury, they are the basis for medical and other professional malpractice cases.

## Civil Law versus Criminal Law

Civil law addresses noncriminal legal matters and involves relationships among individuals and other entities, including a government. Most actions encountered in the healthcare industry are based on civil law. Most often, the remedy for a civil wrong is monetary.

Criminal law addresses the punishment of persons or entities who commit crimes. Crimes are prosecutable wrongful acts against public health, safety, and welfare. Criminal law encompasses both conviction (a declaration of guilt) and punishment. Crimes are either a felony or a misdemeanor as defined by state or federal law. A felony is the more serious of the two categories of crimes (the other being misdemeanor, described below), subject to imprisonment for more than one year. It includes, for example, murder and other homicides, rape, assault, and thefts of items or cash in excess of a certain value set by statute. A misdemeanor is a less severe crime than a felony, subject to imprisonment for up to one year. It includes wrongs such as disorderly conduct and theft of small amounts of property. Information theft crimes (such as hacking, computer destruction, and spamming) can be either misdemeanors or felonies. The criminal provisions of the HIPAA Privacy Rule include only felony crimes.

## The Court System

The American court system is composed of state court systems and the federal court system. The nature of a legal action determines which court has jurisdiction—the power to hear and decide the controversy in each case. Subject matter jurisdiction is a legal doctrine that limits the types of cases—by subject—that a court can decide. In federal court, the first type of subject matter jurisdiction is federal question jurisdiction, which is a claim related to federal law, including federal crimes (for example, racketeering); constitutional issues (for example, interpretations of the US Constitution); and other federal laws (for example, bankruptcy law). The second type of subject matter jurisdiction is diversity jurisdiction, where no plaintiff is from the same state as any defendant in a case. Other civil and criminal cases are brought in the state court systems.

### State Court Systems

State court systems follow a three-level hierarchy. The lowest level is the trial court. State civil and criminal cases are initiated at this level, as it has the authority to first hear a case on a given matter, referred to as original jurisdiction. Some trial courts have limited jurisdiction and may only hear certain types of cases such as probate, domestic, juvenile, traffic, and small claims. Other trial courts have general jurisdiction and may hear various types of cases. Decisions made in a trial court may be appealed to an intermediate court, usually known as an appellate court (or court of appeals). State appellate courts have general jurisdiction.

State legal systems also include a court at the highest level, usually referred to as the supreme court of that state. Supreme courts have general jurisdiction over all cases heard in the state's trial and appellate courts. Decisions coming from the highest state court hearing a case become the law of that state unless a state legislative process enacts a statute to override the court's decision, or unless the decision is overturned by another case.

### Federal Court System

Also following a three-level hierarchy, the 94 trial courts in the federal court system are district courts, which are the lowest tier in the federal court system. District courts hear cases involving federal question jurisdiction or diversity jurisdiction, both described previously. At least one district court is in each state. Specialized federal courts have exclusive jurisdiction over certain matters such as bankruptcy, customs, and claims against the federal government. Cases addressing these matters cannot be filed in a state court.

The federal appellate level is composed of 13 federal courts of appeals, with most courts covering a geographic area known as a circuit (although the federal circuit is based on specialized cases rather than geography) (Rinehart-Thompson 2023a, 452). The US Courts of Appeals are also called circuit courts and they have the power to hear appeals of district courts' final judgments.

The Supreme Court of the United States is the highest court in the federal legal system and hears appeals from the federal courts of appeals and the highest state courts. It most frequently considers cases that have risen through the federal court system. The US Supreme Court has considerable discretion in determining which cases it will and will not hear. A request for the US Supreme Court to consider a case from a lower court is a petition for writ of certiorari. The court will either grant certiorari (that is, it will hear the case) or deny certiorari (that is, it declines to hear the case). Most requests are denied certiorari.

The HIM professional can better serve patient interests by possessing an understanding of the legal process, including how a case moves from filing of a lawsuit or criminal charges toward trial and alternative methods for resolving disputes. This section describes the civil litigation process as well as criminal proceedings, both of which may apply to healthcare legal actions.

## Civil Litigation

The party bringing an action or complaint in a civil case is the plaintiff. The plaintiff or an attorney on the plaintiff's behalf begins the process by filing a complaint, a legal document that sets forth the facts and claims, in the appropriate court. A summons (or notice), an order by a court that requires an appearance or a written response is served along with the complaint to the defendant, the party who is accused of committing the wrong. The defendant or an attorney on the defendant's behalf prepares an **answer** (or response) that addresses the allegations that have been made against the defendant. The answer is filed in the same court where the original complaint was filed. The plaintiff has the burden of proving that a legally recognized wrong occurred, that the defendant committed the wrong, and that the wrong harmed the plaintiff. The plaintiff must also state the expected **restitution**, which is monetary compensation or other actions to make the plaintiff as whole again as possible. At trial the plaintiff presents **evidence**, which is supporting information, before a judge or a jury. It must be compelling enough to meet the **standard of proof**, which is the requisite degree of belief to support the purported claims. The applicable standard of proof varies based on the type of case. For example, the standard of proof is higher in a criminal case than in a civil case because the stakes—jail or prison—are higher than monetary damages, which is the potential consequence in a civil case (Rinehart-Thompson 2023b, 66–67). There may be multiple plaintiffs or defendants in a case. Further, a case may be tried before a jury or before a judge only, which is a **bench trial**. Whether a case is tried before a jury or a judge depends on the nature of the allegations, as not all cases provide the right to a jury trial. Where there is a right to a jury trial, a defendant may waive that right.

Other actions may be taken before a case is resolved. The defendant may bring a claim against the plaintiff (**counterclaim**), one party may bring a claim against another party who is on the same side of the litigation (**crossclaim**), or the defendant may bring a claim against an outsider as a codefendant (**joinder**) (Rinehart-Thompson 2023b, 60).

A case may be resolved in one of five ways. First, a judge can dismiss the plaintiff's case for procedural reasons. The plaintiff's complaint may not set forth a claim recognized by law, the summons and complaint may not have been properly served on the defendant, or the court may not have jurisdiction. Depending on the reason, the judge may permit the plaintiff to correct the error and refile the case. Second, if the defendant fails to file a timely answer, the court will find in favor of the plaintiff and enter a **default judgment** against the defendant. Third, a case may be settled out of court before it goes to trial or at any time during trial before the **trier of fact** (judge or jury) announces the decision. In addition to **settlements**, or official agreements, alternative dispute resolution methods include submitting cases to **arbitration**, where an impartial third party makes a decision, or **mediation**, where an objective third party hears a dispute and brings the parties to a mutual agreement. Fourth, presuming the case does not settle or is not dismissed or no default judgment is entered, the case will proceed with discovery. **Discovery** consists of both the pretrial period and the activities by which both the plaintiff(s) and defendant(s) will obtain information held by other parties to assess the strengths and weaknesses of each party's case (Rinehart-Thompson 2023b, 61). Discovery activities include but are not limited to taking witnesses' **depositions**, or sworn statements; serving **interrogatories**, or written formal questions, on parties to the case; submitting **requests for production**, which are legal requests for documents from the opposing party; and requesting a mental or physical examination of a party. Discovery may be facilitated by the parties issuing **subpoenas**, which are directives to attend or respond to legal proceedings. The judge assigned to the case will set dates according to applicable legal rules by which pretrial discovery must be completed. At the conclusion of this stage, in most cases, one or both parties present **motions for summary judgment**, in which they argue that there are (or are not) any facts remaining in dispute and that one or the other is (or is not) entitled to a judgment being entered without intervention by the trier of fact. If the judge grants this motion, the case ends and has the same effect as if the case had proceeded to trial.

Finally, if a motion for summary judgment is not successful or is not made, the case proceeds to trial before the trier of fact. In most civil cases, the plaintiff must prove his or her case by the standard of proof known as a **preponderance of the evidence**. This "more likely than not" standard means that there is enough evidence to tip the scales, even slightly, in favor of the plaintiff's case. This is a substantially lower standard of proof than a criminal case. Upon conclusion of the trial, a verdict is given. In civil cases, a verdict is a decision of liability or no liability. If a defendant is found to be liable, a determination is made regarding the **damages**, or remedy (often a dollar amount) awarded to the plaintiff. Damages awarded to a plaintiff can be categorized. **Economic compensatory (special) damages** can be objectively verified and are calculable. They include losses such as medical expenses or lost wages. **Non-economic compensatory (general) damages** do not represent an objective monetary loss and, due to their incalculable nature, can be overrepresented by a plaintiff's attorney. These losses include pain and suffering, loss of enjoyment of life activities, and humiliation. Punitive damages, designed to punish a defendant's egregious conduct, are discussed later in this chapter. Tort reform laws have been enacted in a variety of states nationwide to place limits or caps on non-economic compensatory and punitive damages. Either party may appeal the judgment of liability or damages assessed to an appellate court and possibly even to the highest court in that court system. Once a matter has been fully **adjudicated**, or formally decided through the trial court (and, if applicable, appellate courts), the same parties may not pursue the case again under the doctrine of *res judicata*.

## Criminal Proceedings

Although criminal proceedings mirror civil proceedings in many ways, there are important distinctions. Law enforcement agencies investigate alleged crimes. If a **prosecutor** (prosecuting attorney), also known as a district or state attorney (depending on the state) or the US attorney (in the federal court system), determines sufficient evidence is present, he or she files charges against the defendant on behalf of the government. In some states, a **grand jury** must return an **indictment**, or formal charge, for a felony crime to be prosecuted. The grand jury has the authority to issue subpoenas for its investigative process, and all evidence considered by the grand jury remains confidential unless an indictment is returned. At an **arraignment**, the defendant appears before the court, and the prosecutor informs the defendant of the charges. The prosecution team has the burden of proving the charges against the defendant. The standard of proof that the government must meet to establish the defendant's guilt is **beyond a reasonable doubt**, meaning that the jury has virtual certainty that the defendant is guilty because there are no other reasonable explanations than that which the prosecution presented.

The defendant may plead guilty. Alternatively, the defendant may plead not guilty, which results in the case proceeding toward trial. Upon conclusion of the trial, a trier of fact renders a verdict of either guilty or not guilty. When a defendant is found not guilty (**acquittal**), the charges are dismissed. To be found guilty (conviction) or not guilty, all triers of fact (for example, all the members of a jury) must agree on the defendant's guilt or lack of proven guilt. If all individuals cannot agree, this results in a **hung jury**. Whether a defendant pleads guilty or is found guilty by a trier of fact, the defendant may be sentenced to prison (felony), jail (misdemeanor), or placed on probation with or without community service. The defendant may also be ordered to pay a fine. In most jurisdictions, only a defendant who is found guilty at trial can proceed through the appellate process. In certain jurisdictions, criminal cases may be resolved through alternative dispute resolution such as arbitration or mediation.

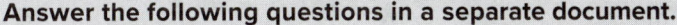

### Check Your Understanding 9.1

**Answer the following questions in a separate document.**

1. What are the four sources of laws in the US and how do they differ?
2. What is the difference between public law and private law?
3. What is the difference between civil law and criminal law?
4. Compare the benefits and drawbacks of each of the types of discovery.
5. Distinguish between the standard of proof required in most civil cases and the standard of proof required in criminal cases. How do they differ, and why is there a different standard of proof for civil versus criminal cases?
6. Describe the three types of alternative dispute resolution described in the chapter.
7. Distinguish the types of federal court jurisdiction described in this chapter.
8. Explain the concept of binding authority in the court system and give an example, distinguishing it from persuasive authority.

## Healthcare Causes of Action

Providers in the healthcare industry may become involved in both civil and criminal cases. Because the federal government continues to pursue investigations into and prosecutions of healthcare fraud, health information privacy violations, and refusal to treat patients based on financial status, criminal cases will occupy an important space in the healthcare area into the future.

However, this chapter focuses on civil actions. The types of civil legal actions that most typically affect the healthcare industry are torts and contracts. The vast majority of tort and contract claims are resolved without court appearances, perhaps without a lawsuit being filed.

## Torts

A tort is a civil, non-criminal wrong. Tort law encompasses actions brought when one party believes another party caused harm through wrongful conduct. The wronged party seeks restitution to become as whole again as possible. In addition to restitution, tort actions are intended to discourage wrongdoers from committing further wrongs. The three categories of tort liability are negligence, intentional torts, and strict liability. This chapter also address product liability, which can occur in any of the three categories of tort liability. Most healthcare incidents are negligence. This section additionally addresses defenses to tort actions and apology statutes.

### Negligence

Negligence is acting in an unreasonable manner or failing to act as a reasonably prudent person would in similar circumstances. Negligence may occur in cases where an individual has evaluated the alternatives and the consequences of those alternatives and has not exercised his or her best possible judgment. A person can also be found negligent when he or she has failed to guard against a risk that he or she knew could happen. Furthermore, negligence can occur in circumstances where it is known, or should have been known, that a particular behavior would place others in unreasonable danger.

Typically, negligence is conduct that is outside the generally accepted standard of care. Standard of care is what an individual is expected to do or not do in each situation. In the healthcare context, the standard of care is the level of care that a reasonably prudent and similarly situated practitioner would have provided in similar circumstances. Standards of care are established by statute or regulation, professional associations or accrediting bodies, or professional practice. Such standards represent expected behavior unless a court rules otherwise. Industry or national standards have generally supplanted inconsistent community standards because the standard of care should not vary by geographic area, especially if patients can be referred to providers where more sophisticated technology exists or consultations can occur via telemedicine, which is often the case.

In addition to direct patient care, the standard of care applies to the physical and emotional safety of patients, staff, visitors, vendors, and members of the public on an organization's premises for myriad reasons. Safety includes being free from physical defects in buildings and grounds, and from being threatened or harmed by patients, staff members, or others.

Negligence can be categorized as one of the following:

- **Nonfeasance**: failure to perform an act that a person has a duty to perform and which a person of ordinary prudence would have done in similar circumstances
- **Misfeasance**: improper performance of a lawful act that causes injury to another
- **Malfeasance**: performance of a wrongful act, and the act may be unlawful (Rinehart-Thompson 2023c, 93)

Further, negligence can be categorized by the degree of wrongdoing. **Ordinary negligence** is failure to do what a reasonably prudent person would do, or doing something that a reasonably prudent person would not do, thus failing to exercise ordinary care. **Gross negligence** is an extreme departure from the ordinary standard of care that shows a reckless disregard toward others. If defined by criminal statute, gross negligence that represents reckless disregard or deliberate indifference to another's safety may constitute **criminal negligence** (Rinehart-Thompson 2023c, 94).

To recover damages caused by negligence, the plaintiff must show that all four elements of negligence are present:

- *Duty of care*. The defendant owed the plaintiff a duty of care. In the healthcare context, there is a duty of care where there is a physician-patient or other provider-patient relationship. A duty of care must be established before a standard of care can exist.
- *Breach of duty of care*. The defendant deviated from their duty of care and did not meet the standard of care, either by committing a negligent act or failing to act per the standard of care.
- *Injury or harm*. The plaintiff suffered injury or harm because of the defendant's breach. Injury includes not only physical harm but also mental suffering, pain, loss of income or reputation, loss of consortium, and the invasion of a patient's rights and privacy.
- *Causation*. The defendant's conduct caused the plaintiff's harm. The plaintiff must prove two types of causation: that the defendant's conduct caused the harm (**actual causation**) and that the breach was also the proximate or foreseeable cause of the harm (**proximate causation**). (57A Am. Jur. 2d Negligence 2022)

When no statute exists to define a standard of care, the trier of fact determines what a reasonably prudent person would have done. Reasonableness is based on relevant current factors including the defendant's physical condition, mental capacity, training, education, and knowledge (Pozgar 2021, 36). The trier of fact assesses the defendant's behavior against the standard of care to determine if there was a breach. If injury or harm resulted, along with actual and proximate (foreseeable) causation, then negligence has occurred (Pozgar 2021, 36).

The burden of proof, which is the obligation to prove a case, generally lies with the plaintiff to meet the four elements of negligence, except in cases where the facts or circumstances allow for an inference of the defendant's negligence. In these cases, the doctrine of *res ipsa loquitur* (the thing speaks for itself) is applied. The elements of *res ipsa loquitur* are as follows:

- Injury would not ordinarily occur unless there was negligence.
- The defendant solely controlled the instrumentality in the incident.
- The plaintiff did not contribute to the incident that caused the injury. (57B Am. Jur. 2d Negligence 2022)

An example of a *res ipsa loquitur* case would be a sponge or an instrument that is left in a patient during surgery.

### Intentional Torts

Although most torts in healthcare are based on negligence, intentional torts are also committed. The element of intent distinguishes intentional torts and negligent torts. Intent means the person committed an act deliberately, intending to cause harm, or knowing that harm would likely occur. Several intentional torts apply to the healthcare, including assault, battery, false imprisonment, defamation of character, fraud, invasion of privacy, and infliction of emotional distress.

**Assault**  Assault is conduct, along with apparent ability, that causes apprehension that physically harmful or offensive contact will occur. For example, a muscular, physically intimidating nurse tells a frail older patient that the nurse will break the patient's arm if the patient does not do what the nurse tells the patient to do. The nurse's comment is a deliberate threat and the nurse's size supports the apparent ability to harm the patient. In this example, the patient does not need to suffer actual damage or even come into physical contact with the nurse. The apprehension that the threat creates is sufficient to constitute assault.

**Battery**  Battery is the intentional and nonconsensual touching of another person (Rinehart-Thompson 2023c, 91). In healthcare, laws regarding battery are especially important because of the consent requirement for medical and surgical procedures. The patient does not need to be aware that battery has occurred. For example, battery occurs to a patient who is sedated and upon whom surgery is performed without either express (stated) or implied (by one's actions) consent. (Note that an emergency situation can qualify either as implied consent or as an exception to the consent requirement.) Thus, the hospital and the treating healthcare professionals may be held liable for harm caused by the lack of a proper patient consent. Even if the outcome of the procedure benefits the patient, touching the patient without proper consent may make the healthcare professional liable for battery.

**False Imprisonment**  False imprisonment is intentional confinement of someone against that person's will. This cause of action includes the defendant's lack of legal authority or justification to confine a person. Thus, there is legal authority and no successful cause of action for retaining an individual who presents a danger to himself or others (for example, a suicide or homicide risk) or who has a contagious disease for which state law permits forced confinement. Healthcare providers must be cautious about preventing a patient from leaving a hospital or other care setting. Physical force is not required for one to be found liable for false imprisonment, but when excessive force is used to restrain a patient, the healthcare provider may be held liable for both false imprisonment and battery. Absent provider's legal authority to retain (that is, to keep a patient in the facility) a patient's insistence on leaving a facility should be honored. It should be documented in the patient's health record, and the patient should be asked to sign a discharge against medical advice (also known as AMA) form that releases the facility from responsibility. If the patient refuses to sign the form, this fact must also be documented in the patient's health record.

**Defamation of Character**  Defamation of character is a false communication about someone to a person other than the subject that may injure the subject's reputation. The communication may be either spoken, which is slander, or written, which is libel. To recover damages in an action for defamation, the plaintiff must prove that the following occurred:

- The defendant made a false and defamatory statement about the plaintiff.
- The statement was not a privileged publication (made appropriately and in good faith to persons with a legitimate reason to know) and was made to a third person.
- The conduct was an act of negligence or contained a higher degree of intent.
- Actual or presumed damages resulted. (Rinehart-Thompson 2023c, 100)

Harm is presumed and a plaintiff is not required to show proof of actual harm to his or her reputation when the defendant allegedly accuses the plaintiff of committing a crime, accuses the plaintiff of having a stigmatic disease, uses words that negatively affect the plaintiff's profession or business, or accuses an individual of being sexually promiscuous.

The defendant has several defenses to a defamation action:

- Truth: There is no defamation liability if the statement was true.
- Privilege: There is no defamation liability if the communication was made in good faith, on the proper occasion, in the proper manner, and to persons who have a legitimate reason to receive the information.
- Lack of publication: If the statement was not disseminated in writing or verbally to a third party, there is no defamation liability.
- Authorization of the disclosure by the plaintiff: A written authorization should be obtained before any communication is made, and maintained thereafter (Rinehart-Thompson 2023c, 100–101).

The defense of privilege is relevant when the person making the communication has an obligation to report such information. For example, healthcare professionals are protected against defamation claims for reporting communicable diseases (and may be held liable for failure to report) if such reporting is required by law (Rinehart-Thompson 2023c, 100).

**Fraud** Fraud is a willful and intentional deception that could result in harm to a person or to property. To prove fraud, the plaintiff must show the defendant knowingly made an untrue statement with an intent to deceive, the victim justifiably relied on the statement being true, and the victim suffered resulting harm (Pozgar 2021, 48).

Fraud is a concern in today's healthcare environment because of the prevalence of deceptive and false claims submitted to Medicare, Medicaid, and private health insurance programs. Identifying and prosecuting it is a priority of the federal government.

**Invasion of Privacy** Invasion of privacy is intrusion on one's solitude. A person's right to privacy, which is "the right to be let alone" (Warren and Brandeis 1890, 193), includes the rights of individuals to be free from surveillance and interference, as well as the right to keep one's information from being disclosed (Rinehart-Thompson and Harman 2017, 78). The US Constitution does not specifically grant the right to privacy; however, courts have interpreted the Constitution to grant privacy rights against government intrusion in various areas (Brodnik 2023a, 7). Likewise, a constitutional right to privacy with respect to health information does not exist, but the privacy of such information has been established through various court decisions, state laws, and federal laws, specifically the HIPAA Privacy Rule (45 CFR 160 and 164)

(Rinehart-Thompson 2023d, 169–170). Causes of action exist to protect patients when their right of privacy is disregarded. One major actionable offense of concern in healthcare involving invasion of privacy is the unlawful disclosure of a patient's health information.

**Infliction of Emotional Distress** The intentional or reckless infliction of emotional distress for which a person can be held liable includes mental suffering resulting from such things as despair, shame, grief, and public humiliation (Pozgar 2021, 49). If the plaintiff shows that the defendant, by inflicting the distress, intended to cause mental distress and knew or should have known that his or her actions would do so, the plaintiff can recover damages (Pozgar 2021, 49). Although this section focuses on the intentional infliction of emotional distress, a plaintiff may have a cause of action for negligent infliction of emotional distress as well, or as an alternative.

The distinction between negligence torts and intentional torts is far from academic and has practical consequences. In most state legal systems, punitive damages—those damages awarded beyond compensation for injury and intended to punish or deter wrongful conduct—are limited in negligence cases and may be capped at a defined dollar amount. However, most states permit punitive damages as a matter of right in cases of intentional torts, and these damages are often outside the scope of state laws capping jury awards or damages. Consequently, it is possible for a battery case involving a failure to obtain surgical consent (an intentional tort) to have more economic value to the plaintiff than a medical malpractice case (a negligence tort) due to punitive damage limitations.

### Strict Liability

Strict liability is liability without fault, or error, and a person or entity is held liable for damages or loss resulting from acts or omissions regardless of whether there was fault. Strict liability is generally limited to highly dangerous activities such as operation of nuclear power plants and zoos, where the law deems the defendant strictly liable for injuries suffered by the plaintiff because of the inherently hazardous nature of the industry (Rinehart-Thompson 2023c, 99).

### Product Liability

Product liability is the legal doctrine under which a manufacturer, seller, or supplier of a product may be liable to a buyer or other third party for injuries caused by a defective product (Pozgar 2021, 50). The injured person may bring an action based in negligence; strict liability; or breach of warranty, either express or implied.

To prevail in a product liability case based on *negligence*, the plaintiff must show all four elements of a negligence case: duty of care; breach of duty; resulting injury or harm; and causation (actual and proximate). The manufacturer will not be held liable for injuries if they resulted from the user's negligent use of the product. However, manufacturers will be held liable for injuries resulting from a bad product design. Thus, manufacturers often provide instructions on the proper use of their product or otherwise face potential negligence liability (Pozgar 2021, 50). Defective packaging and a failure to warn of dangers associated with normal, proper use of the product can also result in the manufacturer being held liable in negligence (Pozgar 2021, 50). The legal principle of *res ipsa loquitur*, discussed earlier, may also apply in product liability cases if a defect existed when the product left the manufacturer, no one had subsequently tampered with it, and it did not perform as intended (Pozgar 2021, 52).

The second basis for a product liability claim is strict liability, regardless of the defendant's fault. To prevail, the plaintiff only needs to show an injury resulted while using the product in the proper manner. The plaintiff does not need to show negligence by the manufacturer. An example would be a defective medical device.

Third, to recover under the theory of **breach of warranty**, or a broken promise, the plaintiff must show there was an express or implied warranty. Through an **express warranty**, the seller makes specific promises to the buyer, whereas an **implied warranty** exists when the facts lead to an inference that such a warranty exists "as a matter of public policy" to protect the public from harm (Pozgar 2021, 51).

### Defenses

Several defenses may be raised in response to a tort lawsuit. A common defense to many types of torts is **consent** by the plaintiff, where the defendant claims that the plaintiff gave permission or agreed to the now-alleged wrongful action. Defenses specific to negligence claims are as follows:

- **Contributory negligence**: If the plaintiff's conduct contributed in any part to the injury the plaintiff suffered, the plaintiff is barred from recovering any damages from the defendant.
- **Comparative negligence**: If the plaintiff's conduct contributed in part to the injury the plaintiff suffered, the plaintiff's recovery is reduced based on his or her percentage of negligence.
- **Assumption of risk**: If the plaintiff, with knowledge and understanding of a danger, voluntarily undertook the risks of that danger, the plaintiff may not recover damages for the resulting injury. The assumption of risk defense has limited application in healthcare cases because voluntariness is generally lacking in a patient seeking medical care.
- **Good Samaritan statutes**: A form of immunity, these statutes protect against liability for ordinary negligence committed by those assisting with emergency care in settings outside of healthcare facilities (such as motor vehicle accident sites, at sporting events, and so forth) where medical equipment is not generally available, and services are not charged. Designed to encourage individuals to provide emergency assistance in good faith, state Good Samaritan statutes can vary based on who they protect (licensed medical providers only versus any rescuer who assists) and the type of assistance protected (all emergency care versus medical emergency care only) (Rinehart-Thompson 2023c, 97–103).

Other defenses that may be raised include the following:

- **Statute of limitations**: If a lawsuit is not brought within a statutory time limit, the plaintiff is barred from pursuing the claim. When the time limit begins can vary. It may be based on factors such as when the alleged wrong occurred, when it was discovered, or when it should have reasonably been discovered.
- **Governmental (sovereign) immunity**: Governments of various levels (federal, state, local and tribal) enjoy a degree of protection from tort lawsuits. Where this protection is limited via qualified immunity, a lawsuit may be brought. There are also situations when governmental immunity can be waived (Legal Information Institute 2020).

Historically, the doctrine of **charitable immunity** was a defense that protected charitable institutions (such as hospitals) from tort liability. Precipitated by the landmark case *Darling v. Charleston Community Memorial Hospital* (1965), however, this doctrine has effectively been extinguished because of the increasing business nature of most healthcare organizations (Rinehart-Thompson 2023c, 98).

### Apology Statutes

Healthcare providers commonly fear apologies or expressions of sympathy made to a patient or patient's family members will be considered an admission of liability and will be used against providers who are named as defendants in lawsuits. Many states have created apology statutes ("I'm Sorry" laws) that protect a healthcare provider's apology from being admitted into evidence as an admission of liability during a court proceeding (Rinehart-Thompson 2023b, 81). While apology statutes are not a type of defense and, instead, protect apologies from being admitted as evidence, their creation has nonetheless served as a defense mechanism for healthcare providers.

## Contract

Contract law addresses the creation of contracts and the resolution of contract disputes. It is the second type of law that is commonly encountered in the healthcare industry. A contract is an agreement that in most cases is enforceable through the legal system. Contracts can be express (written or oral) or implied by the parties' actions. Contracts must not violate state or federal law. The parties to a contract must have the capacity to enter into the agreement, such as being competent adults, being of the age of majority, and not being incapacitated either permanently or situationally (for example, due to the influence of medication or alcohol). Contracts are ubiquitous, and this is also true in the healthcare industry. Contracts are often corporate in nature and include actions such as mergers and acquisitions. However, the provider-patient relationship is also based on a contractual agreement.

The elements of a contract must be stated clearly and specifically. A contract cannot exist unless all the following elements exist:

- There must be an *agreement* between two or more persons or entities.
- The agreement must include a valid offer and an acceptance of the offer.
- There is an exchange of consideration.

In an offer, one party promises to either do something or not do something if the other party agrees to either do something or not do something (Rinehart-Thompson 2023c, 108). The party making the offer must communicate it to the other party so that it can be accepted or rejected.

A contract must be supported by a legal and bargained-for consideration, which is what the parties will receive from each other in exchange for performing the obligations of the contract (Rinehart-Thompson 2023c, 108). There also must be acceptance, which requires a meeting of the minds between the parties about terms that are sufficiently definite and complete (Rinehart-Thompson 2023c, 108).

A contract action arises when one party claims the other party failed to meet an obligation set forth in a valid contract. In other words, the other party has breached the contract. The resolution available is either compensation (monetary damages) or specific performance, which is fulfilling the obligation, or injunction, which is an order to generally stop some action. To succeed in a breach of contract action, the plaintiff must show that parties entered into a valid contract; the plaintiff performed as specified, the defendant did not perform as specified, and the plaintiff suffered an economic loss as a result of the defendant's failure to perform (Pozgar 2021, 75).

The defendant can raise a variety of defenses to a breach of contract action including fraud (the nonperforming party was misled on a material contract term); mistake of fact (both parties relied on a mistake); duress (unlawful threat or pressure was used to execute the contract); impossibility (contract was impossible to perform); or illegality (contract was for illegal purposes or against public policy). A contract provision that places a healthcare provider in a significant position of power over a patient who relies on the provider's services may be deemed an adhesion contract and found to be against public policy (Rinehart-Thompson 2023c, 108–109).

### Check Your Understanding 9.2

**Answer the following questions in a separate document.**

1. Compare the three categories of negligence and give an example of each.
2. Interpret the four elements of negligence and give an example of each in a hypothetical case.
3. Compare the types of intentional torts discussed in the text.
4. Ensure the necessary elements of a contract are present.
5. Describe apology statutes and what purpose they serve.
6. Distinguish the defenses to a breach of contract action, which were described in this chapter.
7. Compare contributory negligence and comparative negligence. How do they differ? Which one is more punitive to a plaintiff that has committed negligence?

# Legal Aspects of Health Information Management

The patient health record is a legal document that serves as evidence of a patient's treatment and continuity of care. Understanding its form and content; identifying it as a legal business record of an organization; and articulating issues associated with the electronic health record (EHR), health record retention, and ownership and access are all important for HIM professionals.

## Form and Content of the Health Record

The health record is a complete, accurate, and current report of the medical history, condition, and treatment that a particular patient receives during an inpatient or outpatient encounter with a healthcare provider. The health record may reflect one episode of care or an accumulation of all episodes of care (a longitudinal record).

The health record is composed of demographic information and clinical information. Most demographic information is collected at the time of admission or registration for treatment. It includes, among other items, the patient's name, legal sex, age, insurance information, and information about the person to contact in case of emergency. The clinical information consists of the patient's complaint, history of present illness, medical history, family history, social history, and physical examination. Documentation of ongoing medical care includes physician progress notes and orders; reports of diagnostic tests, including laboratory and radiology; surgery and other procedure reports, including anesthesia; consultations, if applicable; nursing documentation; graphic representations of the patient's status; and final diagnosis(es).

The content of the health record may be based on multiple external requirements. It is often determined by state statutes and regulations, which may be prescriptive or broad. For example, some laws detail what an appropriate health record must contain and the information to be retained; others specify broad categories of information required; and still others simply require that the health record be accurate, adequate, and complete. Medicare providers must also follow the Medicare CoP, which include minimum requirements for health record content. Third-party payers also dictate how health records for their insured must be maintained for providers to be reimbursed. Accrediting bodies also determine an accredited provider's health record content. The HIM professional must be aware of the most prescriptive definition of the health record content that his or her organization must follow. The following sections outline external forces that impact, to varying degrees, the forms and content of the health record maintained by healthcare providers: licensing agencies, accrediting bodies, and statutory and regulatory law.

### Licensing Agencies

Typically, state legislatures grant authority to designated state administrative agencies to do the following:

- Develop standards hospitals and other healthcare providers must meet
- Issue licenses to hospitals and other healthcare providers that meet the standards
- Monitor continuing compliance with the standards
- Penalize hospitals and other healthcare providers that violate the standards

Licensure is government regulation that is mandatory for hospitals and other healthcare organizations, depending on state law. Licenses are issued to organizations as a whole. Licensure addresses policies and procedures, staffing, and building structural integrity among many other facets of the organization. Some states require additional licenses for specific services. For example, laboratory, pharmacy, radiology, renal dialysis, medical equipment, and substance abuse services in a hospital may require separate licenses in addition to the organization's license.

Depending on state law, healthcare organizations cannot operate without a license or an equivalent type of approval. Those that violate licensure standards may lose their licenses or be penalized in other ways, such as assessment of fines.

### Accrediting Bodies

Accreditation is offered through nongovernmental organizations. Accreditation is considered voluntary and is not legally mandated, but it is very important to healthcare organizations because it indicates high-quality care. The Joint Commission is the most prominent accrediting body for acute-care hospitals. It also accredits organizations in other settings (for example, behavioral health, ambulatory services, and home health). However, other accrediting bodies, such as the Commission on Accreditation of Rehabilitation Facilities (CARF), occupy a larger space in care settings outside the acute-care hospital, such as long-term care.

The Joint Commission develops standards pertaining to all aspects of a healthcare organization that must be met to be accredited. In addition to accreditation surveys that focus on an entire organization, there are also accreditation or certification processes offered by accrediting bodies that focus on specific services such as laboratory and radiology.

An organization applies for accreditation, pays an accreditation fee, and submits to an extensive survey to ensure compliance with the accrediting body's published standards. The Joint Commission, for example, addresses the health record primarily through its Information Management and Record of Care, Treatment and Services chapters. The Joint Commission standards address record content, privacy, information security, confidentiality, ethical behavior, patient rights training, and whether the organization complies with applicable laws, regulations, and standards.

### Statutory and Regulatory Law

An organization must consult state and federal statutes and regulations to determine which ones are applicable. The federal Medicare regulations apply to any provider that participates in the Medicare program. Most providers supply medical services to Medicare beneficiaries, so Medicare patients are significant to most providers because of the volume of services associated with them. To be reimbursed by Medicare, providers must comply with the requirements in the Medicare CoP. The Medicare program also recognizes organizations accredited by the Joint Commission; Health Facilities Accreditation Program (HFAP), which functions within the Accreditation Commission for Health Care (ACHC); DNV GL Healthcare; or the Center for Improvement in Healthcare Quality (CIHQ) as meeting the requirements of the Medicare CoP, and it grants those organizations deemed status, which is a government-recognized designation as an accredited provider. This deeming authority granted by Medicare gives recognized accrediting bodies more power than they would otherwise have as, in addition to Medicare recognition, some states accept accreditation as a basis for partial or full licensure with a limited or no additional survey by a state agency. In addition to Medicare, some states accept Joint Commission or other accreditation as a basis for partial or full licensure with a limited or no additional survey by a state agency.

***Privacy*** Many laws mandate health information privacy. The HIPAA Privacy Rule is a predominant federal regulation. However, HIM professionals must also consult their individual state statutes and regulations for privacy protections in addition to those provided by HIPAA.

Although the US Constitution does not specifically grant a right to privacy, some states, such as California, Arizona, and Florida, have recognized the right to privacy in their state constitutions (California Constitution, Article 1, Section 1; Arizona Constitution, Article 2, Section 8; Florida Constitution, Article I, Section 23).

The Privacy Act of 1974 was an early piece of federal legislation that addressed the right to privacy. This act was written to give individuals some control over the large amounts of information collected about them by the federal government and its contractors (Rinehart-Thompson 2024, 6). While federal healthcare entities such as US Department of Veterans Affairs (VA) facilities are bound by this law, it does not apply to records maintained by private organizations (Rinehart-Thompson 2023d, 172). Under the Privacy Act of 1974, which HIPAA paralleled when it was created, personally identifiable information is protected and individuals are given rights including the right of access and the right to request amendments to their records (Rinehart-Thompson 2024, 6).

The Freedom of Information Act of 1967 (FOIA) is a federal law through which individuals can seek access to information without the authorization of the person to whom the information applies. The underlying premise of FOIA is government accountability and transparency. However, access exceptions exist for medical records to protect patient privacy in most situations. This act, like the Privacy Act, also applies only to federal agencies, so its applicability to healthcare organizations is generally limited to those owned and operated by the VA and the Department of Defense, as most healthcare providers are privately owned.

The Medicare CoP require that healthcare organizations have procedures in place to protect the confidentiality of patient records (Rinehart-Thompson 2023d, 172). This includes the protection of records against unauthorized access and alteration. However, the CoP regulate only providers who receive funds from Medicare and Medicaid (Rinehart-Thompson 2023d, 172).

HIPAA was developed in part to improve the efficiency and effectiveness of the healthcare system. Discussions about these provisions, however, prompted Congress to express concerns about privacy and security of patient information in an electronic environment. Consequently, HIPAA required the US Department of Health and Human Services (HHS) to develop and implement regulations to protect the privacy and security of individually identifiable health information (HIPAA 1996).

The HIPAA Privacy Rule has been in effect since 2003, and the Security Rule has been in effect since 2005. The Health Information Technology for Economic and Clinical Health (HITECH) Act, which was passed in 2009 as part of the American Recovery and Reinvestment Act (ARRA), strengthened the requirements included in the HIPAA Privacy and Security Rules.

## The Health Record as a Business Record

A health record qualifies as a **business record**, which is documentation created and kept in the usual course of business. It is created at or near the time of the event being recorded and made by a person who has knowledge of the events recorded (FRE 803(6)). A significant characteristic of a business record is that it is presumed to be trustworthy. As a result, it has substantial evidentiary value in legal proceedings and is generally admissible in court. The health record is often referred to as a legal health record (LHR), and it is the record that an organization releases upon a valid request. The content of the legal health record may vary as organizations determines what they will disclose pursuant to a legal request. Determining LHR content is complex due to myriad applicable laws and formats (paper, imaged, electronic, hybrid); multiple locations where components of health records are stored; the many ways health information is collected (such as emails and text messages); and the creation of other types of information related to the patient record such as metadata, logs, schedules and patient-generated data. As such, an inventory of all source systems that contribute to the content of the health record should be maintained (Rinehart-Thompson 2023e, 140). When Congress passed the 21st Century Cures Act (Cures) in 2016, it shifted the emphasis on disclosure away from the LHR and toward a prohibition against information blocking of **electronic health information (EHI)**, which is all electronic protected health information (ePHI) in the designated record set (DRS).

Those who use information in the health record rely on it to be correct, accurate, and complete. It must not have been changed either intentionally or accidentally. Reliability and integrity of the health record are critical to meeting the standards of evidence in a court of law and it being recognized as a business record (Rinehart-Thompson 2023e, 140).

Inextricably linked to reliability and integrity is **authenticity**, which means that the record is genuine and "is what it purports to be" (Rinehart-Thompson 2023e, 146; FRE 901(a)). Authenticity relates both to the reliability of the system on which information is created and stored, and to the information itself. System reliability includes such features as user access controls, system security, access tracking and auditing capabilities, and operational stability (dependability and availability). These features are particularly important because of the concern that electronically stored information (ESI) can easily be changed (Rinehart-Thompson 2023e, 146). In both electronic and paper health record environments, information authenticity includes both the content and the identity of authors of health record entries. **Authentication** validates content and proves authorship. In paper records, authentication can be accomplished by a handwritten signature or initials, both in ink. Electronic or digital signatures and computer keys are types of authentication methods in EHRs (Rinehart-Thompson 2023e, 147). Authentication methods must comply with applicable laws and accreditation standards. Other issues that must be considered when maintaining a legally defensible health record include the appropriate uses of abbreviations; legibility; changes such as revisions, additions, deletions, and version management; timeliness and completeness; and control over printing so that paper printouts do not contain more current information than the electronic record (Rinehart-Thompson 2023e, 150–154).

As concerns about inappropriate abbreviations and legibility have lessened with the EHR, another problem has replaced it—the use of the "copy-paste" function enabled in some systems. Because copied and pasted information is often not edited appropriately, patient outcomes can be negatively affected by the presence of outdated information that appears to be current and redundant information that is carried forward. Redundant information leads to lengthy entries and voluminous records that often are not read in their entirety, causing new information to be overlooked. Finally, incorrect information may be copied from one encounter to the next. In addition to negative patient outcomes, there are also legal risks. These include clinical plagiarism, where authorship of the original documentation is not appropriately attributed, and the date of creation is unknown; and the potential for fraud and abuse claims where records are coded based on inaccurate or outdated information.

Alternatives that can safeguard the integrity of the EHR while managing the task of documenting include medical scribes, who are paraprofessionals who accompany healthcare providers and chart for them in real time; voice recognition technology; and EHR features such as drop-down menus and smart phrases.

## Retention of the Health Record

The health record must be retained to meet its many purposes, including patient treatment, communication among providers, and continuity of care; proof of services provided to justify reimbursement; evidence in legal proceedings; evaluation of quality and efficiency of care; source of information for statistics, research, and education; and facilitation of an organization's operations management (Brodnik 2023a, 3). These varied purposes influence health record retention periods. Equally as important as defining retention periods is ensuring information is private and secure during the time it is retained.

Federal and state statutes and regulations often determine retention periods, with the strictest (that is, the longest) retention guidelines to be followed. For example, the Medicare CoP require a five-year retention period for hospital records (42 CFR 482.24(b)(1)). State law may or may not specify a minimum retention period for health records as a whole or for specific portions of the record. Additionally, organizations must take into consideration the applicable statutes of limitations for bringing a legal action (for example, for medical malpractice or breach of contract actions) so the record will still exist if needed for legal proceedings. This consideration is particularly important for retaining the records of minors (should they file lawsuits on their own behalf once they reach the age of majority) or incompetent individuals (should their mental incompetence be lifted by the court system) (Rinehart-Thompson 2023e, 158). The HIM professional must be aware of all applicable retention laws and statutes of limitations at the state level.

In addition to legal considerations, other factors affect retention decisions. Organizations such as accrediting bodies and professional associations (for example, the American Health Information Management Association [AHIMA]) offer guidance. The Joint Commission does not mandate specific retention periods, but instead defers to an organization's applicable laws, its use of records, and hospital policy (Joint Commission 2023). As a result, some organizations opt for longer retention periods than others based on factors such as cost and operational needs including availability of information for statistics, research, and education.

Finally, technology continues to affect retention. The EHR makes it possible for many organizations to retain records for longer periods of time, but retention decisions associated with EHRs are also affected by federal and state e-discovery rules. Organizations must know how long information is stored, in what form(s) it exists, and when it will be destroyed. They must also know where information is stored, including hidden locations such as document drafts, shadow records, and electronic backup systems. Retention schedules must also be developed for metadata (for example, logs showing when electronic documents are created, accessed, and changed) (Rinehart-Thompson 2023b, 64).

## Ownership of and Access to the Health Record

Patients often believe they own their health record. It is true that the information in the record is that of the individual, but the organization that created and maintains the physical record is the legal custodian responsible for its integrity and security. The federal government has made individuals' right of access to their health records abundantly clear through its enforcement of the HIPAA Right of Access Initiative and the information blocking rule that went into effect in 2022. State laws must provide individuals with at least the same degree of access that HIPAA allows. Otherwise, they will be superseded by HIPAA through the principle of **preemption**, which gives federal law precedence over state law. HIM professionals must be able to advise the patient regarding the organization's actual ownership and control of the physical health record and the patient's rights to the information contained in it.

Historically, the physical health record (as a hard copy document) was considered the property of the healthcare provider that maintained it because it was the healthcare provider's business record and there was only one original copy to control. The EHR, along with government initiatives noted above and the creation of patient portals, has caused a paradigm shift. Patients' access to their own health information is ubiquitous, as individuals are not only legally and physically able to access their information but also have been encouraged to do so. First, by meaningful use standards and subsequently by MACRA's Merit-Based Incentive Payment System (MIPS) Promoting Interoperability requirements. Regardless of whether the medical record format is paper or electronic, the organization creates and maintains it is legally responsible for all aspects of it, including its integrity and completeness, elements which make it defensible in a court of law (Rinehart-Thompson 2023e, 146). HIPAA, applicable state laws, and accrediting bodies such as the Joint Commission also enforce this responsibility. In effect, then, the organization that is responsible for the record "owns" it even when it is electronically stored and widely accessible by the individual to whom it pertains.

### Check Your Understanding 9.3

**Answer the following questions in a separate document.**

1. Differentiate licensure and accreditation of healthcare organizations.

2. What are differences between the Privacy Act of 1974 and the FOIA?

3. Assess the types of risks that the copy-paste function presents in EHRs. Determine which risk you believe is the most severe. Why do you believe this?

4. Legally, what factors must be taken into consideration when developing health record retention schedules?

What factors should be taken into consideration? Distinguish internal factors and external factors.

5. Distinguish ownership of and access to the health record, whether it is paper, electronic, or hybrid.

6. The health record serves several purposes. Evaluate each of these purposes, relative to one another.

7. The legal concept of preemption applies with respect to one's access to their own health information. Explain the concept of preemption.

## The Health Record as Evidence

The health record is critical evidence in many types of legal proceedings. It serves as documentation of care provided in civil cases such as medical malpractice (for example, a patient alleges wrongdoing against healthcare providers) or other personal injury (for example, vehicle accidents) and in violent and nonviolent criminal cases against persons and property (for example, rape, homicide, and healthcare fraud). The health record is generally admissible in court as a business record. The health record is also an important repository for consents and advance directives. Other issues associated with the health record as evidence include e-discovery and challenges associated with EHRs as evidence, provider-patient privilege, and the government's right of access to health records.

### Admissibility of the Health Record

The health record can provide valuable evidence in a legal proceeding because of its presumed truthfulness and its permanence. Witnesses may refer to the health record to refresh their recollection. The custodian of records, typically a facility's health information manager, may be called as a witness to identify the record as the one subpoenaed. He or she also may be called to testify regarding policies and procedures relevant to the creation and maintenance of the record, including the system on which it was created and maintained, and mechanisms to prevent improper alteration or access.

Although the health record is considered **hearsay** because it contains out-of-court statements that can be used in court to prove the truth of a claim, the **business records exception** to the prohibition against admitting hearsay evidence will often permit a health record to be admitted (FRE 803(6)). A record is generally admissible under this exception if it is relevant and the record custodian testifies or provides an affidavit that the record was documented and maintained in the normal course of business and made by a person in the business who had knowledge of the events being written about (Rinehart-Thompson 2023b, 78).

For an EHR to be admissible, the court must be confident that the system from which the record was produced is accurate and trustworthy. In 2017, Federal Rules of Evidence (FRE) 902 was amended to include the following as self-authenticating:

- Records generated by electronic systems producing accurate results, as shown by certification of a qualified person complying with the FRE certification requirements
- Data copied from an electronic device, storage medium, or file that is authenticated by digital identification, as shown by certification of a qualified person complying with the FRE certification requirements (FRE 902)

When these self-authenticating measures are present, no testimony or affidavit is required.

### The Electronic Health Record

Despite the provisions of FRE 902, EHRs can present special evidentiary challenges where there is reason for confidence in the system to be questioned. While metadata and the use of audit trails can verify entry creation, revision, and access, other EHR characteristics can lead attorneys and courts to question the integrity of the record, thus influencing its admissibility. As discussed earlier, inappropriate use of the copy-paste function may diminish EHR integrity. Documentation templates and smart phrases, while efficient, may lead to inaccuracies if not used carefully. Version management, and whether the most recent version of a document is present in the EHR, also raises integrity questions. Finally, when printouts of electronic records are provided to attorneys and to the court, documentation may be voluminous (due to copy-paste redundancies) and seemingly inconsistent with the record that one views electronically (Rinehart-Thompson 2023e, 149–150). Nonetheless, laws such as Indiana state law provide that health records made by electronic data processing systems are considered original written records and printouts shall be treated as original records in court for admissibility purposes (Indiana Code Title 34 2021).

Because they contain ePHI, EHR systems must be designed to comply with the HIPAA Security Rule, which addresses the confidentiality, integrity, and availability of PHI. Specifically, covered entities and their business associates (for example, EHR vendors) must ensure the standards and implementation specifications of the administrative, technical, and physical safeguard requirements of the HIPAA Security Rule are met.

## Consent and Advance Directives

It is vital to know an individual's wishes regarding the healthcare they wish to receive, and for those wishes to be documented in the health record. Medical malpractice lawsuits may revolve around whether a patient agreed to medical care that they received or whether they desired not to receive treatment. Thus, consents and advance directives play an important evidentiary role in HIM.

Consent, legally, is one's permission or agreement to an action. Consent can either be express (communicated through words) or implied (communicated through conduct). If consent is express, it can either be written or spoken. Within the broad concept of consent is the consent to receive medical treatment. Express written consent provides greater legal protections because it offers greater proof. One type of implied consent that exists in the healthcare context is emergency consent, where one is presumed to want to receive medical care (unless information is known to the contrary) and would voice this consent if they were conscious or otherwise capable of communicating.

To substantiate one's consent to medical treatment, healthcare organizations obtain **general consent**, also known as battery consent, from patients at the beginning of an encounter to permit providers to perform routine treatment. Failure to obtain general consent can result in legal action, generally for battery. As a treatment or procedure becomes more invasive or risky, it is important that the informed consent process be completed. **Informed consent** ensures the patient has a basic understanding of his or her diagnosis; the nature of the treatment or procedure along with the risks, benefits, and alternatives (to include opting out of treatment); and names of individuals who will perform the treatment or procedure. It is the responsibility of the provider who will be rendering the treatment or performing the procedure to obtain the patient's informed consent and answer the patient's questions. An informed consent document that affirms the outcome of the discussion must be signed and dated by the patient, the provider rendering the treatment, and a witness. This is an important piece of evidence. Failure to obtain informed consent can result in legal action generally based on negligence (Brodnik and Rinehart-Thompson 2023, 117).

An **advance directive** is a special type of written consent that communicates an individual's wishes to be treated or not to be treated, should the individual become incapacitated and unable to communicate on his or her own behalf. A **durable power of attorney for healthcare decisions** is a document in which an adult—while competent—designates another person (proxy) to make healthcare decisions consistent with the individual's wishes and on the individual's behalf if the individual is unable. The term *durable* indicates that the document is in effect when the individual is no longer competent. A **living will** is executed by a competent adult, expressing the individual's wishes to limit treatment should the individual become afflicted with certain conditions (for example, a persistent vegetative state or a terminal condition) and no longer able to communicate on his or her own behalf. Living wills are prescriptive in nature and often address extraordinary lifesaving measures such as ventilator support and either the continuation or removal of nutrition and hydration. The lack of advance directives, where controversy erupted regarding the undocumented wishes of individuals, has sparked such high-profile end-of-life cases as Karen Ann Quinlan, Nancy Cruzan, and Terri Schiavo (Brodnik and Rinehart-Thompson 2023, 130–131).

A third type of document, which always specifies an individual's wish not to receive treatment (specifically, cardiopulmonary resuscitation or CPR) is the **do-not-resuscitate (DNR) order**. Most often used by individuals who are elderly or chronically ill, it directs healthcare providers to refrain from performing the otherwise standing order of CPR should the individual experience cardiac or respiratory arrest. Prior to executing a DNR, the patient and physician should have a discussion, a consent form should be signed by the patient, and the physician is to write an order in the patient's medical record. State law provides the framework for completing DNR orders and forms. Joint Commission-accredited organizations are required to implement policies regarding advance directives and DNR orders (Brodnik and Rinehart-Thompson 2023, 125). Table 9.1 differentiates these three types of advance directive documents.

In 1990, Congress passed the **Patient Self-Determination Act**, which requires healthcare institutions that are Medicare or Medicaid providers to give adult patients information about advance directives; document in the health record whether patients have an advance directive or not; and treat patients equally despite the presence or absence of an advance directive (Brodnik and Rinehart-Thompson 2023, 125–126).

**Table 9.1.** Comparison of advance directives

| Durable power of attorney for healthcare decisions | Executed by a competent adult on his or her own behalf |
| --- | --- |
| | Designates another person (proxy) to make healthcare decisions consistent with the individual's wishes on the individual's behalf |
| Living will | Executed by a competent adult on his or her own behalf |
| | Expresses one's wishes to limit treatment if a medical condition renders the individual unable to communicate on his or her own behalf |
| | May be limited to certain medical conditions (for example, vegetative state), depending on state law |
| **Do-not-resuscitate order** | Most often used by the elderly or chronically ill |
| | Directs healthcare providers to refrain from CPR if the individual experiences cardiac or respiratory arrest |

## E-Discovery

Responsibility for responding to requests for health records involved in litigation, either for depositions or in the courtroom, has long rested with HIM professionals. However, as health records transition to hybrid or completely electronic formats the response process has become much more complex and involves professionals with varying types of expertise. E-discovery is a pretrial process through which parties obtain and review ESI. The e-discovery rules are amendments to the Federal Rules of Civil Procedure (FRCP) (Rinehart-Thompson 2023b, 61). Although the FRCP applies only to cases in federal district courts, states have implemented similar e-discovery rules that apply to state civil and criminal cases.

Issues associated with e-discovery include identifying the locations of all ESI, what information needs to be preserved, the format it will be presented in, legal holds, record retention and destruction policies, disaster recovery, and business continuity (Rinehart-Thompson 2023b, 61–62). In the past, HIM professionals were involved in the pretrial discovery phase by responding to a subpoena for records or by testifying at a deposition. With e-discovery, the HIM professional's involvement begins much earlier in litigation with pretrial conferences, where availability of documents and discussions about document sharing occur among the parties' attorneys. Further, information technology (IT) personnel are involved early on because of the systems platform on which an organization's EHRs reside.

An iconic graphic, the Electronic Discovery Reference Model (EDRM), illustrates the e-discovery process in an iterative process. Its elements include the following:

- Identification (locating ESI sources and determining their scope)
- Preservation (against unauthorized alteration or destruction)
- Collection (for further use, such as e-discovery)
- Processing (volume reduction for manageable review and analysis)
- Review (assessment of information for legal relevance or protection per privilege)
- Analysis (for content and context)
- Production (delivery in appropriate forms and per appropriate mechanisms)
- Presentation (at depositions, hearings, and trial) (EDRM 2023)

The concept of "any and all records" possesses a different meaning with EHRs and e-discovery because the volume of records is certain to be much greater in an electronic record environment than in a paper record environment. As such, e-discovery requests are likely to solicit much more voluminous amounts of information. Any data stored electronically can serve as evidence. This includes emails, voicemails, instant messages, drafts of documents, information on personal mobile devices, calendar files, and websites. Text messages, one type of electronic data, have played a role in many high-profile cases (McCluskey 2022).

HIM professionals must be familiar with documents stored in their original or "native file format," including metadata—electronic data about data that include information not previously available in paper documents, such as time stamps that show when and by whom a document or entry was created, accessed, or changed (Rinehart-Thompson 2023e, 149).

The concepts of legal hold and spoliation continue to be important under the e-discovery rule. A legal hold is typically issued by a court to lock or disengage any editing capabilities to a health record, whether paper or electronic, when there is concern that information relevant to a legal proceeding or an audit could be changed or destroyed. This hold suspends any normal record disposition activities including scheduled destruction. Triggers such as complaints (that is, filing of a lawsuit), subpoenas, notices from opposing counsel, and government investigations should prompt legal hold placement on a health record. **Spoliation** is "intentional destruction, mutilation, alteration, or concealment of evidence" (Rinehart-Thompson 2023b, 63). A trier of fact may reasonably infer that destruction of evidence related to a legal proceeding was done with a consciousness of guilt or nefarious motive; however, courts will generally allow the spoliator to rebut the inference and show there was no bad faith (Rinehart-Thompson 2023b, 63–64).

HIM professionals should understand what is included in EHI, which is subject to the information blocking rule, as well as the LHR and DRS. Knowing where all relevant information resides is also critical. There are many media types and points of entry by which health information can become incorporated into an integrated health information system that is inclusive of an EHR and associated applications, both clinical and administrative. All of these must be accounted for in the e-discovery preservation process. For example, information may be created and stored on laptop and desktop computers, as well as mobile devices such as tablets and smart phones. Storage mechanisms include servers, which may be local, remote, cloud-based, or removable (for example, flash drives).

The location of ESI must also be addressed from the perspective of ancillary services, clinical services, remote access, personal equipment, and email. It is important to know whether ancillary service information is integrated into the EHR or maintained separately. Data residing on devices such as imaging equipment, IV medication pumps, and dictation systems must also be accounted for, both for inclusion in an inventory of ESI that can serve as evidence and due to security risks they can pose if they serve as pathways for a cyberattack on an organization's information system (IS) (Rinehart-Thompson 2024, 192).

Complying with an e-discovery request or subpoena is complex. It is important to understand what electronic information may be discoverable; to have policies, procedures, and a plan in place to respond to litigation; and to recognize that information retained beyond the required retention period may still be subject to e-discovery.

## Privilege

The professional relationship between a patient and each of his or her healthcare providers affects use of the record and its contents as evidence. **Privilege** means that the nature of the relationship is confidential. **Physician-patient privilege** means the information exchanged between patient and physician as part of the professional relationship is a confidential communication that the patient anticipates will be held in confidence, thus encouraging the patient to disclose all relevant information. Privilege provides that the physician is not permitted to testify as a witness about certain information gained because of this relationship without the patient's consent.

The patient holds the privilege, and the information included in the physician-patient privilege is insulated from discovery unless the physician has a legal duty to disclose, the patient authorizes disclosure, or the patient waives the privilege as described below (Rinehart-Thompson 2023b, 800). State laws address the scope of privilege (for example, whether a court can order an examination that is not protected by the privilege and whether the privilege survives if a third party was present during a physician-patient communication) (Rinehart-Thompson 2023b, 80). Depending on the state, a similar privilege exists between other providers such as psychotherapist and patient, sexual assault victim and counselor, and domestic violence victim and counselor, as well as clergy and parishioner, and attorney and client. In states where these professional relationships are recognized, they apply when the provider is being compelled to testify as a witness concerning information obtained because of the treatment relationship. However, these privileges do not preclude the provider from making reports as required by law.

The patient may release the provider from the privilege through words or actions. This release is known as a waiver of privilege. For example, a patient who placed his or her treatment at issue in a trial could not continue to claim a privilege to protect the information. The provider then can testify regarding the information previously considered confidential.

## Government Right of Access to Health Records

Federal and state governments have the right to access health information with or without patient authorization in certain circumstances. For instance, by enrolling in Medicare or Medicaid, the patient gives permission for the healthcare provider to disclose confidential health information to appropriate recipients without patient authorization. Medicare is a federal program that provides medical insurance to the elderly and disabled. Medicaid is a joint federal and state program that provides medical insurance to individuals unable to pay for care. As payers, both programs may request information from the health record to support the healthcare provider's claim for reimbursement. The government also may require access to health information for investigative purposes such as pursuant to federal fraud and abuse statutes.

Another important federal statute for which the government may need access to health information as part of an investigation is the **Emergency Medical Treatment and Labor Act (EMTALA)**. This statute protects any patient seeking emergency care in a Medicare-participating hospital, requiring that they be appropriately evaluated for an emergency medical condition regardless of the ability to pay. Its effort to prevent "patient dumping" stemmed from hospitals that transferred, discharged, or refused to treat patients without stabilizing them if they were unable to pay (Brodnik and Reynolds 2023, 319). However, EMTALA's protections now extend to all patients pursuing emergency care.

---

### Check Your Understanding 9.4

**Answer the following questions in a separate document.**

1. What are the three types of advance directives discussed in this chapter? Compare them to one another.
2. Distinguish general consent and informed consent. In what types of situations would each apply? Why are there situations when general consent is insufficient?
3. Describe what information and locations where information may be housed must be taken into consideration when responding to an e-discovery request.
4. Differentiate at least three examples of metadata. Explain why they are important to e-discovery.
5. Evaluate the importance of the concept of waiver of privilege if a patient sues a physician for medical malpractice.
6. Why is the Patient Self-Determination Act of 1990 significant?
7. Presume that health information was destroyed prior to the end of the retention period required by law, and it was later requested as part of the e-discovery process. Compare spoliation with other types of health record destruction.

---

## Release of Information

Managing the release of information (ROI) requires the HIM professional to be fully aware of federal and state statutes and regulations affecting the use and disclosure of PHI, as well as accreditation standards. In organizations where the ROI function is decentralized and carried out by multiple areas, all departments in the organization that perform the ROI function must follow standardized policies and procedures that adhere to external requirements. ROI staff must also be familiar with the HIPAA authorization requirement by disclosing information pursuant to an authorization when one is required, being aware of authorization exceptions, and understanding when organizational policy mirrors HIPAA's permissiveness (that is, where authorization is not required) or places more stringent authorization requirements on such disclosures. Any alleged HIPAA violations by ROI staff in the disclosure process must be investigated as potential breaches.

### Handling Highly Sensitive Information

Certain types of health information, because of the stigma and sensitivity associated with them, require special protections. Although they are not categorically addressed separately by HIPAA nor subject to a different set of requirements under HIPAA, other laws come into play to protect them. Highly sensitive information includes behavioral health, substance use disorder (SUD), HIV and AIDS, genetic testing, and adoption records.

Behavioral health information is highly safeguarded because of its sensitive nature and the stigma associated with it. HIM professionals should consult their relevant state laws for safeguards provided for behavioral health information. Further, best practice dictates that authorizations for the disclosure of behavioral health information provide a designated area for individuals to authorize the disclosure of that information specifically.

**Confidentiality of Substance Use Disorder Patient Records**, provide special protections for SUD records (42 CFR 2.11 Part 2). Health records that contain one's identity, diagnosis, prognosis, or treatment information where alcohol or drug abuse is either the primary or secondary diagnosis are included in restrictions on disclosure and redisclosure. The regulations apply to organizations that offer a federally assisted drug or alcohol abuse program by either providing alcohol or drug abuse diagnosis, treatment, or referral for treatment. The program may be a standalone, a unit within a general medical facility, or designated personnel within a general medical facility (Brodnik 2023b, 264).

These federal regulations outline disclosures which require patient consent and those that do not require consent; consent form requirements; and reporting of violations. They further limit the acknowledgement of the presence of patients in substance abuse treatment or referral facilities without written patient consent and require that disclosures be accompanied by a notice that generally prohibits redisclosure (42 CFR 2.11 Part 2). Alignment between the requirements of HIPAA and 42 CFR Part 2 has become increasingly important.

HIV and AIDS information is also highly safeguarded because of its sensitive and stigmatic nature. Because it is protected specifically by state law, HIM professionals should be familiar with relevant state laws that safeguard this type of information. Best practice dictates that authorizations for the disclosure of HIV and AIDS information provide a designated area for individuals to authorize the disclosure of that information specifically.

With the availability of genetic testing and information that pertains to one's propensity for developing a certain disease or condition, laws exist at both the federal and state levels to safeguard genetic information. The federal Genetic Information Non-Discrimination Act of 2008 (GINA) protects individuals from being discriminated against by health insurers and employers based on genetic information. State laws provide similar protections. Best practice provides that individuals specifically authorize the disclosure of their genetic information.

Adoption records have historically been sensitive because of closed adoptions. Where closed adoptions still exist, this information must receive special protection. Adoption information is protected by individual state laws. Unless a court order mandates it, the health record is not the usual source from which the identity of a birth parent or birth child should be revealed. Requests for identifying information should be referred to the appropriate agency, such as a state department of health or vital statistics, or the adoption agency that coordinated the adoption (Brodnik 2023b, 268).

## Wrongful Disclosure

Individuals are personally liable for committing unauthorized disclosures of confidential health information. The individual's liability is based on fault because the individual committed a wrong or failed to do something the individual should have done. Employers also may be held liable for any job-related acts of their employees or agents per the doctrine of *respondeat superior* ("let the master answer") (Rinehart-Thompson 2023c, 99). Healthcare organizations are less likely to be found liable for a breach of confidentiality by members of its medical staff if they are not employees or agents of the organization; however, *respondeat superior* has been expanded to often include individuals under the organization's direction and control, even if they are not employees. The organization may also be liable for the consequences of any unauthorized disclosure under the doctrine of *corporate negligence*, whether by employees, agents, or medical staff members, because the organization breached its duty to maintain information in a confidential manner. The injured person benefits from these concepts of fault because the injured person can sue the employer, the employee, or both. Note that the legal theories of *respondeat superior* and corporate negligence are not limited to wrongful disclosure cases.

A plaintiff may bring a claim for wrongful disclosure based on previously discussed intentional tort theories (defamation, invasion of privacy, and intentional infliction of emotional distress). Causes of action for wrongful disclosure may also be based on *breach of confidentiality*, where a *fiduciary duty* exists because of a relationship of trust and obligation between the provider and the patient. A claim for wrongful disclosure can also be based on a negligence inquiry, where the four elements of that cause of action must be met.

Unauthorized disclosure by various healthcare professionals also may be addressed in professional licensure and certification requirements. These provisions subject the professional to potential discipline by the licensing or certifying body for breach of confidentiality or unprofessional conduct.

## Medical Identity Theft

A significant legal challenge facing healthcare organizations, and the HIM profession, is *medical identity theft*. The term was coined by the World Privacy Forum in 2005 (WPF 2022) and introduced nationally through the seminal report "Medical Identity Theft—The Information Crime that Can Kill You" (Dixon 2006). It is the inappropriate or unauthorized use of a person's identity (such as name or insurance information) to do one of two things: (1) obtain medical services or goods (such as medical treatment, including surgery, and prescription drugs); or (2) falsify claims for medical services to fraudulently bill insurance companies (Reynolds and Brodnik 2023, 234). The second type of medical identity theft is most likely to be committed by someone operating within a healthcare organization. In both types of medical identity theft, the individual's health information is either created under the wrong name or altered, leading to potentially deadly consequences.

There are two types of medical identity theft. External medical identity theft is committed by individuals from outside an organization. Perpetrators can include uninsured individuals who use another's insurance to obtain services or technically savvy individuals who gain access to a system. As hacking has increased, with subsequent ransomware and denial-of-service incidents, external threats have created a greater threat for healthcare organizations (Reynolds and Brodnik 2023, 234–235). Internal medical identity theft is committed by individuals inside an organization with access to vast amounts of patient information. These individuals may act alone or as part of a larger crime ring that has intentionally infiltrated the organization to gain access to information (Reynolds and Brodnik 2023, 234–235). The Federal Trade Commission recommends protecting documents containing personal health-related information, such as health insurance cards and records, billing statements, and prescription information (including bottles), as well as medical records (FTC 2021).

What makes medical identity theft unique as compared to other types of identity theft is that it affects both the victim's financial information and medical information. When incorrect information is entered into a victim's health record, improper medical treatment could result. Although laws in the financial industry provide significant protections for victims of financial identity theft, much is left to be done to protect people from medical identity theft. State breach notification laws tailored to health information are limited. The HIPAA breach notification requirement created by ARRA and HITECH provides one way for victims to learn their health information has been compromised due to inappropriate use or disclosure.

## Confidentiality of Quality Improvement Activities

Quality improvement (QI) in healthcare is the process of evaluating and improving medical care and potentially decreasing healthcare costs. QI activities can be carried out on a concurrent review basis (as treatment is being provided) or on a retrospective basis (after an encounter has ended). The healthcare organization is responsible for conducting focused reviews when it detects patterns of questionable care. Questionable care that is deemed to be due to professional practice (that is, it is not at the expected level of care) may result in educational intervention. If warranted, more stringent steps, such as suspension or termination of a physician's medical staff privileges or membership, or termination of a provider's employment, may be taken.

QI review activities involve collecting outcomes and performance data on a healthcare provider. Understandably, the contents of these reviews are potentially of great interest to individuals contemplating or involved in litigation related to medical malpractice or wrongful termination. QI-related records are sought for discovery purposes, with attempts to admit them into evidence. HIM professionals, following relevant state laws, must ensure the privacy and security of data collected and shared as part of the QI process (Brodnik and Reynolds 2023, 318). For example, California Evidence Code Section 1157 protects from discovery the proceedings and records of organized peer review committees responsible for the evaluation and improvement of the quality of care. Without such specific statutory protection, these types of records would generally be discoverable.

### Incident Reports

An occurrence that is inconsistent with the standard of care is generally defined as an *incident*. Standards of care are related to more than direct patient care. Incidents can relate to staff and visitors as well. Any staff member witnessing or involved in an incident should complete an incident report as soon as possible after the incident to capture the details of what happened, collecting information from all involved parties. The *incident report* is one tool staff can use to report unusual incidents to administration, initiate investigations, and provide appropriate feedback to staff involved in the incident, although disciplinary action generally does not result from incident reporting. Blame should be avoided, as the focus of an incident report is improvement of systematic issues. Data should be collected from the incident reports and analyzed for quality improvement purposes to determine if there are trends (Brodnik and Reynolds 2023, 312–313; Rinehart-Thompson 2023b, 65).

Because incident reports contain facts that may be of interest to potential plaintiffs, healthcare organizations strive to protect their confidentiality. Depending on the state, an incident report may or may not be protected by statute or regulation (Rinehart-Thompson 2023b, 65). An incident report could be protected per attorney-client privilege, but this protection might be superseded if the court determines the information is necessary to a plaintiff's case. The protection can be lost entirely if the court decides that the incident report falls outside the scope of privilege or if the defendant provider mentions the incident report in the patient's health record or disseminates copies of the report (Rinehart-Thompson 2023b, 65).

Although the facts regarding an incident and the resolution should be documented in the clinical record, the incident report itself is not part of the health record. It should never be placed in the record nor referred to in the record (Rinehart-Thompson 2023b, 65).

When dealing with incident reports or other events for which documentation has been generated, the health information manager and the risk manager should work together. The risk manager depends on the health information manager to alert him or her to a **potentially compensable event (PCE)**. PCEs could result in a settlement or judgment against the organization, paid either through insurance or directly from the organization's funds. Such events can be identified through coding and abstracting, and various health information review activities conducted by HIM department staff. The health information manager also can advise the risk manager when an attorney requests a copy of a health record. The risk manager can review records identified by any of these methods to determine whether further action is necessary from a risk management standpoint.

### Check Your Understanding 9.5

**Answer the following questions in a separate document.**

1. Compare the types of highly sensitive information discussed in this chapter and explain why each has been identified for specific legal protections.
2. Compare the two legal theories under which employers may be held liable for wrongful disclosure. Which one imposes a higher bar on the employer?
3. Distinguish the types of medical identity theft.
4. What characteristic about medical identity theft distinguishes it from other types of identity theft? Give an example that illustrates this.
5. Compare concurrent and retrospective quality review activities.
6. Differentiate how an incident report may be protected from discovery from how that protection may be lost.
7. Describe the scope of protection provided by the Genetic Information Non-Discrimination Act (GINA).

# References

Administrative Procedure Act. 5 USC 500–576. Law. Co-op. 1989.

Arizona Constitution, Article 2, Section 8. Right to privacy.

Brodnik, M. S. 2023a. "Introduction to the Fundamentals of Law." Chapter 1 in *Fundamentals of Law for Health Informatics and Information Management*. Edited by M. S. Brodnik, L. A. Rinehart-Thompson, and R. B. Reynolds. Chicago: AHIMA.

Brodnik, M. S. 2023b. "Access, Use, and Disclosure of Health Information." Chapter 11 in *Fundamentals of Law for Health Informatics and Information Management*. Edited by M. S. Brodnik, L. A. Rinehart-Thompson, and R. B. Reynolds. Chicago: AHIMA.

Brodnik, M. S. and R. B. Reynolds. 2023. "Risk Management, Quality Improvement, and Patient Safety and Rights." Chapter 13 in *Fundamentals of Law for Health Informatics and Information Management*. Edited by M. S. Brodnik, L. A. Rinehart-Thompson, and R. B. Reynolds. Chicago: AHIMA.

Brodnik, M. S. and L. A. Rinehart-Thompson. 2023. "Consent to Treatment." Chapter 6 in *Fundamentals of Law for Health Informatics and Information Management*. Edited by M. S. Brodnik, L. A. Rinehart-Thompson, and R. B. Reynolds. Chicago: AHIMA.

California Constitution, Article 1, Section 1.

California Evidence Code 1157, Division 9, Chapter 3. 2018.

*Darling v. Charleston Community Memorial Hospital*, 33 Ill.2d 326, 211 N.E. 2d, 253, 14 A.L.R. 3d 860 (1965).

Dixon, P. 2006. *Medical Identity Theft: the Information Crime That Can Kill You*. World Privacy Forum.

https://www.worldprivacyforum.org/2006/05/report-medical-identity-theft-the-information-crime-that-can-kill-you/.

EDRM (Electronic Discovery Reference Model). 2023. "Current EDRM Model." https://edrm.net/edrm-model/current/.

Emergency Medical Treatment and Labor Act (EMTALA). Social Security Act 1867, codified as 42 USC. 1395dd; 42 CFR 489 and others. (Term *active* removed from title in 1989.)

Federal Rules of Evidence (FRE) 803(6): Hearsay Exceptions: Availability of Declarant Immaterial. 2000.

Federal Rules of Evidence (FRE) 901: Requirement of Authentication or Identification. 1975.

Federal Rules of Evidence (FRE) 902: Evidence That Is Self-Authenticating. 2017.

Federal Trade Commission (FTC). 2021. "What to Know About Medical Identity Theft.". https://consumer.ftc.gov/articles/what-know-about-medical-identity-theft.

Florida Constitution, Article I, Section 23. Right of Privacy.

Health Information Technology for Economic and Clinical Health Act. 2009. Public Law 111-5.

Health Insurance Portability and Accountability Act of 1996. Public Law 104-191.

Indiana Code Title 34. 2021 (June 8). Civil Law and Procedure §34-43-1-1. https://codes.findlaw.com/in/title-34-civil-law-and-procedure/in-code-sect-34-43-1-1/.

Joint Commission. 2023. Record of care, treatment, and services. *Comprehensive Accreditation Manual for Hospitals*. Oakbrook Terrace, IL.

Legal Information Institute. 2020 (July). "Governmental Immunity." https://www.law.cornell.edu/wex/governmental_immunity.

McCluskey, M. 2022 (July 18). How your texts can be used as evidence. *Time*. https://time.com/6196754/text-messages-evidence-court-privacy/d.

Pozgar, G. D. 2021. *Legal and Ethical Essentials of Health Care Administration*, 3rd ed. Burlington, MA: Jones and Bartlett.

Reynolds, R.B. and M.S. Brodnik. 2023. "The HIPAA Security Rule and Security Threats." Chapter 10 in *Fundamentals of Law for Health Informatics and Information Management*. Edited by M. S. Brodnik, L. A. Rinehart-Thompson, and R. B. Reynolds. Chicago: AHIMA.

Rinehart-Thompson, L. A. 2024. *Introduction to Health Information Privacy and Security*. Chicago: AHIMA.

Rinehart-Thompson, L. A. 2023a. "The Legal System in the United States." Chapter 3 in *Fundamentals of Law for Health Informatics and Information Management*. Edited by M. S. Brodnik, L. A. Rinehart-Thompson, and R. B. Reynolds. Chicago: AHIMA.

Rinehart-Thompson, L. A. 2023b. "Legal Proceedings and Evidence." Chapter 4 in *Fundamentals of Law for Health Informatics and Information Management*. Edited by M. S. Brodnik, L. A. Rinehart-Thompson, and R. B. Reynolds. Chicago: AHIMA.

Rinehart-Thompson, L. A. 2023c. "Tort and Contract Law." Chapter 5 in *Fundamentals of Law for Health Informatics and Information Management*. Edited by M. S. Brodnik, L. A. Rinehart-Thompson, and R. B. Reynolds. Chicago: AHIMA.

Rinehart-Thompson, L. A. 2023d. "HIPAA Privacy Rule: Part I." Chapter 8 in *Fundamentals of Law for Health Informatics and Information Management*. Edited by M. S. Brodnik, L. A. Rinehart-Thompson, and R. B. Reynolds. Chicago: AHIMA.

Rinehart-Thompson, L. A. 2023e. "Requirements for Legally Defensible Health Records." Chapter 7 in *Fundamentals of Law for Health Informatics and Information Management*. Edited by M. S. Brodnik, L. A. Rinehart-Thompson, and R. B. Reynolds. Chicago: AHIMA.

Rinehart-Thompson, L. A. and L. B. Harman. 2017. "Privacy and Confidentiality." Chapter 3 in *Ethical Health Informatics*. Edited by L. B. Harman and F. H. Cornelius. Sudbury, MA: Jones and Bartlett.

Warren, S. and Brandeis, W. 1890. The right to privacy. *Harvard Law Review* 1890 (Dec. 15).

WPF (World Privacy Forum). 2022 (June 3). WPF urges HHS to clarify the harms of medical identity theft for victims. https://www.worldprivacyforum.org/2022/06/wpf-urges-hhs-to-clarify-the-harms-of-medical-identity-theft-for-victims/.

42 CFR 2.11 Part 2: Confidentiality of substance use disorder patient records. 2017.

42 CFR 482.24(b)(1): Conditions of participation: Medical record services. 2019.

45 CFR 160 and 164: General Administrative Requirements; Security and Privacy. 2013.

57A Am. Jur. 2d Negligence (2022).

57B Am. Jur. 2d Negligence (2022).

# Chapter 10

# Data Privacy, Confidentiality, and Security

*Danika Brinda, PhD, RHIA, CHPS, FAHIMA*
*Amy Watters, EdD, RHIA, FAHIMA*

## Learning Objectives

- Explain the privacy, security, and breach notification requirements of the Health Insurance Portability and Accountability Act (HIPAA) of 1996
- Compare privacy, confidentiality, and security safeguards related to protected health information (PHI)
- Apply the requirements of the Breach Notification Rule to an unauthorized use or disclosure of protection health information
- Demonstrate the appropriate uses and disclosures of protected health information in a given situation
- Explain when an authorization is or is not needed for disclosure and whether the patient has the right to object in a given situation
- Utilize the basic steps of risk analysis and risk management
- Determine best practices for privacy and security in health information exchange
- Apply security measures to safeguard information being accessed on mobile technology
- Apply the HIPAA workforce training requirement and strategies

## Key Terms

Accept the risk
Accounting of disclosures
Actors
Addressable standards
Administrative safeguards
Assessment
Audit
Audit log
Authorization
Biometric authentication
Breach
Breach notification
Breach Notification Rule
Bring your own device (BYOD)
Business associate (BA)
Business associate agreements (BAAs)
Cipher text
Compound authorization
Confidentiality
Contingency plan
Contrary
Covered entity (CE)
Criticality analysis
Cryptographic key
Data at rest
Data backup plan
Data in motion
Decryption
Deidentification
Designated record set
Disaster recovery plan
Disclosure
Emergency mode operation plan
Encryption
Expert determination method
HITECH-HIPAA Omnibus Privacy Act
Individually identifiable health information
Logic bombs
Malware

Minimum necessary
Mitigate the risk
Notice of privacy practices (NPP)
Organizational safeguards
Physical safeguards
Plaintext
Privacy
Privacy Rule
Protected health information (PHI)
Ransomware
Reasonable cause
Recognized security practices
Reidentification
Required standards
Residual risk
Risk analysis
Rootkit
Safe harbor method
Secure information
Security
Security Rule
Social engineering
Stringent
Technical safeguards
Transfer the risk
Trojan horse
Two-factor authentication
Use
User authentication
Virus
Willful neglect
Worms

Effective healthcare requires trusting relationships between patients and their healthcare providers. As the use of health information technology continues to grow, it will improve healthcare delivery and decision-making and reduce costs, but that can only happen if patients trust in the confidentiality and accuracy of their health information. If patients are concerned about the privacy, confidentiality, and security of their information, they may not disclose their health information to their healthcare provider, which can impact patient care or have life-threatening consequences (ONC 2015).

Protecting patient information is a core responsibility for health information management (HIM) professionals. By maintaining knowledge of rules and regulations, establishing and overseeing policies and procedures, and reporting any violations to the proper authorities, HIM professionals ensure patient privacy is maintained, confidential information is protected, and security measures are implemented to prevent unauthorized access to information (Brodnik and Rinehart-Thompson 2023h, 10).

The terms *privacy*, *confidentiality*, and *security* are often used interchangeably; however, there are important distinctions among them in the context of health information:

- **Privacy** generally refers to the freedom from unauthorized intrusion. In healthcare-related contexts it refers to the right of a patient to control disclosure of protected health information.
- **Confidentiality** establishes the healthcare provider's responsibility for protecting health records and other personal and private information from unauthorized use or disclosure. It means that data or information is not made available or disclosed to unauthorized persons or processes.
- **Security** is the means used to control access and protect information from accidental or intentional disclosure to unauthorized persons and from unauthorized alteration, destruction, or loss.

To maintain patient information privacy, confidentiality, and security, HIM professionals must know the applicable standards, rules, and regulations, both at the state and national levels.

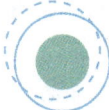

# The Health Insurance Portability and Accountability Act (HIPAA) of 1996

Over the years, the right to privacy and the establishment of requirements to maintain patient confidentiality have been addressed by various state and federal rulings and legislation. The Health Insurance Portability and Accountability Act (HIPAA) of 1996 was originally established to ensure health insurance continuity (also known as portability), set standards for electronic claims and national identifiers, and protect against fraud and abuse. It was subsequently expanded to establish national standards for the protection of privacy and the assurance of the security of health information, which was a significant moment for the healthcare industry. It has had a major impact on the collection and dissemination of information, and it will continue to have this impact long into the future as healthcare organizations ensure compliance with the rules in an increasingly complex electronic environment. This chapter focuses on three of the regulations that provide federal protections for patient health information and give patients rights with respect to that information—the Privacy Rule, the Security Rule, and the Breach Notification Rule, all of which are housed within Title II of HIPAA, known as the Administrative Simplification provisions (ONC 2015, 10–12).

HIPAA's Privacy and Security Rules are focused on ensuring the privacy and security of **protected health information (PHI)** (referred to as ePHI when it is in electronic form), which is individually identifiable health information held or transmitted by a covered entity or business associate (HHS 2013, 16). **Individually identifiable health information** is information that identifies the individual or there is reasonable belief that it can be used to identify the individual, and relates to

- the individual's past, present, or future physical or mental health or condition;
- the provision of healthcare to the individual; or
- the past, present, or future payment for the provision of healthcare to the individual (ONC 2015, 11).

Any documentation that includes a patient's name or any other identifying information would be considered PHI, such as a radiology report, lab results, a hospital bill, or an email communication to a healthcare provider.

Part of the impetus for HIPAA was the development of the electronic health record (EHR). As patient information has moved to the electronic medium, integrated systems across the continuum of care have been developed; thus, standardized federal legislation became imperative as patient information was used and disclosed to many people and organizations needing access to it. HIPAA was designed to guarantee that information transferred and exchanged in this way would be protected. In an electronic environment, protecting privacy is extremely difficult and patients are concerned about the privacy and security of their information. The US healthcare industry has seen an unprecedented increase in cyberattacks as data is moved to an electronic format. Even as one of the most regulated industries within the US, healthcare has seen an increase in the number of data breaches compared to other US industries (HHS 405(d) 2023a). The cost of healthcare data breaches is almost double the amount of any other industry in the US (IBM 2023).

HIPAA applies to specific organizations referred to as covered entities and business associates. A **covered entity (CE)** is defined as a "health plan, healthcare clearinghouse, or healthcare provider that transmits information in electronic form in connection with a transaction" (HHS 2022a). A **business associate (BA)** is a "person or organization, other than a member of a covered entity's workforce, that performs certain functions or activities on behalf of, or provides certain services to, a covered entity that involve the use or disclosure of individually identifiable health information" (HHS 2022a). Whether patient health information is electronic, on paper, or in any other medium, providers are responsible for safeguarding the information by meeting the requirements of the HIPAA Rules (ONC 2015, 11). HIPAA provides only the minimum requirements regarding privacy and security. States are free to adopt more stringent regulations, making it essential that HIM professionals have knowledge of both federal and state requirements to maintain compliance.

## The Privacy Rule

The Standards for Privacy of Individually Identifiable Health Information, commonly known as the **Privacy Rule** (45 CFR Part 160 and Subparts A and E of Part 164), was established to assure the protection of health information. Specifically, the goal of the Privacy Rule is to "address the use and disclosure of PHI as well as standards for individuals' privacy rights to understand and control how their health information is used and shared, including rights to examine and obtain a copy of their health records as well as to request corrections" (ONC 2015, 13). The Privacy Rule was established with three major purposes:

1. To protect and enhance the rights of healthcare consumers by providing them access to their health information and ensure the appropriate use of that information;
2. To improve the quality of healthcare in the United States by restoring trust in the healthcare system; and
3. To improve the efficiency and effectiveness of healthcare delivery by creating a national framework for privacy protection that builds on the efforts of states, health systems and organizations, and individuals (HHS 2013, 74).

The Privacy Rule can be broken into eight primary sections:

1. Uses and disclosures of PHI: General rules (45 CFR 164.502 through 164.512): Identifies how and for what purposes PHI can be used and disclosed and identifies requirements for authorizations. It also establishes the **minimum necessary** standard that requires that a CE or BA make "reasonable efforts to limit protected health information to the minimum necessary to accomplish the intended purpose of the use, disclosure, or request" (HHS 2013, 78). This standard is meant to limit unnecessary or inappropriate access to and disclosure of PHI so that it is only used or disclosed to carry out necessary functions for

treatment, payment, and healthcare operations (TPO). EHR access can also support the concept of minimum necessary by limiting access to ePHI based on responsibilities of the job function or classes of workforce such as nurse, therapist, HIM staff, and others. This is referred to as role-based access (HHS 2013, 78).

2. Uses and disclosures: Organizational requirements (45 CFR 164.504): Establishes requirements for BAs and **business associate agreements (BAAs)**, which are contracts between a CE and a BA that establish the permitted and required uses and disclosures of PHI by the BA (45 CFR 164.504). Examples of scenarios that require a BAA include an attorney providing legal services that require access to PHI, an independent consultant providing services to a facility, or a third party that processes claims for an organization.

3. Notice of privacy practices for protected health information (45 CFR 164.520): Requires the establishment and dissemination of a **notice of privacy practices (NPP)**, which healthcare providers and health plans must give to patients to inform them of how they may use and share the patient's health information and how patients can exercise their health privacy rights (see appendix B) (HHS n.d.a).

4. Rights to request privacy protection for protected health information (45 CFR 164.522): Establishes patients' rights to request alternative means of communication and restrictions for the use and disclosure of their PHI.

5. Access of individuals to protected health information (45 CFR 164.524): Establishes patients' rights to access their health information by allowing them to inspect and obtain a copy of their PHI in a designated record set, which is the group of records maintained by or for a CE (HHS 2013, 105).

6. Amendment of protected health information (45 CFR 164.526): Establishes patients' rights to request that a CE make an amendment to the PHI in the designated record set.

7. Accounting of disclosures of protected health information (45 CFR 164.528): Establishes a patient's right to receive an accounting of disclosures of their PHI made by a CE.

8. Administrative requirements (45 CFR 164.530): Requirements for CEs related to the designation of a privacy official, training of the workforce, the implementation of privacy safeguards, the process for individuals to make complaints, and the establishment of anti-retaliatory standards to ensure there is no intimidation or retaliation for filing a complaint.

As indicated in the Privacy Rule's Administrative Requirements (45 CFR 164.530), organizations "must implement policies and procedures" to address each standard as well as implement a process to ensure those policies and procedures are being followed (HHS 2013, 112–113).

## The Security Rule

The purpose of the Security Standards for the Protection of Electronic Protected Health Information, or the **Security Rule** (45 CFR Part 160 and Subparts A and C of Part 164), is to operationalize the protections identified in the Privacy Rule by addressing the technical and nontechnical safeguards that CEs must put in place to secure individuals' ePHI (HHS 2013, 62). The Security Rule specifies "a series of administrative, technical, and physical security procedures for CEs to use to assure the confidentiality, integrity, and availability of e-PHI" (HHS 2013). It identifies four types of safeguards that organizations must have in place:

- **Administrative safeguards**, such as policies and procedures, to manage administrative actions, policies, and procedures to prevent, detect, contain, and correct security violations
- **Physical safeguards**, such as surveillance cameras and identification badges, to identify measures to protect information systems (ISs), buildings, and equipment from natural and environmental hazards
- **Technical safeguards**, such as automatic log-off and unique user identification, to protect access and control of ePHI
- **Organizational safeguards**, such as BAAs, so that arrangements are made to protect ePHI between organizations as well as the requirement to have written policies and procedures to comply with the HIPAA Security Rule, make sure they are updated on a regular basis and that they are provided to staff (ONC 2015, 27)

All of these safeguards are intended to protect the privacy of health information as CEs continue to adopt new and evolving technologies to improve patient care.

The Security Rule contains two different types of standards—required and addressable. **Required standards** are standards that are mandated, and the organization must implement them as written by the HIPAA Security Rule. **Addressable standards** provide flexibility to the CE and BAs by allowing the organization to implement the standard based on the following:

- The size and complexity of the CE or BA
- The organization's technical infrastructure, hardware, and software security capabilities

- The costs of security measures
- The probability and criticality of potential risks to ePHI (HHS 2022b)

If an organization decides to not implement an addressable standard as written in the regulation, the reason for implementing the standard in a different manner must be documented, including what other safeguards the organization has implemented to protect ePHI (HHS 2022b).

## The HITECH-HIPAA Omnibus Privacy Act

Although organizations were required to comply with the Privacy Rule and Security Rule in 2003 and 2005, respectively, they were impacted in 2009, when the Health Information Technology for Economic and Clinical Health (HITECH) Act was enacted to promote the adoption and meaningful use of health information technology as part of the American Recovery and Reinvestment Act (ARRA). The HITECH Act established more detailed provisions and strengthened the requirements included in the HIPAA Privacy and Security Rules by establishing the following:

- Mandatory reporting requirements and penalties in the event of a breach
- New enforcement responsibilities
- New privacy requirements such as new accounting requirements for the EHR
- Extended requirements to the BAs of CEs (HHS 2013, 59–108)

In response, the US Department of Health and Human Services (HHS) Office for Civil Rights (OCR) published the final omnibus rules in 2013 to address many of the HITECH requirements. The rule is officially titled "Modifications to the HIPAA Privacy, Security, Enforcement, and Breach Notification Rule Under the Health Information Technology for Economic and Clinical Health Act, and the Genetic Information Nondiscrimination Act; Other Modifications to the HIPAA Rule," but is often referred to as the HITECH-HIPAA Omnibus Privacy Act, or the Omnibus Rule.

The Omnibus Rule includes some of the most significant changes to patient privacy since HIPAA was first enacted in 2003. It went into effect on March 26, 2013, and CEs were to ensure compliance by September 23, 2013 (HHS 2013, 17). The Omnibus Rule strengthens the privacy and security of patient health information, modifies the Breach Notification Rule, strengthens privacy protections for genetic information by prohibiting health plans from using or disclosing such information for underwriting, makes BAs of HIPAA-covered entities liable for compliance, strengthens limitations on the use and disclosure of PHI for marketing, research and fundraising, and allows patients increased restriction rights (HHS 2013, 20–21, 75, 85, 78, 85–94, 99–100, 102).

The OCR indicates that more provisions will be established in the future. The Omnibus Rule does not address all HITECH privacy requirements, such as the requirement for accounting of disclosures and access to EHR audit logs.

In January 2021, the HITECH Act was modified to include the use of recognized security practices to help healthcare entities implement strong cybersecurity practices by adopting industry best practices. Recognized security practices are defined as "the standards, guidelines, best practices, methodologies, procedures, and processes developed by the National Institute of Standards and Technology Act, the approaches promulgated under section 405(d) of the Cybersecurity Act of 2015, and other programs and processes that address cybersecurity and that are developed, recognized, or promulgated through regulations under other statutory authorities" (42 USC 17941). The Office of Civil Rights (OCR) is encouraged to consider the implementation and use of recognized security best practices when evaluating compliance with the HIPAA Security Rule through enforcement and audit activities (HHS 2023a).

### The Breach Notification Rule

One of the largest regulation provisions to privacy and security under the HITECH Act were the new requirements related to breach notification, which entails notifying patients if their PHI has been breached (Brodnik and Rinehart-Thompson, 2023 206–207). Unauthorized uses and disclosures of any PHI at any time may be considered a data breach under the updated regulations. The breach notification regulation created a new process for CEs and BAs to investigate and evaluate if a breach occurred from an unauthorized use or disclosure of PHI. The regulation also created a short timeline for investigation, conclusion, and notification of the potential breach (Brodnik and Rinehart-Thompson 2023, 206–207; HHS 2013, 71).

The final HITECH-HIPAA Omnibus Act of 2013 defined a breach as follows:

> An acquisition, access, use, or disclosure of protected health information in a manner not permitted under subpart E is presumed to be a breach unless the covered entity or business associate, as applicable, demonstrates that there is a low probability that the protected health information has been compromised based on a risk assessment. (HHS 2013, 71)

A risk assessment should be conducted to determine if a breach has occurred. The risk assessment should address the following factors at minimum:

1. The nature and extent of the protected health information involved [in the data breach], including the types of identifiers and likelihood of the reidentification;
2. The unauthorized person who used the protected health information or to whom the disclosure was made;
3. Whether the protected health information was actually acquired or viewed [or redisclosed]; and
4. The extent to which the risk to the protected health information has been mitigated (HHS 2023f, 71)

The **Breach Notification Rule** requires CEs and BAs to establish policies and procedures to investigate an unauthorized use or disclosure of unsecured PHI to determine if a breach occurred, conclude the investigation, and to notify affected individuals within 60 days of date of discovery of the breach. Unsecured PHI has not used technology or other destruction methods to render the PHI unusable, unreadable, or impossible to decipher by the individual obtaining the information (Brodnik and Rinehart-Thompson, 2023, 206–206). If the data breach affects 500 or more individuals, the CE or BA must notify the secretary of the HHS within 60 days of date of discovery of the breach. If the data breach impacts fewer than 500 individuals, the CE or BA must annually notify the secretary of the HHS; however, the notification must occur no later than 60 days after the end of the calendar year in which the data breach occurred (45 CFR 164.408). Based on the findings of an investigation into a potential breach, an organization determines whether or not the incident falls into the breach notification process and then take the proper steps to notify those affected. If the number of individuals affected by the breach exceeds 500, a healthcare organization must notify and report the incident to the local media as well as the individuals impacted by the breach and the secretary of the HHS (Brodnik and Rinehart-Thompson, 2023, 206–207; HHS 2023e). The Omnibus Rule defines three exceptions to the Breach Notification Rule requirement.

- The PHI disclosure was not intentional and the individual or individuals that received the information have the requirement to keep the information confidential.
- The access to the PHI was unintentional by a workforce member and the person or persons receiving the information has a right to keep the information confidential.
- The healthcare organization believes in good faith that the protected health information could not have been retained by the person receiving it (HHS 2013, 71).

If the investigation finds any of these to be true, it can be concluded that a data breach did not occur, and the notification requirements of the Breach Notification Rule would not be necessary.

## HIPAA Enforcement under the Omnibus Rule

Included in the HIPAA regulation is the Enforcement Rule, which contains provisions relating to compliance, investigations, penalties for violations, and procedures for hearings (HHS 2023c). Any person or organization who believes a CE or BA is violating the HIPAA Privacy or Security Regulations may file a complaint with the secretary of HHS. The OCR is the enforcement body of HIPAA and is responsible for reviewing all complaints and conducting investigations as necessary. OCR will attempt to resolve the HIPAA noncompliance issue or complaint by obtaining information about the CE or BA through the collection of information and evidence of the issue. The OCR may also open an investigation based on any data breaches reported by the CE or BA. Based on the findings of the investigation conducted by the OCR, the CE or BA may be subject to a corrective action plan (CAP) that may include a civil monetary penalty (CMP) (HHS 2023c).

The Omnibus Rule created a new fine structure for CMP based on a four-tier system for HIPAA violations that occurred after February 18, 2009 (see table 10.1). Tier 1 is the lowest tier and is used for minor violations that have given a CMP. Tier 2 is based on reasonable cause, which was further defined within the HIPAA Omnibus Rule. **Reasonable cause** is "an act or omission in which a covered entity or business associate knew, or by exercising reasonable diligence would have known, that the act or omission violated an administrative simplification provision, but in which the covered entity or business associate did not act with willful neglect" (45 CFR 160.401).

Tier 3 and Tier 4 are based on violations that have been determined to be due to willful neglect. **Willful neglect** is defined as "conscious, intentional failure or reckless indifference to the obligation to comply with the administrative simplification provision violated" (HHS 2013, 23). The difference between falling into a Tier 3 or Tier 4 CMP is when the violation was corrected after the CE of BA became aware of the violation. If the data breach caused by willful neglect is corrected within 30 days from the date of the CE or BA becoming aware of it, it would fall into Tier 3. If the data breach is not corrected within 30 days of discovery and is due to willful neglect, it would fall into Tier 4 (HHS 2023b).

The Omnibus Rule also defined the factors that will be considered for applying a CMP when

**Table 10.1.** Categories of violations and respective penalty amounts effective October 6, 2023

| Violation category—45 CFR 160.404 | Minimum | Maximum | Calendar Year Cap |
|---|---|---|---|
| Tier 1 (A) Did not know | $137 | $68,928 | $2,067,813 |
| Tier 2 (B) Reasonable cause | $1,379 | $68,928 | $2,067,813 |
| Tier 3 (C)(i) Willful neglect–corrected | $13,785 | $68,928 | $2,067,813 |
| Tier 4 (C)(ii) Willful neglect–not corrected | $68,928 | $2,067,813 | $2,067,813 |

*Source:* HHS 2023b.

evaluating a violation of the HIPAA Privacy and Security Regulations. The CMP will be based on the following:

- Nature and extent of the violation (number of individuals affected and time period during which the violation occurred)
- Nature and extent of the harm resulting from the violation (physical harm, financial harm, or reputational harm)
- Covered entity or business associates' prior compliance with the HIPAA regulations (previous violations, previous CAP, response to correct the violation)
- Financial condition of the covered entity or business associate (financial difficulties affecting ability to comply, imposition of CMP would jeopardize the ability to continue business, size of the organization)
- Other such matters as justice may require (HHS 2013, 25)

The OCR will evaluate each violation separately and determine the best CAP, which may include a CMP or just changes in policies, procedures, and practices within the organization. Since 2008, the OCR has initiated 137 CMPs for noncompliance with HIPAA resulting in $136,918,772 in fines (HHS 2023d).

The HITECH revisions of the enforcement law also include the expanded enforcement of HIPAA regulations. ARRA provided state attorneys general with the authority to be enforce HIPAA noncompliance on behalf of state residents. The intent of the expansion of the authority of the state attorneys general was to allow them to "obtain damages on behalf of state residents or to enjoin further violations of the HIPAA Privacy and Security Rules" (HHS 2017b).

The final Omnibus Rule also amended a few other important elements within the HIPAA enforcement regulations. If the OCR determined the CE or BA was not aware of the violation and had been following smart business practices for compliance with the HIPAA regulations, the secretary of HHS may apply a waiver to the penalty (HHS 2013, 26). The new regulations under enforcement were created to make the process more streamlined and transparent for consumers, CEs, BAs, and HHS.

## Proposed Rule Impacting HIPAA and Privacy and Security

The federal government continues to enhance the HIPAA Privacy and Security Regulations to support the changing healthcare industry as well as enhance patient rights and protect the advancement of electronic information. In January 2021, OCR published a Notice of Proposed Rulemaking (NPRM), a notice published in the *Federal Register* intended to receive comments and feedback from the public and industry to help modify and create the final rule making efforts (Rinehart-Thompson 2024, 4). The NPRM modified HIPAA's Privacy Rule in order to expand the individuals' involvement in their healthcare with supporting access to information, remove barriers in the coordination of a patient's care, and reduce regulatory burdens to the healthcare industry while maintaining a focus of the protection of patient's health information in all formats. Specifically, the NPRM focuses on the following:

- Strengthen individuals' rights to access their own health information, including electronic information.
- Improve information sharing for care coordination and case management for individuals.
- Facilitate family and caregiver involvement in the care of individuals experiencing emergencies or health crises.
- Enhance flexibilities for disclosures in emergency or threatening circumstances, such as the Opioid and COVID-19 public health emergencies.
- Reduce administrative burdens on HIPAA covered health care providers and health plans. (HHS 2023g)

The final rule was expected in spring 2023; however, no final rule was published at that time. There is no action on the NPRM until the final rule is published (HHS 2023g).

### Check Your Understanding 10.1

**Answer the following questions in a separate document.**

1. Compare the main sections of the HIPAA Security Rule and give at least three examples of each safeguard.
2. What was the purpose of establishing HIPAA?
3. Analyze the difference between privacy, confidentiality, and security.
4. What is the purpose of a Notice of Proposed Rule Making?
   a. To justify the regulation changes
   b. To provide a heads up to the industry about the regulatory changes
   c. To provide evidence of current regulatory activity
   d. To receive comments and feedback from the public and industry
5. The Breach Notification Rule requires covered entities to do which of the following?
   a. Establish a process for investigating whether a breach occurred
   b. Notify affected individuals when a breach occurs
   c. Establish a policy on minimum necessary
   d. Both a and b

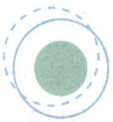

## Privacy and Security Requirements for Disclosure Management

Use and disclosure of patient information is a necessity for day-to-day operations within a healthcare organization. HIPAA distinctly defines the difference between the use and disclosure of PHI. **Use** is defined as "the sharing, employment, application, utilization, examination, or analysis within a covered entity that creates and maintains the PHI" (45 CFR 160.103). **Disclosure** is "the release, transfer, provision of access to, or divulging in any manner of information outside the entity holding the information" (45 CFR 160.103). HIPAA provides specific requirements regarding when PHI can be used or disclosed with and without a signed authorization form by the patient. An **authorization** is "a document that gives covered entities permission to use PHI for specified purposes or to disclose PHI to a third party specified by the individual" (45 CFR 160.103). All CEs and BAs should ensure they have established policies and procedures to manage and govern the use and disclosures of PHI.

One of the foundational elements to the use and disclosure of PHI is the definition of the organization's designated record set. The HIPAA Privacy Rule (45 CFR 164.501) defines a **designated record set** as

> a group of records maintained by or for a covered entity that may include patient medical and billing records; the enrollment, payment, claims, adjudication, and cases or medical management record systems maintained by or for a health plan; or information used in whole or in part to make care-related decisions. (45 CFR 164.501)

The designated record set is used to support a variety of patients' rights under the HIPAA Privacy Rule such as patients' access to PHI, electronic copy of PHI, and amendment of a record (HHS 2013). The privacy and security requirements mandate healthcare facilities to establish procedures to address the use and disclosure of PHI with and without patient authorization, patient identity management, and confidentiality of alcohol and drug abuse patient records.

### Use and Disclosure of Patient Information with Patient Authorization

A valid authorization for use and disclosure of PHI is needed prior to releasing the information unless it is permitted without an authorization under the HIPAA privacy regulation (45 CFR 164.508(a)(1)). A valid authorization of disclosure of health information must be reviewed and evaluated for each specific request received at a CE. The HIPAA Privacy Rule requires a valid authorization be completed for disclosure of information for the following:

- Disclosure of PHI not permitted to be released without an authorization (45 CFR 164.508(a)(1))
- Psychotherapy notes (45 CFR 164.508(a)(2))
- Marketing (45 CFR 164.508(a)(3))
- Sale of protected health information (45 CFR 164.508(a)(4))

Table 10.2 defines the core elements and statements that must be included on an authorization for uses and disclosures of PHI.

Additionally, the authorization must be written in plain language and the CE must provide a copy of the authorization for disclosure to the individual (45 CFR 164.508(3); 45 CFR 164.508(4)). All these elements must be present in order for the disclosure of PHI to be valid. A CE has 30 days to respond and disclose the information from the date the authorization was received (45 CFR 164.524(b)). Prior to the release of any information, all authorizations should be evaluated by the healthcare organization to ensure all required pieces of information are present and appropriate.

An authorization is considered defective under the HIPAA Privacy Rule if any of the following scenarios are true:

- The expiration date has passed, or the expiration event has occurred
- The authorization is not completely filled out
- The authorization has been revoked
- Any required elements defined here are missing
- The authorization is combined with any other documentation to create a compound authorization, except where permitted
- The facility knows the material information included in the authorization is false (HHS 2013, 85)

If an authorization is considered defective, the requestor of the information should be notified in writing, indicating why the authorization is defective and the process for correcting and resubmitting the authorization for disclosure.

Although patient authorization is required for research, the HIPAA Omnibus Rule changed the regulations to strike a better balance between maintaining patient privacy and allowing access to enough information for effective research to occur. The change to the regulation allows for authorization of future research studies with an appropriate and adequate description of how the PHI will be used in the future research through compound authorizations. A **compound authorization** combines the use and disclosure of PHI with other legal permissions such as consent for treatment, which is prohibited by the current HIPAA Privacy Rule. However, this provision was amended by the Omnibus Rule, which permits combining an authorization for the use and disclosure of PHI for a research study with authorization for other permissions for the same study, including informed consent to participate in the study. The Omnibus Rule allows authorization for both conditioned and unconditioned research on one form. This means authorization for multiple research studies may exist on the same form if the authorization form clearly differentiates between the studies and allows the individual to opt in to the unconditioned research activities. A conditioned authorization is used for an individual to consent into the main research study, whereas an unconditioned authorization is used for the individual to consent into additional research studies if the patient elects to be involved. For example, a patient may authorize participation in part

Table 10.2. Authorizations for uses and disclosures: required elements and statements

| Core Elements (45 CFR 164.508(c)(1)): A valid authorization must contain at least the following elements: | Required Statements (45 CFR 164.508(c)(2)): In addition to the core elements, a valid authorization must contain statements notifying individuals of: |
|---|---|
| • A description of the information to be used or disclosed that identifies the information in a specific and meaningful way. | • The individual's right to revoke the authorization in writing, and either: |
| • The name or other specific identification of the person(s), or class of persons, authorized to make the requested use or disclosure. | ○ The exceptions to the right to revoke and a description of how the individual may revoke the authorization; or |
| • The name or other specific identification of the person(s), or class of persons, to whom the covered entity may make the requested use or disclosure. | ○ The extent to which the information is included in the notice of privacy practices |
| • A description of each purpose of the requested use or disclosure | • The ability or inability for the authorization to place conditions on the treatment, payment, enrollment or eligibility for benefits. |
| • An expiration date or an expiration event that relates to the individual or the purpose of the use or disclosure. | • The potential for information disclosed pursuant to the authorization to be subject to redisclosure by the recipient and no longer be protected by this subpart. |
| • Signature of the individual and date. | |

*Source:* HHS 2013.

of a breast cancer research study as the main research study and may elect to be in an additional study on tissue, based on the specific diagnosis of breast cancer. The conditioned authorization would be the consent to participate in the main breast cancer study and the unconditioned authorization would be the tissue research study. In addition, the authorization must give participants an opt-in option; combined authorizations that only allow the individual to opt-out of the unconditioned research are not permitted. This provision applies to all types of research studies except for authorization to use and disclose psychotherapy notes which may not be combined with any other authorization (45 CFR 164.508(b)(3)).

For compliance with the rules around use and disclosure, a CE should have clear policies and procedures that define the requirements for disclosures, when an authorization is needed, when an authorization is valid, signatures and personal representatives, and administrative information such as requiring authorizations be maintained for a minimum of six years (45 CFR 164.530(j)).

## Use and Disclosure of Patient Information without Patient Authorization

The HIPAA Privacy Rule allows CEs to use and disclose PHI for the purpose of TPO (45 CFR 164.506(a)). CEs should clearly define what uses and disclosures of PHI fall into these categories to ensure proper adherence to the regulations. The following are examples of uses and disclosures of PHI where an authorization is not needed:

- Uses and disclosures to BAs
- Uses and disclosures required by law
- Uses and disclosures for public health reporting, and other public health activities
- Disclosures about victims of abuse, neglect, or domestic violence
- Uses and disclosures for health oversight activities such as audits, investigations, and inspections
- Disclosures for judicial and administrative proceedings
- Disclosures for law enforcement purposes
- Uses and disclosures to coroners, medical examiners, and funeral directors
- Uses and disclosures for organ, eye, or tissue donation
- Uses and disclosures for research purposes
- Uses and disclosures to avert a serious threat to health or safety
- Uses and disclosures for specified government functions including military and veterans' activities, national security and intelligence activities, protective services for the president and others, medical suitability determinations, and correctional institutions
- Disclosures for workers' compensation (HHS 2013, 88–96)

Any request for information that falls into these categories should be individually evaluated to verify it meets the criteria of one of the given categories. In addition to having clear guidelines and procedures for releasing information without authorization, healthcare organizations and BAs must ensure they have a process to account for these types of disclosures. Under the HIPAA Privacy Rule, a patient has a right to receive an **accounting of disclosures** for the past six years at any time, which is information that describes a CE's disclosures of PHI other than for TPO; disclosures made with authorization; and certain other limited disclosures (45 CFR 164.528). The accounting must include all disclosures made by the CE or BA, except if the account falls into one of these categories:

- To carry out treatment, payment, and healthcare operations
- To individuals receiving their own protected health information
- Incident to a use or disclosure otherwise permitted or required by the use and disclosure requirements
- Pursuant to an authorization
- For the facility's directory or to persons involved in the individual's care or other notification purposes
- For national security or intelligence purposes
- To correctional institutions or law enforcement officials
- As part of a limited data set
- That occurred prior to the compliance date for the covered entity (45 CFR 164.528(a)(1))

If a patient requests an accounting of disclosures, the CE must respond within 60 days. The accounting report must include (1) date of disclosures, (2) name or entity that received the PHI, (3) a brief description of the PHI, and (4) a brief statement of the purpose of the disclosure (45 CFR 164.528(b)(2)). If during the request time of the accounting, a disclosure was made multiple times to the same recipient for the same purpose, rather than listing each individual disclosure, a CE may list the disclosure one time on the report with the addition of the frequency of the disclosures, number of disclosures, and the date of the last disclosure (45 CFR 164.528(b)(3)). A major change from the HIPAA Privacy Rule of 2003 to the final Omnibus Rule of 2013, was that any accounting of disclosures made by a BA must also be included in the report for accounting of disclosures provided by the CE (HHS 2013, 110–111).

Many of the disclosures being made within healthcare organizations are made from EHRs, which have the capability to track and create a disclosure management log. Even with the use of an EHR, healthcare organizations may still manage and use paper medical records. Policies and procedures should be established to document the process for disclosures of the paper medical records and electronic tracking of the disclosures to meet the expectations of the accounting of disclosures regulation.

PHI can be used and disclosed without permission of the patient if the PHI is deidentified. Under HIPAA, deidentification refers to health information that has had identifiers removed removing the capability to reasonably identify the individual to which the information belongs (45 CFR 164.514(a)). HIPAA regulations define two methods in which information can be deidentified to meet the standard. The first method is using the expert determination method. In this method, data elements that could identify an individual are removed from the data and then an expert the organization hires, such as a statistician, applies scientific methodology to determine the likelihood of identification of the individual and provides documentation of the probability that the information would be identified. If there is low probability that the information can be identified, the information is considered deidentified (HHS 2013, 96). If there is a high probability that the information could be identified, further evaluation of removal of data elements should occur.

The second method of deidentification is the safe harbor method. The safe harbor method requires the CE or BA to remove 18 data elements from the health information. The data elements are defined as the following:

- Names
- All geographic subdivisions smaller than the state (street address, city, county, precinct, zip code, and any other equivalent geocodes, which are geographically referenced data points that have a known position such as a mile marker or a street) (HHS 2024d)
- All elements of dates excluding year (birth date, admission date, discharge date, death date); if over 89 years of age, all elements of dates including year
- Telephone number(s)
- Fax number(s)
- Email address(es)
- Social Security number
- Medical record number
- Health plan beneficiary numbers (insurance information)
- Account numbers
- Certificate and license numbers
- Vehicle identification numbers and series numbers (for example, license plate numbers)
- Device numbers or identifiers
- Web universal resource locator (URL)
- Internet protocol (IP) address
- Biometric identifiers (fingerprints, voice recognition, palm reading)
- Full face photographs
- Any other unique identifiable number, characteristic, or codes (HHS 2013, 97)

All these data elements must be removed from all the health information being deidentified. Challenges arise with this method to ensure all data elements are removed from the entire record. If the organization deidentifying the information wants to reidentify the information for some reason, they are allowed to create a reidentification method. For reidentification, an organization can apply a specific code, or other means, to the data for future reidentification purposes; however, the specific code cannot be derived from any type of data elements that come from the patient's health information. The information regarding reidentification must be kept separate from the deidentified data and should have proper safeguards such as limited access and secure storage to prevent unauthorized reidentification (HHS 2013, 97).

## Use and Disclosure Requiring an Opportunity to Object

A CE has the right to use and disclose PHI for healthcare operations, which can include utilization review, quality improvement, and accreditation activities. However, the Privacy Rule allows the patient to agree or object to disclosure of PHI within the facility directory. For this specific requirement for use and disclosure of PHI, a written authorization is not required, as oral acceptance or objection is acceptable (45 CFR 164.510). A CE must inform a patient that PHI may be included in the directory, and they may disclose the directory PHI to individuals such as clergy. The patient may orally agree to the PHI in the directory or object to the information in the directory. If the patient allows the information to be within the directory, the only PHI that may be allowed and disclosed in the directory is (1) patient name, (2) the individual's location in the covered healthcare provider's facility, (3) individual's condition described in general terms that does not communicate specific medical information about the individual, and (4) religious affiliation (45 CFR 164.510(a)). The general terms that are allowed to be released are undetermined, good, fair, serious, critical, treated and released, or treated and transferred. If a patient has passed away, the healthcare facility would only be able to provide that information to the media if the patient has officially been pronounced dead and the family has been notified (California Hospital Association 2017, 4–5). The disclosure of this information can only be for the purpose of releasing the information to clergy or to an individual who asks for the person by name. A clear process should be established to ensure all patients are given the right to object to PHI being entered in the directory (45 CFR 164.510).

In some cases, the patient is unable to object to the directory information due to being incapacitated or another emergency. In these scenarios, the CE may disclose the information if it is consistent with the patient's previously expressed preferences, or it is in the best interest of the patient based on professional judgment (45 CFR 164.510(a)(3)). A CE should ensure a process regarding the use and disclosure of patient directory information is addressed in their policy and procedure documents.

## Use and Disclosure for Reproductive Health Care

Another big change in the HIPAA regulations was published in April 2024, in response to the Supreme Court's decision in *Dobbs v. Jackson Women's Health Organization* (HHS 2024c). The intent in the proposed rule is to enhance protections to sensitive information regarding women's reproductive healthcare and increase the patient and provider confidentiality. The new privacy regulation strengthens the use and disclosure of protected health information regarding reproductive healthcare in the areas of criminal, civil, or administrative investigations or investigation into liability that an individual may have for seeking reproductive care (HHS 2024c). When a healthcare organization is using or disclosing PHI regarding reproductive care for purposes of health oversight activities, judicial and administrative proceedings, law enforcement request, or disclosures to coroners and medical examiners, the organization must get a signed attestation form identifying that the use or disclosure is not for any prohibited purposes (HHS 2024c). A sample attestation form is located in appendix B. Additionally, a CE or BA must include the information regarding the use and disclosure of reproductive healthcare privacy within the Notice of Privacy Practices (HHS 2024c).

## Patient Identity Management for Use and Disclosure of PHI

When managing the use and disclosure of PHI within a CE or BA, ensuring the correct patient's information is being used or disclosed is vital to preventing data breaches and unauthorized use and disclosure of PHI. Policies and procedures created by the CE or BA to manage the use and disclosures of PHI should address the process for patient identification, including verification of the individual or personal representatives. A clearly defined data dictionary establishes the basic input of patient demographic information to create consistency for input and creation of patients. Basic demographic identifiers include patient name, medical record number, gender, date of birth, social security number, address, city, state, zip code, and telephone number (HealthIT.gov n.d.e). With consistent data input and data collection, the identification of a patient can be made easier to ensure the right patient is being treated and the right information is being used or disclosed.

When verifying the identity of a patient, the Joint Commission recommends verification of a minimum of two different data elements (Joint Commission 2024, 1). However, HIPAA does not mandate a specific form of verification. "The Privacy Rule requires a covered entity to take reasonable steps to verify the identity of an individual making a request for access" (45 CFR 164.514(h)). Generally, using multiple elements such as name, date of birth, and the last four digits of a social security number, is common practice. While this process can be seen as challenging and cumbersome, the process for investigating an unauthorized use or disclosure of PHI or correcting a patient record in which there is incorrect documentation is even more challenging and causes patient safety issues and concerns. Taking the time to verify a patient's identity up front can prevent rework, reduce the likelihood of a data breach, and diminish patient safety issues.

Under the HIPAA Privacy Rule, verification of requestor identity must be completed prior to disclosing any patient information in any format. Verification may come in a variety of different formats, varying by requestor, as shown in table 10.3.

Clearly defined processes for the purpose of patient verification and request verification should be addressed within written policies and procedures for disclosure management within an organization.

**Table 10.3.** Techniques to verify PHI requestors

| Requestor of PHI | Suggested verification documentation |
|---|---|
| Patient | Personal identification: driver's license, passport, state-issued identification |
| Power of attorney | Power of attorney documentation and personal identification |
| Court-appointed guardians | Court paperwork for appointment of guardianship and personal identification |
| Attorney | Request on letterhead, business card, and personal identification |
| Executor of the estate | Legal documentation showing appointment of executor of the estate, personal identification |
| Spouse | Marriage license and personal identification |
| Parent of a minor patient | Personal identification: driver's license, passport, state-issued identification, and verification of address |

*Source:* Adapted from 45 CFR 164.514(h)(1) and 45 CFR 164.514(h)(2).

## Confidentiality of Alcohol and Drug Abuse Patient Records

Alcohol and drug abuse patients' health records must follow the expectations of the HIPAA Privacy Rule and adhere to added safeguards due to the sensitive nature of the patients' care. The Confidentiality of Substance Use Disorder Patient Records, also known as 42 CFR Part 2, was established in 1981, and updated in 2017 and 2024. The regulation was established to help provide additional protections to increase patient privacy and encourage treatment for the vulnerable population (42 CFR Part 2 Subpart B). The goals of the updated regulation in 2024 are to increase the ability to coordinate care for substance abuse patients, increased the confidentiality protections through civil monetary penalties for noncompliance, and enhance the integration of behavioral health information with other health records to improve patient care and patient health outcomes, which are required to be complied with by healthcare organization no later than February 16, 2026 (HHS 2024a).

The substantial changes to the regulations to align with the HIPAA regulations include:

- The use of a single consent form for all uses and disclosures of PHI for purposes of treatment, payment, and healthcare operations
- The ability for a CE and BA that receive records to redisclose the substance abuse records in accordance with the HIPAA regulations
- The ability to discuss PHI with public health authorities without patient consent if the information is deidentified in accordance with the HIPAA regulations
- The restriction of the use of substance abuse records in testimony civil, criminal, administrative, and legislative proceedings against patients without patient consent or a court order
- The removal of criminal penalties of Part 2 violations and replace them with the civil and criminal enforcement authorities that apply to HIPAA violations
- The requirement of Part 2 organizations to follow the HIPAA Breach Notification requirements for impermissible use and disclosures of PHI
- The alignment of the Part 2 patient notice requirements to the HIPAA regulations for the Notice of Privacy Practices.
- The creation of limits to civil or criminal liability for investigative agencies that act with reasonable diligence to determine if a specific provider is required to comply with the Part 2 requirements before making a demand for records during an investigation
- The removal of the requirement that Part 2 records need to be segregated from all other records
- The ability for the patient to file a complaint with the secretary of HHS and the Part 2 Program for any alleged violation of the Part 2 regulations
- The creation of a note type of SUD counseling notes that act as clinician notes analyzing conversations between the clinician and the patient during a session. The SUD counseling notes are given the same protections as psychotherapy notes under the HIPAA regulations
- The creation of a new patient right to opt out of receiving fundraising communication from the Part 2 program.
- The modifications to the patient consent requirements surrounding the use and disclosure of SUD records including:
  - Prohibiting the combining of patient consent for the use of disclosure of SUD records for civil, criminal, administrative, or legal proceeding with any other consent for use and disclosure of SUD records.
  - Creation of the requirement of a separate authorization for consent for any use or disclosure of SUD counseling notes.

○ Require that each disclosure made in response to a patient consent include a copy of the consent or a clear explanation statement of the scope of the consent (HHS 2024a; HHS 2024b).

While there are many changes to the regulations, there are areas of the regulations are unmodified. Any request to access SUD treatment records for the purposes of investigation or prosecuting the patient must be obtained with a patient consent or a court order. In addition, if records are obtained for the purposes of an audit or evaluation, they cannot be used for other purposes, including investigating or prosecuting the patient without a patient consent or a court order (HHS 2024a).

The basic requirement under the 42 CFR Part 2 is that any use and disclosure of patient records should be authorized by the patient or patient's legal representative. While there are a variety of reasons to disclose PHI in health records without a patient's consent, the Confidentiality of Substance Use Disorder Patient Records requirements only allow specific exceptions to the authorization of patient consent:

- Medical emergencies—patient information may be disclosed to medical personnel to meet the medical emergency needs of the patient when consent cannot be obtained. In this exception, the rule of minimum necessary must be applied and only the minimum amount of information should be disclosed to the medical professional (42 CFR Part 2 Subpart D: Section 2.51(a)).
- Food and Drug Administration (FDA)—patient information may be released to FDA medical personnel if there is reason to believe the medical emergency is due to an error in the manufacture, labeling, or sale of the product under the FDA jurisdiction (42 CFR Part 2 Subpart D: Section 2.51(b)).

If any of the above exceptions were applied, the individual disclosing the PHI must document the name of the individual receiving the information, the name of the individual making the disclosure, the date and time of the disclosure, and the nature of the emergency (42 CFR Part 2 Subpart D: Section 2.51(c)).

Another requirement when disclosing substance abuse records in response to a signed patient authorization is the healthcare organization must include one of the following statements with the disclosure:

1. "This record which has been disclosed to you is protected by Federal confidentiality rules (42 CFR part 2). These rules prohibit you from using or disclosing this record, or testimony that describes the information contained in this record, in any civil, criminal, administrative, or legislative proceedings by any Federal, State, or local authority, against the patient, unless authorized by the consent of the patient, except as provided at 42 CFR 2.12(c)(5) or as authorized by a court in accordance with 42 CFR 2.64 or 2.65. In addition, the Federal rules prohibit you from making any other use or disclosure of this record unless at least one of the following applies:

   (i) Further use or disclosure is expressly permitted by the written consent of the individual whose information is being disclosed in this record or as otherwise permitted by 42 CFR part 2.
   (ii) You are a covered entity or business associate and have received the record for treatment, payment, or health care operations, or
   (iii) You have received the record from a covered entity or business associate as permitted by 45 CFR part 164, subparts A and E.

   A general authorization for the release of medical or other information is NOT sufficient to meet the required elements of written consent to further use or redisclose the record" (42 CFR Part 2 Subpart 2: Section 2.32(a)(1)).

2. "42 CFR part 2 prohibits unauthorized disclosure of these records" (42 CFR Part 2 Subpart 2: Section 2.32(a)(2)).

   The authorization for disclosure of alcohol and substance abuse records requires the following information to be completed in order to be valid:

- Name of the patient
- Specific name of the 42 CFR Part 2 program, entity, or individual making the disclosure
- How much and the type of information to be disclosed, including specific language around the disclosure of substance abuse records
- The names of the individual(s) or entity receiving the information
- Purpose of the disclosure
- Statement that the consent is subject to revocation any time
- Date or event when the consent will expire
- Signature of the patient or patient representative, including relationship to patient
- Date of the signature of the consent (42 CFR Part 2 Subpart C: Section 2.31(a))

Organizations with both health and substance abuse records may use the same authorization for disclosure form, but it is extremely important that substance abuse records are requested separately on the authorization form. For example, under the documents to disclose, substance abuse records must be acknowledged separately from all other components of the health record, such as the discharge summary, history and physical, and office visit records. Best practice is to have a separate statement for the disclosure of substance abuse records on the authorization for disclosure form.

Another requirement of 42 CFR Part 2 is to provide an additional notice when an individual becomes a patient. Not only does an organization provide an NPP, but they must also provide a Notice of Confidentiality of Alcohol and Drug Abuse Patient Records (see figure 10.1). This notice is intended to provide the patient's additional information regarding their rights for their alcohol and substance abuse records under federal law (42 CFR Part 2 Subpart B: 2.22).

As with the HIPAA Privacy Rule, physical records must be protected from unauthorized access, use, tampering, and disclosure. 42 CFR Part 2 provides specific details regarding the security of both paper-based records and electronic records. Organizations must establish policies and procedures that define the transfer and removal of paper records, destruction of paper records, the physical security of paper records when not in use, the security of the paper records when in use by the organization, and deidentification of paper records (42 CFR Part 2 Subpart B: 2.16(a)(1)). If the organization creates and stores alcohol or substance abuse records in an electronic format, the organization must create a policy and a procedure that defines how the records will be created, received, maintained and transmitted, how the records will be destroyed in order to render the patient information unreadable and unusable, who can use or access the patient records, and how the electronic records will be deidentified (42 CFR Part 2 Subpart B: 2.16(a)(2)).

**Figure 10.1.** Sample notice for confidentiality of alcohol and drug abuse patient records

---

The confidentiality of alcohol and drug abuse patient records maintained by this program is protected by federal law and regulations. Generally, the program may not say to a person outside the program that a patient attends the program, or disclose any information identifying a patient as an alcohol or drug abuser unless:

1. The patient consents in writing;
2. The disclosure is allowed by a court order; or
3. The disclosure is made to medical personnel in a medical emergency or to qualified personnel for research, audit, or program evaluation

Violation of the federal law and regulations by a program is a crime. Suspected violations may be reported to appropriate authorities in accordance with federal regulations.

Federal law and regulations do not protect any information about a crime committed by a patient either at the program or against any person who works for the program or about any threat to commit such a crime.

Federal laws and regulations do not protect any information about suspected child abuse or neglect from being reported under State law to appropriate state or local authorities.

---

**Source**: 42 CFR Part 2 Section: 2.22(d).

## 21st Century Cures Act and Information Blocking

In 2016, the 21st Century Cures Act (Cures Act) made sharing electronic health information an expectation in healthcare by authorizing HHS to identify "reasonable and necessary activities that do not constitute information blocking" (HealthIT.gov n.d.a). The Office of the National Coordinator for Health Information Technology (ONC) went on to release the *21st Century Cures Act: Interoperability, Information Blocking, and the ONC Health IT Certification Program Final Rule* in 2020, which implements provisions from the Cures Act. The Final Rule aids in the "seamless and secure access, exchange, and use of electronic health information" (HealthIT.gov n.d.b) and encourages patients to access and use their ePHI, helps to support the needs of healthcare providers in providing care to patient, supports and advances innovation in the advancement of patient information. fosters "patient access to their electronic health information, supports provider needs, advances innovation, and addresses information blocking practices" (Anthony 2020).

The Cures Act defines information blocking and establishes exceptions and penalties. Information blocking is a "practice that will likely interfere with the access, exchange, or use of electronic health information, except as required by law or specified in an information blocking exception" (HealthIT.gov n.d.a). There are three categories of **actors** regulated by the information blocking section of the Final Rule, defined as healthcare providers, a health information network (HIN) or health information exchange (HIE), and a Health IT Developer of Certified Health IT (HealthIT.gov 2024). Anyone who experiences or witnesses information blocking by any of the actors can report their concern to the ONC.

In situations where it may be impossible to share electronic health information as requested, or if reasonable and necessary conditions must be met before electronic health information can be shared, there are exceptions to the information blocking law. There are eight exceptions that fall into two categories. Category 1 exceptions involve *not* fulfilling requests to access, exchange, or use EHI to prevent harm, protect privacy and security, or due to infeasibility or health IT performance. Category 2 exceptions involve procedures for fulfilling requests to access, exchange, or use EHI. These exceptions apply to content or manner, fees, and licensing (HealthIT.gov n.d.c).

Upon investigation, if the HHS OIG determines the actor has committed information blocking, penalties may be enforced depending on the actor involved. Health IT developers of certified health IT and HINs and HIEs are subject to penalties of up to $1 million per violation, while a healthcare provider may be subject to "appropriate disincentives," as established by the HHS secretary (Posnack 2020).

## State Privacy and Security Laws

One of the challenges of compliance with privacy and security regulations is navigating between adhering to federal regulations, such as HIPAA, or state law requirements. HIPAA establishes the minimum requirements for application of privacy and security standards under state law. Many states have laws and regulations that are more stringent than HIPAA. This requires a CE to evaluate and apply the regulations based on both federal and state privacy, security, and breach notification requirements for PHI.

HIPAA requirements state that CEs and BAs must comply with both the federal privacy and security regulations as well as state privacy and security regulations (ONC 2015, 11). Preemption is defined as the principle that a statute at one level supersedes or is applied over the same or similar statute at a lower level (45 CFR 160.202). When both laws are unable to be properly complied with, the state law is either considered to be contrary or more stringent. State law is considered **contrary** when (1) a CE determines that it is impossible to comply with both the federal and state privacy regulations or (2) compliance with the state law would create a barrier to compliance with the federal regulations under HIPAA (ONC 2015, 11). If a state regulation is considered to be contrary to the HIPAA regulations, a request to accept a provision of state law can be submitted to the secretary of HHS from an elected official or designee (AHIMA 2013a).

In some cases, state laws are considered more stringent that federal laws. Under HIPAA, state law is considered more **stringent** if the law prohibits or restricts use or disclosure in circumstances under which such use or disclosure would be permitted under federal law. State law is more stringent if it does the following:

- Gives an individual greater rights to acquire, copy, or amend their PHI
- Further prohibits the use and disclosure of PHI
- Provides the individual greater rights of access to the information
- Requires greater authorization requirements for compliance
- Requires more privacy protections
- Requires greater protection with sensitive notes such as mental health or HIV/AIDS (HHS 2013, 19)

For example, under the Minnesota Health Record Act, a patient must sign authorization to release patient information for the purposes of TPO (Revisor of Statutes, State of Minnesota 2015). This is stricter than HIPAA, which states that information can be shared for the purposes of TPO. CEs and BAs must practice due diligence to understand both state law and federal law to ensure they are adequately complying with privacy and security regulations.

For patient records covered by 42 CFR Part 2, the federal law may not preempt the state law. According to the 42 CFR Part 2 regulations, "if a disclosure permitted under the regulations of 42 CFR Part 2 is prohibited under state law, neither the regulations in this part nor the authorizing statute may be construed to authorize any violation of that state law. However, no state law may either authorize or compel any disclosure prohibited by the regulations in this part" (42 CFR 2.20).

### Check Your Understanding 10.2

**Answer the following questions in a separate document.**

1. HIPAA allows patients to access their records except for psychotherapy notes. In the state of Vermont patients are allowed access to psychotherapy notes. Which should be adhered to, HIPAA or state law?
2. What are the exceptions to the authorization of patient consent allowed by the Confidentiality of Substance Use Disorder Patient Records requirements?
3. Refer to the Privacy Rule's requirements for use and disclosure of PHI to develop a response to a patient who requests an explanation of how their information may be used and disclosed in the hospital directory.
4. Develop a policy related to a healthcare organization's process for responding to a patient who objects to their information being included in the facility directory.
5. If an attorney for the plaintiff requests health records for a malpractice case that he or she is assigned to, what documentation requirements are necessary to release the records, and what type of verification should be completed prior to releasing the records?
6. When releasing substance abuse records for the purposes of investigating or prosecuting a patient, what are the only two ways to appropriately disclose these records?

## Managing an Effective Security Program

Managing all the patient data and information a healthcare organization creates, receives, maintains, or transmits can be a challenge; however, it is a necessity to ensure the confidentiality, integrity, and availability of health information. The HIPAA Security Rule requires organizations to implement a variety of physical, technical, and administrative safeguards to protect patient data. As healthcare data becomes predominantly electronic, security safeguards are essential to protect and control the confidentiality, integrity, and accessibility of PHI. Cybersecurity has become a focal point of the healthcare industry. The HHS 405(d) (2023a) workgroup found that cyberattacks on healthcare organization directly impact the ability to provide healthcare safely and effectively. Recent cyberattacks on healthcare organizations have caused the inability to access patient records, inability to provide care, and diverting of patients to different healthcare organizations resulting in a delay of care (HHS 205(d) 2023).

A seven-step approach for creation of an effective security program within the guide provides the following steps:

- Step 1: Lead your culture, select your team, and learn.
- Step 2: Document your process, findings, and actions.
- Step 3: Review existing security of ePHI.
- Step 4: Develop an action plan.
- Step 5: Manage and mitigate risks.
- Step 6: Attest for Meaningful Use security-related objects (if applicable).
- Step 7: Monitor, audit, and update security on an ongoing basis. (ONC 2015, 37)

As part of security governance, policies and procedures create consistency in processes across the organization. Supporting the organization's goals and objectives and properly creating policies and procedures that directly link the organization's objectives and mission are key steps toward building an effective security management program (HHS 405(d) 2023a). It is a necessary part of the oversight and governance structure of security management that the policies and procedures are evaluated and monitored on a regular basis to ensure compliance and enforcement within an organization (HHS 405(d) 2023a; ONC 2019, 27).

## Risk Analysis and Risk Management

Under HIPAA, both CE and BAs must comply with the entire HIPAA Security Rule. CEs and BAs must execute and complete a HIPAA risk analysis by conducting a complete and accurate *assessment* of the potential risks and vulnerabilities to the confidentiality, integrity, and availability of ePHI at their organization (45 CFR 164.308(a)(1)(ii)(A); CMS 2007a, 3). A *risk analysis* is a systemic process for reviewing all systems, applications, and processes to identify potential threats and vulnerabilities, document current controls, and understand the likelihood of the impact (45 CFR 164.308(a)(1)(ii)(A); NIST 2024, 15–23). Commonly, the HIPAA security officer will lead the HIPAA risk analysis process with a multidisciplinary team made up of administration, legal, HIM, information technology, clinicians, human resources, and any others are identified as part of the risk analysis process.

HIPAA does not define the methodology for how to conduct the risk analysis due to the vast difference in healthcare organizations and CEs, nor does the regulation define how often a risk analysis needs to be completed. It is up to each individual CE and BA to create and establish a policy, procedure, and process for regularly conducting a risk analysis. To assist with the process of the risk analysis, the ONC published a free security risk assessment tool available to CEs and BAs (ONC n.d.b). A common methodology for risk analysis is based on the framework defined by the National Institute of Standards and Technology (NIST), as presented in figure 10.2.

While no specific methodology must be followed, a complete and accurate risk analysis includes some basic steps. One of the most important steps of the risk analysis process is to properly scope out and prepare for the risk analysis. This includes identifying:

- The location where all ePHI is generated
- Where and how ePHI enters the organization
- Where and how ePHI flows through the organization and systems
- Where ePHI is stored
- Who accesses ePHI and where do they access it
- Where the ePHI leaves the organization (NIST 2024, 16)

While this information creates a foundation to understand the flow of ePHI throughout an organization, it is also important to understand and include in the scope of the assessment the physical aspect of the organization. This includes the location where ePHI is being stored, and how ePHI is accessed (NIST 2024, 16). These steps are foundational to ensuring the correct evaluation of threats and vulnerabilities to ePHI.

In addition to conducting a risk analysis, the HIPAA security officer should establish a plan for the

**Figure 10.2.** NIST risk analysis methodology

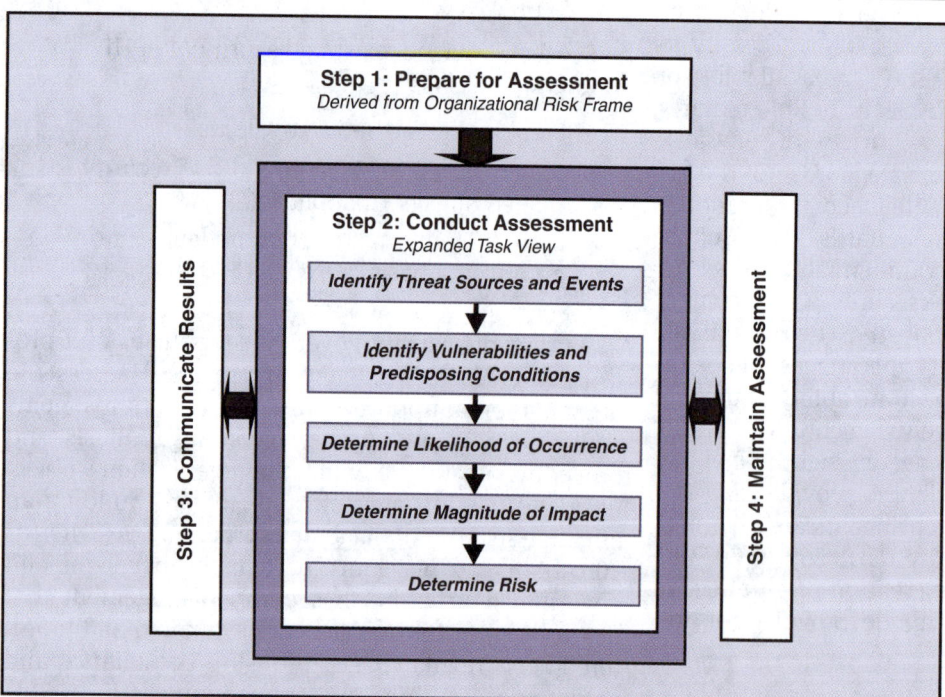

**Source:** Ross 2012, 23.

risk management component of the HIPAA requirements, which mandate CEs and BAs implement security measures sufficient to reduce risks and vulnerabilities to a reasonable level (45 CFR 164.308(a)(1)(ii)(B)). See table 10.4 for the five security components for risk management. Based on the findings from the risk analysis, CEs and BAs need to evaluate and implement adequate and appropriate security measures and controls that sufficiently reduce or eliminate the risks and vulnerabilities to an organization. There are three basic methods for addressing risks: **mitigate the risk**, which refers to the process of reducing or eliminating the risk by implementing a control; **transfer the risk** by outsourcing or insuring the risk against any potential loss to the organization; and **accept the risk** by taking no action, understanding that **residual risk**, which is the risk(s) that remain even with the current safeguards and controls applied, will exist as no additional controls would be implemented (NIST 2024). No risks should be left unaddressed or unevaluated. Each risk should be evaluated and fall into one of the basic methods for addressing risks defined previously.

The Medicare Promoting Interoperability (PI) Program has continued the focus on the HIPAA risk analysis and risk management by requiring a risk analysis be conducted in accordance with the HIPAA security rule when providing information regarding the Merit-Based Incentive Payment System (MIPS) (HHS 2024). The PI Program requires eligible hospitals and critical access hospitals to attest they have conducted a security risk analysis during the calendar year in which the EHR reporting period occurs, referred to as the performance period. It is important to have clearly written risk analysis reports and risk management documentation that show supporting dates and evidence that the work was completed prior to the end of a specific performance period.

**Table 10.4.** Five security components for risk management

| Security component | Examples of vulnerabilities | Examples of security mitigation strategies |
|---|---|---|
| Administrative safeguards | • No security officer is designated<br>• Workforce is not trained or is unaware of privacy and security issues<br>• Periodic security assessment | • Security officer is designated and publicized<br>• Workforce training begins at hire and is conducted on a regular and frequent basis<br>• Security risk analysis is performed periodically and when a change occurs in the practice or the technology |
| Physical safeguards | • Facility has insufficient locks and other barriers to patient data access<br>• Computer equipment is easily accessible by the public<br>• Portable devices are not tracked or not locked up when not in use | • Building alarm systems are installed<br>• Offices are locked |
| Technical safeguards | • Poor controls allow inappropriate access to EHR<br>• Audit logs are not used enough to monitor users and other EHR activities<br>• No measures are in place to keep electronic patient data from improper changes<br>• No contingency plan exists<br>• Electronic exchanges of patient information are not encrypted or otherwise secured | • Secure user IDs, passwords, and appropriate role-based access are used<br>• Routine audits of access and changes to EHR are conducted<br>• Anti-hacking and anti-malware software is installed<br>• Contingency plans and data backup plans are in place<br>• Data are encrypted |
| Organizational standards | • No breach notification and associated policies exist<br>• Business associate (BA) agreements have not been updated in several years | • Regular reviews of agreements are conducted and updates made accordingly |
| Policies and procedures | • Generic written policies and procedures to ensure HIPAA security compliance were purchased but not followed<br>• The manager performs ad hoc security measures | • Written policies and procedures are implemented and staff is trained<br>• Security team conducts monthly review of user activities<br>• Routine updates are made to document security measures |

**Source:** ONC 2015, 45.

## Audit Logs and Monitoring

As electronic data grows more prevalent, HIPAA regulations play an important data safety role. The HIPAA Security Rule requires an organization to (1) implement a process for regular review of system activity, and (2) implement hardware, software, and such to allow the ability to track and review activity on an IS (45 CFR 164.308(a)(1)(ii)(D)). Reviewing electronic system activities during security audits can help a healthcare organization proactively ensure the information they store and maintain is only accessed during the normal course of business. An **audit** is a function that allows retrospective reconstruction of events, including who executed the events in question, why, and what changes were made as a result. To have the EHR certified for the PI Program, EHR vendors must provide an **audit log**—a chronological record of electronic system activities of individual user activity over a period of time—and record actions a user takes within the system (NIST 2024, 70). The core steps of an effective audit and monitoring program are as follows:

Establish a process and document a policy and procedure for auditing and monitoring activity within electronic systems.

- Define and determine who will conduct the audits and the frequency.
- Define and determine who and what will be audited.
- Select the tools that will be deployed for auditing and system activity reviews.
- Define how the audit's findings will be analyzed and reported.
- Define and document the process for documenting audits and how long the data will be kept (NIST 2024, 33, 70).

By establishing an effective program, an organization protects patient information and meets the requirements of HIPAA.

HIPAA also mandates monitoring log-ins (45 CFR 164.308(a)(5)(ii)(C); CMS 2007a). CEs and BAs must ensure procedures are established for review of system logins and that a process exists for reporting and reviewing any potential discrepancies. Some systems are set up with capabilities to produce alerts or warnings when several failed logins have occurred. In other cases, a user may be locked out of the system or require a password reset if they fail a log-in for a predetermined number of times (CMS 2007a, 16). Clear policies and procedures should be written to address how login discrepancies are reviewed and evaluated.

Recent large-scale data breaches were reported due to hacking into systems with usernames and passwords of credentialed people. Evaluation from these large data breaches indicates many systems and servers are not equipped with robust log file audit reports and software that helps to assist and manage login monitoring. While these systems may not block hackers and malware that access the system, they assist in identifying suspicious activity based on logins and potential activity happening (HHS 405(d), 2023a; NIST 2024, 33). They can assist in an early detection of a potential security incident or data breach.

## Contingency Planning

A **contingency plan**, also known as a disaster plan, prepares organizations for a potential event that could impact the ability to access patient information, the integrity of the information, or the confidentiality of the information. The contingency plan requires all CEs and BAs to adequately plan for an event that disrupts normal day-to-day operations (45 CFR 164.308(a)(7); CMS 2007a; NIST 2024, 47). In recent years several situations across the US occurred where contingency planning needed to be enacted. For example, when Hurricane Idalia hit Georgia and Florida in 2023, the 2024 Change Healthcare cyberattack, or the 2024 cyberattack at Ascension Healthcare System (CNN 2024). The HIPAA Security Rule requires healthcare organizations to create a contingency plan in the case of such events so a strategy is in place to ensure ePHI is available when needed.

### Data Backups

The first requirement under the contingency planning regulation is data backup (45 CFR 164.308(a)(7)(ii)(A)). This HIPAA requirement mandates that organizations create and store exact copies of ePHI (CMS 2007a, 19; NIST 2024, 48–49). This requirement exists to ensure that, in the event of a loss of data, the data can be restored to support continuity of care and business operations. Every organization should have a thorough and robust data backup strategy that includes backup processes for all mission-critical assets and systems, including the EHR (HHS 405(d) 2023c). For example, the server that houses the EHR, file system, and PACs system should be backed up daily to a cloud-based server that allows for an exact, retrievable copy. To properly understand backup processes, it is important to evaluate the organization to know all existing systems that store and maintain PHI. Each of the electronic systems should have a documented **data backup plan** that defines how the system is being backed up, the method of backing up the data, location of the backup, frequency of the backup, and testing of the backup (HHS 405(d) 2023b). Table 10.5 represents an example of documentation that should be maintained as part of a data backup plan.

**Table 10.5.** Examples of data backup documentation

| System name | Purpose of system | Location of system | Backup process | Backup location | Frequency of backup | Testing frequency |
|---|---|---|---|---|---|---|
| ABC Health System | Electronic health record (EHR) | Onsite Server #1A | Backup Cloud System–Cloud Based | Cloud-Based System in Austin, TX | Continuous backup | Data tested monthly |
| ABC Health System | Lab information system | Onsite Server #2A | Weekly Tape Backup | On-site Backup, stored in fireproof safe in the Ambulance Garage | Weekly backup | Data tested monthly |

*Source:* HHS 405(d) 2023c.

Backup storage must be considered for all backup systems. Additionally, healthcare organizations should evaluate the process of encrypting backup media to know they are properly secured in the event of lost or stolen backup (HHS 405(d) 2023c, 50; NIST 2024, 48–49). Healthcare organizations should make certain that only authorized staff have access to the data backups (NIST 2024, 48–49). To support the backup process, AHIMA recommends a functional backup plan that includes the following:

- Processes for backing up all data on all systems, as well as steps for recreating all components of the health information system
- Description and location of all components of the electronic, hybrid, or paper records, and the configuration of any networked device including hardware and software deployed
- Processes for recreating data tables, contracts, licenses, and policies and procedures
- Assignment of responsibility for each component that identifies backup personnel if key individuals are inaccessible or incapacitated
- An estimate of how long the organization or provider can continue to function at various stages of recovery (AHIMA 2016, 9)

A well-defined data backup plan with well-established physical controls is critical to helping an organization restore data in the event of an emergency.

### Disaster Recovery Plan

The second requirement of the contingency planning regulation is that CEs and BAs should have a **disaster recovery plan** that defines the processes for recovery of data in the event of a disaster. Stated in 45 CFR 164.308, procedures should be created to restore any loss of data that may have occurred (CMS 2007a, 20). The disaster recovery plan should be specific to each hospital unit or clinical location and allow guidance and support for decision-making processes regarding the data created during a disaster (AHIMA 2016, 8).

The disaster recovery plan should also address how data created during a downtime will be restored in the electronic format. When defining data restoration, healthcare organizations must address what information will be back-entered into the electronic system and the steps and processes for entering data, including sequence of events, communication regarding data restoration, and verification and checks on the integrity of the restored data (AHIMA 2016, 8; CMS 2007a, 20). The back-entered information will be based on patient care needs, reimbursement requirements, and organization workflow. A clearly defined plan for the restoration of data should be written and kept within the contingency planning documentation.

### Emergency Mode Operation Plan

As part of contingency planning, all CEs and BAs need to anticipate how they will conduct day-to-day operations in the event of an emergency (45 CFR 164.308(a)(7)(ii)(C)). An **emergency mode operation plan** creates processes and procedures to support the continuation of critical business and patient care operations while protecting the security of ePHI in the event of a disaster (CMS 2007a, 20; NIST 2024, 49). The plan should include how the CE or BA will protect the confidentiality, integrity, and accessibility of the ePHI; what additional security measures need to be implemented to provide protection; processes and procedures for collection of data and protection of the data; and contact information for key people involved in the emergency mode operations plan (NIST 2024, 49). The plan should be easily accessible to everyone who needs it in the event of an emergency.

The emergency mode plan may include the following:

- Detailed communication plan including scope of disaster, extent of resources disabled, and recovery and restoration process as it occurs

- Documentation requirements needed at a minimum
- Emergency registration sets including patient identification
- Emergency paper chart
- Downtime procedures for paper documentation
- Stickers or other processes for alerts of allergies
- Filing procedures that will allow information to be accessed at a later date and time (AHIMA 2016, 10)

Creating a plan and training staff for this process is essential. During an emergency, the day-to-day operations can become frantic. With proper planning and an established emergency plan, an organization's workforce will feel confident and the likelihood of ePHI being mishandled will be reduced.

## Emergency Access

Another area to address within a contingency plan is how the organization will manage and provide emergency access to systems (45 CFR 164.312(a)(2)(ii)). CEs and BAs should ensure that procedures exist for obtaining access to necessary ePHI in an emergency. Procedures should define instructions and practices for providing and obtaining access to pertinent ePHI in the event of an emergency (CMS 2007b, 5; NIST 2024, 67). The procedures should evaluate various emergency scenarios, determine what workforce members might need access to ePHI, what ePHI they will need access to, how the access will be obtained, and who is responsible for providing access (CMS 2007b, 5).

## Software Criticality Analysis

Under the HIPAA Security Rule, CEs and BAs should assess all current systems and applications defined in the contingency plan that interact with patient information and conduct a criticality analysis for each individual application (45 CFR 164.308(a)(7)(ii)(E); CMS 2007a). A criticality analysis consists of evaluating each of the different systems of the organization to determine how crucial the information in the system is to day-to-day healthcare operations and patient care (CMS 2007a; NIST 2024, 47). The goal of this addressable requirement is to create a list that prioritizes all systems to allow for the successful restoration of critical systems more efficiently after an unexpected or expected downtime. Having clear, established processes in the event of a disaster or interruption to systems is critical to data management.

## Data Security Methods

Data security is the process in which organizations implement tools that help protect and safeguard PHI.

The Security Rule allows healthcare organizations to be flexible with the implementation of different data security methods depending on the needs of the organization. Common types of data security methods include authentication, malicious software protection and evaluation, data encryption, and other methods.

### Authentication

User authentication is the front-line process for protecting sensitive information an organization has ownership over, including patient health and business information. User authentication is the process where an end user logs into an electronic system using specific credentials defined by the organization. Some common forms of authentication are a username, a common form of user identification (ID), and password (the most common in healthcare), a username and personal identification number (PIN), and biometric log-in, such as a fingerprint. Through the push of government regulations, password management is becoming a requirement and justifies organizations focusing on and funding password management initiatives. For most computer systems, the user ID and password is the first step in the authentication process to access a network (HHS 403(b) 2023; CMS 2007b, 4; NIST 2023, 73–74). A user ID is a unique name or number used to identify a specific user of an information system. With the user ID and password being used to access all information on an information network, organizations must ensure they are effectively and efficiently managing passwords.

The first step to building an effective password management process is to create a systemwide policy. The policy should include standards regarding the length of the password, the type of characters to be included in the password, the process of password expiration, the process of password reuse, sharing of passwords, and potential sanctions or penalties for policy violations (HHS 403(b) 2023b; NIST 2020, 73–74). With a standard policy used systemwide, organizations are better able to govern and use passwords within their systems and protect their information against hackers.

Password strength is an important factor for effective password management. Users are always encouraged to use unique and unpredictable passwords. While length alone does not make a strong password, it is recommended that a password be a minimum of eight characters (HHS 403(b) 2023, 44). In addition to password length, strong passwords consist of three of the four characters from the following categories: numeric, alphabetic, capitals, and symbols (HHS 403(b) 2023, 44). One example of a strong password is "Health2024!" A common way to create a strong password is to use passphrases in place of passwords.

Passphrases combine multiple words to create a more complex password that is difficult to guess. An example of a passphrase is "SummerTimeSunshineBeach." Additional complexity can be added to the passphrase by adding characters, symbols, and numbers. The following is one way to make the above passphrase more secure: "$ummerT!meSun$h1neBeaCh." Using passphrases decreases the ability to guess a password and hack into a system.

Requiring that passwords expire regularly is another important process for password management. This allows organizations to properly reduce the ability for hackers to gain and maintain access to systems with proprietary and personal information (NIST 2024, 42). Best practice in the industry suggests that passwords change every 120 to 180 days.

To enhance the complexity of authentication, organizations may implement multi-factor authentication, which requires the user to have an additional requirement for authentication beyond the username and password, to gain access to systems. For example, a randomly generated PIN sent to a mobile device or a security question (HHS 405(d) 2023a; NIST 2024, 42). Based on the sensitivity of the system, an organization can implement different levels of multi-factor authentication (HHS 405(d), 2023a, 16; NIST 2024, 47). The most common multifactor authentication is **two-factor authentication**, which provides additional security to the authentication process as it requires one additional step to verify the user's identification. For example, a user must input a username and password plus a generated PIN to be allowed into a system (HHS 405(d) 2023a; NIST 2024, 61). For systems containing extremely sensitive data or access to sensitive parts of a system such as the program code, tri-factor authentication may be used. This involves adding a third identification to the authentication process. One example of tri-factor authentication is a username and password, randomly generated PIN sent to a mobile device, and security questions (HHS 405(d) 2023a).

Another form of authentication is the use of biometric identifiers. **Biometric authentication** allows a user to be uniquely identified and access the system based on one or more biometric traits such as fingerprints, hand geometry, retinal pattern, or voice waves. The most common and oldest form of biometrics is fingerprint scanning and recognition, which is based on the specific ridges and characteristics of a person's fingerprint. Since the fingerprint is unique and detailed to each specific person, it is difficult to duplicate (HHS 405(d) 2023a). Fingerprint scanning is also the most cost-effective biometric authentication process available. Not only are devices for scanning fingerprints more reasonably priced, the space needed to store the fingerprint data and information is small (HHS 405(d) 2023a).

Voice recognition is another popular biometric technology. Voice recognition technology is based on different vocal characteristics individuals possess. Like fingerprint technology, voice recognition technology is relatively cost-effective and nonintrusive to the end users. A disadvantage of voice recognition technology is that it is easier to hack and has a low reliability standard because it is easier to duplicate the sound of another person's voice. In addition, a recording of someone's voice could create the ability to authenticate into a system (HHS 405(d) 2023b). Organizations that implement voice recognition should have a good security and governance structure to manage and protect the data files containing the voice recognition.

The most reliable biometric technology available for use is retina scan technology. This technology tends to cost the most due to the space required to store the data and the cameras required to scan the retina, and it also has the lowest acceptability among end users as it is the most invasive biometric technology (HHS 405(d) 2023b). Since it is the costliest and the most challenging to convince people to use, it is the least common type of biometric use for authentication purposes.

Authentication prevents unwanted access to electronic patient information. Even though organizations might not be able to limit access to patients, they can limit what patient information a user can see with properly set up role-based access. In some cases, patients' records need additional security due to the sensitivity of the information or interest in the information, such as high-profile cases or celebrities. Most electronic systems offer the option to provide an additional authentication requirement referred to as "break the glass" (Primeau 2017, 19). Breaking the glass requires the user to authenticate an additional time and select a reason for accessing the patient's record. This creates an audit log that can be evaluated to make sure access was necessary to support treatment, payment, or healthcare operations (Primeau 2017, 19).

### Encryption and Decryption of ePHI

Under HIPAA, encryption of data is defined in two separate requirements: the encryption of data at rest and the encryption of data in motion (45 CFR 164.312(a)(2)(iv); 45 CFR 164.312(e)(2)(ii)). **Data at rest** are data in storage within a database or on a server and are no longer being used or accessed. **Data in motion** are data in the process of being transmitted from one location to another location, such as an email. Under HIPAA, both are addressable requirements, which allows the CE and BA to evaluate and determine if they are going to implement the technical safeguard. If the CE chooses not to implement the encryption safeguards, other safeguards to protect the information need to be documented, including the reason for not implementing the encryption (CMS 2007b, 6–7).

**Encryption** is a mathematical method for the transformation of data from plaintext into cipher text, allowing no individual or machine to get access and decipher the original information (45 CFR 164.304). **Plaintext** is the original text that has not been altered and **cipher text** is unreadable or indecipherable due to encryption. The process of transforming the information from cipher text to plaintext is referred to as **decryption** (NIST 2020, 4). To encrypt the information, the plaintext is changed into cipher text using a cryptographic key. A **cryptographic key** is the tool applied to the data to turn the information into cipher text as well as convert the data from cipher text back to plaintext (NIST 2020, 5). Figure 10.3 depicts the process when data are encrypted and when the data are decrypted.

Under the final HIPAA Omnibus Rule, information is considered secure if it is encrypted. **Secure information** is considered unreadable, unusable, and indecipherable (HHS 403(b) 2023b). Under the Breach Notification Rule, if the information is considered secure PHI, then an investigation does not need to take place, and the determination that a breach did not occur can be applied to most scenarios. Essentially, encryption allows the assumption that the data are secured and therefore no risk to the data or patient has occurred (HHS 403(b) 2023b). The final HIPAA Omnibus Rule of 2013 also added a few standards regarding encryption into the regulations. While it did not change any of the regulations from the HIPAA Security Rule, it did call out a few examples of use of encryption. The HIPAA Final Omnibus Rule of 2013 allows patients to access PHI in an electronic format if the PHI is part of the organization's designated record set and is stored in an electronic format. While encryption of the medium used to provide the electronic copy is not required, CEs should implement proper safeguards to ensure the ePHI protections are in place, including encryption of information (HHS 2022c). Email is an acceptable method for producing the electronic copy of information; however, if the CE is using unencrypted email, the patient must be advised and agree to the risks to the data while being sent in an unencrypted format (HHS 2022c). CEs should create a policy and procedure for electronic access to ePHI to address this requirement and establish how the information will be protected.

Recently, CEs and BAs have seen a significant increase in the number of data breaches due to hacking into systems as well as lost and stolen devices. HHS reported that 75 percent of data breaches in 2021 that affected 500 individuals or more were caused by hacking and IT incidents (HHS 2022d, 10). If encryption technology had been implemented on laptops

**Figure 10.3.** Encryption function and decryption function

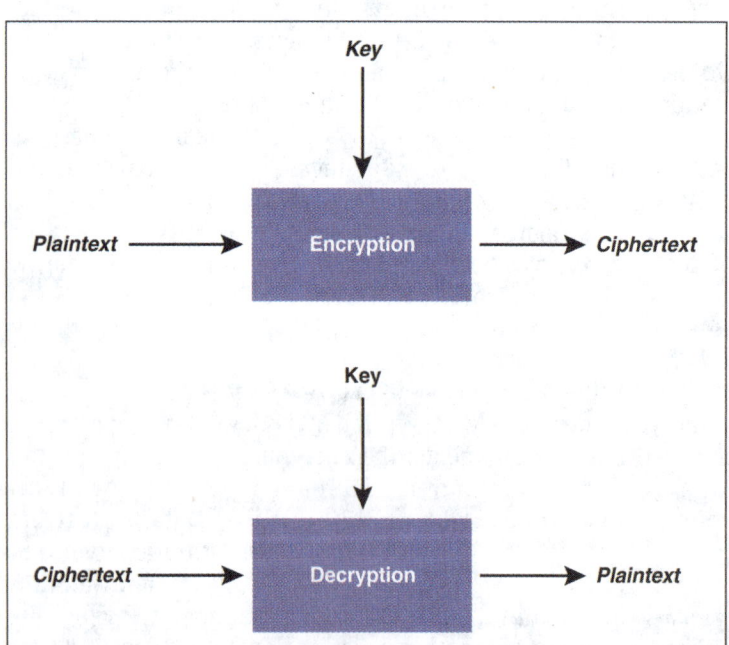

*Source:* NIST 2020, 32.

and other portable media, some of the large-scale data breaches could have been prevented as the data would have been inaccessible (HHS 2023h). One of the best tools for preventing and fighting data breaches is the implementation of encryption of data at rest and data in motion. All ePHI should be evaluated to determine if encryption is appropriate to protect data.

## Malicious Software Management and Cybersecurity Threats

HIPAA requires CEs and BAs to protect all ePHI from malicious software, also known as malware, by implementing policies and procedures for guarding against, detecting, and reporting malicious software within their organization (45 CFR 164.308(a)(5)(ii)(B)). **Malware** is any program that causes harm to systems by unauthorized access, unauthorized disclosure, destruction, or loss of integrity of any information.

Some of the common types of malware that healthcare organizations encounter are as follows:

- **Viruses**: Programs that search out other programs and infect them by embedding a copy of itself. This type of malware has the capability to spread to other computers by attaching itself to programs shared through a network.
- **Worms**: Programs that reproduce on their own that have no need for a host application; they are self-contained programs.
- **Trojan horses**: Programs that are disguised as a normal program to trick users to download the file.
- **Ransomware**: Programs that lock a device or files by deploying encryption technology that demands a ransom payment to restore access.
- **Logic bombs**: Malware that will execute a program, or a string of code, when a certain event happens.
- **Rootkit**: A type of malware that will remotely access or control a computer without being detected by users or security programs (Stouffer 2021).

Frequent methods of malware infiltration include email attachments, downloaded programs, social media sites, inappropriate websites, and lack of updating security patches (CMS 2007a, 15). The challenges that healthcare organizations face regarding malware and its impact on ePHI are as follows:

- Data breaches
- Unauthorized access or disclosure of ePHI
- Increased central processing unit (CPU) use
- Slowed computer response time
- Modified or deleted files
- Additions or changes to ePHI being stored. (Stouffer 2021)

Ransomware attacks have become increasingly common in healthcare. In some cases, even when the organization or user pays the ransom, the hacker does not provide the encryption key, and the data are permanently locked and unavailable to the user. There can be legal consequences for organizations that fall prey to such attacks. In October 2023, the OCR settled the first HIPAA resolution agreement with a fine in response to a ransomware attack. Doctor's Management Services (DMS), Inc., reported that in April 2017, they experienced a ransomware attack that was not detected until December 2018 when the attack made files inaccessible. Upon investigation, OCR determined that the lack of a risk analysis and a risk management plan, failed implementation of information activity review, and insufficient HIPAA policies and procedures were the root cause of the ransomware attack that went undetected for 20 months (HHS 2023i). In addition to a $100,000 fine, DMS also has entered a two-year CAP with HHS.

Another type of threat for healthcare organizations is social engineering. **Social engineering** "is an attempt to trick someone into revealing information (e.g., a password) that can be used to attack systems or networks or taking an action (e.g., clicking a link, opening a document)" (HHS 405(d) 2023b, 18). The most common type of social engineering are phishing attacks. Phishing attacks are a version of a cybersecurity attack and involve an attempt to gather sensitive information, such as a username and password or credit card number, from a user by masquerading as a trustworthy entity in an electronic communication (HHS 405(d) 2023b). For example, an individual may receive an email that appears to be from a provider asking them to enter personal information prior to the appointment. However, the email is actually from a third party posing as the provider to get the patient to enter sensitive data. If the patient enters information into the false website, it can be used to steal the patient's identity or open fraudulent credit cards.

CEs and BAs should establish policies and procedures to manage malware within the organization. At a minimum, the policies and procedures should define security patch updating, antivirus software process and review, reporting processes for malware infestations, containment and removal processes, verification of ePHI integrity after a malware attack, and workforce education on malware (HHS 405(d) 2023a; HHS 405(d) 2023b). Written policies and procedures help to create consistent management over malware within organizations.

The patch management process includes ensuring the application of security patches for operating systems on all computers, servers, and applications within an organization. Organizations should create a process for promptly testing and applying hardware and software security updates to prevent malware from being implemented on the organization's network. In addition, antivirus software should be applied to all hardware within the organization (HHS 405(d) 2023c, 74). Antivirus software reviews and checks all the files on the computer or server to ensure there is no malware that can be identified within the system. Antivirus software can also provide real-time evaluation and blocking of potential threatening software from being applied to a computer or server. Additionally, organizations should ensure all attachments received through email are subject to security verification. Some systems can be applied to email to scan the attachment for potential threats prior to downloading. These systems will alert the end user that there is potential harm if the attachment is downloaded. Staff training is crucial for ensuring that malware cannot enter an organization's network.

### Check Your Understanding 10.3

**Answer the following questions in a separate document.**

1. Distinguish between the three methods for addressing risks and rationalize when each method would be appropriate. Provide an example of each.
2. Explain the situations in which the HIPAA Security Rule requires an organization to review system activity.
3. Explain the HIPAA encryption requirement and distinguish between the encryption of data at rest and the encryption of data in motion.
4. An organization is currently using a four-digit PIN to log into the EHR. During a recent review of security practices for obtaining cybersecurity insurance, a finding indicated that the organization had to implement a more robust authentication process for gaining access to the EHR. You are the security officer, and you have been tasked with developing a more effective and secure method for authentication. Develop a plan to change the process for authentication and to make it more secure and effective.
5. Explain the main purposes of the creation of a system and data criticality analysis document.

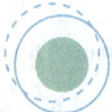

## Management of Privacy and Security in Health Information Exchange

HIE is the electronic exchange of health information between providers and others with the same level of interoperability. It allows healthcare professionals and patients to access and securely share a patient's electronic health information (HealthIT.gov 2023). HIE can help improve quality of care and reduce healthcare costs for the patient and healthcare organization by improving access to a patient's health information and reducing duplicate testing, for example. With a combination of government mandates and financial incentives and the desire to improve patient care, many healthcare organizations want to electronically exchange information. However, HIE comes with concerns regarding the privacy and security of patient information.

Exchanging health information has many benefits and challenges. A properly established HIE allows for many benefits to the patient and the healthcare organization. If health information is available electronically, it can help facilitate coordinated patient care, reduce duplicative treatments and avoid costly mistakes (HealthIT.gov n.d.d). Maintaining the privacy and security of information in HIE is one of the major challenges to address. Pursuing HIE requires that organizations evaluate the benefits and risks to the organization. With the implementation of an HIE, CEs must evaluate current HIPAA privacy and security practices to ensure adequate safeguards are established to control access to the information and provide adequate security.

One challenge the healthcare community faces with HIE is the assurance of the correct patient identity. Challenges related to data quality, completeness, and lack of standardization make patient matching in HIEs very difficult (Eramo 2019). The Government Accountability Office (GAO) concluded in its report that no one effort will solve the problem. Rather, patient matching requires a combination of methods such as algorithms, unique patient identifiers, or a manual review (HIMSS 2023). Patient matching for HIE refers to the techniques used to identify and match the data about patients held by one healthcare provider with the data about the same patients held either within the same system or by another system (HHS 2017a, 1). Incorrect patient matching can cause errors in treatment, care delivery, and patient safety, payment and resource issues, and data sharing and interoperability challenges (Riplinger et al. 2020).

Although sometimes cost prohibitive, advances in technology have created additional methods for patient matching within HIE, which include the following:

- Advanced algorithm methods
- Plastic identification cards
- Subscriber identity models for mobile phones and electronic passports
- Biometric identification (fingerprint, facial recognition, iris scanning, voice recognition)

However, if not all healthcare organizations can implement the technology, it reduces the technology's efficacy at patient matching.

Additional issues challenging HIE are the risk of data breaches and ensuring consumer privacy of exchanged information. HIPAA regulates patients' rights to information, patient restriction of information, and adequate privacy safeguards to protecting patient information. Although privacy laws are intended to ease the process of sharing health information among treating providers, some perceive them to be barriers to HIE growth and point to the challenge of finding balance between allowing information to flow easily to improve healthcare, while protecting patient privacy (Mello et al. 2018).

In a national survey, 86 percent of community HIEs indicated privacy concerns related to patient consent and patient matching as particular barriers to progress (Mello et al. 2018). The most important perceived legal barriers to HIE are:

- The HIPAA Privacy Rule
- Differing state law requirements for patient consent for disclosure
- Special federal and state law protections for specific types of sensitive health information, such as substance abuse records
- Failure to implement a uniform patient identifier
- Insufficient measures to prevent information blocking (Mello et al. 2018)

Efforts to overcome these perceived barriers are ongoing. For example, the Coronavirus Aid, Relief, and Economic Security (CARES) Act directs the ONC to continue to issue "guidance on common legal, governance, and security barriers" to HIE, and HHS to further educate providers about engaging in HIE when caring for patients (Mello et al. 2018). HIPAA security regulations related to HIEs are challenging to healthcare organizations as well. Conducting a risk analysis is one step to ensure adequate security safeguards for HIE. This should include an analysis of all potential risks associated with the confidentiality, integrity, and accessibility of the data transmitted and stored in the HIE to identify common risks such as access management and audit trail evaluation. Without the establishment of basic principles that align with the HIPAA security regulations, HIEs can be an easy target for unauthorized use and disclosure of PHI. In addition to mitigating the risks identified in the security risk analysis, a healthcare organization should create a policy and procedure to manage HIE and to establish consistent practices across the organization for access and use of the HIE. At a minimum, the policy and procedure should define the following:

- Consent and authorization processes
- Patient identification and matching processes
- User access management processes
- Termination of user processes
- Access of patient information processes
- Breach notification processes (if through HIE)
- Secondary use of HIE data into the organization's record
- Audit trail review process and functionality
- BAA processes
- Data integrity management processes (AHIMA and HIMSS 2011; Landsbach and Just 2013)

Having clearly defined processes help create a HIE governance structure within an organization that clearly identifies how and when the HIE is to be used, and protects the confidentiality, integrity, and accessibility of the information.

Another recommendation for managing privacy and security of HIE is to dedicate a person or team to manage the internal processes of when, how, and by whom the data in the HIE can be used. This will help alleviate some of the challenges and stresses that come with no oversight and management of a system (AHIMA and HIMSS 2011; Landsbach and Just 2013). This individual or team should be responsible for the creation of the policy and procedure, access management, review of audit trails, user termination processes, and overall evaluation of HIE use within the organization. By having dedicated staff to manage the process and the development of a clear governance structure, the ability to successfully implement and manage HIE privacy and security within an organization is more easily attained.

The last recommendation for best practice of HIE is education of the workforce. Proper education should be provided to those individuals who will be using or interacting with the HIE or the data from the HIE in any manner to meet the requirements of their job responsibilities (AHIMA and HIMSS 2011). At minimum, training should cover the following areas:

- Process for consent and authorization
- Process for education to patients and families
- Process for adequate patient searching and patient matching
- Process for assurance of selection of the correct patient
- Process for patient information to be utilized to support care
- Process for processing patient information if used to support care
- Process for reporting any issues or concerns with the HIE and data being used
- Information regarding the organization's evaluation of audit trails and supporting of patient care for accessing PHI in the HIE (AHIMA and HIMSS 2011)

Regular ongoing training should be a requirement. If there are concerns and issues with the way the HIE is utilized for supporting patient care, additional education should be provided.

One growing technology that hopes to break down barriers to HIE is blockchain. Blockchain technology is "a distributed digital ledger of cryptographically-signed transactions that are grouped into blocks. Each block is cryptographically linked to the previous one (making it tamper evident) after validation and undergoing a consensus decision" (NIST n.d.). This technology disrupts existing architecture by providing an efficient and decentralized data management platform (Poquiz 2022). Blockchain technology was originally created to be the public transmission ledger for the cryptocurrency Bitcoin. However, blockchain has many potential applications within the healthcare industry, particularly in the management of EHRs, revenue cycle management, and system interoperability (Poquiz 2022). Blockchain-based health record systems can be linked into existing health record software and serve as an overarching, single view of a patient's record without placing patient data on the blockchain. Each new record can be appended to the blockchain in the form of a unique hash function, which is only decoded if the person who owns the data (that is, the patient) gives consent. Blockchain is expected to provide the healthcare industry with improved confidentiality and increased access to more comprehensive data: better quality and more trustworthy goods and services; and less fraud, cheaper prices, and more innovation (HHS, 2021).

## Mobile Health Technology and HIPAA

With the increased use of technology within our healthcare organizations, health data are on the move now more than ever. To encourage the implementation and use of health information technology, many different mobile devices are used within healthcare organizations. Common types of mobile devices in use include laptop computers, tablets, smart phones, USB drives, wearable technology, and external hard drives (HHS 405(d) 2023a, 24). **Bring your own device (BYOD)** refers to personal devices that are allowed to be used within a healthcare organization and interact with ePHI (HHS n.d.d.; NIST 2024). As more mobile devices are used in healthcare, risks emerge affecting PHI and ePHI's privacy and security. If organizations choose to implement and use mobile technology, proper safeguards should be established for mobile technology management, compliance with HIPAA, and protection of the security and privacy of patient information.

Healthcare organizations should evaluate and implement proper security measures to safeguard information accessed on mobile technology. The ONC recommends five steps every healthcare organization should take to implement an effective mobile device management program defined in table 10.6.

Policies and procedures should be established to safeguard mobile technology used within the organization. The security management measures discussed earlier in this chapter should also be evaluated and implemented on mobile technology, as appropriate, to protect ePHI

With the increased use of mobile technology in healthcare and the increased cybersecurity risks, it is recommended that healthcare organizations implement mobile device management technology (MDM). Mobile device management technologies "manage the configuration of devices connected to the MDM system, which allows organizations to have oversight

**Table 10.6.** Steps to implementing an effective MDM program

| Step | Description |
|---|---|
| Decide | Decide whether mobile devices will be used to access, receive, transmit, or store patients' health information or used as part of your organization's internal networks or systems (for example, your EHR system). |
| Assess | Consider how mobile devices affect the risks (threats and vulnerabilities) to the health information your organization holds. |
| Identify | Identify your organization's mobile device risk management strategy, including privacy and security safeguards. |
| Develop, Document, and Implement | Develop, document, and implement the organization's mobile device policies and procedures to safeguard health information. |
| Train | Conduct mobile device privacy and security awareness and training for providers and professionals. |

*Source:* Adapted from ONC n.d.a.

and governance over all applications enrolled" (HHS 405(d) 2023c, 27). For example, this could allow a healthcare organization to track the number of devices in a department and their charging status, and permit the organization to deploy alerts and system updates. Additionally, organizations can implement mobile application management (MAM) solutions, which manage specific applications installed on a device versus the entire device (HHD 405(d) 2023, 27–28). Both solutions enforce security policies—MDM at the device level, and MAM at the application level. Having the ability to remotely manage mobile devices and applications provides healthcare organizations with more control over their security practices. In addition, regular employee education should be conducted on the risks of mobile technology and the processes and safeguards for managing mobile technology use in the organization.

### Check Your Understanding 10.4

**Answer the following questions in a separate document.**

1. Determine the privacy and security risks when PHI is accessed with devices permitted under a BYOD policy.
2. Recommend two safeguards to implement to protect patient information for systems that contain PHI. Explain your rationale.
3. Evaluate the benefits and risks of HIE to an organization and determine potential impacts of the benefits and risks.
4. Identify and describe two common best practices related to privacy and security for the use of mobile technology in healthcare.
5. You are tasked with creating employee training for privacy and security of the HIE implemented at your hospital. Recommend areas to cover in training.

## Workforce Training

The HIPAA Privacy and Security Rules require formal workforce education and training to ensure ongoing accountability for the privacy and security of PHI. The Privacy Rule defines the workforce as "employees, volunteers, trainees, and other persons whose conduct in the performance of work for a covered entity or business associate is under the direct control of such" (HHS 2013).

CEs are not responsible for training the BAs' workforce. However, they should conduct due diligence to ensure the appropriate privacy and security training has been completed and documented (Alder 2023). The Security Rule states that training must be applied to "all members of its workforce (including management)" (HHS 2013). The rules are not prescriptive so organizations have flexibility in implementation, and each rule independently addresses training requirements. The training component of HIPAA is one of the most critical elements in achieving compliance; therefore, it is especially important to examine the

Privacy and Security Rules before planning a training program to gain a comprehensive understanding of the requirements needed to create a compliant training program in the most efficient manner possible. The Privacy Rule requires the following:

> A covered entity must train all members of its workforce in policies and procedures with respect to protected health information required by this subpart, as necessary and appropriate for the members of the workforce to carry out their function within the covered entity. (HHS 2013)

This includes general training of HIPAA concepts and job-specific training for new employees, and ongoing training for established employees (often conducted annually), particularly for those whose job functions are affected by a change in policy or procedure.

The Security Rule mandates that entities "implement a security awareness and training program for all members of its workforce (including management)" (HHS 2013). Although this portion of the Security Rule is more abstract than the Privacy Rule, the underlying message is the same—the workforce must be trained effectively on the entity's policies and procedures as they relate to HIPAA, and the entity must have a program in place to address this on an ongoing basis. The security awareness and training standard identifies four addressable topics:

1. Periodic security updates and reminders to the workforce.
2. Procedures to guard against, detect, and report malware.
3. Procedures for monitoring login attempts and reporting discrepancies.
4. Procedures for creating, changing, and safeguarding passwords. (Alder 2023)

Between the Privacy Rule and the Security Rule, it is clear that an entity must have a training program that is presented to all members of the workforce. The training program must cover information about privacy and security, how the two concepts relate to the employee's job and their workplace, and how they are addressed in the organization's policies and procedures. The program must also provide training on an ongoing basis, and all of this must be documented by the entity. HIPAA requires that training be "as necessary and appropriate" as possible for the members of the workforce to carry out their duties, so a reasonable approach, based on the size and needs of the organization, is appropriate (HHS 2013). The entity needs to use its best judgment to decide what is "reasonable" for them and what type of training program will work for their organization.

## HIPAA Training Components

The Privacy and Security Rules can be further broken down to discern three distinct components of a compliant HIPAA training program. First, a program for training new employees should be in place. The Privacy Rule indicates that training on policies and procedures related to PHI needs to take place "within a reasonable period of time after the person joins the covered entity's workforce" (HHS 2013); and although the Security Rule does not specify a timeframe or impetus for training, one can infer that training new employees on security policies and procedures is required and should be done within a reasonable timeframe. This first category of training should include general privacy and security requirements as well as information on the entity's particular policies and procedures regarding PHI and system security. Then, specific training should be provided based on the employee's job "as necessary and appropriate for the members of the workforce to carry out their function within the covered entity" (HHS 2013).

The second component of a HIPAA training program includes ongoing training and awareness-building. The Security Rule specifies "awareness" as a requirement of a training program that, although not specified in the Privacy Rule, should be expanded to include privacy for continued workforce compliance (HHS 2013). The ongoing awareness and training on privacy and security should include everything that was addressed in initial training, which includes core concepts, policies and procedures, and job-specific information. This ongoing portion of the training program will reinforce the initial training and ensure that the behaviors expected by the workforce will become an automatic part of their daily activities.

The third component of a HIPAA training program addresses the inevitable changes that occur in any organization on a regular basis. For example, retraining must occur when job duties change, reorganization happens, or new rules or regulations are issued. Furthermore, policies and procedures are continually being evaluated and changed, and new policies emerge. The Privacy Rule requires that as policies and procedures change over time, employees be kept apprised of these changes. In addition, employees are required to be trained on how the changes affect their job functions. Although this specification is not made in the Security Rule, one can deduce that retraining of the workforce on changing policies and procedures and the effects on job-specific functions is a requirement of ongoing compliance with the Security Rule as well.

The HIPAA Privacy Rule states that "a covered entity must document that the training...has been provided" (HHS 2013). The Security Rule requires the maintenance of policies and procedures as necessary to comply with the standards. It further states, "if an action, activity, or assessment is required by this subpart to be documented, maintain a written (which may be electronic) record of the action, activity, or assessment" (HHS 2013).

## HIPAA Training Principles and Strategies

The HIPAA Privacy and Security Rules address minimum training standards that require scalability. Organizations should customize training programs to fit their operational needs and individual job responsibilities. Some of the privacy and security standards apply to a universal audience; however, other portions of the rules may not. Taking the time to develop a comprehensive HIPAA training program can reduce the cost and administration of training by addressing audience overlap, reducing redundancies, and preventing multiple or conflicting messages. One approach to HIPAA workforce training is to consider creating levels of training. For example, level 1 would address the topics universal to the entire workforce, while level 2 would include training on topics specific to a role or job position. Often the training process is prioritized so those who require training most urgently, such as clinicians who need regular and immediate access to sensitive information, receive it as soon as possible. Whether one's job duties require extensive handling of PHI (such as nurses) or minimal contact with it (such as maintenance staff), all members of the workforce must receive the appropriate level of training.

The following best practice guidance is recommended regarding HIPAA privacy and security training procedures:

- Provide general training for all workforce members, including contract workers.
- Establish timelines for training new employees according to their date of hire before the employee's first day of work in the department.
- Require annual training for all employees.
- Develop a training and awareness program that becomes part of the culture of the organization.
- Include in-depth education and ongoing awareness that includes training on PHI in all forms, including verbal, written, and electronic.
- Develop a regular communication process to address questions that arise after training and on an ongoing basis.
- Develop continuously updated reference materials of policies and procedures.
- Develop a procedure for evaluating training program effectiveness, reliability, and validity.
- Develop a process to verify employees have completed privacy and security training before they receive access to paper and electronic PHI (AHIMA 2013a).

An important aspect of workforce training is documenting such training has occurred, including content, dates, and attendee names.

It is essential that CEs and BAs document training and program assessments on an ongoing basis. Revisions to training programs and methods must occur regularly and be based on assessment results. All documents created should be maintained for six years, in accordance with HIPAA's retention requirement (AHIMA 2013a).

### Check Your Understanding 10.5

**Answer the following questions in a separate document.**

1. Identify the types of roles included in the definition of workforce in the HIPAA regulations.
2. When establishing a HIPAA training strategy for an organization, recommend the appropriate timeframe to perform training for the workforce.
3. Identify each requirement for training under the HIPAA regulations and describe the training requirements for each regulation.
4. Analyze workforce training to ensure compliance with the Privacy and Security Rules.
5. What are the four addressable topics identified in the security awareness and training standard?

# References

AHIMA and HIMSS. 2011. *The Privacy and Security Gaps in Health Information Exchange*. http://library.ahima.org/xpedio/groups/public/documents/ahima/bok1_049023.pdf.

AHIMA (American Health Information Management Association). 2016. *Disaster Planning and Recovery Toolkit* (2016 version). http://bok.ahima.org/doc?oid=301964.

AHIMA (American Health Information Management Association). 2013. Privacy and security training (2013 update). *Journal of AHIMA* 84(10).

Alder, S. 2023 (May 21). HIPAA training requirements. *The HIPAA Journal*. https://www.hipaajournal.com/hipaa-training-requirements/.

Anthony, E. S. 2020 (March 6). "The Cures Act Final Rule: Interoperability-focused Policies That Empower Patients and Support Providers." https://www.healthit.gov/buzz-blog/21st-century-cures-act/the-cures-final-rule.

Brodnik, M. S., L. A. Rinehart-Thompson, and R. B. Reynolds. 2023. *Fundamentals of Law for Health Informatics and Information Management,* 4th Edition. Chicago: AHIMA.

California Hospital Association. 2017. Release of Patient Information to the Media: A Guide for Hospital Public Relations Professionals and the News Media as Specified by California Law and HIPAA. https://www.calhospital.org/sites/main/files/file-attachments/guide_to_release_2017_web.pdf.

CMS (Centers for Medicare and Medicaid Services). 2007a. HIPAA Security Series: Security Standards: Administrative Safeguards. https://www.hhs.gov/sites/default/files/ocr/privacy/hipaa/administrative/securityrule/adminsafeguards.pdf.

CMS (Centers for Medicare and Medicaid Services). 2007b. HIPAA Security Series: Security Standards: Technical Safeguards. https://www.hhs.gov/sites/default/files/ocr/privacy/hipaa/administrative/securityrule/techsafeguards.pdf.

Eramo, L. A. 2019 (October). Close doesn't count: Patient matching challenges in HIEs. *Journal of AHIMA* 90(9): 14–17.

HHS (Department of Health and Human Services). 2024a. "Fact Sheet 42 CFR Part 2 Final Rule." https://www.hhs.gov/hipaa/for-professionals/regulatory-initiatives/fact-sheet-42-cfr-part-2-final-rule/index.html.

HHS (Department of Health and Human Services). 2024b. Confidentiality of substance use disorder (SUD) patient records. *Federal Register* 89(33). https://www.govinfo.gov/content/pkg/FR-2024-02-16/pdf/2024-02544.pdf.

HHS (Department of Health and Human Services). 2024c. "HIPAA Privacy Rule Final Rule to Support Reproductive Health Care Privacy: Fact Sheet." https://www.hhs.gov/hipaa/for-professionals/special-topics/reproductive-health/final-rule-fact-sheet/index.html.

HHS (Department of Health and Human Services). 2024d. Guidance Regarding Methods for De-identification of Protected Health Information in Accordance with the Health Insurance Portability and Accountability Act (HIPAA) Privacy Rule. https://www.hhs.gov/hipaa/for-professionals/special-topics/de-identification/index.html.

HHS (Department of Health and Human Services). 2017. "Research." https://www.hhs.gov/hipaa/for-professionals/special-topics/research/index.html.

HHS (Department of Health and Human Services). 2023a. "Request for Information (RFI) on Recognized Security Practices and Sharing Civil Money Penalties and Monetary Settlements with Harmed Individuals Under the HITECH Act." https://www.hhs.gov/hipaa/for-professionals/regulatory-initiatives/hitech-rfi/index.html.

HHS (Department of Health and Human Services). 2023b. Annual civil monetary penalties inflation adjustment (final rule). *Federal Register*, 88(193), 69531–69553. https://www.govinfo.gov/content/pkg/FR-2023-10-06/pdf/2023-22264.pdf.

HHS (Department of Health and Human Services). 2023c. "How OCR enforces the HIPAA Privacy and Security Rules." https://www.hhs.gov/hipaa/for-professionals/compliance-enforcement/examples/how-ocr-enforces-the-hipaa-privacy-and-security-rules/index.html.

HHS (Department of Health and Human Services). 2023d. "HIPAA Enforcement Highlights." https://www.hhs.gov/hipaa/for-professionals/compliance-enforcement/examples/how-ocr-enforces-the-hipaa-privacy-and-security-rules/index.html.

HHS (Department of Health and Human Services). 2023f (April 25). "HHS Proposes Measures to Bolster Patient-Provider Confidentiality around Reproductive Health Care." https://www.hhs.gov/about/news/2023/04/12/hhs-proposes-measures-bolster-patient-provider-confidentiality-around-reproductive-health-care.html.

HHS (Department of Health and Human Services). 2023g. "HIPAA Privacy Rule and Care Coordination."

https://www.hhs.gov/hipaa/for-professionals/regulatory-initiatives/hipaa-care-coordination/index.html.

HHS (Department of Health and Human Services). 2023h. "Breach Notification Rule." https://www.hhs.gov/hipaa/for-professionals/breach-notification/index.html.

HHS (Department of Health and Human Services). 2023i. "Doctors' Management Services, Inc. Resolution Agreement and Corrective Action Plan." https://www.hhs.gov/hipaa/for-professionals/compliance-enforcement/agreements/dms-ra-cap/index.html.

HHS (Department of Health and Human Services). 2022a. "Summary of the HIPAA Privacy Rule." https://www.hhs.gov/hipaa/for-professionals/privacy/laws-regulations/index.html.

HHS (Department of Health and Human Services). 2022b. "Summary of the HIPAA Security Rule." https://www.hhs.gov/hipaa/for-professionals/security/laws-regulations/index.html.

HHS (Department of Health and Human Services). 2022c. "Individuals' Right under HIPAA to Access their Health Information." https://www.hhs.gov/hipaa/for-professionals/privacy/guidance/access/index.html.

HHS (Department of Health and Human Services). 2022d. "Annual Report to Congress on Breaches of Unsecure Protected Health Information for Calendar Year 2021." https://www.hhs.gov/sites/default/files/breach-report-to-congress-2021.pdf.

HHS (Department of Health and Human Services). 2021 (October 7). *Blockchain for Healthcare*. https://www.hhs.gov/sites/default/files/blockchain-for-healthcare-tlpwhite.pdf.

HHS (Department of Health and Human Services). 2017a. "HHS Names Patient Matching Algorithm Challenge Winners." https://www.hhs.gov/about/news/2017/11/08/hhs-names-patient-matching-algorithm-challenge-winners.html.

HHS (Department of Health and Human Services). 2017b. "State Attorney General." https://www.hhs.gov/hipaa/for-professionals/compliance-enforcement/state-attorneys-general/index.html.

HHS (Department of Health and Human Services). 2013. HIPAA Administrative Simplification Regulation Text. https://www.hhs.gov/sites/default/files/ocr/privacy/hipaa/administrative/combined/hipaa-simplification-201303.pdf.

HHS (Department of Health and Human Services). n.d.a. "Notice of Privacy Practices." Accessed October 16, 2024. http://www.hhs.gov/ocr/privacy/hipaa/understanding/consumers/noticepp.html.

HHS (Department of Health and Human Services). n.d.b. "The HIPAA Enforcement Rule." Accessed October 16, 2024. http://www.hhs.gov/ocr/privacy/hipaa/administrative/enforcementrule/index.html.

HHS (Department of Health and Human Services). n.d.c. "Breach Portal: Notice to the Secretary of HHS Breach of Unsecured Protected Health Information." Accessed October 16, 2024. https://ocrportal.hhs.gov/ocr/breach/breach_report.jsf.

HHS (Department of Health and Human Services). n.d.d. "You, Your Organization, and Your Mobile Device." Accessed October 16, 2024. https://www.healthit.gov/topic/privacy-security-and-hipaa/you-your-organization-and-your-mobile-device.

HIMSS (Health Information Management Systems Society). 2023. "Immunization Integration Program (IIP) Collaborative Patient Matching Brief." https://www.himss.org/resources/patient-matching-and-impact-immunization-community.

HealthIt.gov. 2024. *Information Blocking* Actors. https://www.healthit.gov/sites/default/files/2024-04/IB_Actors_Fact_Sheet_508_0.pdf.

HealthIt.gov. n.d.a. "Information Blocking." https://www.healthit.gov/topic/information-blocking.

HealthIt.gov. n.d.b. "ONC's Cures Act Final Rule." https://www.healthit.gov/topic/oncs-cures-act-final-rule.

HealthIT.gov. n.d.c. Cures Act Final Rule: Information Blocking Exceptions. https://www.healthit.gov/sites/default/files/2022-07/InformationBlockingExceptions.pdf.

HealthIT.gov. n.d.d. "HIE Benefits." https://www.healthit.gov/topic/health-it-and-health-information-exchange-basics/hie-benefits.

HealthIT.gov. n.d.e. "Patient Demographics/Information." https://www.healthit.gov/isa/uscdi-data-class/patient-demographicsinformation#uscdi-v3.

HHS 405(d). 2023a. Hospital Cyber Resiliency Initiative Landscape Analysis. https://405d.hhs.gov/Documents/405d-hospital-resiliency-analysis.pdf.

HHS 405(d). 2023b. Health Industry Cybersecurity Practices: Managing Threats and Protecting Patients 2023 Edition. https://405d.hhs.gov/Documents/HICP-Main-508.pdf.

HHS 405(d). 2023c. Health Industry Cybersecurity Practices: Managing Threats and Protecting Patients 2023 Edition. https://405d.hhs.gov/Documents/HICP-Main-508.pdf.

IBM Security. 2023. *Cost of a Data Breach: Report 2023*. https://www.ibm.com/resources/downloads/cost-data-breach-report?

Joint Commission. 2024. "Hospital National Patient Safety Goals." https://www.jointcommission.org/-/media/tjc/documents/standards/national-patient-safety-goals/2024/npsg_chapter_hap_jan2024.pdf.

Landsbach, G. and B. H. Just. 2013. Five risky HIE practices that threaten data integrity. *Journal of AHIMA* 84(11):40–42. http://library.ahima.org/xpedio/groups/public/documents/ahima/bok1_050474.hcsp?dDocName=bok1_050474.

Mello, M. M., J. Adler-Milstein, K. L. Ding, and L. Savage. 2018. Legal barriers to the growth of health information exchange—Boulders or pebbles? *The Milbank Quarterly* 96(1).

NIST (National Institute of Standards and Technology). 2024. "Implementing the Health Insurance Portability and Accountability Act (HIPAA) Security Rule: A Cybersecurity Resource Guide." NIST Special Publication: 800 NIST SP 800-66r2. https://doi.org/10.6028/NIST.SP.800-66r2.

NIST (National Institute of Standards and Technology). 2020. "Guideline for Using Cryptographic Standards in Federal Government: Cryptographic Mechanisms." NIST Special Publication: 800-175B Revision 1. https://nvlpubs.nist.gov/nistpubs/SpecialPublications/NIST.SP.800-175Br1.pdf.

NIST (National Institute of Standards and Technology). n.d. "Blockchain." https://csrc.nist.gov/glossary/term/blockchain.

ONC (Office of the National Coordinator for Health Information Technology). 2015. *Guide to Privacy and Security of Electronic Health Information*. http://www.healthit.gov/sites/default/files/pdf/privacy/privacy-and-security-guide.pdf.

ONC (Office of the National Coordinator for Health Information Technology). n.d.a. Five steps organizations can take to manage mobile devices used by health care providers and professionals. https://www.healthit.gov/topic/privacy-security-and-hipaa/five-steps-organizations-can-take-manage-mobile-devices-used.

ONC (Office of the National Coordinator for Health Information Technology). n.d.b. "Security Risk Assessment Tool." https://www.healthit.gov/topic/privacy-security-and-hipaa/security-risk-assessment-tool.

Posnack, S. 2020 (December 16). "Pssst…Information Blocking Practices, Your Days Are Numbered…Pass It On." https://www.healthit.gov/buzz-blog/information-blocking/pssst-information-blocking-practices-your-days-are-numberedpass-it-on.

Poquiz, W. A. 2022. Blockchain technology in healthcare: An analysis of strengths, weaknesses, opportunities, and threats. *Journal of Healthcare Management* 67(4).

Primeau, D. 2017. How small organizations handle HIPAA compliance. *Journal of AHIMA* 88(4): 18–21. http://library.ahima.org/doc?oid=302074#.XEST5M9KjfY.

Rinehart-Thompson, L. A. 2024. *Health Information Privacy and Security*, 3rd Edition. Chicago: AHIMA.

Revisor of Statutes, State of Minnesota. 2023. Minnesota Health Record Act 144.293: Release and Disclosure of Health records. https://www.revisor.mn.gov/statutes/?id=144.293&format=pdf.

Riplinger, L., J. Piera-Jimenez, and J. P. Dooling. 2020. Patient identification techniques–Approaches, implications and findings. https://www.ncbi.nlm.nih.gov/pmc/articles/PMC7442501/.

Ross, R. 2012. *Guide for Conducting Risk Assessments, Special Publication (NIST SP), National Institute of Standards and Technology* (updated January 27, 2022). Accessed December 10, 2023. https://doi.org/10.6028/NIST.SP.800-30r1.

Stouffer, C. 2021 (August 27). "10 Types of Malware + How to Prevent Malware from the Start." *Norton*. https://us.norton.com/blog/malware/types-of-malware.

42 CFR Part 2 Subpart B: General provision. 2017 (Jan. 18).

42 CFR Part 2 Subpart C: Disclosures with patient consent. 2017 (Jan. 18).

42 CFR Part 2 Subpart D: Disclosures without patient consent. 2017 (Jan. 18).

42 USC 17941. Recognition of security practices (2021).

45 CFR.160.103: Definitions. 2013 (Jan. 25)

45 CFR 160.202: Preemption definitions. 2013 (Jan. 25).

45 CFR 160.401: Imposition of Civil Money Penalties: Definitions. 2013 (Jan. 25).

45 CFR 164.304. Definitions. 2013 (Jan 25).

45 CFR 164.308: Administrative safeguards. 2013 (Jan. 25).

45 CFR 164.312: Technical safeguards. 2013 (Jan. 25).

45 CFR 164.408: Notification to the secretary. 2013 (Jan. 25).

45 CFR 164.501: Privacy of individually identifiable health information definitions. 2013 (Jan. 25).

45 CFR 164.502: Uses and disclosures of protected health information: General rules. 2013 (Jan. 25).

45 CFR 164.504: Uses and disclosures: Organizational requirements. 2013 (Jan. 25).

45 CFR 164.506: Uses and disclosures to carry out treatment, payment, or health care operations. 2013 (Jan. 25).

45 CFR 164.508: Uses and disclosures for which an authorization is required. 2013 (Jan. 25).

45 CFR 164.510: Uses and disclosures requiring an opportunity for the individual to agree or to object. 2013 (Jan. 25).

45 CFR 164.514: Other requirements relating to uses and disclosures of protected health information. 2013 (Jan. 25).

45 CFR 164.520: Notice of privacy practices for protected health information. 2013 (Jan. 25).

45 CFR 164.522: Rights to request privacy protection for protected health information. 2013 (Jan. 25).

45 CFR 164.524: Access of individuals to protected health information. 2013 (Jan. 25).

45 CFR 164.526: Amendment of protected health information. 2013 (Jan. 25).

45 CFR 164.528: Accounting of disclosures of protected health information. 2013 (Jan. 25).

45 CFR 164.530: Administrative requirements. 2013 (Jan. 25).

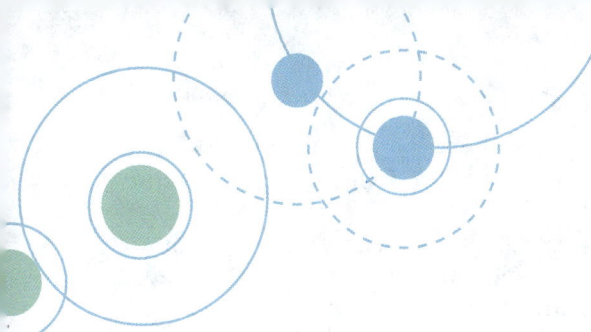

# Clinical Quality Management

*Rosann M. McLean, DHSc, MS, RHIA, CDIP*

## Learning Objectives

- Evaluate quality and performance improvement efforts in healthcare
- Identify current and emerging issues affecting clinical quality
- Evaluate how both internal and external functions and mechanisms influence clinical quality
- Describe tools, measures, and processes used to evaluate and improve clinical quality
- Analyze provider practice requirements related to clinical quality

## Key Terms

Accreditation
Adverse event
Benchmarking
Business continuity plan (BCP)
Care coordination
Case management
Change management
Clinical Laboratory Improvement Amendments (CLIA)
Clinical pathways
Clinical privileges
Contingency Planning
Credentialing
Emergency Medical Treatment and Active Labor Act (EMTALA)
Evidence-based clinical practice guideline
Evidence-based practice
Explicit knowledge
External benchmarking
Health data stewardship

Health Care Quality Improvement Act of 1986 (HCQIA)
Hospital Value-based Purchasing Program
Institute for Healthcare Improvement
Institute of Medicine
Internal benchmarking
Interprofessional education
Leadership
Learning health system
Managed care
Medical malpractice liability
Medicare Prescription Drug, Improvement, and Modernization Act of 2003
National Academy of Medicine
National Practitioner Data Bank (NPDB)
Organizational culture
Outcomes and effectiveness research (OER)

Patient Protection and Affordable Care Act of 2020 (ACA)
Peer review
Performance
Performance improvement
Performance measures
Plan-do-check-act (PDCA)
Quality
Quality indicators
Quality management
Quality professional
Regulation
Remote patient monitoring device
Risk management
Root cause analysis
Sentinel event
Tacit knowledge
Tracer methodology
Triple Aim
Value-based payments

Quality management and performance improvement are important concepts in the delivery of healthcare services. In healthcare literature, a definition of **quality** is "the degree to which health services for individuals and populations increase the likelihood of desired health outcomes and are consistent with current professional knowledge" (IOM 2001). Healthcare quality is influenced by a variety of factors, including effective and knowledgeable clinicians and staff, processes and systems that support patient care, engaged leaders, and the ongoing evaluation of clinical care to identify opportunities for improvement.

**Quality management** refers to the evaluation of the quality of healthcare services and delivery using standards and guidelines developed by various entities, including the government and independent accreditation organizations. It includes efforts to assess, measure, and evaluate the quality of care provided to patients. Quality management is interprofessional and multidisciplinary in nature, and no single health profession is solely responsible. Instead, quality management is the responsibility of all health professionals. Emerging healthcare professionals should appreciate that upon entering the healthcare workforce, their daily work is influenced by organizational efforts, initiatives, and requirements focused on quality management. Quality management efforts produce data and information to assist an organization and its units of operation with understanding how well it performs any given task or function; these efforts provide an objective mechanism to identify opportunities for improvement. Effective quality management programs include a complimentary focus on performance improvement.

Defined in a basic sense, **performance** is the execution of a task. In the context of clinical care, a complex assortment of actions, tasks, decisions, and functions occur involving a multidisciplinary and interprofessional team of health professionals. The complex nature of patient care is precisely why quality is managed and opportunities to improve performance are identified. Without concerted focus on quality and performance in healthcare organizations, little would be known about outcomes of care or patient satisfaction. **Performance improvement** refers to the continuous study and adaptation of a healthcare organization's functions and processes to increase the likelihood of achieving desired outcomes.

Today's healthcare environment is increasingly driven by stakeholder expectations for safe and effective care. All the while, numerous policy changes, regulations, and the need to reduce costs influence day-to-day operations in healthcare. Health information professionals must possess an understanding of quality management and performance improvement, as well as the context of their professional contributions and roles in these areas. This chapter examines historical and current trends related to quality; considers the role of organizational influence and uses of tools and processes to affect quality and performance; describes professional certifications and roles related to healthcare quality; and discusses emerging topics influencing health service provision and quality.

## Historical Perspectives in Healthcare Quality

Patient care should be provided with a focus on quality. In the context of the entire history of medicine and healthcare, quality management is a more recent development. A lack of focus on quality was not because of a historical disregard for patients. Instead, the evolution of science and technology brought forth an understanding that certain protocols and evidence-based approaches reduce the risk of death, injury, and unfavorable outcomes among patients.

### Patient Safety Concerns Emerge

Some of the most significant threats to quality of care stem from infections and the lack of infection control processes. For example, surgical procedures were noted as occurring hundreds of years before risks of infection were understood and even before anesthesia was available (Alexander 1985, 423–424). It was not until the mid-18th century that pioneers in medicine and nursing began to identify infections as primary culprits to unfavorable patient care outcomes.

As an increasing body of knowledge emerged about opportunities to reduce mortality in healthcare settings in the early 1900s, the American College of Surgeons (ACS)—a professional association of surgeons formed to improve the quality of surgical care—began advocating for sweeping changes to healthcare in the US. By the 1920s, the ACS championed a variety of initiatives to improve healthcare. These included recommendations that complete health records be created and maintained for all patients, implementation of peer-review processes, and the development of uniform approaches to medical education (ACS n.d.). The need for a health record of each patient is underscored by the importance of clinical documentation therein, which depicts the care and treatment provided and complications or other factors arising from this care and treatment, all of which assist in evaluating care quality and reducing medical errors. Related to patient safety, an accurate and complete record is necessary to ensure care provided to patients is clearly documented, communication among the care team is depicted, and other factors about the patient's health status are evident to the care team. These factors are important in ensuring appropriate care is provided to any given patient based on their individual health status and risk factors. Peer review, described later in this chapter, provides an objective evaluation of healthcare professional performance. Improvements in medical education, such as standardized curriculum and requirements, provided a mechanism to better ensure physicians were prepared to safely practice medicine.

## Legal Implications Related to Quality of Care

Following the conclusion of World War II, healthcare services in the US became more expansive to support a growing population. As US healthcare infrastructure grew, it developed initially with limited regulatory requirements or standards. Legal issues and liability related to patient care were among the earliest indicators that an increased focus on quality would inform the future of American healthcare.

One court case discussed in educational, healthcare, and legal venues is *Darling v. Charleston Community Memorial Hospital*, for which a final decision was rendered in appellate court in 1965 (Wiet 2005, 402–403). In *Darling*, a young man broke his leg while playing football. Upon receiving emergency services and being admitted to Charleston Community Memorial Hospital, a series of clinical errors and miscommunication among Darling's care team ensued. The young man who entered the hospital with a broken leg was later transferred to another hospital because of a series of errors, including an unidentified infection of the broken leg inside a cast and inadequate oversight in care processes by improperly trained clinicians who directed care decisions. This resulted in extensive necrosis and damage to the leg requiring specialty care at an academic medical center. After a series of surgical procedures performed at the receiving hospital, the leg could not be restored and required amputation (*Darling v. Charleston* 1965).

*Darling* was a landmark case in healthcare law because the final legal judgment found both the treating physician as well as Charleston Community Memorial Hospital liable for the harm caused to Darling. Prior to *Darling*, never in the history of medical malpractice liability had a healthcare organization been held legally responsible for clinical errors occurring in the care of a patient. **Medical malpractice liability** refers to instances where a civil claim for damages against a healthcare provider successfully proves that the provider was negligent in their care of the patient leading to injury or death. From this point forward, a legal precedent was set that healthcare organizations and healthcare professionals had a shared responsibility for patient care and safety, and healthcare organizations were no longer immune to liability for medical errors occurring within the walls of a healthcare facility (Wiet 2005, 403–405). Drivers of quality and safety in patient care began to develop, such as federal requirements and regulations, accreditation standards, and quality and safety advocacy groups.

## Toward Systematic Quality and Performance Initiatives

While the *Darling* case was underway in 1965, another significant change occurred in the US healthcare system. Title XIX of the Social Security Amendments of 1965 (Public Law 89–97) created the Medicare and Medicaid programs—the former providing health insurance coverage to Americans aged 65 and older as well as those with disabilities and certain medical conditions, and the latter providing insurance coverage to low-income individuals and families. As the Medicare and Medicaid programs became operational and began providing insurance coverage to populations with unique vulnerabilities, a variety of standards and requirements were set forth by the federal government to promote safe care environments for Medicare and Medicaid beneficiaries. While providers and healthcare entities providing services to beneficiaries must adhere to numerous regulations, the baseline requirements stem from the Conditions of Participation (CoPs). These conditions are those that "healthcare organizations must meet in order to begin and continue participating in the Medicare and Medicaid programs" (CMS 2023a). These conditions describe the administrative and operational guidelines and regulations under which facilities are allowed to take part in the Medicare and Medicaid programs; they are published by the Centers for Medicare and Medicaid Services (CMS), a federal agency under the Department of Health and Human Services (42 CFR 482).

The CoPs are health and safety standards for each applicable provider setting. The following types of healthcare organizations are subject to CoPs created specifically for the respective settings:

- Ambulatory surgical centers
- Community mental health centers
- Comprehensive outpatient rehabilitation facilities

- Critical access hospitals
- End-stage renal disease facilities
- Federally qualified health centers
- Home health agencies
- Hospices
- Hospitals
- Hospital swing beds
- Intermediate care facilities for individuals with intellectual disabilities
- Organ procurement organizations
- Portable x-ray suppliers
- Programs for all-inclusive care for the elderly organizations
- Clinics, rehabilitation agencies, and public health agencies as providers of outpatient physical therapy and speech-language pathology services
- Psychiatric hospitals
- Religious nonmedical healthcare institutions
- Rural health clinics
- Long-term care facilities
- Transplant centers (CMS 2023a)

Manuals that define applicable standards by healthcare setting are available on the CMS website (CMS 2023a). These standards address multiple topics ranging from environment of care standards to health record requirements. The standards required of healthcare organizations accepting Medicare and Medicaid patients help ensure that all aspects of an organization focus on quality management to promote a safe care environment for patients and promote clinical documentation as a mechanism to capture factual details about care provided.

Another driving influence on quality management in healthcare includes the patient advocacy movement, which arose because of the recognition that patients are due certain rights in their pursuit of health services. In 1973, the American Hospital Association published *A Patient's Bill of Rights* to frame the rights of patients receiving hospital-based care and treatment; this bill of rights also addressed expectations of patient-provider relationships (Olejarczyk and Young 2024). The current iteration of the previously mentioned bill of rights is known as the *Patient Care Partnership* (AHA n.d.). Because the intent of the *Patient Care Partnership* is to demonstrate the rights and responsibilities of patients in their pursuit of quality healthcare services, many hospitals share the *Patient Care Partnership* with patients as a brochure, as signage in heavy traffic areas of the facility, or posted on their website.

Patient advocacy, driven by healthcare consumers, commonly focuses on promoting safety. One example is an organization known as Consumers Advancing Patient Safety, which "envisions a partnership between consumers and providers to create global healthcare systems that are safe, compassionate, and just" (Consumers Advancing Patient Safety 2017). Another such organization is the Josie King Foundation, whose "mission is to prevent patients from dying or being harmed by medical error" (Josie King Foundation n.d.). As patients increasingly voice concerns about medical harm, third-party payers for health services are also vocal about quality in patient care.

Changes in health insurance plans, especially those in the 1970s related to managed care models, introduced new stakeholder expectations and emphases related to healthcare quality. Managed care is a payment method in which the third-party payer has implemented some provisions to control the costs of healthcare while maintaining quality. An early example of a managed care model are health maintenance organizations (HMOs), which came about following the passage of the Health Maintenance Organization Act of 1973. This legislation provided federal funding in the exploratory implementation HMOs. The government believed that HMOs, through their emphasis on patient referrals to specialists occurring only at the request of primary care physicians and predetermined fixed rates of prepayment to providers, had the ability to influence healthcare delivery by lowering costs and increasing quality. Under the Act, organizations receiving funding to establish HMOs were required to have a quality assurance program that "must emphasize health outcomes and provide for physician review and for review by other health professionals" (SSA 1974, 37).

In the 1990s and 2000s, patient safety was a forefront topic in American healthcare. An increasing body of evidence suggested that healthcare delivery was suboptimal at best (IOM 2003, 2001). Various challenges existed within healthcare, such as high rates of patient safety issues, lacking mechanisms for care coordination, increasingly high healthcare expenditures, and inequity in access to health services.

Originally known as the Institute of Medicine (IOM) and established in 1970, the present-day National Academy of Medicine, a branch of the National Academy of Sciences, exists "to advance science, inform policy, and catalyze action to achieve human health, equity, and well-being" (National Academy of Medicine n.d.). During the 1990s, the then IOM collaborated with healthcare quality and patient safety experts to conduct an exhaustive analysis of the US healthcare system (IOM 2001). At the time, there was an awareness about medical errors, but little was occurring systematically to improve safety in healthcare. The first publication related to the IOM's work was titled *To Err Is Human: Building a Safer Health System*. This publication was an eye-opening analysis of the numbers of lives lost and billions of dollars wasted in US healthcare due to ineffective care and processes causing harm to patients. It became increasingly evident that until safety improved, quality of care would remain lackluster (Kohn et al. 2000).

The healthcare industry took note, and the IOM continued advocacy efforts for improved patient safety as a mechanism to enhance clinical quality. By 2001, the IOM followed up its previous work with a publication titled, *Crossing the Quality Chasm: A New Health System for the 21st Century* (IOM 2001). This publication was a formal call for complete redesign of the US healthcare system. Redesign in this context was not a roadmap for healthcare organizations. Instead, IOM recommendations centered on approaching healthcare from a "new perspective on the purpose and aims of the healthcare system, how patients and clinicians should relate, and how care processes can be designed to optimize responsiveness to patient needs" (IOM 2001). The IOM findings were timely because healthcare industry stakeholders, legislators, and health policy specialists were increasingly concerned that the current infrastructure of US healthcare delivery was not sustainable and left room for improvement. The IOM offered evidence about the shortcomings suspected by most stakeholder groups and its findings provided a basis for informed dialogue about necessary improvements and opportunities.

*Crossing the Quality Chasm: A New Health System for the 21st Century* outlined that healthcare ought to be safe, effective, patient-centered, timely, efficient, and equitable (IOM 2001). Its authors argue that 10 redesign components are necessary for improvements in patient safety and clinical quality to occur:

1. Care should be based on continuous healing relationships.
2. Care should be customized to align with individual patient preferences and values.
3. The patient should serve as the central source of control on the care team.
4. Information should flow freely to bolster knowledge and communication.
5. Decision-making ought to be evidence-based.
6. The healthcare system should focus on safety as a hallmark priority.
7. Increased transparency is needed.
8. Needs of patients should be anticipated versus addressed reactively.
9. Waste should be consistently and continuously decreased.
10. Collaboration and cooperation among clinicians is essential. (IOM 2001)

Around the year 2015, when the IOM became the NAM, the focus of the organization expanded. While at one time, the organization focused near exclusively on patient safety and health system redesign, its present strategic plan encompasses goals related to application and advancement of science in health and medicine, action on issues related to society and health, health system transformation, equity, and national readiness for the future of health and medicine (NAM n.d., 3–9). Inherent to the NAM's current goals and strategic plan are elements which pertain to patient safety and healthcare quality.

Another organization that has continuously influenced healthcare quality is the **Institute for Healthcare Improvement (IHI)**, a healthcare improvement organization that focuses on the "values of courage, love, equity, and trust to improve health and health care worldwide so that everyone has the best care and health possible" (IHI n.d.a). The IHI has worked on a variety of issues in healthcare and presently frames their efforts as improvement areas. Patient safety is one improvement area. The concept of the **Triple Aim** is another. The Triple Aim indicates that vast and systematic improvements are needed to improve experiences for patients in their pursuit of healthcare, enhance health among the population, and lower per capita costs (IHI n.d.b).

## Today's Drivers of Healthcare Quality

Healthcare today is delivered with a keen focus on quality. Rarely does a new healthcare regulation or policy occur at the national level without significant quality elements at its core. While concepts, initiatives, and groups influence quality management efforts such as those previously described, a few key drivers are introduced as particularly noteworthy at the present, such as accreditation standards, regulatory requirements, advocacy groups focused on safe and effective care, quality indicator reporting and transparency, value-based payment efforts, and consumer engagement from patients.

## Accreditation Standards

**Accreditation** refers to a voluntary process of organizational review in which an independent body created for this purpose periodically evaluates the quality of the entity's work against preestablished written criteria. Although seeking and maintaining accreditation for a healthcare facility or specific programs within a facility is optional, there are compelling reasons to do so. For example, accreditation is one way to demonstrate a commitment to quality and continuous improvement to patients, communities, and other stakeholders. Additionally, accreditation is a pathway for ongoing participation in the Medicare and Medicaid programs. Regardless of the accrediting body, the healthcare organization must meet standards to illustrate organizational compliance with an array of requirements related to patient safety, the environment of care, information management and governance, medical staff obligations, staffing, and others.

In today's environment, a healthcare organization cannot avoid undertaking accreditation. Stakeholder groups that expect healthcare organizations to be accredited include third-party payers, professional liability insurance providers, healthcare professionals, and patients, to name a few. Accreditation is worth its investment because it helps portray a healthcare organization as committed to meeting high standards, and accreditation status can be used in marketing strategies to attract patients. In addition, as previously noted, accreditation is a pathway for healthcare organizations to maintain their participation in the Medicare and Medicaid programs. The federal government is the largest single payer for health services in the US. Because many patients are covered with insurance through programs such as Medicare and Medicaid, it makes strategic and business sense for a healthcare organization to accept patients with such insurance coverage or else they would lose a large market share of patients. It should be understood, however, that being an accredited healthcare organization does not automatically indicate excellence in patient care is achieved without quality issues arising. Instead, accreditation illustrates a commitment of striving to meet standards that promote quality and safety in patient care. See table 11.1 for examples, although not a complete listing, of accreditation organizations for a variety of facility types.

## Regulatory Requirements

Various federal regulations influence healthcare. A **regulation** is a rule established by an administrative agency of government. All federal regulations affecting healthcare stem from federal law, including the following examples:

- **Emergency Medical Treatment and Active Labor Act (EMTALA)**, which was enacted to "ensure public access to emergency services regardless of ability to pay" (CMS 2024a)
- **Clinical Laboratory Improvement Amendments (CLIA)**, which was enacted to "ensure quality laboratory testing" (CMS 2024b)

**Table 11.1.** Examples of accreditation organizations

| Name of accreditation organization | Description |
| --- | --- |
| Joint Commission | An independent, not-for-profit organization, the Joint Commission accredits and certifies more than 22,000 healthcare organizations and programs in the United States. Joint Commission accreditation and certification is recognized nationwide as a symbol of quality that reflects an organization's commitment to meeting certain performance standards (Joint Commission n.d.a.). |
| Accreditation Association for Ambulatory Health Care (AAAHC) | A professional organization that offers accreditation programs for ambulatory and outpatient organizations such as single-specialty and multispecialty group practices, ambulatory surgery centers, college/university health services, and community health centers (AAAHC n.d.) |
| American College of Radiology (ACR) | The ACR accredits radiology facilities and offers specialty accreditations in breast ultrasound, computed tomography, mammography, magnetic resonance imaging, nuclear medicine and position emission tomography, radiation oncology practice, stereotactic breast biopsy, and ultrasound (American College of Radiology n.d.) |
| Commission on Accreditation of Rehabilitation Facilities (CARF) | An international, independent, nonprofit accreditor of health and human services that develops customer-focused standards for areas such as behavioral healthcare, aging services, child and youth services, and medical rehabilitation programs and accredits such programs based on its standards (CARF n.d.) |
| DNV | Provides hospital accreditation services to acute care, critical access, and psychiatric hospitals (DNV n.d.) |

- **Medicare Prescription Drug, Improvement, and Modernization Act of 2003**, which was enacted to provide prescription drug coverage within the Medicare Program and to modernize the Medicare Program with additional options to better support Medicare beneficiaries (Medicare Prescription Drug, Improvement, and Modernization Act 2003).
- Health Information Technology for Economic and Clinical Health (HITECH) Act, which was created to promote the adoption and meaningful use of health information technology (HIT). It also provides for additional privacy and security requirements. These requirements will develop and support electronic health information, facilitate information exchange, and strengthen monetary penalties (Public Law 111-5 2009).
- **Patient Protection and Affordable Care Act of 2020 (ACA)**, which was enacted to reform healthcare. It was designed to increase the rate of health insurance coverage for Americans and reducing the overall costs of healthcare (Public Law 111-148 2010).

When considering each of the previously mentioned federal laws, two things are noticeable. The first is that the major issue addressed in each one is unique from the others. The second is that each includes requirements pertaining to quality or safety, which in turn influences healthcare organizations' quality management undertakings. Healthcare workers should continue to expect quality-related requirements embedded into forthcoming laws and regulations as various stakeholders—such as patients and their families, payers, advocacy groups, regulators, and accreditation organizations—expect that safety and effectiveness in care is achieved and continues to improve.

As the costs of healthcare continue to soar (CMS 2023c), room for improvement exists throughout the healthcare system; advocates and researchers argue that a total systems approach to safety is necessary rather than continuing to only focus on specific safety topics (IHI 2022). There are also growing expectations from advocacy groups and government agencies that science and technology support improved quality when used intelligently and in accordance with established evidence-based guidelines (AHRQ n.d.b).

## Quality Indicator Reporting and Transparency

Quality indicators are reported from healthcare providers and organizations to various government agencies, nonprofit organizations, accreditation bodies, and payers to illustrate performance with meeting quality measures. **Quality indicators** are standards against which actual care may be measured to identify a level of performance for that standard. When healthcare organizations collect quality indicator data, the data are analyzed internally for performance improvement benchmarking. When the data are reported to external bodies, external stakeholders also use the data to evaluate and compare healthcare providers and organizations.

A significant amount of quality-related data is available online for public viewing. See table 11.2 for a list of sources of publicly available quality indicator data.

**Table 11.2.** Sources of publicly available quality indicator data

| Organization name | Organization website | Overview of quality indicator data provided |
|---|---|---|
| Centers for Medicare and Medicaid Services (CMS) | https://www.medicare.gov/care-compare/ | Quality data reported from various healthcare settings to the Medicare program as required by law. Examples of quality data available for consumers to review include readmission rates, infection rates, staff-to-patient ratios, and patient satisfaction scores. |
| The Leapfrog Group | https://www.hospitalsafetygrade.org/ | Quality data submitted voluntarily from hospitals to the Leapfrog Group. Examples of data available include details on the use of computerized medication ordering, presence of specialty trained ICU physicians, processes used to avoid harm, management of errors when they occur, maternity care, high-risk surgeries, and hospital-acquired conditions. |
| National Committee on Quality Assurance (NCQA) | https://www.ncqa.org/hedis/health-plan-ratings/ | Quality data about health plans (including public and private insurance plans) regarding quality of care received by patients, patient satisfaction, and health plan efforts related to performance improvement. |

A healthcare organization's willingness to be transparent in sharing quality-related data is important. Healthcare professionals, patients, and policy makers alike recognize the public has the right to transparent data about healthcare providers and organizations, so they are most informed as patients and consumers.

## Value-Based Care Reforms

Payment for healthcare services by third-party payers has been based more on the quantity of services provided instead of the quality of care rendered. This model offers little incentive for improved quality and is an ineffective use of limited financial resources available to pay for health services. A variety of value-based care models are currently in use or being explored. Accountable care organizations are an example of a value-based care model; although they vary in specifics, accountable care organizations aim to avoid fee-for-service reimbursement for patient care, rely on voluntary membership and coordination of patient care among groups of clinicians and healthcare facilities, and emphasize avoidance of duplicative tests and procedures.

Value-based care methods focus on paying for quality in patient care versus quantity. **Value-based payments** can be thought of as any method of healthcare reimbursement that either financially incentivizes providers for good quality and outcomes or penalizes providers for inadequate quality and unfavorable outcomes. In the Hospital Value-Based Purchasing Program, an example of value-based payments, acute-care hospitals are eligible to earn incentive payments for the quality of patient care provided. This program allows Medicare to adjust payments to hospitals through the Inpatient-Prospective Payment System, a Medicare program reimbursement methodology. This program emphasizes improved quality of care and hospitalization experiences for patients with Medicare (CMS 2023d).

The previously described reimbursement methods will continue to influence quality management efforts throughout healthcare. In an environment where payment is increasingly linked to the quality of care instead of the quantity of care provided, healthcare organizations and providers must increasingly focus their efforts on enhanced quality and performance or experience significant losses in revenue. This paradigm shift in payment also challenges the current healthcare system to move toward more continuous follow-up and engagement with patients after they complete an episode of care to ensure their needs are met and their health is positively progressing.

## The Patient as a Consumer

Patients are increasingly more savvy consumers of healthcare and are essential influencers on healthcare quality. The internet provides unfiltered access for a patient to compare providers and insurance plans, and to research any healthcare topic for which they have an interest. In a competitive healthcare market, the stakes are higher for healthcare providers and organizations to attract and retain patients. One way healthcare providers and organizations attract patients is to be known for excellence in clinical quality and patient safety. While accreditation is one way to become known for quality and safety, healthcare providers and organizations can also increase their community engagement activities and patient outreach efforts to maintain a good reputation. Because the influences on clinical quality are growing, healthcare organizations must continually focus on quality management.

### Check Your Understanding 11.1

**Answer the following questions in a separate document.**

1. The nurse manager in the oncology unit noticed a delay in receiving medications from the pharmacy during the afternoon shift. She scheduled a meeting with a representative from the pharmacy, the charge nurse for the afternoon shift on that floor, and the health unit coordinator. What term best describes this scenario?
   a. Quality
   b. Quality management
   c. Performance
   d. Performance improvement

2. A patient on a nursing unit of a hospital falls while using the bathroom unattended. A review of facts after the incident shows that the patient was not correctly assessed or determined to be at risk for falls, and therefore fall risk protocols were not used with the patient. Legal action is brought against the physician in charge of her care. Can legal action be brought against the hospital, and could it possibly be liable? Please explain.

3. Which of the following is an example of an adverse event?
   a. A patient develops a post-operative surgical site infection.
   b. A nurse administers an ordered medication to a patient and the patient has a severe allergic reaction to the medication.
   c. A patient developed a pressure ulcer on their hip during an inpatient hospitalization.
   d. All the above could be considered an adverse event.

4. Why is accreditation important?
    a. Maintaining accreditation demonstrates an organizational commitment to quality.
    b. Maintaining accreditation is one way to remain eligible to treat Medicare and Medicaid patients.
    c. In recent years, it has been argued that accreditation is not that important.
    d. Answer choices a and b are both correct answers.

5. Physician reimbursement is slightly reduced by a payer because the physician's patients' score fell below an expected measurement on outcomes measures. Describe how this is a value-based care scenario.

## Organizational Influence on Healthcare Quality

Everything within an organization is interrelated; the sum of all its parts influences the whole of an organization. One way to consider this is to imagine a hospital in which every employee might indicate on a survey that they are committed to safe and effective care. However, if these same employees work for an organization that does not truly embrace within its culture a commitment to safety and quality, clinical quality will be difficult to achieve, and quality management efforts will appear futile. An organization and its members must wholeheartedly embrace quality and performance improvement throughout the enterprise for it to be a meaningful undertaking. Organizational mission and vision, leadership, organizational culture, interprofessional education and practice, change management, and risk management play roles in influencing quality and performance improvement.

### Organizational Mission and Vision

The mission and vision of an organization represent more than words depicted in marketing content or organizational reference materials. The purpose (or mission) of an organization and how it hopes to exist in the future (the organization's vision), are necessary areas of understanding for employees and providers within an organization. In the example of healthcare organizations, it is common for mission and vision statements to indicate quality as a tenet. What is sometimes overlooked about mission and vision statements is that for them to have any meaning, the statements must be conducted daily within the organization and embraced by staff and providers at all levels of the organization.

A mission statement defines an organization's core philosophies and purpose for existing, whereas a vision statement refers to what an organization sees as its ideal future state.

An example of a mission and vision statement follows:

- *Mission*: Above all else, we are committed to the care and improvement of human life.
- *Vision*: Together, we will be the premier healthcare destination for all we serve (Overland Park Regional Medical Center n.d.)

Organizational mission and vision relate to quality in that they go beyond being statements advertised to the public. Instead, mission and vision are created based on the organizational goals, strategic initiatives, and organizational culture. In the previous example statements, the mission succinctly articulates that the organization commits itself to the care and improvement of human life, and the vision articulates that the organization hopes to become a premier destination for patients to seek health services. If the mission and vision are carried out and pursued daily in all areas of a healthcare organization, quality is more tangible and achievable. While everyone within an organization must share in the commitment to quality, those in formal and informal leadership positions play essential roles in inspiring organizational commitment to quality.

### Influence of Leadership

**Leadership** is the "activity of guiding a group of people to a definite result" (Kelly and Greenstone 2019, 913). Leadership occurs within organizations through two primary groups of leaders. These groups include those in formal management roles who are expected to provide leadership because of their position in the organization, as well as personnel from all ranks of the organization who naturally exhibit leadership qualities and are regarded as leaders by their peers.

Managers in healthcare organizations have the authority and obligation to commit to quality and safety as core values. Leadership actions should embed themes of safe, equitable, and reliable care within organizational mission, professional core competencies, and workplace standards (IHI 2022, 6). Because the management infrastructure of hospitals and other types of healthcare organizations is uniquely complex, individuals designated as managers within these organizations are most effective when they possess leadership attributes and skills. Without them, managers likely find themselves unable to influence staff and provider commitment to quality.

As previously mentioned, there are also leaders within organizations without a formal job title placing them in a leadership role. They may, however, have considerable influence on and respect from others. Considering the aims of quality management and related performance improvement, it is evident why leadership from within all ranks and titles in a healthcare organization is essential. Healthcare professionals often relate well to their peers, and leadership demonstrated among peers provides a respected avenue and basis to improve collaboration and efforts focused on improved clinical quality.

## Organizational Culture

An organization's mission and vision, leadership influence, and human resources work in concert to inform the organizational culture. The culture may have many attributes and can change over time. Organizational culture refers to an organization's norms, beliefs, and values. It is what is felt by staff on any given day that is intangible but influences how employees feel about their job and the environment in which they perform it. In relationship to quality in patient care, the ability for staff to perform duties with a focus on quality is in part dependent on working in an environment that is positive, supports goals of excellence, and promotes teamwork.

## Interprofessional Education and Practice

Historically, when healthcare professionals provided their services to patients in patient care settings, the various health professions worked in silos, meaning they worked in isolation from one another. While these types of challenges remain, there are efforts underway to reshape the ways health professionals work together and view one another's contributions to patient care. The IOM was one of the first organizations to vocalize that having silos in place, which prevent connecting all the moving parts of clinical care, is unacceptable. Released in 2003, the report *Health Professions Education: A Bridge to Quality* called for changes to education in the health professions (IOM 2003). The premise of this publication centers on the need for enhanced opportunities for health professions students to receive education alongside their peers in other specializations to promote teamwork. This approach to education also allows for those entering the healthcare workforce to better understand the various professions versus only possessing an understanding of one's own professional role (IOM 2003).

Collaboration and teamwork among the various health professions can positively influence quality and safety in patient care. For this reason, many bodies responsible for accrediting academic programs in the health professions now incorporate standards requiring interprofessional education into the curriculum. Interprofessional education occurs when "two or more professions learn about, from, and with each other to enable effective collaboration to improve health outcomes" (WHO 2010, 15).

A benefit to introducing interprofessional education to students is that they can enter the workforce and influence it by implementing interprofessional practice into daily work. Without interprofessional teamwork, clinical quality is compromised in a variety of ways. If those working for the care of a patient do not understand how all the needs of the patient are met, this diminishes the ability to provide optimal care. Lacking teamwork also negatively influences communication among the variety of professionals who support and provide patient care. Organizations that promote teamwork and interprofessional practice are often noted as experiencing less staff turnover. More consistency among staff and reduced turnover leads to a team of professionals more comfortable with each other and familiar with internal processes in the care of patients. In healthcare organizations that have not achieved interprofessionalism, silos can be broken down, and change management techniques offer approaches to do so.

## Change Management

Change management is the formal process of introducing change, getting it adopted, and diffusing it throughout the organization. Effectively instituting change can be challenging, and some aspects of change management relate to psychology and behavior. Change presents potential challenges among staff because even if change is needed, the idea of change can be perceived as counterintuitive to the basic need for humans to feel stable in their environment (Nilsen et al. 2020). While there is widespread understanding among healthcare stakeholders that change is needed to improve quality and safety, progress toward these improvements seems slow at times. Evidence is mounting that current ways of working in healthcare must change to actualize needed improvements. Increased expectations for the healthcare industry to improve quality, safety, and value exist from various influential stakeholders including state and federal governments, accreditation organizations, and third-party payers. If an organization cannot improve quality and patient care, or meet the varied expectations previously noted, the organization risks lost funding or reduced reimbursement and can lose its accredited status.

In some organizations, a culture that embraces quality forms naturally. Other organizations may experience challenges in achieving a culture that that supports consistent execution of high-quality patient care due to limitations in leadership and staff morale. Regardless of the organization, to maintain an existing culture or initiate a new culture focused on quality, ongoing change management techniques may be useful.

## Risk Management

Risk is the possibility of a bad or good event occurring, and the purpose of a risk management program is to protect an organization and its assets against negative risks, including accidental losses. **Risk management** is a comprehensive program of activities intended to minimize the potential for injuries to occur in a facility and to anticipate and respond to ensuring liability for those injuries that do occur. Present-day healthcare organizations operate under this comprehensive approach to managing risks focused on investigative and compliance strategies to reduce future risk, protect organizational assets, and negate major financial losses.

To appreciate the scope of risk concerns in healthcare, there are eight categories of risk and associated considerations impacting healthcare organizations to consider. Operational risks often result from inadequate or failed internal processes, people, or systems. Clinical and patient safety risks may include failure to follow evidence-based practice guidelines, medication errors, hospital-acquired conditions, and serious safety events. Strategic risks arise when an organization heads in a strategic direction that does not meet the needs of stakeholders. These risks are associated with reputation, competition, healthcare reform, ability to adapt to change, and customer priorities. Financial risks affect the organization's financial sustainability. They include losses arising from malpractice, litigation, insurance premiums, lack of adequate revenue, and various financial concerns. Human capital risks are associated with workforce including staffing, retention and turnover, absenteeism, work-related injuries, and productivity, among others. Legal and regulatory risks include failure to identify and manage legal, regulatory, and statutory mandates on the local, state, and federal levels. These risks are associated with fraud and abuse, accreditation, and licensure. Technology risks include those related to hardware, software, and systems including the use of technology for clinical diagnosis and treatment, information storage and retrieval, and education and training. Hazards are risks to assets such as facility infrastructure and may occur due to human-created events or natural or natural disasters (ASHRM n.d.).

When a risk-producing incident occurs, prompt and accurate reporting is critical. An incident report is used to record these occurrences in detail. In these reports, it is important to capture any dates, times, and locations of incident occurrences. Each incident report is reviewed individually or used to create report data that is tabulated and analyzed to identify trends and establish probable cause. Tabulated incident report data can include types of occurrences, severity of the injuries, frequencies and patterns, demographics, and effectiveness of corrective measures. Incident reporting within a healthcare organization occurs within the framework of established policies and procedures. These policies and procedures address factors such as events that must be reported, the reporting process, and identification of the reporting channels.

While many types of incidents are reported, examples of common reportable events include patient complaints, medication errors, security incidents, and adverse events. An **adverse event** is when a medical event causes injury (AHRQ n.d.a). It is a clinical and patient safety risk in which the care or treatment provided to a patient produces an unanticipated and unfavorable outcome or injury. A patient developing a postoperative surgical site infection while in the hospital is one example of an adverse event. Adverse events are subject to an organization's reporting policies. Often, reporting occurs through the organization's risk management reporting system to determine if additional review or steps are necessary to remedy the situation and prevent its recurrence.

All reportable risk incidents are evaluated by all parties within the organization that have a stake or role in the incident. The most serious type of incident which can occur in healthcare is a *sentinel event*. A **sentinel event** is an unexpected occurrence involving death or serious physical or psychological injury, or the risk thereof. Such events are called "sentinel" because they signal the need for immediate investigation and response (Joint Commission n.d.b). In healthcare risk management, the occurrence of a sentinel event triggers a process known as a *root cause analysis*. A **root cause analysis** is an analysis of a sentinel event from all aspects (human, procedural, machinery, material) to identify how each contributed to the occurrence of the event and to develop new systems that will prevent recurrence.

## Business Continuity and Contingency

In times of crisis or unexpected emergencies beyond a healthcare facility's control, its ability to continue patient care services (ideally uninterrupted) is essential and has a relationship to care quality and patient safety. Healthcare organizations must proactively evaluate how patient care and business practices will continue during unexpected situations. Contingency planning is one tool to evaluate and plan accordingly. **Contingency planning** is one component of a broader emergency preparedness process that includes an understanding of business practices, operational continuity requirements, and disaster recovery planning (HHS n.d.). A comprehensive contingency plan needs to highlight potential vulnerabilities and threats as well as identify the approaches to either prevent them or, at least, minimize the impact. There are three major categories or types of threats:

- Natural threats (for example, floods or earthquakes)
- Technical/manmade (that is, mechanical, biological, or the like)
- Intentional acts (namely, terrorism, computer security, and such) (HHS n.d.)

Contingency planning includes processes to follow to continue normal business operations in any emergency situation. The National Institute of Standards and Technology (NIST) Special Publication SP800-34 defines seven components to a viable contingency planning program. HHS identifies that the following NIST steps are "to be integrated throughout a project's life cycle to help guide stakeholders in the planning, development, implementation, key success factors and maintenance of contingency plans" (HHS n.d.):

1. Identify specific regulatory requirements related to contingency planning.
2. Conduct a business impact analysis to prioritize critical systems, business processes, and components.
3. Identify and implement preventive controls and measures.
4. Develop recovery strategies.
5. Develop contingency plans with guidance and procedures.
6. Plan and implement testing and training to both validate and identify gaps, as well as prepare staff.
7. Maintain contingency plans, updating regularly.

The goal is to become a resilient organization that can continue its mission-essential functions during any type of disruption. The core of HIM principles, such as managing records and maintaining confidentiality, are at risk during disasters.

One key component of planning for a disaster includes the development of a **business continuity plan (BCP)** which incorporates policies and procedures for continuing business operations during computer system downtime. This plan covers downtime, disaster recovery, and backup procedures. The overall goal of the plan is to reduce interruptions while lessening the impact on the organization's ability to carry out its mission and to remain in compliance with laws and regulations.

## Quality Management Tools and Processes

While an organization itself has influence on clinical quality, it is important to appreciate the ongoing processes and mechanisms that support operational oversight of quality. It is also crucial to determine the level of quality through identified performance measures, developed and used both internally and externally, and to generate knowledge from the results of such measurements. Process improvement methodologies such as the plan-do-check-act (PDCA) cycle, peer review, and the Joint Commission's tracer methodology are all tools that identify, address, monitor, and maintain or improve the level of clinical quality in a healthcare organization.

### Performance Measures

**Performance measures,** sometimes referred to as *quality measures,* "measure or quantify healthcare processes, outcomes, patient perceptions, and organizational structure and/or systems that are associated with the ability to provide high-quality health care and/or that relate to one or more quality goals for health care" (CMS 2023b). Within a healthcare organization, a variety of reviews continuously occur to evaluate the quality of care provided to patients. Reviews of patient care are often performed by reviewing a patient's health record and extracting necessary data to identify performance or nonperformance of established quality measures. In the instance of CMS quality measures, a healthcare organization may abstract health record data and submit necessary data to CMS. CMS may also collect data to evaluate performance of quality measures from other sources such as claims data. Table 11.3 provides two examples of data abstracted from patient records to identify clinical quality from the Hospital Inpatient Quality Reporting Program.

Data collected during reviews to measure quality are often based on the needs of the organization, the type of organization, and requirements from accreditation standards, regulatory requirements, or payer guidelines. For example, the quality measures noted in table 11.3 relate to various Medicare program elements such as value-based purchasing and impact payment rates to hospitals. These results are publicly available on

**Table 11.3.** Examples of data abstracted from patient health records to identify clinical quality

| Description of CMS quality measure | Data abstracted from the health record to identify compliance |
|---|---|
| Percentage of patients who received appropriate care for severe sepsis and/or septic shock | Analysts may review documentation in the record such as progress notes, consultation notes, medication orders and administration records, and the discharge summary. |
| Percentage of patients who came to the emergency department with stroke symptoms who received brain scan results within 45 minutes of arrival. | Analysts may review documentation in the health record such as the emergency department report, physician orders for imaging, and imaging reports. |

*Source:* CMS 2024c.

the Medicare Hospital Compare website, which helps consumers understand the choices among hospitals in their area.

Stakeholders to clinical quality such as the Agency for Healthcare Research and Quality (AHRQ), National Quality Forum, and Joint Commission promote the development and use of quality measures through research and monitoring (Shaw and Carter 2019). As previously noted, a variety of factors indicate which quality measures a healthcare organization will evaluate. It is also important to understand that the widespread support from stakeholders regarding quality measures stems from the fact that these measures are established because they have been scientifically validated and are evidence-based approaches to quality.

Data collected for quality reviews are used by providers and organizations to conduct internal and external benchmarking. **Benchmarking** is the systematic comparison of the products, services, and outcomes of one organization with those of a similar organization, or the systematic comparison of one organization's outcomes with regional or national standards. There are two types of benchmarking—internal and external. **Internal benchmarking** compares similar processes, services, or outcomes across internal departments of an organization; it may also track changes within the organization over time (Altan et al. 2022). An example of internal benchmarking would be to compare rates of hospital-acquired pressure ulcers among nursing units within the same hospital. This type of comparison may yield valuable information for understanding which units are experiencing fewer pressure ulcers and why their rates are low. From this, best practices to reduce instances of pressure ulcers can be identified and implemented throughout the hospital.

**External benchmarking** occurs when an organization compares similar processes, services, or outcomes with other organizations (Altan et al. 2022). Data is readily available for external benchmarking through a variety of online dashboards. For example, hospitals must report data during billing to CMS to identify if patient diagnoses are hospital-acquired. Hospitals might choose to compare their rates of hospital-acquired conditions with those from similar hospitals to identify how they are performing in comparison.

## Quality and Knowledge Generation

Quality management efforts are comprehensive and ongoing, and require time, money, and human resources. Data obtained through quality management activities must be used in meaningful ways. If an organization collects vast amounts of data but does nothing meaningful with it, then its efforts are unproductive. However, if the organization uses the data to evaluate its performance, identify areas for improvement, and provide a basis for action and improvement, more people within the organization will appreciate the efforts and buy in to the rationale for quality management activities.

One might consider the potential value of quality measurement data through the lens of the hierarchical relationship between data, information, knowledge, and wisdom. Without data and information, organizations cannot generate knowledge to understand the current state of quality nor the wisdom to recognize necessary future efforts to improve it. Knowledge exists in two forms—explicit and tacit. **Explicit knowledge** includes documents, databases, and other types of recorded and documented information; and **tacit knowledge** is the actions, experiences, ideals, values, and emotions of an individual that tend to be highly personal and difficult to communicate. This hierarchy indicates the following:

- Data in crude format have little meaning (for example, raw facts stored as characters, symbols, measures, and statistics).
- Information is the convergence of data with relevant and meaningful details (for example, processed data in the form of a report).
- Knowledge depicts that which is known based on available information (for example, information combined with experience and context).
- Wisdom is the ability to translate knowledge into informed actions, behaviors, and changes (for example, actionable and long-term application of knowledge). (Cato et al. 2020)

As healthcare organizations enhance their knowledge about internal successes and opportunities in the context of quality, long-term efforts to improve in necessary areas will occur from an informed perspective. The hierarchy from data to wisdom illustrated in figure 11.1 shows that the vast amounts of data collected and reported during performance measure review holds potential value that can transform a healthcare organization and improve quality and safety in patient care.

## Plan-Do-Check-Act Cycle

A commonly used process in clinical quality management is the plan-do-check-act (PDCA) cycle. PDCA is also referred to as the plan-do-study-act (PDSA) cycle, the Deming Wheel, or the Deming Cycle. PDCA is an ongoing process entailing "a systematic series of steps for gaining valuable learning and knowledge for the continual improvement of a product or process" (W. Edwards Deming Institute n.d.). Healthcare organizations frequently use the PDCA cycle within quality and performance improvement activities.

This four-step process is cyclical in nature and intended to be never-ending. See figure 11.2 for an illustration of this cyclical process. The basis for the PDCA cycle is that constant evaluation of activities and processes should occur to ensure quality and identify when change or improvement is necessary. The W. Edwards Deming Institute describes the PDCA cycle as follows:

The cycle begins with the Plan step. This involves identifying a goal or purpose, formulating a theory, defining success metrics and putting a plan into action. These activities are followed by the Do step, in which the components of the plan are implemented, such as making a product. Next comes the Study step, where outcomes are monitored to test the validity of the plan for signs of progress and success, or problems and areas for improvement. The Act step closes the cycle, integrating the learning generated by the entire process, which can be used to adjust the goal, change methods, or even reformulate a theory altogether. These four steps are repeated over and over as part of a never-ending cycle of continual improvement. (n.d.)

The PDCA cycle can be used, for example, to reduce errors in clinical documentation. Assume a healthcare organization becomes concerned about clinical documentation quality in the electronic health record (EHR).

Figure 11.1. Hierarchy of data, information, knowledge, and wisdom

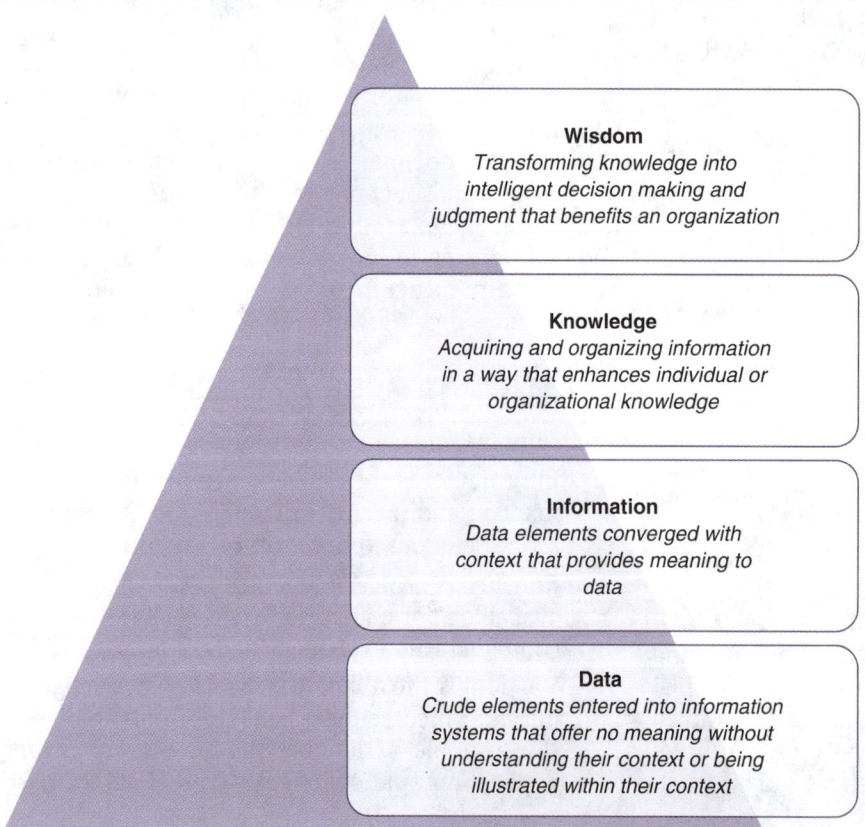

**Figure 11.2.** PDCA cycle

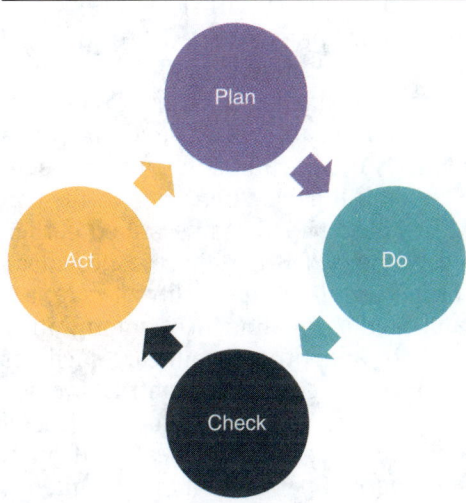

One area of concern is that documentation about the stage of pressure ulcers is often insufficient, even when the documentation indicates the presence of a pressure ulcer on a patient. An interprofessional committee determines that documentation of pressure ulcer stages must improve, and the committee develops an educational activity that all nursing staff in the organization are required to complete. The committee members train all nursing staff. Two weeks after all nursing staff undergo the training, health information management (HIM) analysts conduct retrospective record reviews on patients with pressure ulcers. The record review identifies that all but two nursing units have improved pressure ulcer staging documentation. The next step of action is to retrain the two nursing units still struggling with documentation. The PDCA cycle is as follows:

- Plan—identify pressure ulcer documentation issues, form an interprofessional committee to evaluate the problem, and create a training program to comprise the plan.
- Do—conduct the required training session for all nursing staff.
- Check—perform retrospective record review to gauge documentation quality after training concludes.
- Act—retrain two deficient nursing units.

The PDCA cycle is used to comprehensively identify an issue, create and implement a plan of action, check to ensure the plan is working, and continue to improve. In some cases, the PDCA process concludes once a certain goal or metric is achieved; however, PDCA can also be iterative in nature when appropriate.

## Peer Review

While many quality management efforts, techniques, and tools focus on evaluating systematic processes, there are instances in which the actions and behaviors of clinical staff are evaluated. One example of a method to evaluate clinical staff is peer review. **Peer review** is a review by like professionals, or peers, established according to an organization's medical staff bylaws, organizational policy and procedure, or the requirements of state law. The peer review system allows medical professionals to candidly critique and criticize the work of their colleagues without fear of reprisal.

Physicians were the first professional group in healthcare to grapple with the concept of peer review (Vyas and Hozain 2014). Medical malpractice lawsuits occurred at high rates during the 1970s and, over time, a growing concern emerged that physicians could move freely around the country and reestablish their practice with little question after having been found liable for injury, death, or other harm experienced by patients under their care. During this time, there were concerns that without legal protections in place for healthcare providers to participate in peer-review activities, physicians would be reluctant to evaluate peers even when doing so was necessary. The **Health Care Quality Improvement Act of 1986 (HCQIA)** is a federal law that established standards and requirements related to peer review among physicians. In the legislation, peer review is also referred to as *professional review*. When an incident has occurred and it is believed that peer review is necessary, healthcare organizations must follow standards to ensure that any actions taken against the physician are appropriate and justifiable. This includes that the review is occurring to advance quality, that reasonable efforts to obtain all relevant facts pertaining to the incident have been made, that the physician under review is given advance notice and is afforded a fair hearing, and that any actions taken are justified based on facts (HCQIA 1986). An example of when peer review may be used is when a patient dies from a surgical complication. In this example, it may be determined by hospital policy that a team of peer physicians review the performance of the surgeon to ensure standards of care were met.

The HCQIA also provides legal immunity to other physicians who participate in peer-review activities. This ensures competent physicians willingly participate in review of their peers without the threat of legal implications when the review occurs in accordance with the law. This legislation also describes a variety of reporting requirements when malpractice occurs, other reportable actions occur, or payments are made related to malpractice (HCQIA 1986).

The National Practitioner Data Bank (NPDB) is "an information clearinghouse [. . .] to collect and release certain information related to the professional competence and conduct of physicians, dentists, and, in some cases, other healthcare practitioners" (HHS 2018, A-2). The NPDB was mandated under the HCQIA to provide a database of medical malpractice payments; adverse licensure actions including revocations, suspensions, reprimands, censures, probations, and surrenders of licenses for quality-of-care purposes only; and certain professional review actions (such as denial of medical staff privileges) taken by healthcare entities such as hospitals against physicians, dentists, and other healthcare providers (NPDB 2006).

Information that details reportable events in the NPDB is provided to the federal government through a required reporting mechanism. Entities that make malpractice payments—including insurance companies, boards of medical examiners, and entities such as hospitals and professional societies—must report to the NPDB. Information reported to the NPDB includes details about the involved practitioner, the reporting entity, and any related judgment or settlement (when applicable). Information on physicians must be reported, and the law requires entities such as private accrediting organizations and peer review organizations to report adverse actions to the databank (NPDB 2006). In addition, adverse licensure and other actions against any healthcare entity must be reported. Monetary penalties and other sanctions may be assessed for failure to report qualifying events to the NPDB.

The NPDB also allows eligible entities to query for provider information housed within the database. Among those considered eligible entities are "medical malpractice payers, hospitals and other health care entities, professional societies, health plans, peer review organizations, private accreditation organizations, quality improvement organizations, and certain federal and state agencies. Health care practitioners, entities, providers, and suppliers are authorized to query on themselves for information reported to the NPDB" (HHS 2018, A-1).

In settings such as hospitals, physicians undergo rigorous screenings before they are appointed to the medical staff. *Medical staff* refers to physicians and other approved practitioners granted rights and responsibilities to admit patients into a healthcare facility for medical care. CMS specifies that the medical staff must include members who are doctors of medicine and osteopathy, and may also include doctors of dental medicine or surgery, podiatry, optometry, and chiropractic medicine. Further, CMS indicates that if states grant certain privileges to other practitioners such as nurse practitioners, these professionals may be included in the medical staff infrastructure (CMS 2014).

If physicians or other practitioners hope to join a hospital medical staff and are eligible to do so, they must undergo the credentialing process. Credentialing is a screening process to evaluate and validate a healthcare provider's qualifications for medical staff membership. One tool utilized extensively in the credentialing process is the NPDB. As described earlier, details included in the NPDB pertain to a provider's historical performance related to quality of care, adverse issues, and medical malpractice, among other details. As hospitals and other healthcare facilities strive to maintain a talented medical staff to provide the best possible care, the NPDB is an important tool in the credentialing process and medical staff management. For the safety of patients and in the interest of adhering to various federal requirements, clinical privileges are not granted to healthcare providers by hospitals and other care settings until the rigorous screening of their professional background successfully concludes. Once a physician or other healthcare provider is deemed appropriate to provide care in a hospital or other facility, they do so in accordance with defined clinical privileges. Clinical privileges refer to the authorization granted by a healthcare organization's governing board to a member of the medical staff that enables the physician to provide patient services in the organization within specific practice limits.

## Tracer Methodology

Healthcare organizations often replicate accreditation surveyor processes. In replicating surveyor processes, an organization can conduct internal evaluations of daily operations and clinical care to identify compliance with accreditation standards that focus on quality and patient safety. Tracer methodology is one such example of a process used by surveyors who conduct on-site accreditation surveys for the Joint Commission that is replicated within a healthcare organization to evaluate performance. Tracer methodology is

> a process the Joint Commission surveyors use during the on-site survey to analyze an organization's systems, with particular attention to identified priority focus areas, by following individual patients through the organization's healthcare process in the sequence experienced by the patients; an evaluation that follows (traces) the hospital experiences of specific patients to assess the quality of patient care; part of the new Joint Commission survey processes. (Joint Commission n.d.c)

Healthcare organizations using tracer methodology, sometimes referred to as *tracers*, allow for peers within an organization to assess care processes, evaluate the environment of care, and conduct benchmarking of performance in the context of accreditation standards. Staff participation from all units within an organization is particularly useful when conducting tracers. This type of interprofessional involvement best ensures various professionals of differing expertise in healthcare can thoroughly evaluate the who, what, where, when, why, and how of clinical care, with the understanding that each professional provides a unique and valuable point of view.

## Check Your Understanding 11.2

**Answer the following questions in a separate document.**

1. A quality analyst at a hospital identifies that needle sticks among nurses from unit A occur 10 percent more often than they do among nurses on unit B. Is this an example of external benchmarking?

2. Assume a healthcare organization is working on a quality initiative and is using the PDCA cycle. Read this example and then choose from the answers below to indicate which step of the PDCA cycle is being reflected in the example:

   An ad hoc team of employees conduct an accreditation tracer exercise. When reviewing the notes and findings from this process, it is determined that nurses and other professionals on some units are entering and exiting patient rooms without using sanitizing foam on their hands consistently. The director of patient safety meets with a team to develop strategy for addressing this issue.

   a. Plan
   b. Do
   c. Check
   d. Act

3. In your own words, describe why a healthcare organization hiring a new physician would be interested in reviewing details about the physician regarding state licensure actions as reported to the NPDB.

4. Medical malpractice insurance premiums continue to rise for obstetricians who staff the labor and delivery unit of ABC Hospital. Regardless of whether errors in care processes have or have not contributed to these rising costs, in what way is this a financial risk to the hospital?

5. In healthcare, what type of patient safety event is serious enough that it requires immediate investigation and response?
   a. Sentinel event
   b. Adverse event
   c. Reportable adverse event
   d. None of the above are correct

6. Which federal law provides immunity to physicians who participate in peer-review activities?
   a. Emergency Medical Treatment and Active Labor Act
   b. Healthcare Quality Improvement Act of 1986
   c. National Practitioner Data Bank Law
   d. There is no federal law that addresses this, but states may have laws to this effect.

## Assessing Outcomes and Effectiveness of Healthcare

**Outcomes and effectiveness research (OER)** "describes, interprets, and predicts the impact of healthcare interventions on endpoints that matter to patients, families and caregivers, providers, private and public payers and purchasers of healthcare, regulatory agencies, healthcare-accrediting organizations, and society generally" (NIH 2023). There is no single methodology for assessing outcomes and effectiveness in healthcare. Depending on what is being assessed, these types of inquiries may be performed by analyzing large data sets, reviewing health records, conducting randomized controlled clinical trials, or conducting literature reviews of published scholarly research, as examples. This type of research may be conducted at the patient, institutional, community, or system level. The following section examines current approaches and topics that relate to assessing outcomes and effectiveness in healthcare.

### Healthcare Quality Measures

A significant aspect of quality and performance improvement efforts is establishing measurements to objectively and accurately assess if changes implemented within performance improvement processes produce the intended results. The IHI posits that there are three general categories of measures used in healthcare—outcome, process, and balancing measures. In addition, the Agency for Healthcare Research and Quality indicates that structural measures are another pertinent category of measurement in healthcare quality (AHRQ 2015). Table 11.4 summarizes these types of measures.

In instances where known quality indicators require measurement, a healthcare organization will conduct ongoing measurement accordingly. In other instances, an organization may determine specific things unique to the organization that it sees value in measuring.

## The Role of the Agency for Healthcare Research and Quality

While analyzing outcomes and effectiveness in healthcare through research and measurement methods is common in present-day US healthcare, this was not always the case. These ideas began gaining momentum in the 1980s, when the prospective payment system (PPS) for Medicare inpatient care was implemented. At that time, the public and policymakers were concerned that Medicare patients were being discharged from hospitals too quickly for financial reasons. The fear was that patients were being discharged based on their length of stay rather than when they were clinically ready. In response, Medicare databases were promoted and used to monitor the quality of care through measurement of mortality rates, readmission rates, and other adverse outcomes.

Simultaneously, others were advancing the outcomes movement, which contained elements of research, measurement, and management. Other research efforts on geographic variations in medical practice, appropriateness of care, and the inferior quality of medical evidence to support various interventions and treatments resulted in the establishment of the Agency for Health Care Policy and Research (AHCPR) in 1989. The Healthcare Research and Quality Act of 1999 changed the agency's name to the AHRQ. The mission of the AHRQ is "to produce evidence to make health care safer, higher quality, more accessible, equitable, and affordable, and to work with the U.S. Department of Health and Human Services and with other partners to make sure that the evidence is understood and used" (AHRQ 2024).

A component of AHRQ is the AHRQ quality indicators (QIs) (AHRQ n.d.c). QIs are measures that address various aspects of quality. The various types of AHRQ QIs include the following:

- *Prevention QIs* identify access issues to high-quality outpatient care and ensure appropriate follow-up care after inpatient discharge.
- *Inpatient QIs* focus on the quality of care inside hospitals, including inpatient mortality and proper utilization of procedures.
- *Patient safety indicators* provide information related to potentially avoidable safety events to identify opportunities for improvement.
- *Pediatric QIs* focus on potentially avoidable events for pediatric inpatients and on preventable hospitalization for pediatric patients. (AHRQ n.d.c)

Emergency department prevention quality indicators are in beta testing stage and may be included as an AHRQ PI in the future. Examples of AHRQ QIs appear in table 11.5.

In addition to quality indicators, the AHRQ supports the Healthcare Cost and Utilization Project (HCUP). This project includes publicly available databases and software tools; the data within the databases represent various aspects of healthcare cost and utilization, including that which is "derived from administrative data and contain encounter-level, clinical and non-clinical information including all-listed diagnoses and procedures, discharge status, patient demographics, and charges for all patients, regardless of payer, beginning in 1988" (AHRQ 2022a). Through these databases, researchers can explore a variety of topics related to healthcare quality, including cost and quality of care, medical malpractice patterns, and health outcomes.

**Table 11.4.** Types of healthcare quality measures

| Type | Description | Example |
| --- | --- | --- |
| Outcome measure | How the values, health, and well-being of patients are affected | Measuring the number of adverse drug events per 1,000 doses of administered medication |
| Process measure | How a system performs in relation to established processes | Average number of hours available each day for a provider to see patients for appointments |
| Balancing measure | How changes in one area of a system may cause issues in another part of a system | Ensuring that efforts to reduce patient length of stay are not occurring in a way that discharges patients too early and results in readmissions |
| Structural measure | How the capacity, existing systems, and established processes influence the ability for high-quality care to be delivered | Nurse-to-patient staffing ratios or number of board-certified physician specialists available |

*Source:* Adapted from AHRQ 2015.

**Table 11.5.** AHRQ QIs

| Type of indicator | Measure | Description |
|---|---|---|
| Prevention | Urinary tract infection admission rate | "Hospitalizations with a principal diagnosis of urinary tract infection per 100,000 population, ages 18 years and older" (AHRQ 2023a) |
| Inpatient | Acute stroke mortality rate | "In-hospital deaths per 1,000 hospital discharges with a principal diagnosis of acute stroke for patients ages 18 years and older" (AHRQ 2023b) |
| Patient Safety | Pressure ulcer rate | "Stage 3 or 4 (or unstageable) pressure ulcers (secondary diagnosis does not present on admission) per 1,000 hospital discharges of surgical or medical patients ages 18 years and older" (AHRQ 2023c) |
| Pediatric | Neonatal bloodstream infection rate | "Hospital discharges with healthcare-associated bloodstream infection per 1,000 discharges for newborns and outborns with birth weight of 500 grams or more but less than 1,500 grams; with gestational age between 24 and 30 weeks; or with birth weight of 1,500 grams or more associated with an operating room procedure, mechanical ventilation, transfer from another hospital within two days of birth, or death" (AHRQ 2023d) |
| ED Prevention | ED visits for nontraumatic dental conditions | "Emergency Department (ED) visits with a principal (first-listed) diagnosis of a non-traumatic dental condition per 100,000 population, for individuals ages 5 years and older" (AHRQ 2023e) |

*Source:* AHRQ 2023a; 2023b; 2023c; 2023d; 2023e.

## Check Your Understanding 11.3

**Answer the following questions in a separate document.**

1. A hospital treats an appropriate number of hip fracture patients; however, the same hospital has a higher mortality rate among hip fracture patients than a comparable competitor hospital. What might a quality analyst be looking for in their analysis of health record documentation among hip fracture patients who expired in the hospital?

2. Why is a significant variance of cesarean section delivery rates noteworthy when reviewing quality indicator data on cesarean section rates among comparable hospitals in the same geographic location?

3. Provide an example of a topic a healthcare administrator might review in the Health Care Utilization Project (HCUP) database and explain why the HCUP database is a good resource for reviewing the topic.

4. Assume a healthcare facility identifies an overly high rate of pressure ulcers among inpatients. Provide an example of documentation from the health record to evaluate and better understand instances of pressure ulcers.

5. Which of the following is true about the Healthcare Cost and Utilization Project (HCUP)?
    a. It is supported by the AHRQ.
    b. It is supported by the ONC.
    c. Its databases contain various administrative and clinical data elements.
    d. Answer choices a and c are both correct.

# Systematic and Process-Driven Focus to Improve Performance

While it is important to appreciate quality management approaches and techniques, it is equally valuable to examine concepts related to supporting improved performance in patient care. The following sections describe approaches and processes used in healthcare to support quality and improve performance.

## Evidence-Based Care and Treatment

The expansive nature of clinical research and scientific discovery in the health sciences benefits patient care in many ways. Applying the scientific method to study clinical endeavors shows certain approaches, methods, protocols, and treatments are proven to produce the best results for patients. The care and treatment of patients based on proven approaches is considered evidence-based practice.

**Evidence-based practice** is the "integration of clinical expertise, patient values, and the best research evidence into the decision-making process for patient care" (Sackett et al. 1996). An **evidence-based clinical practice guideline** is an explicit statement that guides clinical decision-making and has been systematically developed from scientific evidence and clinical expertise to answer clinical questions. The ability of healthcare professionals to identify and apply evidence in patient care requires them to possess knowledge and skills related to information appraisal and research. Because of early concerns that evidence-based medicine thwarted physician autonomy, some providers opposed the concept and suggested it was an unfavorable approach because it negated the role of physician judgment in patient care (Gerber and Lauterbach 2005). However, increased knowledge and understanding has led to widespread support for evidence-based practice. It not only provides a more proven basis for clinical judgments among providers it also relies on provider expertise and patient engagement in care decisions. Some evidence-based practice protocols are illustrated in CMS quality measures. The following are a few examples of evidence-based care that are also CMS quality measures:

- Appropriate treatment for upper respiratory infection—This measure evaluates if treatment protocols were followed in which patients three months of age or older diagnosed with an upper respiratory infection were ordered or prescribed antibiotics (CMS 2024d).
- Antidepressant medication management—This measure examines prescribing trends and ongoing treatment with antidepressants among patients aged 18 and older with a diagnosis of major depression (CMS 2022).

## Clinical Pathways

**Clinical pathways**, also sometimes referred to as critical pathways, guide evidence-based care and help "translate clinical practice guideline recommendations into clinical processes of care within the unique culture of a healthcare institution" (Rotter et al. 2019). Clinical pathways aim to standardize patient care for common conditions, when appropriate (Lehman 2022). Clinical pathways have gained momentum in healthcare organizations because the concept relates to quality improvement initiatives; used consistently, evidence suggests they can improve patient outcomes and organizational efficiency, while also promoting cost containment (Lawal et al. 2016, 2).

Clinical pathways expand the concept of a care plan because the pathway is established with the intent that the care plan accounts for the patient's needs and promotes the interdependent nature of the health professions to achieve more cohesive patient care. Clinical pathways and their relationship to evidence-based practice illustrate the changing landscape in healthcare in which efforts to facilitate patient care are enhanced by scientific discovery, collaboration, and communication.

## Case Management

Another process-driven concept in healthcare that benefits patients and improves performance in clinical care is case management. **Case management** refers to the ongoing, concurrent review performed by clinical professionals to ensure the necessity and effectiveness of the clinical services being provided to a patient. The unique needs of each individual patient must be accounted for to maximize outcomes—during an episode of care and afterward. The complexity of the US healthcare system poses significant challenges to patients and families when they must navigate it after a complex acute illness. For example, research has shown that patients with chronic health conditions see a primary care provider less frequently, even though research suggests primary care management of chronic conditions optimizes continuity of care (Ladapo and Chokshi 2014). However, seeking primary care services and maintaining a patient-provider relationship in a primary care setting can be complicated by a variety of factors such as inadequate access to care in rural or underserved locations, lack of health insurance coverage, or changes to health insurance plans. Because the US healthcare system is not intuitive to navigate, patients discharged from healthcare facilities find themselves at risk when follow-up care, ongoing services, and medication management are necessary.

Case management offers a solution to help ensure patients' needs are met during a hospitalization or other care episode and after they are discharged from a healthcare setting. Often healthcare organizations, such as hospitals, psychiatric hospitals, and long-term care facilities, staff a team of case managers. These case managers evaluate the appropriateness of hospital admissions against preestablished criteria, are assigned to a patient during their stay, remain with the patient during their care to ensure their medical and psychosocial needs are appropriately being met, and assist in facilitation of ongoing needs after discharge. Without these coordinated efforts, patients are at greater risk for readmission, poor medication management, or not receiving necessary ongoing care.

## Care Coordination

Care coordination is reflected in clinical pathways as well as case management. In addition, healthcare providers engage in care coordination in the scope of ongoing management of a patient. **Care coordination** is the act of "organizing patient care activities and sharing information among all of the participants concerned with a patient's care to achieve safer and more effective care" (AHRQ 2018).

Care coordination is necessary to ensure a patient is provided care at the appropriate level, and to ensure care is coordinated in thoughtful and proactive ways. Care coordination reflects an opportunity to provide healthcare services in a way that is proactive versus reactive in nature; for example, care coordination relies on better communication among health professionals and early identification of a patient's current and future healthcare needs. If care is coordinated more effectively, oversights that could pose risks to the patient are reduced.

The AHRQ argues that there is an important role for primary care medical homes (also known as patient-centered medical homes) in case management and care coordination. Care increasingly occurs in ambulatory settings and primary care is foundational to quality, accessibility, and efficiency in US healthcare. In medical home models, comprehensive care, patient-centeredness, care coordination, service accessibility, and quality and safety are essential focus areas (AHRQ 2022b).

## Effective Deployment and Use of Information Technology

EHRs and other health information systems (HISs) include features and mechanisms that support patient care improvements. Some functionalities in EHRs and other HISs include visual and audio alerts when a patient has a known drug allergy, visual and audio alerts when a patient has a do-not-resuscitate order, as well as mechanisms to identify when ordered medications may be contraindicated by a patient's existing medications. Varieties of evidence-based guidelines are available as references within these systems and can be configured to produce reminders and alerts within EHRs and HISs. The ability for healthcare providers to have these resources available at their fingertips while they are already documenting in and reviewing a patient's health record is beneficial. Immediate and easy access to current evidence in the care and treatment of patients assists in creating a more appropriate plan of care.

EHRs and HISs also support clinical pathways, case management, and care coordination. Clinical pathways rely on interprofessional and multidisciplinary collaboration based on evidence to maximize patient outcomes. Case management requires the appreciation for a patient's social and cultural needs, and a comprehensive understanding of a patient's emotional and physical health status and future needs. Care coordination occurs when decisions related to ongoing or next levels of care are made proactively and timely. When functionalities of EHRs and other information systems (ISs) are continually optimized and used to their fullest potential with a focus on thorough documentation and effective information sharing, there is a potential for improved care coordination because decisions regarding care can be based on meaningful real-time information.

Artificial intelligence (AI) applications are becoming commonplace in daily life and are increasingly piloted for use in healthcare settings. While the extent to which AI is presently adopted within healthcare organizations varies, its known capabilities provide new possibilities related to patient safety. For example, AI can scan electronic records to identify patients who may be at higher risk for falls or infections. Some posit several potential influences which AI may have on quality and safety in patient care settings. Table 11.6 summarizes examples of the possible impact of AI on patient care. Some of the summarized impacts are positive or potentially positive, while others pose valid questions about risks related to AI.

**Table 11.6.** Potential of AI to impact quality and safety

| Factors in Quality and Safety | How AI May Support Quality and Safety |
| --- | --- |
| Using incident management systems to monitor and track safety or other issues that negatively impact quality of care | AI can identify safety risks in real-time or outliers that may indicate deviations from the norm in patient care. |
| Ensuring the roles and responsibilities among the clinical care team are clearly defined within clinical governance. | AI may pose some risks related to an overreliance in trusting suggestions or plans proposed by AI systems. |
| Diagnosing diseases and conditions with accuracy to ensure proper care and treatment. | AI shows significant promise in helping clinicians render diagnoses, especially when clinicians drive the decision-making and rely on AI for support. |

**Source:** Adapted from Phelps and Cooper 2020.

# Professional Designations and Roles in Healthcare Quality

It is important for emerging professionals to familiarize themselves with credentials and roles related to all areas of professional specialization within healthcare, including those related to healthcare quality. Upon entering the workforce, many in HIM perform work that overlaps with organizational quality management efforts, serve on organizational quality-related committees, and sometimes choose to work in a quality management role. Therefore, understanding credentials, roles, and functions of quality management are important for workforce preparation. Appreciating the variety of designations related to quality management is important for navigating one's career as well as working in the interprofessional environment of healthcare.

## Certifications Related to Quality Management

In 1928, the ACS established the American Association of Medical Record Librarians, which is today known as the American Health Information Management Association (AHIMA). The creation of a professional association related to health records helped ensure that health records in patient care settings remained a high priority and that support was available for those working with health records. It was around this time that hospitals and other care settings in the US increasingly began creating and maintaining health records on patients to document care provided. Health records have evolved in their requirements and mediums throughout the years, and as such, so has the profession which is known today as *health information management*.

Health information managers credentialed as a registered health information administrator (RHIA) or registered health information technician (RHIT) who are working in quality management and related roles find value in adding the CPHQ, HCQM, or CPHRM credentials to their resume. Because so many functions and roles related to quality management rely on professionals understanding healthcare data, care processes, and data science, HIM professionals are uniquely equipped to work in roles related to quality management.

Some professionals who work in quality management roles may choose to or are required to obtain certifications related to their work. The following provides an overview of several professional certifications related to quality.

### Certified Professional in Healthcare Quality

The certified professional in healthcare quality (CPHQ) designation is commonly obtained by those with experience in healthcare quality. The CPHQ is a certification exam offered by the National Association for Healthcare Quality (NAHQ). A quality professional is one who possesses a variety of knowledge and skills including those related to data analytics and information management, quality and performance improvement, leadership, and patient safety and risk management (NAHQ n.d.). Any healthcare professional is eligible to take the CPHQ, although the NAHQ indicates that possessing at least two years of experience in healthcare quality is a general rule of thumb for readiness to take the CPHQ and notes that the CPHQ is not an entry-level certification exam (NAHQ 2019).

### Certification in Health Care Quality and Management

The certification in health care quality and management (HCQM) is another certification option for health professionals working in roles related to quality. The HCQM is offered by the American Board of Quality Assurance and Utilization Review Physicians. This certification option focuses on the typical tenants of quality management. It also allows those obtaining the certification to optionally complete subspecialty certifications in categories such as physician advisor, transitions of care, managed care, patient safety and risk management, case management, or workers' compensation (ABQAURP n.d.).

### Certified Professional in Healthcare Risk Management

Those employed in risk management roles in healthcare work with issues related to healthcare quality each day. Among the duties of risk managers are evaluating instances of potential or actual medical errors and other patient safety issues that produce risk to a healthcare organization. Those working in risk management may also be certified as a certified professional in healthcare risk management (CPHRM). The CPHRM is administered by the American Hospital Association's Certification Center. Two eligibility pathways to the CPHRM certification exam exist. One is based on education and healthcare experience with the other solely based on risk management experience (ASHRM 2022).

## The Health Information Manager Role in Healthcare Quality

The ability to effectively evaluate the quality of care provided to patients and measure performance related to quality indicators hinges on an understanding of documentation in health records as well as an understanding of healthcare data and information science. The health record, and documentation therein, is considered the keeper of truth in recording care provided to patients. Health information managers possess a unique understanding and insight into diminished quality in documentation and how that relates to various uses of data. For these reasons, many HIM professionals pursue careers in or related to quality management.

Some with health information backgrounds fill positions in departments of healthcare organizations in positions ranging from a data analyst to a manager in departments such as quality management or quality improvement, performance improvement, or risk management. Others with health information expertise may choose to apply their understanding of quality management to roles related to the quality assurance of functions performed in HIM and information technology departments. Regardless of the way a health information manager applies their knowledge and skills to quality functions, they possess several underlying areas of expertise that are highly valued in healthcare and applicable to quality management.

## Data Stewardship and Information Governance

As uses of EHRs expand, data stewardship and information governance are increasingly important in today's healthcare environment given the digital nature of EHRs and health information systems. Data stewardship and information governance are strategic concepts in the management of health information. **Health data stewardship** pertains to responsibilities that best ensure appropriate use of health data (NCVHS 2009). The concept of data stewardship in healthcare relates to information governance. Information governance is an organizational-wide framework for managing information throughout its life cycle and supporting the organization's strategy, operations, regulatory, legal, risk, and environmental requirements (IG Advisors 2017).

Effective data stewardship and information governance are necessary to maximize the value of health information available in health records used to evaluate and measure quality of care. Without a robust framework focused on the quality, usability, and availability of healthcare data and information, evaluation of clinical care through data analysis is challenging and limits the potential for generating knowledge.

## Data Analytics

The increasing volume of data created each day in healthcare provides opportunities to better understand quality of care, clinical outcomes, and performance related to quality standards and metrics. As end users grapple with technologies such as EHRs and other ISs, there are growing expectations that meaningful data can be garnered from these systems.

While health information managers working in quality management roles historically focused many of their efforts on extracting data from health records to help identify performance in meeting quality measures, health information managers today and in the future will assume roles performing data analytics. In relationship to measuring quality and evaluating performance in clinical care, data analytics affords opportunities to examine large amounts of data to identify trends, opportunities, and probabilities in the care and outcomes of patients.

Application of data analytics to measure quality and performance offers great potential to strategically assess and improve all aspects of care delivery. Effective data analytics only occurs when those performing the analysis fully comprehend the complexity, limitations, meaning, and uses of healthcare data. To this end, the health information manager has the necessary skills and knowledge to lead in the era of big data.

## Regulatory Compliance

Another area in which health information managers may provide expertise related to quality management is leadership in regulation compliance. Within a healthcare organization, there is a need for professionals who can understand sources of regulation, interpret regulation, and operationalize compliance with regulations.

This chapter describes the environment of healthcare in which regulations fully or partially focus on improving healthcare quality; these ongoing requirements and oversights influence the need for organizations to staff appropriately with personnel who can navigate, monitor, and report on these types of requirements. Often, these types of regulations require that specific measurements of quality and performance are conducted or that new quality management efforts are initiated in healthcare settings. HIM professionals possess knowledge and skills related to health information and its regulated uses, and have backgrounds in quality management. These complimentary domains afford health information professionals many opportunities to provide leadership in quality programs and processes to best ensure regulatory compliance.

# Trends Impacting Healthcare Quality

Various concepts in health service delivery are increasingly relevant to the topics of clinical quality, quality management, and performance improvement. Among such concepts are reputation, identity, and social media; increased utilization of telehealth services; and learning health systems.

## Reputation, Identity, and Social Media

The impact of social media on healthcare organizations is evidenced by information sharing in these mediums by patients about their experiences, including providing ratings about satisfaction with health services. Healthcare is not immune from the transparent and accessible nature of immediate information that becomes viral.

Today, healthcare organizations and providers are active on social media. Even if a healthcare organization or provider chose not to have a social media presence, the reality is that the public is very active on social media. Social media provides immediate information sharing including instances in which patients express either satisfaction or dissatisfaction with care they have received. To this end, continually improving quality and safety in patient care is not only an ethical imperative, but also necessary to maintain good relations and ratings among patients and consumers.

## Telehealth Services

The internet, apps, and smart devices are revolutionizing patient care. Telehealth "lets your healthcare provider care for you without an in-person office visit. Telehealth is done primarily online with internet access on your computer, tablet, or smartphone" (HHS 2024). Prior to the COVID-19 pandemic, telehealth was available but not widely embraced by health insurance companies; as a result, widespread adoption was not commonplace. However, the pandemic necessitated embracing telehealth so patient care could continue while it was unsafe for patients to come into healthcare facilities for nonemergent care and treatment. Telehealth services include but are not limited to virtual appointments with a healthcare provider, exchanging secure messages with a healthcare provider via patient portals to address care and treatment concerns, and remote patient monitoring. A **remote patient monitoring device** is one that enables a healthcare provider to monitor and treat a patient from a remote location. Some of the earliest uses of remote patient monitoring focused on measuring things such as blood pressure, pulse oximetry, and glucose levels. Remote patient monitoring has expanded greatly, however. Some health systems operate virtual intensive care units (ICUs) to serve patients not in close proximity to an acute-care hospital with ICU beds yet require that level of care and monitoring.

Telehealth provides convenience to patients and expands access to health services. One concern about telehealth pertains to how quality management will apply to virtually provided healthcare services, particularly in instances when the care is ad hoc and offered as a one-time patient-provider exchange through an app and webcam. As telehealth expands and changes the way health services are delivered, organizations offering these services must consider a variety of factors related to quality management such as the following:

- What processes are used to identify appropriate physician partners from remote locations to offer clinical services through telehealth?
- Are health services beyond traditional medical care—such as consultations from physical therapists, occupational therapists, and audiologists— of use to patients?
- How are telehealth services documented and how are health records pertaining to these encounters managed?
- Will patient satisfaction be measured for patients seen in telehealth settings?
- How does telehealth affect care continuity?
- Through which mechanisms can a patient submit a complaint related to the quality of service they received?

Reimbursement for telehealth services is expanding, which is another indicator telehealth use will increase. The future of measuring clinical quality in this environment provides opportunities and challenges, and emerging leaders in healthcare must consider how they will contribute to advancing goals of safe and effective care in these settings.

## Learning Health Systems

Another concept supported by the AHRQ is that of *learning health systems*. A **learning health system** is "a health system in which internal data and experience are systematically integrated with external evidence, and that knowledge is put into practice" (AHRQ 2019). While an organization may not label itself as a learning health system per se, the tenets of working towards operating as this type of facility include organizations which do the following:

- Commit to continuous learning and improvement.
- Apply and gather evidence in real-time to guide care.
- Promote IT as mechanism to share new evidence with clinicians.
- Include patients as vital members of the care team.
- Collect and analyze data to improve care.
- Assess outcomes and continually refine processes and training to promote learning and improvement (AHRQ 2019).

The healthcare ecosystem is rapidly changing. All indications suggest that clinical quality management and performance improvement will remain embedded in all that is done throughout healthcare. As healthcare changes and more patients access health services through a variety of avenues, emerging professionals must be prepared to identify new and innovative approaches to improving the quality of care provided to patients.

### Check Your Understanding 11.4

**Answer the following questions in a separate document.**

1. How can interprofessional education positively influence patient safety? Give an example.
2. Assume you are a performance improvement specialist for a company that provides app-based primary care dealing with acute minor health issues. What challenges might you have in collecting patient satisfaction data?
3. Provide one reason clinical pathways relate to clinical quality.
4. Evaluate how an HIM professional is uniquely qualified to work in roles related to quality in healthcare organizations.
5. If an HIM professional with the RHIA credential begins working as a risk management analyst in a hospital, which additional credential might they want to obtain?

# References

AAAHC (Accreditation Association for Ambulatory Health Care). n.d. "About Us." Accessed August 7, 2024. https://www.aaahc.org/about-us/.

AHRQ (Agency for Healthcare Research and Quality). 2024. "Mission and Budget." https://www.ahrq.gov/cpi/about/mission/index.html.

AHRQ (Agency for Healthcare Research and Quality). 2023a. "Technical Specifications for Prevention Quality Indicators." https://qualityindicators.ahrq.gov/measures/PQI_TechSpec.

AHRQ (Agency for Healthcare Research and Quality). 2023b. "Technical Specifications for Inpatient Quality Indicators." https://qualityindicators.ahrq.gov/measures/IQI_TechSpec.

AHRQ (Agency for Healthcare Research and Quality). 2023c. "Technical Specifications for Patient Safety Indicators." https://qualityindicators.ahrq.gov/measures/PSI_TechSpec.

AHRQ (Agency for Healthcare Research and Quality). 2023d. "Technical Specifications for Pediatric Quality Indicators". https://qualityindicators.ahrq.gov/measures/PDI_TechSpec.

AHRQ (Agency for Healthcare Research and Quality). 2023e. "Technical Specifications for Emergency Department Prevention Quality Indicators." https://qualityindicators.ahrq.gov/measures/ED_PQI_TechSpec.

AHRQ (Agency for Healthcare Research and Quality). 2022a. "Healthcare Cost and Utilization Project." https://www.ahrq.gov/data/hcup/index.html.

AHRQ (Agency for Healthcare Research and Quality). 2022b. "Patient Centered Medical Home (PCMH)." https://www.ahrq.gov/ncepcr/research/care-coordination/pcmh/index.html.

AHRQ (Agency for Healthcare Research and Quality). 2019. "About Learning Health Systems." https://www.ahrq.gov/learning-health-systems/about.html.

AHRQ (Agency for Healthcare Research and Quality). 2018. "Care Coordination." https://www.ahrq.gov/ncepcr/care/coordination.html.

AHRQ (Agency for Healthcare Research and Quality). 2015. "Types of Health Care Quality Measures." https://www.ahrq.gov/talkingquality/measures/types.html.

AHRQ (Agency for Healthcare Research and Quality). n.d.a. "Adverse Events." Accessed August 10, 2024. https://psnet.ahrq.gov/glossary-0?f%5B0%5D=glossary_az_content_title%3AA.

AHRQ (Agency for Healthcare Research and Quality). n.d.b. "Evidence-Based." Accessed August 10, 2024. https://psnet.ahrq.gov/glossary-0?f%5B0%5D=glossary_az_content_title%3AA.

AHRQ (Agency for Healthcare Research and Quality). n.d.c. "AHRQ Quality Indicators." Accessed June 11, 2024. http://www.qualityindicators.ahrq.gov/.

Alexander, J. W. 1985. The contributions of infection control to a century of surgical progress. *Annals of Surgery* 201(4). http://www.ncbi.nlm.nih.gov/pmc/articles/PMC1250728/pdf/annsurg00110-0033.pdf.

Altan D., V. Ahuja, C. M. Kelleher, and D. C. Chang. 2022 (July 19). Look in the mirror, Not out the window: In favor of internal benchmarking. *Annals of Surgery Open* 3(3). https://www.ncbi.nlm.nih.gov/pmc/articles/PMC9508963/.

ABQAURP (American Board of Quality Assurance and Utilization Review Physicians). n.d. "Health Care Quality Management (HCQM) Certification." Accessed August 10, 2024. https://www.abqaurp.org/ABQMain/Certification/HCQM_Certification/Overview_of_HCQM/ABQMain/Certification.aspx?hkey=b6edc3b2-6da9-49d0-a824-3399badf629e.

American College of Radiology. n.d. "Accreditation." Accessed January 1, 2024. https://www.acr.org/Clinical-Resources/Accreditation.

AHA (American Hospital Association). n.d. "The Patient Care Partnership." Accessed January 1, 2024. https://www.aha.org/other-resources/patient-care-partnership.

ASHRM (American Society for Health Care Risk Management). 2022. *Certified Professional in Health Care Risk Management Candidate Handbook*. Accessed June 12, 2024. AHA_CC-CPHRM-Handbook.pdf.

ASHRM (American Society for Health Care Risk Management). n.d. "Enterprise Risk Management." Accessed June 11, 2024. https://www.ashrm.org/system/files?file=media/file/2019/06/ERM-Tool_final.pdf.

Cato, K. D., K. McGrow, and S.C. Rossetti. 2021. Transforming Clinical Data into Wisdom. *Nurse Management*. 51(11). https://www.ncbi.nlm.nih.gov/pmc/articles/PMC8018525/.

CMS (Centers for Medicare and Medicaid Services). 2024a. "Emergency Medical Treatment and Active Labor Act (EMTALA)." https://www.cms.gov/Regulations-and-Guidance/Legislation/EMTALA/.

CMS (Centers for Medicare and Medicaid Services). 2024b. "Clinical Laboratory Improvement Amendments (CLIA)." https://www.cms.gov/Regulations-and-Guidance/Legislation/CLIA/index.html?redirect=/clia/.

CMS (Centers for Medicare and Medicaid Services). 2024c. "Hospital Compare." https://www.cms.gov/medicare/quality-initiatives-patient-assessment-instruments/hospitalqualityinits/hospitalcompare.html.

CMS (Centers for Medicare and Medicaid Services). 2024d. "Appropriate Treatment for Upper Respiratory Infection." https://cmit.cms.gov/cmit/#/MeasureView?variantId=1163&sectionNumber=1

CMS (Centers for Medicare and Medicaid Services). 2023a. "Conditions for Coverage and Conditions of Participation." http://www.cms.gov/Regulations-and-Guidance/Legislation/CFCsAndCoPs/index.html.

CMS (Centers for Medicare and Medicaid Services). 2023b. "Quality Measures." https://www.cms.gov/Medicare/Quality-Initiatives-Patient-Assessment-Instruments/QualityMeasures/index.html.

CMS (Centers for Medicare and Medicaid Services). 2023c. "National Health Expenditures 2022 Highlights." Accessed June 12, 2024. https://www.cms.gov/newsroom/fact-sheets/national-health-expenditures-2022-highlights.

CMS (Centers for Medicare and Medicaid Services). 2023d. "Hospital Value-Based Purchasing Program." Accessed June 12, 2024. https://www.cms.gov/medicare/quality/initiatives/hospital-quality-initiative/hospital-value-based-purchasing.

CMS (Centers for Medicare and Medicaid Services). 2022. "Antidepressant Medication Management." https://cmit.cms.gov/cmit/#/MeasureView?variantId=1542&sectionNumber=1.

CMS (Centers for Medicare and Medicaid Services). 2014. "CMS Manual System. Pub. 100–07 State Operations. Provider Certification." https://www.cms.gov/Regulations-and-Guidance/Guidance/Transmittals/downloads/R122SOMA.pdf.

CARF (Commission on Accreditation of Rehabilitation Facilities). n.d. "Accreditation." Accessed August 7, 2024. http://www.carf.org/Accreditation/.

Consumers Advancing Patient Safety. 2017. "About Us." https://www.patientsafety.org/about-us/.

*Darling v. Charleston Community Memorial Hospital*, 33 Ill.2d 626, 211 N.E. 2d, 253 (1965).

HHS (Department of Health and Human Services). n.d. *Practices Guide: Contingency Plan.* Accessed August 10, 2024. https://www.hhs.gov/sites/default/files/ocio/eplc/EPLC%20Archive%20Documents/36-Contingency-Disaster%20Recovery%20Plan/eplc_contingency_plan_practices_guide.pdf.

HHS (Department of Health and Human Services). 2024. "Why Use Telehealth?" https://telehealth.hhs.gov/patients/why-use-telehealth#what-does-telehealth-mean.

HHS (Department of Health and Human Services). 2018. *NPDB Guide Book.* http://www.npdb.hrsa.gov/resources/NPDBGuidebook.pdf.

DNV. n.d. "Hospital Accreditation." Accessed June 12, 2024. https://www.dnv.us/services/hospital-accreditation-218999.

Fahrenholz, C. G. 2013. Purpose of health record documentation. Introduction in *Documentation for Health Records.* Edited by C. G. Fahrenholz and R. Russo. Chicago: AHIMA.

Gerber, A., and K. Lauterbach. 2005. Evidence-based medicine: Why do opponents and proponents use the same arguments? *Health Care Analysis* 31(1).

Healthcare Quality Improvement Act of 1986 (HCQIA). Public Law 99-660.

IHI (Institute for Healthcare Improvement). 2022. National Steering Committee for Patient Safety Declaration to Advance Patient Safety. Boston, MA: Institute for Healthcare Improvement.

IHI (Institute for Healthcare Improvement). n.d.a. "Vision, Mission, and Values." Accessed June 12, 2024. https://www.ihi.org/about/vision-mission-values.

IHI (Institute for Healthcare Improvement). n.d.b. "Triple Aim and Population Health." Accessed January 1, 2024. http://www.ihi.org/Topics/TripleAim/Pages/default.aspx.

IOM (Institute of Medicine). 2003. *Health Professions Education: A Bridge to Quality.* Washington, DC: National Academies Press.

IOM (Institute of Medicine). 2001. *Crossing the Quality Chasm: A New Health System for the 21st Century.* Committee on Quality of Health Care in America. Washington, DC: National Academies Press.

Joint Commission. n.d.a. "Facts About the Joint Commission." Accessed August 7, 2024. https://www.jointcommission.org/who-we-are/facts-about-the-joint-commission/.

Joint Commission. n.d.b. "Sentinel Event." Accessed August 7, 2024. https://www.jointcommission.org/resources/sentinel-event/.

Joint Commission. n.d.c. "Tracer Methodology Fact Sheet." Accessed August 7, 2024. https://www.jointcommission.org/resources/news-and-multimedia/fact-sheets/facts-about-tracer-methodology/.

Josie King Foundation. n.d. "About Josie King Foundation." Accessed August 10, 2024. https://josieking.org/about/.

Kelly, J. R. and P. S. Greenstone. 2019. *Management for the Health Information Professional.* Chicago, IL: AHIMA.

Kohn, L. T., J. M. Corrigan, and M. S. Donaldson. 2000. *To Err Is Human: Building a Safer Health System.* Washington, DC: National Academies Press.

Ladapo, J. and D. Chokshi. 2014. *Continuity of Care for Chronic Conditions: Threats, Opportunities, and Policy.* Health Affairs Blog. http://healthaffairs.org/blog/2014/11/18/continuity-of-care-for-chronic-conditions-threats-opportunities-and-policy-3/.

Lawal, A. K., T. Rotter, L. Kinsman, A. Machotta, U. Ronellenfitsch, S. D. Scott, D. Goodridge, C. Plishka, and G. Groot. 2016. What is a clinical pathway? Refinement of an operational definition to identify clinical pathway studies for a Cochrane systematic review. *BMC Medicine* 14(35).

Medicare Prescription Drug, Improvement, and Modernization Act of 2003. Public Law 108-173.

Lehman, C. 2022. *Clinical Pathways: Leading the Way to Better Outcomes.* Medbridge Blog. https://www.medbridge.com/blog/2022/02/clinical-pathways-leading-the-way-to-better-outcomes/.

NAM (National Academy of Medicine). n.d. *NAM Strategic Plan.* https://nam.edu/wp-content/uploads/2024/01/NAM-Strategic-Plan-2024-2028.pdf.

NAHQ (National Association for Healthcare Quality). n.d. "CPHQ Certification." Accessed August 10, 2024. https://nahq.org/certification/certified-professional-healthcare-quality.

NAHQ (National Association for Healthcare Quality). 2019. *2019 Domestic Candidate Examination Handbook.* https://nahq.org/UPLOADS/certification/US_Handbook.pdf.

NCVHS (National Center on Vital and Health Statistics). 2009. *Health Data Stewardship: What, Why, Who, How—a NCVHS Primer.* http://www.ncvhs.hhs.gov/wp-content/uploads/2014/05/090930lt.pdf.

NIH (National Institutes of Health). 2023. "Outcomes and Effectiveness Research Interest Group." https://oir.nih.gov/sigs/outcomes-effectiveness-research-interest-group.

NPDB (National Practitioner Data Bank). 2006 (March 21). National Practitioner Data Bank for adverse information on physicians and other health care practitioners: Reporting on adverse and negative actions. *Federal Register* 71 FR 14135.

Nilsen, P., I. Seing, C. Ericsson, S. Birken, and K. Schildmeijer. 2020. Characteristics of Successful Changes in Health Care Organizations: An Interview Study with Physicians, Registered Nurses, and Assistant Nurses. *BMC Health Services Research* 20(147). https://bmchealthservres.biomedcentral.com/articles/10.1186/s12913-020-4999-8.

Olejarczyk, J., and M. Young. 2024. "Patient Rights and Ethics." *StatPearls*. https://www.ncbi.nlm.nih.gov/books/NBK538279/.

Overland Park Regional Medical Center. n.d. "About Us." Accessed August 10, 2024. https://www.hcamidwest.com/locations/overland-park-regional-medical-center/about-us/.

Patient Protection and Affordable Care Act of 2010. Public Law 111-148.

Phelps, G., and P. Cooper. 2020. Can artificial intelligence help improve the quality of healthcare? *Journal of Hospital Management and Health Policy* 4(December 2020).

Rotter, T., L. Kinsman, E. L. James, A. Machotta, H. Gothe, J. Willis, P. Sno, and J. Kugler. 2010. Clinical pathways: Effects on professional practice, patient outcomes, length of stay, and hospital costs (review). *The Cochrane Library* 7. https://www.ncbi.nlm.nih.gov/pubmed/20238347.

Sackett, D., W. M. C. Rosenberg, J. A. M. Gray, R. B. Haynes, and W. S. Richardson. 1996. Evidence-based medicine: What it is and what it isn't. *BMJ* 312:71–72.

Shaw, P. L., and D. Carter. 2019. *Quality and Performance Improvement in Healthcare: Theory, Practice, and Management*. Chicago: AHIMA.

SSA (Social Security Administration). 1974. *Notes and Briefs Report: Health Maintenance Act of 1973*. http://www.ssa.gov/policy/docs/ssb/v37n3/v37n3p35.pdf.

Vyas, D. and A. Hozain. 2014. Clinical peer review in the United States: History, legal development, and subsequent abuse. *World Journal of Gastroenterology* 20(21): 6357–6363.

W. Edwards Deming Institute. n.d. "PDSA Cycle." Accessed August 10, 2024. https://deming.org/explore/pdsa/.

Wiet, M. J. 2005. *Darling v. Charleston Community Memorial Hospital* and its legacy. *Annals of Health Law* 14(2). http://lawecommons.luc.edu/cgi/viewcontent.cgi?article=1196&context=annals.

WHO (World Health Organization). 2010. *Framework for Action on Interprofessional Education and Collaborative Practice*. https://iris.who.int/bitstream/handle/10665/70185/WHO_HRH_HPN_10.3_eng.pdf?sequence=1&isAllowed=y.

# PART III
# Informatics, Analytics, and Data Use

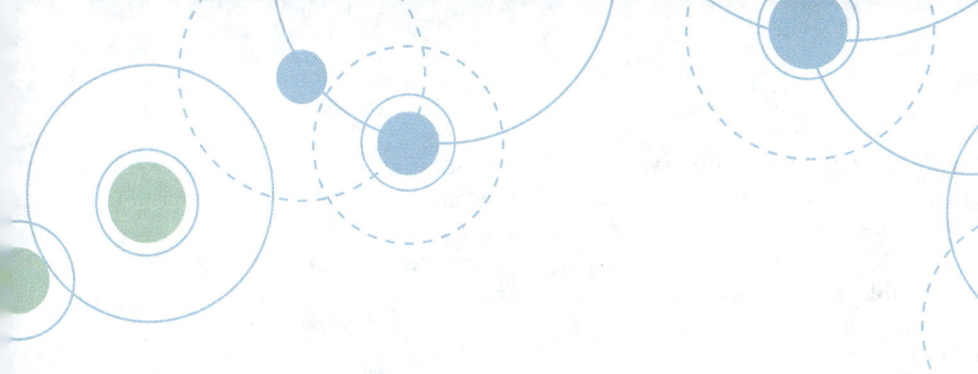

# Health Information Technologies

*Scott B. Lee-Eichenwald, MSDD*

## Learning Objectives

- Assess the field of information technology as applied to healthcare
- Assess the types of current and emerging technology used for data collection, storage, analysis, and reporting of information
- Evaluate the challenges associated with computerizing health data and information
- Assess how interoperability and health information exchange can transform healthcare delivery
- Articulate the characteristics of different architectures and models used in health information exchange
- Describe the stages of a health information exchange implementation.

## Key Terms

Administrative applications
Admit-discharge-transfer (ADT) message
Ancillary systems
Artificial intelligence (AI)
Automated drug dispensing machines
Bar-coding technology
Centralized model
Clinical decision support (CDS) systems
Clinical Document Architecture (CDA)
Clinician web portal
Cloud computing
Computerized provider order entry (CPOE) system
Consumer-mediated exchange
Continuous speech input
Data repository
Data use and reciprocal support agreement (DURSA)
Data warehouse
Directed exchange
eHealth Exchange
Electronic document/content management (ED/CM) system
Electronic health record (EHR)
Electronic medical record (EMR)
Enterprise master patient index (EMPI)
E-Rx (e-prescribing)
Extranets
Federated model
Gesture recognition technology
Health informatics
Health information exchange (HIE)
Health Information Technology for Economic and Clinical Health (HITECH) Act
Health Level Seven International (HL7)
Health Level 7 Fast Healthcare Interoperability Resources (HL7 FHIR)
Health record banking model
Human–computer interface (HCI)
Hybrid model
Informatics
Information management
Intelligent document recognition (IDR) technology
Interoperability
Intranet
Internet of Medical Things (IoMT)

Multimedia
Natural language processing (NLP) technology
Open-source technology
Optical character recognition (OCR) technology
Patient portals
Physiological signal processing system
Point-of-care information systems
Query-based exchange
Radio frequency identification (RFID)
Record locator service (RLS)
Redundancy
Software as a Service (SaaS)
Source systems
Speech recognition technology
Text mining
Trust community
Usability
Vector graphic data
Virtualization
Web content management system
Web portal
Web service
Wireless systems

Healthcare organizations focus on controlling costs and improving efficiency. At the same time they experience demands to ensure patient safety, improve the quality of care, promote access to healthcare services, and ensure compliance with privacy and security regulations. Many healthcare organizations look to technology to help them respond to these pressures to provide high-quality services in a cost-effective manner. The use of technology to manage data and information means that well-trained, skilled individuals with healthcare and computerized information technology knowledge are required to manage (that is, design, develop, select, and maintain) health data and information systems. It also means healthcare organizations must prioritize which computer technologies and information systems to deploy in their institution.

In 2009, the **Health Information Technology for Economic and Clinical Health (HITECH) Act** was passed. This legislation was created to promote the adoption and meaningful use of health information technology (HIT) in the US. Subtitle D of the Act provides for additional privacy and security requirements to develop and support electronic health information, facilitate information exchange, and strengthen monetary penalties. It was signed into law February 17, 2009, as part of the American Recovery and Reinvestment Act of 2009 (ARRA) (Public Law 111-5 2009). The legislation's objectives are to explore innovations in reimbursement; provide guidance on HIT standards, certification, and interoperability; and present incentives to healthcare providers to adopt electronic health record (EHR) systems. It was created to launch initiatives that could prove the benefits of information technology (IT) in relation to better healthcare delivery and coordination of services to the patient.

The Centers for Medicare and Medicaid Services (CMS) established the EHR Incentive Programs in 2011 to encourage meaningful use of EHRs and the exchange of healthcare data. A few iterations of this program have been implemented and retired. The program is currently known as the Medicare Promoting Interoperability Program. These programs support high-quality, high-value care through the use of certified health IT (ONC 2024a). The 2015–2020 Nationwide Interoperability Roadmap has been revised to the 2020–2025 Federal Health IT Strategic Plan. The aim of this 2020–2025 Federal Health IT Strategic Plan is to outline concrete steps federal partners can take to improve health through health IT. The goals, objectives, and strategies within this plan highlight the importance not only of electronic health information, but also of the capabilities enabled by health IT, including public health initiatives, telehealth, and remote monitoring (ONC 2020, 1–2). The plan framework is in figure 12.1.

This chapter introduces the field of informatics as currently applied in the healthcare industry. It also describes the current and emerging technologies used to support the delivery of healthcare and the management and communication of patient information.

## The Field of Informatics

**Informatics** is a field of study that focuses on the use of technology to improve access to, and utilization of, information. It uses computers to manage data and information and support decision-making activities. **Information management** includes the generation, collection, organization, validation, analysis, storage, and integration of data, as well as the dissemination, communication, presentation, utilization, transmission, and safeguarding of information.

The healthcare industry is information intensive. A large percentage of healthcare professionals' activities relate to managing massive amounts of data and information. This includes obtaining and documenting information about patients, consulting with colleagues, staying abreast of the current literature, determining strategies for patient care, interpreting laboratory data and test results, and conducting research. Health information is largely electronic, so the study of informatics and its focus on utilizing technology to manage information is critical for patient care. Informatics comes into play in healthcare in this way. **Health informatics**

**Figure 12.1.** 2020–2025 Federal Health IT Strategic Plan Framework

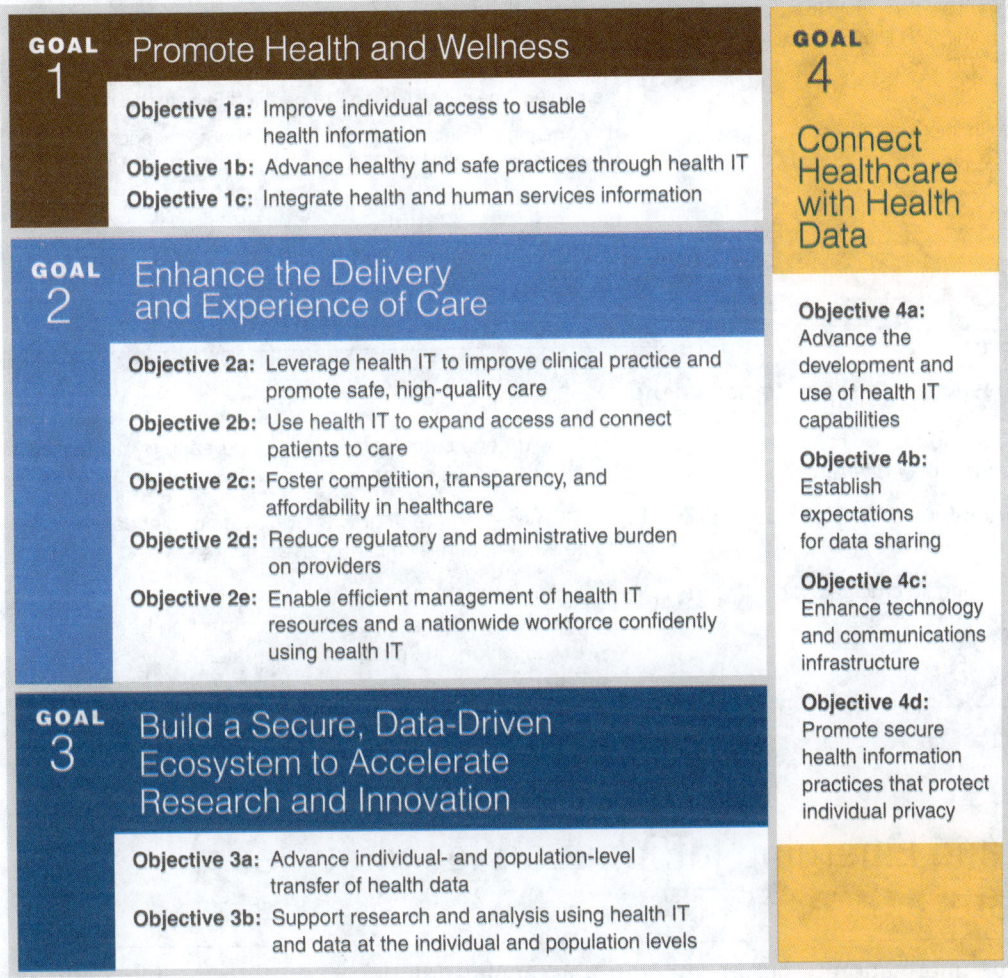

*Source:* ONC 2020, 5.

is a scientific discipline concerned with the cognitive, information-processing, and communication tasks of healthcare practice, education, and research, including the information science and technology to support these tasks. Health informatics is also an interprofessional field that analyzes biomedical data, information, and knowledge for decision-making to improve human health (Jen et al. 2023). Overall, it is concerned with the management of all aspects of health data and information through the application of computers and computer technologies.

The use of information technologies to improve the healthcare delivery system gained attention in the early 1990s and has continued to the current time with the publication of several reports, implementation of initiatives, and passing of legislation. See table 12.1 for a summary of these efforts.

Examples of informatics success have steadily grown over the ensuing years. Charge collection and billing, automated laboratory testing and reporting, clinical documentation, computerized provider order entry (CPOE), patient and provider scheduling, diagnostic imaging, and secondary data use make up a distinguished list of health informatics successes, proving what is doable and supporting further investment. Today's task for informatics is to design, develop, and implement computer information systems that enable healthcare organizations to accomplish visions for providing the highest-quality care in the most effective way.

**Table 12.1.** HIT initiatives

| Year | Initiative | Purpose |
|---|---|---|
| 2000–2001 | Institute of Medicine (IOM) reports published | To highlight concerns regarding patient safety and role of HIT in improving healthcare delivery |
| 2004 | Office of the National Coordinator of Health Information Technology (ONC) established | To oversee and support the adoption of a national HIT infrastructure |
| 2008 | Federal Health Information Technology Strategic Plan developed | To guide the advancement of HIT throughout the federal government through 2012 |
| 2009 | HIT for Economic and Clinical Health (HITECH) provision of ARRA passed | Authorized the (CMS) to provide reimbursement incentives for eligible professionals and hospitals who are successful in becoming "meaningful users" of certified EHR technology |
| 2015–2025 | Federal Health Information Technology Strategic Plan updated | To continue advancement of HIT throughout the federal government for 2015–2025 |

### Check Your Understanding 12.1

**Answer the following questions in a separate document.**

1. How are the disciplines of information management and informatics related? How are they different?
2. What are the two provisions of the HITECH Act? Explain why they are important to the field of HIT.
3. Why are data and information so crucial to a healthcare professional's daily work?
4. Provide one example of how using health IT can benefit healthcare organizations.
5. Give an example of how the government influences the level of health IT utilized in healthcare.
6. Using table 12.1, HIT initiatives, which initiative listed do you think had the most financial impact on healthcare organizations? Explain your rationale.

## Current and Emerging Information Technologies in Healthcare

To examine the information resources and systems that enable healthcare organizations to accomplish their visions in the most effective way, health information management (HIM) professionals must possess fundamental knowledge of computer-based information systems' components. This includes knowledge of system hardware, software, and service components; communication and networking components; the internet and its derived technologies; and system architectures. In addition to fundamental knowledge, the HIM professional must also remain informed about emerging topics in health IT.

Artificial intelligence (AI) is emerging as a valuable asset within healthcare delivery organizations. AI is comprised of high-level information technologies used in developing machines that imitate human qualities such as learning and reasoning. Research in the application of AI in healthcare continues to advance quickly, including in the areas of drug discovery, virtual clinical consultation, disease diagnosis, prognosis, medication management and health monitoring. AI related technologies such as speech recognition and natural language processing (NLP) are also helping healthcare organizations increase their efficiencies and engagement with patients.

It is appropriate that HIM professionals review some of the current and emerging technologies used to support the delivery of healthcare and the management and communication of health data and information within the healthcare setting. HIM professionals' involvement includes supporting capture of various data types and formats; supporting efficient access to and flow of data and information; and supporting diagnosis, treatment, and care of patients.

# Technologies Supporting the Capture of Different Types of Data and Formats

The IT currently in use for healthcare applications and the new technologies being developed support the capture of many data types and formats. All are used to support the clinical services and administrative functions performed in every healthcare setting.

Data formats may be structured or unstructured. For example, the demographic data elements and laboratory results in a patient's record are coded and alphanumeric. The fields are predefined and limited in format and length. The type of data is discrete, and the format is structured. This means when a healthcare professional searches a database for one or more coded, discrete data elements based on the search parameters such as a patient name or cholesterol level, the search engine can easily find, retrieve, and manipulate the element. However, the format of the data contained in a patient's transcribed history and physical (H&P) report, for example, is unstructured. Free-text data, as opposed to discrete, structured data, are not predefined and limited. Therefore, data embedded in unstructured text are not easily retrieved by the search engine. About 70 to 80 percent of clinical data is unstructured and found in narrative clinical reports, medical images, and patient notes (Rahman and Khatun 2023, 9). See figure 12.2 for an illustration of structured and unstructured data in healthcare.

When more than one unstructured data type is present in an information system, the data and system they represent are referred to as **multimedia**. The EHR system is multimedia. (See table 12.2 for examples of EHR unstructured data types and sources.)

## Speech Recognition Technology

As the need for immediately available healthcare documentation increases, the development and application of different forms of speech recognition technology have evolved.

Today, **speech recognition technology**, which translates speech to text, is speaker independent with

**Figure 12.2.** Structured and unstructured data in healthcare

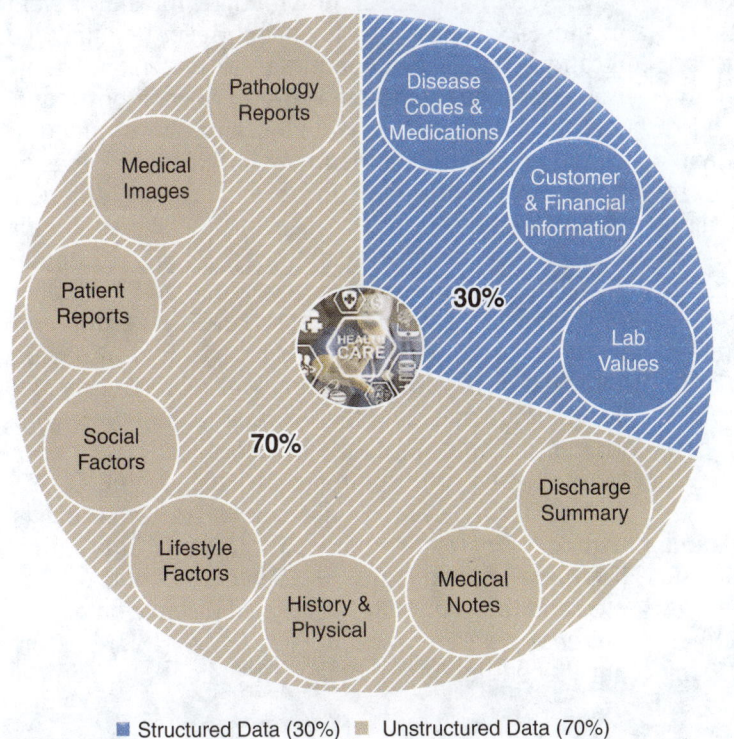

■ Structured Data (30%)  ■ Unstructured Data (70%)

*Source:* Rahman and Khatun 2023, 9.

**Table 12.2.** EHR unstructured data types and sources

| Data category | Unstructured data type | Source |
|---|---|---|
| Diagnostic Image Data | Bitmapped | CT scan, magnetic imaging (MRI), digitized (scanned) x-ray film images |
| Document Image Data | Bitmapped | Scanned (digitized) paper-based documents or photographs |
| Audio Data | Sound bites; signal processing (vector graphic) | Electrocardiogram (ECG), electroencephalogram (EEG), fetal heart rate (FHR) |

continuous speech input. Speaker independence does not require extensive training. The software is already trained to recognize generic speech and speech patterns. Continuous speech input does not require the user to pause between words to let the computer distinguish between the beginning and ending of words. However, the user must be careful to enunciate when speaking.

Although speech recognition vocabularies are expanding due to faster and more powerful computer hardware, only limited clinical vocabularies have been developed. Limited vocabulary–based speech recognition systems require the user to say words known or taught to the system. In healthcare, limited clinical vocabulary-based specialties such as radiology, emergency medicine, and psychiatry have realized significant benefits for dictation from the technology.

The goal in speech recognition technology is the ability to talk to a computer's central processor and rapidly create vocabularies for applications without collecting speech samples (in other words, without training). It includes the ability to speak at natural speed and tone and in no specific manner. It also includes having the computer understand what the user wants to say (the context of the word or words) and then apply the correct commands or words as coded data in a structured format. Finally, it includes identifying a user's voice and encrypting the voiceprint. In the coming decades, clinical vocabularies and algorithms will improve, true speaker independence will be achieved, and natural language understanding will ultimately make structured dictation a reality.

AI has found a place within speech recognition technology. These technologies have the potential to enhance usability and efficiency and reduce provider workload related to the clinical documentation process within EHR systems. Voice-enabled AI advances speech recognition, seeking to interpret a provider-patient conversation and capture important clinical information for the electronic patient record. However, the maturity of voice-recognition tools in a clinical setting needs more time to evolve. Voice recognition in healthcare is complex and difficult to capture. A human must identify and capture important clinical terminology from general conversation (Padmanabhan 2022).

## Natural Language Processing Technology

Natural language processing (NLP) technology is a technology that converts human language (structured or unstructured) into data that can be translated then manipulated by computer systems. It is considered a branch of AI. As such, it differs from simple Boolean word search programs (simply combining search terms with *and*, *or*, *not*, or *near*) that often complement speech recognition technology–based systems. For example, the narratives "no shortness of breath, chest pain aggravated by exercise" and "no chest pain, shortness of breath aggravated by exercise" look the same to a Boolean word search engine when looking for occurrences of *chest* and *pain* in the same sentence.

NLP technology can differentiate the narratives' meanings. For example, for health record coding applications, it teaches computers to understand English well enough to "read" transcribed reports and notes and then find certain key concepts (not merely words) by identifying the many different phrasings of the concept. By normalizing these concepts, different phrases of the same content can be compared with one another for statistical purposes. For example, "the patient thinks he had a seizure" and "the doctor thinks the patient had a seizure" have different meanings from a coding perspective. By employing statistical or rules-based algorithms, NLP technology can compare and code these similar expressions with different meanings accurately and quickly.

Autocoding and computer-assisted coding (CAC) are the terms used to describe NLP technology's method of extracting and subsequently translating dictated and then transcribed free-text data, or dictated and then computer-generated discrete data, into *International Classification of Diseases* (ICD) or Current Procedural Terminology (CPT) codes for clinical and financial applications such as patient billing and health record coding. AI-powered autonomous medical coding is an upcoming advancement that will enhance the ability to code with little to no human intervention. Text mining and data mining are the terms commonly used to describe the process of extracting and then quantifying and filtering free-text data and discrete data, respectively.

NLP is an important tool in the efforts to transform unstructured healthcare data into useable information. NLP can capture unstructured data elements from the EHR, analyze and obtain meaning from their grammatical structure, and summarize information for use in further analysis (Shah and Khan 2020, 136951). See figure 12.3 for an illustration.

## Electronic Document and Content Management Systems

Care delivery organizations may use bridge technology to enhance access to patient information when they do not have a full complement of source systems or have source systems that cannot support the major clinical components of an EHR. In some cases, providers interact well with the bridge technology applications. In other cases, the applications primarily enhance financial and administrative processes.

Electronic document management (EDM) systems greatly improve financial and administrative processes after discharge, where many departments need access to the patient's record, where there are record completion responsibilities for several providers, and where access to clinical information may be needed in immediate outpatient or emergency department (ED) follow-up. It is also possible to add workflow technology to these systems, which can be used to queue work among staff or between departments.

A document is any analog or digital, formatted, and preserved "container" of data or information, collectively referred to as content. The document is a well-worn and very useful construct, but unless data contained within documents are formatted and accompanied by print-like qualities, such as headings or bolding, data are difficult to interpret.

An electronic document/content management (ED/CM) system is any electronic system that manages an organization's analog and digital documents and content (that is, not just the data) to realize significant improvements in business work processes. Like most ISs, the ED/CM system consists of several component technologies that support both digital and analog document and content management. These component technologies are discussed in table 12.3.

**Figure 12.3.** Example of NLP and EHR data

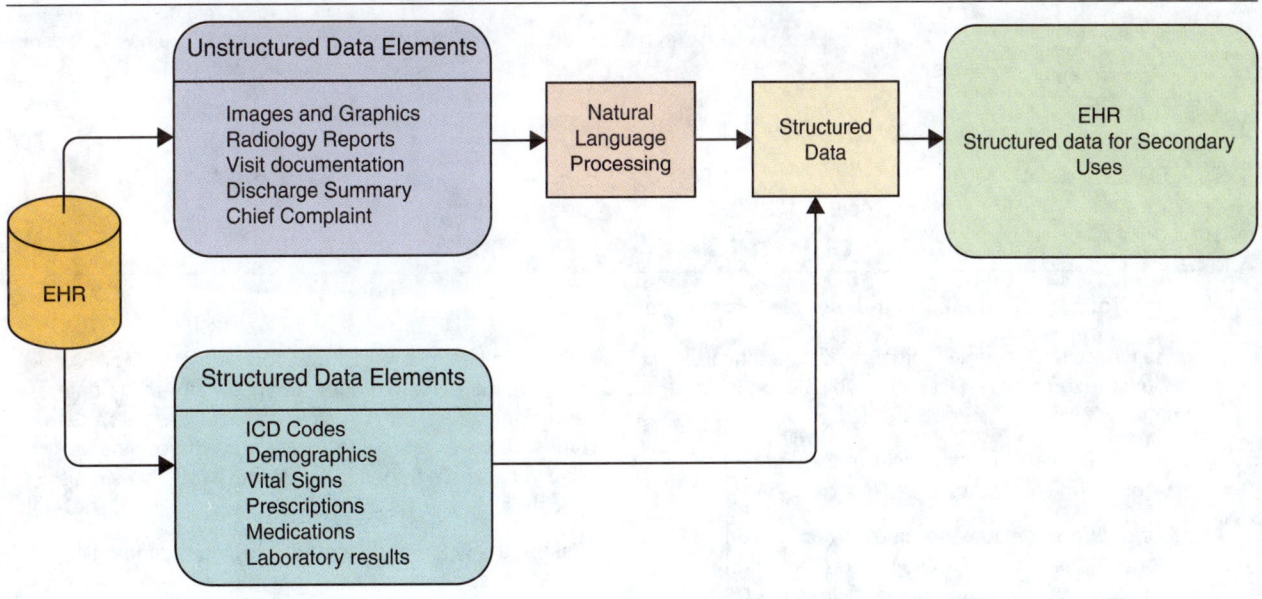

*Source:* Shah and Khan 2020, 136951.

**Table 12.3.** Component technologies of ED/CM systems

| Technology | Function | Application |
|---|---|---|
| Document imaging technology | Electronically captures, stores, identifies, retrieves, and distributes documents not generated digitally or that are generated digitally but stored on paper for distribution purposes | Handwritten physician problem lists and notes; "fill-in-the-blank" typeset nursing forms; preprinted Conditions of Treatment forms; and documents external to the organization |
| Document management technology | Automatically organizes, assembles, secures, and shares documents | Document version control, check in–check out control, document access control, and text and word searches |
| Electronic records management (ERM) technology | Allows mass storage of structured and unstructured data and a variety of documents which comprise electronic records; properly classifies content using appropriate categories so that applicable legal and regulatory retention rules can be applied | Components that ensure the long-term authenticity, security, and reliability of an organization's electronic records |
| Workflow technology | Assigns, routes, activates, and manages document flow based on business rules | Automatic routing of electronic documents into electronic inboxes of its department staff for work assignment |
| Enterprise report management technology | Electronically stores, manages, and distributes documents that are generated in a digital format and whose output data are report formatted and print-stream originated | Viewing digitally generated documents such as emails, transcription files, e-faxes, voice files |
| Automatic forms-processing (e-forms) technology | Allows users to electronically enter data into online forms and electronically extract the data from the online forms for various data-manipulation purposes | Electronic data entry and viewing within structured forms |
| Digital signature management technology | Offers both signer and document authentication for analog or digital documents. Signer authentication is the ability to identify the person who digitally signed the document. | Allows for digital signature verification |
| Picture archiving and communication systems (PACS) | Capture images of the human body that can be used for clinical decision-making. | An integrated computer system that obtains, stores, retrieves, and displays digital images, e.g., diagnostic imaging technology where images taken from multiple sources (CT scans or MRIs ultrasounds, etc.) |

### Check Your Understanding 12.2

**Answer the following questions in a separate document.**

1. Describe why it is challenging to have most healthcare data as unstructured data. Describe one solution for this challenge.
2. How can workflow technology assist in the completion of records following discharge?
3. What is the difference between speech recognition technology and NLP technology? What is the difference between NLP technology and Boolean searching? Explain the benefits or drawbacks of using these three technologies within the EDM.
4. Provide a healthcare example for each of the following data types: real audio data, motion or streaming data, and signal or vector graphic data. How can these data types be used to provide care across the population? Use your own perspective or research to answer this question.
5. Assess the value of document imaging technology, workflow and business process management (BPM) technology, automated forms technology, and digital signature management technology, and provide a practical example of how each could be used.

# Technologies Supporting Efficient Access to and Flow of Data and Information

Many current and emerging information technologies are used to support efficient access to and flow of healthcare data and information. This chapter highlights automatic recognition technologies, enterprise master patient indices, identity management, and cloud-based technologies and applications, which are instrumental in the daily management and maintenance of medical equipment and systems.

## Automatic Recognition Technologies

Several types of automatic recognition technologies exist, which can be grouped into two categories. Character and symbol recognition technologies recognize electronically scanned characters or symbols from analog items, such as tangible materials or documents, enabling the identified data to be quickly, accurately, and automatically entered in digital systems. Character and symbol recognition technologies include bar coding, optical character recognition, and gesture recognition technologies. Technologies that identify actual items include radio frequency identification (RFID) and intelligent document recognition (IDR) technologies. These technologies do not require a character or symbol for recognition. They can track an item using an embedded chip or recognize form types by remembering patterns in the form.

### Bar-coding Technology

Decades ago, the barcode symbol was standardized for the healthcare industry, making it easier to adopt and realize the potential of bar-coding technology. **Bar-coding technology** is a method of encoding data that consists of parallel arrangements of dark elements, referred to as *bars*; light elements, referred to as *spaces*; and interpreting the data for automatic identification and data collection purposes. Since then, bar-coding applications have been adopted for labels; patient wristbands; specimen containers; business, employee, and patient records; library reference materials; medication packages; dietary items; paper documents; and more. Benefits have been realized by the uniform consistency in the development of commercially available software systems, fewer procedural variations in healthcare organizations using the technology, and the flexibility to adopt standard specifications for functions while retaining current systems. Because virtually every tangible item in the clinical setting, including the patient, can be assigned a barcode with an associated meaning, it is not surprising to find barcoding as the primary tracking, identification, inventory data-capture, and even patient safety medium in healthcare organizations.

When bar-coding systems are interfaced to healthcare ISs, the barcode can be used to enter the data, especially repetitive data, saving additional processing time and paper generation. More importantly, the data input error rates with bar coding are close to zero. Bar-coded data, with an error rate of approximately three transactions in one million, can be considered error free. Thus, it is a most effective remedy for medication errors when used to ensure that the right medication dose is administered to the right patient.

### Optical Character Recognition Technology

Like bar-coding, **optical character recognition (OCR) technology** was invented to reduce manual data input, or hand-keying. OCR technology recognizes machine-generated characters (for example, preprinted numbers and letters) by interpreting the scanned, bitmapped shapes of the characters' images and then converting the characters into computer-processable codes. OCR technology was initially used to automatically identify financial accounts consisting of preprinted Arabic numbers and Roman letters using a standardized font on thousands of paper-based documents, such as bank checks.

OCR has been perfected to recognize the full set of preprinted typeset fonts as well as point sizes. The best OCR systems compensate for imperfectly formed characters and scanned pages by employing characteristics such as deskewing ("straightening" oblique characters), broken character repair ("fixing" incomplete characters), and redaction ("hiding" superfluous characters). OCR is used to perform everything from indexing scanned documents to digitizing full text. Its ability to dramatically reduce manual data input, or hand-keying, while increasing input speed represents the best aspect of this technology.

### Gesture Recognition Technology

The recognition of constrained or unconstrained, handwritten, English-language free text (print or cursive, upper- or lower-case, characters or symbols) typically stored on paper-based, analog documents, is known as intelligent character recognition (ICR) technology. ICR technology is adopted primarily for activities that use digital pens to enter data. For example, documenting nurses' notes or progress notes. ICR technology may also be used for translating forms completed manually, such as a patient registration or insurance forms, to text. The recognition of hand-marked characters in defined areas of, typically, paper-based analog documents is known as mark sense technology. Consequently, it is used for processing analog questionnaires, surveys, and tests, such as filled-in circles with number two pencils on standardized tests. Collectively, these technologies (ICR and mark sense) are referred to as **gesture recognition technology**.

### Radio Frequency Identification Technology

**Radio frequency identification (RFID)** is an automatic recognition technology that uses a device attached to an object to transmit data to a receiver and does not require direct contact. The technology works in the following manner: Chips that emit radio signals are embedded in analog items and products. The signals are read and captured by receivers. The receivers act as data collectors and send the signals to PCs on a network, allowing the items and products to be tracked.

RFID's applicability in the healthcare industry is limited only by the imagination. Like barcodes, it is being used to track moveable patients, clinicians, medications, and equipment. As such, in a wireless environment, RFID could replace barcodes for these applications. RFID technologies can be removable units or embedded within the technology.

### Intelligent Document Recognition Technology

**Intelligent document recognition (IDR) technology** trains itself to identify document or form types and to sort the information accordingly for subsequent data entry, eliminating the need for barcodes or other identifying characters and symbols. This training process requires a period of continuously scanning each type of document or form. As such, the pattern of document and form layouts and information locations educates the system to recognize the document or form for future recognition situations.

## Enterprise Master Patient Indices and Identity Management

As healthcare organizations continue to come together into integrated delivery networks (IDNs), it is increasingly likely that identifying information about a patient is spread across multiple databases and in multiple formats. Consequently, healthcare organizations are developing strategic initiatives for the **enterprise master patient index (EMPI)**. In the broad sense, this involves the increasingly important service referred to as identity management.

EMPIs provide access to multiple repositories of information from overlapping patient populations that are maintained in separate systems and databases. This occurs through an indexing scheme to all unique patient identification numbers and information in all the organizations' databases. As such, EMPIs become the cornerstones of healthcare system integration projects.

EMPIs work in two ways, as shown in figure 12.4. At the back end, EMPIs coordinate recordkeeping. The EMPI receives information from multiple systems that need no modification. The receiving process is often performed through an integration gateway or engine. The enterprise index tests to see whether the patient is identified in all the systems. If not, it may assign a unique identification number or other, related identifier and correlate records throughout the enterprise.

At the front end, EMPIs receive requests from existing registration systems to send data to these systems. Usually, these existing registration systems need some reprogramming to enable them to request and receive data from the EMPI. Currently, there is no consistent accepted trigger event and standard data format to do this.

EMPI building is complex. Variations in IS, data capture, and organizational goals and objectives present multiple challenges to integrating patient data. For example, EMPI building involves a multitude of decision points. These include deciding whether to employ centralized or distributed data storage; whether to maintain limited, additional information such as allergies or robust information such as problem lists, which include a full list of medical conditions; and whether to establish batch processing or real-time communication between the registration system and the EMPI.

In addition, EMPIs include complex capabilities. These capabilities include merging records pertaining to the same person using probabilistic matching and algorithms, maintaining source systems' pointers, removing duplicate records, and providing a common user interface. Finally, after technical and organizational issues are overcome, the purely operational tasks of linking patients across multiple entities and episodes of care and maintaining these linkages are difficult and can be costly.

## Cloud-Based Technologies and Applications

Within healthcare, there is significant movement toward the adoption of cloud technologies. It is becoming

**Figure 12.4.** EMPI functionality

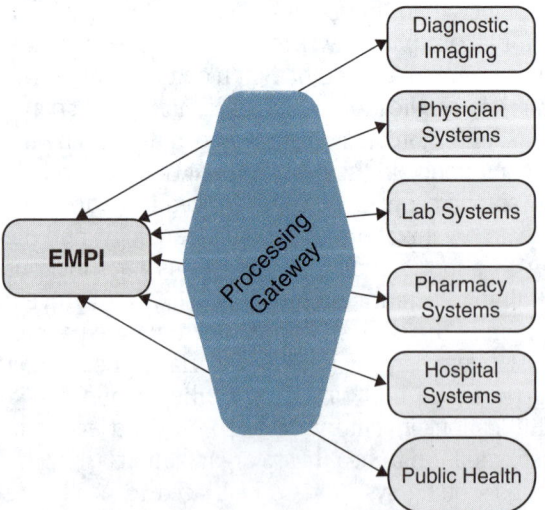

common for organizations to migrate from legacy on-premises infrastructure to cloud hosted applications which support the digital transformation initiatives happening in healthcare. The capabilities of **cloud computing**, in which servers that may be located anywhere in the world supply data and functionality through the internet, are useful in implementing EHRs and other healthcare technologies in a variety of contexts. Cloud computing benefits include the ability for efficient upgrades, easy data sharing, and strong control over patient privacy and information security. For example, upgrading cloud-based programs is efficient because each cloud computing program on any of the computers in the organization can individually process updates. Cloud data sharing is easily available for all devices connected to the server at any location and in any form. Increased security exists because the nature of the cloud infrastructure does not allow the consumer to manage and control it. In the cloud infrastructure model, healthcare software developers are responsible for protecting the privacy and security of patients (Ahmadi and Aslani 2018). There are a variety of cloud-based health information technologies needed for healthcare organizations to accomplish their digital initiatives. This section will provide detailed information on web portals, intranets and extranets, web content management systems, web services, and open-source technology.

## Web Portals

A **web portal** is a single point of personalized access (an entryway) through which one can find and deliver information (content), applications, and services. Web portals began in the consumer market as a pathway to an array of internet services and information found on websites.

Consequently, **clinician web portals**, sometimes referred to as physician web portals, first were seen as a way for clinicians to easily access (through a web browser) the healthcare organizations' multiple sources of structured and unstructured data from any network-connected device. Clinician web portals evolved into an effective medium for providing access to multiple applications and the data. And because clinician portals are cloud-based technologies, they became the access points to sources of data and applications both internal and external to the organization. With the success of clinician web portals and the trend toward improving patient engagement in healthcare through technology, a growing number of healthcare provider and payer organizations have established web portals for their patients and members. Each participant creates an account on the web portal with a unique login and password. Typical payer-based portal uses include accessing membership information and choosing a primary care physician. Typical provider-based portal uses include requesting prescription renewals, scheduling appointments, and asking questions of providers through secure messaging. Patients increasingly use internet entryways called **patient portals** to pay their bills online and to securely view all or portions of their provider-based EHR, such as current medical conditions, immunization records, medications, allergies, and test results.

Although patients or payer members access the portals over the internet, all the information, including the secure messaging applications, resides on the provider's or payer's secured servers. These portals dovetail well with privacy and security regulations, which empower patients with the authority to determine who can have access to their healthcare information. Also, patients can use the portal to notify providers if their EHR is incorrect. As consumers seek to take a larger role in their healthcare, such patient "entryways" to information (content), applications, and services are common practice.

## Intranets and Extranets

Cloud-based information systems and applications cannot continue to proliferate without a cloud-based **intranet**, which uses internet technologies but are protected with security features and designed to enhance communication among an organization's internal employees and facilities only; and a cloud-based **extranet**, designed to enhance communication among an organization's external business partners. Intranets link every employee within an organization through an easy-to-navigate, comprehensive network devoted to internal business operations, while extranets link an organization's external business partners with the same comprehensive network but one that is devoted to external business operations. For example, private, secure networks provide every healthcare organization employee with basic information such as message boards, employee handbooks, manuals, mail, cafeteria menus, newsletters, directories, and contact lists. Also, they are used for the development of the organization's EHR. Restricted access to intranets by authorized users provides assurances the general internet public cannot access this private, secure network. However, through its intranet, a healthcare organization can access the internet's servers for general internet mail and messaging.

Extranets connect intranets that exist outside an organization's firewall. For example, typically, an IDN's autonomous care facilities (for example, acute care, long-term care, home healthcare), each with its own intranet, need to communicate between and among themselves through secure email or other collaboration tools. The facilities connect the various intranets and form an extranet.

## Web Content Management Systems

**Web content management systems** label and track the information that is placed on a website so that the information can be easily located, modified, and reused. These systems are a critical component in personalizing an organization's web-based intranet and extranet, web portal, and page content for site users and visitors. They also provide crucial versioning and globalization capabilities. Versioning enables the website's content components to be tracked individually. As the content changes, each version of the content can be identified, and the overall website can be recreated as it existed at any specific point in time. Globalization enables the look and feel of an organization's website to be managed centrally, while specific content is managed for local requirements.

## Web Services

**Web services** technology is a platform for software applications (or services) whose basic communication mechanism is XML, the universal language of the web and the accepted format for data exchange over the internet. In addition, web services technology uses web-based infrastructure protocols, such as Hypertext Transfer Protocol (HTTP), Hypertext Transfer Protocol Secure (HTTPS), and transmission control protocol/internet protocol (TCP/IP). As such, web services technology allows programs written in different languages and on different operating systems to communicate with each other in a standards-based way. In short, web services technology is an open, standardized way of integrating disparate, web browser–based and other applications.

By using XML messages to format and tag data, web services technology allows for data interchange without the need for translation. In addition, the messages use system-independent vocabularies and protocols, such as simple object access protocols (SOAP) to transfer the data; universal description, discovery, and integration (UDDI) to list what services are available; and web services description language (WSDL) to describe the services available. Healthcare organizations have been gradually installing web services to ease integration of disparate web-based and legacy applications, often written in incompatible languages. This ensures the organizations' applications interoperate and that healthcare organizations can more easily choose tools for important interorganizational and regional data sharing.

## Open-Source Technology

Open-source software products are applications whose source (human-readable) code is freely available to anyone who is interested in downloading the code. Advantages of **open-source technology** include its availability, its ability to be customized, and the collaborative nature of the product in which a community of developers and users can interact, review, and improve upon each other's ideas. Disadvantages of open-source technology include the need for skilled developers within an organization to take advantage of the benefits noted earlier and a lack of dependable technical support.

### Check Your Understanding 12.3

**Answer the following questions in a separate document.**

1. Considering yourself as a patient, identify five features or functions you would like in your patient portal?

2. Evaluate how healthcare organizations can utilize automatic recognition technologies. Provide a healthcare example for each of the following: barcoding, OCR, ICR, RFID, and IDR. In addition, please provide your thoughts on the effectiveness of at least one of these technologies based on personal experience or additional research.

3. How might an on-call physician use a clinical portal to respond to a patient suffering from a sudden anxiety attack outside of clinic hours?

4. What is the difference between an intranet and an extranet? Provide an example of how each can be used in healthcare. From your experience (or research, if no experience) using an intranet or extranet personally or professionally, what issues can you identify with each?

5. ABC Clinic is planning to purchase a new EHR. The clinic manager is investigating several options keeping the budget in mind with the only two IT staff members at the clinic. They have been told to investigate open-source software. Describe the benefits and drawbacks of open-source technology and make a recommendation to ABC Clinic regarding whether or not to use an open-source product.

6. Explain what advantages and disadvantages providers may experience when providing patient portals.

# Technologies Supporting the Diagnosis, Treatment, and Care of Patients

Many current and emerging information technologies are used to support the diagnosis, treatment, and care of patients. In this chapter, the following technologies are highlighted:

- Physiological signal processing systems
- Point-of-care information systems
- Mobile and wireless technology and devices
- Automated care plans, clinical practice guidelines, clinical pathways, and protocols
- Telehealth systems
- EHR systems

These healthcare technologies are commonly implemented because they are expected to yield a high return on investment in terms of increased efficiency, and provider and patient satisfaction.

## Physiological Signal Processing Systems

The human body is a rich source of signals that carry vital information about underlying physiological processes. Traditionally, such signals have been used in clinical diagnosis and in the study of the functional behavior of internal organs.

**Physiological signal processing systems**, such as ECG and EEG systems, store data based on the body's signals (such as heart activity and brain waves) and create output based on the lines plotted between the signals' points. The data type used by these systems is referred to as signal tracing or **vector graphic data**.

Physiological signal processing systems measure biological signals. Also, they help to integrate the medical science of analyzing the signals with such disciplines as biomedical engineering, computer graphics, mathematics, diagnostic image processing, computer vision, and pattern recognition. The integration of these disciplines allows these systems to electronically compile measurement equations, estimate the signals' parameters, and characterize the feedback elements. For example, the computer-based analysis of the neuromuscular system, the definition of cardiovascular system models, the control of cardiac pacemakers, the regulation of blood sugar levels, and the development of artificial organs not only serve patient diagnostic and care purposes but also support the development and simulation of instrumentation for physiological research and clinical investigation.

## Point-of-Care Information Systems

**Point-of-care information systems** allow healthcare providers to capture and retrieve data and information at the location where the healthcare service is performed. Functionally, almost every type of patient clinical and administrative application has been introduced to provide care services at the bedside, in the exam room, at the home, or even on the patient, as in medical monitoring. Technologically, massive changes have occurred in these systems' platforms, footprints, and networking capabilities.

For example, many acute-care facilities installed clinical point-of-care information systems that, among other services, provide online medication order entry, profiles, administration schedules, and records. The records include information about medications not given (with reasons) and related information such as fluid balances, physical assessments, laboratory test results, and vital signs. All medications, including unit doses, are barcoded and scanned at or near the patient's bedside along with the patient's wristband and the caregiver's identification badge. This prompts a safety edit, documents administration of the medication, and generates the charge. Other acute-care facilities have installed administrative point-of-care (or service) systems that eliminated admitting areas. Inpatients are greeted at the door with their room assignments, and roving admissions representatives visit patients in their assigned rooms to complete admission procedures.

Typically, point-of-care information systems use portable, handheld, wireless devices to enable data entry with a barcode scanner, keypad, digital pen, or touch screen. Wireless devices are also used to upload and download information to and from hardwired workstations. Data retrieval occurs at the wireless device or on wall-mounted or portable, cart-based computers. The data also can be entered and retrieved on hardwired workstations located in areas outside the point of care, such as central areas at patient care units, back offices, central or satellite pharmacies, and physician lounges, homes, and offices.

## Mobile and Wireless Technology and Devices

Perhaps the biggest influence on, and challenge for, point-of-care information systems and their use comes from significant advances in wireless technology and smaller, mobile devices. For the healthcare industry, the successful integration of wireless technology and smaller, mobile devices with point-of-care software supports and enhances the clinician's decision-making processes.

True **wireless systems** use wireless networks and wireless devices to access and transmit data in real time. At the basic level, wireless technology is based on the use of radio waves. For years, healthcare organizations have used in-building wireless point-of-care information systems, such as telemetry systems. These systems were based on existing technologies and use a portion of the radio spectrum reserved for industrial, scientific, and medical purposes (ISM band). Individual licenses are not required for these types of systems.

Also, provider organizations have long used wide-area wireless technology to support information systems such as point-of-care systems. This technology involves microwave systems that are based on fixed, point-to-point wireless technology used to connect buildings in a campus network. Microwave systems are regulated and require licenses and compliance with Federal Trade Commission procedures.

It is the widespread adoption of cellular telephone technology that has significantly advanced the development of wireless technology and, consequently, its support for point-of-care systems. A brief look at healthcare organizations today shows mobile phones, two-way pagers, smartphones, and tablets in use.

Mobile devices improve point-of-care systems by allowing clinicians to use a device personalized to their individual workflows, such as clinical (for example, e-prescribing), documentation, and billing workflows. In addition, mobile devices provide clinicians the information they need anytime, anywhere, and on any network-addressable device.

Another important technology to recognize is the **Internet of Medical Things (IoMT)**, which describes a network of physical objects or "things" integrated to exchange healthcare data between devices and systems over the internet. IoMT is important because medical devices and systems need to connect with systems within healthcare delivery organizations. Digital health initiatives, system integration, and interoperability require medical technology to connect and transfer data bidirectionally between information systems such as EHRs, which is most often the official record for patient information (Dwivedi et al. 2022).

## Automated Clinical Care Plans, Practice Guidelines, Pathways, and Protocols

Providers recognize enormous variation in how they diagnose, treat, and care for patients. Consequently, providers increased their use of guidelines, formalized pathways, and protocols emerging from clinical research (evidence-based medicine [EBM]) to reduce variation and improve care outcomes. Automating these guidelines, pathways, and protocols for providers to easily access them is a first step. As automated clinical documentation systems are implemented, there is a trend to incorporate automated clinical pathways and care plans into providers' notes.

Clinical care plans, guidelines, pathways, and protocols, drug formularies, and other clinical knowledge bases, are being automated for easier access and use by healthcare providers, updating, and maintenance. Many healthcare organizations purchase subscriptions from agencies, societies, or research companies to gain access to peer-reviewed libraries of clinical practice guidelines and clinical knowledge bases. They do so to efficiently download periodic updates of this content into their transaction-based or analytic systems.

The challenge for automated care plans, practice guidelines, pathways, and protocols is that—like clinical workstations and web portals—no one form of clinical documentation or one view of the information suits everyone or all situations. Therefore, automated plans, guidelines, pathways, and protocols require customization capabilities to help individuals and groups better share knowledge to reach similar decisions about patient care.

## Telehealth Systems

Interactive, electronic patient-provider consultations for clinical care, patient education, public health, and health administration across a geographic distance represent what is often referred to as telehealth (sometimes called telemedicine). However, the field has always encompassed a multitude of strategies for moving clinical knowledge and expertise instead of moving people. As such, telehealth systems, like EHR systems, are concepts made up of several cost-effective technologies used to bridge geographic gaps between patients and providers. Telehealth services range from teleradiology (interpreting a scan from a distance) to telepsychiatry (consultations at a distance) to telesurgery and robotics (surgery from a distance).

Telehealth systems utilize clinically adequate, interactive media conferencing (for example, video conferencing) integrated with other technologies. Telehealth systems include telecommunications and remote control–based biomedical technologies. Telehealth utilizes in-room systems, mobile systems, desktop systems, and handheld units. Often it is integrated with component technologies of the EHR system and derived technologies of the internet. The access and ability to transmit patient records and the integration with reference databases on the internet all play into the telehealth model. The use of telehealth systems centers on "education, consultation (including decision support), psychosocial/cognitive behavioral therapy (including problem solving training), social support, data collection and monitoring, and clinical care delivery" (Chi and Demiris 2015, 37).

As both a clinical and technological endeavor, telehealth systems play a key role in the integration of managing patient care and in the more efficient management of the information systems that support it. Telehealth experienced a rise in necessity and popularity during the COVID-19 pandemic as it helped expand access to care. Once the pandemic passed and activities returned to pre-pandemic healthcare models, the need for telehealth remained as it provided a convenient option for care without leaving home. However, overcoming multiple technical challenges remains a concern. These challenges include the lack of systems interoperability and network integration as well as metropolitan broad bandwidth limitations. Other challenges that require overcoming complex behavioral, economic, and ethical constraints are physician resistance; lack of consistent, proven cost-effectiveness; lack of consistent, proven medical effectiveness; concerns for safety; and challenges related to reimbursement for services provided.

## Electronic Health Record Systems

EHRs have been around since the late 1960s., They consist of several integrated component information systems and technologies. The EHR is more than a digital version of a patient's paper chart (ONC 2017). An EHR is an electronic record of health-related information about an individual conforming to nationally recognized interoperability standards. Authorized clinicians and staff across many healthcare organizations can create, manage, and consult EHRs, allowing information to be recorded by and available instantly and securely to authorized users involved in a patient's care—such as specialists, primary care providers, therapists, pharmacies, and more. The EHR includes not only the current encounter; it is inclusive of a patient's entire continuum of care and can be shared across multiple healthcare organizations as needed (ONC 2017). The intent of EHR technology is to capture clinical data from multiple sources for use at the point of care in clinical decision-making. Also, to exchange such data across the continuum of care for care coordination.

As with any revolutionary system, the EHR has suffered somewhat from multiple different interpretations and rapid development of products that failed to fully meet the vision. EHR functionality continues to be optimized to provide the most efficient and effective patient care.

Ultimately, the EHR should be able to do the following:

- Improve the quality of healthcare through data availability and links to knowledge sources
- Enhance patient safety with context-sensitive reminders and alerts, computerized clinical decision support (CDS), automated surveillance, chronic disease management, and drug and device recall capability
- Support health maintenance, preventive care, and wellness through patient reminders, health summaries, tailored instructions, educational materials, and home monitoring and tracking capability
- Increase productivity through data capture and reporting formats tailored to the user; streamlined workflow support; and patient-specific care plans, guidelines, and protocols
- Reduce frustration and improve satisfaction for clinicians, consumers, and caregivers by managing scheduling, registration, referrals, medication refills, and work queues, and by automatically generating administrative data
- Support revenue enhancement through accurate and timely eligibility and benefit information, timely claims adjudication, cost-efficacy analysis, clinical trials recruitment, rules-driven coding assistance, external accountability reporting and outcomes measures, and contract management
- Support predictive modeling and contribute to development of evidence-based healthcare guidance
- Maintain patient confidentiality and exchange data securely among all stakeholders (IOM 1991, 37–46)

Overall, the EHR should help clinicians and other healthcare professionals provide safer, more efficient, and more cost-effective care by providing information and decision support to end users.

### EHR Terms

As the EHR has evolved, various terms have been used to describe it. Considerable confusion has arisen between the terms electronic *health* record and electronic *medical* record (EMR). Hospitals sometimes say they have an EMR, which is an EDM system, and an EHR, which is composed of applications used by clinicians at the point of care.

In 2008, the federal government asked the National Alliance for Health Information Technology (NAHIT) to develop a set of terms and definitions to help the industry avoid confusion and achieve consensus on terminology. While NAHIT no longer exists, the definitions it published serve as the foundation for the government's adoption of the term *EHR* and are distinguished as follows:

- Electronic health record (EHR) is defined as "an electronic record of health-related information on an individual that conforms to nationally recognized interoperability standards and that can be created, managed, and consulted by authorized clinicians and staff across more than one healthcare organization" (NAHIT 2008).
- Electronic medical record (EMR) is defined as "an electronic record of health-related information on an individual that can be created, gathered, managed, and consulted by authorized clinicians and staff within one healthcare organization" (NAHIT 2008).

The key difference between the terms *EHR* and *EMR* as suggested by NAHIT is in EHR being interoperable and EMR not. Interoperability refers to the ability of two different systems to communicate and exchange data with each other. Unfortunately, many healthcare organizations are challenged with systems not being as interoperable as desired within their own organization, let alone with other organizations.

## EHR Complexity

The EHR remains a complex system to implement. Its many elements must work together to achieve specific goals. For an EHR, these system elements must include not only hardware and software but also attention to people, policy, and process.

Even for clinicians who use computers frequently, the EHR may represent a different way of practicing their professional skills, depending on their training and experience. For instance, some clinicians are taught to quickly assess a patient, take immediate action to stabilize them in an emergency, and then gather further information about the patient through referencing previous records of care, interviewing the patient, and obtaining data diagnostic studies. Only after most fact-finding is complete is information documented in narrative.

As EHRs are required within the healthcare practice workflow, the clinician is expected to document and even practice in different ways. Data must be entered as captured at the point of care, and in standardized and structured form rather than unstructured data or narrative form. This often takes longer to enter than the typical dictation of a report without the ability to express nuances important to clinicians (Ford et al. 2016). The result of this structured data (data that can be captured in a fixed field) often is a bulleted list of findings that clinicians do not find very user-friendly. The clinician is expected to receive and be guided by CDS systems that process the structured data against a drug knowledge database (DKB) and other EBM into alerts, reminders, and context-sensitive templates for data capture, although the volume of these alerts is frequently ignored (Ford et al. 2016).

### Check Your Understanding 12.4

**Answer the following questions in a separate document.**

1. Provide at least five distinct examples of diagnostic tests that involve physiological signal processing. Propose why these types of tests are valuable as assessment tools in diagnosis.
2. What patient data are typically collected and viewed (accessed) by care providers using point-of-care systems? How does this benefit them in providing care?
3. Describe the barriers to advancing telehealth systems.
4. Evaluate how the EHR may impact the way physicians care for patients. What issues may arise? Provide an example that you have experienced, read, or heard about related to the use of an EHR in the care setting. It can be positive, negative, or neutral.
5. Analyze the definitions offered by NAHIT. What is the key difference between the definition of EHR and EMR, and what impact does it have?

# EHR Functionality and Technology

An EHR is not a single application or computer device but a complex set of software and hardware. It consists of source systems such as administrative and financial systems, ancillary and departmental clinical systems, and the core EHR applications which are used at the point of care. The EHR also incorporates peripherals such as medical devices, supporting infrastructure such as interface engines and AI, and connectivity systems such as the cloud and telehealth. Figure 12.5 displays a conceptual model that depicts these components.

## Source Systems

The ability to communicate data with multiple sources is an important element of the EHR. Hence there must be ISs in many, if not all, hospital departments. Although physician practices will have fewer systems with which they must communicate, such systems may more commonly be external to the practice. Collectively these are called source systems, and there are several types.

### Financial and Administrative Systems

Hospitals have numerous financial and administrative applications. These are no longer solely the domain of the finance department or patient financial services (PFS). HIM professionals have long provided input on the revenue cycle management (RCM) process through diagnostic and procedural codes and sometimes charge master management. This link between clinical and financial systems is becoming more and more important as there is increasing convergence of claims data (information required to be reported on a healthcare claim for service reimbursement) with health data. As claims data and clinical data are used together, healthcare quality and cost improvements can be made. Improved business intelligence (BI) is available to support better decisions by both the administrative and clinical leadership of healthcare organizations. For example, with more complete clinical information available at the time of admission, a hospital can better verify a patient's eligibility for health plan benefits so it does not receive a denied claim later. An order placed for a potentially duplicate diagnostic study or therapy can be flagged for physician review, potentially displaying the previous study results simultaneously. Conducting a duplicate study or treatment is potentially hazardous for the patient and costly to the healthcare delivery system overall; it may also be cause for a payer denial after the service is provided.

Financial systems use technology to organize data collected for the purpose of managing the assets and expenses of the business. They include both general accounting systems (such as general ledger, accounts payable, contract management, procurement, and others), and systems specific to patient accounting—often called PFS systems. PFS systems support RCM processes. RCM starts with eligibility verification to determine if a patient's health plan will provide reimbursement for services to be performed. Sometimes prior authorization is required by health plans to review and approve a procedure (or referral) before performing the service. Once patient care commences, charge capture collects information from ancillary systems and the EHR about services performed; and claims are generated for reimbursement. Checking claims status, posting remittance advice reflecting actual fees reimbursed to the organization, receiving electronic funds transfers (EFTs), sending explanations of benefits (EOBs) to patients, challenging denials, and managing collection are all RCM functions after claims have been sent.

Administrative systems use technology to gather and organize data and information used for administrative and healthcare operations, such as billing and quality oversight. Administrative data include patient identification data, diagnosis and procedure codes,

**Figure 12.5.** EHR system technical components

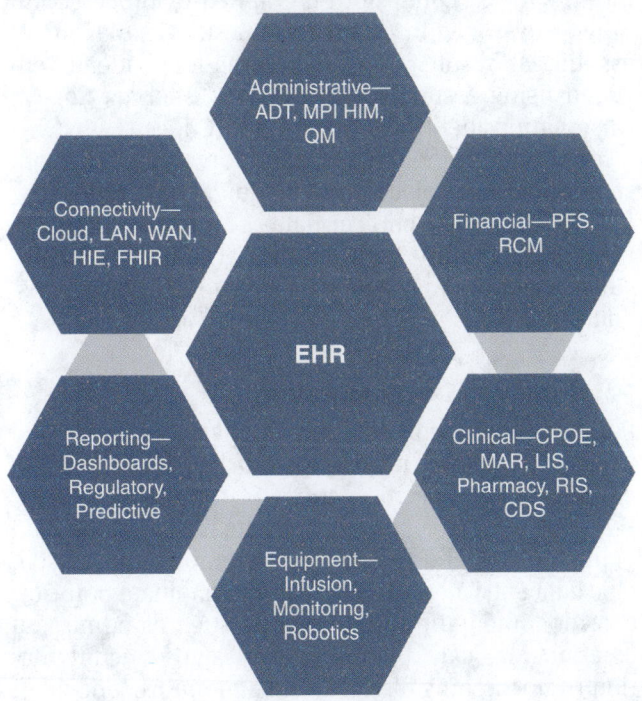

and insurance data, such as eligibility information, claims information, and managed care encounters. **Administrative applications** are the technologies and software used to gather and organize administrative data. These applications include registration-admission, discharge, transfer (R-ADT); EMPI or master patient index (MPI); encoders, record tracking, record deficiency management, release of information; order communication/results reporting (OC/RR); quality management—including core quality measures abstracting and reporting—and many others. Physician practices may have a practice management system (PMS) that provides patient registration, appointment scheduling, and the same PFS a hospital performs.

### Ancillary or Clinical Departmental Systems

**Ancillary systems** (clinical department applications) collect and organize tests and procedures ordered by a practitioner to provide information for use in patient diagnosis or treatment; they include laboratory information systems (LISs), radiology information systems (RISs), pharmacy information systems, and others. When considering an EHR, it is important to recognize the primary purpose of ancillary systems—to help manage the operations of the departments in which they are used. For example, while LISs produce lab results, they do many other things to achieve that outcome. They must receive the order for the test, assign an accession number to the order and specimen if the specimen accompanies the order, generate a specimen collection list and barcode labels for the specimen collection vials, schedule phlebotomists to collect the specimens from the patient, and interface with auto analyzers that run the tests to download the results. Once the test results are available and quality checked, the system prints the results or otherwise makes them available for viewing by the ordering provider. In addition to these basic features, LISs manage workload balancing; manage supplies inventories; manage Medicare medical necessity checking, billing, and public health reporting; and generate custom reports for clinical or quality management. RISs perform equivalent functions for the radiology department. While the clinical pharmacy in a hospital does not produce diagnostic studies results as do the LISs and RISs, it must receive orders for medications, track and maintain inventory, perform quality checks, manage staff, and perform other departmental management functions. In addition, there are other departments that may have their own applications, such as a blood bank, nutrition and food services, housekeeping, and others. These may all ultimately have a connection to the EHR through ordering meals, special services, or other functions.

### Specialty Clinical Systems and Smart Peripherals

In addition to ancillary systems, there are specialty clinical applications. These include many systems for hospitals, and also some for physician practices. Examples include intensive care, perioperative or surgical services, cardiology, oncology, emergency medicine, obstetrics, infection control, behavioral health, dentistry, and others.

Hospitals and physician practices are also acquiring smart peripherals, which are medical instruments that have information processing components including auto-analyzers for lab testing, medication dispensing devices, robotics, smart infusion pumps, and vital signs monitoring equipment.

## Core Clinical EHR Applications

Core clinical EHR applications are those used directly by clinicians at the point of care. Although there may be many specific applications, they are organized in five major categories: results management, point-of-care documentation, medication management, CDS, and reporting.

### Results Management

Results management systems are applications that enable diagnostic studies results to be processed according to the needs of the users. In the past, results review systems enabled clinicians to view lab results in print file format. While abnormal results were flagged in these reports, the data were not structured, so they could not be graphed or processed in other ways or with other data. Results management assume lab results are in structured form, ideally encoded using a standard vocabulary, such as Logical Observation Identifiers Names and Codes (LOINC)—a common terminology for laboratory and clinical observations—and placed into a clinical data repository (CDR) with other clinical data. The results management functionality then enables graphing of lab results over time and against medications, vital signs, and other data.

### Point-of-Care Documentation

Point-of-care documentation applications guide the user through the necessary data to collect in the context of the specific patient (often using context-sensitive templates that react to the nature of the data being entered and that tailor the template to the specific data entry needs). Hospitals often initiate point-of-care documentation with records such as admission assessments, care planning, vital signs documentation (if not coming directly from a monitoring device), intake and output records, and other documentation. As with lab results, nursing documentation is aided by standard vocabularies such as NANDA International, which exists to develop, refine, and promote terminology that accurately reflects nurses' clinical judgment (NANDA 2017).

Physician documentation occurs largely through voice recognition and use of structured templates within the EHR. Physicians must enter problems on the problem list using the *International Classification of Diseases, Tenth Revision, Clinical Modification* (ICD-10-CM) or Systematized Nomenclature of Medicine-Clinical Terms (SNOMED-CT) to achieve standardization of terminology. Point-of-care documentation is intended to capture patient data as the care encounter occurs, allowing for complete and accurate documentation immediately available to the care team.

### Medication Management

Applications that support the closed-loop medication management process, where patient safety is ensured through proper drug ordering, dispensing, administering, and monitoring of reactions, are special forms of point-of-care documentation. These systems include CPOE, e-Rx as a special type of CPOE, electronic (EMAR) or barcode medication administration record (BCMAR), medication reconciliation systems, and automated drug dispensing.

***Computerized Provider Order Entry*** A **computerized provider order entry (CPOE) system** enables ordering of everything from patient admission, laboratory tests, x-rays and other diagnostic studies, dietary and food and nutrition, therapies, nursing services, and consults to discharge of patient, referrals, and even building personal task lists, as well as entering orders for medications. In the past, physicians typically handwrote these orders, which were faxed to the respective departments or transcribed by nursing personnel into an order communication system. These order communication systems, however, only enabled transmission of the order to various departments' information systems; and there was no CDS in the order communication system. CPOE systems today have at a minimum drug-allergy checking and drug-drug contraindication checking. There may be resistance to CPOE from physicians because:

- they see order entry as a clerical task,
- there can be an excessive number of unnecessary alerts, causing alert fatigue, and
- CPOE systems are based on standard order sets, which often need to be modified for unique patients.

For acceptance and satisfaction with CPOE, alerts must be meaningful so they are not ignored, and standard care sets must be easily modified to avoid errors or unintended consequences.

***e-Prescribing*** **E-Rx (e-prescribing)** is a special type of CPOE application used to write prescriptions and transmit them to retail pharmacies through the National Council for Prescription Drug Programs (NCPDP) SCRIPT standard sent through a pharmacy information exchange. E-Rx is used in physician practice, in hospital outpatient departments or clinics, and when a patient is discharged from the hospital or emergency service with a prescription. The e-Rx system includes medication alerts and reminders just like the hospital-based CPOE system. It also includes formulary information from pharmacy benefit managers that identifies whether the patient's health plan covers the cost of a drug and what co-pay may be required. E-Rx systems benefit physicians by including the availability of a medication list. This reduces calls from pharmacies unable to read handwriting, needing to advise them an ordered drug is off formulary for a patient, and facilitating electronic communications from retail pharmacies for renewal approvals.

***Electronic Medication Administration Record*** The medication administration record is used by hospital nurses to document drugs given to patients. The frequency and care required to ensure a nurse administers the right drug is critical to avoid medication errors. In response, computerized systems have been created. Early electronic medication administration record (EMAR) systems were simply electronically generated paper lists of medications from the pharmacy information system after it processed physician orders. Later, the lists were retained on the computer and nurses were expected to post the date and time of medication administration. Any exceptions to or issues with medication administration, however, were still included in handwritten nurses' notes. Most importantly, these systems, while providing a legible list of medications, did not fully address the medication five rights—right patient, drug, route, time, and dose (Hanson and Haddad 2023).

Today, many hospitals use BCMAR systems. These require the hospital to have each patient identified with a barcode (usually on a wristband) and to package (or buy prepackaged) drugs in unit dose form, each with a barcode or RFID tag that identifies the drug, dose, and intended route of administration. At the time the drug is to be administered to a patient, the nurse logs onto the BCMAR system and scans the patient's wristband and unit dose package. The system automatically dates and timestamps the entry. As a result, the medication five rights have been followed. Most BCMAR systems also enable notes to describe exceptions, such as the fact that the patient was in surgery at the time the next dose was to be administered. BCMAR systems provide some CDS, as do CPOE systems, often including links to additional information about drugs.

Although nurses value the more legible medication lists and patient safety assurances that are part of EMAR or BCMAR, there are issues to be overcome. One issue is that to use a BCMAR system, nurses must bring a computer, barcode device, and medication to the patient's bedside. Some hospitals use wireless workstations on wheels (WOWs) that include these devices as well as a drug dispensing drawer (and a long-life battery). Once fully loaded, these can be heavy to push. A tablet computer outfitted with a barcode device may be carried as an alternative to a WOW. Walking around all day with such equipment on one's person, however, is not comfortable. Bedside terminals may be used, although many hospitals express privacy concerns with respect to implementing these. The bags that contain specially compounded drugs administered intravenously require special labels, which not all hospital pharmacy information systems can accommodate, resulting in a patient safety gap.

A medication list is generated from the closed-loop medication management applications. The Promoting Interoperability (PI) program requires that the medications be documented using an RxNorm terminology. While this is a standard expression of drug names in clinical form, pharmacy information systems typically utilize the National Drug Code (NDC), which is an inventory coding system. For example, a drug may be described in the NDC with respect to its package size, such as 100 bottles of 100 pills per bottle—information not relevant to clinical administration of the drug. Translations must be able to be made throughout the closed-loop medication management process, so drug naming conventions are followed appropriately.

***Medication Reconciliation*** The medication reconciliation process may also be automated, although not as easily as other elements of medication management. Each time a patient is transferred across levels of care—when admitted, transferred into an intensive care unit, sent to surgery, and so on—a special review of medications must be performed. This is because, very often, certain medications are discontinued or a dose is altered due to the change in level of care. Additionally, clinicians working with the patient are different at different levels of care. Connecting all systems at the different levels of care is a challenge few hospitals have achieved.

***Automated Drug Dispensing*** Finally, with respect to medication management, automated drug dispensing machines are available that are secure and make drugs specific to patient orders readily available to nursing staff. These machines are typically filled by pharmacy department staff based on the physician orders.

## Clinical Decision Support

Clinical decision support (CDS) systems are interactive programs designed to assist clinicians in making patient care decisions. The utilization and value of CDS systems are an important reason for documenting at the point of care and is the functionality that most clearly distinguishes an EHR from paper records.

When CDS systems were introduced in the 1970s, usability and value were questioned along with ethical and legal issues around the use of computers in medicine, physician autonomy, and liability. Currently, CDS systems often use web-applications or integrate with EHRs and CPOE. CDS systems can be administered through desktop, tablet, smartphone, and other devices such as biometric monitoring and wearable health technology (Sutton et al. 2020).

The most common CDS systems are knowledge-based. Knowledge-based CDS systems use logical rules to produce results and subsequently recommendations to guide clinicians. They consist of two main components, a knowledge base and inference engines. A knowledge-based system provides facts, or evidence, concerning a domain of practice, such as drug knowledge, and has rules that are a generic set of "if...then..." statements drawing from the knowledge base. An inference engine is the software controlling how the rules are applied to specific facts about the patient. It runs the built-in logic based on pre-defined rules and entered patient data. Common outputs from knowledge-based CDS systems include the following:

- Guidance and advice for physicians
- Patient-specific recommendations
- Integration into EHRs
- Alerts or reminders (Gholamzadeh et al. 2023)

CDS systems use alerts and reminders to improve patient safety through prevention of medication errors including drug-drug interactions, dosage errors, or missed dosages; increase in adherence to clinical guidelines; and improved documentation. Other considerations for use of CDS systems include clinician workflows and the level of disruption affecting time with patients; the design and frequency of alerts, which may cause alert fatigue due to unnecessary or inappropriate alerts; and the level of computer literacy and training required to ensure effective use (Sutton et al. 2020).

While the rewards of CDS use are great, it must be implemented carefully and regularly maintained. CDS systems must be kept current, so they do not grow obsolete or fail to function. For example, if a rule directs a clinician to perform certain diagnostic examinations or studies based on best practices and the best practices change, the rule must change as well. In addition to keeping rules current, each rule requires the correct information to process. For example, in an emergency where a patient presents with chest pain, there are several possible diagnoses, each based in a different body system, including cardiac, respiratory, digestive, and so forth. If a CDS system requires a specific set of data to be collected for every patient presenting with chest pain and all data requirements are met, the system will operate properly. However, if one data element is not entered, the rule either may not fire when it should or it may fire when unnecessary, causing an annoyance. If clinicians routinely override the rule and identify such inconsistencies in the rule firing, they will lose trust in the CDS. Many organizations will not permit a required field to be overridden for this reason. Other organizations allow the override but have the EHR produce an alert indicating the CDS has been negated due to lack of information. Users are advised they are on their own in making the applicable decision.

However, even in cases where all necessary data are entered and a rule fires appropriately, physicians may need to override a CDS rule. For example, it may be that a patient is allergic to a medication. Having tried other medications, and in consultation with the patient, it is agreed to give a lower dose of the medication with heightened monitoring. This is a legitimate clinical reason for the override. The EHR should enable a pop-up for the rationale to be recorded. It is also possible, however, to fire rules in accordance with classes of users. For example, when a house staff member logs on, he or she could have more CDS than when an attending physician logs on. Certain specialties may want more rules than others. Overdependence on alerts raises some concerns where professional judgment may not be applied. For example, always assuming a drug-allergy alert must be obeyed could lead to delayed or less effective treatment.

### Reporting and Analytics

Reporting and analytics are considered core clinical EHR applications because they previously required manual abstraction of data—even from electronic systems. As a result of the increasing availability of patient data in the EHR, healthcare routinely uses advanced analytics in clinical decision-making. These analytics allow healthcare professionals to make data-driven decisions that can improve patient outcomes, such as reduced hospitalization. Health plans are starting to use predictive modeling to evaluate what their future costs will look like in order to develop products accordingly, reduce cost, and ensure adequate resourcing.

### Supporting Infrastructure for EHR

Some elements of the EHR require special attention once the core clinical EHR components are acquired. These include the nature of the databases used in managing EHR data, storage management and e-discovery, special software to support application software, human-computer interfaces (HCIs), and enhanced security controls.

***Databases*** Databases are the means to hold data for processing. Every application has its own database. But the integration of data from multiple independent systems into a central database is generally considered essential to a comprehensive EHR. Integration provides access to data in a manner that facilitates processing in real time and for CDS. For example, the CPOE system can process drug-allergy and drug-drug contraindication alerts in its own database (although in this case it taps into a separate drug knowledge base to do so). The CPOE database, however, does not retain lab results. To support drug-lab checking, such as whether a patient will tolerate a drug known to be contraindicated in patients with poor liver function, there must be the ability to use both drug and lab data. Collecting and processing data in this integrated manner requires a special open-structure database called a **data repository**. The data repository is not dedicated to the software of any specific vendor or data supplier. It stores data from diverse sources to achieve an integrated, multidisciplinary view. This database incorporates special indexing and management functions to capture, sort, process, and present information back to users—specific to a patient and in a split second of time. To distinguish repositories that focus on clinical information (instead of financial or administrative data), the term CDR is used. The CDR is a component of the EHR that captures clinical data. CDRs are relational databases optimized to perform online transaction processing (OLTP). Every time a user enters data, retrieves data, views data, and is supplied an alert specific to a given patient, that action is considered a transaction.

A CDR is typically used for processing transactions, and even though they may be very complex, each transaction does not require processing an immense amount of data at one time. When complex reporting and analytics are to be performed, a clinical data warehouse (CDW) may be the more appropriate database structure to use. Data warehouses are databases that make it possible to access data from multiple databases and combine the results into a single query and reporting interface. Data warehouses are often hierarchical or multidimensional and are designed to receive very large volumes of data (often as an extraction of data from a repository) and perform complex, analytical processes on the data. This processing is referred to as online analytical processing. Data can be mined and processed in many ways. For example, a data warehouse may be used for clinical quality improvement and best practice guideline development. This does not suggest reports can't be generated from any individual application or a CDR. However, complex, analytical processing degrades the processing power of the CDR and frustrate users. Hence, small organizations without a CDW generate fewer complex reports, process them at night or on weekends when the CDR is less active, or rely on external CDWs they send data to for processing.

**Storage Management and e-Discovery** Storage management is important in an EHR. The volume of data captured by information systems in general and EHRs, is immense. In addition, the industry expects data to be accessible in real time for very long periods. Clinicians depend on the computer for all their data, and they will not tolerate downtime or delays for retrieving archived data. As a result, managing data storage is critically important. Many hospitals have created specific storage management service units within IT departments. Storage management is the process of determining the type of media to use to store data, deciding how rapidly data must be accessible, arranging for replication of storage for backup and disaster recovery, and determining where storage systems should be maintained. Storage management requires an understanding of the nature of the data to be maintained and its potential future use.

New technologies should aid storage management. Many healthcare organizations use storage area networks, which have the sole purpose of transferring data between computers and storage elements (Tate et al. 2017). Some healthcare organizations are considering virtualization to reduce both processing and storage hardware costs. Virtualization is the emulation of one or more computers within a software platform that enables one physical computer to share resources across other computers (Blokdijk 2012). Healthcare's data storage strategy is quickly moving to cloud computing, which is not limited to storage management. Some EHR vendors provide EHRs as Software as a Service (SaaS)—a subscription service to EHRs delivered over the cloud. Although more than storage, redundancy in servers must be part of contingency planning that includes backup, emergency mode operations, and disaster recovery. Redundancy is the concept of building a backup computer system that is an exact version of the primary system and that can replace it in the event of a primary system failure. As data is entered and processed by one server, data is simultaneously being entered and processed by a second server. These may be new strategies for many care delivery organizations as they adopt mission-critical EHR component systems.

In accordance with an organization's review of their EHR functionality, the retention schedule for electronic data should be determined. An element of the retention schedule should be to understand the impact of e-discovery and address what will be retained for what period. E-discovery refers to a pretrial process through which parties obtain and review electronically stored information.

**Support Software** Special software to support applications are increasingly needed in an EHR environment. Such software includes interfaces and interface engines and their associated data exchange standards, in addition to the previously described inference engines, registry systems, and knowledge bases.

Because an EHR relies on exchanging data with multiple source (and destination) systems, communication across these systems is essential. But few of these systems are fully integrated, and improving the integration capabilities across disparate systems is gaining importance so the realization of e-health exchange can be achieved universally across the country. Integration in this context means the systems seamlessly exchange data without the need for an interface, or special software to negotiate the exchange. In most cases, however, source systems are from different vendors, or from vendors who have acquired different products and merged them with a strong interface. The result is often that applications do not exchange data easily with one another, or with a CDR into which much of the data should be placed for ease of EHR use. For an interface to be designed, however, the applications' software must be written to conform to a data exchange standard protocol. HL7 is the predominant standards development organization that creates standards for exchange of clinical data. Founded in 1987, **Health Level Seven International (HL7)** is a not-for-profit, ANSI-accredited standards-developing organization dedicated to providing a comprehensive framework and related standards for the exchange, integration, sharing, and retrieval of electronic health information that supports clinical practice and the management, delivery, and evaluation of health services (HL7 2017). Likewise, the Accredited Standards Committee X12 develops standards for exchange of the HIPAA Transaction Code Sets. Digital Imaging and Communications in Medicine (DICOM) develops standards for exchange of clinical images, and the NCPDP develops standards for exchange of retail pharmacy financial and administrative data and for prescriptions. Where a hospital may have hundreds of applications and a growing number of medical devices to connect to ISs, there are potentially even more interfaces needed so applications can communicate with one another. (Physician practices will have fewer applications, but the potential still exists to have at least two or more interfaces.) Consider only the R-ADT application that must communicate with virtually every other clinical system. The result, then, could be that hospitals may have hundreds of interfaces. While many vendors write their software to comply with standard protocols, there can be nuances. The interfaces must be kept up to date as changes are made to both the underlying applications and the standards themselves. Hence, an interface engine is a tool to manage the multiplicity of interfaces and track changes.

Recall that data exchange standards only focus on syntax, the structure and format, of the data. Data exchange standards are often called message format standards for this reason. The interoperability achieved through application of message format standards is often referred to as technical interoperability. Technically, the data from one application can be exchanged with another application. Technical interoperability, however, does not address semantics, or the meaning of the data. Semantic interoperability requires use of a standard vocabulary to ensure that when data are exchanged the meaning of the data is understood.

***Human-Computer Interface*** Data capture and retrieval technology must also be reassessed considering the EHR and its clinical users. The term **human–computer interface (HCI)** is used to describe these technologies because they are the construct that enables exchange of data between the human and the computer. That interface is improving, but still challenging. HCIs must direct data capture in a clear and concise manner for both the novice and the power user. Data capture and visualization techniques have a significant impact on patient safety. Consideration must be given to screen size and effective use of screen space; the nature of icons and the universality of their meaning; and even sound, animation, and color with respect to the healthcare environment, which features many different sounds and types of lighting. Clinicians are mobile and often work in teams that must simultaneously view the same information. Structured data entry can be counterintuitive to clinicians, so these tools must be easy to use. Clinicians may prefer to be able to read narrative, especially for documentation of progress notes, so structured data entry must be convertible to a narrative output. Different techniques, each with its own benefits and risks, are available. These include the computer wrapping narrative around structured data to produce sentences or paragraphs, NLP, or through macros or copy and paste techniques that reuse standard phraseology.

**Usability**, or the overall ability of a user to capture and retrieve data efficiently and effectively to achieve results from health information systems, has been an increasingly recognized issue of importance. For example, EHR vendors must include evidence of user-centered design and user test results in their submission for ONC EHR certification. They must follow a formal User Centered Design (UCD) process and perform in depth usability testing on specific areas of their product (ONC n.d.a.). Usability is also important in medical devices:

> For medical devices, the most important goal of the human factors/usability engineering process is to minimize use-related hazards and risks and then confirm that these efforts were successful and users can use the device safely and effectively.

Specific beneficial outcomes of applying human factors/usability engineering to medical devices include:

- Safer connections between device components and accessories (e.g., power cords, leads, tubing, cartridges),
- Improved controls and displays interaction,
- Better user understanding of the device's status and operation,
- Better user understanding of a patient's current medical condition,
- More effective alarm signals,
- Easier device maintenance and repair,
- Reduced user reliance on user manuals,
- Reduced need for user training and retraining,

- Reduced risk of use error,
- Reduced risk of adverse events, and
- Reduced risk of product recalls. (FDA 2022)

The Federal Drug Administration (FDA) mandates usability testing documentation as a component to their medical device clearance process.

***Enhanced Security Controls*** Enhanced privacy and security controls are needed in an EHR environment, as recognized by the HIPAA Privacy and Security Rules in HITECH. Although most of HIPAA's privacy requirements are accomplished through administrative and operational activities, EHR technology can support a few of the privacy and security standards.

### Check Your Understanding 12.5

Match the category of EHR system components to the specific functionality and technology (components may be used more than once):

1. _____ Storage area network
2. _____ E-prescribing
3. _____ Eligibility verification
4. _____ Nutrition and food services system
5. _____ Data repository
6. _____ Laboratory Information System
7. _____ Interface engine
8. _____ Practice management system

   a. Financial and administrative system
   b. Ancillary or clinical departmental system
   c. Core clinical EHR applications
   d. Data quality management
   e. Supporting infrastructure
   f. Systems to provide connectivity

## Health Information Exchange

**Health information exchange (HIE)** is the exchange of health information electronically between providers and others with the same level of interoperability. It is "the electronic movement of health-related information among organizations according to nationally recognized standards" (Vest and Miller 2011). It enables healthcare providers and patients to "appropriately access and securely share a patient's vital medical information electronically—improving the speed, quality, safety and cost of patient care" (ONC 2020). HIE is culture, process, and technology directed to deliver added value to patients, providers, healthcare organizations, and the public. It is the natural outcome of over 50 years of advances in biomedical knowledge, and the digitization of data to enable information to be accessible when and where it is most needed.

Stakeholders in healthcare reason it is possible to achieve advances in healthcare delivery through better management of the vast amounts of data generated during a healthcare event. Greater management and accessibility of health information are assumed to hold the key to better population health insights and higher quality of care. By making a patient's information available when needed and through data aggregation of best outcomes, a foundation for fact-based diagnosis and treatments is provided. It is assumed by many policy makers and diverse professionals in the healthcare industry that the aggregation of diagnostic and therapeutic processes will lead to a reduction of practice and diagnostic variability, providing more consistent treatment based on best practices mined from large amounts of collected data.

Although there are continuous enhancements to healthcare data exchange, a great deal of knowledge is not shared among practitioners and systems that could provide benefits for patients, healthcare providers, payers, and other stakeholders in the health information continuum. Analysis of information and data points on best practices in surgeries and treatments across a wide range of ailments may be aggregated into new knowledge available to the industry, making many treatments safer and more efficient. Researchers' data mining of health information may also lead to new human health insights and treatment discoveries. HIE can enable health information to become accessible and shared healthcare knowledge.

Individually, EHRs provide a longitudinal patient record to better inform a patient's providers. In aggregate, EHRs create knowledge for population health and individual treatment. A shareable health record reduces treatment variability and minimizes redundant testing. The overarching goal is to provide better and more current information at the point of care to inform diagnostic decision-making.

HIT infrastructure can potentially manage the complexity of the healthcare delivery system. Computer applications, processing power, networked workstations, and storage facilitate the management of the abundance of patient information. Adopting HIT in the full range of healthcare providers and organizations is a foundational step in the creation of the value chain HIE represents.

HIE is an essential advancement in healthcare delivery that can improve patient outcomes. Major opportunities remain for expanded use of HIE, including the active engagement of clinical and patient stakeholders (Sarkar 2022).

## Interoperability and Its Challenges

**Interoperability** is the ability of different information technology systems and software applications to communicate; to exchange data accurately, effectively, and consistently; and to use the information that has been exchanged. In healthcare, the variability of services, products and systems, and the lack of motivation to share information to achieve a common purpose, continues to confound healthcare's efforts for interoperability. Some challenges to interoperability include variations in medication information, variability in document structure and format, numerous protocols and standards, and a lack of commitment and trust among organizations.

### Medication Variability

A single medication has a clinical, branded, generic, and chemical name. That same medication may have multiple forms in which it can be administered, different strengths in which it is available, and a combination of names, forms, and strengths. The same medication may also be described using ingredient names and strengths, and through multiple ingredient names—either clinical, branded, or generic. For example, acetaminophen has seven different forms; eight different strengths; eleven different clinical, branded, and generic names; and six different combination names, forms, and strengths (Shrestha and Gudivada 2015). This is only a small sample of the level of variability in descriptors for this common pharmaceutical. This example, compounded by numerous others, illustrates the interoperability challenges created by medication variability alone.

### Document Structure and Format

Another area of information complexity is the document structure used to share patient information at transitions of care between providers. The organizations behind the ASTM Continuity of Care Record and the HL7 International Clinical Document Architecture (CDA) collaborated to create the Continuity of Care Document (CCD) to bring together the benefits of two complementary but incompatible XML document formats to better serve the purpose of HIE. The CCD is a more interoperable version of the two formats, providing flexibility between systems while maintaining message context and accuracy (Rhapsody Health n.d.). The formatting flexibility making the CCD a valuable standard is also an attribute contributing to a lack of interoperability when seeking to send messages outside the originating organization's network.

### Protocols and Standards

Additional elements that challenge interoperability include EHR vendors' implementations of protocols for information transmission, messaging and document frameworks such as Extensible Markup Language (XML), External Data Representation (XDR), Transmission Control Protocol (TCP), Health Level 7 International Admit Discharge Transfer message (HL7 ADT), Health Level 7 International Consolidated Continuity of Care Document (HL7 C-CCD), **Health Level 7 International Fast Healthcare Interoperability Resources (HL7 FHIR)**, to name just a few document formats, metadata descriptors, and transmission protocols. FHIR is quickly becoming the HL7 gold standard that is being adopted.

The HL7 FHIR "standard defines how healthcare information can be exchanged between different computer systems regardless of how it is stored in those systems" (ONC n.d.b). It supports secure access to healthcare information and data for those with the right to access it. FHIR's development began in 2012, in response to growth in the availability of healthcare data. Clinicians and consumers needed to share data using modern internet technologies and standards for the benefit of patient care (ONC n.d.b).

FHIR is based on internet standards used by industries outside healthcare. By adopting existing standards and technologies already familiar to software developers, FHIR allowed for a smooth transition for new software developers to support healthcare needs. The FHIR standard provides the ability for fast and easy implementation of interfaces; it is free to use, has support from major EHR vendors, has a strong foundation in web standards, and offers many downloadable tools and resources (ONC n.d.b). Since FHIR was launched, it has been used to implement healthcare applications across the globe (ONC n.d.b).

Healthcare delivery is highly fragmented in its knowledge base and, consequently, in its analysis and treatment of various diagnoses. It is challenging and expensive to integrate older computer hardware and software with newer technology for interoperability. Individual healthcare systems frequently customize their technology to better serve their internal constituents. Customizations can occur even with terminology standards such as LOINC, used for medical laboratory observations. Also, SNOMED-CT is used for general medical terminology in EHR systems, which are deployed within individual institutions' information systems. Any customization of a standard renders it a nonstandard deployment and not interoperable with others using the standard.

## Commitment and Trust

Achieving interoperability with another entity requires a cultural commitment and a strong trust relationship. Before the IT departments ever get involved there must be committed governance of the standards for classifications, terminologies, vocabularies, and other such structures used. Building a governance structure and agreeing upon the standards and how they are to be implemented for successful mapping between systems is the most difficult work to be accomplished in any HIE implementation. Despite the funding provided by ARRA to incentivize digitizing health records, the federal government only provides guidance and some incentives to motivate progress toward its regional, state, and national goals of interoperability in support of HIE. The ONC relies on the industry and individual users to work out the details and make interoperability work for the benefit of healthcare delivery organizations and the consumer.

Being able to guarantee privacy and security of patient health information at rest and in transit is a primary concern of all stakeholders. Despite the significant regulations around privacy and security that exists within HIPAA, there remains significant variability within HIE implementation across the industry. The nationwide privacy and security framework is designed as guidance to industry participants on the consistent adoption and implementation of standards that address cyber security, encryption, ID validation, and permissions to collect, share, and use PHI. Figure 12.6 illustrates the Fair Information Practice Principles, which guide the nationwide privacy and security framework. Addressing the issues of trust for the exchange and use of regular and sensitive information across regional, state, and national boundaries remains one of the more challenging issues facing the adoption of HIE.

### Check Your Understanding 12.6

Answer the following questions in a separate document.

1. Explain some of the benefits HIE is expected to deliver to the healthcare industry. Give an example of when HIE is of benefit to a patient.

2. Identify and rank in order of most important to least important three reasons why you feel the HL7 FHIR standard is attractive to healthcare system developers. Explain your rationale.

3. What is interoperability? Aside from the technical aspects, what is critical to the success of an HIE project between two or more organizations?

4. Evaluate the complex healthcare industry and determine why it is difficult to achieve interoperability between HIT providers.

5. Provide an example of an interoperable medical device system used commonly within the healthcare arena. What are the benefits of this type of system?

**Figure 12.6.** The privacy and security framework

> **Nationwide Privacy and Security Framework (based on the FIPPs)**
>
> 1. **INDIVIDUAL ACCESS:** Individuals should be provided with a simple and timely means to access and obtain their individually identifiable health information in a readable form and format.
> 2. **CORRECTION:** Individuals should be provided with a timely means to dispute the accuracy or integrity of their individually identifiable health information and to have erroneous information corrected or to have a dispute documented if their requests are denied.
> 3. **OPENNESS AND TRANSPARENCY:** There should be openness and transparency about policies, procedures and technologies that directly affect individuals and/or their individually identifiable health information.
> 4. **INDIVIDUAL CHOICE:** Individuals should be provided a reasonable opportunity and capability to make informed decisions about the collection, use and disclosure of their individually identifiable health information.
> 5. **COLLECTION, USE, AND DISCLOSURE LIMITATION:** Individually identifiable health information should be collected, used, and/or disclosed only to the extent necessary to accomplish a specified purpose(s) and never to discriminate inappropriately.
> 6. **DATA QUALITY AND INTEGRITY:** Persons and entities should take reasonable steps to ensure that individually identifiable health information is complete, accurate and up-to-date to the extent necessary for the person's or entity's intended purposes and has not been altered or destroyed in an unauthorized manner.
> 7. **SAFEGUARDS:** Individually identifiable health information should be protected with reasonable administrative, technical and physical safeguards to ensure its confidentiality, integrity and availability and to prevent unauthorized or inappropriate access, use, or disclosure.
> 8. **ACCOUNTABILITY:** These principles should be implemented and adherence assured, through appropriate monitoring and other means and methods should be in place to report and mitigate non-adherence and breaches.

*Source:* FPC n.d.

## Models for Health Information Exchange

There are several conceptual models for public HIE. The basic models are the centralized model, the federated or decentralized model, and the hybrid model (McCarthy et al. 2014). Participants, or members, in an HIE have the responsibility of making the HIE economically viable and governing the numerous details that define the relationships that comprise an HIE organization. Each model has pros and cons of sustainability, privacy and security, liability, interoperability, and development to consider in the early stages of planning. All of the models described have the potential to provide labs, imaging, medication lists, notes, and demographic information at the point of care delivery.

### The Centralized Health Information Exchange Architecture

In the centralized model, all data are stored in a shared data repository. Figure 12.7 illustrates at a high level how data are pushed to the centralized database and received through queries to the database. The governance policies between the participants in the data warehouse dictate the scope of data usage, patient consent for data sharing, and the specific standards and information that are exchanged. Some of the advantages of this architecture are uniformity of data, quick response times to queries, and consistency in data accessibility. Disadvantages include increased chances of data duplication, information not being current due to scheduling of data transfers from participants, and increased costs for the development of a data warehouse and the supporting software.

### The Decentralized Health Information Exchange Architecture

In the decentralized or federated model there is not a centralized database of patient information. Figure 12.8 illustrates the decentralized model, indicating that the record locator service (RLS) is the focal point for a query on a patient. An RLS provides the

**Figure 12.7.** The centralized HIE model

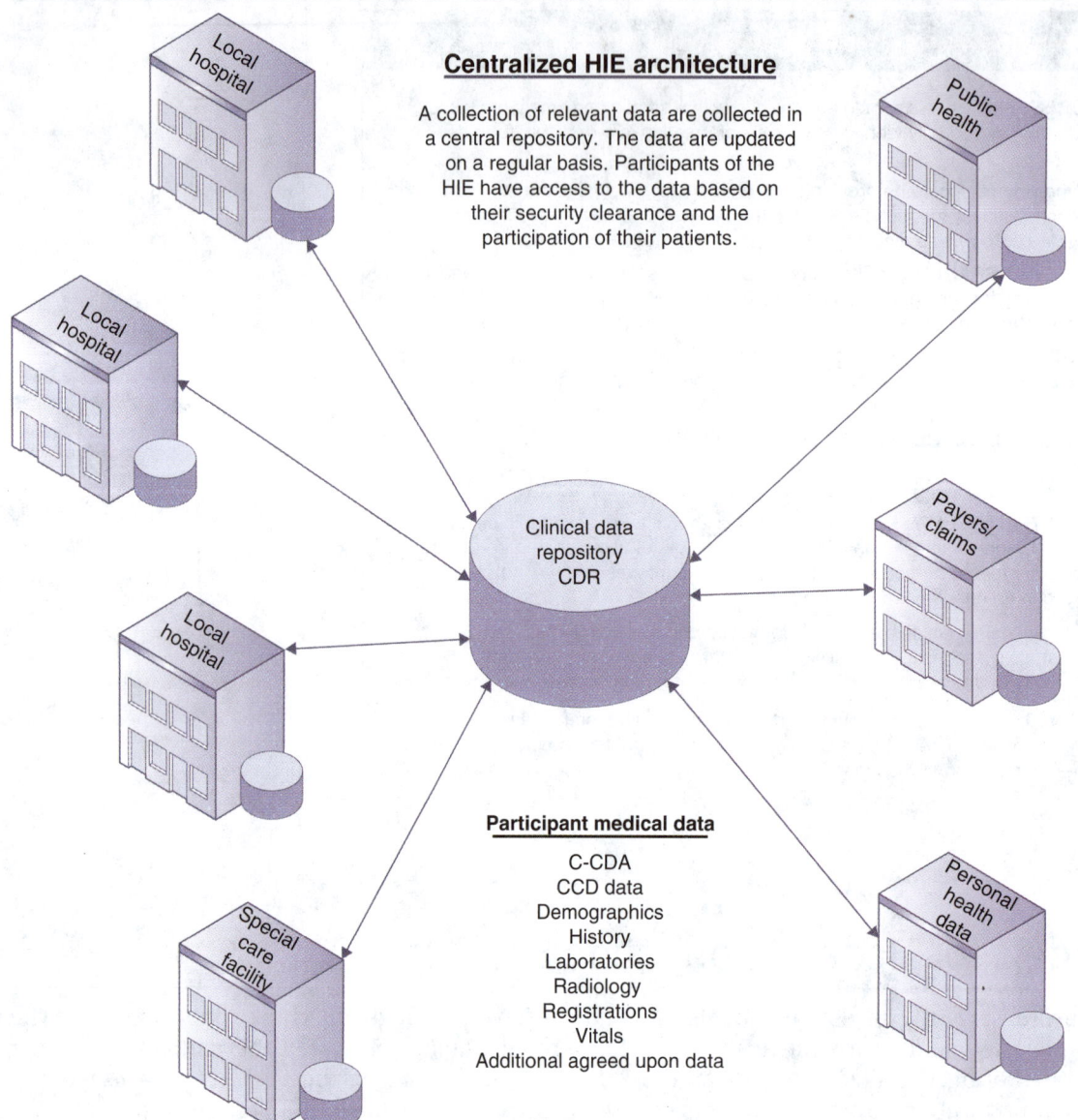

ability to identify where records are located based upon criteria such as a person ID and record data type, and provides functionality for the ongoing maintenance of this location information (HL7 n.d.a). Data and information remain on the facility's servers until called for through a query. The HIE's RLS manages the pointers to the information on the servers of the HIE participants. The pointers in an RLS can include a person identification number (person ID) and metadata. The RLS does not provide information about the record, it merely points to where it might be found (HL7 n.d.a). Data are not stored in a centralized database and records are only provided when queried. Some advantages of the federated model include data remaining under the control of the HIE participant until needed, redundancy in the event of a disaster because multiple systems mitigate the risks caused by a single point of failure, and data potentially being more current. Disadvantages include data potentially not being available when needed due to technical challenges with a participant, a potential lack of data sharing for purposes or research, and incomplete data because a patient has records across several participants.

## The Hybrid Health Information Exchange Architecture

The **hybrid model** is a cross between the centralized and the decentralized models. Figure 12.9 illustrates

**Figure 12.8.** The decentralized HIE model

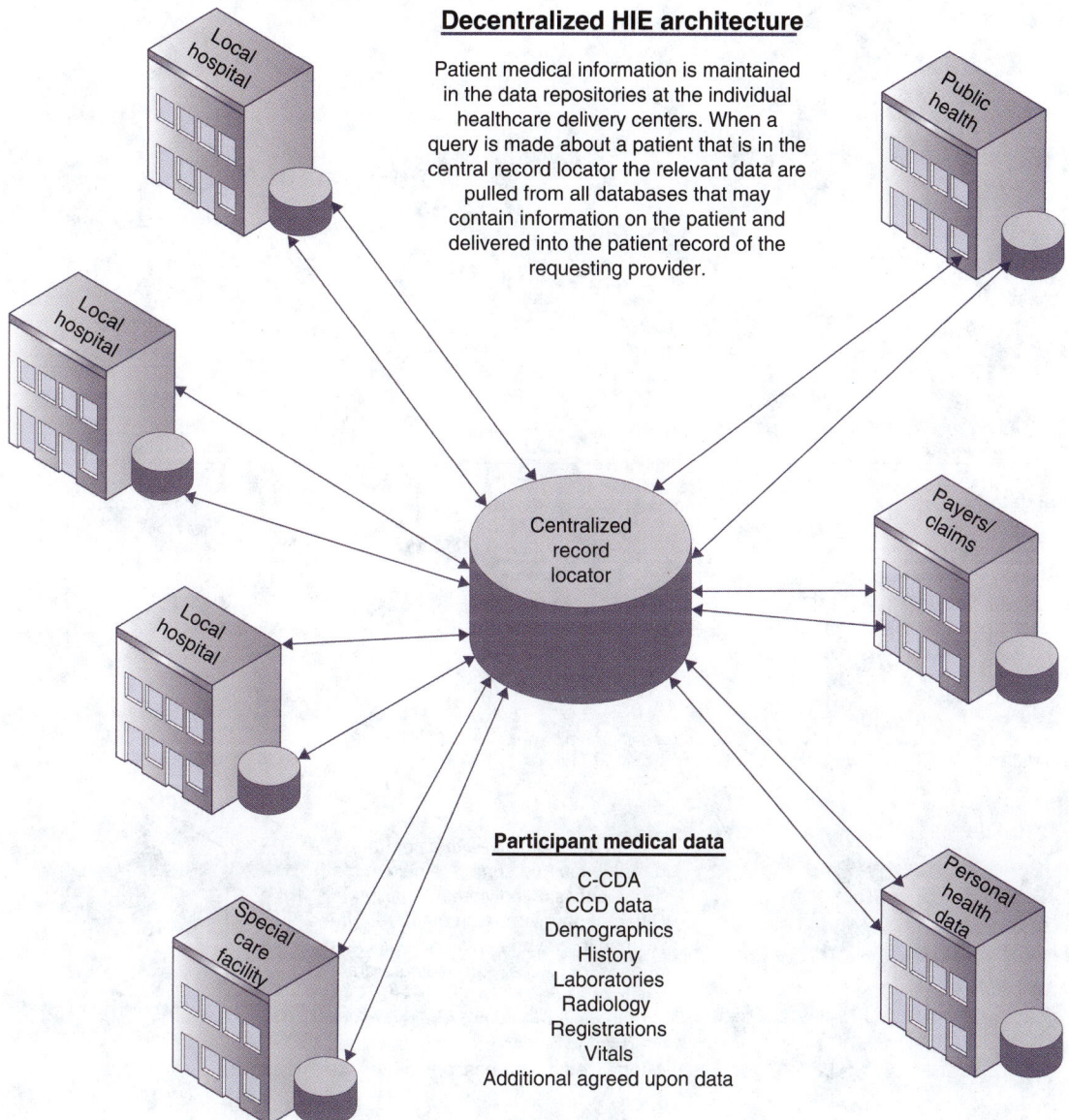

the hybrid model, which combines the functionality of an RLS and a centralized data repository. In a hybrid model, some data are stored in a centralized database, and some remain on the HIE participants' servers until queried. In many respects, the hybrid is the best of two models. A centralized database enables the data for research queries from HIE participants and entities that have contracted for de-identified data for research purposes. A centralized warehouse makes the data available faster and potentially more readily available to patients through a common patient portal tethered to the HIE instead of one hospital. The decentralized aspects of the model provide more current data resident in each participant's EHR, and enhanced security for patient records that remain within the systems of the most recent participant. Information also remains tied to the individual participants, creating a redundant data element that enhances data availability and integrity.

## The Health Record Banking Health Information Exchange Architecture

The health record banking model is an organization with information-sharing agreements between a group of healthcare providers that enables the

**Figure 12.9.** The hybrid HIE model

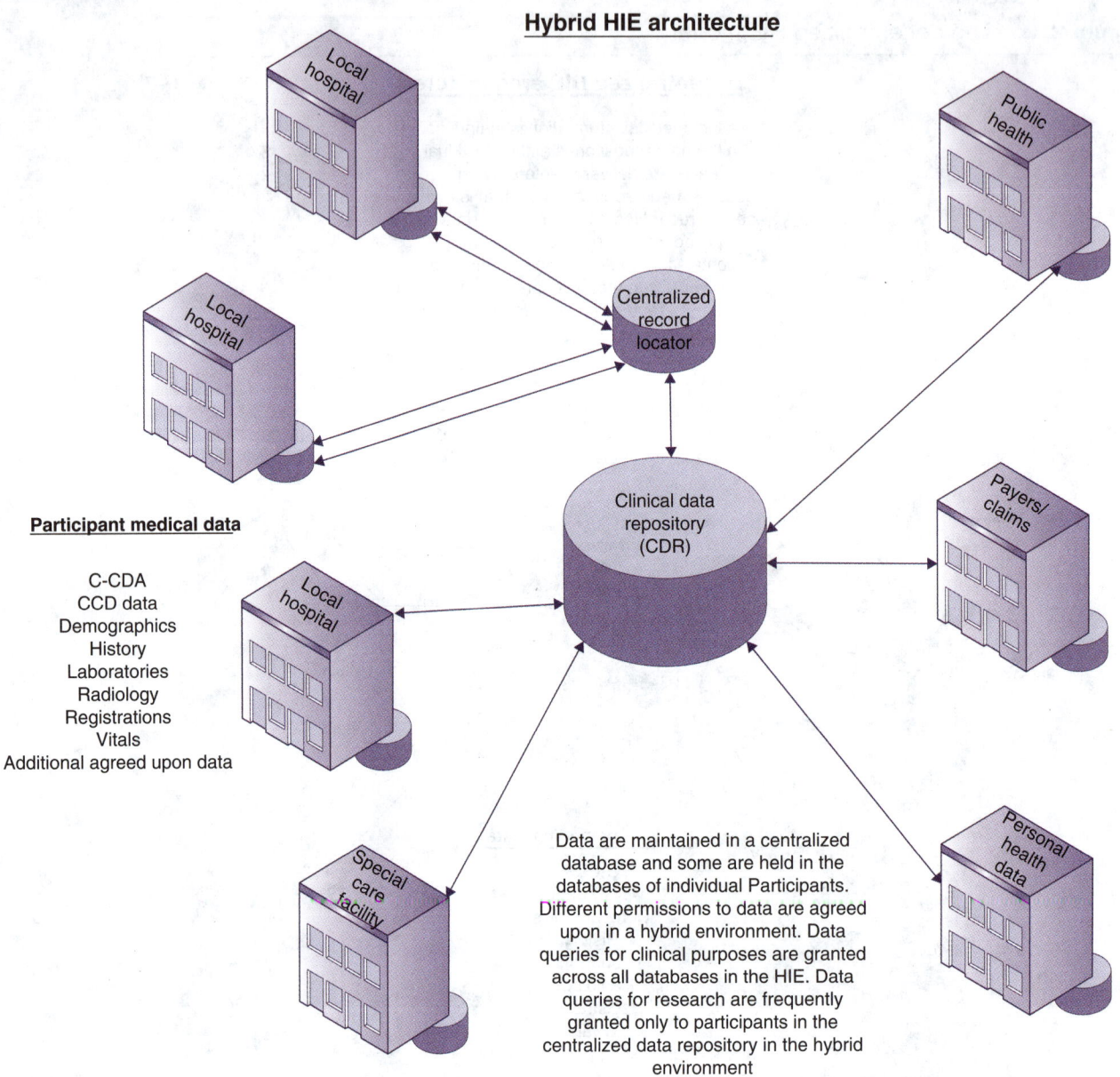

aggregation and delivery of patient information to the patient under the control of the patient. A health record bank (HRB) uses a centralized data repository that receives patient information from organizations that participate within the HIE. Instead of the patient information being owned and controlled by the participant, individual patient information is controlled by the patient (consumer). HIE organizations push patient information out to the patient portal as they encounter the patient. The patient is delivered a standardized set of information they can deliver to care providers on an as-needed basis, negating issues of patient privacy and ownership of the patient record.

An HRB creates a record that stores a consumer's longitudinal health record. The HRB's focus is on collecting all the necessary patient data instead of select data sets (Health Record Banking Alliance n.d.).

The architectural models for HIE mask the issues a lack of interoperability creates, which permeate every HIE discussion between technology vendors and healthcare organizations. HIE can exist with minimal technology if there is an agreement between organizations beneficial to all involved. Technological interoperability can be developed between participants in stages once a shared vision and trust relationship is established.

## Legal Issues in the Exchange of Electronic Protected Health Information

HIE relies on the patient to both opt in and agree to participate in the HIE or opt out by choosing not to participate. A patient's decision not to share health information is protected by HIPAA and can have critical consequences for the healthcare provider if the decision is not respected. Fines may be significant if a complaint is filed with the Office of Civil Rights and it finds the provider was negligent or cavalier in their compliance with HIPAA privacy regulations. HIPAA (45 CFR 164.522) mandates that a covered entity that has agreed to restrict access to patients' information—except for emergency and other authorized purposes—must maintain that restriction or risk violating HIPAA privacy laws. Because of the HIPAA privacy regulations, significant resources and time are committed to coordinating the accurate documentation of a patient's choice to participate or not participate in HIE.

Many states legislate whether the decision to participate in an HIE is default-in or default-out. In a default-in decision state, when a patient visits a healthcare provider in an HIE, the provider must provide the patient with meaningful disclosure of the right not to participate in the HIE and ask the patient if they prefer not to participate. In a default-out decision state, healthcare providers in an HIE provide the patient an opportunity to join the HIE. Choosing to join the HIE makes the patient's information available to other participants in the HIE on an as-needed basis, to be used in good faith for the patient's benefit. Opting into the HIE makes information immediately available through the HIE if the patient visits another participant facility for care or emergency treatment. A patient's historical health record can influence readmissions, treatments, and administered pharmaceuticals by providing the treating medical team with insight on the patient's medical history.

In organizations where the HIE interface is integrated into the EHR, a decision whether to participate in the HIE is communicated to the exchange through transmission of admit-discharge-transfer (ADT) messages coded at the time of registration. ADT messaging capabilities are built into many patient registration, administration, and EHR systems. ADT messages are generated during the registration process. If an organization does not use computerized PMSs or has chosen a specialty EHR that does not generate ADT messages, a consent portal should be accessible through a web browser and a virtual private network (VPN) to register the patient's decision to opt in or out of the HIE. Registering the correct patient decision is critically important to avoid noncompliance with HIPAA privacy rules and the possibility of fines. Informing patients about the choices available to them is vital to the final outcome. Registration staff have scripts to read to patients, informing them of their right to choose to participate or not participate in the HIE. This right to choose differs according to state regulations. The organization's legal staff must assist with scripting the language, so information is not missed and registration staff have a standardized process to follow. Each state has their own governance that determines the rules about HIE participation.

Whether patients have chosen to opt in or opt out of an HIE sharing agreement, they may always reverse their decision the next time they present at an HIE-participant facility. The public has mixed feelings about the privacy of their personal health information, and some will frequently change their consent-to-share status. HIE participant organizations go to great lengths to ensure they correctly document consumers' preference. Because of the high stakes involved and the threat of legal sanctions, significant resources are allocated to testing, implementation, and training of personnel regardless of the participant's technology solution for documenting consent. ADT feeds are tested over an extended period to ensure the feed and the transmitted data conform to the agreed-upon specifications.

## Exchange Methodologies

An HIE does not contain the legal health record. The legal health record of participant patients is maintained separately by each HIE participant organization. Many exchanges are merely conduits of data facilitating the transmission, translation, and mapping of electronic protected health information (ePHI) between participant EHRs in the HIE. The medical information acquired through an HIE will be a collection of available information about the patient. It is the requesting organization's responsibility to format the patient's information, so it is meaningful and easily readable to the requesting provider.

For the exchange to be meaningful, a minimum required data set must be agreed upon among the HIE participants. If the HIE aspires to connect to the eHealth Exchange, it will be required to conform to that network's minimum data set requirements. The eHealth Exchange is a group of federal agencies and nonfederal organizations that came together under a common mission and purpose to improve patient care, streamline disability claim benefits, and improve public health reporting through secure, trusted, and interoperable HIE (Sequoia Project 2017). Participants mutually agree to support a common set of standards and specifications. Additionally, multiple transmission protocols are considered. HL7 International is an organization focused on creating comprehensive frameworks and standards for integrating, sharing, exchanging, and retrieving ePHI. Many of its frameworks provide a structure for sharing and exchanging information like race and other demographics, in addition to other medical-related details such as allergies, medications, immunizations, labs, documents, radiology images, procedures, and language.

One of the main issues between providers is requests for or the sending of too much information about a patient. The information shared must be relevant and specific so that only necessary details are exchanged. For this reason, participants in an HIE must agree on what information is valuable in specific situations and what minimum set of information should be collected and shared during ordinary operations. For example, the information needs of an ED encounter can be vastly different than the information needs of a cardiologist seeing a patient for a maintenance visit. HIM staff or care coordinators will acquire the needed information on a patient based on the provider's and organization's predetermined requirements for the unique circumstances of the patient visit.

Currently available exchange methodologies provide access to HIE across the economic spectrum of providers. Directed exchange can be available to any provider with access to an internet connection. Query-based and consumer-mediated exchange requires a more sophisticated technology infrastructure. It is important to remember all HIE relies on documenting the correct patient decision for participation or nonparticipation in the HIE.

## Directed Exchange

Directed exchange is used by providers to easily and securely send patient information directly to another healthcare provider over the internet, similar to sending a secured email (ONC 2020). Directed exchange is used for patient referrals, transmission of discharge summaries to primary care physicians, transmission of lab results to ordering physicians, and the transmission of various continuity of care documents. This form of information exchange enables coordinated care among trusted healthcare professionals, benefitting both providers and patients. Directed exchange is also used to send immunization data to public health organizations or to report quality measures to the CMS (ONC 2020). Directed exchange is important because it is accessible to large and small providers.

## Query-Based Exchange

Query-based exchange is "used by providers to search and discover accessible clinical sources on a patient" (ONC 2020). A query asks a question of the database and pulls information based on the keywords used. This type of exchange is often used when delivering unplanned care such as ED visits (ONC 2020). Query-based exchange, depending on the technology vendor, uses Boolean search queries to locate patient information in either a centralized data repository or across a federated network of providers. In a Boolean search engine, the application combines the keywords used in the search string to retrieve an index of possible solutions from the queried database based on the keyword and the hierarchy in which those keywords appear in the search string.

Participant organizations with the appropriate patient permission can prepare a patient's health record in advance of their visit. This way, the organization can monitor if the patient has received treatment they should be aware of from another provider in a different facility. This use has positive implications for coordination and quality of care. A query-based search can be used in emergency situations where the query is performed by staff seeking medication, allergies, and medical problems on a patient presenting at the ED.

HIE is a significant cultural and process reengineering project. Use cases and their workflows must be established in advance and shared with departmental staff expected to effectively use the new technological capabilities. Query-based capabilities are frequently integrated into an organization's EHR system, making it easier to add queried information to the patient record. Standardizing data field specifications (data normalization) between the participants in the HIE enables queried data to be easily shared and used by all participant providers.

## Consumer-Mediated Exchange

Consumer-mediated exchange provides patients with access to their health information, allowing them to manage their healthcare online in a similar fashion to how they might manage their finances through online banking (ONC 2020). An example of consumer-mediated exchange is the Blue Button initiative. Blue Button is a public-private partnership based within the ONC. It was developed by the Office of Veteran's Affairs (VA) in close partnership with CMS and the Department of Defense (DOD) along with the Markle Foundation's Consumer Engagement Workgroup. "The Blue Button represents a national movement that enables consumers to have easy access to their own health information in a format they can use" (VA 2021). Consumer-mediated exchange provides the ultimate solution to patient privacy by giving consumers control of who has access to their protected health information (PHI) and when they have access to it.

# Health Information Exchange Initiatives

Innovation projects and programs, private and public, begin with an assumption of an end goal and then proceed to test various ways of attaining that objective. The innovation process typically initiates numerous projects (prototypes) to test their viability and to attain the quick wins and failures informing the knowledge base and decisions in later stages of their initiative. An example of such an initiative is the Sequoia Project, which resulted in additional programs and organizations such as the eHealth Exchange and CareQuality. The Trusted Exchange Framework and Common Agreement (TEFCA) further enables assurance and trust for data and information sharing. Table 12.4 illustrates recent HIE initiatives.

As health IT evolved, it was clear multiple health information networks were needed to interconnect, not just one network to serve the entire country. To address this need, The Sequoia Project convened stakeholders, such as EHR vendors and HIEs, across the private and government sectors to develop a common interoperability framework to enable exchange among health data sharing networks. They collaborated to determine technical and policy agreements enabling data exchange among the various networks and platforms across the nation. This led to the creation of Carequality. Carequality also had immense success and became an independent nonprofit in 2018 (David and Swenson 2022).

## The Sequoia Project

The Sequoia Project is an independent advocate for nationwide health information exchange. It builds and supports new programs and initiatives focused on information exchange and educates the community on interoperability and more. The Sequoia Project supported both the eHealth Exchange and Carequality initiatives until they were able to become independent companies (Davis and Swenson 2022).

In 2012, The Sequoia Project assumed responsibility for the nationwide health information network exchange, NwHIN Exchange, from the Office of the National Coordinator for Health Information Technology (ONC), which later was renamed eHealth Exchange. Under The Sequoia Project, the eHealth Exchange network quadrupled in size, connecting participants across the country. Recognizing the maturity and sustainability of the network, eHealth Exchange became independent from The Sequoia Project in 2018 (Davis and Swenson 2022).

## Trusted Exchange Framework and Common Agreement

Under the purview of the ONC, the Trusted Exchange Framework is a common set of principles designed to facilitate trust between health information networks (HIN) that voluntarily agree to enable widespread information exchange. The Common Agreement defines the legal and technical requirements for secure information sharing on a nationwide scale. It also sets the infrastructure and governance to enable users in different HINs to securely share information with each other under mutually agreed upon expectations. The Trusted Exchange Network and Common Agreement (TEFCA) has three goals: (1) to establish universal governance, policies, and technical requirements for nationwide interoperability; (2) to simplify connectivity for organizations to securely exchange information to improve patient care, population health, and healthcare value; and (3) to enable individuals to obtain their healthcare information (ONC 2024b).

## Table 12.4. HIE initiatives

| Title | Origination | Purpose |
|---|---|---|
| American Health Information Community (AHIC) | Chartered in 2005. as an advisory committee to the US Department of Health and Human Services (HHS) | To initiate a common, open, transparent, collaborative framework for achieving interoperability between technology vendors by using a process of advisory committee guidance and competition between technology companies within the industry |
| Beacon Community Cooperative Agreement | Funded in 17 communities throughout the US | To test the potential for building and strengthening HIE infrastructure, to streamline and modify workflows, and to adjust organizational culture sufficiently to leverage HIT tools to improve population health and improve the quality of care while reducing costs |
| Nationwide Health Information Network (NHIN) | Established by ONC in 2004 | To create a governance structure for HIE information exchange across organizational, regional and state boundaries. |
| American Recovery and Reinvestment Act (ARRA)—Meaningful Use | Legislation passed in 2009 | Stage 1—To exchange with another organization<br>Stage 2—To exchange between EHR systems from different vendors<br>Stage 3—To improve interoperability between EHR systems and access to health information for patients |
| ONC sponsored state HIE program | Established by ONC in 2010 | To provide funding to nurture HIE within the states and enable statewide exchange using DIRECT and query-based exchange methods |
| The Sequoia Project | Founded in 2012, and launched as its first initiative, a federal health information network | To identify barriers to interoperability and develop processes to help HIE at a national level (The Sequoia Project n.d.) |
| eHealth Exchange | Established by ONC in 2012, under The Sequoia Project; it became independent in 2018 as an exchange network that spans across 50 states, 70,000 medical groups, 5 federal agencies, and 75 percent of US hospitals (eHealth Exchange n.d.) | To utilize the standards, governance, and legal agreements of the NHIN as a foundation for an exchange network |
| CareQuality | Developed under The Sequoia Project; became independent in 2018 | To connect existing and future data sharing networks to each other using an interoperability framework (The Sequoia Project n.d.b). |
| CommonWell Health Alliance | CommonWell was founded in 2013 by a handful of health IT companies | To help solve the longstanding problem of interoperability in the healthcare industry. Traditionally competitors, these seven companies set aside their differences to focus on this simple vision. |
| Trusted Exchange Framework and Common Agreement (TEFCA) | Established by ONC in 2023 | To facilitate trust between health information networks (HIN) which voluntarily agree to enable widespread information exchange |

### Check Your Understanding 12.7

Answer the following questions in a separate document.

1. Evaluate the recent HIE initiatives and offer your assessment of the level of progress being made. Consider the successes and the challenges in your assessment.
2. If Sandy is a very private person and wants control over who accesses her health information, which HIE model would she be most in favor of?
3. If Sandy is a very private person and says she does not want to be included in an HIE at all, what HIE model option would you recommend to her? What benefit of being a part of an HIE would you want her to know before making her decision?
4. What are the key differentiators between a centralized and a federated HIE model?
5. Describe one similarity and one difference between The Sequoia Project and TECFA.

# Health Information Exchange Implementation Considerations

There is no prescriptive formula for the successful implementation of HIE practices. Vision and planning are essential for organizations that choose to pursue cross-organizational information exchange. The business goals and strategic plans of all HIE participants must be in alignment for the services and products they will collaborate on through the implementation of the HIE. When implementing an HIE, considerations should include the identification of a trust community, the development of a governance committee, identification of the technology platform, development of contracts and participant agreements, development of operational policies, development of vendor and participant project teams, a plan for data governance, and the creation of a sandbox for system testing.

## Identification of a Trust Community

A **trust community** is a group of organizations that identified a set of mutual goals and dependencies that, through collaborative effort, led to mutual benefit. HIE depends upon the formation of a trust community. Many times, trust communities are formed among members of an IDN to facilitate sharing of resources and to formalize the network connections they have for referrals and transitions of care. In the context of HIE outside of a single enterprise or IDN, a group of regional healthcare organizations can collaborate to facilitate cross-organizational exchange of patient information in support of better patient care, quality of healthcare delivery, and population health. A trust community has common interest and goals and opportunities for collaboration that provide benefits for all involved.

## Development of Governance Committees

Once the trust community is identified, governance must be considered. Like any large infrastructure investment, it is important to identify and engage as many stakeholders as possible and actively involve them in the planning and decision-making to minimize objections once the program is initiated. HIE implementations are dominated by a company's IT department, similar to the implementation of EHRs in the early stages of the Meaningful Use program. Considering that HIE is a trust agreement between competing organizations, identifying return on investment and other organizational benefits is challenging. Early involvement of the organizational and HIM teams may make the transition to HIE practices a smoother migration for all participants.

## Identification of the Technology Platform

Once governance is in place, the selected committees should do the research necessary to determine what technology features are most important to their HIE operational needs. Teams should read about and benchmark the experiences of other operational HIEs and interview organizations to understand potential barriers to success and determine the best paths. After the research and interviews are conducted, a request for proposal (RFP) is issued to vendors that provide the required technology and service capabilities. Selection of the final vendor is a function of the governing committees and a rigorous search in the HIE platform technology market through the RFP process. Preparing an RFP involves researching the desired specifications in a technology purchase and putting those specifications into a structured document so the applicants answer questions designed for easy analysis. Once the RFP responses are reviewed by the committee, the answers are scored, and the interview candidates are chosen. Committee interviews with candidate executives and technologists lead to the final selection of a vendor.

## Contracts and Participant Agreements

The eHealth Exchange has the **Data Use and Reciprocal Support Agreement (DURSA)**, a legally binding contract that draws from federal and local laws and defines the requirements for participation in the eHealth Exchange national network (eHealth Exchange 2019). The HIE participants should develop a legally binding agreement, like the DURSA, among all members. The participant agreement provides granular details of all members' obligations and responsibilities. The agreement also addresses the sanctions for violations of the contract. Once a technology platform is chosen, the participants should also create an equally binding contract between their HIE entity and the vendor.

## Operational Policies

Agreements reached in the participant agreement and vendor contract should be developed into operational policies and procedures. Once created, they are distributed to all participants as a reference for the staff handling integrating technology and workflows into member organizations.

## Development of Vendor and Participant Project Teams

The various governance committees created by the trust community initiate the planning cycle for the project. Project managers are designated, and plans are developed. Technology implementations, as well as organizational change management projects, are deployed in stages. For the IT team, the initial step is to coordinate communications from the participants' HL7 ADT feeds from their EHR interfaces to the HIE interface engine.

## Data Governance

Data governance and normalization should be ongoing throughout the technology implementation. One of the initial projects requiring collaboration and governance will be the HL7 **admit-discharge-transfer (ADT) message**, which is used to communicate patient demographics and visit information and to track patient status at a healthcare facility. Data governance is important when sharing ADT messages between organizations to ensure the exchanged data are interoperable between IT systems created by different manufacturers. The HL7 ADT represents a flexible standard modified to create greater efficiencies within a closed organizational system. Once that system is opened to sharing information, the affiliated organizations must work to normalize how they are using the standard so information can be shared. The ADT is a patient tracking mechanism transmitted from numerous systems within a healthcare facility as a patient moves through the system. An ADT message contains demographic and other information. Payer systems, registration systems, and EHRs can all send an ADT message.

## The Creation of the Sandbox for System Testing

A virtual sandbox is an isolated electronic environment that simulates the production environment used once testing is completed. Connecting to the sandbox and thoroughly testing and adjusting systems and applications to discover flaws in development and execution is a necessary step in the implementation cycle. Nothing leaves the sandbox before it is completely tested and proven to be 100 percent compatible with the live production environment. Once ADT feeds are proven reliable in the sandbox, the project managers schedule a date for go-live in the production environment.

## Stages of HIE Implementation

An HIE project has three stages of implementation. They include ensuring proper connectivity and the aggregation of data, the exchange of clinical data, and making the exchange available to participants.

## Stage 1 of Implementation

Once a participant is transmitting messages and data to the HIE's interface, the aggregation of data that enables the creation of the registry that allows the system to identify patients begins. Depending upon the HIE system, there are locator systems and structures that allow retrieval of information on individual patients.

### Master Patient Index

The MPI is a patient-identifying directory referencing all patients related to an organization, which also serves as a link to the patient record or information, facilitates patient identification, and assists in maintaining a longitudinal patient record from birth to death. In the context of an HIE, the MPI will rely on algorithms that match elements of patient demographic information to determine relationships in patient identity. During the testing stages of the implementation, these algorithms and criteria are adjusted until a designated performance metric for accuracy is met.

### Record Locator Service

The RLS provides the ability to identify where records are located based upon criteria such as a person's ID and record data type, and functionality for the ongoing maintenance of this location information (HL7 n.d.a). The locator service maintains the following knowledge:

- At a minimum, given an identity, the RLS retrieves all appropriate locations with information associated with that identity.
- Provides for context-sensitive information location based on matching metadata

requirements. It also allows for labeling technology like extensible metadata that can be embedded within the file.

- Retains what categories or registered patterns of information (HL7 Templates) a given location knows about.
- Recognizes what categories of information (topics) a given location wants to receive messages.
- Identifies individuals for which information is stored. (HL7 n.d.a)

In many HIE environments, it is desirable to measure how many patients move between facilities within the participant trust community. ADT messages are monitored (de-identified) to build reports on the patients' movements between facilities. ADT messages can also capture the information needed to track patient opt-in or opt-out status either initiating or terminating participation in the HIE. The patient consent profile is often updated every time the patient presents at an HIE participant organization, depending upon relevant state legislation. Stage 1 is also when connection to public health and disease registries occur, and directed exchange is implemented. Stage 1 operations will run long enough for the technology and project management teams to mitigate any challenges arising with any participant or the vendor before moving to stage 2.

## Stage 2 of Implementation

Stage 2 of implementation will initiate the exchange of clinical data (labs, radiology reports, medications, CCDs, discharge summaries, physician notes, and others). HL7 **Clinical Document Architecture (CDA)** is used as the standard for document exchange. HL7 defines the CDA as "a document markup standard that specifies the structure and semantics of 'clinical documents' for the purpose of exchange between healthcare providers and patients" (HL7 n.d.b). The CDA framework is both human- and machine-readable. A CDA document can include text, images, and even multimedia content. This level of flexibility enables it to contain any type of clinical content. Discharge summaries, imaging reports, admissions and physicals, pathology reports, and more are common uses for a CDA document (HL7 n.d.b). The CDA framework has enabled several additional document standards and architectures that have improved and stabilized some elements of interoperability across multiple technology vendors.

All the governance, normalization, and testing activities conducted in stage 1 implementation will be repeated for stage 2 because the information exchange and standards conformity must be exact to enable interoperability between EHR and information location systems. Issues that can arise include nonconforming use of coding systems like LOINC, SNOMED CT, and medication nomenclatures and vocabularies.

## Stage 3 of Implementation

In stage 3 of implementation, the HIE is made available to the ambulatory care facilities and providers that refer patients to the acute-care facilities. In this phase, the HIE is considered a community. Adding value to the enterprise and to the consumer experience is what differentiates a great business from the rest of the competitors in its marketplace. HIE provides timely and secure sharing of important patient information at the point of care resulting in a more complete patient health record and an increased ability for better decision making. It offers the potential for providers to avoid readmissions and medication errors, improve diagnoses, and decrease duplicate testing among other improvements (ONC 2020).

## Health Information Management in HIE

Inside a healthcare organization, the creation of an HIE is traditionally viewed as just another large-scale IT implementation. Because of the scarcity of resources many organizations experience, the desire to minimize the involvement of employees not directly related to the IT department frequently arises. The extreme compartmentalization occurring within healthcare has made information about HIE invisible because of a lack of proximity or access. Many who would get involved do not because they have no knowledge of an internal implementation, may not want to increase their workloads unnecessarily, or they may think they lack knowledge to add value to the project. However, HIM professionals have so much information to share with the organization. Involvement in a data governance or data normalization committee or workgroup is clearly within their expertise. The HIM professional can add great value in user groups when information about the benefits of HIE workflows is distributed to multiple departments within the organization. An HIM professional may also serve as a project manager, working with clinical units, registration, and IT to create functional workflows for the correct processing of patient opt-in and opt-out decisions. HIM professionals also add value as an organizational bridge between the IT team and the clinical teams. These teams ultimately determine the value of the HIE to the organization by facilitating the integration of its capabilities into the daily routines of the different clinical domains.

It is important that any professional who wants to become involved asks for the opportunity. Like the implementation of EHRs and other business ISs, HIE implementation requires the involvement of many organizational disciplines. Asking to participate is a good place to start. HIM professionals' knowledge of informatics, codes, business practices, and vocabularies makes them a valuable asset to any project management team.

### Check Your Understanding 12.8

Answer the following questions in a separate document.

1. Reflect on the benefits of HIE. Choose one that strongly resonates with you as a critical aspect for improving the delivery of healthcare. Describe the reasons for your choice, including an example.
2. What roles can or should an HIM professional play within HIE implementation?
3. Explain the importance of MPI and how it is important to the HIE implementation.
4. Why is trust the most important requirement for an HIE to be successful? Explain why and how you would ensure sensitive patient information is secured.
5. What role does governance play in the successful deployment of an HIE?

# References

Ahmadi, M., and N. Aslani. 2018. Capabilities and advantages of cloud computing in the implementation of electronic health record. *Acta Informatica Medica* 26(1):24–28. https://www.ncbi.nlm.nih.gov/pmc/articles/PMC5869277/.Blokdijk, G. 2012. *Virtualization—The Complete Cornerstone Guide to Virtualization Best Practices*, 2nd ed. Newstead, Australia: Emereo Pty Ltd.

Chi, N. C., and G. Demiris. 2015. A systematic review of telehealth tools and interventions to support family caregivers. *Journal of Telemedicine and Telecare* 21(1):37–44.

Davis, B., and A. Swenson. 2022. How Carequality, The Sequoia Project, and eHealth Exchange support the interoperable exchange of health data in the USA. *Journal of Digital Imaging* 35(4):812–816. https://www.ncbi.nlm.nih.gov/pmc/articles/PMC9450827/.

Dwivedi, R., D. Mehrotra, and S. Chandra. 2022. Potential of internet of medical things (IoMT) applications in building a smart healthcare system: A systemic review. *Journal of Oral Biology and Craniofacial Research* 12(2):302–318. https://www.ncbi.nlm.nih.gov/pmc/articles/PMC8664731/.

eHealth Exchange. n.d. "Our Network." Accessed on June 16, 2024. https://ehealthexchange.org/.

eHealth Exchange. 2019. "Data Use and Reciprocal Support Agreement (DURSA)." https://ehealthexchange.org/onboarding/dursa/.

FDA (Food and Drug Administration). 2022 (May 2). "Human Factors and Medical Devices." https://www.fda.gov/medicaldevices/deviceregulationandguidance/humanfactors/.

Ford, E., J. A. Carroll, H. E. Smith, D. Scott, and J. A. Cassell. 2016. Extracting information from the text of electronic medical records to improve case detection: A systematic review. *Journal of the American Medical Informatics Association* 23(5):1007–1015. https://doi.org/10.1093/jamia/ocv180.

Gholamzadeh, M., H. Abtahi, and R. Safdari. 2023. The application of knowledge-based clinical decision support systems to enhance adherence to evidence-based medicine in chronic disease. *Journal of Healthcare Engineering*. https://www.ncbi.nlm.nih.gov/pmc/articles/PMC10241579/.

Hanson, A., and L. Haddad. 2023 (September 4). *Nursing Rights of Medication Administration*. StatPearls Publishing. https://www.ncbi.nlm.nih.gov/books/NBK560654/#article-34518.s1.

Health Record Banking Alliance. n.d. "What Is a Health Record Bank?" Accessed October 17, 2024. http://www.healthbanking.org/.

HL7 (Health Level Seven International). n.d.a. "Record Locator Service." Accessed June 16, 2024. https://www.hl7.org/documentcenter/public/wg/servicesbof/Record%20Locator%20Integrated%20Description%20v0.9.doc.

HL7 (Health Level Seven International). n.d.b. "CDA Release 2." Accessed October 17, 2024. http://www.hl7.org/implement/standards/product_brief.cfm?product_id=7.

IOM (Institute of Medicine). 1991. *The Computer-Based Patient Record: An Essential Technology for Health Care*. Washington, DC: National Academies Press.

Jen, M. Y., O. J. Mechanic, and D. Teoli. 2023 (September 4). "Informatics." *StatPearls*. https://www.ncbi.nlm.nih.gov/books/NBK470564/.

McCarthy, D. B., K. Propp, A. Cohen, R. Sabharwal, A. Schacter, and A. Rein. 2014. Learning from health information exchange technical architecture and implementation in seven beacon communities. *The Journal for Electronic Health Data and Methods* 2(1): 1060. https://www.ncbi.nlm.nih.gov/pmc/articles/PMC4371446/.

Mellowood Medical. n.d. "IDEAS EMR Clinical Mobile App and Web Portal." Accessed June 14, 2024. https://mellowoodmedical.com/clinical-portal/.

NAHIT (National Alliance for Health Information Technology). 2008 (April 28). "Defining Key Health Information Technology Terms." https://tigerstandards.pbworks.com/f/HITTermsFinalReport.pdf.

NANDA. 2017. "About NANDA." http://www.nanda.org/.

ONC (Office of the National Coordinator for Health Information Technology). 2024a. "Promoting Interoperability Programs." https://www.cms.gov/medicare/regulations-guidance/promoting-interoperability-programs?redirect=/EHRIncentivePrograms.

ONC (Office of the National Coordinator for Health Information Technology). 2024b. "Trusted Exchange Framework and Common Agreement (TECFA)." https://www.healthit.gov/topic/interoperability/policy/trusted-exchange-framework-and-common-agreement-tefca.

ONC (Office of the National Coordinator for Health Information Technology). 2020. "What Is HIE?" https://www.healthit.gov/topic/health-it-and-health-information-exchange-basics/what-hie.

ONC (Office of the National Coordinator for Health Information Technology). 2020 (October). *2020–2025 Federal Health IT Strategic Plan*. https://www.healthit.gov/sites/default/files/page/2020-10/Federal%20Health%20IT%20Strategic%20Plan_2020_2025.pdf.

ONC (Office of the National Coordinator for Health Information Technology). 2017. "Benefits of EHRs." https://www.healthit.gov/topic/health-it-and-health-information-exchange-basics/benefits-ehrs.

ONC (Office of the National Coordinator for Health Information Technology). n.d.a. "Healthcare Usability." Accessed June 16, 2024. https://www.healthcareusability.com/article/onc-meaningful-use-and-usability-testing.

ONC (Office of the National Coordinator for Health Information Technology). n.d.b. *What is FHIR?* Accessed June 15, 2024. https://www.healthit.gov/sites/default/files/2019-08/ONCFHIRFSWhatIsFHIR.pdf.

Padmanabhan, P. 2022. "Why Voice Recognition is the New Competitive Battleground in Healthcare's Digital Transformation." https://www.healthcareitnews.com/blog/why-voice-recognition-new-competitive-battleground-healthcares-digital-transformation.

Rahman, M., and F. Khahtun. 2023. "Challenges and Prospective of AI and 5G Enabled Technologies in Emerging Applications during the Pandemic." Chapter 2 in *Industry 4.0 Perspectives and Applications*, edited by M. Gordan, K. Ghaedi, and V. Saleh. https://www.intechopen.com/chapters/85738.

Rhapsody Health. n.d. "The Continuity of Care Document." Accessed June 15, 2024. https://rhapsody.health/resources/continuity-care-document-ccd-changing-landscape-healthcare-information/.

Sarkar, I. 2022. Transforming health data to actionable information: Recent progress and future opportunities in health information exchange. *Yearbook of Medical Informatics* 31(1):203–214. https://www.ncbi.nlm.nih.gov/pmc/articles/PMC9719753/.

Shah, S. M., and R. A. Khan. 2020. Secondary use of electronic health record: Opportunities and challenges. *IEEE Access* 8:136947–136965. https://ieeexplore.ieee.org/document/9146114.

Schnitzer, G. 2000. Natural language processing: A coding professional's perspective. *Journal of AHIMA* 71(9):95–98.

The Sequoia Project. n.d.a. "About Us: The Sequoia Project." Accessed August 21, 2024. https://sequoiaproject.org/about-us/The Sequoia Project.

The Sequoia Project. n.d.b. "CareQuality, and eHealth Exchange: What's the Difference?" Accessed August 21, 2024. https://sequoiaproject.org/whats-difference-ehealth-exchange-carequality-sequoia-project/.

Shrestha, R., and R. C. Gudivada. 2015. Beyond the Hype: Achieving True Semantic Interoperability in Healthcare. Presented at the HIMSS Annual Conference, Chicago, IL, April 2015.

Sutton, R. T., D. Pincock, D. C. Baumgart, D. C. Sadowski, R. N. Fedorak, and K. I. Kroeker. 2020 (February 6). An overview of clinical decision support systems: Benefits, risks, and strategies for success. *npj Digital Medicine* 3(17). https://doi.org/10.1038/s41746-020-0221-y.

Tate, J., P. Beck, H. Hugo Ibarra, S. Kumaravel, and L. Miklas. 2017. *Introduction to Storage Area Networks*, 9th ed. IBM Redbooks. http://www.redbooks.ibm.com/redbooks/pdfs/sg245470.pdf.

VA (Department of Veterans Affairs) 2021. "Blue Button." https://www.healthit.gov/topic/patient-access-information-individuals-get-it-check-it-use-it/blue-button.

Vest, J. R., and T. R. Miller. 2011. The Association between Health Information Exchange and Measures of Patient Satisfaction. *Applied Clinical Informatics* 2(4):447–459. https://www.ncbi.nlm.nih.gov/pmc/articles/PMC3612996/.

45 CFR 164.522: Rights to request privacy protection for protected health information. 2011 (Oct. 1).

# chapter 13

# Health Information Systems Planning

*Braden Tabisula, MBA, RHIA, CHDA*

## Learning Objectives

- Participate in planning the systems development life cycle for health information systems
- Facilitate the design, implementation, and ongoing maintenance of health information systems
- Evaluate health information systems from a utilization perspective to optimize their use
- Assess health information systems from an information and data governance perspective to help ensure their value

## Key Terms

Administrative data
Administrative metadata
Adoption
Application software
Application service provider (ASP)
Benefits realization
Best of breed
Best of fit
Change control
Chart conversion
Chief financial officer (CFO)
Chief information officer (CIO)
Chief medical informatics officer (CMIO)
Chief operating officer (COO)
Chief technology officer (CTO)
Clinical data
Clinical data analyst
Clinical transformation
Contract negotiation
Data administrator
Data conversion
Data model
Data provenance
Data quality measurement
Database administrator
Decision support
Dependency
Descriptive metadata
Due diligence
End users
Environmental scan
Financial data
Go-live
Governance
Health data
Health information
Health information system (HIS)
Health information technology (HIT)
Implementation
Implementation plan
Installation
Interface
Legacy system
Migration path
Personal health data
Planning horizon
Population health data
Project communication plan
Project plan
Project risk management
Public health data
Request for proposal (RFP)
Requirements analysis
Requirements specification
Research data
Return on investment (ROI)
Scribe
SMART goals
Steering committee
Stewardship
Strategic plan

Structural metadata
Sunsetting
Super users
System
System customization
System development life cycle (SDLC)
System integrator
System optimization
Systems view
Tactical plan
Thoughtflow
Turnover plan
Turnover strategy
Workflow

Many people, including healthcare professionals, use computers and other types of electronic systems daily, almost without thought. However, ensuring accurate and complete health information can be shared electronically across the continuum of healthcare continues to be a challenge.

Administrative and financial uses for computers have existed in healthcare since the early 1970s. Information systems, which consist of a set of components for collecting, processing, storing, and presenting data, have been deployed more recently for clinical uses. Systems to support laboratory testing, pharmacy management and dispensing, radiology studies, and prescription writing were among the earliest uses of information systems. Electronic health records (EHRs) are among the most recent information systems to aid documentation and provide clinical decision support for physicians, nurses, and other clinical users. There remain, however, many providers who view EHRs as burdensome and do not take full advantage of their benefits.

In 2010, the federal government incentivized using EHRs to encourage both acquisition and support for improved quality of care. In 2018, these efforts were renamed Promoting Interoperability (that is, the ability to communicate and exchange data across separate systems), and the federal government now focuses less on incentives and more on value-based care (VBC) programs. These programs aim to achieve better quality of care, improvement in population health, and reduction in healthcare costs by paying providers for value (that is, quality and cost outcomes) rather than paying a fee for every service provided (CMS 2023). VBC requires information systems to be interoperable so data sharing across the continuum of care and with patients can be accomplished (Bresnick 2018). The healthcare system as a whole—from primary and specialty care physicians and hospitals to skilled nursing, rehabilitative, and home care—remains in the process of fully acquiring, implementing, and adopting information systems for use within a given setting; for exchanging data with other providers, health plans, and patients; and for health research. As such, a **health information system (HIS)** is a set of many individual information systems focused on various aspects of health services that must work together to support delivery of quality healthcare, at a reasonable cost, and with a positive experience for both users and patients. HISs inherit the components of information systems and are applied to achieve specific objectives in the delivery of healthcare. Figure 13.1 models the relationship between HISs and information systems.

The life cycle of information technology (that is, the equipment that supports information systems) evolves so rapidly that what we buy today practically becomes obsolete tomorrow. HISs and their technology are expensive, complex, and time-consuming to implement. Their life cycle is somewhat longer than other technologies—but they still require upgrades, enhancements, and sometimes replacements. This chapter focuses on components of planning for this life cycle. This includes identification, requirements specification, acquisition, implementation, adoption, maintenance, and monitoring of results to ensure HISs address current needs. If at any point an HIS does not address current needs, the systems development life cycle begins again with new strategies for optimizing the HIS.

**Figure 13.1.** Health information systems versus information systems

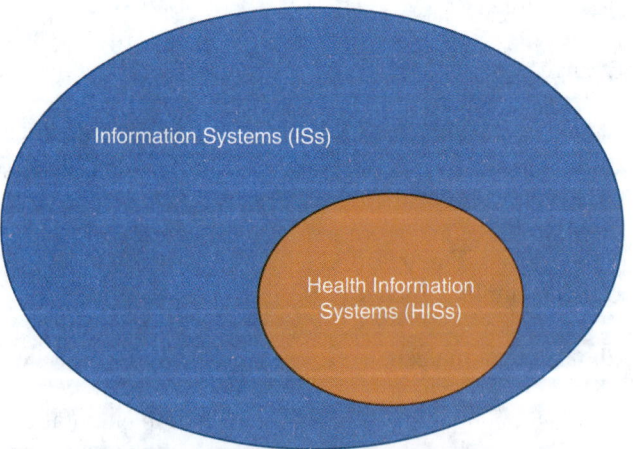

# A Systems View

In general, a **system** is a set of components that work together to achieve a common purpose. For example, a transportation system is comprised of cars, trains, airplanes, and other mechanisms to move people and goods; roads, train tracks, and other forms of routing for effectiveness and efficiency; and rules of the road and other forms of guidance to provide oversight for safety and security. In healthcare delivery, professionals, hospital structures, medical equipment, policies and procedures, and much more must work together to provide a functioning system to care for the sick and injured, and to help maintain health and wellness. Figure 13.2 diagrams an example of how HISs work together to provide a functioning healthcare system. An HIS is comprised of many computer (software applications and other HIT) and human (people, policy, and process) components. A local HIS exists in an individual organization, including in provider settings, insurance companies, health plan offices, and data warehouses of various types.

Computers are systems of devices programmed to translate electrical pulses to represent and process data. However, an information system includes computers and humans. Humans build the computer hardware, write software so that computers process data, connect applications to one another, and address the operational issues relating to people, policy, and process. Such operational elements include, for example, training on use of the various information system applications, establishing policy for how applications will be used and when data can and should be shared, and improving associated processes and workflows. As a result, information systems are comprised of various IT, professionals, standards, and more that enable useful information to be available when and where it is needed.

A system has many components that are required to work together, so all of its components must be considered when making any changes to improve its outcomes; this is referred to as taking a **systems view**. If a system is not achieving its desired purpose, focusing on only selected components will not ensure all components will work together effectively. If an HIS is not achieving its intended purpose, taking a systems view ensures all components are considered and adjusted accordingly to achieve improvement. Figure 13.3 models aspects of an HIS system from a systems view.

An entire discipline is devoted to systems analysis and design, but many healthcare professionals

**Figure 13.2.** Health information system example

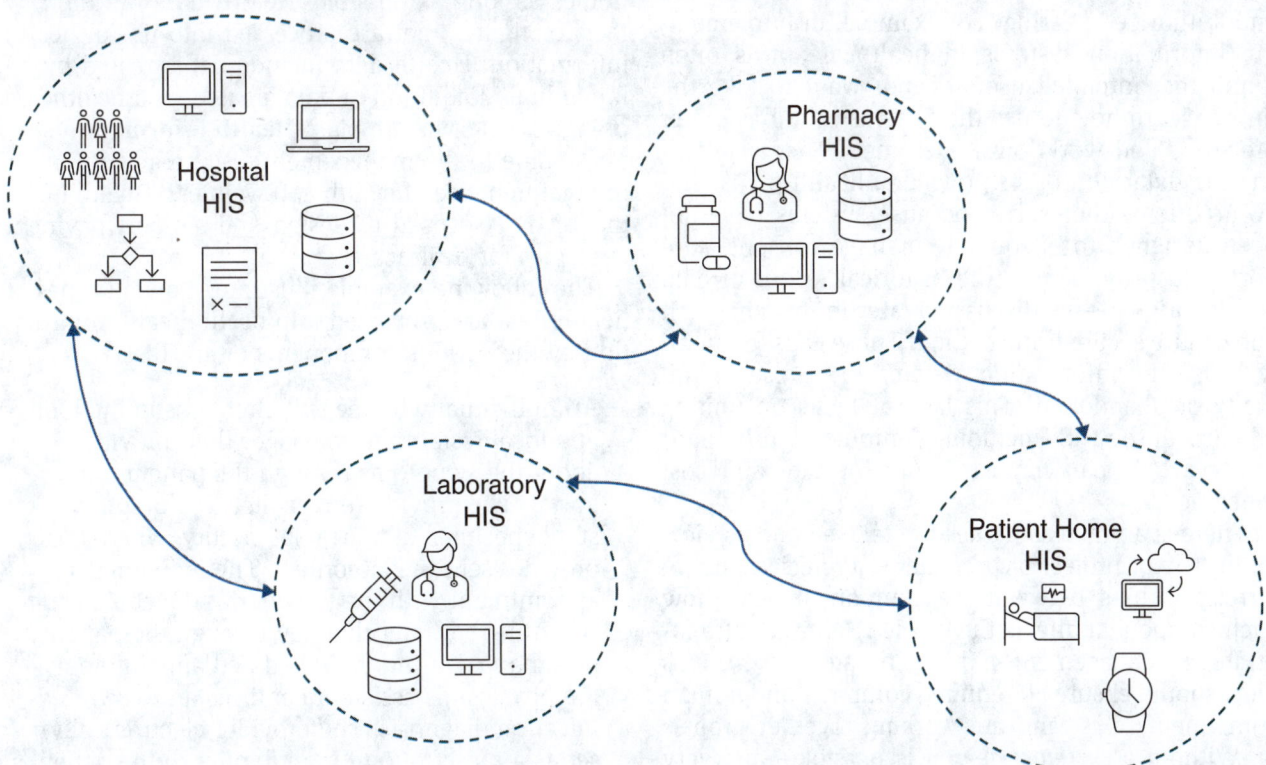

**Figure 13.3.** HIS scope

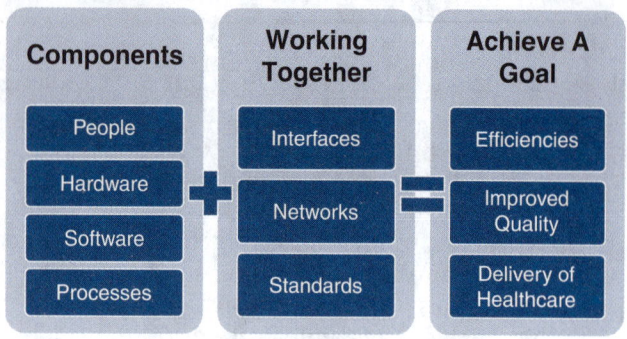

are not trained to look at all system elements and how they must work together to be successful in their mission. Additionally, many healthcare organizations have not previously had to consider with whom they must share data, and vendors have had limited ability to work together due to proprietary interests in IT components. This has often resulted in a narrow perspective focused on implementing IT for just one specialty of care (for example, primary care or orthopedics) or one type of organizational structure (for example, a clinic, hospital, or laboratory). Individuals involved in design, implementation, or use of ISs often do not think about the components as part of an overall system and how all the parts must work together to achieve the desired result.

Increasingly, the human element is not sufficiently considered in system design to support optimal use and authorized sharing. For example, in implementing information systems in healthcare, it is often found that intended users do not want to take the time to learn how to use the systems or to have their processes and workflows redesigned. They also fear sharing data with other providers, health plans, and even patients themselves because systems have not been designed to adequately manage consent, support data provenance (the historical record of data and its origins—see discussion later in this chapter), and ensure secure transmission. These gaps frequently cause the information systems to be used minimally or abandoned. This lack of focus on uniting all parts of the HIS (including computer and human) into a whole can impact quality of care and cost outcomes.

There is an increasing need to take a systems view of any major project or program to appreciate the interrelationships between the components and how each component affects the whole (Haines Centre for Strategic Management n.d.). Ultimately, a systems view should ensure all required computer and human components exist and are working together properly. Without a systems view, it is possible—and very likely—that components will not work well together. Ideally, the result of taking a systems view of information systems is that one can improve the quality of care, patient safety, access to care, cost of care, efficiency of care processes, patient experience of care, and the health of the nation in general.

Healthcare industry members sometimes use the terms *health information system* and *health information technology* synonymously. However, their meanings are distinct. HIS refers to all the components, human and computer, that ensure health data are processed into useful health information. Health information technology (HIT) is reserved to describe computer systems and associated components such as networks, software, and end-user devices used to process health data into health information.

Increasingly, data warehouses, health information exchange services, and health data repositories from various vendors are being used to aid information exchange across care settings and with health insurers and patients. They enable sharing and analysis of the data within them to support health research and to create new forms of evidence-based clinical decision support. Data analysis uses machine learning and artificial intelligence for population health management and precision medicine. Components of these systems must also consider healthy individuals, caregivers, and patients who want to connect with care delivery systems that enable them to be more informed and engaged, and even receive care in their homes as long as possible. Health data are the raw facts or figures that are processed into useful health information. Health data include data created by an individual in addition to data created by a healthcare organization or health plan. Health information supplies value to the management of illness or injury or the maintenance of health and wellness. Health information is also used to design and support payment strategies for healthcare.

The following example illustrates how all types of health data are processed into useful health information by the various components of an HIS.

> An individual who feels ill after consuming food at a local restaurant, messages their provider about the symptoms through the patient portal. The provider directs her to drop off a stool specimen at a local laboratory, where the provider sent the lab orders. The individual's appointment with the provider at the clinic is scheduled for later that day through the patient portal app. During the scheduled appointment, the physician's assistant confirms an *E. coli* infection diagnosis. The provider electronically sends a prescription for antibiotics to the patient's

pharmacy of choice. The patient's insurance covers part of the cost of the drug, and the patient documents a record of the co-pay for income tax purposes. The laboratory conveys the potential for food contamination and the provider's system sends a confirmation of the diagnosis to the local public health department, which will manage further contamination. If the food contamination spreads, an entire region's population may be affected.

Until very recently in healthcare, the sharing of health information across disparate systems was not valued. With a new focus on VBC and accountability for the quality and cost of healthcare delivered, the ability to share information across the continuum of care has become essential.

## System Development Life Cycle

As suggested by the fast pace at which HIT changes and the many processes and components entailed in processing health data, it should be clear that HISs have life cycles that, when fully understood, can be used to manage changes so the system continues to produce the desired results. The **system development life cycle (SDLC)** refers to the steps taken from an initial point of recognizing the need for a desired result, through the steps taken to ensure all components needed for the system to achieve the desired result are addressed, to repeating this cycle whenever the system fails to produce the desired result (Radack 2009). The applicability of the SDLC is not limited to information systems; the outcomes of any major project (for example, construction of a new building) can be improved with a systems view. Failure of a system to produce the desired result may be due to internal or external changes. For example, if an HIS was acquired several years ago, and there is a new federal mandate for a change in a code system or the operating system software is no longer being supported, the healthcare organization must address needed changes in the system or acquire a replacement to continue to produce desired results. The general nature of an SDLC is illustrated in figure 13.4.

There may be variations in how the steps in the SDLC are described depending on the context in which it is used. For example, a hardware or software developer may go through the SDLC when creating a new product. The vendor may identify a need for a new product; then determine the feasibility of creating the new product with specifications that would satisfy the new product needs; design the product; develop it for mass production; maintain the product as small changes in the environment may impact it; and monitor sales to justify continued maintenance or sunsetting (no longer selling or supporting) the product. As another example, when a provider identifies a need for HIS support, the provider will specify the requirements, acquire the new system, implement the new system, maintain it, and monitor that it continues to meet needs over time. Sometimes the SDLC identifies that an HIS may need to be replaced, in which case the SDLC of acquiring a new product is repeated.

Each of the major steps in the SDLC generally includes several smaller steps. For example, when an upgrade to a provider's HIS becomes available from the vendor, a provider may determine if it wishes to accept the upgrade (identify need); develop a plan for implementation (specify requirements such as when the upgrade should occur and who will perform the implementation); acquire the upgrade; implement it; and continue to use it for its operations (maintain it) until monitoring proves the need for another upgrade, replacement, staff retraining, or other action.

The SDLC is most often applied when information systems are being developed or acquired. However, the SDLC should also be applied as part of a continuous improvement process to ensure systems meet ongoing and any new needs. If a system is not being adopted, the SDLC can help identify whether there are issues with how the system was developed (for example, there may be a "bug" in the system that the vendor needs to address); how the system was implemented (for example, one-size-fits-all or tailored

**Figure 13.4.** System development life cycle

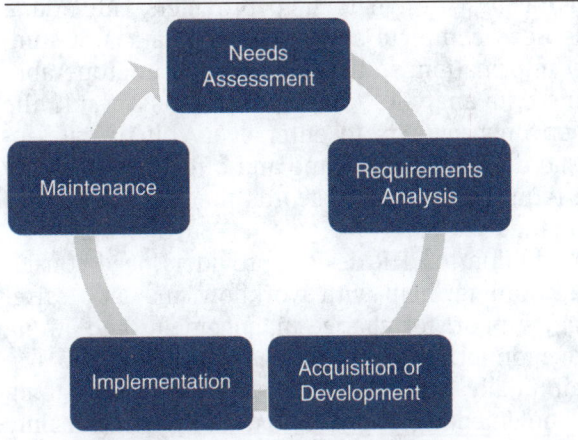

to unique needs of individuals); whether there was sufficient attention to process improvement and workflow redesign; and even if there was appropriate training for each user type. The key value of the SDLC is to apply a formal, logical process to any new program, expanded service offering, or other project to ensure that all necessary components are in place for a system to optimally achieve its value.

## Strategic Planning for Health Information Systems

An SDLC view, in which all components are expected to work together to achieve the desired goal, can be especially useful when developing any strategic plan, and especially for HISs. Generally, a strategic plan is long term, covering a period of at least three to five years, and focused on the organization's mission, vision, and goals to help set the organization's direction.

Computer systems tend to have a short life cycle; therefore, many organizations develop plans for information systems that are often only one or two years. This is a tactical plan (short-term, focused on one component or project) rather than a strategic plan. Tactical plans often do not fully address the SDLC, resulting in a short-term project focused on one component of the larger HIS that does not work well with its other components. In this section we discuss the purpose and preparation of a strategic plan for HISs.

### Purpose of HIS Planning

Strategic planning is necessary to address all parts of an HIS, especially as new hardware and software components are continuously developed. Many HISs expand beyond organizational boundaries to connect large systems with other large systems, such as connecting a health system to a large payer or pharmacy system. Individual patient applications, such as those that may stream vital signs data to a provider or help maintain a patient's health diary, are included. Application software is the set of instructions that cause the computer hardware to perform tasks. Applications for the EHR can be immense. Apps are smaller applications, more limited in scope, and browser-based, such as those designed to run on smartphones and other mobile devices. Most providers find the timeline for planning a major information system implementation or enhancement is at least three to five years, and many have exceeded 10 or more years, especially when considering all of the components that must be addressed. For example, to implement an EHR, most providers need, at a minimum, a patient registration system to supply patient demographic data to the EHR. Hospitals need many additional systems, such as laboratory information systems, nursing documentation systems, food and nutrition systems, human resource systems, patient financial systems, and many others. Figure 13.5 depicts a few additional HISs and their categories.

Most hospitals have upwards of 100 systems, and very large healthcare delivery networks may have several hundred systems. The smallest physician office may have as many as 10 different types of HISs, including the EHR and systems for patient registration, patient billing, medical coding, payroll, disease registry, and others. Even when most of the HISs are acquired from the same vendor and look like one cohesive system, they comprise many components, often installed separately over time.

If an HIS, as defined previously, includes human and computer components, then both human and computer components must be planned for. Technology affects people in different ways. In a physician's office, for example, a practice management system (PMS) is primarily used by practice administrators for patient registration and billing processes. Administrators often have considerable experience using these functions as standalone systems, and providers rarely, if ever, use the PMS. However, both practice administrators and providers are affected when an EHR integrates with the PMS to acquire EHR functionality.

Many factors may contribute to today's EHR issues. Vendors, concerned that providers might have difficulty using EHRs, initially designed them to look like paper records, even though this may not have been the best design to help providers enter data. EHRs need complete and structured data, not summary information, to best support the interoperability and data analytics functionalities. As a result, the burden on providers to enter every bit of data increased documentation time and often increased the time required to review records that do not contain summaries.

In addition to EHR design, providers need considerable training, help with workflow and process redesign, support for change management, and strong usage monitoring to ensure they are using the system optimally. Taking a systems view when designing and implementing any information system not only

**Figure 13.5.** Examples of health information systems and their categories

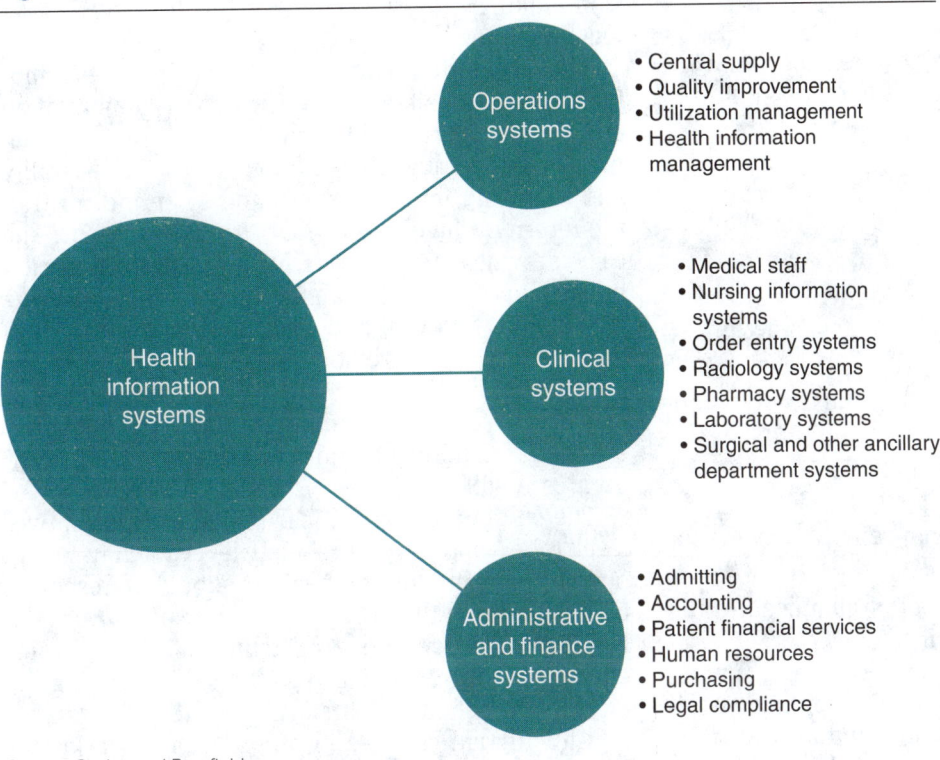

*Source:* Sayles and Barefield

ensures the technology is addressed but also that "people, policy, and process" factors are addressed to ensure users achieve value from the technology.

Another planning consideration from a systems view is the need to sequence implementation of technical components within the HIS and the need to recognize the impact of sequencing on people, policy, and process. Such sequencing includes the initial implementation and ongoing updates, upgrades, and additions.

For example, in the early stages of implementing EHRs, many hospital leaders decided to implement barcode medication administration record (BCMAR) systems nurses use to ensure the right medication is given to the right patient at the right time. From a strategic planning perspective, these same leaders often thought nurses would learn these systems easily and assist physicians when computerized provider order entry (CPOE) systems were implemented. However, the result of not addressing the full SDLC led to nurses finding these systems difficult to use. For example, when a barcode reader is tethered to a computer by cable, the cable may not comfortably reach the patient's barcoded wristband to be scanned. As a result, many hospitals found that nurses were printing extra copies of the patient wristbands and scanning them at the nurses' station, then going to the bedside to administer the medications; this workaround defeated the ability to positively identify the patient and document at the exact time of medication administration. Those tasked with acquiring and implementing the technology may not have considered how the barcode reader would be used in practice.

Nurses were also concerned about what appeared to be an increase in medication "errors" that resulted from using the system. Some of these errors were previously impossible to track manually, or, potentially, the error indicators were set too stringently when first implemented. For example, the default policy for medication timeliness in many BCMAR systems was to record any delay of more than a few minutes in administering medication as an error. An error would be recorded even if the patient was in surgery at the originally programmed medication administration time. Without planning from a systems view to identify the need to evaluate policy, many nurses created workarounds such as scanning copies of the patient's wristband at the nursing station and later administering the medications when the patient was available.

HISs are major investments and complex systems that require extensive preparation, time to implement, and attention to human factors to get people to use them correctly and achieve intended results.

# Designing a Health Information Systems Plan

An HIS strategic planning life cycle reflects the SDLC. In preparation, organizational leadership should recognize the following as necessary steps:

- Create governance for the system.
- Specify the planning horizon for the system.
- Translate needs to goals for the system.
- Use an environmental scan to identify system challenges to address in the system's design requirements.
- Document the design of the HIS in a migration path that provides a reference point for acquiring, implementing, gaining adoption, and optimizing use of the HIS' components.
- Establish system maintenance requirements for the system.
- Develop a monitoring program that ensures the goals for the system are met.
    - If they are not met, take steps to examine new needs, specify requirements to address new needs, design and implement changes in the system, and keep those changes current and appropriate for continuous goal achievement.

Once the scope of strategic planning is understood, organizational leadership is responsible for creating a governance structure and monitoring its work through each of the steps.

## Governance

Governance of the HIS strategic planning process should be established before planning begins. **Governance** is the establishment of policies and the continual monitoring of their implementation for managing an organization's assets. For example, in an HIS, governance would involve policies relating to the human, computer, and information components. Effective governance results from interactions among key stakeholders who are accountable to one another and who follow a transparent, responsive, equitable, and inclusive process to make decisions about how an organization will use its assets to achieve a specific goal or set of goals (McDonald 2022).

Therefore, the strategic planning process for an HIS will be governed by representatives from senior management (financial, operational, and clinical) and the leadership of IT and enterprise health information management (HIM). The individual who chairs the governance process should be neutral, meaning the individual has no vested interest in any particular function. The following senior managers with decision-making authority should be involved in HIS strategic planning:

The **chief financial officer (CFO)** is the senior manager responsible for the fiscal management of an entity. The CFO should participate in strategic planning to impart knowledge about financial feasibility and financing for the system, and to be informed of the return on investment (ROI) from the system. The CFO provides insight into how health information must converge with financial information, ensuring that patient financial and cost information integrates with clinical data. Providers must be aware of the financial implications of their care recommendations, as patients are also becoming much more consumer-oriented to healthcare and want to know how much their care will cost them.

The **chief operating officer (COO)** is an executive-level role responsible at a high level for day-to-day operations of an entity. The COO should be responsible for ensuring that all applicable persons within the healthcare delivery process use the HIS. Input provided by this representative regarding the planning for an HIS can help anticipate and prepare the organization for myriad changes in processes and workflows as part of HIS adoption and the broader context of health reform.

Senior clinical officers, including the chief medical officer (CMO) and chief nursing officer (CNO), represent the primary users of the clinical components of HISs. Their contributions to strategic planning for an HIS are vital to getting grassroots adoption of the systems to be implemented. They provide input and gain understanding to generate their peers' trust in the systems.

Leaders of IT and information management are also involved in HIS strategic planning. Such individuals have the technical knowledge and skills to direct the implementation of the HIS being planned.

A **chief medical informatics officer (CMIO)** is a physician with a special interest in technology implementations and advanced analytics (Rucker, 2023). They typically are practicing physicians who can put policy into practice. While the CMO represents the medical staff on all matters relating to their practice of healthcare, the CMIO is the bridge between the medical staff and the administration of a healthcare entity implementing an HIS. They are enlightened advocates and strong proponents of system usability—the efficiency, effectiveness, and satisfaction with which users achieve results from HISs (Pfister and Ingargiola 2014)—and patient safety, that is, the absence of and reduction of risk for preventable harm to a patient (WHO 2023). The modern-day CMIO optimizes patient care with the use of data analytics tools and the latest technology (Mena 2023). The **chief**

**information officer (CIO)** is responsible for the management, implementation, and usability of information and computer technologies for an entity (Rouse 2022a). The CIO should participate in the strategic planning process as a key subject matter expert, both with respect to the current state of the HIT already in place and in level-setting for the planning timeline over which changes and new technology can realistically be implemented. The CIO manages many of the staff members who play important roles in incorporating HIT into the entity's HIS strategic plan.

A **chief technology officer (CTO)** is responsible for overseeing current technology and creating relevant policies for its use (Rouse 2022b). The CTO contributes information regarding the current state of IT and its relevance to healthcare.

Other critical informatics professionals exist within healthcare, including those with clinical experience and have paired their domain knowledge and experience with informatic skills and interests. For example, pharmacy informaticists may be a liaison or project manager for a new pharmacy system being implemented, provide domain knowledge and validation for a pharmacy terminology server, or be given the responsibility to design new pharmacist workflows in the EHR. Public health informaticians focus on populations and society. These professionals may provide one or more representatives to the strategic planning process for an HIS depending on the size of the organization and the status of building a robust HIS.

Other key individuals whose input is vital throughout the strategic planning process include the following:

- **Clinical data analysts** ensure protocol is followed when research data is collected and analyzed. These professionals also provide reporting and share results of the analysis while also ensuring the data management processes are followed.
- **Database administrators** are technical staff members within IT departments who design and manage the technical implementation and maintenance of databases.
- **Data administrators** are people who apply domain expertise to the logical design of a database, establish policies and standards governing creation and use of data, maintain data dictionaries, and manage data quality. Data administrators may have backgrounds in HIM or health informatics.
- The HIM professional complements the CIO's perspectives in planning HIS strategy. Where the CIO addresses the technical components of health information as processed by HIT, the HIM professional provides information and data governance perspectives. These focus on managing the input (data) and output (information) of the HIS. They specifically address the components of data design, such as data models, data capture, data security, data quality, information access and use, information retention and disposal, documentation requirements, legal and regulatory compliance, ethical use of information, and the intellectual property ownership of information (Kloss 2015, 40).

### Planning Horizon

The **planning horizon** for strategic planning of an HIS refers to both the scope of the system to be addressed and the number of years estimated for planning, acquiring, implementing, adopting, and optimizing use of the components identified. The planning horizon helps anticipate the resources that will be needed and the feasibility of carrying out the plan. If resources are insufficient, the planning horizon may need to be lengthened, the scope narrowed, or alternatives considered.

### Translate Needs into Goals

Needs for the entity that an HIS can address are most commonly expressed as goals. Goals for what and how the HIS will achieve desired results reflect current and anticipated needs and should drive all subsequent elements of the planning process. **SMART goals** are statements that identify results that are:

- **S:** Specific. Provide details of who the responsible party is and what it is that the entity is trying to achieve.
- **M:** Measurable. Incorporate benchmarks and metrics to keep track of progress.
- **A:** Achievable. Identify resources available to meet the goal or determine limitations and dependencies up front.
- **R:** Relevant. Determine the reason for setting this goal, whether it be to meet a larger goal of the organization or a specific need of a determined population
- **T:** Time-based. Define a timeframe to complete the goal or set milestones.

Any organization will have several SMART goals for its HIS. For example, a physician office may include the following goal in its planning:

Physicians (specific) will aid in reducing unnecessary diagnostic tests (relevant) by

10 percent (measurable) over the next two years (time-based) through the interoperability capability of the system (achievable), making available, at the time an order is placed for a test, the results from previous tests performed across the enterprise within a period specific to the type of test and schedule for the patient (specific).

SMART goals incorporated into an HIS strategic plan should address all system components, including desired functionality, specific technology requirements to support the desired functions, and the expectations for people to adopt new policies and processes to ensure the goals' achievement and, therefore, provide value back to the organization for its investment (Amatayakul 2017, 86–87).

### Identify Challenges

Challenges are inevitable elements that pose barriers to achieving success with an HIS. Without recognizing them early in the planning process, it becomes very difficult to overcome them. An **environmental scan** is part of the strategic planning process where an organization identifies external opportunities and threats that could impact the business in the future (SHRM 2012). Reviewing published data, conducting surveys, and interviewing are a few of the many ways to collect information about the environments.

Published data can help identify lessons learned from others. For example, determining how many hospitals already had an EHR prior to implementing the Meaningful Use (MU) incentive program may have been the trigger for the federal government to implement such a program. However, in its strategic planning for the incentive program's timeline, the federal government did not apply the fact that most hospitals took much longer to implement their systems than outlined in the government's timeline. A hospital seeking to implement an EHR under the incentive program would recognize the opportunity for help with funding an EHR, but in its environmental scan may have identified as a challenge the average cost of EHRs and average timelines for implementation. Looking to overcome these barriers led some hospitals and physicians to acquire EHRs matching the incentive funding and timeline—only later to find that these vendors were struggling to implement Stage 2 requirements at low cost. Many of these healthcare entities are now faced with replacing their systems because they are not fully meeting their present needs and, in some cases, because the vendors have gone out of business.

Surveys are another important way to understand the potential challenges to be addressed in planning for an HIS. A simple survey of all hospital staff, including clinicians might have identified that, on average, low numbers of potential users regularly use a computer. This is factual data. Perceptions are also important to understand. If a survey of potential users finds concerns about using an EHR, immediate work can begin on helping overcome the challenge of EHRs being burdensome to new users.

Anecdotal information from observations and interviews is also important to help identify challenges. Before the EHR incentive program, articles published about the unintended consequences of EHR use described issues with the system's design, lack of user training, and the like. All these issues could be overcome by paying attention to people, policy, and process issues; but the headlines only added to providers' distrust of EHRs, which to this day is a challenge to address. The sources of information gathered about the environment should be many and varied. This ensures a comprehensive understanding of the environment and reduces bias.

### Design Documentation

Design refers to a picture or framework for how a planned HIS is expected to appear. It is a high-level outline of all components the organization has identified as required to achieve its goals. General statements of goals for each part of the timeline and the general nature of the applications (software), technology (computer systems), and operational elements (people, policy, and process) are documented. This documentation of the plan may be referred to as a **migration path** (Amatayakul 2017, 63–70).

The migration path should reflect the IT architecture of hardware and software and the operational elements to address improvements in clinical quality, patient safety, evidence-based practices, cost of care, productivity, user satisfaction, patient experience of care, and more.

The migration path is supported by documentation that provides the SMART goal statements; describes the detailed nature of the IT infrastructure; and addresses the policies, procedures, training, workflow changes, and other operational elements that need to be put into place. Staffing, budgets, detailed requirements specifications, and detailed plans follow from the migration path. Figure 13.6 provides an example of a strategic plan with three phases, and each phase includes plans related to the successful completion of the phase. Upon completion of a phase, the strategic plan moves to the next phase with new implementation plans and details.

Some healthcare organizations question the need for a migration path when either their vendor heavily dictates the components and implementation sequence,

**Figure 13.6.** Example strategic plan with implementation plans

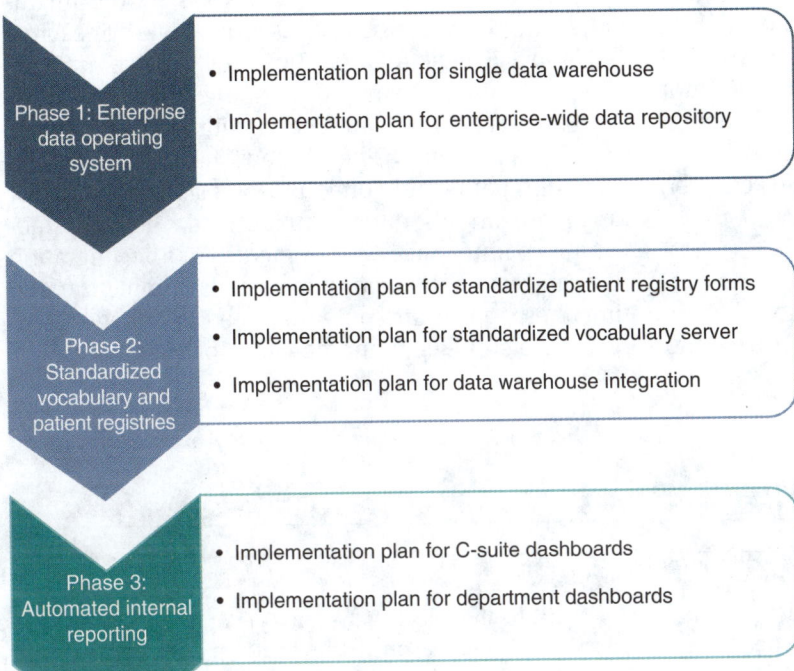

or the federal incentive program directs required EHR elements. While these circumstances provide a framework for a strategic plan for HISs, they do not create a complete picture of all the major elements a healthcare organization may need in its strategic plan.

For example, an EHR vendor may not supply all the software an organization desires, such as that for integrating clinical and financial data needed to analyze the level of risk that may be entailed in participating in a VBC contract. In such a contract, providers need data and analytics tools that can supply information on the quality of care they are providing and its cost to reduce their risk. In addition, most HIS vendors will acknowledge that the people, policy, and process issues associated with gaining adoption and optimizing system use are very important, but they consider these issues to be the healthcare organization's responsibility. Organizations must determine when certain types of staff are needed, what policies are needed, and how processes and workflows must change to ensure goal achievement.

Timelines and sequencing decisions should be made by the healthcare organization. An example is an alert that a health plan authorization is needed prior to a specific type of surgery or for a referral to a certain kind of specialist. Another example is a delay in treatment often results because the need for prior authorization was not discovered until after the patient left the clinic. Also, a hospital could implement a BCMAR system sometime before or concurrent with CPOE. An organization constructing its HIS strategic plan determines the timeline and sequencing, considering all factors identified in its environmental scan.

There are also dependencies between applications, technology, and operational elements. A **dependency** exists when one component cannot operate without another component. An example is when software cannot be used without hardware. Not all dependencies are obvious. For example, a nurse acuity system, which supports scheduling nurses for shift duty based on historical patient volumes and how acutely ill the patients are, requires administrative data from a human resource system to identify nurse credentials, a patient acuity classification system, clinical data to classify patients, and a scheduling system that tracks patient volumes by type of patient acuity. Another example many experts recognize is that it is advisable for EHR users to review the clinical decision support (CDS) system rules prior to their implementation. This gives users the opportunity not only to customize the system to their needs but also to learn how the CDS system is constructed, develop trust in the rules or modify them per local practices and policies, and, as a result, be more inclined to use the CDS system effectively.

It is important to note that a migration path is a high-level view of the strategic plan, not an implementation plan for each component. **Implementation plans** are used to manage the thousands of tasks involved in selecting, acquiring, implementing, adopting, and optimizing the use of the various hardware, software, and operational components of the HIS. Implementation plans are tactical, relatively short term, and often repeated with only slight variation for every system component implemented. Implementation plans are condensed versions of project plans, which are discussed in the next section of this chapter.

### Maintenance and Monitoring

Once the migration path is developed, it should be reviewed regularly and updated as needed. It becomes the road map for all decisions relative to going forward with HISs. Achieving consensus on the migration path keeps organizations from making reactive decisions. Except for unanticipated changes in current applications, technology, or operations, or unexpected external mandates, the migration path should be relatively stable. There is no one right or wrong migration path—only one that is most appropriate for an organization's given situation and goals. Establishing maintenance requirements for the migration path and using it to monitor both its completion and timeliness, given any potential need to change, completes the strategic planning cycle for HISs.

## Check Your Understanding 13.1

**Answer the following questions in a separate document.**

1. Provide three examples of how the SDLC may be used in each of the following different contexts in a healthcare delivery organization:
   a. Implementing a clinically integrated network
   b. Planning a merger or acquisition of another healthcare provider
   c. Renovating an aging facility

2. For each of the following individuals, describe why the individual would or would not be best to lead the strategic planning process for promoting interoperability.
   a. Chief information officer
   b. Chief operating officer
   c. Chief medical informatics officer

3. For each of the following, identify if it belongs on a migration path for HISs and, if so, under which section it belongs (applications, technology, or operations):
   a. $100,000 for patient housing assistance
   b. Customer relationship management system
   c. Opening a project management office
   d. Writing direct-to-consumer apps
   e. Health insurance provider network

4. Create a table differentiating the roles (for instance, leader, compliance, subject matter expert, and potentially others) and scope (for instance, all staff, all physicians, subject matter experts, or others) of the following individuals in HIS strategic planning for an organization:
   a. Chief medical officer
   b. Chief medical informatics officer
   c. Chief technology officer
   d. Chief nurse informaticist

5. Describe the role(s) of the health information manager in health information system strategic planning, including specifying which applications, technology, and operations are affected.

6. Write a SMART goal for developing a dashboard for the health information department.

7. Conducting an environmental scan as part of strategic planning may help identify:
   a. Barriers to using HIT due to staff inexperience with computers
   b. Challenges with respect to organizational goals
   c. Operational elements needed to support application software and technology
   d. Which vendors sell products that meet the organization's requirements and specifications

8. The SDLC step in which it may be found that an IT component is no longer of value is which of the following?
   a. Needs assessment
   b. Requirements analysis
   c. Acquisition
   d. Maintenance

# Strategic Plan Execution

The strategic plan becomes a tool to identify components of an IS to add to those the organization has in place. Each component is implemented, often as one or more projects, each with a project manager and project plan. A project represents a specifically defined scope of work. This work includes specifying detailed requirements for each component, acquiring and putting in place the appropriate resources, implementing the components, gaining user adoption through monitoring the components' use, optimizing use of the components so they are well-integrated within the organization's workflows and processes, providing ongoing maintenance, and determining when it is appropriate to upgrade, enhance, or replace a component.

From a systems view, as each component is implemented and ongoing monitoring occurs, reference to the strategic plan ensures that the components are still contributing to the goals and fit with the remaining acquired and implemented components. As this assessment occurs, and especially if new components need to be added, the HIS strategic plan may need to be modified or enhanced, pushing forward into further planning horizons.

## Project Management

Project management generally includes appointing a steering committee and project manager, constructing a project plan, and developing policies and procedures associated with maintaining the plan, managing risk in the project, and reporting on the completion status of the project plan.

The steering committee is a representative group of key stakeholders who provide advice and guidance in the acquisition of the HIS components under consideration. The steering committee members are managers and representative users from the departments most affected by the given component or components of the acquired and implemented HIS.

Although some organizations do not identify a project manager until implementation of a new HIS is underway, many find it necessary to initiate project planning earlier. In addition, the project manager gets engaged sufficiently early in the process so there is no learning curve at the critical juncture of implementation readiness. Planning for acquisition and implementation are significant project components. Thus, the organization typically appoints a project manager and project team for large organizations or projects.

The project manager is responsible for developing a detailed project plan and ensuring all tasks within the project scope are successfully performed on time and on budget. A project plan is a tool that aids in carrying out a specific set of tasks that lead to the completion of a specific goal. The project plan serves to document what needs to be done, when, and by whom. It helps control task timing and sequencing, schedule and allocate resources, manage risk, and celebrate success. The plan includes a list of tasks, their start and end dates, dependencies associated with each task, and resources required to complete each task. There will likely be hundreds, if not thousands, of tasks on a project plan for any given HIS component. For large organizations, some system components may be phased in over time. For example, in implementing an EHR, the BCMAR may have been implemented before CPOE. As another example, an EHR may be required to be in place before a personal health record. In some cases, phasing of components is not always easy or clear, such as when participating in a health information exchange service does not necessarily require an EHR but would benefit from an EHR component being in place.

Each system component may also have a turnover plan, which is a plan that specifies how and when each part of an information system component is to be implemented for different users. A hospital with many nursing units might implement BCMAR on only one or two units simultaneously until all are fully adopted. A multispecialty clinic may decide primary care physicians will be trained to use the EHR before specialists. This type of staging is often referred to as a turnover strategy that considers which users may be the easiest to train, which users are most interested in using the system, and which components are not dependent on other components not yet implemented.

The project manager is also responsible for the project resources, generally specified in a project budget; managing all contractors involved in the project and the internal project team; identifying and resolving all issues that occur during the implementation; and performing risk management. Contractors would predominantly be the vendor's team but might also include other contractors who assist with special activities, such as workflow and process redesign, coaching physicians, building special databases, or writing interfaces not supplied by the primary vendor, and others.

The project team consists of dedicated IT staff from the organization (or contracted for the project specifically), super users, and operations staff who assist with workflow and process redesign, policy development, and other tasks. **Super users** are typically staff members who will ultimately be end users who have agreed to help with the implementation, testing, training, and post go-live troubleshooting. **End users** are those using the system for everyday tasks. Super users may be trained and, sometimes, certified by the vendor for the specific product being implemented.

During any implementation, several risk factors arise. The project manager must be skilled in risk management. **Project risk management** is a process in an HIS project that identifies and reduces the possibility that a key step or series of steps may not be performed on time, where a component of the system may not work properly potentially delaying other aspects of the implementation or be costly to fix, and other risks.

Communication is a vital role for the project manager and is essential throughout the entire project life cycle. Regular communication about the project's status, invitations to contribute to requirements specifications, announcements about vendor selection, progress on implementation, and regular expressions of appreciation for support and celebration of accomplishments help reduce stress in the highly demanding experience of HIS adoption. Many project managers use a **project communication plan** specifying the types of communications needed at various stages of the project, who should deliver the communications, the medium for the communications, and the communication that was undertaken, and any feedback or lessons learned from it.

## Requirements Analysis

**Requirements analysis** is the step that identifies, in detail, the precise requirements needed for both HIT (that is, hardware and software) and operational components (people, policy, and process) of the HIS to meet the goals specified in the strategic plan. It is not enough to say, "we want an EHR," or even something expressed as a SMART goal, such as "we want to provide patients easy, electronic access to their health information within 24 hours of their encounter with the healthcare system." It is necessary to specifically describe what functionality the organization means by EHR or patient access to health information.

Functionality requirements include those relating to data entry, information retrieval, data and information storage, alerts, data analytics, data quality management, security and privacy protection of the data and information, data integrity, access to information, sharing of data and information, and others. The following are important areas that impact functionality and should be addressed in a requirements specification that is provided to potential vendors: scope of EHR certification, potential gaps and variations in technology, and workflow and process improvement opportunities.

### EHR Certification

The federal government specified the standards an EHR must have to be certified under federal government requirements (ONC 2015). Despite these standards, buyers must know that not all certified EHRs are identical. The certification standards specify the minimum functionality for the minimum components comprising an EHR. From there, the possibilities are virtually endless.

For example, EHR certification does not include automation of every conceivable piece of health information that is captured in the course of caring for a patient. It does not address anesthesia records, nurses' notes, the patient's required diet, documentation of vital signs, a physical therapy plan, and other information that currently may be captured on paper or automated in standalone systems. EHR certification does not address document management, transcription of notes and reports, and incorporation of referral letters and consultations. Some healthcare organizations have not recognized these gaps in their haste to acquire an EHR and earn incentives. The result is a hybrid record of paper and electronic, or electronically scanned paper and electronic. In many cases, the vendor that sells an EHR does not address these other components, leaving the organization to integrate them itself.

### Gaps and Variations in Technology

The previously identified gaps are only those related to technology. Gaps are also likely to be present in operational elements. Some vendors supply extensive training on their system, including providing professional certification to super users who help implement and provide ongoing training on the system. Other vendors offer a website that intended users can visit for training as needed.

As previously noted, many vendors acknowledge the importance of, but do not address, changes in workflow and processes. Few vendors will highlight the policy implications of implementing the technology. For example, suppose a physician uses a **scribe**, an individual who performs data entry functions at the point of care. What authority does the scribe have to document, sign a note, or override an alert? CMS, the Joint Commission, and the American Health Information Management Association (AHIMA) have all published guidelines and requirements for using scribes. These organizations' recommendations should be considered as part of the healthcare organization's due diligence in deciding how scribes will be used.

Recognizing gaps is not to criticize any given vendor but to ensure an organization decides what to do about them. For example, one organization may scan all health information on paper and not plan for more than that. Another organization may prioritize automating all health information through direct entry of pertinent data currently on paper so that, ultimately, scanning paper is eliminated.

Gaps are not the only variations in EHRs or other HIS components. Looking at the internal workings of HIS components could also lead to identifying important variations. For example, investigating the type of audit logging performed by the system is important. Does the system review who accessed what record, at what time, and what part of the record was viewed, added to, or changed? Do the audit logs help determine if access was to a relative's record, done retrospectively of the care rendered, or given concurrently at the point of care? Another example is to investigate how data about documentation is retained and made visible to the users. Most HISs incorporate a process to correct a documentation error, but not all systems display that there was an error correction made, when it was made, or by whom. These errors could potentially affect the patient. For example, an order for the wrong patient could have been entered, then recognized a few hours later and changed. While there should be failsafe policies and procedures for others to apply professional judgment in carrying out all orders, it is possible that the incorrect order could have been carried out before the correction was made. Not only may this have an immediate negative effect on the patient, but it also may be missed later by the person making the correction (or another person), which could compound the potential for negative impact.

### Workflow and Process Improvement for Effective Health Information Systems

Considering how an HIS will fit into the organization's workflow is also important. If workflows and processes are currently problematic and automation might improve poor productivity, some assistance with workflow and process redesign may be necessary. Additionally, the HIS may need to be flexible enough to accommodate applicable changes. An example is a physician who wanted an EHR that supports improvement in preventive service offerings for patients. The physician anticipated staff would address some preventive services, such as flu shot receipt, at the point of registration; nurses would speak to patients about other preventive services, such as mammograms or prostate exams either before or after the patient's examination; and the physician would address more targeted preventive services with the patient at the conclusion of a patient visit. While evaluating various vendor products, the physician found that not one met this requirement. One vendor, however, recognized that the physician was describing the ideal workflow for preventive services and offered to redesign the product. This vendor was then successful in selling this change to several other clients.

Once all the requirements to be acquired from a vendor are identified, they are put into a **requirements specification**, which is a formal document detailing a list of functionalities that the system should be able to do and conveyed to vendors. Operational requirements should be treated similarly, though they are brought to senior management to ensure they are available as appropriate.

## Acquisition

Acquisition of the HIS is a process that encompasses many considerations, including a vendor strategy that considers the type of vendors to be considered, issuing a request for proposal (RFP) that includes the requirements specifications, and narrowing the field of vendors to the one with whom the organization negotiates a contract.

### Vendor Strategy

Many organizations go through a process of considering whether they will select one or many vendors for the various components of their HIT. Most healthcare organizations are currently leaning toward engaging a single vendor for most of the needed technology, but almost always find they need to fill in gaps with other vendors. The situation in which the goal is to minimize the number of vendors is referred to as a **best of fit** approach to acquisition. Alternatively, selecting a vendor for each type of technology throughout the migration path potentially resulting in several different vendors is referred to as **best of breed**. A best of fit approach ensures the technology components will work together, whereas the best of breed approach acquires the very best any vendor has to offer. Unfortunately, the best of breed approach has required the organization to acquire software that works between two or more systems to enable the two systems to share data. This software is referred to as an **interface**. The Fast Healthcare Interoperability Resources (FHIR), developed by HL7, can enable the exchange of data among components of HISs without the elaborate interface software used in the past. "The standard is now widely used in mobile applications, cloud communications, EHR-based data sharing, and server communications across the healthcare industry" (HealthITAnalytics 2023).

Realistically, however, best of fit solutions do not necessarily work as smoothly as might be hoped. Sometimes a best of fit vendor is nothing more than a **system integrator**—a company that acquires products and develops permanent interfaces between them, selling them then as a single technology offering. This is not true of all best of fit vendors, but it is important to determine how a given vendor compiles its technology offerings so that one can anticipate potential issues. For example, a system integrated from multiple different vendors may exchange data well, but each component may have a different look and feel. This could be an issue for users having to learn various components. The trade-off must be considered before going to market.

Another consideration with respect to how HIT may be acquired is the organization's financing needs and preference for how products can be acquired. In the past, most healthcare organizations used client-server technology. The organization purchased computers that served as the location where software and data were stored and from which data and functionality were delivered to users' computers. The computers were often housed on-site, at or near the healthcare organization, and maintained by the organization's staff. As small provider organizations acquired more HIS components but did not have the resources to maintain the equipment themselves, use of **application service provider (ASP)** vendors became popular. These vendors provided the servers, loaded the organization's software and data on these servers, and provided the organization's users with the data and functionality through a secure connection. Over time, EHR vendors offered the ASP model so the healthcare organization did not need to acquire its own software. Cloud computing, which refers to using remote servers hosted on the internet, has become more popular and is at least as secure as client-server technology, housed either on-site or at a vendor site. Software as a service (SaaS), which also provides server hosting and software, has become popular. In general, the ASP and SaaS models are a somewhat less expensive acquisition strategy than the traditional client-server model. It should be noted that where the ASP or SaaS offers software in addition to hosting servers, the degree of software configuration may be limited. Generally, such changes should be left to the software vendor. However, most EHR and other HIT vendors today offer sufficient tools for IT staff, and in some cases, users themselves, to customize input screens, data displays, reports, clinical decision support rules, and other functions to meet users' needs without changing the underlying software.

### Request for Proposal

Once all requirements are determined for functionality, vendor strategy, and other elements being sought from a vendor, an organization typically compiles all this information into a **request for proposal (RFP)**. This solicitation to vendors usually also includes basic information about the healthcare organization, such as how many users will access the system, the timeline for implementation, and any special contractual issues that must be addressed. RFPs typically are sent to four to six vendors the organization has prescreened during preliminary investigations, such as at trade shows, through referrals from other organizations, and sometimes in a formal request for information (RFI) process. If a healthcare organization is in the early stages of acquiring an HIS, the RFP may be lengthy and cover all, or nearly all, of the HIT desired over the planning horizon. When a healthcare organization is in the middle of rolling out its strategic plan and finds it needs to fill a gap not covered by existing vendors, the RFP will be more focused. Even when the existing vendor could fill such gaps, some organizations will issue an abbreviated RFP to several vendors, especially to compare functionality. Such an RFP should include information about what other vendors are involved in the mix of existing components so that the vendor can determine what may be needed for system integration.

### Request for Proposal Response Evaluation

Evaluating responses to an RFP for a major HIS acquisition generally follows several steps:

1. An internal analysis of the proposal against the requirements specification and other components of the RFP should be conducted by the steering committee. The steering committee should also thoroughly analyze all components of the proposal, not just the price to avoid bias. The price may, though not always, reflect quality of the HIT itself and the included associated operational elements, such as timeliness of implementation completion, responsiveness of ongoing maintenance and upgrades, and other factors.

2. Once the internal review is complete, the steering committee should narrow the field by dropping from consideration any vendors whose bids are deficient.

3. Remaining vendors, often three or four who meet the requirements specified in the RFP, should be invited to conduct a demonstration of their products. Ideally, this should be an in-person demonstration so intended users can see firsthand what the system can do and the vendor can get a better understanding of the organization. While it is not expected that the vendor will attempt to sell more than requested, there may be gaps the organization did not consider. There may also be other challenges the vendors identify that narrow or broaden their scope of response.
4. Following the demonstration, the vendor may be asked by the organization (or may ask the organization) to return a revised proposal. If this is not necessary, generally the next step is again narrowing the field. Any vendor whose product did not demonstrate well is dropped from consideration. Typically, two or three viable vendors remain.
5. Remaining vendors from the second cut may be further analyzed by conducting various forms of **due diligence**, steps taken to confirm various facts about the product. Due diligence for HIS components acquisitions almost always includes reference checks, frequent site visits to see how the products work in a real-life setting, and for very big acquisitions, corporate site visits and investigations. The extent to which an organization takes these steps is often determined by the scope of what is acquired. Reference calls may be sufficient when acquiring a single component, such as a blood banking system, food and nutrition system, or respiratory therapy system.
6. Once all information is accumulated, the steering committee, potentially with the assistance of the finance department or procurement officer, should consider all findings to date in light of the price and contract terms. At this point a contract issues checklist should be started. This can be a simple spreadsheet on which every issue is identified and then sent to the vendor to be addressed. An example of an issue might be that a desired function is missing, and the healthcare organization wants to know if it will be provided in the next upgrade or, if not, what it would cost to include it today. Another common issue with vendor contracts is that they can be weak in their obligations to implement federally mandated changes. For example, many providers found vendors unwilling to implement and test *International Classification of Diseases, Tenth Revision* (ICD-10) changes immediately when the mandate first came out. Some vendors attempted to make the change contingent upon buying other components unnecessary for ICD-10. Stronger contractual language may have prepared more organizations earlier. Price may also be an issue for negotiation, although asking for discounts or competitive bidding should wait until all other issues are addressed. Financing may be an exception, if not already included in the RFP. Most healthcare organizations have the contract issues checklist reviewed by their legal counsel prior to using it in contract negotiation (Amatayakul 2017, 206–207).

## Contract Negotiation

**Contract negotiation** is the process of identifying and discussing issues with the vendor until all are resolved to the satisfaction of both parties. It is not advisable to start a negotiation discussing price, as the vendor typically addresses all other negotiable factors with price increases. Once all factors other than price are addressed, the payment schedule, discounts, end-of-year concessions, and other price-cutting tactics should be discussed.

One very important issue related to price is the payment schedule. The payment schedule should include a small down payment, a small payment upon installation, a larger payment upon completion of implementation, a small payment upon completion of training and go-live, and a final payment once it is ensured no unforeseen implementation issues exist. For example, an organization could make a small down payment of 10 percent; another 10 percent on installation; 40 percent on completion of implementation; 20 percent upon completion of training and go-live; and the remaining 20 percent 90 days after go-live.

Interfaces are one place where price cuts are often successful. For example, if both the system being acquired and the system that must be interfaced are mainstream, chances are high the vendor has already written many such interfaces and should not charge for this, or should charge only a modest fee for minor adjustments and testing.

Another way to cut costs is for the healthcare organization to acquire its own hardware. IT vendors typically mark up the prices of hardware, and most organizations may buy in bulk at a discount. In general, organizations negotiating price should consider that expecting a vendor to deeply discount a price puts the vendor, and ultimately the organization, at risk. If a vendor loses too much money on deep discounts, the vendor may not stay in business or may need to cut staff, and hence services. Unfortunately, this was an all-too-frequent occurrence during stage 1 of the MU incentive program. Such vendors either found it very difficult to modify the systems for stage 2 on a timely basis, putting their clients at risk for not earning the next stage of incentives, or simply went out of business, leaving the healthcare organization with no support or ongoing upgrades. Some providers simply gave up while others waited out the delays and were grateful for the federal extensions. Still other organizations sought to remove the old system and replace it with a new system. The latter is a costly and time-consuming process. However, some found that it resulted in acquiring a better system and users more willing to adopt the system.

## Implementation

**Implementation** follows acquisition and is the process in which hardware is installed; software is loaded to the organization's servers, to the ASP environment, the SaaS environment, or a combination of these; special tools supplied by the vendor are used to customize the system in order to meet a specific organization's needs; data from a preexisting system are converted and loaded to the new system; paper chart conversion is performed via scanning or direct data entry; and policies and procedures are updated with new process and workflow requirements.

### Installation

**Installation** is the process used to set up hardware and to load software onto the acquired hardware. While technically a part of implementation because it is not performed until after a contract has been negotiated, installation is usually performed by the vendor, not the implementing organization itself.

### System Customization

A significant part of implementation is system customization. It is often referred to as system build or system configuration. **System customization** includes loading data tables and master files (for example, files of all the names of staff members and their permissions for access to the system), adjusting decision support rules for transitioning, writing interfaces, customizing screens, and numerous other tasks that make the system work for the specific organization. For example, coder screens can be customized to incorporate the view of a patient's chart alongside the encoder to optimize the collection of data and minimize the number of clicks performed when coding a chart. Another example of customization would be to provide the ROI analyst screens with a pre-sorted drop-down menu or list to have the most frequently accessed request types at the top of the list. Customization differs from configuration, which refers to changing the underlying software. Vendors do, and should, reconfigure their software to provide updates and upgrades. However, most vendors do not allow organizations to reconfigure their software; instead, they provide tools that enable the existing software to meet the unique needs of each organization that acquires the software. Much of the time spent on implementation is related to customization, and many healthcare organizations hire the software vendor or another vendor to help them do the customization.

### Data Conversion

Implementation may also include **data conversion**, which is the process of taking data already in one automated system and putting it into a new system. Many organizations evaluate the quality of their data, the cost of the conversion, and the extent of differences between the old and new system when deciding whether data conversion will be performed or if data will be reentered into the new system. For example, many new practice management systems for physician offices have far more revenue cycle management functions than old systems. Many old systems also do not have very good data quality (for example, duplicate patients or old account information). As a result, many clinics have decided to use the new system implementation to enter all new patient information so there are fewer issues with data quality, and there are no issues regarding whether the data from the old system can accurately populate the fields in the new system.

### Chart Conversion

Another conversion issue, often called **chart conversion**, refers to moving from paper to an electronic system. It most often impacts physician offices and clinics moving from paper-based health records to EHRs. Chart conversion considers how much of the paper should be moved into the electronic system and in what form: scanned images or structured data manually entered from the paper files. Most organizations find providers need less of the old information on paper than they initially thought. The clinics make the paper files available for the first one or two uses of the electronic system, at which time users enter only the data needed for ongoing care. Thereafter, the paper file is provided only on request.

### Workflow and Process Improvement

Implementation almost always entails considerable involvement by the organization. If workflow and process improvement steps were not started prior to implementation, during implementation is when it is essential to address the types of changes that can be made with the IT to meet the organization's strategic goals for its HIS. A process is work performed; **workflow** is the sequence of steps in the process. Workflows and processes are often depicted in workflow diagrams, which are tools that illustrate what process steps are performed by whom and when, often including information about the decision factors that play a role in the process. HIT can often help automate these decision factors. Computers are tireless, and, once programmed correctly, they follow the rules and do not forget. For example, reminders and alerts integrated through workflows help patients improve adherence to their treatment plans (Butte 2020).

In healthcare, the concept of thoughtflow applies to most healthcare professional processes (Ball and Bierstock 2007). **Thoughtflow** refers to a process and its sequence when the process is largely conducted mentally. Thoughtflows are unique because they are not visible to others who might be tasked with helping identify workflow and process improvements. Thoughtflows are also unique to the individual, and are a health professional's primary asset. If thoughtflow must be changed without the individual internalizing and creating the change themselves, it can be extremely difficult to adjust. For this reason, many healthcare professionals have a difficult time adapting to EHRs and other HISs.

### Policies and Procedures

Policies and procedures about how to use the IT must be reviewed during EHR and HIS implementations. In some cases, existing policies, which refer to the general action to be taken, can be improved upon because of the greater level of precision with which HIT capture and measure the quality of care and other areas for improvement. In other cases, HIT introduces the need for new policies. For example, scribes who assist healthcare professionals with documentation in HIT are increasingly popular with some providers. How scribes are used, and their scope of authority, should be codified in policy. Procedures are step-by-step guides in how to carry out a process. Procedures performed through IT almost always need updating.

### Testing

Testing the system to ensure it is working as intended should be performed as part of implementation and prior to training. Testing may be conducted in phases during implementation. Individual elements of the system should be tested as they are installed. Comprehensive system testing should be performed once all system parts have been implemented. This is a formal process where test scripts or use cases are created and used by super users and others to verify that all processing can be performed as expected. As with any issues that arise during the project, any testing failures should be documented in an issues log and corrected by the vendor before the system is released for training.

### Training

Training for all end users is the final step of implementation before system go-live. Two key issues with respect to training are pertinent. First, training must be done after testing. It is not fair to new users to attempt to learn the system while also having to identify system issues. Physicians may not tolerate this, and some may resist using such a system. Second, everyone must be trained. HISs are complex tools configured to the specific organization in which they have been implemented. It is advisable to consider developing policy in advance of system acquisition relating to training compliance.

### Go-Live

**Go-live** is the final step in turning over the information system to the end users. Go-live should be planned as carefully as the entire project itself. The day of go-live can be stressful for everyone and is usually a time when all-hands-on-deck is required. Usually, no vacations are permitted in areas where go-live is occurring. In many cases, all available super users are brought to this area to support new users. "At the elbow" support, where someone is immediately available to help a new user having a problem, is essential for healthcare professionals starting to use a new information system. Many project managers set up a hotline for calls of concern, set up a command center for support staff to wait for issues, and sponsor a break area where new users can relax, get a special treat, vent, relax and reflect, or even celebrate that they made it through their first use with no problems. The project manager should frequently check how things are going and be prepared to adjust as needed. Many healthcare organizations find it helpful for senior management and executives to have a visible presence, especially for implementation of major system components that impact patient safety. These individuals are not expected to troubleshoot system issues, but their presence shows support for the system and the ability to mobilize staff or take other critical actions at any point. Finally, there should be a debriefing at the end of the first day or at the first half and the end. The debriefing should celebrate success even when there may be outstanding issues. Everyone should be thanked for their support, especially the new end users. A simple reward like giving gold stars to any user who logs on or views one thing on the system can maintain the morale and motivation needed for a successful go-live.

Go-live activities will gradually taper off. Generally, most major issues are identified and hopefully resolved within the first week of use. Super users will be needed for a while, but the project manager should monitor ongoing use to determine if there are any areas or persons with unique difficulties. It is important to determine and address the root cause of any problem. The project manager should have the authority to require retraining, make workflow changes, or take other steps to ensure the system is both suitable for use and is being used.

## Continued Information System Review and Support

Once the major aspects of implementation are completed, several steps must be taken to ensure the system works as intended. These include ongoing monitoring of use, ensuring adoption of the system, checking that intended benefits are realized, ensuring the system is properly maintained, installing upgrades, making enhancements as applicable, and replacing elements of the system as necessary. These components of the SDLC are discussed in the following section.

### Ongoing Monitoring of Information System

Ongoing monitoring refers to evaluating the level of usage and the value it achieves. This should be a routine task starting immediately after go-live. If a user is not using the system, this should be investigated. If a report is produced inconsistent with expectations, this should be evaluated. Formal complaints should be recorded in the issues log and addressed. The task of ongoing monitoring is often turned over from the project manager to a staff person at this time, as the project manager will likely move on to managing another project. The staff person assigned to this function should convene a task group to address any issues that are multidisciplinary or crosscutting throughout an organization.

Many organizations find it helpful to hold weekly, then monthly, and potentially even ongoing quarterly informal or social events as part of ongoing monitoring of all systems. These events convey the notion of openness and equality among all who are implementing and learning to use new HIT, and aid in spotting when an older system may need to be replaced or phased out. The CMIO, nurse informaticist, health informaticist, or other person involved in day-to-day operations of the HISs and who can bridge communications between users and IT staff should attend, listen, and investigate. Many new ideas can come from such events. Persistent issues can often be resolved. An organization with many different locations or remote workers may not distinguish implementation from adoption, or adoption from optimization. This is unfortunate because, where implementation is performed by IT staff, adoption is a function of trainers, super users, and end users. It is the point in time when all end users are trained, the system has gone live, and there has been time to acclimate and embrace as much of the process changes and functionality as possible. It is an important milestone to recognize and celebrate.

### Benefits Realization for Information Systems

Benefits realization is a formal process of studying whether the value (for example, cost savings, productivity improvements, revenue enhancements, improved quality of care and patient safety, and patient and provider experience of care satisfaction) was worth the investment of time, energy, and money. Benefits realization, however, can be a powerful motivator to keep pressing ahead and value even small gains. It should start during ongoing monitoring of any new system and ideally continue through to optimization when the SDLC begins again.

Benefits realization begins with a review of the original SMART goals to determine whether the organization believes they have been met. Some goals may be in the form of financial rewards with a specific ROI to be achieved. Many goals for EHRs are related to patient safety and quality. These are often considered more qualitative than quantitative, yet still measurable. Some goals depend on perception surveys, such as patient and provider experience of care satisfaction. Other goals may be recognized as achieved based on anecdotal evidence.

Goal achievement may be staged over time. For instance, in a physician office, the office may set a goal to reduce transcription by 50 percent within the first year of adoption then to 85 percent within the second year. In a hospital, it may be that 75 percent of all medication orders and 30 percent of all other orders are entered into the CPOE system within three months of go-live, with full utilization by the end of the first year. If these milestones are not met, the organization needs to determine why, and take steps to correct the course. Is it a system problem, user training issue, resistance to change, or technology issue? For example, an organization may not have correctly anticipated the bandwidth necessary to support all the new users. System configuration may need changing or additional bandwidth acquired, even after careful system configuration tasks have been performed. In other cases, the goals may have been unrealistic, in which case they should be modified.

A solid management theory that "you cannot manage what you cannot measure" is very true in an HIS project. If an organization cannot determine whether goals have been met, there is a management issue. Some organizations include in their benefits realization a formal ROI analysis. **Return on investment (ROI)** determines if the system has paid for itself, comparing the financial benefits to the total costs of the system. This is difficult in an IS environment.

HISs are expensive. The cost of the EHR component for a hospital is very difficult to generalize because an EHR is a shared system across the organization. Source systems and other applications also must be connected to these components. The Department of Veterans Affairs reported estimating the cost of its EHR to be around $10 billion in 2018 and now estimates that cost will increase to $50 billion (Muoio 2023). For physician practices, the cost of an EHR is somewhat easier to estimate because the purchased components are generally more integrated. However, costs vary considerably by size of practice, adoption of functionality beyond the minimum required for EHR certification, and deployment methodology. Larger practices will generally have more source systems to interface, and often, the practices want greater customization and more comprehensive functionality. An EHR implementation costs $162,000 for a multiphysician practice plus an additional $85,500 for the first year of maintenance (Green 2024). Costs for physician practices described here do not include other direct and indirect costs for the organization necessary to implement the system, such as labor, contractors, consultants, training materials, staff time spent in training, and such.

In addition to the challenge of identifying the complete cost of an HIS, many other variables may influence whether a system returns its investment or not. Systems take a long time to implement, and costs may have been spread out over a long period of time. Some costs may be shared between systems or with other types of expenditures. For example, medical devices are increasingly incorporating information system components—are they costs of the process of care or information technology? Other factors may have caused expenditures or investment opportunities to be different than initially planned. Many CFOs have dropped formal ROI analyses but still want to see changes that demonstrate achievement of other important goals.

### Information System Maintenance

System maintenance refers to ongoing tasks that keep the system current with minor software fixes supplied by vendors to correct system bugs, new hardware requirements, patches for security updates, and many other potential needs based on continuous monitoring by the organization and the vendor. While system maintenance has been viewed more as a technology issue, applying a systems view should also recognize that maintenance of workflows, policy compliance, and other operational elements should be addressed. Technical system maintenance includes ensuring continuous system backups, installing updates to antivirus software, or adding new drug information to clinical systems. Workflow maintenance should investigate whether there are workarounds to the use of an HIS. Even proactive investigation as to whether the clinical decision support rules reflect current, evidence-based medical knowledge should be a routine part of ongoing maintenance. Continuing maintenance, then, requires a variety of staff skills as well as a plan and checklist.

### Upgrades to Information Systems

Upgrades to information systems are more formal processes, generally supplied by the vendor when there is a major change. Vendors typically push major updates annually along with minor updates throughout the year. Upgrades released by vendors are intended to fix system glitches that may have been identified by their clients or user groups; or there may be federal mandates such as ICD-10, new versions of Health Insurance Portability and Accountability Act of 1996 (HIPAA) transaction standards, and others.

For example, the modernization or replacement of an organization's existing HIT entails a huge undertaking and requires time, labor, and a significant financial commitment; organizations like the Indian Health Services and VA have gone through modernization and would be considered a major upgrade (Amlung et al. 2020). A minor upgrade is smaller in scope, affects fewer systems, or has a system downtime for a short period of time from a few minutes to a few hours. A minor upgrade example would be a security patch for the operating system on a smartphone or laptop.

### Enhancements to Information Systems

Enhancements to the HIS may be new functionality provided by the vendor to an existing system or expansion of the HIS within the organization by adding an additional system component. New functionality provided by the vendor may be considered an upgrade and included in regular maintenance fees; or it may be considered a separate product that is optional and therefore is priced as a new product. It is very important to distinguish between what is an upgrade and what is optional. Vendors often require their clients to keep current with at least a certain level of upgrades. If this is not done, new upgrades, including those required by federal mandates, may be excluded from regular maintenance and a fee paid for their installation and implementation. This fee covers the cost of installing all previous upgrades so the latest upgrade works properly. New system components continue to be common changes to an organization's HISs. In fact, many of these may be included in the strategic plan as components specifically reserved for later implementation. Others may arise out of new demands in the industry. It is anticipated that health reform will require several new types of IT support.

### Replacements for Information Systems

The healthcare industry is at the point where many organizations have a significant amount of HIT already in place. By 2021, about 88 percent of office-based physicians in the US adopted some form of EHR, with approximately 78 percent using a certified EHR system. This adoption rate has been steadily increasing since 2015. Since 2008, the adoption of EHRs by office-based physicians has more than doubled, rising from 42 percent to 88 percent. Additionally, since the ONC and CDC started tracking certified EHR adoption in 2014, the percentage has grown from 74 percent to 78 percent (ONC n.d.). While this is good news, it also means the time has come for replacement of older and out-of-date systems, referred to as **legacy systems**. In some cases, there is recognition that poorly performing systems need replacement; in other situations, a need exists to replace systems sunset by the vendor. **Sunsetting** refers to the action taken by a vendor to no longer support ongoing maintenance or upgrades for a legacy system.

Replacement often means a reselection must be performed. Reselection is the process undertaken to acquire a replacement for an existing system. Reselection should reflect lessons learned from the primary selection, especially for replacement of poorly performing systems. For example, many EHRs were selected in haste to help the organization meet the MU incentive program requirements. Such systems may have been acquired without any formal selection process. Many of these systems were implemented by IT staff with minimal or no input from end users. Workflows and processes were not changed, components may not have been configured properly, and policy on use may have been haphazard. Contracts may not have been well-negotiated, upgrades not installed, or users not trained.

A reselection does not need to start with a totally clean slate. The strategic plan's components, requirements specifications, RFP, and other elements should be reviewed and updated based on lessons learned.

### Check Your Understanding 13.2

Evaluate the process of carrying out the strategic plan for implementing an HIS and match the activity to the process in which the activity is performed.

1. \_\_\_\_\_ Use cases are created and performed by super users
2. \_\_\_\_\_ Adjust decision support rules
3. \_\_\_\_\_ Step after testing
4. \_\_\_\_\_ Moving data from paper files to an electronic system
5. \_\_\_\_\_ Set up hardware and load software
6. \_\_\_\_\_ Moving data from an automated system to the new system
7. \_\_\_\_\_ Step-by-step guides on how to carry out a process are updated
8. \_\_\_\_\_ Diagrams depicting sequence of steps are developed
9. \_\_\_\_\_ The day when all-hands-on-deck is needed

a. Installation
b. System customization
c. Data conversion
d. Chart conversion
e. Workflow and process improvement
f. Policies and procedures
g. Testing
h. Training
i. Go-live

# Planning for Health Information System Optimization

Just as strategic planning addresses the full SDLC, distinguishing between the degrees to which users employ the information system is important to ensure full use. A variety of maturity models for HIS components are available from HIMSS Analytics (see figure 13.7). A simpler maturity model might consider three key stages: implementation, adoption, and optimization.

## EHR System Implementation Level of Maturity

As previously described, implementation is the process of putting a new system into place for an organization. During the implementation, users are trained to use the system. While it would be desirable for everyone to be prepared to fully use the system immediately after training, this is rarely the case. Initial use is often slow. Sometimes organizations encourage new users of HISs to perform only certain, limited functions on the computer initially, gradually increasing these functions over time. Some elements of training may need reinforcement. Altered workflows and processes may need to be changed again to better fit a personal style while producing the intended results. In some cases, not all components of the information system are fully implemented, and the degree of use depends on their implementation status. A key point to bear in mind from this distinction is that even though a system has been implemented, it does not necessarily mean all users are fully using the system.

## EHR System Adoption Level of Maturity

Adoption, as previously described, refers to the stage where every intended user is fully using the basic functionality of the system. Adoption requires a period of acclimation where users work through how they will use the system, identify what configuration may be necessary, acquire retraining and further redesign of workflows and processes, and have changes reinforced. Providers who are new to HISs often need time to see for themselves that there has been improvement in quality of care, timeliness of treatment, and other benefits with use of the system.

Some users may never reach the adoption stage, in which case counseling, workarounds, sanctions, terminating employment or medical staff privileges, or other strategies may be necessary to achieve the results needed by all.

Figure 13.7. Adoption model for analytics maturity (AMAM) from HIMSS

| | |
|---|---|
| 7. | Personalized medicine & prescriptive analytics |
| 6. | Clinical risk intervention & predictive analytics |
| 5. | Enhancing quality of care, population health, and understanding the economics of care |
| 4. | Measuring and managing evidence based care, care variability, and waste reduction |
| 3. | Efficient, consistent internal and external report production and agility |
| 2. | Core data warehouse workout: centralized database with an analytics competency center |
| 1. | Foundation building: data aggregation and initial data governance |
| 0. | Fragmented point solutions |

*Source:* Adapted from HIMSS n.d.

## EHR System Optimization Level of Maturity

**System optimization** refers to the activities that extend use of information systems beyond the basic functionality that characterizes adoption. The term *power user* may be applied to users who know how to perform all or close to all the available functions in the system. Optimization focuses on using an HIS to improve the clinical practice of medicine. **Clinical transformation** requires "assessing and continually improving the way patient care is delivered at all levels in an organization" (Sensmeier 2011). For example, if a physician has always prescribed a certain medication for a given condition, the physician who has optimized use of CPOE will follow evidence-based medicine guidelines in selecting the appropriate medication. New knowledge coming from multiple sources, including the organization's own HIS, can be made available at the point of care. Typically, optimization also includes the integration of clinical and financial data. For example, if there is a choice of medications but some are more expensive for the patient than others, provider and patient are given a more informed choice.

Optimization often leads to acquisition of additional technology, such as more sophisticated clinical decision support, different input devices, medical device integration, data analytics, or additional applications as they become available on the market. It could be said that optimization is the continuous state of quality improvement that derives from the monitoring results stage of the SDLC.

# Planning for Ongoing Management of Health Information

In the context of strategic planning for the ongoing management of health information, management of health information refers to the process of ensuring the quality of data and information. While the HIM professional should be engaged in strategic planning for the HIS and the acquisition and implementation of information system components, data governance and information governance are also key roles and responsibilities for HIM professionals.

Data governance is distinguished from information governance. In data governance, the data input into an information system is the governed asset. Information governance focuses on the control and use of the actual documents, reports, and records created from this data (Smallwood 2020). Both data and information should be treated as strategic organizational assets. When viewed in this way, the importance of data and information is elevated to the same level as any other organizational assets, such as land, buildings, furnishings, and equipment. Without these assets, it would not be possible for the organization to run.

Unfortunately, health data and information are often not treated with the importance they deserve. There are several reasons for this. While providers value health information, some find documenting health data to be cumbersome and time-consuming. Another reason for not treating data and information as strategic assets is that traditionally health data and information have been in stacks of paper that are very difficult and laborious to process. Privacy and security protections on health data and information often further contribute to not making health data and information as available for use as appropriate. Finally, some question the accuracy and completeness of health data and information. The purpose for which certain data (such as diagnoses and procedure data for claims) are collected may be inconsistent with other purposes for which that same data are needed (such as to determine the value of performing a given procedure for a specific diagnosis). To improve the value of healthcare, it is recognized that the industry must become a learning health system. A learning health system integrates experience, internal data, and research data to create knowledge that is put into practice (AHRQ 2019). These considerations should be addressed in a health data and information governance plan that is part of the strategic plan for the HIS.

## Health Data and Information Governance Plan

Strategic planning for ongoing management of health information must address the governance of all types of health data and information for which the organization is responsible, and all processes performed on this data and information, such as their capture, use, storage, sharing, and disposal as applicable. It is essential for there to be governance and **stewardship**, which includes data owners, data stewards, and data users all playing a role to maintain accuracy, security, and accessibility of data (MediQuant 2022).

ARMA International has established Generally Accepted Recordkeeping Principles for information governance. The principles include accountability for the governance program, integrity assurance so data and information are not altered during the course of their processing, protection of the data and information, compliance assurance for adherence to applicable laws and other requirements in collecting and using the data and information, assurance of the availability of the data and information for all authorized users and uses, appropriate retention and disposition of the health data and information, and transparency with respect to how the governance program operates (ARMA International 2017).

In addition to a focus on recordkeeping, data and information governance for healthcare must also ensure the data and information contained in records (of any type—EHR, accounting, personnel, and others) are accurate, comprehensive, consistent, current, used according to a standardized definition of the data, granular, precise, relevant, and timely (Davoudi et al. 2015). The content of the record must also support effective patient care. Just as medication has five rights, EHR content also requires right actions. The right clinical data must be captured. The data must be presented in a usable manner. Right decisions must be able to be made from the data. Right work processes help support the right collection and use of the data. These "rights" should yield the desired outcomes for quality and cost-effective care.

## Types of Health Data and Information

Health data and information are a healthcare organization's strategic assets over which governance is needed. Several types of data and information in healthcare delivery settings require governance.

**Administrative data** are facts associated with identifying patients, location of care, healthcare professionals, and more. These data are vital for organizational operations and ensuring accurate patient documentation.

**Clinical data** are facts produced by healthcare providers when diagnosing and treating patients. While the bulk of clinical data are processed within the EHR set of HIS components, clinical data may reside in standalone components. Some of this may be temporary data. An example of temporary data may be preliminary findings found on the electronically read EKG that are later confirmed or modified by the cardiologist. Other clinical data should ultimately be incorporated into the EHR. These data require the same level of governance as all other data.

**Financial data** are facts associated with healthcare produced by and often exchanged between healthcare providers and health plans, including eligibility and benefits information, healthcare claims, and the like. Increasingly, financial and clinical data are being merged to assess healthcare value. As a result, there is an increasing need to ensure common data definitions across what are often disparate financial and clinical components.

**Research data** are facts that may be the same as any previous data listed, plus additional data associated with a specific research protocol. For example, a research protocol may require a patient to document and submit to the researcher diet, sleep, and other information not normally collected during a treatment episode to evaluate the pharmacodynamics of a new drug. Such research data are often housed in separate databases, but also must be governed in the same way as all other information assets of the organization.

**Personal health data** are facts maintained by an individual, often in a personal health record. Much of this data will come from various healthcare organizations that treat the patient, but some of the data may be compiled by the patient directly, such as a diabetic blood sugar diary. Some healthcare organizations offer HIT to support an individual's compilation of personal health data. Whatever data is supplied to a patient or directly to a patient's personal health record should be governed with the same due diligence as data that may be maintained only by the healthcare organization itself.

**Population health data** are facts about the quality, cost, and risk associated with the health of a specific set of individuals (Esterhay et al. 2017). This set of data may concern all patients seen by the healthcare organization, a subset of the patients seen, and, increasingly, a set of data about many more patients than a single healthcare organization treats. Various data contribute to the larger data set. Health plans as well as information exchange organizations (HIOs) in a state or region may also compile population health data. The primary use of population health data is to study trends in clinical data, and often financial data, to determine best practices that can be fed back to the providers in the community to improve the quality and cost of care.

**Public health data** are facts used to prevent the spread of disease. Public health data are generated by providers, public health nurses, social workers, and others. A healthcare organization should maintain any public health data it generates in the applicable component(s) of the HIS. Public health departments are obligated to govern their data following the same principles as healthcare organizations.

While addressing virtually every possible form of health data and information, a formal governance program is key to ensuring the quality of such data and information.

## Metadata

Metadata are a special type of data associated with all data and information in an HIS. Many define metadata as data about data. There are three types of metadata: descriptive, structural, and administrative (Mosha and Ngulube 2023). Essentially, any data about data in an information system is metadata. It is important to note that metadata is generally not considered part of the legal health record but may be subject to compulsory discovery in a court of law under the Amendments to Federal Rules of Civil Procedure and Uniform Rules Relating to Discovery of Electronically Stored Information (referred to as e-discovery). It is important to understand what metadata exist within the HIS, to establish policies for retention and about who may have access to the metadata, and to ensure these policies are being followed.

### Descriptive Metadata

Descriptive metadata describes each data element to be captured and processed by IT. A data dictionary is typically used for this purpose. For example, the term *principal diagnosis* would be something commonly collected in an EHR. The data put into the field called "principal diagnosis" should conform to the definition in the data dictionary. Data dictionaries are often maintained in databases. Table 13.1 provides an example of part of a data dictionary entry for the data element principal diagnosis.

### Structural Metadata

Structural metadata describes how the data for each data element are captured, processed, stored, and displayed. A data model is used to describe how data elements are used in processing data, including the various attributes and relationships between data. A data model ultimately contributes to the ability to write software to process data as described in the model. The data model is also used to troubleshoot issues with data entry, processing, or information generation after the software implementation. An example of a process that would be modeled for an EHR is the basic function "physician enters an order." *Physician* can be defined in a data dictionary; *order*, however, is a broader concept; and different types of orders will likely be processed differently in an HIS. For example, a medication order will be sent to a clinical pharmacy application in a hospital. An order for a laboratory test will be sent to a laboratory application. A series of data models are required, one for a drug order, another for a lab test order, and more. Even then, "drug order" would have several data elements, such as "drug name," and "dose." Each of these data elements would be defined in the data dictionary.

Figure 13.8 provides examples of the high-level form of a data model and the more detailed version of the same data model, with labels identifying the various features of the model. These data models are depicted in an entity relationship diagram type of data model. The model helps describe relationships between entities. For instance, the example here indicates that a patient has an appointment in the high-level form, but the detailed version provides attributes that belong to the patient and the appointment entity along with a definition of the relationship between these entities. A patient has zero or many appointments, and an appointment has one and only one patient; these relationships are identified by the markings at the end of each relationship line.

### Administrative Metadata

The third type of metadata is administrative metadata. This type of metadata is programmed to be generated

**Table 13.1.** Example of part of a data dictionary entry

| Table | Field Name | Long Name | Data Type | Description | Allowable Values |
|---|---|---|---|---|---|
| Patient | DOB | Date of Birth | Date | The patient's date of birth | YYYY-MM-DD |
| Patient | AdmtDt | Admit Date | Date | The date the patient is admitted | YYYY-MM-DD |
| Patient | MRN | Medical Record Number | Number | The patient's medical record number | |
| Patient | VisitType | Visit Type | Code | The patient's visit type for the encounter | I – Inpatient<br>O – Outpatient<br>E – Emergency |
| Patient | PDx | Principal Diagnosis | Text | Condition determined to be chiefly responsible for a patient's admission to a healthcare facility or for a particular episode of care. | |

Figure 13.8. Examples of a basic and more complete version of a data model

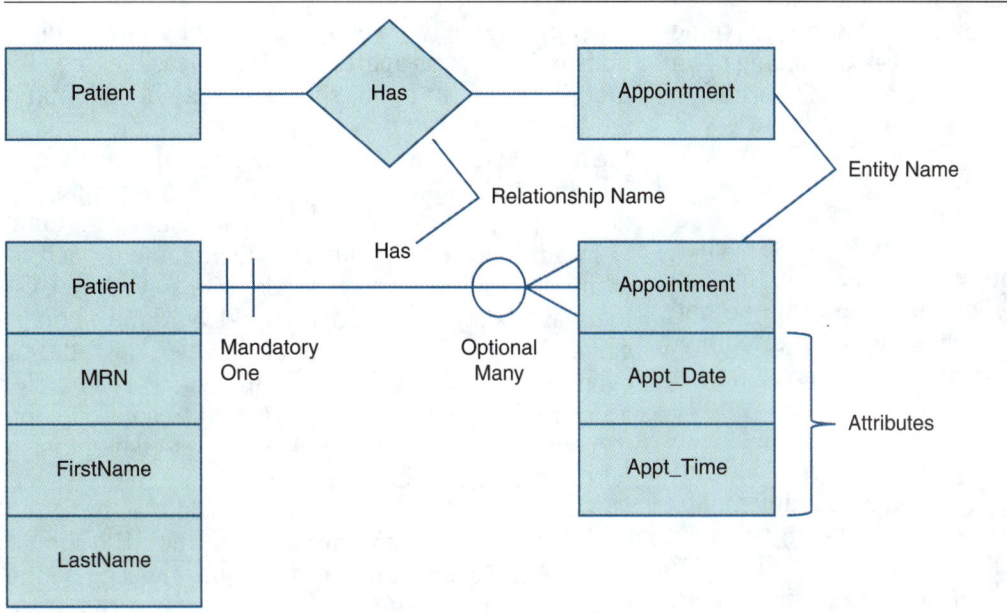

by IT. It provides information about how and when data were created and used. It also is a record of the instructions given to users about actions to be taken with the IT and what the user response was.

Audit logs and information system activity review (ISAR) logs are examples of administrative metadata. Audit logs are records of actions taken on data within IT. The content of audit logs ranges from basic—such as only identifying who accessed what component of the HIS—to complex—such as recording who accessed what data when and what process (for example, view, copy, enter, or delete) was performed on the data. Audit logs are often used as a security control but may also help determine how a data entry error was made, when it was corrected, and who may have accessed information about the error. Audit logs are sometimes used to evaluate the timeliness of actions performed, such as what time a drug was administered. ISAR logs (as required by the HIPAA Security Rule) document the events that impact IT, such as attempted hacks, system crashes, and others.

Another example of administrative metadata is decision support. **Decision support** rules are programmed into software to recognize various combinations of data that are being captured in IT and to generate various types of actions by the technology according to the rule requirements. For instance, when a data dictionary defines a data element as required to be entered, if a user does not enter data in this field, the software will display an alert to the user to enter data into this field. In HISs there are many types of decision support, especially clinical decision support, in an EHR.

Data provenance is another type of administrative data and refers to where data originated and where data may have moved between databases (Sembay et al. 2023). This is becoming increasingly important as the healthcare industry shares data across many stakeholders. For example, a discharge summary's original author and originating facility name would be provenance data.

## Data Quality Management

Another element of strategic planning for ongoing management of health information is the assurance of the quality of the various types of data being used and the types of processes performed on the data. Data quality management, in the context of HIT, is "the business processes that ensure the integrity of an organization's data during collection, application (including aggregation), warehousing, and analysis" (Davoudi et al. 2015). AHIMA also distinguishes data quality management from **data quality measurement**, in which "a data quality measure is a mechanism to assign a quantity to quality of care by comparison to a criterion" (Davoudi et al. 2015). Both data quality management and measurement are important. However, the former ensures good data and the later ensures good care. It is believed that good care is not fully feasible without good data. AHIMA offers a data quality management model and characteristics of data quality, including a checklist to assess data quality management efforts (Davoudi et al. 2015).

With respect to strategic planning for HISs, data and information governance must address how data quality issues can be discovered, how corrective action should be taken, and the necessary change controls that should reflect any changes made because of the corrective action.

## Data Quality Discovery Process

Data entry errors are easy to make, such as by clicking the wrong item, entering too many or too few digits in a number, copying narrative from one note to create another and not changing all the required variables, underusing structured data in favor of comments fields, or overriding CDS system alerts and reminders. HIM professionals should assist their care delivery organizations in updating policies and procedures that describe the required documentation practices for the organization's HIS. The organization should also require checks and balances in the HIS to support data quality (such as valid values for a field, alerts to enter data for a required field, checks for internal consistency for right and left, and so on) and utilize regular data quality audits.

In the data quality discovery process of auditing unstructured data, one focus is the common practice of data reuse in computer-based systems. Because it is easy to copy and paste, providers soon learn to use this capability where it exists. As mentioned earlier, such a practice often results in not fully addressing all the required variables within the documentation. Even if the data element copied from one record to another does not contribute to a medical error, the inconsistency or incomplete documentation can result in questioning the entire record's integrity if the record is brought to court. Many organizations are disabling this capability where they can, or monitoring for it with applicable sanctions. Yet others have found the practice sufficiently useful, so they put users on notice they are individually at risk for errors. Each organization should do a risk analysis to address such issues for itself.

Another factor to consider, which focuses on the EHR, is that providers may not realize that the EHR is more than an automated chart. There are many other benefits that rely on structured data. However, if the findings of the audit reveal the value placed in the comment field is one not on the drop-down menu and occurs frequently, there should be consideration for adding the choice or identifying it as a synonym, as applicable. Again, new users may assume they must work with what they are given and not think about improving the system.

Documentation audits within the EHR should look for completeness, timeliness, internal consistency, and other factors that have typically been evaluated in paper documentation. For example, when reviewing patients' data within the EHR, do all patients on a unit appear to have been given their morning medications only seconds apart? This is not feasible in walking from room to room, so nurses may have found a workaround where they are scanning all the meds at the nursing unit instead of at the point of care, defeating the medication five rights of ensuring right patient, right drug, right dose, right route, and right time.

In addition to reviewing the EHR content itself, it is important to do walkarounds to observe how systems are being used. This should be done periodically, not just after go-live but also when upgrades or even slight modifications are applied. For example, a desired fix may necessitate a slight change in the placement of a data entry field on an assessment form within the EHR, which then may cause an unexpected workflow and process change. While a change to the placement of data entry field in the EHR should be communicated through a pop-up message at the time of login for affected users, choosing the same day of that change to do a walkaround provides the extra emphasis on the commitment and support the organization is making in its EHR and to the clinical transformation initiative, and it provides an opportunity to observe any unexpected impact on workflow that the EHR users may reveal. Walkarounds also demonstrate that those responsible for the technology and compliance are approachable. Documentation audits and walkarounds should not be punitive but serve to enhance the EHR's usefulness.

Finally, a common cause of data error is a result of heightened use of core clinical applications where source systems are either not connected or an audit of all changes in one application is not traced to the potential impact on other applications. Common medication dispensing errors, like improper dosing or route of administration, are caused by distortions that originate from abbreviations or improper translations; an example would be when an unavailable medication is substituted by a nonprescribing clinician (Tariq et al. 2024).

When technology, software applications, and workflow processes throughout the organization are synchronized to support the work of the system's many end users, the organization has achieved process interoperability, a situation where all its subsystems can process data in like manner, with similar access controls and other policy and process constraints.

## Corrective Action

For many of the examples used in this discussion, corrective action has been suggested. Discovering issues with data quality must lead to corrective actions, or the same errors will be repeated, and users' frustration will continue if they do not see their concerns addressed. Corrective actions generally entail making decisions about changes in data elements or pieces of software that generate CDS system alerts and reminders, reports, and more. Such corrective actions should always be done in a formal manner. Some corrective actions simply entail retraining staff or revising procedures to make them clearer. These actions should be documented. If the data quality issues continue, other forms of corrective action may be needed.

Where corrective action entails a specific change in the information system, a work group of stakeholders to the issue should be convened to review the corrective action needed, agree and formally approve the best approach to correction, ensure the corrections are carried out, and monitor that the corrections are effective.

### Change Control

**Change control** is a formal process of documenting what change in an information system is needed, the rationale for the change, necessary approvals (for example, the stakeholder workgroup's approval to turn off a specific CDS system alert), when the change was made, who made the change, that related documentation (for example, data model, data dictionary, policy, and procedure) has been updated to reflect the change, and that monitoring for a period of time was performed. It is important to note that changes to ISs reflect metadata. Such a change could significantly impact patient care. For this reason, a CDS system rule that is turned off or changed in some way, for example, should have a risk analysis performed: What is the likelihood that the change could result in significant harm? Is there evidence that providers apply sufficient professional judgment that such an event would be very unlikely? The answers to these and similar questions as applicable to the specific issue being studied should lead to appropriate action. HISs can be powerful tools; but as with any tool, the tool must be properly built, the user of the tool must be properly trained, and the tool may need to be updated or replaced as the SDLC enfolds.

---

### Check Your Understanding 13.3

**Answer the following questions in a separate document.**

1. Quality measurement staff in a hospital report that several physicians are documenting part of their medication orders in comment fields included in the CPOE system. This resulted in inconsistencies between the order generated in structured form from the CPOE system and the comments, which can pose a patient safety issue, and also resulted in the inability of the quality data extraction system to pull accurate medication data from the EHR into the quality measurement data registry. What methods of discovery should staff use to determine the full nature and extent of the issue and its impact?

2. Complete table 13.1 with four additional data fields you may find in a patient table and provide the additional metadata for each field.

3. Differentiate between public health data and population health data by supplying a specific example of each.

4. With reference to population health data, should such data be included in the EHR? Provide a rationale for your answer. If your answer is yes, identify where such data might be recorded and how and by whom it should be entered. Provide specific examples. If your answer is no, identify where such data should be compiled and how the information derived from such data could be provided to healthcare professionals caring for a specific patient as applicable.

5. The organization's information privacy and security officer is investigating a potential breach to a local government official's health record. Which type of metadata should be reviewed? Explain why.

---

## References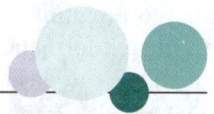

AHRQ (Agency for Healthcare Research and Quality). 2019 (May). "About Learning Health Systems." https://www.ahrq.gov/learning-health-systems/about.html.

Amlung, J., H. Huth, T. Cullen, and T. Sequist. 2020. Modernizing health information technology: lessons from healthcare delivery systems. *JAMIA Open*

3(3):369–377. https://doi.org/10.1093/jamiaopen/ooaa027.

Amatayakul, M. K. 2017. *Electronic Health Records: A Practical Guide for Professionals and Organizations*. Chicago: AHIMA.

American College of Surgeons. 2019 (December 4). "Joint Contracting under Antitrust Laws: An Overview." https://www.facs.org/for-medical-professionals/news-publications/news-and-articles/bulletin/2019/12/joint-contracting-under-antitrust-laws-an-overview/.

ARMA International. 2017. "Generally Accepted Recordkeeping Principles." https://cdn.ymaws.com/www.arma.org/resource/resmgr/files/Learn/2017_Generally_Accepted_Reco.pdf.

Ball, M. J., and S. Bierstock. 2007. Clinician use of enabling technology. *Journal of Healthcare Information Management* 21(3):68–71.

Boogaard, K. 2023 (December 26). "How to Write SMART goals (with Examples)." https://www.atlassian.com/blog/productivity/how-to-write-smart-goals.

Bresnick, J. 2018. "CMS Renames Meaningful Use to Highlight Interoperability Goals." HealthIT Analytics. https://healthitanalytics.com/news/cms-renames-meaningful-use-to-highlight-interoperability-goals.

Butte, N. 2020 (January 23). "Health Information and Technology and Its Impact on Digital Health." HIMSS Iowa Chapter. https://iowa.himss.org/resources/health-information-and-technology-and-its-impact-digital-health.

Cea, B. 2018. "Population Health Exchange Insights Report: A New Era for Telemedicine." *Health Leaders Media*. https://www.healthleadersmedia.com/report/exchange-insight/six-considerations-advancing-telemedicine.

CMS (Centers for Medicare and Medicaid Services). 2024. "Promoting Interoperability (PI)." https://www.cms.gov/Regulations-and-Guidance/Legislation/EHRIncentivePrograms/index.html?redirect=/EHRIncentivePrograms/.

CMS (Centers for Medicare and Medicaid Services). 2023. "What Are the Value-Based Programs?" https://www.cms.gov/medicare/quality-initiatives-patient-assessment-instruments/value-based-programs/value-based-programs.html.Darling, G. 2011. "What Does a Clinical Informatics Data Analyst Do, Exactly?" http://healthcareittoday.com/2011/11/08/clinical-informatics-data-analyst/.

Das, R. 2016. "Five Technologies That Will Disrupt Healthcare by 2020." *Forbes*. https://www.forbes.com/sites/reenitadas/2016/03/30/top-5-technologies-disrupting-healthcare-by-2020/#4ee536426826.

Davoudi, S., J. A. Dooling, B. Glondys, T. L. Jones, L. Kadlec, S. M. Overgaard, K. Ruben, and A. Wendicke. 2015. Data quality management model (2015 update). *Journal of AHIMA* 86(10): expanded web version. https://bok.ahima.org/topics/healthcare-data-lifecycle/data-quality-management-model-2015-update/.

Esterhay, R. J., L. S. Nesbitt, J. H. Taylor, and H. J. Bohn, Jr., eds. 2017. *Population Health: Management, Policy, and Technology*. 2nd ed. Virginia Beach, VA: Convurgent Publishing.

Green, J. 2024. "How Much EHR Costs and How to Set Your Budget. EHR In Practice." https://www.ehrinpractice.com/ehr-cost-and-budget-guide.html.

Haines Centre for Strategic Management. n.d. "A Systems View of the Organization." Accessed June 7, 2024. http://hainescentreasia.com/concepts/systems_view_of_organization.htm.

HealthIT.gov. 2015. "Connecting Health and Care for the Nation: A Shared Nationwide Interoperability Roadmap, DRAFT Version 1.0." https://www.healthit.gov/sites/default/files/hie-interoperability/nationwide-interoperability-roadmap-final-version-1.0.pdf.

HealthITAnalytics. 2023 (December 27). 4 basics to know about the role of FHIR in interoperability. HealthITAnalytics. Accessed May 30, 2024. https://healthitanalytics.com/news/4-basics-to-know-about-the-role-of-fhir-in-interoperability.

HIMSS (Health Information and Management Systems Society). n.d. Advanced model for assessing maturity (AMAM). DHI HIMSS. https://dhi.himss.org/rapid/img/AMAM.png.

Kloss, L. 2015. *Implementing Health Information Governance: Lessons from the Field*. Chicago: AHIMA.

McDonald, S. 2022 (November 25). "9 principles of good governance." *BoardPro* (blog). https://www.boardpro.com/blog/principles-of-good-governance.

MediQuant. 2022 (June 1). "Data stewardship in healthcare: A who's who." *MediQuant* (blog). https://www.mediquant.com/data-stewardship-in-healthcare-a-whos-who/.

Mena, A. 2023 (November 8). "The evolution of the CMIO role in hospitals and health systems." *Symplr* (blog). https://www.symplr.com/blog/evolution-of-cmio-role-hospitals-health-systems.

Miliard, M. 2017 (March 17). "FHIR Holds Big Promise for Interoperability, but Will Need to Co-exist with Other Standards for the Foreseeable Future." *Healthcare IT News*. https://www.healthcareitnews.com/news/fhir-holds-big-promise-interoperability-will-need-coexist-other-standards-foreseeable-future.

Mosha, N. F. and P. Ngulube. 2023. Metadata standard for continuous preservation, discovery, and reuse of research data in repositories by higher education institutions: A systematic review." *Information* 14(8):427. https://doi.org/10.3390/info14080427.

Muoio, D. 2023 (May 3). VA renegotiates $10B EHR contract with stronger performance metrics, bigger penalties. *Fierce Healthcare*. https://www.fiercehealthcare.com/health-tech/va-renegotiates-10b-ehr-contract-stronger-performance-metrics-bigger-penalties.

ONC (Office of the National Coordinator for Health Information Technology). n.d. "National Trends in Hospital and Physician Adoption of Electronic Health Records." Accessed August 2, 2024. https://www.healthit.gov/data/quickstats/national-trends-hospital-and-physician-adoption-electronic-health-records.

ONC (Office of the National Coordinator for Health Information Technology). 2019a. "EHR Incentives and Certification: How to Attain Meaningful Use." https://www.healthit.gov/providers-professionals/how-attain-meaningful-use.

Pfister, H. R., and S. R. Ingargiola. 2014. "ONC: Staying Focused on EHR Usability." iHealthBeat. https://www.healthcareusability.com/article/onc-staying-focused-ehr-usability.

Radack, S., ed. 2009. "The System Development Life Cycle (SDLC)." http://csrc.nist.gov/publications/nistbul/april2009_system-development-life-cycle.pdf.

Rouse, M. 2022a. "Chief Information Officer (CIO) Definition." TechTarget. http://searchcio.techtarget.com/definition/CIO.

Rouse, M. 2022b. "Chief Technology Officer (CTO) Definition." TechTarget. https://searchcio.techtarget.com/definition/Chief-Technology-Officer-CTO.

Rucker, L. 2023 (March 1). *CMIO 30: Top 30 most influential CMIOs*. Healthcare Innovation. https://www.hcinnovationgroup.com/clinical-it/electronic-health-record-electronic-medical-record-ehr-emr/article/21250442/cmio-30.

Sembay, M. J., D. D. J. de Macedo, L. P. Júnior, R. M. M. Braga, and A. Sarasa-Cabezuelo. 2023. Provenance data management in health information systems: A systematic literature review. *Journal of personalized medicine* 13(6):991. https://doi.org/10.3390/jpm13060991.

Sensmeier, J. 2011 (October). Clinical transformation: Blending people, process, and technology. *Nursing Management* 42(10): 2–4. https://www.nursingcenter.com/journalarticle?Article_ID=1239188&Journal_ID=54013&Issue_ID=1239187.

Smallwood, R. F. 2020. *Information Governance: Concepts, Strategies, and Best Practices*, 2nd ed. Hoboken, NJ: John Wiley and Sons.

SHRM (Society for Human Resource Management). 2012. "Strategic Planning: What Are the Basics of Environmental Scanning?" https://www.shrm.org/resourcesandtools/tools-and-samples/hr-qa/pages/basics-of-environmental-scanning.aspx.

Tariq, R. A., R. Vashisht, A. Sinha, and Y. Scherbak. 2024 (February 12). "Medication Dispensing Errors and Prevention." StatPearls Publishing. https://www.ncbi.nlm.nih.gov/books/NBK519065/.

WHO (World Health Organization). 2023 (September 11). "Patient Safety." https://www.who.int/news-room/fact-sheets/detail/patient-safety.

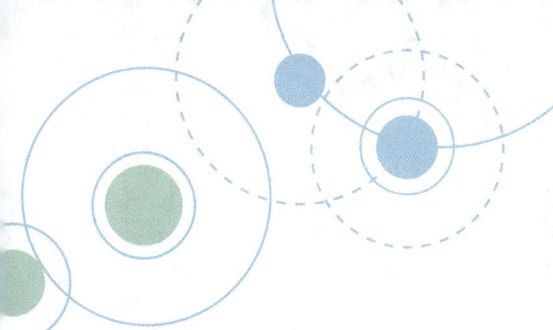

# Public Health and Consumer Engagement

*Ryan H. Sandefer, PhD*

## Learning Objectives

- Explain consumer health informatics
- Differentiate patient portals, personal health records, and personalized medicine
- Assess methods for promoting patient and family engagement
- Evaluate the impact of social determinants of health
- Analyze patient-centered care

## Key Terms

Consumer health informatics
Continuity of care record (CCR)
Internet forum
Learning health system
mHealth
Organizational health literacy
Patient activation measure (PAM)
Patient engagement
Patient portal
Patient-centered care
Patient-centered medical home (PCMH)
Patient-generated health data (PGHD)
Personal health literacy
Personal health record (PHR)
Precision medicine
Secure messaging
Social determinants of health (SDOH)
Telehealth

The personal use of web-based technology and information is proliferating across nearly every dimension of modern life. Individuals bank, purchase books and music, and socialize using the internet. Healthcare is not different in this respect. A growing number of individuals interact with some aspect of healthcare delivery by using technology. Individuals may seek information regarding their symptoms using the internet, track their eating habits with a mobile application, access their clinical information through a secure web portal, or have a remote encounter with a healthcare provider through video technology. All of these examples are considered consumer health informatics. **Consumer health informatics** is largely focused on developing tools and processes to empower patients. By creating, using, and sharing health information, consumers are more engaged in their health and healthcare, which can lead to overall improvements in individual and population health outcomes.

To emphasize the importance of consumer engagement in the healthcare delivery process, the Office of the National Coordinator for Health Information

Technology (ONC) produced a federal Health IT Strategic Plan that puts the consumer at the center of improving care quality, lowering costs, and improving population health (see figure 14.1). The 2020–2025 Federal Health IT Strategic Plan has four goals: (1) promote health and wellness; (2) enhance the delivery and experience of care; (3) build a secure, data-driven ecosystem to accelerate research and innovation; and (4) connect healthcare with health data. Consumer health informatics objectives and tactics are woven throughout the plan, such as using health IT to expand access and connect patients to care (ONC 2020).

The model described in the federal health IT strategic plans has been called the learning health system. The **learning health system** is

a health system in which internal data and experience are systematically integrated with external evidence, and that knowledge is put into practice. As a result, patients get higher quality, safer, more efficient care, and health care delivery organizations become better places to work…. [These Systems]

- Have leaders who are committed to a culture of continuous learning and improvement.
- Systematically gather and apply evidence in real-time to guide care.
- Employ IT methods to share new evidence with clinicians to improve decision-making.
- Promote the inclusion of patients as vital members of the learning team.
- Capture and analyze data and care experiences to improve care.
- Continually assess outcomes and refine processes and training to create a feedback cycle for learning and improvement. (AHRQ 2019)

**Figure 14.1.** Health IT strategic plan goals

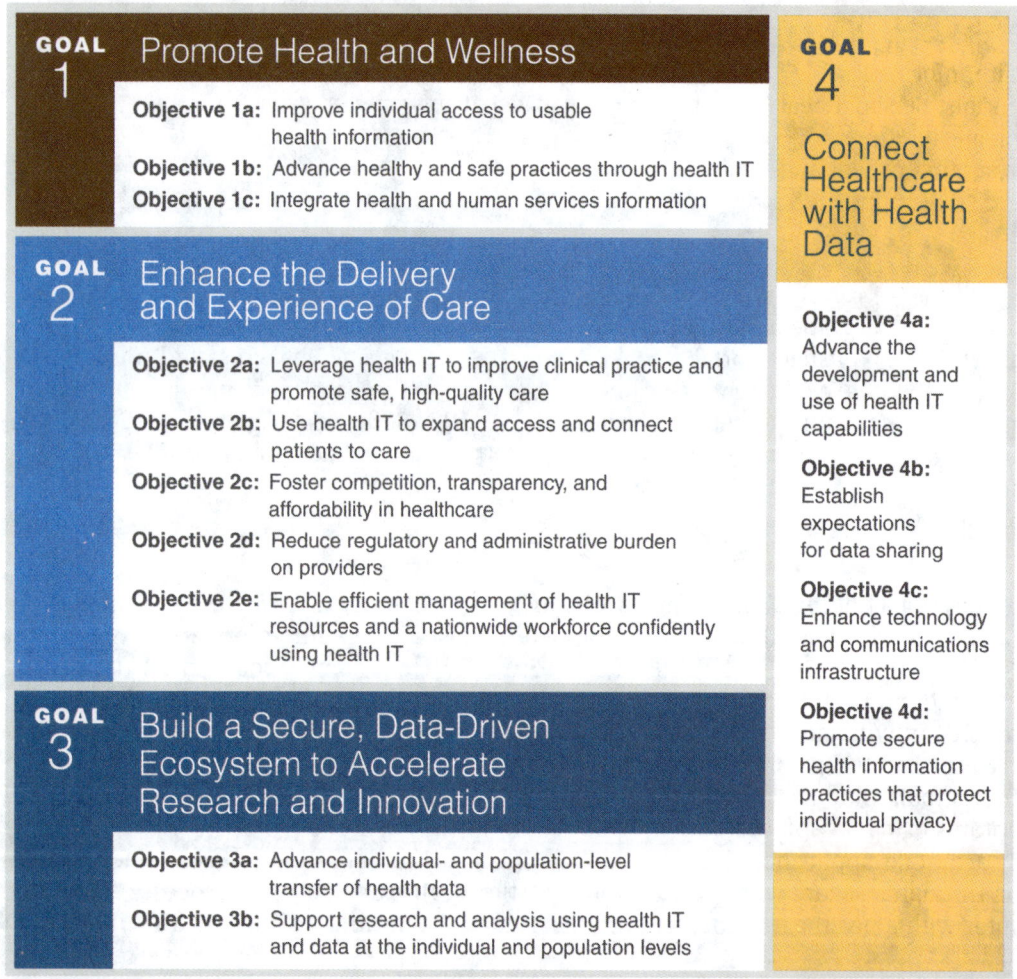

*Source:* ONC 2020, 5.

Because the consumer is the central stakeholder in this care delivery model, it is essential that consumers can effectively contribute and use information for decision-making purposes. Figure 14.2 illustrates how continuous learning cycles work across the healthcare continuum by showcasing how information collected throughout the care process can be used to inform care at each level.

This chapter examines the various aspects of consumer health informatics and discusses recent research shaping the future of the discipline. Ultimately, the goal of consumer health technology is for individuals to become more engaged in their health and healthcare, thereby improving the overall health experience and potentially health outcomes.

**Figure 14.2.** The learning health system

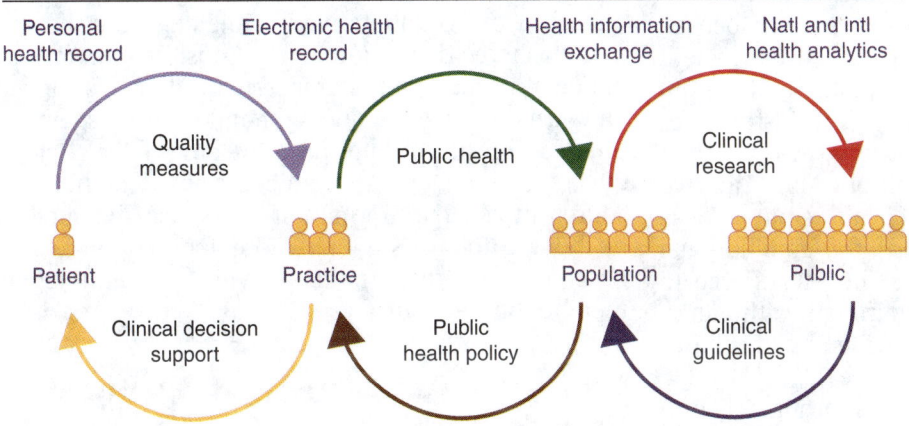

*Source:* ONC 2015, 19.

## Consumer Health Informatics and Consumer Engagement

Informatics is a field of study that focuses on the use of technology to improve access to, and utilization of, information. Focusing informatics on the patient, consumer health informatics is the "field devoted to informatics from multiple consumer or patient views. These include patient-focused informatics, health literacy, and consumer education. The focus is on information structures and processes that empower consumers to manage their own health" (AMIA n.d.). Where clinical or health informatics primarily focuses its attention on healthcare providers or organizations, the intent of consumer health informatics is to focus specifically on the needs of the consumer, whether the consumer is formally interacting with a healthcare provider or not. Because the needs of consumers are unique from those of other health informatics stakeholders (for example, providers), the design of products, services, and information displays must be customized to ensure the greatest impact on engaging the patients in managing their health.

Consumer health informatics' focus on consumer needs and preferences speaks to its inherent link to consumer and patient engagement. **Patient engagement** is defined as "the desire and capability to actively choose to participate in care in a way uniquely appropriate to the individual, in cooperation with a healthcare provider or institution, for the purposes of maximizing outcomes or improving experiences of care" (Higgins et al. 2017).

Patient engagement is related to more than healthcare and is not limited to informatics or technology. Patient engagement is patient-centered as opposed to clinician- or organization-centered. It represents a shift in the way health and healthcare are viewed. It is focused on patient activities that support improved health and therefore health outcomes, rather than simply healthcare-related activities. As the former US surgeon general, Dr. Regina Benjamin, stated, patient engagement occurs "not just in the doctor's office. It's got to be where we live, we work, we play, we pray" (Brown 2011). This is evident when considering that healthcare and managing one's health is increasingly interconnected with our daily lives. Information about one's health is central to promoting one's wellness, and this information is accessed and used via multiple technology-enabled devices and systems across the continuum of our modern experience.

The application of consumer health informatics to consumer engagement is not limited to the formal interactions between patients and clinicians, but rather encompasses a much wider view of how individuals work with technology and information to improve health understanding and health outcomes. The focus on consumer engagement is critical to the Institute for Healthcare Improvement's Triple Aim initiative, which has a goal to optimize health system performance. The Triple Aim initiative revolves around improving care outcomes and patient experience, and reducing healthcare costs. The aim focused on patient experience is intended to address patient experience from both the clinical quality and patient satisfaction perspectives (IHI n.d.). The Institute for Healthcare Improvement has proposed transitioning from the Triple Aim to the Quintuple Aim. The two additions relate to workforce and health equity. These two additional areas underscore the foundational component of having a highly skilled workforce to drive outcomes, as well as maintaining health equity central to the discussion to avoid widening the chasm in outcomes across populations (Mate 2022).

Models were developed to illustrate consumer health informatics that position consumers at the center of a process that involves inputs, integrating processes, and outputs (see figure 14.3). The model depicts how the consumer is affected by various factors, such as psychosocial status and the environment, and how available information such as digital health information can personalize and impact a consumer's health status. Digital health information such as health-related websites, patient portals, and patient generated health information through mobile technology can influence consumers' level of health literacy and, subsequently, their health status.

## The Evolution of Consumer Engagement in Healthcare

Historically, the healthcare delivery system placed the provider at the center of care. The providers determined the diagnosis, created the care plan, managed the care team, and delivered the care according to their objectives. This is known as medical paternalism. (Pomey et al. 2019). A patient-centered care approach is gradually replacing this focus on the provider and requiring clinicians and the entire care team to work collaboratively while engaging the patient in shared decision-making. Consideration for the patients' needs and preferences as well as a stronger emphasis on patient education and self-management intends to result in improved outcomes (Clavel et al. 2021). While this reliance on clinicians to be the sole source of health information was once the model, healthcare today is much more focused on team-based care where the patient is viewed as an integral member of the team.

## Consumer Assessment of Healthcare Providers and Systems

An early attempt to evaluate consumer perception with health plans was launched in 1995, through a partnership between the Agency for Healthcare Research and Quality (AHRQ), Harvard Medical School, RAND Corporation, and the Research Triangle Institute. This partnership eventually led the Centers for Medicare and Medicaid Services (CMS) to adopt the Consumer Assessment of Healthcare Providers and Systems (CAHPS). CAHPS is a standardized assessment of consumer perspectives regarding healthcare access and quality. CMS required certified organizations to evaluate the

**Figure 14.3.** Model of consumer health informatics

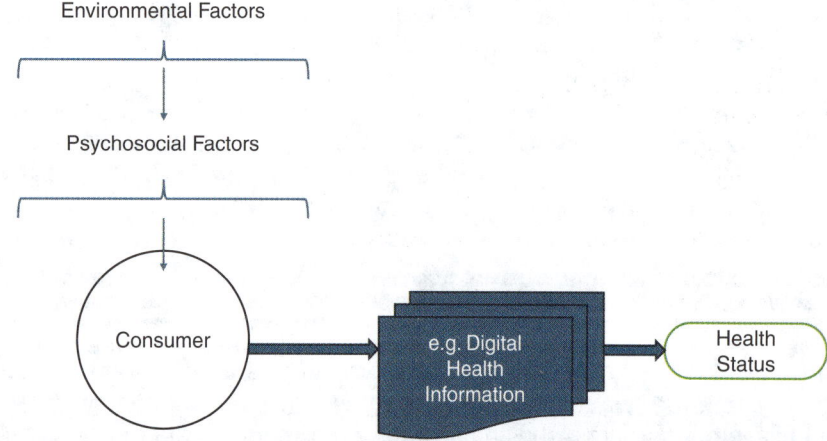

patient experience since the implementation of the Hospital Consumer Assessment of Healthcare Providers and Systems (HCAHPS) in 2002. Similarly, CMS required clinicians and ambulatory care groups to survey patients on their experience since 2007, with the Clinician and Group CAHPS (CG-CAHPS) survey tool. There are also CAHPS surveys focused on the following healthcare settings: health plans, surgical care, dental plans, home health, hospice, nursing homes, and others (AHRQ 2024). The rise of the internet, patient-focused websites, information sharing portals, and other similar tools for tracking and sharing patient and organization-generated data has rapidly transformed this domain of informatics.

Numerous research studies show a clear link between patient engagement and improved clinical outcomes, including diabetes control, cancer screening, and depression follow-up care. Patients who engage in using personal health information also have higher rates of satisfaction, health management, and loyalty to healthcare organizations (Vat et al. 2020).

## Patient-Centered Medical Home

With an increased focus on quality outcomes and patient satisfaction, and a changing healthcare reimbursement environment, healthcare organizations and payers focus more attention on viewing patients and families as full members of the healthcare team and providing **patient-centered care**, which is relationship-based primary care with an orientation toward the whole person (AHRQ 2022). The **patient-centered medical home (PCMH)**, for example, is a model that attempts to improve care outcomes and reduce care costs by reorganizing how primary care is delivered. There are five pillars to the PCMH model: a patient-centered orientation; comprehensive, team-based care; coordinated care; superb access to care; and a systems-based approach to quality and safety (AHRQ 2022).

## Promoting Interoperability Programs

The Promoting Interoperability (PI) Programs is another federal initiative attempting to improve consumer engagement in healthcare. CMS created the EHR Incentive Program in 2011 and adopted the goals of the National Priorities Partnership and its National Quality Strategy when creating the goals and objectives for meaningful use of electronic health records (EHRs). One of the goals is to "engage patients and families" by providing them with "timely access to data, knowledge, and tools to make informed decisions and to manage their care" (Tavenner and Sebelius 2012). The focus of the program has been providing access to health information in electronic format and increasing the proportion of patients who must engage in the use of these technologies to meet the threshold. For example, the proportion of patients expected to participate in secure messaging increases from 5 percent in stage 2 to 25 percent in stage 3 (CMS 2017).

The EHR Incentive Program included additional measures related to patient engagement apart from providing patients and families with their health information. The program required changes in the way demographic information was collected, including preferred language, and it also required that demographic information be captured in structured format. The program also introduced measures related to sending patient reminders, using data analytics to create patient lists, utilizing the EHR to identify patient-specific educational resources, and requiring patient family history to be recorded as structured data (CMS 2017).

The EHR Incentive Program was modified into the PI Program in 2016, changing many of the measures of the EHR Incentive Program related to consumer health informatics. These programs indicate ways patient engagement is used to impact care outcomes, access, and cost. The current PI Program requires eligible professionals and hospitals to adopt certified technology and provide at least one patient electronic access to their health information (CMS 2024).

## Hospital Value-Based Purchasing Program

The CMS Hospital Value-Based Purchasing (VBP) Program is another program that has placed significant value on patient experience. The Hospital VBP Program provides financial incentives for hospitals that perform well. The total performance score that determines the incentive is based on four domains—clinical outcomes, safety, efficiency and cost reduction, and person and community engagement. The person and community engagement domain accounts for 25 percent of the total performance score. In other words, patient engagement as measured by nurse and physician communication with patients, discharge information, and other patient-centered measures are critically important for reimbursement of each hospital that participates in the program (CMS 2019). Similarly, other programs related to healthcare reform, such as accountable care organizations, aim to improve how care is coordinated across the continuum of care. They are required to engage patients in the care process, and patient engagement is seen by healthcare leaders as critical to the success of the delivery and payment model (Taylor et al. 2011).

### Check Your Understanding 14.1

**Answer the following questions in a separate document.**

1. Propose ways in which organizations encourage and enhance patient engagement.
2. A learning health system is "an ecosystem where all stakeholders can securely, effectively, and efficiently contribute, share, and analyze data and create new knowledge that can be consumed by a wide variety of electronic health information systems to support effective decision-making leading to improved health outcomes." Present what this concept means in your own words. Consider the learning health system diagram in your response.
3. Compare the concepts of medical paternalism and patient-centered care and describe the main motivator for the shift in approach to patient care.
4. Assess care coordination and how it relates to the PCMH model.
5. Evaluate why patient experience accounts for a large percentage of the Hospital VBP Program?

## Social Determinants of Health

Consumers' engagement in their healthcare has been noted in several groundbreaking Institute of Medicine (IOM) reports (such as Page 2004; Knebel and Greiner 2003; IOM 2001; Kohn et al. 2000; Wunderlich and Kohler 2001) as key to addressing the issues of healthcare access, cost, and quality. One of the central challenges facing the US healthcare system is the disparity in health outcomes based upon a variety of socioeconomic factors such as age, race, ethnicity, income level, education level, and healthcare access. These factors have been labeled by the World Health Organization (WHO) as the **social determinants of health (SDOH)**, defined as

> the conditions in which people are born, grow, work, live, and age, and the wider set of forces and systems shaping the conditions of daily life. These forces and systems include economic policies and systems, development agendas, social norms, social policies, and political systems. (WHO n.d.)

The federal government initiated multiple projects aimed at researching and promoting patient engagement. HealthyPeople and a focus on health literacy are major initiatives.

### HealthyPeople 2030

HealthyPeople 2030, an initiative sponsored by the US Department of Health and Human Services (HHS), has organized the social determinants of health into five domains (see figure 14.4):

1. Economic stability
2. Education access and quality
3. Healthcare access and quality
4. Neighborhood and built environment
5. Social and community context (HHS n.d.a)

These domains reflect the SDOH that ultimately impact health outcomes. By developing this model, HHS goals and objectives may be developed within each domain. All the SDOH have an impact on consumer engagement.

The HealthyPeople initiative determines goals and objectives for each of the five domains, collects information to determine a baseline measure, and monitors this measure against the target. For example, one of the measures related to health and healthcare is the number of individuals with a "usual primary care provider." The rate in 2017 was 76 percent and the target is 84 percent (HHS n.d.c). There is a clear divide between those who report having a usual primary care provider and those who do not. Overall, the percentage of individuals reporting a usual primary care provider increased by 0.4 percent between 1996 and 2017 (HHS n.d.b). There are disparities in healthcare outcomes based upon social determinants. White respondents generally report higher levels of usual care providers, and living in a state with expanded Medicaid further increases the divide. By better understanding the disparities and setting goals and objectives to address them, health disparities can be addressed.

**Figure 14.4.** HealthyPeople 2030 model of social determinants of health

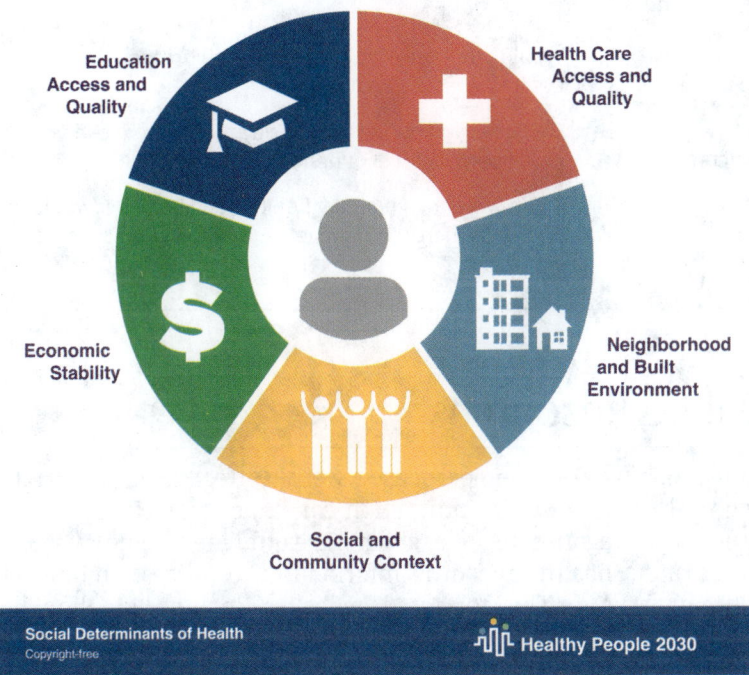

*Source:* HHS n.d.a.

## Health Literacy

One of the SDOHs outlined by HealthyPeople 2030 is health literacy. There are two types:

- **Personal health literacy** is the degree to which individuals have the ability to find, understand, and use information and services to inform health-related decisions and actions for themselves and others.
- **Organizational health literacy** is the degree to which organizations equitably enable individuals to find, understand, and use information and services to inform health-related decisions and actions for themselves and others. (HHS n.d.b)

Consumer health informatics is focused on empowering patients by effectively communicating with them using a variety of methods, including health information in various formats. The communication of health information, whether in verbal or written format, relies on the ability of the individual to understand the information to achieve its desired purpose. However, the IOM reports that approximately half of the American adult population may "have difficulties acting on health information" (Sørensen et al. 2012). A recent study found that approximately 94 percent of patients initiated secure messages while only 53 percent replied to a clinician's message (Huang et al. 2022). While individuals may search for health information online or obtain their own health information from providers, they may not fully understand the information or use it for behavioral change. Research shows that individual health literacy level is a predictor of health outcomes, including medication adherence, self-management skills, and knowledge of disease (Sørensen et al. 2012). Every percentage increase in health literacy levels results in a two percent increase in health status (Sentell et al. 2014). Because consumer health informatics largely involves developing technology for consumers to more effectively engage in healthcare, especially through the capture and use of health information, health literacy must be a key factor when developing tools and techniques to engage patients.

There are numerous valid and reliable measures of health literacy, including the Short Assessment of Health Literacy—Spanish and English (SAHL–S&E) and the Rapid Estimate of Adult Literacy in Medicine—Short Form. The AHRQ produced a resource guide with access to validated tools that provide the ability to assess the health literacy of individuals. The tools can be used for research, clinical, or programmatic purposes. For example, the SAHL–S&E instrument instructions and information regarding training are available for download. This measurement of health literacy includes 18 test terms meant to assess an individual's vocabulary and comprehension. The assessment takes approximately two to three minutes to complete and, depending upon the individual answers, the results are presented as a score. The score is indicative of the individual's health literacy (AHRQ 2022).

### Check Your Understanding 14.2

Answer the following questions in a separate document.

1. Propose your own definition of health literacy from what you have read or experienced yourself or with a family member. Provide examples for your rationale.
2. How does an initiative like HealthyPeople help increase consumer engagement?
3. Would you rate yourself as having high, medium, or low health literacy? Explain why.
4. Considering your answer to question 3, how can you increase your level of health literacy?
5. If you were a community health educator, how would you approach increasing the level of health literacy in your community?

## Health Information Online Resources

One of the most basic forms of consumer engagement is the use of the internet for seeking health information online. According to research conducted in 2013 by the Pew Research Center's Internet and American Life Project, 72 percent of American adults searched the internet for information related to a health issue in the past 12 months, including 55 percent who searched for information regarding a specific medical diagnosis; 43 percent for a specific procedure or treatment; 27 percent for information regarding how to lose or manage weight; and 25 percent for information regarding health insurance. Interestingly, of those individuals who use the internet for seeking health information, 60 percent reported that the information found online affected the decision regarding how to treat the illness or condition; 56 percent reported that it changed the approach to maintaining their health; and 53 percent reported that the information led them to ask a doctor new questions or seek a second opinion (Rainie 2013). There are many options for patients to access online resources, including websites, forums, and other tools.

### Healthcare-Focused Websites

There are many examples of health information maintained on the internet and available for consumption. The Mayo Clinic has developed one of the most utilized patient education-focused websites. Its website receives more than 127 million visitors per month (O'Connor 2021). The website allows users to access thousands of patient education materials, including content focused on symptoms, diseases and conditions, treatments and procedures, medications, research, and various other topics and services. There are numerous healthcare-focused websites where consumers seek information and guidance. The Medical Library Association's Consumer and Patient Health Information Section (CAPHIS) annually ranks the top 100 consumer-focused websites regarding their ability to provide information consumers can trust. The categories include general health, men's and women's health, and drug information resources, among others. The top-rated websites include MedlinePlus, Centers for Disease Control and Prevention, Mount Carmel Consumer Health Information, and the Ohio State University Wexner Medical Center "Patient Education" (CAPHIS 2019).

### Internet Forums

In addition to general health-related searches and healthcare-focused websites, another aspect of consumer health informatics is internet-based forums. An internet forum is a "web application for holding discussions and posting user-generated content, also commonly referred to as web forums, newsgroups, message boards, discussion boards, bulletin boards or simply a forum" (Ho 2009, 187). Internet forums are frequently used by individuals who share a common interest. One of the most popular healthcare internet forums is PatientsLikeMe. PatientsLikeMe was created in 2004 and has a goal of connecting patients in a forum that allows them to better understand and manage their conditions by sharing their experiences and learning from others with similar conditions. Additionally, the website has a research mission. Members of PatientsLikeMe can provide data regarding their condition and experience to track and manage their health, and this data can be used in research studies. Currently, PatientsLikeMe.com has more than 850,000 members, representing 2,900 conditions. The website boasts that more than 100 research studies have been published using member data (PatientsLikeMe n.d.). There are numerous general internet forums (like PatientsLikeMe), but there are other, more focused ones, such as IHadCancer.com (focused on cancer patients), and CureDiva.com (focused on breast cancer patients). Internet forums provide a venue for individuals to safely connect with each other to discuss health concerns. For individuals with rare conditions or who live in rural areas, for example, these forums allow them to pose questions, share stories, and generally connect with other individuals who had similar health-related experiences. This ability to create communities through technology adds value to the individual in terms of addressing the isolation that oftentimes accompanies clinical diagnoses and has resulted in improved healthcare outcomes.

## Patient Activation Measure

Given the association between the level of health literacy and the overall level of engagement in healthcare and clinical outcomes (Sørensen et al. 2012), the patient activation measure (PAM) was developed as a way to be able to predict the patient's level of engagement in healthcare, including the knowledge, beliefs, skills, and behaviors necessary to manage one's health (Hibbard et al. 2004). The PAM is a 13-item Likert survey instrument (a Likert item is a statement that allows an individual to respond based upon their level of agreement with the statement) that scores patients on a scale of 1 to 100 and classifies patients as falling into one of four categories based upon their total score. The levels describe four progressive domains of activation—from passive health consumer to active health advocate. The PAM provides a useful tool for measuring one's level of engagement as it is a predictor of health outcomes:

Those who are activated [based upon the results of the survey] believe patients have important roles to play in self-managing care, collaborating with providers, and maintaining their health. They know how to manage their condition and maintain functioning and prevent health declines; and they have the skills and behavioral repertoire to manage their condition, collaborate with their health providers, maintain their health functioning, and access appropriate and high-quality care. (Hibbard et al. 2004, 1010)

The four levels of the PAM are (1) disengaged and overwhelmed; (2) becoming aware, but still struggling; (3) taking action; and (4) maintaining behaviors and pushing further (Insignia n.d.).

Research has shown that the PAM works to accurately predict a patient's level of activation (overall level of engagement in managing one's health), yet a patient's activation is minimally impacted by socio-economic and demographic factors. Thus, the PAM score can be increased over time (Hibbard et al. 2013, 2005, 2001). Moreover, increasing PAM scores among patient populations has shown significant impact on improved healthcare outcomes and reductions in cost. For each percentage point increase in the PAM score, there is a two-point reduction in hospital readmission rates and a two-point increase in medication adherence rates (Insignia n.d.). Organizations purchase the PAM, survey their respective patient populations, and can use the PAM scores as a tool for more effectively partnering with patients to meet their care goals.

### Check Your Understanding 14.3

Answer the following questions in a separate document.

1. Why are so many internet searches health-related?
2. What are some potential implications of high rates of health-related web searches for patient engagement?
3. Assess the meaning of level four of the PAM.
4. What are a few areas of a health-focused website that provide value to consumers, and what is one area that may pose a challenge for users?
5. Offer one reason why care providers may not want to promote the use of online health information resources.

## Patient Portals, Personal Health Records, and Telehealth

The federally sanctioned definition of EHR includes the requirement for use of nationally recognized interoperability standards so data can be shared across more than one healthcare organization. The PI program's criteria require the ability to exchange key clinical information not only with providers but also with patients and includes the provision of electronic copies of discharge instructions, clinical summaries for office visits, and timely electronic access (CMS 2017). Coordinating care across the continuum and consumer empowerment are key principles of the federal government's focus on building a better health system. The consumer health informatics tools that have been garnering significant attention in recent years are patient portals, personal health records (PHRs), and telehealth encounters between patients and providers. The use of patient portals and PHRs has a significant impact on clinical outcomes, patient satisfaction, and professional and organizational efficiency (Dorr et al. 2007; Sequist et al. 2011; Simon et al. 2011).

## Patient Portals

A patient portal is an internet entryway that allows patients to pay their bills online and to securely view all or portions of their provider-based EHR, such as current medical conditions, immunization records, medications, allergies, and test results. Patient portals allow patients to view information from recent clinical visits, hospital discharge summaries, medications, immunizations, allergies, and lab results. Depending on the vendor or the organization, patient portals may allow patients to request prescription prefills, schedule appointments, make payments, send secure messages, and view educational materials.

Clinical messaging was an early form of connectivity, most commonly between providers. If any protected health information (PHI) was exchanged, encryption was sometimes deployed—although the lack of interoperability between encryption software products sometimes made that difficult to do. Web portals are more commonly used today to provide secure connectivity. This technology is a step up from clinical messaging because messages may be exchanged securely and direct access to certain applications may be provided. For example, there may be a patient portal set up by a healthcare organization for use by patients. Patients may be able to exchange secure email messages with their providers—for example, to request an appointment, for access to lab results, to obtain access to a patient health summary, or for tailored instructions for taking medications, wound care, and so on. E-visits are online provider encounters that provide reimbursement and which can save patients an office visit.

A continuity of care record (CCR) is a core data set of the most relevant administrative, demographic, and clinical information about a patient's healthcare, covering one or more healthcare encounters. It provides a means for one healthcare practitioner, system, or setting to aggregate all the pertinent data about a patient and forward it to another practitioner, system, or setting to support the continuity of care. The CCR was originally conceived by the Massachusetts Medical Society to standardize referral information and was ratified as a standard under ASTM International (ASTM 2012) with assistance from the Health Information Management and Systems Society (HIMSS) and other medical societies. A continuity of care document (CCD) is the result of the CCR standard content from the American Society for Testing and Materials (ASTM) being represented and mapped into the Clinical Document Architecture/Consolidated Clinical Document Architecture (CDA or C-CDA) specifications from Health Level Seven (HL7) to enable transmission of referral information between providers; also frequently adopted for PHRs. Fast Healthcare Interoperability Standards (FHIR) is also an HL7 data format that allows for the formatting and exchange of information that impact patient engagement programs. The CCR, CCD, and FHIR standards are forms of connectivity, required in the federal EHR adoption programs.

Figure 14.5 provides an illustration of a patient portal offered by the US Department of Veterans Affairs. The application is called MyHealtheVet. The web-based application allows a patient to access a variety of personal health information through one centralized repository, including information related to vital signs and readings, labs and tests, and health history (VA n.d.). The figure also illustrates one of the key features of patient portals—secure messaging. Because of the requirements of the EHR Incentive Program, organizations or professionals are required to make patient portals available to patients, and the portals must allow for secure messaging between patients and providers. Secure messaging enables

> a user to electronically send messages to, and receive messages from, a patient in a manner that ensures: (1) both the patient (or authorized representative) and EHR technology user are authenticated; and (2) the message content is encrypted and integrity-protected in accordance with the standard for encryption and hashing algorithms. (NIST 2013)

## Personal Health Records

PHRs are yet another form of connectivity popular with some patients and the federal government, health plans, and employers who are promoting their use for value-driven healthcare. PHRs are like patient portals. Whereas patient portals are typically tethered to and maintained by a healthcare organization on behalf of a patient, PHRs are created and maintained by the consumer. A personal health record (PHR) has been defined as an electronic or paper health record

**Figure 14.5.** Example of web-based patient portal

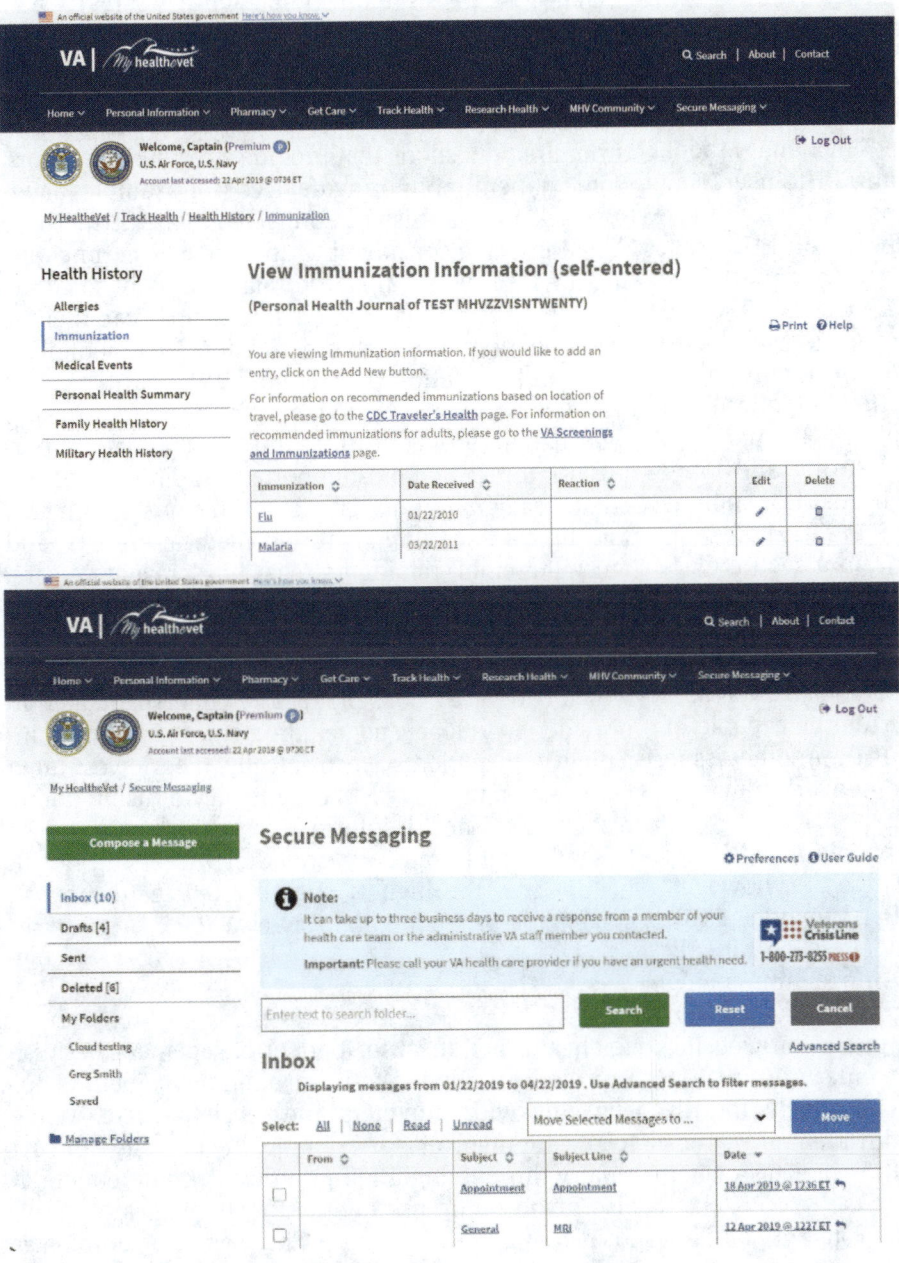

*Source:* VA n.d.

maintained and updated by an individual for himself or herself; a tool that individuals can use to collect, track, and share past and current information about their health or the health of someone in their care.

Detailed elements that are potentially available in a PHR vary. PHRs can include calendars and reminders, health record organizers, communication portals, cost management tools, wellness programs, and educational resources. The Mayo Clinic developed the following list of elements to include in a PHR as a means of helping individuals manage their health:

- Your doctors' names and phone numbers
- Allergies, including drug allergies
- Your medications, including dosages
- List and dates of illnesses and surgeries
- Chronic health problems, such as high blood pressure
- Living will or advance directives
- Family history
- Immunization history

- Home blood pressure readings
- Exercise and dietary habits
- Health goals, such as stopping smoking or losing weight (Mayo Clinic 2022)

HL7 has adopted the PHR-System Functional Model, which offers standard content for PHR use (HL7 n.d.). PHRs come in many forms. PHRs electronically populate elements or subsets of PHI from provider organization databases into the electronic records of authorized patients, their families, other providers, and sometimes health payers and employers. A range of people and groups maintain the records, including the patients, their families, and other providers. The development of PHRs parallels the consumer-centrism described earlier and long-evident in other vertical market industries, such as banking, where consumers can maintain and examine their activities 24 hours a day in a secure electronic environment.

Several issues are at stake. The first is whether a provider organization is willing to work with a PHR. For example, increasing consumer demand for useful PHRs requires that an EHR system be capable of sending and receiving data from a PHR. Another issue is whether a patient can trust the network transmitting his or her information.

Although fewer than expected, people are adopting PHRs (Ruhi and Chugh 2021). There are, however, an increasing number of EHRs that support a PHR, as well as commercial PHR vendors selling directly to consumers. In general, PHRs range from being fairly unsophisticated (for example, where patients can direct providers to send a fax to a given website, or they can upload documents or enter information themselves), to quite comprehensive (including direct feeds from a provider or health plan and structured templates for the individual to enter his or her own data).

Health plans are particularly interested in populating PHRs they support with problem lists and medication lists from claims data. While there are concerns about how clinically relevant diagnosis information may be from claims data, the fact that the health plan can provide this information across all providers is attractive. The health plan can then provide direct disease management support to patients.

Similarly, PHRs linked or tethered to EHRs enable the provider to direct specific information to the patient's PHR and to retrieve information from it (Mayo Clinic 2022). In more comprehensive forms of PHRs, the source of the data is identifiable, and the data entered by any given source is only able to be altered by that source—maintaining the integrity of all data. Although these tethered forms of PHR may only contain the information from the one provider that supports the PHR, the patient's ability to enter his or her own data can be an aid to the provider. The patient can login before a visit or at a kiosk in the waiting room and enter his or her own medical history, family history, and history of present illness and respond to structured questions that provide a review of systems. Some patient monitoring devices (for example, activity trackers) may also be connected to the PHR. These functions save considerable documentation time during the visit, where this information only needs to be reviewed and validated. The time savings can then be spent on more thorough examination, treatment planning, and education (Kim et al. 2019).

Patients and caregivers want access to personal health information through features in PHRs and patient portals. Features rated most important by patients included accessing an up-to-date health history, summaries for clinical encounters, current medication lists, and receiving email reminders regarding preventive care. The highest-rated feature by patients was the ability to email providers. Yet emailing providers was one of the lowest-rated features by providers themselves, which can partly be explained by concerns related to provider workload and reimbursement in communicating with patients electronically. The lowest-rated feature by patients was the frequency of using online resources for health information in the past year, yet this was highly rated by providers. Accessing health history was the highest overall rated feature by all stakeholders (Fricton and Davies 2008).

## Telehealth

Telehealth is critical for patient engagement because it provides patients with an alternative method for engaging with providers and receiving care. While telehealth involves, for example, the provision of psychiatry through high-definition video conferencing, it also involves the use of smart technologies to monitor patients in their homes. These smart technologies include devices for collecting vitals, tracking medication adherence, tracking movement and dietary habits, or glucometers. The use of telehealth expanded significantly during the COVID-19 pandemic. According to one study, percentage of visits increased by 68 percent (Andino and Boxer 2023).

Unlike patient portals and PHRs, telehealth is not a web-based application to provide timely access to health-related information. **Telehealth** is "the use of electronic information and telecommunications technologies to support long-distance clinical health care, patient and professional health-related education, health administration, and public health. Technologies include videoconferencing, the internet, store-and-forward imaging, streaming media, and land and wireless communications" (HRSA 2022). Telehealth may be considered a form of connectivity. Telehealth is not new and does not require an EHR. Telehealth supplements a healthcare organization's capabilities such as for remote intensive care unit monitoring (Young et al. 2011). However, there are also questions as to whether critical care outcomes are improved (Kahn 2011) or are only supplements to staffing. Telehealth can be used to provide emergency care, offer consultations across great distances (or in limited access areas, even including inner-city areas), monitor local patients with chronic disease, track progress in recovery of certain types of illnesses or injuries (Melville 2012), and bring sign language to the hearing impaired during a local healthcare encounter (Hirsch and Marano 2007).

### Check Your Understanding 14.4

**Answer the following questions in a separate document.**

1. Sally is completing a wellness questionnaire so she can receive a discount on her health insurance next year. She needs to find out what her cholesterol level was at her clinic visit in June. Would you recommend she refer to a patient portal or a PHR?

2. If Jane accessed her patient portal offered through her local health system and accessed the secure message feature to send a message to her primary care provider regarding the results of her lab test and prescribed medications, what standard would be used to send the secure message electronically?

3. Joe manages a group home with five residents who have chronic medical conditions. He would like to ensure he has documentation of daily behavioral and physical occurrences available for each of the resident's routine clinic appointments. What recommendation do you have for Joe?

4. Consider your health priorities and develop a model for your own PHR including information that you feel is important to your health. For example, is it important to track your A1c or glucose, your water intake, minutes of exercise, weight, hours of sleep, calorie intake, steps in a day, heart rate, and the like? Also determine the best modality for your PHR. For example, is it a web-based PHR, a paper record, your own electronic device, an electronic document on your own computer, and so on. Explain your response.

5. Give an example of how telehealth can improve consumer engagement?

## Patient-Generated Health Data

The ONC defines **patient-generated health data (PGHD)** as "health-related data created, recorded, or gathered by or from patients (or family members or other caregivers) to help address a health concern" (ONC n.d.). PGHD can include "health history, symptoms, biometric data, treatment history, lifestyle choices, and other information" (Deering 2013). PGHD collection has increased with the proliferation of smart phone adoption and development of mobile applications (Omoloja and Vundavalli 2021). PGHD can improve the efficiency of healthcare entities by reducing the frequency of office visits, improving the overall understanding of health conditions among patients, improving the treatment of chronic conditions, improving patient-provider relationships, and generally improving the patient experience of care (Lordon et al. 2020; Deering 2013). As opposed to other types of clinical data generated by healthcare organizations, patients (or their caregivers) are responsible for recording this information and for determining who gets access to the generated information and when they are provided access to the information. PGHD is converging with the traditional medical record in new and innovative ways.

Figure 14.6 illustrates the process of recording PGHD and how the information could be used in the clinical process. First, the patient (consumer) either enters data into an electronic device or the information is captured by a remote monitoring device or wearable (a technology a patient wears that collects and transmits data). Second, the person grants access to the information to a third party and transfers the data to them, in this case to a provider organization and a particular physician and staff member. The third step in the process is for the provider and staff to review and document the information, potentially within the EHR but not necessarily (it could be through a third-party system access through an API, for example) and,

**Figure 14.6.** Patient-generated health data flow

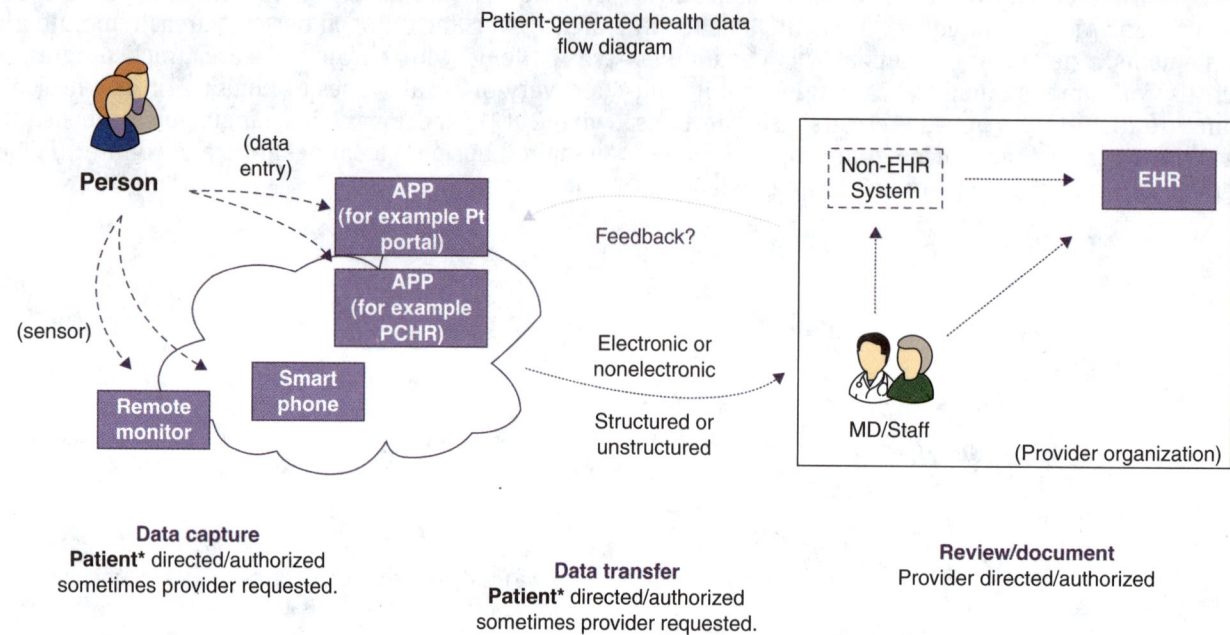

*Patient, person, designee     Abbreviations: APP=application; PCHR=personally controlled health record; EHR=electronic health record

*Source:* Shapiro et al. 2012.

depending on the type of information provided, they could provide feedback to the person. APIs are application programming interfaces—they allow different systems to talk to one another by sending information between them. Examples of PGHD that could use an API are cardiac monitoring or blood pressure tracking.

In addition to the recording and collecting of data that can be used for routine engagements with healthcare providers, there is a global movement that promotes and supports the collection and use of large amounts of information regarding personal activity—diet, physical activity, psychological states and traits, mental and cognitive traits, environmental variables, and social variables (Swan 2013). The explosion of mobile cellular devices and other wireless personal devices focused on health and fitness monitoring has facilitated the growth of this movement. The use of these devices for health-related purposes has been labeled **mHealth** and has been defined by HIMSS as "the generation, aggregation, and dissemination of health information via mobile and wireless devices" (HIMSS n.d.). For example, mobile phones have the capability to serve as a pedometer, connect with other wearable devices, and track weight, heart rate, respiration, sleeping activity, calories burned, and much more. There are also a variety of additional wearable devices that have made quantifying daily activity extremely easy—both for data collection and data analysis. The adoption and use of mobile device fitness applications continues to grow and is expected to grow by 18 percent between 2024 and 2033 (Market. Us 2024). Individuals are engaging with health-related information at unparalleled rates. This engagement is altering expectations regarding the types of information that can be collected, how it is displayed, and how it can be used.

## Precision Medicine

**Precision medicine** has been defined by the US Food and Drug Administration (FDA) as tailoring "disease prevention and treatment for individual variability (e.g., genetic and lifestyle differences among patients)" (FDA 2022). Precision medicine focuses on utilizing very specific attributes of patients as a basis of providing treatment. One of the driving forces of precision medicine is the collection and use of genetic information. For example, the FDA has approved a drug that treats cystic fibrosis caused by a specific gene mutation (the G551D mutation). The drug restores function to a specific protein that is affected by the gene mutation (FDA 2022). This ability to sequence or partially sequence patient genomes has the potential to revolutionize healthcare delivery by providing treatments tailored to these specific genetic markers. The Human Genome Project, which involved the sequencing of the 3 billion base pairs of the human genome, took 13 years to complete and approximately $3 billion (NIH 2024). This project has opened the door to using genetics to predict risks of future illnesses. Today, the cost for a complete genome sequencing is approximately $1,000, down from more than $5,000 in 2014 (NIH 2023) (see figure 14.7 for a detailed breakdown of sequencing costs over time). As it becomes less expensive to learn more about our genes and how they influence our health, consumers will be able to engage with this information (and their providers) to create customized care plans that potentially influence major decisions regarding healthcare interventions. The progress made on genome sequencing has also opened multiple options for at-home genetic testing allowing individuals to learn about their family history and also some health risk factors.

**Figure 14.7.** Cost per genome from 2001 to 2022

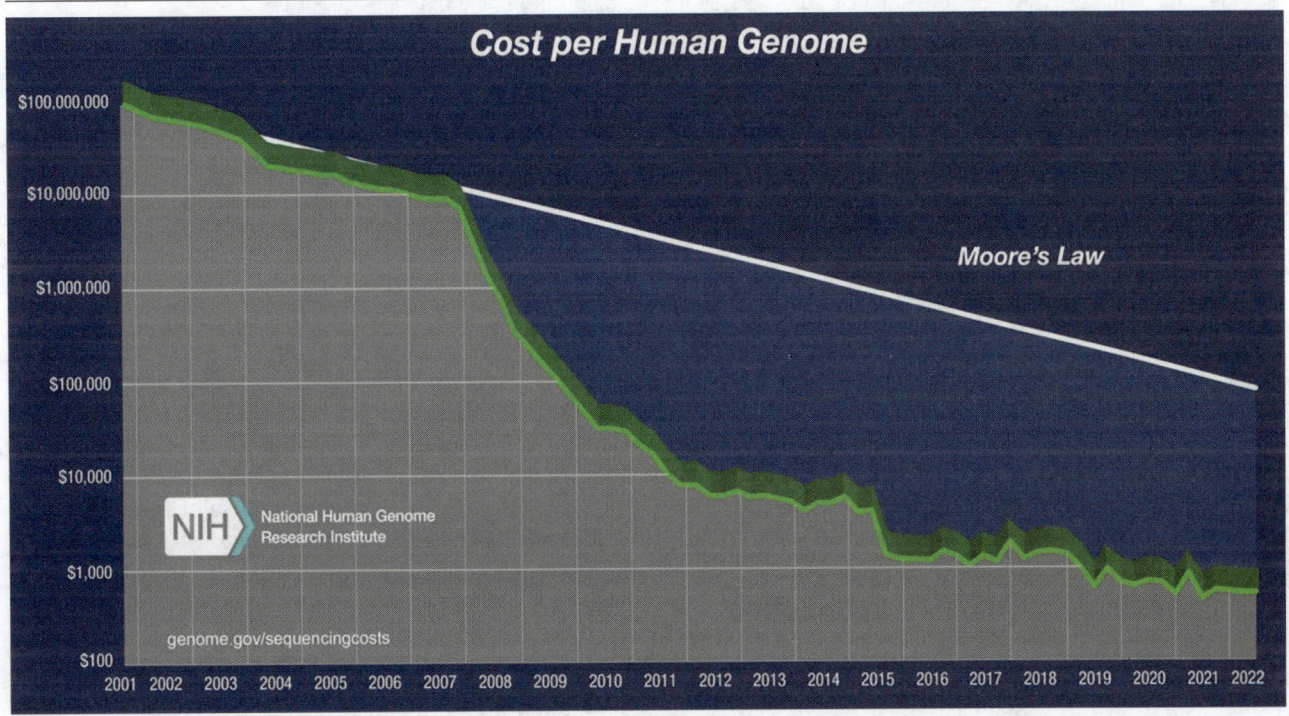

*Source:* NIH 2023.

## Consumer Health Informatics and Next Steps

The transition from the organization-focused system characterized by silos of care to a patient-centered system has been challenging. The patient-centered system with teams of care delivery using informatics, research, and evidence-based guidelines, including patients as key members of the team, is referred to as the learning health system. Consumer health informatics plays a critical role in the learning health system. Consumers who access and use health information report improved health outcomes and patient satisfaction levels, yet there are wide disparities in terms of populations who use the tools that offer access to health information. Consumer health informatics professionals will be responsible for designing tools and resources that provide access to health information, collect and report data, and engage with providers and caregivers. These tools and resources are designed in such a way that the consumer's needs and preferences are integrated to address the disparities that have impacted the adoption of tools in the past.

## Check Your Understanding 14.5

Answer the following questions in a separate document.

1. How do PGHD and the PHR work together?
2. How do PGHD and precision medicine work together?
3. How can personalized medicine be of value to an individual? Develop your own personalized medicine plan.
4. Phyllis collects PGHD and wants to share it with her provider, so she goes through the process of entering the data into an electronic device and then transferring the data to the provider. Her provider, Dr. Jones, says she did not receive the data. Why do you think Dr. Jones did not receive it?
5. As the community health educator, you have been tasked with increasing the number of patients using their provider's patient portal in the community in which you live. Using your community as an example, assess the challenges related to the local population (such as age barriers, economic levels, level of education, resources, cultural issues, and such) and develop a plan that may promote use of a patient portal.

# References

AHRQ (Agency for Healthcare Research and Quality). 2024. "CAHPS Patient Experience Surveys and Guidance." https://www.ahrq.gov/cahps/surveys-guidance/index.html.

AHRQ (Agency for Healthcare Research and Quality). 2022. "Defining the PCMH." https://www.ahrq.gov/ncepcr/research/care-coordination/pcmh/define.html.

AHRQ (Agency for Healthcare Research and Quality). 2019. "About Learning Health Systems." https://www.ahrq.gov/learning-health-systems/about.html.

AMIA (American Medical Informatics Association). n.d. "Consumer Health Informatics." Accessed May 11, 2024. https://www.amia.org/applications-informatics/consumer-health-informatics.

Andino, J., N. Eyrich, and R. Boxer. 2023. Overview of telehealth in the United States since the COVID-19 public health emergency: A narrative review. *mHhealth* 15(9):26. https://mhealth.amegroups.org/article/view/115704/html.

ASTM International. 2012. "ASTM E2369-05 Standard Specification for Continuity of Care Record (CCR)." https://www.astm.org/e2369-05.html.

Baumgartner, J. C., S. R. Collins, and D. C. Radley. 2023. "Inequities in Health Insurance Coverage and Access for Black and Hispanic Adults. The Impact of Medicaid Expansion and the Pandemic." The Commonweath Fund. https://www.commonwealthfund.org/publications/issue-briefs/2023/mar/inequities-coverage-access-black-hispanic-adults.

Brown, E. 2011 (March 13). Surgeon general discusses health and community. *Los Angeles Times*. http://articles.latimes.com/2011/mar/13/health/la-he-surgeon-general-20110313.

CAPHIS (Consumer and Patient Health Information Section). 2019. "CAPHIS' Most Trusted Health Websites." https://www.mlanet.org/d/do/13143.

Clavel, N., J. Paquette, V. Dumez, C. Del Grande, D. Ghadiri, M. Pomey, and L. Normandin. 2021. Patient engagement in care: A scoping review of recently validated tools assessing patients' and healthcare professionals' preferences and experience. *Health Expect* 24(6):1924–1935. https://www.ncbi.nlm.nih.gov/pmc/articles/PMC8628592/.

CMS (Centers for Medicaid and Medicare Services). 2024. "Requirements for Previous Years." https://www.cms.gov/medicare/regulations-guidance/promoting-interoperability-programs/requirements-previous-years.

CMS (Centers for Medicaid and Medicare Services). 2019. "Step-by-step Calculations for Value-based Purchasing." https://www.qualityreportingcenter.com/globalassets/iqr_resources/july-2019/vbp_fy2020_ppsrrelease_scoring_qrg_vfinal508.pdf.

CMS (Centers for Medicaid and Medicare Services). 2017. "Eligible Professional Medicaid EHR Incentive Program Stage 3 Objectives and Measures Objective 6 of 8." *Centers for Medicaid and Medicare Services*. https://www.cms.gov/Regulations-and-Guidance/Legislation/EHRIncentivePrograms/Downloads/MedicaidEPStage3_Obj6.pdf.

Deering, M. J. 2013. "Issue Brief: Patient-Generated Health Data and Health IT." http://wanghaisheng.github.io/images/pghd_brief_final122013.pdf.

Dorr, D., L. M. Bonner, A. N. Cohen, R. S. Shoai, R. Perrin, E. Chaney, and A. S. Young. 2007. Informatics systems to promote improved care for chronic illness: A literature review. *Journal of the American Medical Informatics Association* 14(2):156–163.

FDA (Food and Drug Administration). 2022. "Focus Area: Individualized Therapeutics and Precision Medicine." https://www.fda.gov/science-research/focus-areas-regulatory-science-report/focus-area-individualized-therapeutics-and-precision-medicine.

HHS (Department of Health and Human Services). n.d.a. "Social Determinants of Health." Accessed August 30, 2024. https://health.gov/healthypeople/priority-areas/social-determinants-health.

HHS (Department of Health and Human Services). n.d.b. "Health Literacy in Healthy People 2030." Accessed August 30, 2024. https://health.gov/healthypeople/priority-areas/health-literacy-healthy-people-2030.

HHS (Department of Health and Human Services) n.d.c. "Increase the Proportion of People with a Usual Primary Care Provider—AHS-07." Accessed September 4, 2024. https://health.gov/healthypeople/objectives-and-data/browse-objectives/health-care-access-and-quality/increase-proportion-people-usual-primary-care-provider-ahs-07.

HIMSS (Health Information Management and Systems Society). n.d. "mHealth." Accessed September 4, 2024. https://lib.digitalsquare.io/server/api/core/bitstreams/c19059b4-a342-4a0a-aa90-10512c79130f/content.

HL7 (Health Level Seven). n.d. *EHR and PHR System Functional Models—Record Lifecycle Events Implementation Guide*. Accessed on January 16, 2024. https://build.fhir.org/ig/HL7/ehrs-rle-ig/.

HRSA (Health Resources and Services Administration). 2022 (March). "What is Telehealth." https://www.hrsa.gov/telehealth/what-is-telehealth.

Hibbard, J. H., J. Greene, and V. Overton. 2013. Patients with lower activation associated with higher costs; Delivery systems should know their patients' "scores." *Health Affairs* 32(2):216–222.

Hibbard, J. H., E. R. Mahoney, J. Stockard, and M. Tusler. 2005. Development and testing of a short form of the patient activation measure. *Health Services Research* 40(6 Pt 1):1918–1930.

Hibbard, J. H., J. Stockard, E. R. Mahoney, and M. Tusler. 2004. Development of the patient activation measure (PAM): Conceptualizing and measuring activation in patients and consumers. *Health Services Research* 39(4 Pt 1):1005–1026.

Hibbard, J. H., M. Geenlick, H. Jimison, J. Capizzi, and L. Kunkel. 2001. The impact of a community-wide self-care information project on self-care and medical care utilization. *Evaluation and the Health Professions* 24(4):404.

Higgins, T., E. Larson, and R. Schnall. 2017 (January). Unraveling the meaning of patient engagement: A concept analysis. *Patient Education and Counseling* 100(1):30–36.

Hirsch, J. and F. Marano. 2007. "Better Patient Care through Video Interpretation." https://www.hcinnovationgroup.com/home/article/13000339/better-patient-care-through-video-interpretation.

Ho, J. 2009. Consumer health informatics. *Studies in Health Technology and Informatics* 151:185–194.

Insignia. n.d. "Patient Activation Measure." Accessed on August 14, 2019. http://www.insigniahealth.com/products/pam-survey.

Huang, M., J. Fan, J. Prigge, N.D. Shah, B. A. Costello, and L. Yao. 2022. Characterizing patient-clinician Communication in secure medical messages: Retrospective study. *Journal of Medical Internet Research* 24(1).

IHI (Institute for Healthcare Improvement). n.d. "The IHI Triple Aim." Accessed June 10, 2024. http://www.ihi.org/Engage/Initiatives/TripleAim/pages/default.aspx.

IOM (Institute of Medicine). 2001. *Crossing the Quality Chasm: A New Health System for the 21st Century*. Washington, DC: National Academies Press.

Kahn, J. M. 2011. The use and misuse of ICU telemedicine. *Journal of the American Medical Association* 305(21):2227–2228.

Kim J. W., B. Ryu, S. Cho, E. Heo, Y. Kim, J. Lee, S. Y. Jung, and S. Yoo. 2019. Impact of personal health records and wearables on health outcomes and patient response: Three-arm randomized controlled trial. *JMIR Mhealth Uhealth* 4;7(1):e12070. doi: 10.2196/12070. PMID: 30609978; PMCID: PMC6682299.

Knebel, E. and A. C. Greiner, eds. 2003. *Health Professions Education: A Bridge to Quality*. Washington, DC: National Academies Press.

Kohn, L. T., J. M. Corrigan, and M. S. Donaldson. 2000. *To Err Is Human: Building a Safer Health System*. Washington, DC: National Academies Press.

Lordon, R., S. Mikles, L. Kneale, H. Evans, S. Munson, U. Backonja, and W. B. Lober. 2020. How patient-generated health data and patient-reported outcomes affect patient-clinician relationships: A systematic review. *Health Informatics Journal* 26(4):2689–2706. doi: 10.1177/1460458220928184. Epub 2020 Jun 20. PMID: 32567460; PMCID: PMC8986320.

Market.Us. 2024. "Fitness App Market Surges Towards USD 25.9 Billion by 2033: Growth Driven by Increasing Health Consciousness." https://www.globenewswire.com/en/news-release/2024/01/29/2818703/0/en/Fitness-App-Market-Surges-Towards-USD-25-9-Billion-by-2033-Growth-Driven-By-Increasing-Health-Consciousness.html#:~:text=Wearable%20Medical%20Devices%20Market%20size,at%20a%20CAGR%20of%2016.60%25.

Mate, K. 2022. On the quintuple aim: "Why Expand Beyond the Triple Aim?" Institute for Health Improvement. https://www.ihi.org/insights/quintuple-aim-why-expand-beyond-triple-aim.

Mayo Clinic. 2022. "Personal Health Records and Patient Portals." https://www.mayoclinic.org/healthy-lifestyle/consumer-health/in-depth/personal-health-record/art-20047273.

Melville, N. A. 2012 (January 18). Teledermatology sessions improve diagnoses, outcomes. *Medscape Medical News*. https://www.medscape.com/viewarticle/757108.

NIST (National Institute for Standards and Technology). 2013. *Test Procedure for §170.314(e)(3) Secure Messaging—Ambulatory Setting Only*. http://healthit.gov/sites/default/files/170.314e3securemessaging_2014_tp_approvedv1.3.pdf.

NIH (National Institutes of Health). 2024. "Human Genome Project." https://www.genome.gov/about-genomics/educational-resources/fact-sheets/human-genome-project.

NIH (National Institutes of Health). 2023. "The Cost of Sequencing a Human Genome." https://www.genome.gov/about-genomics/fact-sheets/Sequencing-Human-Genome-cost.

O'Connor, K. 2021. "Top 10 Healthcare Websites by Organic Traffic." https://www.scripted.com/content/top-10-healthcare-websites-by-organic-traffic.

ONC (Office of the National Coordinator for Health Information Technology). 2020. "2020–2025 Federal Health IT Strategic Plan." https://www.healthit.gov/sites/default/files/page/2020-10/Federal%20Health%20IT%20Strategic%20Plan_2020_2025.pdf.

ONC (Office of the National Coordinator for Health Information Technology). 2017. "What Is a Patient Portal?" http://www.healthit.gov/providers-professionals/faqs/what-patient-portal.

ONC (Office of the National Coordinator for Health Information Technology). 2015. "Connecting Health and Care for the Nation: A Shared Nationwide Interoperability Roadmap." https://www.healthit.gov/sites/default/files/nationwide-interoperability-roadmap-draft-version-1.0.pdf.

ONC (Office of the National Coordinator for Health Information Technology). n.d. "Patient-Generated Health Data." Accessed September 4, 2024. https://www.healthit.gov/topic/health-it-health-care-settings/patient-generated-health-data.

Omoloja, A., and S. Vundavalli. 2021 (November). Patient generated health data: Benefits and challenges. *Current Problems in Pediatric and Adolescent Health Care* 51(11):101103. https://pubmed.ncbi.nlm.nih.gov/34799255/. Epub 2021 Nov 16. PMID: 34799255.

Page, A., ed. 2004. *Keeping Patients Safe: Transforming the Work Environment of Nurses*. Washington, DC: National Academies Press.

PatientsLikeMe. n.d. "PatientsLikeMe: Live Better, Together." Accessed on January 16, 2024. https://www.patientslikeme.com.

Pomey, M., J. Denis, and V. Dumez. 2019. *Patient Engagement: How Patient-provider Partnerships Transform Healthcare Organizations*. Switzerland: Palgrave Macmillan.

Rainie, L. 2013. "E-patients and Social Media." Pew Research Center. https://www.slideshare.net/PewInternet/2013-101013-epatients-and-social-media-pdf.

Ruhi, U., and R. Chugh. 2021. Utility, value, and benefits of contemporary personal health records: Integrative review and conceptual synthesis. *Journal of Medical Internet Research*. 23(4):e26877. doi: 10.2196/26877. PMID: 33866308; PMCID: PMC8120425.

Sentell, T., W. Zhang, J. Davis, K. K. Baker, and K. L. Braun. 2014. The influence of community and individual health literacy on self-reported health status. *Journal of General Internal Medicine* 29(2):298–304.

Sequist, T. D., A. M. Zaslavsky, G. A. Colditz, and J. Z. Ayanian. 2011. Electronic patient messages to promote colorectal cancer screening: A randomized controlled trial. *Archives of Internal Medicine* 171(7):636–641.

Shapiro, M., D. Johnston, J. Wald, and D. Mon. 2012. "Patient-Generated Health Data: White Paper." Office of the National Coordinator for Health Information Technology. http://www.healthit.gov/sites/default/files/rti_pghd_whitepaper_april_2012.pdf.

Simon, G. E., J. D. Ralston, J. Savarino, C. Pabiniak, C. Wentzel, and B. H. Operskalski. 2011. Randomized trial of depression follow-up care by online messaging. *Journal of General Internal Medicine* 26(7): 698–704.

Sørensen, K., S. Van den Broucke, J. Fullam, G. Doyle, J. Pelikan, Z. Slonska, and H. Brand. 2012. Health literacy and public health: A systematic review and integration of definitions and models. *BMC Public*

*Health* 12(80). https://bmcpublichealth.biomedcentral.com/articles/10.1186/1471-2458-12-80.

Swan, M. 2013. The quantified self: Fundamental disruption in big data science and biological discovery. *Big Data* 1(2):85–99.

Tavenner, M., and K. Sebelius. 2012. Medicare and Medicaid programs; Electronic health record incentive program–Stage 2. *Federal Register* 77(171):53968–54162.

Taylor, E. F., T. Lake, J. Nysenbaum, G. Peterson, and D. Meyers. 2011. Coordinating care in the medical neighborhood: Critical components and available mechanisms. Mathematica Policy Research.

Turley, M., T. Garrido, A. Lowenthal, and Z. Y. Yvonne. 2012. Association between personal health record enrollment and patient loyalty. *American Journal of Managed Care* 18(7):e248–e253.

VA (Department of Veterans Affairs). n.d. "MyhealtheVet." Accessed September 4, 2024. https://www.myhealth.va.gov/mhv-portal-web/anonymous.portal?_nfpb=true&_nfto=false&_pageLabel=mhvHome.

Vat, L. E., T. Finlay, J., T. Jan Schuitmaker-Warnaar, N. Fahy, P. Robinson, M. Boudes, A. Diaz et al. 2020. Evaluating the "return on patient engagement initiatives" in medicines research and development: a literature review. *Health Expectations* 23(1):5–18.

WHO (World Health Organization). n.d. "Social Determinants of Health." Accessed July 11, 2024. http://www.who.int/social_determinants/en/.

Wunderlich, G. S., and P. O. Kohler. 2001. *Improving the Quality of Long-Term Care* (Institute of Medicine Committee on Improving the Quality of Long Term Care). Washington, DC: Division of Health Care Services. https://www.nap.edu/read/9611/chapter/1.

Young, L. B., P. S. Chan, X. Lu, B. K. Nallamothu, C. Sasson, and P. M. Cram. 2011. Impact of telemedicine intensive care unit coverage on patient outcomes: a systematic review and meta-analysis. *Archives of Internal Medicine* 171(6):498–506.

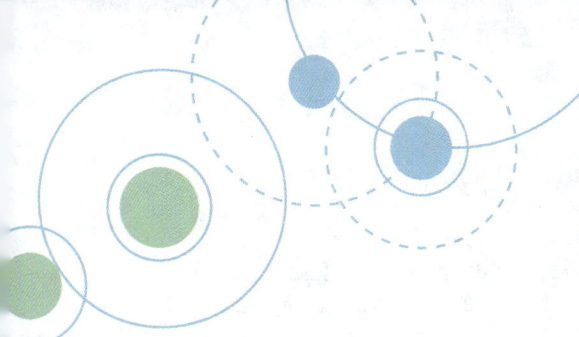

# chapter 15

# Healthcare Statistics

*Cindy Edgerton, MEd, MHA, RHIA*

## Learning Objectives

- Differentiate between inferential statistics and descriptive statistics
- Calculate and interpret statistical data related to volume of service, utilization, clinical services, and patient care
- Recommend ways healthcare administrators can use statistical data for decision-making
- Differentiate between diagnosis-related groups (DRGs) and case mix
- Identify vital statistics and evaluate how they are used
- Analyze how epidemiology and public health statistics influence patient care initiatives

## Key Terms

A&C
A&D
Autopsy
Average daily census
Bed count
Bed turnover rate
Descriptive statistics
Direct maternal death
Epidemiology
Fetal death
Fetal death rate
Gross autopsy rate
Gross death rate
Health statistics
Hospital autopsy rate
Hospital death rate
Hospital inpatient
Hospital newborn inpatient
Hospital outpatient
Incidence rate
Indirect maternal death
Infection rates
Inferential statistics
Inpatient admission
Inpatient bed occupancy rate
Inpatient census
Inpatient discharge
Inpatient service day (IPSD)
Length of stay (LOS)
Maternal death
Mean
Median
Mode
Morbidity
Mortality
National Vital Statistics System (NVSS)
Net autopsy rate
Net death rate
Newborn death rate
Nosocomial infection rate
Notifiable diseases
Population-based statistics
Prevalence rate
Rate
Ratio
Statistics

All healthcare entities depend on accurate, reliable, and robust data to report outcomes and make important decisions. Many of the data used in the decision-making process are presented as statistics in tables, spreadsheets, reports, or graphs. These data should be readily available and usable by healthcare managers and other staff who use data in their job.

Health information management (HIM) professionals are often at the heart of the data collection process that provides data to other departments and administrators who gather those data and organize them into valuable information. Because much of the data collected in the healthcare environment are abstracted from patient health records, the HIM department plays an important role in the process. HIM professionals ensure patient data are complete and accurate so that statistics and information used throughout the organization are reliable.

Statistics can be intimidating. This chapter intends to make healthcare statistics less scary and show how they can be easily calculated to assist with management of healthcare entities and become a part of day-to-day organizational decision-making.

## Introduction to Healthcare Statistics

**Statistics** can be defined as "a branch of mathematics concerned with collecting, organizing, summarizing, and analyzing data" (White 2023, 1). In the healthcare environment, statistics are usually referring to clinical data but can also involve data that assists with the operations of a healthcare entity. The US Library of Medicine (n.d.) describes **health statistics** as providing information for understanding, monitoring, improving, and planning the use of resources to improve the lives of people, provide services, and promote their well-being. Healthcare statistics are an important source of information for daily operations and decision-making by administrators and supervisors. Even staff use statistics in their daily work at times, to report information and make decisions.

### Use of Statistics

In many ways, health statistics help to improve healthcare quality and improve business operations. Statistical data are used by a wide variety of healthcare professionals, from administrators to providers and caregivers, to ancillary departments, department managers, researchers, and many others. With such a wide variety of users come a wide variety of uses and needs for healthcare statistics.

Healthcare administrators and department managers use healthcare statistics to make operations and business decisions every day. Budgets, capital expenditures, staffing, and strategic plans all involve complex decisions supported by data and statistical analysis. Clinical care statistics are also used to report on quality-of-care issues and patient care outcomes.

An example of using data and healthcare statistics for operational decision-making follows. A hospital chief financial officer (CFO) has been closely monitoring the budget because the hourly wage expense has spiked over the last couple of months. However, admissions and revenue has increased at the same pace. The CFO has been speaking with the departments affected to determine if the increased hourly wage expense is because of a need for more staffing due to increased admissions. For three months, the CFO graphed the three sets of data (hourly wage, admissions, and revenue) to illustrate the relationship between the data in each month as seen in figure 15.1.

This graph in figure 15.1 shows that as admissions increased, so did hourly wage and revenue, at about the same pace. For example, in January as admissions increased 15 percent over budget, revenue increased 21 percent and hourly wages increased 11 percent. February and March also show corresponding increases over budget between the three variables that provides evidence that the variables are related. The CFO will continue to monitor this to be sure that a

**Figure 15.1.** Analysis of hourly wages in relation to admissions and revenue

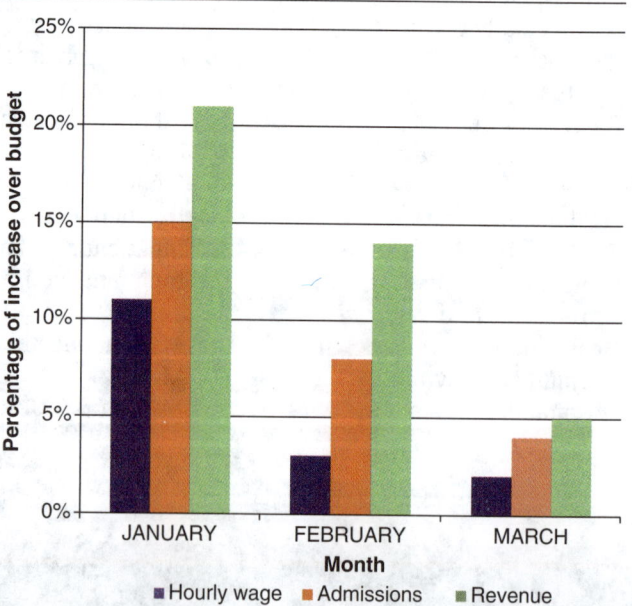

decrease in admissions and revenue is matched with a decrease in hourly wage.

In another example, clinical analysis can be used to make decisions that may impact quality of patient care. The nursing manager collects infection data each week and monitors hospital-acquired infections by computing statistics that show daily, weekly, monthly, quarterly, and then yearly numbers of these infections. If the statistical information indicates an infection rate higher than the standard, the nursing manager will work to find trends and issues and put processes into place to improve the infection rates. The nursing manager graphs the data to report to the nurses at their monthly staff meeting and provides the graphs and data to the infection control committee for their quarterly meetings.

Ancillary departments such as lab, radiology, and pathology use similar statistical data to make the same types of decisions. They use the data to make decisions about budget and staffing, and they use statistics to monitor quality within their department. All departments have goals and standards, and the statistical data are needed to measure if those standards are met. For instance, if the lab has a process standard that all hematology lab results are placed on the patient's chart within three hours of the blood draw, then statistical data regarding turnaround time must be collected and monitored to determine if the department is meeting that standard.

Researchers use existing data to compute statistics for their research studies or they collect their own data for statistical analysis. These statistics help them determine if their hypothesis is supported by the data or if the results are not what they were hoping for. Statistics are used in pharmaceutical studies and studies that are done to find treatments or cures for diseases. Researchers must be experts in data collection and analysis. Public health agencies, such as the Centers for Disease Control and Prevention (CDC), rely on statistics to inform them of disease trends, survival rates, and other public health concerns. These data are used to direct public health education initiatives and make decisions about which areas will receive the most financial support. For example, during the height of the COVID-19 pandemic, healthcare entities, providers, public health officials, the public, and government entities all relied on the CDC for statistics regarding infection rates, hospitalization rates, symptoms, and vaccination rates.

Another example of how statistics are used to improve patient health comes from the CDC's Morbidity and Mortality Weekly Report (MMWR). "Since 1961, when CDC began publishing MMWR, the publication has been considered to be the 'voice of CDC,' with a focus on communicating timely, authoritative, accurate, and objective scientific reports to guide public health action" (Rasmussen et al. 2020). MMWR focuses on the value of electronic quality data to public health reporting. "With greater EHR use, more health data are linked with available patient demographic information in a format that is easily retrievable and collected at the point of care" (Heisey-Grove et al. 2015). One example provided in the report was on the use of electronic clinical quality measures (eCQM). There were 63,000 healthcare providers who submitted data to the Medicare Electronic Health Records Incentive Program so the data could be analyzed with the goal of improving blood pressure control for hypertension patients. In a three-year reporting period, it was found that 62 percent of the patients achieved controlled blood pressure. These statistical data are being used to evaluate nationwide progress toward public health improvement goals (Heisey-Grove et al. 2015). It is through public health agencies' work that the news can report how many people had a heart attack last year, for example, and how many people were diagnosed with lung cancer.

## Sources of Data

In any study of statistics, it is important to consider the sources of the data used for statistical analysis. As mentioned earlier, the patient health record tends to be the most used source for statistical information in a healthcare organization. The health record is usually a primary data source as it is a "record that was developed by healthcare professionals in providing care or services to a patient" (White 2023, 3). It is the first place the data were recorded. Secondary data sources are created using the information from a primary data source. Some examples of secondary data sources are indices, registries, and reports created within the healthcare organization to manage data and assist with operations and decision-making. To create secondary data sources, data and information are abstracted from the primary data source. This means the data are pulled from the primary data source and placed in a database or in a special form used to collect data.

## Descriptive versus Inferential Statistics

When conducting statistical analysis, it is important to understand the difference between the two classifications: descriptive statistics and inferential statistics. **Descriptive statistics** are meant to *describe* a large amount of data by illustrating the data with charts, graphs, and tables in a way that the data are summarized and organized. Descriptive statistics are *not* used to draw conclusions about the population the data describe. An example is a graph showing how many patients at a specific medical clinic got the flu shot in 2023, based on age group.

On the other hand, **inferential statistics** are used to test a hypothesis and draw conclusions about the population. The conclusions are used to *infer* that the conclusions about the sample are reflective of the whole population from which the sample was taken. Consider the previous example about flu shots. A researcher might want to learn why people choose not to get the flu shot. Doing so would require research in the form of surveys or interviews of a sample of the population to come to conclusions about the whole population and why they choose not to get the flu shot.

## Basic Calculations and Descriptive Statistics

Before anyone can learn to use statistical formulas or understand statistical analysis, knowledge and review of some basic mathematical calculations is important. Mathematical calculations are the basis for many statistical formulas.

### Ratio

A **ratio** is a comparison of two numbers of the same type of data. The ratio is spoken as "a to b" but is usually written as a:b. For instance, an analysis of adult to pediatric patients at a local clinic finds that the ratio is five adult patients for every two pediatric patients. The ratio would be spoken as "five to two" and would be written as 5:2.

For small numbers in a population or set of data, the ratio can be seen without any mathematical calculation, but for large numbers there is a simple division equation, shown in the following formula, to ensure the ratio is stated in the lowest numbers possible. For example, a clinic has 5,000 adult patients and 2,000 pediatric patients. One way to show the ratio would be 5,000:2,000; however, that is cumbersome. In this case, both numbers are divisible by 1,000, as shown in the formula:

$$\text{Ratio} = \frac{x}{y} = \frac{5000}{2000} = \frac{5000/1000 = 5}{2000/1000 = 2}$$

The ratio is 5 : 2

### Rate

A **rate** is a type of ratio where the two numbers are representing different things. For example, a rate may compare the total number of patients with the number of patients who have a certain disease. Another example is the comparison of the total number of discharges with the number of discharges that were due to death. Rates are usually expressed as a percentage. For this reason, most rates should include the percent sign (%) after the value.

To calculate a rate, it is important to remember one formula. Once this formula is known, any type of rate can be easily calculated. The general rate formula is as follows:

$$\frac{\text{The number of times something happened}}{\text{The number of times it could have happened}} \times 100$$

Multiplying the rate by 100 puts the decimal point in the right place for a percentage. It means the difference between 0.305 percent (forgetting to multiply by 100) and 30.5 percent. This is a critical difference, so it is a step that must not be skipped.

Most often, the smaller number is divided by the larger number. For example, a health information manager wants to know the productivity rate of the coders in the HIM department this week. There were 239 discharges this week, so potentially, the coders could have coded all 239 discharged charts. However, they actually coded 192 of the charts. To calculate the rate, the HIM manager divides 192 (the number of times something happened) by 239 (the number of times something could have happened) and multiplies it by 100, for a rate of 80.33 percent:

$$\frac{192 \,(\text{Number of discharges coded this week})}{239 \,(\text{Total number of discharges this week})} \times 100 = 80.33\%$$

When reporting rates in healthcare, it is important not to round to less than two decimal places; it is often meaningful to show more detail than less because 5.09, 5.37, and 5.49 can signify important differences even though they could all be rounded down to 5. For instance, if these were lab results, the small differences could mean the difference between a normal and abnormal level.

## Average

The average is also referred to as the arithmetic average, the mean, or the arithmetic mean. The **mean** is the most common type of average. To calculate the mean, the sum of all numbers in a group of data is divided by the number of items in that group of data. For example, there may be a need to know the average age of the patients who attended a small diabetes seminar at the clinic. Eleven patients attended:

- *Step 1*: Add all the ages of the attendees. 49 + 62 + 68 + 54 + 42 + 31 + 62 + 48 + 38 + 36 + 28 = 518
- *Step 2*: Divide the total by the number of items in the data. 518/11 = 47

The average age of attendees at the diabetes seminar is 47.

Although the arithmetic mean is the most commonly reported type of average, there are two other types of average—median and mode. The **median** is the middle number in a set of scores, or the midpoint in a list of numbers or data. Values are listed in order and then the middle number is located, and that is the median. It is used instead of the mean when there is an extreme low or high score (outliers) that would skew the results in a way that they would not be valid or realistic (Salkind and Frey 2019).

To calculate the median in the previous example, do the following:

1. Place the list of numbers in the set of data into numerical order.
   The set of data: 49, 62, 68, 54, 42, 31, 62, 48, 38, 36, 28
   Listed in numerical order: 28, 31, 36, 38, 42, 48, 49, 54, 62, 62, 68

   Note: When there are multiple instances of the same number, each instance of that number is included in the list. See the above example and notice how 62 is listed twice because there were two instances of 62 in the data set.

2. Choose the number in the middle of the list: 28, 31, 36, 38, 42, **48**, 49, 54, 62, 62, 68
3. The median in this set of data is 48. If there is an even number of values in the data, then two numbers will be in the middle. If this is the case, the mean of those two numbers must be calculated. That will be the median.

The **mode** is the value with the highest frequency of occurrence. It is calculated by counting which number in a set of data occurs most often. Calculate the mode as follows:

1. List the numbers in the set of data in numerical order.
   The set of data: 5, 7, 9, 8, 9, 5, 6, 4, 2, 2, 3, 2, 5, 9, 8, 5, 5, 7, 5, 6, 5
   Listed in numerical order: 2, 2, 2, 3, 4, 5, 5, 5, 5, 5, 5, 5, 6, 6, 7, 7, 8, 8, 9, 9, 9
2. Count how many times each number occurs in the list:
   2–3
   3–1
   4–1
   5–7
   6–2
   7–2
   8–2
   9–3
3. The value of 5 occurs more times than any other of the values, so 5 is the mode.

The mode is used to find the most common or frequent value. For example, the mode may be used to find the most frequent Medicare severity diagnosis-related group (MS-DRG) for patients admitted in the month of December.

### Check Your Understanding 15.1

**Answer the following questions in a separate document.**

1. If there were 30 adult patients seen on a given day at City Clinic, and 10 pediatric patients, what is the ratio of adult patient visits to pediatric patient visits? How might this ratio be used by the clinic administrator?
2. Midwest Hospital admitted 780 patients for cancer diagnosis procedures in 2022. Of those patients, 430 were diagnosed with cancer. What is the rate of cancer diagnosis for this group of admissions? How might this information be used?
3. What is the average (mean) age for the following group of OB/GYN patients? How might this information be helpful to the hospital administrator and OB/GYN medical staff?

| Admission | Discharge | Department | Patient age |
|---|---|---|---|
| 6/15/23 | 6/16/23 | OB/GYN | 26 |
| 6/15/23 | 6/17/23 | OB/GYN | 32 |
| 6/15/23 | 6/17/23 | OB/GYN | 29 |
| 6/16/23 | 6/20/23 | OB/GYN | 36 |
| 6/17/23 | 6/18/23 | OB/GYN | 28 |
| 6/17/23 | 6/20/23 | OB/GYN | 40 |
| 6/18/23 | 6/20/23 | OB/GYN | 32 |

4. For the same group of patients in this table, what is the median of the patient ages? Why is the median important?

5. For the same group of patients in this table, what is the mode of the patient ages? What does the mode indicate?

6. If the medical staff quality committee wants to determine if prediabetic women who take Ozempic are less likely to be diagnosed with diabetes, would they use descriptive or inferential statistics? Explain your rationale.

## Terminology Related to Healthcare Statistics

Studying any topic requires commitment to learning the topic's terminology. The study of statistics is no different. HIM professionals must be familiar with many statistical terms related to healthcare statistics. HIM professionals may assist with the calculations of these types of statistics or the collection and reporting of the data.

- **Hospital inpatient**: "A patient who is provided with room, board, and continuous general nursing service in an area of an acute-care facility where patients generally stay at least overnight" (IHS n.d.).
- **Hospital outpatient**: A patient who receives hospital services without being admitted for inpatient care. An outpatient may be classified as either an emergency outpatient, an observation patient, or a clinic outpatient.
    - An emergency outpatient is admitted to the emergency department of a hospital for diagnosis and treatment of a condition that requires immediate medical, dental, or other emergency services.
    - A clinic outpatient is admitted to a clinical service of the clinic or hospital for diagnosis and treatment on an ambulatory basis.
    - An observation patient is defined as "one who presents with a medical condition that imposes a significant degree of instability and disability and who needs to be monitored, evaluated, and assessed to determine whether he or she should be admitted for inpatient care or discharged for care in another setting" (White 2023, 53). The process for reporting or counting these patients will vary depending on hospital policy.
- **Hospital newborn inpatient**: A patient born in the hospital at the beginning of the current patient hospitalization.
    - Newborns are usually counted separately because their care is so different from that of other inpatients.
    - Infants born on the way to the hospital or at home are considered hospital inpatients, not hospital newborn inpatients.
- **Inpatient admission**: An acute-care facility's formal acceptance of a patient who is to be provided with room, board, and continuous nursing service in an area of the facility where patients generally stay overnight.
- **Inpatient discharge**: The termination of hospitalization through the formal release of an inpatient by the hospital.
    - The term includes patients who are discharged alive (by a healthcare provider's order), who are discharged against medical advice (AMA), or who died while hospitalized.
    - Unless otherwise indicated, inpatient discharges include deaths.
- **Inpatient service day (IPSD)**: The unit of measure denoting the services received by one inpatient in one 24-hour period. The term is often shortened and referred to simply as patient day.
- **Inpatient census**: Indicates the number of inpatients present in the hospital at a particular point in time.

# Statistics Related to Volume of Service and Utilization

Monitoring the volume of service is an important factor in managing healthcare services at any type of facility. In other words, how many patients are served in a specific period and the type of services each patient receives should be monitored. It is important for administrators to keep a constant watch on numbers of patients, numbers and types of services provided, and utilization of resources. The collected data related to volume of service are critical to making daily operational decisions that affect staffing and budgeting, inventory of supplies, space needs, and technology needs.

## Inpatient Census

Inpatient census is an important volume measure tracked in the hospital environment. The inpatient census indicates the number of inpatients present in the hospital at a particular point in time. Before hospitals had robust automated systems for tracking inpatients' status, census reporting was a manual process. Today, it is an automated process because the movement of patients from nursing unit to nursing unit, or from inpatient status to discharged, is entered into the computer and the software can be used to pull census data at any given time.

Because during the course of any given day, patients are discharged, new patients are admitted, and patients are transferred between units within the hospital, the census data can vary throughout the day. For instance, at 9:00 a.m. six patients are discharged, but at the same time two patients are admitted. Between 9:15 and 10:00 a.m., three more patients are admitted. This would make the census data at 9:00 a.m. different than census data at 10:00 a.m. This will change throughout the day. For this reason, each hospital must decide on a consistent time to take the census and use that time every day. This ensures consistent and valid data. Midnight is a common census-taking time.

### Daily Inpatient Census

The daily inpatient census is the technical name for the census data reported at midnight or other official census-taking time. The daily inpatient census will include all patients present as inpatients at midnight, plus any patients admitted and discharged during the same day. These patients are referred to as **A&D**, which symbolizes patients admitted and discharged on the same day. These patients are not present at midnight for the census-taking time, but they must still be counted because they were classified as an inpatient at some point during that day. For example, a patient is admitted through the emergency department at 6:49 p.m. on June 15, but the patient dies at 9:22 p.m. on the same day. Because this patient was an inpatient and received inpatient services, they must be counted in the daily inpatient census. Forgetting to include the A&D patients in the census would not accurately reflect service volume. The daily inpatient census should reflect all the patients treated as inpatients during the 24-hour period. In table 15.1, a daily census report is illustrated. Notice there is a separate column labeled NB for newborn reporting as well as a column labeled **A&C** for adults and children. In a daily census, newborns are reported separately because they require a different type and volume of service and care compared to inpatient adults and children.

Also note that the daily census indicates numbers transferred in and transferred out. When case managers and healthcare providers talk about transferring a patient at discharge, they are usually discussing a transfer to another facility. In the case of the daily census, transfers are simply patients transferring from one nursing unit in the hospital to another, or intra-hospital transfers. For instance, an 89-year-old patient was admitted to the intensive care unit (ICU) after suffering a heart attack, but three days later was moved out of the ICU to the cardiac care unit. This patient has been transferred out of the ICU and transferred into the cardiac care unit. In this 24-hour period, this would count as one transfer out and one transfer in. In the daily census, the totals for transferred in and transferred out should be equal. Any transfer to another facility would be a discharge and recorded in the daily census as such.

### Inpatient Service Days

An IPSD is a unit of measure reflecting the services received by one inpatient during a 24-hour period

**Table 15.1.** Daily census

| Line # | | Newborns | A&C |
|---|---|---|---|
| 1 | Remaining last report | 11 | 159 |
| 2 | Admitted | 5 | 42 |
| 3 | Transferred in | 0 | 8 |
| 4 | Total (sum of lines 1, 2, 3) | 16 | 209 |
| 5 | Transferred out | 0 | 8 |
| 6 | Discharged | 8 | 49 |
| 7 | Died | 0 | 2 |
| 8 | Total (sum of lines 5, 6, 7) | 8 | 59 |
| 9 | **Remaining midnight** (Line 4 — Line 8 =) | 8 | **150** |

(White 2023, 35). An IPSD can be thought of as one for each patient treated. Therefore, the daily inpatient census will be equal to the number of IPSDs for that day. The IPSD is an important measure of volume of services provided by the facility. IPSDs will be reported on a daily, weekly, monthly, quarterly, and annual basis to track volume of service that has a direct correlation to amount of revenue. CFOs will be very interested in IPSD reports, as the reports are one reflection of the facility's financial condition because IPSDs are included in calculations determining cost per patient and revenue totals per patient.

### Census Calculation

As seen in table 15.1, calculating the daily census consists of counting the patients who remained at the previous midnight, adding the admissions for the next 24-hour period, and subtracting the discharges in that same period. This is typically automated, and a report similar to table 15.1 could be generated daily if needed. Another important calculation in daily census reporting is the average daily census. The *average daily census* is the mean number of hospital inpatients present in the hospital each day for a given period. The formula for calculating the average daily census is as follows:

$$\text{Average daily census} = \frac{\text{Total number of inpatient service days for a given period}}{\text{Total number of days in the period}}$$

Just as newborns (NBs) and adults and children (A&C) are reported separately on the daily census report, they can be reported separately for the average daily census as well. This helps managers and administrators with planning for the different levels of services and budgeting for the newborn unit separately from other nursing units. The formula for calculating the average daily census for adults and children is as follows:

$$\text{Average daily census for } A \text{ Cs} = \frac{\text{Total number of inpatient service days for A \& Cs for a given period}}{\text{Total number of days in the period}}$$

The formula for calculating the average daily census for newborns is as follows:

$$\text{Average daily census for NBs} = \frac{\text{Total number of inpatient service days for NBs for a given period}}{\text{Total number of days in the period}}$$

### Using Census Reports

In addition to the daily census report shown in table 15.1, other census reports such as monthly, quarterly, and annual census reports are created to give managers and administrators a bigger picture of the census activity. While daily and monthly census reports are used to react to current budget needs, quarterly and annual reports are used for future staffing and budgeting considerations. The census data are also used in strategic planning when deciding on areas for expansion or development. The following examples illustrate real-life scenarios where census data are used daily.

***Hospital Census in Practice***  Liz Taylor, MS, RHIT, former health information director at Sharon Hospital in Sharon, CT, explains that

> As part of the daily organizational safety huddle, we review the patient census statistics to determine our patient volume for the day, what departments may be overburdened or at full capacity as well as address any immediate or urgent staffing and/or resource needs. This discussion also provides an opportunity for other departments and ancillary services to know and be prepared for downstream effects of an overburdened or full capacity unit. Quick discussions and requests for assistance are held, opportunities to address or elicit assistance for other resources or needs for a particular service or assessments/resources can be noted and more detailed discussions held as appropriate outside of the huddle.
>
> The patient statistics discussion at the huddle alerts other departments and services of volume, resources, critical patients, needs for staffing and/or opportunities for service and/or service recovery. Patient engagement and patient satisfaction is known to be an outgrowth (at times) of patient census (high volume, staffing shortages, resources) and helps the organization to recognize such trends and take appropriate action. Patient census statistics and patient engagement (satisfaction) is crucial to the future of value-based purchasing initiatives for healthcare organizations. First and foremost, the patient census statistics discussion at the daily morning huddle is a safety-first initiative and brings patient safety to the forefront of every discussion every day. (Taylor 2015)

This is an example of how the census is used daily by various departments in a hospital. It shows how the census data are used to make both operational and patient care decisions. This hospital's daily census huddle equips staff with data and knowledge from which decisions can be made throughout the day.

**The Important Use of a Daily Census Report** Jen Hoefs, CRHCP, Patient Care Coordinator at Burnett Medical Center, a critical access hospital in Grantsburg, WI, explains how a daily census report is used in various areas of the hospital:

> The utilization of the daily census report is a vital component of patient case management by key staff members in the healthcare setting. It serves as an overall snapshot of how many patients are in the hospital at a given moment in time and under what type they have been registered (inpatient, observation, swing bed, hospice, respite).
>
> The census report is generated by a designated patient access staff member each morning after ensuring that all overnight registrations to an inpatient observation, swing bed, respite, and hospice status have been completed. This report is verified against a hard copy of the current patients on the medical-surgical (med-surg) floor that was created by the med-surg nursing station health unit coordinator. This report is then distributed to key staff members involved in the patients' care/management.
>
> Listed are a few examples of how some of these key staff members utilize and rely on this report.
>
> - Utilization review (UR) coordinator: This staff member utilizes the report to keep track of the number of days patients have been in the hospital, to which doctor they have been admitted, and what type of patient status they fall under; for example, inpatient medical, inpatient respite, inpatient hospice, inpatient surgery, observation, or OB observation. The UR coordinator also uses this to prep for the daily patient planning meeting to ensure that the length of stay is correct and in line with the patient's insurance guidelines for that specific diagnosis and treatment currently taking place.
> - Dietitian/dietary department: The dietary department uses this report to determine how many meals they will need to prepare while working closely with the dietitian on staff to ensure the patients' specific diet requirements are being met. The dietitian uses this report to review the patients' records regarding their diets that are ordered by the providers; for example, a diabetic diet, gluten-free diet, low-sodium diet, cardiac diet, or a liquid diet.
> - Business office manager: This staff member uses this report to track who is placed in a bed currently and under what patient type class they fall; for example, inpatient, observation, or swing bed. They use this report to prepare for the daily patient care planning meeting looking at it from the facility's financial perspective to ensure that the proper steps are being completed to bill the patients' insurance appropriately, accurately, and promptly. This staff member works closely with the UR coordinator.
> - Social services: These staff members utilize this report to visit with the patients and determine and assist the patient in arranging and discussing any services that may be needed upon discharge; for example, a nursing home placement, in-house assistance once returning to home, questions related to living wills and advance directives for healthcare, and medical power of attorney.
> - Infection control: This staff member uses this report to review patient records to determine if appropriate infection control precautions are in place, being followed, and if there are any cases of infection that need to be reported.
> - Emergency department: This team uses this report to determine bed availability for patients who may need to be admitted
> - Ancillary department (radiology, pharmacy, and physical/occupational therapy): These departments use this report as a case management tool in determining the patient's name, room number, patient class status, and to verify if any of the current orders are for procedures, therapies, or medications for patients who are currently in-house.
>
> (Hoefs 2015)

This is another example of how patient census is used by various departments to make crucial decisions throughout the day. Census data are much more than numbers posted in the system each day. These data are tracked, analyzed, used, and discussed within healthcare teams daily and are a very important statistic.

## Occupancy Data

Along with inpatient census, another important measure of volume of service and utilization is inpatient bed occupancy. Bed occupancy is monitored, and occupancy rates are used for decisions about staffing, materials, and other budget items. Occupancy rate, or percentage of occupancy, is an important indicator of the hospital's financial picture. The **inpatient bed occupancy rate** is the percentage of official beds occupied by hospital inpatients for a given period. Hospitals strive for a high occupancy rate because that usually equates with higher revenues.

## Bed Count

To calculate occupancy rate, the bed count must be known. The **bed count** is the number of inpatient beds set up and staffed for use on a given day. These beds are included whether they are occupied or not. Bed count is one way a hospital is classified. For example, it is likely that bed count will be indicated in the overview of the hospital on a hospital website. For instance:

> Valley Hospital is a 129-bed acute-care hospital with a 72-bed skilled care nursing home, and a 156-bed assisted living facility. Valley Hospital also operates three outpatient multispecialty clinics within the Valley community.

There are also times when a hospital may need to set up temporary beds, especially during a disaster or an epidemic when the need for care in the community is greater than the normal number of existing beds. The hospital's licensing body allows it to set up beds as needed. In these unusual cases, the temporary beds do not count as part of the official bed count.

## Calculating Inpatient Bed Occupancy Rate

When calculating inpatient bed occupancy rate, the numerator is the total number of IPSDs for the given period and the denominator is the total possible IPSDs for the given period. The maximum number of IPSDs indicates that every available bed in the hospital is occupied every single day (White 2023, 35). The occupancy rate compares the number of patients treated daily to the number of patients who could have been treated. The formula for calculating the inpatient bed occupancy rate is as follows:

$$\text{Inpatient bed occupancy} = \frac{\text{Total number of inpatient service days for a given period}}{\text{Total number of inpatient bed count for the same period}} \times 100$$

For example, if 325 patients occupied 370 beds on July 25, the inpatient bed occupancy rate would be 87.8 percent (325/370 × 100). If the rate were for more than one day, the number of days would have to be factored in, so the number of beds would be multiplied by the number of days in the given time. For instance, if the occupancy rate was being calculated for a week, the number of beds would be multiplied by seven for the seven days in the week. If the same hospital wanted to measure occupancy rate for the week of July 25, 370 (number of beds) would be multiplied by 7 (number of days in the week). Therefore, there are a possible 2,590 IPSDs in a week at this hospital. In this given week, there were 2,190 IPSDs. To calculate the occupancy rate, the equation would look like this: ([2,190/{370 × 7}] × 100). The occupancy rate at this hospital for the week of July 25 would be 84.55 percent.

It is possible that a hospital could report an occupancy rate of greater than 100 percent. When a hospital is full and uses temporary beds, the temporary beds are not added to the denominator when calculating occupancy rate. If the inpatient bed count at the hospital is 290 and 5 temporary beds are used for a certain period, the total number of inpatient bed count is still 290. For example, on October 2, Community Hospital has 279 patients occupying their 290 inpatient beds. But a tragic train derailment occurs in the afternoon and 16 patients are rushed to the hospital and temporary beds are set up to serve all the patients. The IPSDs for October 2 is 295 (279 + 16). The occupancy rate for the day would be calculated as 295/290 × 100, which equals 101 percent. If an occupancy rate is greater than 100 percent, it can be concluded that all the hospital beds are occupied with the addition of temporary beds.

## Hospital Bed Turnover

Another important measure of volume of service and utilization at a hospital is the **bed turnover rate**. This measure indicates how many times each bed was occupied in a given period. This information is a statistic that helps administrators make decisions about budgeting and staffing, as well as strategic planning. For instance, if the hospital has a high turnover rate, this means that it experiences many short stays. Administrators know that every time a patient leaves, the room and bed must be cleaned and sterilized at a higher level than the daily cleaning that happens when a patient remains in the room. This means that high turnover requires a higher level of cleaning staff, which increases the budget for housekeeping. High turnover also increases the workload for case managers, nurses, and many other staff throughout the hospital. The formula for the bed turnover rate is as follows:

> Bed turnover rate =
> $\dfrac{\text{Number of discharges for the time period}}{\text{The bed count for the time period}}$

For example, City Hospital had 1,899 discharges and deaths for the month of July. The bed count is 420. Therefore, the bed turnover rate is 4.5 percent (1,899/420). This illustrates that, on average, each bed had 4.5 patients occupying the bed during the month of July.

## Length of Stay

Length of stay (LOS) is an important measure of utilization and volume of service at any hospital. When a patient is discharged, the LOS is indicated. **Length of stay (LOS)** is the number of days a patient occupied a hospital bed. An important thing to remember when counting LOS is that the day of discharge is not counted. If patient A was admitted on August 4 and discharged on August 7, his or her LOS is three days. To calculate this using a mathematical equation, the day of admission is subtracted from the day of discharge. For patient A, this would be calculated as (7 − 4 = 3). There is a slightly different approach when the patient is discharged in a different month than the admission. The day of admission is subtracted from the last day of the admission month, the first day of the discharge month is subtracted from the discharge date, and one transition day between the months is added (White 2023, 68). For example, if the patient is admitted on July 28 and discharged on August 4, the LOS is ([July 31−July 28 = 3 days] + [August 4 − August 1 = 3 days] + [1 transition day between July and August]), 3 + 3 + 1 = 7.

Another way to think of this is to count the days the patient was in the hospital, but do not count the day of discharge. In the example above where the patient was admitted on August 4 and discharged on August 7, August 4, 5, and 6 are counted for a total of three days. The final day, August 7, is not counted.

It is common for a patient to be admitted and discharged on the same day. In this case, regardless of how many hours they were an inpatient, the LOS is one day. Remember, the day of discharge is not counted when figuring LOS, so a patient who is admitted one day and discharged the next is also counted as an LOS of one day. The LOS for a patient who is admitted on November 5 at 6:30 a.m. and discharged on November 5 at 4:50 p.m. is one day. The LOS for a patient who is admitted on November 5 at 6:30 a.m. and discharged on November 6 at 11 a.m. is also one day.

In a given period of time, the LOS for all of the patients is added up for a total LOS. For example, if the chief of staff would like to know the total LOS for the ICU for the patients who were either discharged or died on July 15. Table 15.2 may be assembled as an illustration of this total LOS.

This total LOS indicates the number of days care was provided to these patients who were either discharged or died. It is typical that LOS will be calculated for each department or nursing unit, and then for the hospital.

The hospital administration may also want to know the average length of stay (ALOS) for each day, each week, each month, each quarter, and then the annual LOS. ALOS is calculated from the total LOS data collected each day. The total LOS is divided by the number of patients discharged in the same period. Using table 15.2, the average length of stay for the six patients discharged from the ICU on July 15 is 5.33 (32/6). The general formula for calculating ALOS is as follows:

> Average length of stay =
> $\dfrac{\text{Total length of stay for a given period}}{\text{Total number of discharges, including deaths, for the same period}}$

Along with the measures discussed earlier, the ALOS for adults and children (A&C) would be reported separately from the newborn ALOS.

Table 15.3 is an example of a summary report that illustrates all the statistics discussed in this section. The HIM department may be responsible for compiling this type of report periodically for meetings and planning sessions.

**Table 15.2.** Total length of stay

| Patient | LOS |
|---|---|
| 1 | 2 |
| 2 | 7 |
| 3 | 5 |
| 4 | 9 |
| 5 | 6 |
| 6 | 3 |
| **Total LOS** | 32 |

Table 15.3. Statistical summary, Community Hospital, period ending July 20XX

| Admissions | July 20XX Actual | July 20XX Budget | Year-to-Date 20XX Actual | Year-to-Date 20XX Budget |
|---|---|---|---|---|
| Medical | 1,022 | 916 | 8,116 | 7,864 |
| Surgical | 629 | 645 | 4,259 | 4,264 |
| OB/GYN | 590 | 650 | 4,870 | 4,510 |
| Psychiatry | 211 | 205 | 1,640 | 1,700 |
| Physical medicine and rehab | 69 | 60 | 420 | 410 |
| Other adult | 241 | 214 | 1,810 | 1,690 |

| Admissions | July 20XX Actual | July 20XX Budget | Year-to-Date 20XX Actual | Year-to-Date 20XX Budget |
|---|---|---|---|---|
| Total adult | 2,762 | 2,690 | 21,115 | 20,438 |
| Newborn | 480 | 502 | 3,410 | 3,620 |
| Total admissions | 3,242 | 3,192 | 24,525 | 24,058 |

| Average length of stay | July 20XX Actual | July 20XX Budget | Year-to-Date 20XX Actual | Year-to-Date 20XX Budget |
|---|---|---|---|---|
| Medical | 5.6 | 5.8 | 5.7 | 5.9 |
| Surgical | 6.5 | 6.5 | 6.8 | 6.9 |
| OB/GYN | 1.5 | 1.8 | 2 | 2.1 |
| Psychiatry | 12.2 | 12.4 | 11.8 | 11.5 |
| Physical medicine and rehab | 28.2 | 26 | 24 | 25.5 |
| Other adult | 4.6 | 4.4 | 4.2 | 4.4 |
| Newborn | 3 | 3.4 | 3.5 | 3.5 |
| Total ALOS | 5.5 | 5.3 | 5.5 | 5.3 |

| Patient days | July 20XX Actual | July 20XX Budget | Year-to-Date 20XX Actual | Year-to-Date 20XX Budget |
|---|---|---|---|---|
| Medical | 4,760 | 4,890 | 33,290 | 32,980 |
| Surgical | 4,320 | 4,500 | 34,650 | 34,800 |
| OB/GYN | 1,420 | 1,720 | 12,120 | 12,210 |
| Psychiatry | 1,767 | 1,554 | 9,800 | 9,223 |
| Physical medicine and rehab | 1,219 | 1,210 | 9,987 | 9,722 |
| Other adult | 744 | 756 | 4,920 | 4,968 |
| Total adult | 14,230 | 14,630 | 104,767 | 103,903 |
| Newborn | 2,210 | 2,087 | 15,120 | 14,863 |
| Total patient days | 16,440 | 16,717 | | |

| Other key statistics | July 20XX Actual | July 20XX Budget | Year-to-Date 20XX Actual | Year-to-Date 20XX Budget |
|---|---|---|---|---|
| Average daily census | 545 | 569 | 562 | 562 |
| Average beds available | 687 | 670 | 687 | 670 |
| Clinic visits | 24,631 | 21,621 | 165,281 | 157,523 |
| Emergency visits | 3,952 | 3,890 | 32,242 | 31,404 |
| Inpatient surgery patients | 621 | 554 | 4,023 | 3,690 |
| Outpatient surgery patients | 829 | 789 | 5,120 | 4,675 |

## Check Your Understanding 15.2

**Answer the following questions in a separate document.**

1. A patient is admitted through the emergency department at 1:23 p.m. on December 2, but the patient dies at 7:52 p.m. on the same day. Should this patient be included in the daily census? Why or why not?

2. What is the average daily census for A&C for March if the total IPSDs was 6,256? Explain how you reached your answer.

3. What is the daily inpatient census for July 16 if the census at midnight for July 15 was 239 and there were 59 discharges, 67 admissions, and 24 A&Ds? Explain how you reached your answer.

4. For the following table, calculate the length of stay for each patient.

|  | Admission | Discharge | Length of stay |
|---|---|---|---|
| Patient A | June 5 | June 8 |  |
| Patient B | June 6 | June 6 |  |
| Patient C | June 11 | June 17 |  |
| Patient D | June 29 | July 3 |  |
| Patient E | June 15 | June 16 |  |
| Patient F | June 21 | June 28 |  |
| Patient G | June 26 | July 1 |  |

5. For the following table of patient data, calculate the average length of stay statistics.

| Date | Number of patients discharged | Discharge days | Average length of stay |
|---|---|---|---|
| June 2 | 16 | 86 |  |
| June 3 | 22 | 119 |  |
| June 4 | 12 | 54 |  |
| June 5 | 19 | 109 |  |
| June 6 | 15 | 45 |  |
| June 7 | 24 | 128 |  |
| June 8 | 18 | 68 |  |

## Statistics Related to Clinical Services and Patient Care

Along with the many calculations this chapter has introduced to measure utilization and volume of service, there are many other important statistical calculations in the healthcare environment that indicate levels of clinical services and patient care. These statistics often relate to quality of patient care, or the severity of illness of each facility's patient demographics. Each hospital reports morbidity and mortality rates for all patients discharged within a certain period. Epidemiologists define **morbidity** as being symptomatic of an illness or disease and **mortality** as another word for an incidence of death in a specific population. These data help identify opportunities for improvement, trends, and any issues that may need immediate attention. These types of statistics can be reported as a whole for the hospital, but can also be broken down by department, nursing unit, or individual healthcare provider to determine if any cases of excellence or any issues are isolated to just one certain area, or if they are hospital-wide.

### Death Rates

An important measure of quality of care and patient demographic for each hospital is the **hospital death rate**. This is calculated using the number of patients discharged from the hospital (both alive and dead) during a specific period. As discussed earlier, deaths are always counted as discharges because it is one way to end a patient's hospitalization. Following are the types of death rates that may be calculated for each hospital.

## Gross Death Rate

The **gross death rate** is the number of all hospital discharges compared to the number of deaths from that same group of patients. It indicates the proportion of deaths, or mortality, that the hospital experiences in a period. The gross death rate is calculated by dividing the total number of deaths occurring in that time by the total number of discharges, including deaths, for the same time period. The formula for calculating the gross death rate is as follows:

$$\text{Gross death rate} = \frac{\text{Total number of inpatient deaths (including NBs) for a given period}}{\text{Total number of discharges, including A\&C and NB deaths, for the same time period}} \times 100$$

For example, Midwest Hospital reported 19 deaths (both A&C and NB) during the month of August. There were 689 total discharges, including deaths. The gross death rate is 2.75 percent ([19/689] × 100).

## Net Death Rate

The **net death rate** is a death rate that is adjusted so that certain deaths are not counted against the hospital. The net death rate does not include any deaths that occurred within 48 hours of the patient's admission to the hospital. This is an important measure because 48 hours is not usually enough time to improve the patient's health. Especially if the patient was admitted to the hospital gravely ill and died within 48 hours, it is assumed that the care providers did all they could, but the patient was so ill upon admission that there was not enough time to treat them to result in a positive outcome. The formula for calculating the net death rate is as follows:

$$\text{Net death rate} = \frac{\text{Total number of inpatient deaths (including NBs) minus deaths} < 48 \text{ hours of admission for a given period of time}}{\text{Total number of discharges (includings NBs) minus deaths} < 48 \text{ hours for the same period}} \times 100$$

Using the data from the previous example of gross death rate, Midwest Hospital reported 19 deaths (both A&C and NB) during the month of August. Six of those were within 48 hours of admission. There were 689 total discharges. Therefore, the net death rate is 1.9 percent ([{19 − 6} / {689 − 6}] × 100). It is important to report the net death rate because it will usually be a lower death rate and may be a more accurate indicator of quality care.

## Newborn Death Rate

Although newborn deaths are included in a hospital's gross death rate and net death rate calculations, it can also be valuable to calculate a newborn death rate separately. This measure can give important information about mortality and morbidity of newborns at each individual hospital. The number of newborns at a hospital includes only those born alive at the hospital. The **newborn death rate** is the number of newborns who died in comparison to the total number of newborns discharged, alive and dead. To be counted as a newborn death, the newborn must have been delivered alive (White 2023, 98). A stillborn infant is not counted in any death rate statistics because, by definition of *stillborn*, the infant was not born alive. The formula for calculating the newborn death rate is as follows:

$$\text{Newborn death rate} = \frac{\text{Total number of NB deaths for a given period}}{\text{Total number of NB discharges (including deaths) for the same period}} \times 100$$

For example, Midwest Hospital reported three newborn deaths during the month of August. There were 69 newborn discharges (including these three deaths). The newborn death rate is 4.34 percent ([3/69] × 100).

## Fetal Death Rate

Fetal death rates are tracked and reported to help understand the prevalence and causes of these events. Per the American Academy of Pediatrics, **fetal death** is "death before the complete expulsion or extraction from the mother of a product of human conception, irrespective of the duration of pregnancy that is not an induced termination of pregnancy" (Barfield et al. 2016). It is important to understand that a fetal death classification indicates that the fetus did not have a heartbeat or was not breathing at the time of expulsion or extraction.

Fetal deaths are categorized according to the number of weeks of gestation and "for statistical purposes, fetal deaths are further subdivided as 'early'

(20–27 weeks' gestation) or 'late' (≥28 weeks' gestation)" (Barfield et al. 2016). Stillbirth is a term that is also used to describe fetal death using these parameters of gestation. A fetal death in utero, prior to 20 weeks gestation, is classified as a miscarriage (Barfield et al. 2016)

Hospitals and public health agencies calculate fetal death rates for reporting purposes. There are varying reporting requirements depending on the state. To calculate the fetal death rate, divide the total number of early and late fetal deaths for the period by the total number of live births and early and late fetal deaths for the same period. Remember that pregnancy loss prior to 20 weeks is not included in the calculation for fetal death rate. The formula for calculating the fetal death rate is as follows:

$$\text{Fetal death rate} = \frac{\text{Total number of early and late,}}{\text{fetal deaths for a given period}} \times 100$$
$$\frac{\text{Total number of live births plus total}}{\text{number of early and late fetal}}$$
$$\text{deaths for the same period}$$

For example, Midwest Hospital reported 329 live births and 8 early and 2 late fetal deaths during the month of August. The fetal death rate is 2.94 percent ([8 + 2/{329 + 8 + 2}] × 100).

## Maternal Death Rate

Another specific area of death rates that hospital administrators and managers find important to track is the hospital maternal death rate. A maternal death is the death of any woman while pregnant or within 42 days of delivery from any cause related to, or aggravated by, pregnancy or its management, regardless of the duration of the pregnancy or the site of the death. Maternal deaths that are not related to the pregnancy, such as a car accident, are not counted in the maternal death rate.

Maternal deaths are referred to as either direct or indirect. A direct maternal death is the death of a woman resulting from obstetrical (OB) complications of the pregnancy state, labor, or puerperium (the period within 42 days following delivery). Direct maternal deaths are included in the maternal death rate. Some examples of direct maternal causes of death would be infection, hemorrhage, obstructed labor, and hypertensive disorders such as eclampsia. An indirect maternal death is the death of a woman from a previously existing disease or a disease that developed during pregnancy, labor, or the puerperium that was not due to obstetric causes, although the physiologic effects of pregnancy were partially responsible. Indirect maternal deaths are not included in the maternal death rate. Maternal death rates are tracked as an indicator of quality of care, but they can also help researchers and public health agencies understand trends in prenatal care and conditions that may be increasing in prevalence. The statistics can identify prenatal care needs in certain communities that will lead to public health initiatives.

The formula for calculating the hospital maternal death rate is as follows:

$$\text{Hospital maternal death rate} = \frac{\text{Total number of direct maternal deaths for a given period}}{\text{Total number of maternal (OB) discharges, including deaths, for the same period}} \times 100$$

As an example, in August, Midwest Hospital reported 330 maternal discharges. Two of these patients died. The maternal death rate for August is 0.60 percent ([2/330] × 100).

## Autopsy Rates

An autopsy, also known as a postmortem examination, is the examination and study of a dead body to determine the cause of death. Although autopsies are not performed for every death, they are very helpful in the education and training of medical and other clinical care students. They are also valuable for continued research of the human body and cause of disease. Family members also find autopsy results very useful in identifying diseases that are hereditary so that family members can be proactive in disease prevention and treatment. Autopsies in the hospital are usually conducted by pathologists or another physician trained in this area. When the autopsy is complete, the autopsy report is created and documented in the patient's health record. The next sections discuss the different types of autopsies that are commonly conducted in a hospital.

## Gross Autopsy Rate

The gross autopsy rate includes all deaths that occurred with inpatients, and it indicates the proportion of those on which an autopsy was performed. The formula for calculating the gross autopsy rate is as follows:

$$\text{Gross autopsy rate} = \frac{\text{Total number of autopsies on inpatient deaths for a given period}}{\text{Total number of inpatient deaths for the same period}} \times 100$$

For example, at Midwest Hospital during the month of September, the hospital reported 18 deaths. Autopsies were performed on five of those patients. The gross autopsy rate is 27.7 percent ([5/18] × 100).

## Net Autopsy Rate

The **net autopsy rate** is calculated in the same way, but the bodies of patients who were not available for autopsy are removed from the denominator. The reason some bodies may not be available for autopsy is that there are times the coroner or medical examiner may remove the body from the premises. This is usually done for legal reasons, such as a patient who was involved in a crime that led to their death. Using the same example for the gross death rate, where there were 18 deaths and five autopsies, in calculating the net autopsy rate the numerator will still be five because five autopsies were performed at the hospital. However, one body was removed from the premises by the medical examiner. Therefore, that person would be removed from the denominator. The net autopsy rate would be 29.4 percent ([5/(18 − 1)] × 100). The formula for calculating the net autopsy rate is as follows:

$$\text{Net autopsy rate} = \frac{\text{Total number of autopsies on inpatient deaths for a given period}}{\text{Total number of inpatient deaths minus unautopsied coroner or medical examiner cases for the same period}} \times 100$$

## Hospital Autopsy Rates

Another type of autopsy rate is the **hospital autopsy rate**. This autopsy rate includes anyone who had an autopsy at the hospital. While the gross autopsy rate and net autopsy rate only include those patients who died while an inpatient at the hospital, the hospital autopsy rate includes any former patients who died anywhere other than as a hospital inpatient. Upon death, if an autopsy is needed, these former patients are brought to the hospital for the autopsy.

The formula for hospital autopsy rate is as follows:

$$\text{Hospital autopsy rate} = \frac{\text{Total number of hospital autopsies, including former patients who did not die at the hospital for a given period of time}}{\text{Total number of deaths of hospital patients whose bodies were available for autopsy for the same time period}} \times 100$$

## Newborn Autopsy Rate and Fetal Autopsy Rate

The newborn autopsy rate and the fetal autopsy rate would be calculated in the same way as the gross autopsy rate.

The formula for the newborn autopsy rate is as follows:

$$\text{Newborn autopsy rate} = \frac{\text{Total number of autopsies on NB deaths for a given period}}{\text{Total number of NB deaths for the same period}} \times 100$$

The formula for the fetal autopsy rate is as follows:

$$\text{Fetal autopsy rate} = \frac{\text{Total number of autopsies on intermediate and late fetal deaths for a given period}}{\text{Total number of intermediate and late fetal deaths for the same period}} \times 100$$

## Hospital Infection Rates

Although hospital **infection rates** have been calculated for a very long time, in today's healthcare environment where patient care outcomes are emphasized more than ever, infection rates are a focus of healthcare entities, such as the Joint Commission, CMS, and public health agencies. Infections are a major focus because they can lead to other complications, longer inpatient stays, and even death. A low infection rate can be an indicator of quality care.

## Hospital-Acquired Infection Rates

Hospital-acquired infection (HAI) rates, or **nosocomial infection rates**, indicate the rate of infections that were acquired during the hospital stay. These rates are calculated for the entire hospital but will also be calculated for each unit to monitor any issue affecting a certain unit. Hospitals want to have a hospital-acquired infection rate of 0.0 percent, but it is common to have a very low infection rate. A spike in the infection rate will warrant immediate attention of administrators, medical staff, and nurses who will work to determine a reason for the sudden increase. In 2022, the WHO released their first global report on HAI infection rates. It found that "out of every 100 patients in acute-care hospitals, seven patients in high-income countries and 15 patients in low- and middle-income countries will acquire at least one health care-associated infection (HAI) during their hospital stay. On average, 1 in every 10 affected patients will die from their HAI" (WHO 2022). Hospitals are tasked with tracking statistics in this area and striving to make improvements.

The formula for calculating hospital-acquired infection rates is as follows:

$$\text{Hospital-acquired infection rates} = \frac{\text{Total number of hospital – acquired infections for a given period}}{\text{Total number of discharges, including deaths for the same period}} \times 100$$

For example, if there were 196 discharges last week and two hospital-acquired infections were reported, the hospital-acquired infection rate would be (2/196) × 100 = 1.02 percent.

### Postoperative Infection Rates

Another important indicator of quality care is the postoperative infection rate. A postoperative infection is one that occurs after a clean surgical case, meaning that there was no infection before the surgery. A postoperative infection could indicate poor wound care or some type of surgical contamination.

The formula for calculating postoperative infection rate is as follows:

$$\text{Postoperative infection rates} = \frac{\text{Number of infections in clean surgical cases for a given period}}{\text{Total number surgical operations for the same period}} \times 100$$

For example, if there were 582 surgical operations performed in March, and three postoperative infections were reported for March, the postoperative infection rate would be calculated as (3/582) × 100 = 0.515 percent.

---

## Check Your Understanding 15.3

**Answer the following questions in a separate document.**

1. Determine the death rate in the following cases. Which death rate is more representative of the quality of care and why?

| Cases | Gross death rate | Net death rate |
|---|---|---|
| City Hospital reported 49 deaths in June. There were 489 discharges. Eight of those deaths occurred within 48 hours of admission. | | |
| County Hospital reported 62 deaths in May. There were 524 discharges. Seventeen of those deaths occurred within 48 hours of admission. | | |

2. Determine the autopsy rate in the following cases. What is the key difference between the gross and net autopsy rates?

| Cases | Gross autopsy rate | Net autopsy rate |
|---|---|---|
| City Hospital reported 49 deaths in June. Twelve of those bodies were autopsied. Four of the 49 bodies were removed from the hospital for examination by the medical examiner. | | |
| County Hospital reported 62 deaths in May. Sixteen of those bodies were autopsied. Nine of the 62 bodies were removed from the hospital for examination by the medical examiner. | | |

3. Community Hospital admitted 1,619 patients for orthopedic procedures in 2023. Twenty of those patients developed a postoperative infection. What is the postoperative infection rate for this group of admissions? Why is this rate important, and how can it be used to assess care quality?

## Ambulatory Care Statistics

Although the statistics discussed so far have focused on hospital inpatients, all healthcare environments have statistics monitored on a regular basis. Ambulatory care, or outpatient care, must track the number of patients, volume of service, quality of care, and many related rates. For example, while hospitals calculate and report census, ambulatory facilities track the number of daily visits or encounters. While hospitals track LOS and average length of stay, clinics track length of appointments and average length of appointments.

It has become increasingly common for hospitals to provide ambulatory or outpatient services, such as labs, radiology, and same-day surgery. This requires tracking of the outpatient services in the same way that inpatient services are tracked. Each visit may be referred to as one of the following, which were developed for hospital outpatient visits but can be applied to other ambulatory settings as well:

- Occasion of service: Identifiable acts of service involved in the care of outpatients (for example, lab test, x-ray, PT treatment, chemotherapy injection). Does not include direct encounters with a provider.
- Encounter: Face to face contact between the patient and a provider who has primary responsibility for assessing and treating the patient and exercises independent judgment in the care of the patient. This is understood to be a contact between the patient and the physician or other provider responsible for the patient's care. It does not include nurses or allied health practitioners who give treatment at the direction of the physician.

For volume of service statistics, the average daily outpatient census can be calculated. First, outpatient service days should be determined. Outpatient service days = occasions of service + encounters. Next, the outpatient service days would be divided by the number of days in the period. Remember that clinics are not typically open seven days a week, so only the number of days of operation should be used. For example, City Clinic was open 6 days per week in the month of March for a total of 26 days. The outpatient service days came to 1,040. Average outpatient service days would 40. (1,040/26 = 40).

Administrators in all ambulatory settings use these data for decision-making, staffing, and budgeting, just as hospital administrators do for inpatient services. Regardless of the setting, statistical reporting is crucial to the success of healthcare service and financial stability. Monitoring a variety of statistical data lends valuable information for strategic planning.

## Statistics in Revenue Cycle Management

As discussed throughout this chapter, statistics are used for decision-making in all healthcare environments. Statistics are also used in revenue cycle management, which is directly related to the budget and the financial success of a healthcare organization. Some examples of important areas administrators monitor in relation to reimbursement are coding and billing errors, clinical documentation improvement queries and responses, accounts receivable, level of care and resources used per case, claims turnaround time, and claims denial rate.

## Case-Mix Analysis

The case-mix index (CMI) at each hospital informs administrators about resources consumed for patients with similar diagnoses and treatments. CMI is "a single number that compares the overall complexity of the healthcare organization's mix of patients with the complexity of the average of all hospitals" (Casto and White 2024, 92). Case mix gives details about how complex the patient cases are at each hospital or a picture of the severity of illness typical at each hospital. This information is important because the complexity of the hospital's patients reflects on the cost of treating those patients.

Along with CMI, diagnosis-related groups (DRGs) "were developed as a patient classification scheme consisting of classes of patients who were similar clinically and in terms of their consumption of hospital resources" (CMS n.d., 3). The DRG method assigns a numeric value to an acute-care inpatient hospital episode of care, which serves as a relative weighting factor intended to represent the resource intensity of hospital care of the clinical group that is classified to that specific DRG. As a reimbursement system, the DRG assignment determines the payment level the hospital will receive (Comfort et al. 2017).

CMI is calculated by adding the DRG weights for all Medicare discharges and dividing by the number of discharges. Using the data in table 15.4, if the total of the MS-DRG weights for the top 10 MS-DRGs at Community Hospital Neurology Center is 2,726.269, this total would be divided by the number of discharges. If the number of discharges were 2,439, the calculation would be 2,726.269 divided by 2,439 for a CMI of 1.1177. The MS-DRG system is the current CMS inpatient reimbursement methodology system which became effective October 1, 2007. The MS stands for Medicare severity.

## Example One of Case-Mix Analysis

The Huron Consulting Group gives the following example of how CMI might be used:

> The case-mix index (CMI) can be used to adjust the average cost per patient (or day) for a given hospital relative to the adjusted average cost for other hospitals by dividing the average cost per patient (or day) by the hospital's calculated CMI. The adjusted average cost per patient would reflect the charges reported for the types of cases treated in that year.
>
> For example, if Hospital A has an average cost per patient of $1,000 and a CMI of 0.80 for a given year, their adjusted cost per patient is $1,000/0.80 = $1,250. Likewise, if Hospital B has an average cost per patient of $1,500 and a CMI of 1.25, their adjusted cost per patient is $1,500/1.25 = $1,200.
>
> Therefore, if a hospital has a CMI greater than 1.00, their adjusted cost per patient or per day will be lowered and conversely if a hospital has a CMI less than 1.00, their adjusted cost will be higher. (Birg n.d.)

**Table 15.4.** Calculation of case-mix index for the top 10 MS-DRGs at Community Hospital Neurology Center

| MS-DRG | Number (N) | MS-DRG weight | N × MS-DRG weight |
|---|---|---|---|
| 056 | 223 | 1.7368 | 387.3064 |
| 058 | 560 | 1.6027 | 897.512 |
| 059 | 419 | 1.0399 | 435.7181 |
| 060 | 166 | 0.7899 | 131.1234 |
| 073 | 129 | 1.3014 | 167.8806 |
| 074 | 242 | 0.0786 | 19.0212 |
| 053 | 319 | 0.8746 | 278.9974 |
| 054 | 83 | 1.3195 | 109.5185 |
| 055 | 229 | 1.0100 | 231.29 |
| 089 | 69 | 0.9406 | 64.9014 |
| **TOTAL** | 2,439 | | 2,726.269 |
| **CMI** | | | 1.1177 |

## Example Two of Case-Mix Analysis

The State of California provides the following example of how their Office of Statewide Health Planning and Development uses case-mix and MS-DRG data:

> To calculate the CMI, the California Department of [Health Care Access and Information] (HCAI) uses Medicare Severity-Diagnosis Related Groups (MS-DRG) and their associated weights, assigned to each MS-DRG by the Centers for Medicare & Medicaid Services (CMS). Each patient record is assigned an MS-DRG based on the principal and secondary diagnoses, age, procedures performed, the presence of co-morbidities and/or complications, and discharge status. Each MS-DRG has a numeric weight reflecting the national "average hospital resource consumption" by patient for that MS-DRG, relative to the national "average hospital resource consumption" of all patients. Although the MS-DRG weights are based on resource consumption by Medicare patients, HCAI applies them to all patient discharge data reported by hospitals in California during the course of a calendar year. (HCAI n.d.)

# Public Health and Epidemiology Data

Vital statistics are based on the reporting of the vital events of births, deaths, marriages, divorces, and fetal deaths. All 50 states are required to register all births, deaths, marriages, divorces, and fetal deaths; and this information is shared between various governmental organizations. Each state's government is responsible for keeping a registry of vital events and for issuing birth, death, marriage, and divorce certifications (CDC 2018).

The National Vital Statistics System (NVSS) is used to collect the nation's vital statistics information. It is the data-sharing organization to which each state disseminates their vital statistics registry data. Traditionally, all vital event information is registered with the NVSS using standardized forms. However, electronic reporting will certainly become the norm as work continues on developing secure electronic reporting systems.

Through the eVitals Standards Initiatives, the CDC, in collaboration with other agencies, implemented eVitals Standards for reporting birth and fetal death, and all other deaths so these vital statistics are reported electronically in the same way by all users (CDC 2018). This standardization was necessary to ensure the electronic reporting system would produce accurate and valid information and was the first step in the modernization process.

The National Vital Statistics System Modernization initiative is working to promote interoperability among all jurisdictions and others interested in vital statistics to create a robust, interoperable, quality-oriented database (CDC 2023). This project aims to make nationwide vital statistics reporting fast and efficient. The CDC states that "reducing processing time for vital records from years to months—or even from weeks to days—can help identify, monitor, track, and potentially predict the course of diseases and other urgent events. Faster and more accurate vital statistics data will bolster our nationwide capacity to answer both longstanding and emerging health challenges" (CDC 2023).

Secure reporting systems will be important for access to real-time data rather than having to wait until an annual report is published. As-needed data will help public health agencies, government entities, and researchers move forward with reporting and studies without delaying their work until the data are available.

## Epidemiology Statistics

Epidemiology statistics are based on large populations through public health agencies. According to the World Congenital Disorders of Glycosylation Organization, "epidemiology is the study of the distribution and determinants of health related states or events in specified populations and the application of this study to control health problems" (Piedada 2021). Populations may include a city, a county, a neighborhood, a school, or any other entity to be studied (CDC 2016). These studies assist health researchers in assessing current health issues. The data collected in the studies lead to public health education initiatives.

Epidemiologists conduct research studies on a public health issue for a certain population and collect large amounts of data. These data are analyzed with statistical formulas used by researchers to determine if the data and information they have gathered in their research has significance. Any significant findings may be researched further, and results are used to create initiatives to impact the issues that were identified. For instance, if research and statistics show that one city has a significantly higher prevalence of skin cancer, public health agencies may wish to launch an education campaign about the use of sunscreen and other skin protections. These statistics are referred to as population-based statistics because they track the mortality and morbidity of a population.

Some typical population-based statistics reported are birth rates, infant mortality rates, general death rates, and cause-specific death rates. Disease-specific data are also collected, and rates are reported regarding the frequency, or incidence rate, of disease, along with reports of specific diseases and their prevalence rates. Prevalence rates report the proportion of persons with a certain disease to the number of persons in a population. Prevalence rates are used to track severity of diseases and can indicate whether a disease may be at an epidemic proportion. These statistics help public health professionals plan where research dollars will be allocated, where community education is needed, and what initiatives should be a focus in future public health initiatives. Figure 15.2 is a graph of the prevalence of cancer in males from 1973 to 2017, to illustrate an example of the use of public health statistics. This type of public health data can inform decisions about cancer treatment and research.

## Community-Based Disease Tracking

Another important mechanism for tracking disease incidence and prevalence is the National Notifiable Diseases Surveillance System (NNDSS). Like the NVSS, it is managed by the CDC. The system tracks notifiable diseases. Notifiable diseases are those that a state must report to the CDC when the diseases are identified by hospitals or other healthcare facilities. The list of notifiable diseases changes over time and can vary by state. The information reported is specific to the disease and demographics of the patient, but patient identifiers are not reported.

**Figure 15.2.** Age-adjusted cancer incidence rates in the US, 1973–2017: Top 10 cancers in males of all ages

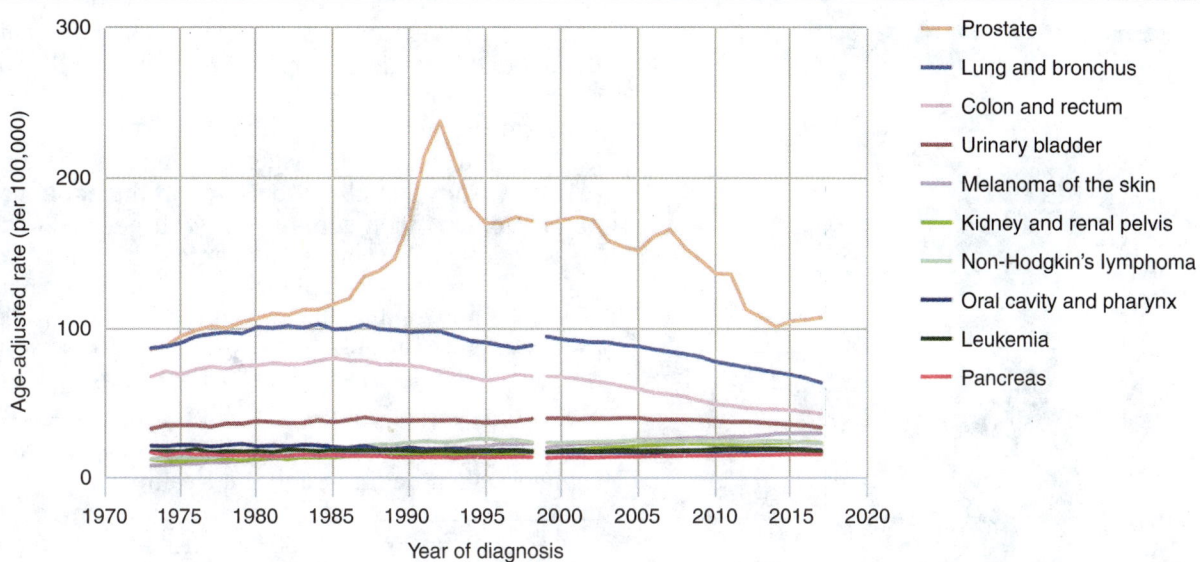

Due to differences in the data sets used to estimate cancer incidence, data from 1973–1998 (NCI, 2018, 2020) should not be directly compared with data from 1999–2017 (CDC and NCI, 2020).

Rates are age-adjusted to the 2000 U.S. standard population.

Information on the statistical significance of the trends in this exhibit is not presented here. For more information about uncertainty, variability, and statistical analysis, view the technical documentation for this indicator.

**Data source:** CDC and NCI, 2020; NCI, 2018, 2020

*Source:* EPA n.d.

National morbidity data are reported to the CDC each week. These timely data are used by public health administrators to act quickly on any data that may signify an epidemic or a crisis. The data are analyzed on a regular basis to find trends, changes, and patterns that should be monitored and investigated. Each annual list of notifiable diseases can be found on the website for the CDC. If needed, past years' lists can also be downloaded on the site.

## Finding and Using Healthcare Statistics

Healthcare statistics are widely used in the healthcare environment. HIM professionals are often involved in the data collection process, but they must know how to calculate various statistics to use in their day-to-day decision-making and reporting. HIM professionals may be responsible for calculating or finding statistical information for administrators who need the information for strategic planning, budgeting, and staffing decisions.

Researchers know they do not always have to do their own data collection studies because many databases and statistics already exist. Healthcare managers may also use existing data for reports, presentations, decision-making, justifications, and benchmarking. Online search engines have made it possible to find valuable statistics easily. It is also important for HIM professionals and other healthcare administrators to be able to locate existing statistics and use them in projects, studies, decision-making, and benchmarking. There is a wealth of valuable healthcare data available, and becoming a practiced researcher is important. Figure 15.3 illustrates helpful steps to take in a search for statistics. The researcher would first need to determine the purpose and goals for the research project, then search publications and the internet for existing research and data found in publications. Next, the researcher should go to the original sources and analyze the information and collect the data. If they find they need more information or different types of data, they must reassess their needs, and go back to the beginning

**Figure 15.3.** Steps in searching for existing health statistics

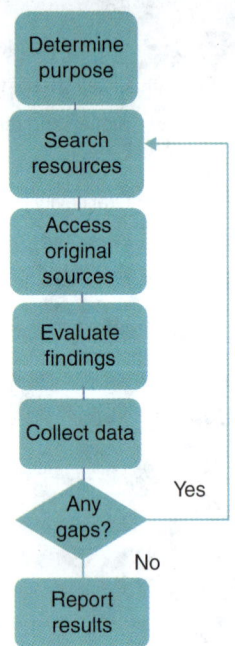

of the process to find even more data. Searching publications and the internet can help the researcher find valuable information. However, time must be taken to evaluate the data found to assess its value and validity and determine if the source can be used or if more sources should be sought.

As an example of the value of existing statistics, a health information manager has volunteered to be part of a team at a clinic focusing on the adolescent population in their community. The goal is to increase adolescent visits at the clinic, with a focus on well visits for health maintenance. The project manager asks for a volunteer to find some national data of how many adolescents typically have well visits in any given year. This information will be used as a benchmark that your clinic will try to exceed. The HIM manager has volunteered for this task and finds some excellent data through the Healthy People 2030 initiative (HealthyPeople.gov n.d.). Since one of the goals of Healthy People 2030 is to increase the proportion of adolescents who have had a wellness visit in the past 12 months, the HIM manager is able to find national data on this topic for the past seven years. These data can be taken to the next project meeting. The project manager may decide that the team can use these data as the benchmark.

 **Check Your Understanding 15.4**

Answer the following questions in a separate document.

1. Differentiate DRGs from case mix. How can a CEO use these indicators?
2. How could DRGs and case mix be used in budgeting decisions?
3. National statistics have been released that identify cities with the highest mortality rate due to lung cancer. How might the public health officials in those cities respond to those data if they want to improve that statistic?
4. How are ambulatory care statistics similar to inpatient hospital statistics? How are they different?
5. Summarize how vital statistics data can be used in public health initiatives

# References

Barfield, W. D., K. Watterberg, W. Bennitz, J. Cummings, E. Eichenwald, B. Poindexter, D. Stewart, S. Aucott, K. Puopolo, and J. Goldsmith. 2016. Standard terminology for fetal, infant, and perinatal deaths. *PEDIATRICS* 137(5). https://doi.org/10.1542/peds.2016-0551.

Birg, G. 2016. *Case Mix Index: Analyzing Case Mix Index and the Impact on CDI Programs* [White paper]. The Huron Group. https://www.huronconsultinggroup.com/-/media/Resource-Media-Content/Healthcare/cdi-casemix-whitepaper.pdf.

Casto, A., and S. White. 2024. *Principles of Healthcare Reimbursement*, 8th ed. Chicago: AHIMA.

CDC (Centers for Disease Control and Prevention). 2023. "Modernizing the National Vital Statistics

System." https://www.cdc.gov/nchs/nvss/modernization.htm.

CDC (Centers for Disease Control and Prevention). 2018. "National Center for Health Statistics. How to Access e-Vital Standards." https://www.cdc.gov/nchs/nvss/evital/accessing_evital_standards.htm.

CDC (Centers for Disease Control and Prevention). 2016. "What Is Epidemiology?" http://www.cdc.gov/EXCITE/epidemiology.html.

CMS (Centers for Medicare and Medicaid Services). n.d. "Design and Development of the Diagnosis Related Group (DRG)." Accessed September 17, 2024. https://www.cms.gov/icd10m/version37-fullcode-cms/fullcode_cms/Design_and_development_of_the_Diagnosis_Related_Group_(DRGs).pdf.

Comfort, A., D. Rugg, and M. Ward. 2017 (June). Evolution of DRGs (2017 Update). *Journal of AHIMA* 88 (6):48–51.

EPA (Environmental Protection Agency). n.d. "Cancer Incidence." Accessed August 10, 2024. https://cfpub.epa.gov/roe/indicator.cfm?i=73#.

HCAI (California Department of Health Care Access and Information). n.d. "Inpatient Discharges: Case Mix Index." Accessed December 15, 2023. https://hcai.ca.gov/data-and-reports/healthcare-utilization/inpatient/#case-mix-index.

HealthyPeople.gov. n.d. "Healthy People 2030." Accessed May 28, 2024. https://health.gov/healthypeople.

Heisey-Grove, D., H. K. Wall, A. Helwig, and J. S. Wright. 2015 (May). "Using Electronic Clinical Quality Measure Reporting for Public Health Surveillance." http://www.cdc.gov/mmwr/preview/mmwrhtml/mm6416a3.htm.

Hoefs, J. 2015 (May). Personal communication with author.

IHS (Indian Health Service). n.d. *Indian Health Manual*. Accessed August 12, 2024. https://www.ihs.gov/ihm/index.cfm?module=dsp_ihm_pc_p3c3.

Piedada, A. 2021. "Worldwide CDG Organization. What Is Epidemiology and Why Is It Important?" https://worldcdg.org/research/epidemiology.

Rasmussen S. A., J. W. Ward, and R. A. Goodman. 2020. Protecting the editorial independence of the CDC from politics. *JAMA* 324(17):1729–1730. doi:10.1001/jama.2020.19646.

Salkind, N., and B. Frey. 2019. *Statistics for People Who (Think They) Hate Statistics*, 7th ed. Thousand Oaks, CA: SAGE Publications, Inc.

Taylor, L. 2015 (May). Personal communication with author.

US Library of Medicine. n.d. "Finding and Using Health Statistics." Accessed August 10, 2024. https://www.nlm.nih.gov/oet/ed/stats/index.html.

White, S. 2023. *Calculating and Reporting Healthcare Statistics*, 7th ed. Chicago: AHIMA.

WHO (World Health Organization). 2022 (May 6). "WHO Launches First Ever Global Report on Infection Prevention and Control." https://www.who.int/news/item/06-05-2022-who-launches-first-ever-global-report-on-infection-prevention-and-control.

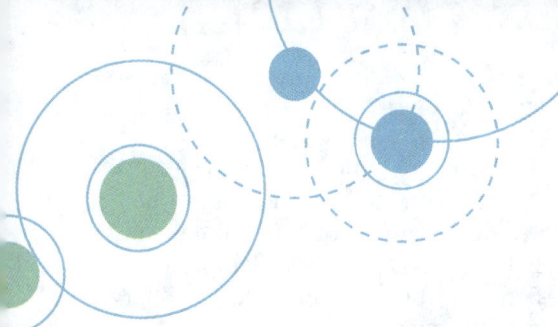

# Healthcare Data Analytics

Susan White, PhD, RHIA, CHDA

## Learning Objectives

- Determine the role of data analytics in healthcare operations
- Determine and apply the proper statistical techniques to questions related to healthcare data
- Apply statistical inference and interpret the results
- Calculate and assess hypothesis tests and confidence intervals
- Evaluate the role of health information management professionals in healthcare data analytics
- Interpret the results of statistical analysis to drive data-informed decisions

## Key Terms

Alternative hypothesis
Cluster sampling
Coefficient of determination
Confidence interval
Continuous data
Continuous variables
Correlation
Data analytics
Data mining
Dependent variable
Discrete data
Healthcare data analytics
Hypothesis test
Independent variable
Indirect standardization
Interval data
Nominal data
Normal distribution
Null hypothesis
One sample t-test
Ordinal data
Predictive modeling
p-value
QualityNet
Range
Ratio data
RAT-STATS
Simple linear regression (SLR)
Simple random sampling
Standard deviation
Stratified random sample
Systematic random sampling
Type I error
Type II error
Value-based programs
Variance

The term **data analytics** describes a variety of approaches to using data to make business decisions. **Healthcare data analytics** is, therefore, the practice of using data to make business decisions in healthcare. More specifically, healthcare data analytics is the application of statistical techniques to allow informed decisions to be made based on the data. A variety of descriptive statistics are used in healthcare, including rates and proportions as well as measures of central tendency, such as the mean, median, and mode. Inferential statistics include techniques such as confidence intervals and hypothesis testing and are used to determine if a provider's performance is significantly better or worse than national norms. In this chapter, both types of statistical techniques will be applied in the healthcare operations and business context.

The business of healthcare requires the management of both clinical and financial decisions. Healthcare is rich with a wide variety of data sources that may be analyzed to drive those decisions. Professionals working in the field of analytics do not typically collect data for the purpose of a research study or design experiments to prove or disprove theories. The field of analytics often involves the use of secondary data already collected by others for various purposes. Sampling and experimental design may be used to collect primary data to answer specific business analysis needs, but that is often a time-consuming and expensive task. The healthcare industry produces a tremendous amount of clinical and operational data. The secondary use of that data is often for analytic projects to measure and improve the performance of healthcare entities.

## Healthcare Initiatives and the Impact on Data Analytics

Electronic health records (EHRs) bring a flood of data into the already data-rich healthcare environment. The true value of that data may only be realized through applying analytic techniques to distill the raw data into information that can support decision-making. The results of data analytics can have a significant impact on both the clinical and financial outcomes of the healthcare system. Many federal initiatives have put the spotlight on the importance of data analytics in healthcare. A few samples of these initiatives are discussed here.

Value-based programs are based on data-driven metrics to measure both the quality and efficiency of a healthcare provider. Bonus payments may be awarded, or penalties imposed on providers, depending on their level of performance. The Centers for Medicare and Medicaid Services (CMS) implemented the first stage of their value-based payment programs in July 2003, with the National Voluntary Hospital Reporting Initiative (CMS 2009). The five original value-based programs include:

- End-Stage Renal Disease Quality Incentive Program (ESRD QIP)
- Hospital Value-Based Purchasing (VBP) Program
- Hospital Readmission Reduction Program (HRRP)
- Value Modifier (VM) Program (also called the Physician Value-Based Modifier or PVBM)
- Hospital Acquired Conditions (HAC) Reduction Program (CMS 2023a)

Each of these programs are supported using healthcare data and analytic techniques. CMS is in various stages of the implementation of these programs throughout the Medicare system. In the hospital setting, both the inpatient prospective payment system (IPPS) and the outpatient prospective payment system (OPPS) include a penalty for providers that do not report the required quality indicators.

In the area of financial analytics, the Healthcare Financial Management Association (HFMA) developed a set of indicators to measure revenue cycle performance. These so-called MAP (measure, apply, perform) indicators include financial metrics that may be derived from healthcare data. They provide a framework for benchmarking the ability of a healthcare provider to collect the money owed for the treatment of patients. The MAP indicators measure performance in four key areas—patient access, revenue integrity, claims adjudication, and management (HFMA n.d.).

Accountable care organizations (ACOs) tie together the use of clinical and financial analytics throughout the healthcare delivery system. The ACO is an integrated delivery system that includes physicians, hospitals, and other providers all focused on the delivery of care to a particular geographic segment of the Medicare population. The ACO receives incentive payments for delivering care in an efficient manner and providing a level of preventive care and education that may avoid subsequent treatment for chronic diseases. The intent of the ACO program is to improve the efficiency of care delivered to Medicare beneficiaries. To do so effectively, the ACO must have a robust database regarding the care delivered to the beneficiaries the ACO serves as well as a broad spectrum of analytics to understand the patterns of care and chronic diseases present in the population.

All the examples presented in this section highlight the growth of analytics in the healthcare setting. The demand for professionals with solid analytic skills, and the ability to interpret the results of analysis to nonanalytic staff, is currently outpacing availability. Health information management (HIM) professionals who can demonstrate these skills will become invaluable resources in their organization.

## Types of Data

Data can be characterized in several ways. The broadest categorization is structured versus unstructured. Structured data are data comprised of values that can be stored as either numbers or a finite number of categories. Healthcare data such as height, weight, age, gender, and Medicare severity diagnosis-related groups (MS-DRGs) are all examples of structured data. Conversely, unstructured data cannot be expressed as numbers or categories. The provider notes recorded in an EHR are a classic example of unstructured data in healthcare. The notes often contain valuable data regarding treatment protocols and documentation of comorbid conditions or symptoms, but they are recorded as freeform text and are therefore difficult to use in analyses. Analytic tools such as natural language processing (NLP) or other methods of characterizing key words or concepts may be used to analyze unstructured data. For example, NLP engines are used in computer-assisted coding programs to identify key medical terms found in clinical documentation such as nursing notes.

Structured data may further be broken down into levels of measurement. Care should be taken to understand the level of measurement of each data element that may be analyzed so the proper statistical method is applied. The four basic levels of measurement are displayed in table 16.1. Ordinal and nominal data are both **discrete data** types. They take on categorical values and cannot be added together or divided. **Nominal data** are expressed as categories that represent names of items, but do not have a natural order. Examples of data with a nominal measurement level include gender, color, MS-DRGs, Current Procedural Terminology (CPT) codes, and *International Classification of Diseases* (ICD) codes. **Ordinal data** are also expressed as categories, but in this case the categories have a natural order. Patient severity level, trauma center level, and trimester of gestation are all examples of ordinal data found in healthcare.

Ratio and interval data are both considered **continuous data**. This type of data can take on a continuum of values, such as fractions and decimals, as opposed to discrete categories. Their values may be added and subtracted for comparison. **Ratio data** examples include length of stay, charges, and hemoglobin levels. **Interval data** are also continuous, but do not have a meaningful zero value. An example of interval data is temperature. The temperature may be zero, but that does not represent the absence of temperature, only that it is very cold. Another distinction between ratio and interval data is that the concepts of "half of" or "twice" have meaning. For instance, if the average length of stay at one unit is 5 days and the average length of stay in another unit is half as long, the value is 2.5 days. The concept of twice as cold does not have a practical interpretation. The interval between two temperature values does have an interpretation. This is where the term *interval* was derived. If the difference or interval between two data values has meaning, then the measurement level is interval. If the ratio or multiplication of two data values has meaning, then the measurement level is ratio.

Table 16.1. Basic levels of measurement

| Data type | Examples | Appropriate descriptive statistics |
| --- | --- | --- |
| Nominal—categorical data where the categories are mutually exclusive, but do not have a natural order | Gender, HCPCS codes, department or unit | Frequency counts, proportions, mode |
| Ordinal—categorical data where the categories are mutually exclusive, and they do have a natural order | Patient satisfaction scores, severity scores, trauma center level, surveys measured on a Likert scale | Frequency counts, proportions, mode, range |
| Interval—naturally numeric data where the distance between two values has meaning, but multiplying values and zero value has no interpretation | Temperature, pH level, dates | Mean, median, standard deviation, range |
| Ratio—naturally numeric data where zero has an interpretation and the values may be doubled or multiplied by a constant and still have meaning | Charges, length of stay, age | Mean, median, standard deviation, range, geometric mean, coefficient of variation |

## Descriptive versus Inferential Statistics

The science of statistics is segmented into two broad categories—descriptive and inferential. Descriptive statistics are used to describe the distribution of the variable of interest. Inferential statistics are used to test hypotheses or make decisions. These hypotheses have a probability or risk of making an error based on the data collected. This probability is referred to as the type I error or p-value. Inferential statistics help analysts trend and summarize the data to determine whether they are observing significant results in the sample or simply observing an event that occurred due to chance.

The appropriate descriptive statistic is determined by the type of data analyzed. If the intent is to describe how often an event of interest occurs, then rates and proportions are often used. For instance, a mortality rate is used to measure how many patients died compared to the total number of patients. A proportion is the appropriate statistic to use when describing the breakout of MS-DRG cases without complications or comorbidities (w/o CC), complications or comorbidities (CC), and major complications or comorbidities (MCC). If the intent is to analyze a variable that is interval or ratio in nature, then the appropriate descriptive statistic is the mean, median, or mode. For instance, length of stay for inpatient services is described using mean (average) or median. Table 16.1 lists types of data and the appropriate descriptive statistics.

The appropriate inferential statistic method is determined by the hypothesis to be tested or the question to be answered. An analyst may be asked to compare their facility's length of stay or mortality rate to a state standard or to determine if the MS-DRG change rate is different from the value typically observed at the facility. These questions may be answered using inferential techniques. The appropriate statistical method is dependent on the question and the type of data available for analysis.

Basic healthcare operations questions may often be analyzed using confidence intervals or hypothesis tests. A **confidence interval** is a range of values, such that the probability of that range covering the true value of a parameter is a set probability or confidence. A **hypothesis test** allows the analyst to determine the likelihood that a hypothesis is true given the data present in the sample with a predetermined acceptable level of making an error.

For instance, suppose the goal of a study is to determine the typical wait time in a hospital's emergency department (ED). A random sample of patients is selected from the population of patients visiting the ED during the previous month. The average wait time, 53.5 minutes, is a statistic that describes the typical wait time, but that statistic alone does not give any information about the precision of the estimate or how certain it is that the true population ED wait time is a range of around 53.5 minutes.

A confidence interval may be used to provide that additional information. A 95 percent confidence interval for the ED wait time was calculated and found to be: (50.1, 56.9). The value 95 percent is the confidence level or the probability that the confidence interval contains the true population average. In this case, there is a probability of 95 percent that the interval (50.1, 56.9) includes the true population average ED wait time. Confidence intervals may be reported as a value plus or minus the margin of error. In the ED example, this would be 53.5 +/- 3.4 minutes. Recall that these figures are based on a sample, and we do not know the entire population value. The sample is used to make inferences or conclusions about the population. The width of the confidence interval is a measure of the precision of the estimate. A narrower interval is more precise.

Continuing with this same ED wait time example, suppose the goal was to test to determine if the average wait time was meeting the facility standard of 60 minutes. In this case, a hypothesis test is the correct statistical method. Hypothesis testing requires the definitions of the null hypothesis to be tested versus an alternative hypothesis. The **null hypothesis** is typically the status quo (White 2021, 76). The **alternative hypothesis** is sometimes called the research hypothesis and is a conclusion that typically requires some action to be taken (White 2021, 76). The null hypothesis is that the ED wait time is less than or equal to 60 minutes; the alternative hypothesis is that the ED wait time is greater than 60 minutes. In hypothesis testing, an acceptable type I error level should be selected prior to calculating the result. **Type I error** is the probability of incorrectly rejecting the null hypothesis when it is true given the values present in the sample. In this example, type I error is making the conclusion that the wait time is longer than 60 minutes when it is truly less than or equal to 60 minutes. Analysts must also be aware of type II error in hypothesis testing. **Type II error** occurs when the null hypothesis is not rejected when it is actually false (White 2021, 76). Type II error may be controlled by adjusting the sample size used for the study; a larger sample will decrease the likelihood of committing a type II error.

The practical implication of making a type I error in this situation is the expense that may be incurred to study the root cause of the long wait times and make operational corrections. For this example, the type I error is set to be 5 percent or 0.05. The probability of making a type I error may be calculated using the sample data and the appropriate test statistic. The probability of making a type I error based on a particular set of data is called the p-value. If the p-value or probability of making a type I error is less than the type I error level set prior to testing, then the null hypothesis may be rejected. After calculating the test statistic and determining the p-value is 0.03, the null hypothesis is rejected, and the conclusion is made that the ED wait time is longer than the standard.

The first step in any analytic study is to identify the research question. Many data analysis projects start without a clear idea of the exact question to be answered. The analyst becomes so concerned with summarizing the data and producing reports that they forget their efforts may be wasted if the question is not well defined at the outset. Examples of some of the applied research questions that may be of interest include the following:

- What is the typical ED wait time?
- Does our ED wait time meet our facility standard?
- What is the percentage of lab orders that are not signed by a physician?
- What is the coding accuracy rate for secondary diagnosis codes?

Once the research question is defined, the unit of analysis must also be determined. For example, to determine the percentage of lab orders that are not signed by a physician, the unit of analysis is the entire set of lab orders for the period of interest. This set of lab orders serves as the population of interest. It is practically impossible to collect the entire population of lab orders to definitively answer the questions posed. The data required is often selected through a sampling plan and then analyzed to make inferences or conclusions about the percentage of lab orders unsigned in the population.

In practice, it is sometimes difficult to determine the unit of analysis. For instance, in determining the coding accuracy rate for secondary diagnosis codes, should the unit of analysis be each code or the claim on which the code appears? There is a critical difference between the two units of analysis. If the unit of analysis is the code, then the resulting rate would be the proportion of correct codes and not the proportion of correct claims. If the research question is to estimate the number of claims correctly coded, then the claim should be the unit of analysis.

## Impact of Sampling

If the entire population of units of analysis were available for a study, then there would be no reason to use inferential statistics. Consider the previous lab order example. If the entire population of lab orders submitted at the facility during the period of interest could be profiled, then the signature rate could be calculated exactly and compared to a standard. Unfortunately, the availability of the population or the time required to review the population is often not practical.

The most common types of random sampling are simple, stratified, systematic, and cluster sampling. In simple random sampling, every member of the population has an equal probability of inclusion in the sample. A stratified random sample is selected by first dividing the population into subsets or strata. A simple random sample is then selected from each stratum of the sample. Cluster sampling is like stratified sampling in that the population is divided into subsets—called clusters here. The clusters are then randomly selected. All units within the randomly selected clusters are included in the sample. Systematic random sampling is a method used to determine a simple random sample. In systematic random sampling every N/$n$th record is selected from the population. N is the number of units in the population and $n$ is the sample size (White 2021, 152).

The statistical techniques used are dependent on the sampling method used to collect the data. Stratified and cluster sampling require a more complex set of statistical methods than simple random sampling.

Sampling techniques are used frequently in the healthcare setting. For instance, CMS allows hospitals to report many of the required quality indicators based on a sample of claims and not the full population. Figure 16.1 is an example of the sample size requirements outlined in the QualityNet Hospital Inpatient Measures Specification Manual (QualityNet 2023). QualityNet is a CMS website that provides information about quality measurement and serves as the basis for communication between CMS, their contractors, and healthcare providers regarding quality data and metrics. Note that the sample size is dependent on the quarterly patient population at the reporting hospital. For the XYZ Measure Set in the example, the sample size will range from n = 16 to n = 48.

CMS reports the sample size and rate for measures based on samples rather than full population statistics. Notice that University Hospital's statistics displayed in figure 16.2 are based on a sample of n = 275 for the death rate and n = 258 for the payment for pneumonia patients.

**Figure 16.1.** Example quarterly sample size

Quarterly sample size
Based on Hospital's Initial Patient Population for the XYZ Measure Set

| Average Quarterly Stratum Initial Patient Population "N" | Minimum Required Stratum Sample Size "n" |
|---|---|
| ≥471 | 48 |
| 161–470 | 10% of Initial Patient Population |
| 16–160 | 16 |
| <16 | No sampling; 100% of the Initial Patient Population is required |

*Source:* QualityNet 2023, 4–5

CMS also includes guidance on how to calculate a confidence interval for rates based on samples. These instructions are found in table 16.2 (CMS n.d.).

Using the guidance in table 16.2 and the data presented in figure 16.2, confidence intervals may be formed for the example quality indicators. For example, a 95 percent confidence interval for the death rate for pneumonia patients for University Hospital is 14.2 percent +/− 3.75 percent. The 3.75 percent comes from table 16.2 looking up the value for the row with a sample size of 275 or 226–275 and the column for the observed rate of 10 percent (rounding the observed 14.2 percent down to 10 percent). Based on the sample selected, one can be 95 percent sure that the population compliance with this quality indicator is between 10.45 percent and 17.95 percent at University Hospital. Notice that the confidence interval is completely below the national death rate of 18.2 percent. This is why the comparison to the national rate in figure 16.2 states "better than the national rate."

Notice the pattern of the values presented in table 16.2. The values in the table represent the half widths of the confidence interval or the amount to be added and subtracted from the observed rate to formulate the 95 percent confidence interval. For a fixed value of the observed rate (column in the figure), the half-width values decrease as the sample size increases. This makes intuitive sense. As the sample size increases, the analyst knows more about the population and therefore may formulate narrower or more precise intervals for the rate. For a fixed sample size (row in the figure), the half-width values increase until the observed rate is 50 percent and then decrease across the row as the observed rate decreases. This pattern is because the standard deviation of the rate statistic is equal to the rate multiplied by one minus the rate, which is maximized at 50 percent. If an event has an equal chance of occurring or not, like flipping a coin, then it is difficult to make precise estimates; and therefore, the confidence interval must be wider or less precise for a fixed sample size.

## Tools for Sampling and Design

The sample size for a study is determined by the amount of precision desired for the study. There are several tools available to assist analysts in calculating the required sample size. Traditional statistical software packages such as SAS or R offer a module for sample size calculation. G-Power is a public domain software application that may be used to calculate sample size for several statistical methods (Buchner et al. n.d.). The Office of the Inspector General (OIG) offers a statistical package called RAT-STATS that is free to download (OIG 2019). RAT-STATS can be used

**Figure 16.2.** Example hospital comparison based on a sample

Pneumonia

| Death rate for pneumonia patients | **14.2%** |
| | Better than the national rate |
| | National result: 18.2% |
| | Number of included patients: 275 |

| Payment for pneumonia patients | **$20,036** |
| | No different than the national average payment |
| | National average payment: $20,362 |
| | Number of included patients: 258 |

*Source:* CMS 2023.

**Table 16.2.** Guide to calculating confidence intervals for rates based on samples

| Estimating confidence intervals for the process of care measures: Estimated values for proportion data | | | | | | | | | |
|---|---|---|---|---|---|---|---|---|---|
| Sample size | Observed rate | | | | | | | | |
| | 10% | 20% | 30% | 40% | 50% | 60% | 70% | 80% | 90% |
| <25 | – | – | 24.9% | 26.6% | 27.2% | 26.6% | 24.9% | – | – |
| 25–75 | 8.3% | 11.1% | 12.7% | 13.6% | 13.9% | 13.6% | 12.7% | 11.1% | 8.3% |
| 76–125 | 5.9% | 7.8% | 9.0% | 9.6% | 9.8% | 9.6% | 9.0% | 7.8% | 5.9% |
| 126–175 | 4.8% | 6.4% | 7.3% | 7.8% | 8.0% | 7.8% | 7.3% | 6.4% | 4.8% |
| 176–225 | 4.2% | 5.5% | 6.4% | 6.8% | 6.9% | 6.8% | 6.4% | 5.5% | 4.2% |
| 226–275 | 3.75% | 5.0% | 5.7% | 6.1% | 6.2% | 6.1% | 5.7% | 5.0% | 3.7% |
| 276+ | 2.9% | 3.9% | 4.5% | 4.8% | 4.9% | 4.8% | 4.5% | 3.9% | 2.9% |

Note: CMS/OCSQ/QIG: The values in the table are the approximate amount to add and subtract from the observed rate to estimate a 95 percent confidence interval for the given sample size. (Interpolation between the values in the table is appropriate.) Estimates of an interval in these cells exceed the natural limits for proportions.

Source: CMS n.d.

for both sample size determination and the generation of the random numbers required for sampling.

The OIG developed RAT-STATS to help providers select samples for audits required for those under corporate integrity agreements to resolve compliance issues. The OIG also requires random sample audits to support the estimation of amounts subject to repayment under self-disclosure agreements. The claim error rate and overpayment per claim is estimated from the sample and then extrapolated to determine the repayment amount. CMS Medicare integrity contractors use a similar methodology to determine amounts of over- or underpayments during their audits (CMS 2023).

Suppose a health data analyst at a recovery audit contractor (RAC) is asked to select a sample of medical records to determine if a provider is accurately coding the CC and MCC for their congestive heart failure (CHF) cases for discharges from October 1, 2022, to September 30, 2023. The analyst knows that CHF groups to MS-DRGs 291, 292, and 293. It is also known that the provider of interest submitted 953 claims for these MS-DRGs during the period. The RAC's medical record reviewers will make a correct or incorrect coding determination for each claim and then estimate the total amount of payment error for this MS-DRG set. The Program Integrity Manual suggests that contractors use a one-sided lower 90 percent confidence interval to determine the amount of the payment error (CMS 2023). They claim this is a conservative estimate of overpayment since there is a 90 percent probability that the true overpayment amount is more than the one-sided lower 90 percent confidence bound.

The unit of analysis in this study is the claim. The population to be sampled is the 953 claims that the provider submitted during the study period for the MS-DRGs of interest. The research question is to determine the average amount of payment error for claims assigned to an incorrect MS-DRG. In RAT-STATS this is referred to as a variable study since the goal is to measure a continuous variable such as currency or time for each sampling unit (OIG 2019).

To determine the sample size required for this audit, the analyst must set a precision range and confidence level. Suppose the analyst wishes to draw a simple random sample, with a precision range of +/− 5 percent and a confidence level of 80 percent. This level is selected since an 80 percent confidence level in RAT-STATS results in the same sample size as the one-sided 90 percent confidence interval suggested for RAC use in the CMS Program Integrity Manual (CMS 2023). The sample size calculation also requires a prior estimate of the overpayment amount average and standard deviation. These statistics are typically determined via a probe sample or pilot study, which is a version of the study performed using a small sample. From previous studies the analyst knows that the typical provider audit yields an average overpayment of $500 with a standard deviation of $150.

To determine the required sample size within RAT-STATS, perform the following steps:

1. Open RAT-STATS. Click Variable Using Probe Sample
2. Enter the Universe or Frame Size and select all confidence and precision levels (figure 16.3)
3. The mean ($500) and standard deviation ($150) from the probe sample should be entered when requested in the appropriate cells.
4. Click Process
5. The required sample sizes are then presented (See figure 16.4.)

**448** Chapter 16 **Healthcare Data Analytics**

**Figure 16.3.** RAT-STATS variable sample size determination screen

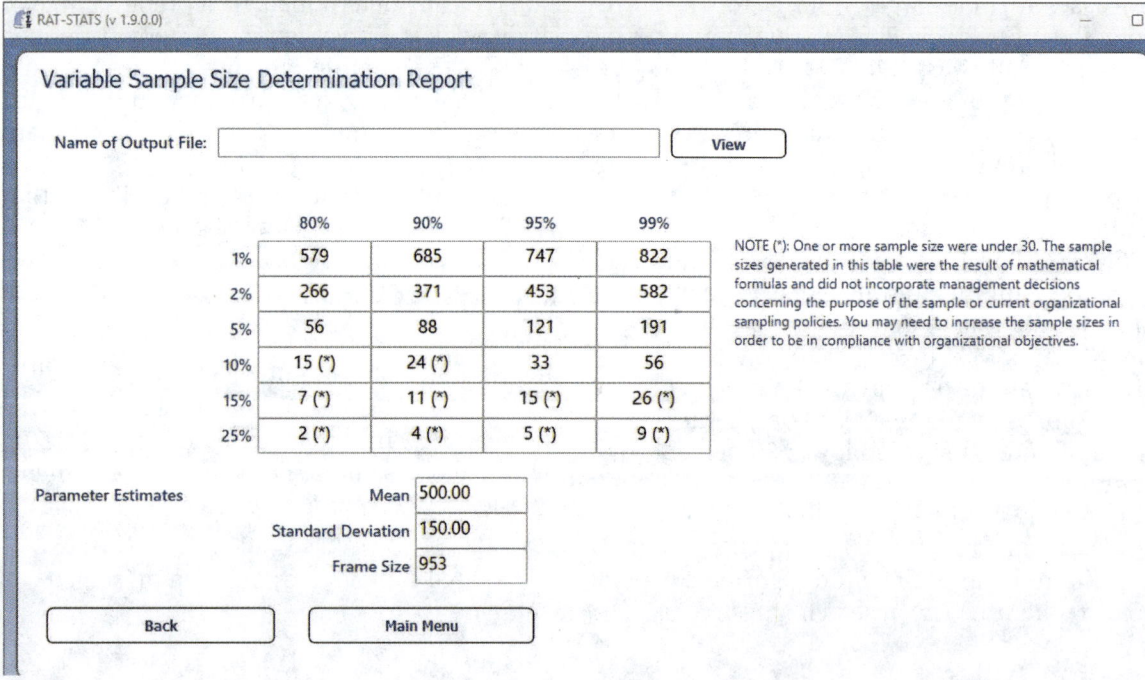

*Source:* OIG 2019.

**Figure 16.4.** RAT-STATS variable sample size output

|  | 80% | 90% | 95% | 99% |
|---|---|---|---|---|
| 1% | 579 | 685 | 747 | 822 |
| 2% | 266 | 371 | 453 | 582 |
| 5% | 56 | 88 | 121 | 191 |
| 10% | 15 (*) | 24 (*) | 33 | 56 |
| 15% | 7 (*) | 11 (*) | 15 (*) | 26 (*) |
| 25% | 2 (*) | 4 (*) | 5 (*) | 9 (*) |

NOTE (*): One or more sample size were under 30. The sample sizes generated in this table were the result of mathematical formulas and did not incorporate management decisions concerning the purpose of the sample or current organizational sampling policies. You may need to increase the sample sizes in order to be in compliance with organizational objectives.

Parameter Estimates
Mean 500.00
Standard Deviation 150.00
Frame Size 953

*Source:* OIG 2019.

The sample size required for the audit to result in the desired confidence level of 80 percent and the desired precision of 5 percent is 56. Notice that the required sample size increases as the confidence level increases and as the desired precision decreases. Decreasing precision levels are equivalent to narrower or more precise confidence intervals. This is the same pattern noted in the CMS confidence interval guidance presented in table 16.2.

## Check Your Understanding 16.1

**Answer the following questions in a separate document.**

1. If an analyst does not reject the null hypothesis that a hospital's average length of stay is greater than or equal to a benchmark of three days when the true population length of stay is two and a half days, what type of error is committed?
   a. Type II
   b. Type I
   c. This is not an error
   d. Type IV

2. If an analyst wishes to test a hypothesis and limit the type I error to 0.05, which of the following p-values would result in rejecting the null hypothesis?
   a. 0.01
   b. 0.06
   c. 0.1
   d. 5

3. Patient gender is classified as what type of data?
   a. Ordinal
   b. Interval
   c. Nominal
   d. Ratio

4. If the health data analyst using figure 16.4 to determine the audit sample size decided that a conservative value would be appropriate to complete an audit with 95 percent confidence and 5 percent precision, what would be the required sample size?
   a. 453
   b. 88
   c. 292
   d. 121

## Analyzing Continuous Data

Interval and ratio scales of measurement are also referred to as continuous data. Examples of **continuous variables** in healthcare include length of stay, charges, reimbursement, wait time, patient body mass index (BMI), and minutes to code a health record. Descriptive statistics such as the arithmetic mean, geometric mean, median, standard deviation, and standard error may all be used to describe the distribution of continuous data.

### Measures of Central Tendency

The center of the distribution of a continuous variable is typically described by the mean (arithmetic average), median, or mode. Each of these statistics has properties that make them the correct choice in a particular situation. The mean is the most common statistic used in practice. The mean is found by adding up all the values and dividing by the number of observations in the sample. The median is the middle value in the sample. To find the median, the data are sorted from smallest to largest value and the center value is chosen as the median. If the sample has an even number of observations, then the two middle values are averaged to determine the median. The mode is the value with the highest frequency of occurrence. There may not be a unique mode for some continuous variables such as charges since each value may be different in the sample.

The mean can be heavily influenced by extreme values. If the sample has extreme values on either the high or low end of the scale, then the median may be the better choice for describing the center of the distribution. The median is less influenced by outliers. For example, consider the mean length of stay for a set of patients with the following values: 2, 5, 9, 1, and 6 days. The mean length of stay is 4.6 days, and the median length of stay is 5 days. If the patient who stayed 9 days is replaced by a patient with a 20-day stay, the mean length of stay becomes 6.8 days while the median is still 5 days. The outlier value of 20 pulls the mean higher, but the median is unchanged by the extreme value. The mode is most often used when summarizing categorical data, since the values in continuous variables may not repeat. For instance, multiple patients are not likely to have the same charge for an admission or the same blood pressure measure. Since the number of possible values for categorical variables is typically limited to a relatively small set, for example gender or trauma level, repeating values are more likely, and the mode is a more meaningful statistic.

## Measures of Spread

The most common measures of spread of a continuous variable are the variance, standard deviation, and range. In sampling, **variance** refers to a measure of variability which is calculated as the average squared deviation from the mean. The formula for the sample variance is as follows:

$$s^2 = \frac{\sum (y - \bar{y})^2}{n - 1}$$

In this equation, subtract the sample mean (y with a bar over it) from each value in the sample (y). Each of these differences from the mean are then squared and summed up. The resulting summation is then divided by the sample size (n) minus 1.

In the length of stay example with values 2, 5, 9, 1, and 6 days, the variance calculation is as follows:

$$s^2 = \frac{(2-4.6)^2 + (5-4.6)^2 + (9-4.6)^2 + (1-4.6)^2 + (6-4.6)^2}{5-1} = 10.3$$

The **standard deviation** is the square root of the variance. In the example, the standard deviation is the square root of 10.3 or 3.2. The value 3.2 is a measure of variability or consistency in the lengths of stay for this population of patients. This may be compared to other patient populations to determine if the lengths of stay are variable. The variance and standard deviation are both influenced by outliers. The median absolute deviation is occasionally used as an alternative measure of spread if the data includes extreme outliers, but the variance and standard deviation are the most common measures of spread used in practice.

The **range** is the difference between the minimum and maximum values. The range is very sensitive to outliers, since it is calculated as the difference between the two most extreme values. The range in our example data is the maximum value (9) minus the minimum value (1) or 9 − 1 = 8.

## Inferential Statistics for Continuous Data

The presentation of the full spectrum of inferential techniques used with continuous variables is beyond the scope of this text. However, the following sections present two common methods that demonstrate the utility of statistical inference in the healthcare setting.

### Inference Example: One Sample t-Test

Hypothesis tests are a common technique used to determine if the results for the sample are truly significant or if they are simply due to random chance. The **one sample t-test** is used to compare a population to a standard value. The example regarding the wait times in an ED is an application of the one sample t-test.

The first step in performing any hypothesis test is to determine the null and alternative hypotheses. Suppose in the ED wait time example, the ED director is concerned that the wait times exceed the standard of 60 minutes. The marketing director would like to run a new campaign that touts ED wait times that are significantly shorter than the standard of 60 minutes. In this case, the research question is to determine if the ED wait times are significantly shorter or longer than 60 minutes and a two-sided alternative hypothesis will be used. The null and alternative hypotheses are as follows:

$$H_0 : \mu = 60$$
$$H_1 : \mu \neq 60$$

The lowercase Greek letter $\mu$ (mu) represents the true population mean. This is a two-sided hypothesis test since the alternative is not equal. The next step is to determine the acceptable level of type I error. Recall that type I error is the probability of rejecting the null hypothesis when it is true. In this example, the type I error level is set to be 5 percent. Since type I error or rejecting the null hypothesis when it is true may cause the analyst to reach a conclusion that may cause a change in process or patient care, the level of type I error or alpha level for a statistical test should be selected based on the context of the test. If an error would be costly, then the type I error should be set to a very small value. Many researchers use 5 percent or 0.05 as the acceptable level of type I error.

A sample of 20 patients is selected and the sample mean ED wait time is 53.5 minutes with a standard deviation of 7.23 minutes. The null hypothesis may be tested using the following formula:

$$t = \frac{(\bar{x} - \mu_0)}{s / \sqrt{n}}$$
$$t = \frac{(53.5 - 60)}{7.23 / \sqrt{20}}$$

Studying the anatomy of the t-test can help formulate the intuition regarding hypothesis tests in general.

In general, the null hypothesis is rejected when the test statistic, t in this case, is an extremely large positive value or extremely small negative value. The numerator of the t statistic is the difference between the sample mean ($\mu_0$) and the null hypothesis ($H_0$) value. If that difference is large (positive or negative), then the t statistic is large. The denominator of the t statistic is the standard error, or the standard deviation ($s$) divided by the square root of the sample size ($n$). This value is directly proportional to the standard deviation and indirectly proportional to the sample size. In other words, the standard error increases if the standard deviation is larger and decreases as the sample size grows. The t statistic increases as the standard error decreases. The t statistic is comparing the difference between the sample mean and the null hypothesis value relative to the spread in distribution and the sample size.

The determination of the value of the t statistic that is extreme enough to reject the null hypothesis is dependent on the t distribution and the acceptable level of type I error. The t statistic is compared to the t distribution, which is similar in shape to the standard normal distribution. Using the t distribution, a cutoff or critical value can be determined so that the probability of observing a value that large by chance is the type I error level. The critical value is determined by the type I error level and the degrees of freedom or the sample size minus one ($n - 1$). The degrees of freedom for a statistical test is the number of observations ($n$) minus the number of parameters estimated when calculating the test statistic. In this case, the sample mean is estimated and then used to calculate the t-test value. Therefore, the degrees of freedom for the one sample t-test is $n - 1$. In this example, the degrees of freedom are $20 - 1 = 19$ and the error level is 0.05. The test statistic must be greater than 2.09 or less than −2.09 to reject the null hypothesis. This value may be derived from a table of the t distribution found in most statistical tests or from Microsoft Excel by using the TINV function: = TINV(0.05,19). TINV is a function in Excel that returns the inverse of the t distribution given the alpha or type I error level and degrees of freedom for a two-sided t-test. Figure 16.5 shows the shape of the t distribution, and the probability represented by the 2.09 and −2.09 critical values. The probability of observing a value outside of −2.09 and 2.09 on the t distribution with 19 degrees of freedom is 2.5 percent + 2.5 percent = 5 percent.

Based on the sample, the t statistic is as follows:

$$t = \frac{(53.5 - 60)}{7.23 / \sqrt{20}} = \frac{-6.5}{1.62} = -4.01$$

Since −4.01 is less than −2.09, the null hypothesis is rejected, and the conclusion is that the ED wait time is less than the 60-minute standard. (Note: In hypothesis testing, the null hypothesis is either rejected or not rejected. The null hypothesis is never accepted.)

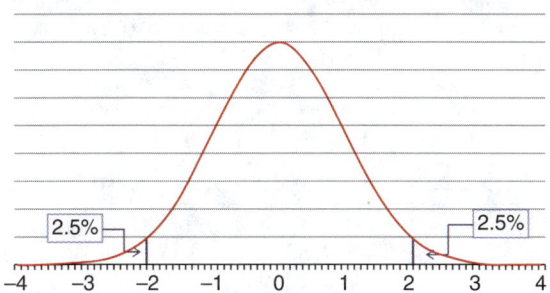

**Figure 16.5.** T distribution with 19 degrees of freedom

### Inference Example: Confidence Interval for Mean

Since the null hypothesis was rejected in favor of the alternative that the ED wait times are significantly lower than the standard, the marketing director is interested in finding out how far below the standard the ED wait times might be. The marketing director is interested in publishing a figure in the new campaign but needs to be sure the value is defensible. A confidence interval will result in a range of values with an associated level of confidence that the interval contains the population average ED wait time. The confidence level is designated to be 95 percent. The formula for the 95 percent confidence interval for the mean is as follows:

$$\left( \bar{x} - t_{\frac{\alpha}{2}, n-1} \times \frac{s}{\sqrt{n}}, \bar{x} + t_{\frac{\alpha}{2}}, n - 1 \times \frac{s}{\sqrt{n}} \right)$$

Where $\bar{x}$ is the sample mean, $t_{\frac{\alpha}{2}, n-1}$ is the critical value from the t distribution at $\alpha/2$ with $n - 1$ degrees of freedom, $s$ is the sample standard deviation, and $n$ is the sample size.

The confidence interval is centered at the sample mean. The width of the confidence interval is a function of the t distribution (confidence level), the sample standard deviation and the sample size. To calculate a 95 percent confidence interval, we set $\alpha = 0.05$ to determine the critical value of $t_{\frac{\alpha}{2}, n-1}$. Notice that a larger standard deviation results in a wider interval. A larger sample size results in a narrower or more precise interval. Recall that the earlier discussion about sample size selection was dependent on the sample standard deviation, the desired precision, and the confidence level. The concept of sample size selection is directly related to the width or precision of the desired confidence interval. $t_{\frac{\alpha}{2}, n-1}$ is the value from the t distribution with $n - 1$ degrees of freedom where there is an $\alpha/2$ chance of observing a value that extreme by chance. A 95 percent confidence interval may also be expressed as a $(1 - \alpha)$ percent confidence interval. In this case $\alpha$ is 0.05 and the degrees of freedom are $20 - 1 = 19$.

$$t_{\frac{\alpha}{2}, n-1} = 2.09$$
$$\frac{(53.5 - 2.09 \times 7.23)}{\sqrt{20}}, \frac{(53.5 + 2.09 \times 7.23)}{\sqrt{20}}$$
$$(53.5 - 3.4, 53.5 + 3.4)$$
$$(50.1, 56.9)$$

The result of this analysis is that the marketing director can be 95 percent sure that the true population average ED wait time is between 50.1 and 56.9 minutes.

Two-sided hypothesis test and confidence interval for the population mean are related. The formulas contain the same sample statistics and if the confidence level is one minus the type I error rate, then the null hypothesis will be rejected for any value outside of the confidence intervals. For the ED wait time example, notice that the 95 percent confidence interval does not contain 60 minutes. The null hypothesis that the ED wait time was equal to 60 minutes was rejected at the 5 percent level. The confidence interval end points tell us that any null hypothesis greater than 56.9 minutes or less than 50.1 minutes would be rejected at the 5 percent level since those values are outside of the upper and lower bounds of the 95 percent confidence interval.

## Normal Distribution

The distribution of data values may be described with statistics. The **normal distribution** is the formal name of the distribution known as the bell-shaped curve. The shape of the normal distribution is symmetric around its mean and uniquely defined by its mean and standard deviation. Figure 16.6 shows the standard normal distribution, which is a special case where the mean is zero and the standard deviation is equal to one. All normally distributed variables may be transformed to the standard normal distribution by subtracting the mean and dividing by the standard deviation.

The normal distribution is often used to describe the approximate distribution of variables. It is used in quality control charts and other tools because the percentage of the distribution within multiples of the standard deviation is easily defined. For instance, 66 percent of the distribution is concentrated between one standard deviation below to one standard deviation above the mean; 95 percent of the distribution is concentrated between two standard deviations below to two standard deviations above the mean; and over 99 percent of the distribution is concentrated between three standard deviations below the mean to three standard deviations above the mean.

**Figure 16.6.** Standard normal distribution function

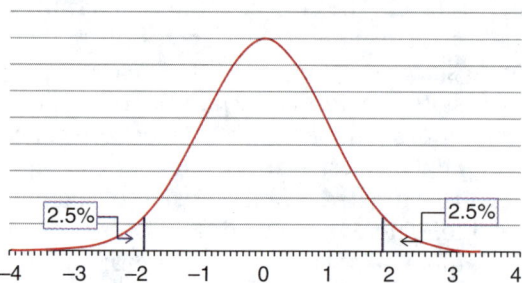

 **Check Your Understanding 16.2**

**Answer the following questions in a separate document.**

1. Which of the following describes the center of distribution for a variable such as length of stay?
   a. Variance
   b. Mean
   c. Standard deviation
   d. Range

2. When describing the typical length of stay for patients admitted for CHF, which is the most appropriate measure of central tendency, given the following values for lengths of stay are (3, 4, 5, 2, 3, 9, and 10)?
   a. Minimum
   b. Mean
   c. Median
   d. Mode

3. The one sample t-test may be used to do which of the following?
   a. Determine if the length of stay in a hospital is highly variable
   b. Determine if the length of stay for normal deliveries is shorter than the standard negotiated in a commercial contract
   c. Determine the most likely value of the hospital's overall mean length of stay
   d. Define a range of likely values for the hospital's overall mean length of stay

4. Which of the following is a not a characteristic of the normal distribution?
   a. Mean and median are equal
   b. The distribution is skewed to the left.

c. Half of the distribution is greater than the mean
d. The probability of a value being more than two standard deviations from the mean is about 95 percent

5. An analyst provides a 95 percent confidence interval for the mean length of stay for hip replacement patients: 2.3 to 4.7 days. If the utilization review committee requests a more precise or narrower interval, what is the best option for the analyst to pursue?
   a. Collect a larger sample
   b. Repeat the analysis for a later time
   c. Provide an interval with a higher level of confidence
   d. Suggest that the surgeons reduce the variance in length of stay

6. If the average length of stay for a sample of 15 patients is 2.3 days and the standard deviation is 1.5 days, which of the following statements is true?
   a. A 90 percent confidence interval will be narrower than a 95 percent confidence interval.
   b. A 95 percent confidence interval and 90 percent confidence interval will be the same.
   c. A 95 percent confidence interval will be narrower than a 90 percent confidence interval width.
   d. Not enough information is provided to answer.

# Analyzing Rates and Proportions

Rates and proportions are summary statistics based on either a sample or population. A rate is the number of times an event of interest occurs divided by the number of times that event could have occurred. The event and the number eligible must be carefully defined so that the calculations of rates are valid and reproducible.

## Descriptive Statistics for Rates and Proportions

Rates may be reported as percentages, counts per 1,000, or as a fraction, as in $x$ out of $y$. When calculating a rate, the numerator (top number in a fraction) is the number of subjects with the trait of interest. The denominator (bottom number in a fraction) is the number of subjects that could have had the trait of interest.

Consider the example of measuring the mortality rate at a facility. The mortality rate may be interpreted as the probability of any one of the 100 patients dying. In other words, in the context of this analysis each patient has two outcomes—living or dying. The mortality rate calculated from a sample is an estimate of the population probability of dying, or $p$.

It is always good practice to not only estimate the probability or $p$ of an event, but to also estimate the variance or spread around the sample proportion estimate. If our sample of size $n$ produces a proportion estimate of $p$, denoted as $\hat{p}$, then standard error of a proportion estimate is as follows:

$$SE_p = \sqrt{\frac{\hat{p} \times (1-\hat{p})}{n}}$$

The standard error of the sample proportion is the standard deviation divided by the square root of the sample size. In this formula, $\hat{p}$ is the estimated proportion based on the random sample. Therefore, both the mean and the standard error of the sample proportion depends on the estimated value. Notice that the standard error decreases and the sample size increases. The value of $SE_p$ is maximized when the sample proportion is 0.5 or 50 percent. Recall from the discussion of the CMS quality indicators that the confidence intervals using their guidance were the widest when the observed rate was 50 percent.

## Inferential Statistics for Rates and Proportions

The most common types of inferential statistical techniques used with rates and proportions are hypothesis tests to compare rates to a standard or confidence intervals. If an analyst is trying to determine if a rate is higher or lower than a standard, then a hypothesis is the correct statistical technique. In hypothesis testing, the first step is to define the null hypothesis (status quo) ($H_0$) and the alternative or research hypothesis ($H_1$).

$$H_0: p = p_0$$
$$H_1: p \neq p_0$$

The test is performed to determine if the analyst should reject the null hypothesis at a given error level. This is called the type I error level. The error level should be set low (0.01 or 0.05) as the action to be taken is costly in terms of money, time, or patient lives. If the question is less critical, then the error level may be set higher. The test statistic used in this situation is a z-test. A z-test should be used to test hypotheses regarding proportions:

$$z = \frac{(\hat{p} - p_0)}{\sqrt{p_0 \times (1 - p_0)/n}}$$

In this formula, $n$ is the sample size, $p_0$ is the null hypothesis value, and $\hat{p}$ is the estimated proportion based on the random sample. If the test statistic $z$ is greater than $z_{\alpha/2}$ or less than $-z_{\alpha/2}$ where $\alpha$ is the predefined type I error level, then the null hypothesis will be rejected. For this test, the standard normal distribution is used to determine a critical value beyond which the null hypothesis should be rejected. If the error level of the test is 0.05 or 5 percent, then the critical value or $z_{\alpha/2}$ is 1.96. This may be derived from the standard normal table found in most statistics textbooks or from using the following formula in Excel: = NORMSINV(0.025). NORMSINV(0.025) will return a z score that represents the point for which 2.5 percent of the curve is outside +/− that point. The argument 0.025 is used because the type I error level was set to 0.05 and this is a two-sided test (0.05/2 = 0.025). Figure 16.6 shows the critical values on the probability curve of the standard normal distribution. As with the t-test, one half of the type I error is allocated to each side of the curve. Notice that the critical value for the standard normal distribution is slightly smaller than that from the t distribution with 19 degrees of freedom. As the degrees of freedom for the t distribution increases, it becomes closer to the standard normal distribution.

One of the CMS quality indicators measures the proportion of pneumonia patients assessed and given influenza vaccination. A facility may wish to compare their rate to the national vaccination rate. If 80 percent of the patients out of a sample of 74 eligible patients received a flu vaccine at University Hospital, can we conclude that their vaccination rate is significantly different from the national rate of 91 percent?

The hypothesis to be tested here is as follows:

$$H_0: p = 0.91$$
$$H_1: p \neq 0.91$$

The test statistic is as follows:

$$z = \frac{(0.80 - 0.91)}{\sqrt{0.91 \times (1 - 0.91)/74}} = \frac{-0.110}{0.033} = 3.33$$

Since the test statistic, $z = -3.33$, is less than the critical value, $-1.96$, the null hypothesis is rejected. The conclusion is that University Hospital's flu vaccine rate for pneumonia patients is significantly lower than the national rate.

The $z_{\alpha/2}$ is the same critical value identified for the two-sided hypothesis test presented. A 95 percent confidence interval for the flu vaccine rate at University Hospital is as follows:

$$\left(\hat{p} - z_{\alpha/2} \times \sqrt{\frac{\hat{p} \times (1-\hat{p})}{n}}, \hat{p} + z_{\alpha/2} \times \sqrt{\frac{\hat{p} \times (1-\hat{p})}{n}}\right)$$

$$\left(0.80 - 1.96 \times \sqrt{\frac{0.80 \times (1-0.80)}{74}},\right.$$
$$0.80 + 1.96 \times \sqrt{\frac{0.80 \times (1-0.80)}{74}}$$
$$0.80 - 1.96 \times \sqrt{\frac{0.80 \times (1-0.80)}{74}},$$
$$\left.0.80 + 1.96 \times \sqrt{\frac{0.80 \times (1-0.80)}{74}}\right)$$

$(0.80 - 0.09, 0.80 + 0.09)$ or $(0.71, 0.89)$

The 95 percent confidence interval for the population pneumonia patient flu vaccine rate is from 71 percent to 89 percent. This precision for this interval is +/− 9 percent. If a more precise interval is desired, then a large sample size should be collected for the next measurement period.

### Check Your Understanding 16.3

**Answer the following questions in a separate document.**

1. The standard error of a sample proportion is dependent on which of the following?
   a. The estimated proportion
   b. The sample size
   c. a and b
   d. The population size

2. What value of a proportion results in the widest confidence interval?
   a. 50%
   b. 100%
   c. 5%
   d. 95%

3. If we wish to test the hypothesis that a facility's mortality rate is significantly different than the state average of 5 percent, which of the following null and alternative hypotheses are appropriate?
   a. $H_o: p \leq 5\%$; $H_1: p \geq 5\%$
   b. $H_o: p = 5\%$; $H_1: p \neq 5\%$
   c. $H_o: p > 5\%$; $H_1: p \leq 5\%$
   d. $H_o: p \neq 5\%$; $H_1: p = 5\%$

4. If a 95 percent confidence interval for the proportion of postoperative infections is (0.9 percent, 1.5 percent), what is the precision of that interval?
   a. ±1.5%
   b. ±0.6%
   c. ±0.9%
   d. ±0.3%

5. If the test statistic for testing the hypothesis that the readmission rate at General Hospital is different from zero is $z = 3.45$, what would the conclusion of the test be at the 0.01 level?
   a. Accept $H_o$
   b. Reject $H_1$
   c. Reject $H_o$
   d. Do not reject $H_o$

## Analyzing Relationships between Two Variables

A data analyst may need to explore the relationship between two variables. Examples include the relationship between length of stay and charges, patient age, and mortality, or number of coding staff members and number of records coded per shift.

### Correlation

**Correlation** is the statistic that is used to describe the association or relationship between two variables. In the healthcare setting, we may note that length of stay, and charges are highly related or correlated. Since charges increase as length of stay increases, it is said the two variables are positively correlated. An example of two negatively correlated variables may be years of coder experience and time to code a medical record. If the more experienced coders have shorter review times, then the two variables are negatively correlated.

Pearson's correlation coefficient or $r$ measures the strength of the linear relationship between two variables. The statistic can range from $-1$ to $+1$. Negative one is perfect negative correlation while positive one is perfect positive correlation. The formula for calculating Pearson's correlation coefficient is

$$r = \frac{\sum_{i=1}^{n}(X_i - \bar{X}) \times (Y_i - \bar{Y})}{\sqrt{\sum_{i=1}^{n}(X_i - \bar{X})^2} \times \sqrt{\sum_{i=1}^{n}(Y_i - \bar{Y})^2}}$$

where $\bar{X}$ and $\bar{Y}$ are the mean of the variables $X$ and $Y$ respectively and $n$ is the number of data points.

Notice that the numerator of the statistic will determine the sign of the correlation. Confidence intervals and hypothesis tests may be performed to make inference about the strength of association between two variables. Pearson's $r$ is a measure of correlation and not causation. Causation is far more difficult to prove through data and really requires a carefully designed and controlled experiment to prove.

Suppose an analyst wishes to study the relationship between number of years of coding experience and time required to code an outpatient medical record. The analyst selects a random sample of seven coders and collects the data presented in table 16.3 (answers are rounded to two decimal places).

The Pearson's $r$ for experience and time is as follows:

$$r = \frac{\sum_{i=1}^{n}(X_i - 3.0) \times (Y_i - 41.6)}{\sqrt{\sum_{i=1}^{n}(X_i - 3.0)^2} \times \sqrt{\sum_{i=1}^{n}(Y_i - 41.6)^2}}$$

$$r = \frac{-56.93}{\sqrt{21.50} \times \sqrt{286.00}} = -0.83$$

The interpretation of the negative value of the correlation coefficient is that time to code records decreases as experience increases. A scatter plot of two variables is a useful tool for exploring the relationship. Figure 16.7 shows the decreasing trend in coding time as the years of experience increase for each subject in the sample.

Pearson's $r$ may be converted to the **coefficient of determination** or $r^2$. The $r^2$ measures how much of the variation in one variable is explained by the second variable. In this example, $r^2 = (-0.83)^2 = 0.68$. Therefore, 68 percent of the variance in coding time may be explained by the years of experience.

Table 16.3. Example calculation of Pearson's correlation coefficient

| Subject | X: Experience (yr) | Y: Time (min) | $(X_i - \bar{X}) \times (Y_i - \bar{Y})$ | $(X_i - \bar{X})^2$ | $(Y_i - \bar{Y})^2$ |
|---|---|---|---|---|---|
| 1 | 5.00 | 30.00 | (20.94) | 3.72 | 117.88 |
| 2 | 1.00 | 55.00 | (29.30) | 4.29 | 200.02 |
| 3 | 2.50 | 45.00 | (2.37) | 0.33 | 17.16 |
| 4 | 4.50 | 35.00 | (8.37) | 2.04 | 34.31 |
| 5 | 3.50 | 45.00 | 1.78 | 0.18 | 17.16 |
| 6 | 2.00 | 39.00 | 1.99 | 1.15 | 3.45 |
| 7 | 3.00 | 37.00 | 0.28 | 0.01 | 14.88 |
| Total | 21.50 | 286.00 | (56.93) | 11.71 | 404.86 |

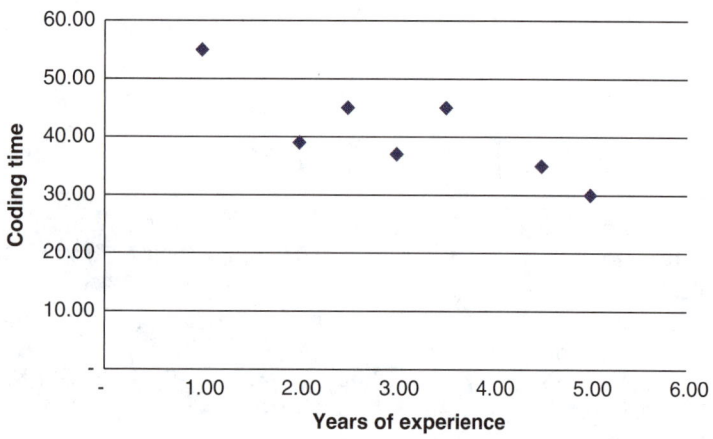

Figure 16.7. Example of relationship between two continuous variables

## Simple Linear Regression

**Simple linear regression (SLR)** is another type of statistical inference that not only measures the strength of the relationship between two variables, but also estimates a functional relationship between them. SLR may be used when one of the two variables of interest is dependent on the other. For instance, the total charge incurred during an inpatient stay is often dependent on the length of time spent in the hospital. Regression may also be used to describe the relationship between coder experience and time per record beyond simply stating they have a negative correlation or inverse relationship. In general, the variable that is used to predict is called the **independent variable**. The outcome or variable to be predicted is called the **dependent variable** (White 2021, 132).

SLR is typically performed by fitting a line through a least squares algorithm. Basically, the least squares method selects the line that minimizes the vertical (Y) distance between all points and the selected line. The result is a line that may not actually go through any points but comes as close as possible to all points.

The least squares line for this example is displayed in figure 16.8.

The slope of the least squares line is always the same sign as the correlation between the two variables. The formula for the least squares line for this data is as follows:

$$[Coding\ time] = -4.86 \times [Experience] + 55.78$$

The SLR line represents the predicted or expected values of the dependent variable given various values of the independent variable. The interpretation of this relationship is that the predicted coding time for a coder with no experience is 55.78 minutes. This value, 55.78, is referred to as the y-intercept of the line. Each year of experience reduces the predicted time to code records by 4.86 minutes. This value, −4.86, is referred to as the slope of the line. The slope is an estimate of the change in the dependent variable, $y$, which is expected for each one unit change in the independent variable, $x$. The line displayed in figure 16.8 states that the expected coding time for a coder with four years of experience is y = −4.86 × 4 +

55.78 = 36.34 minutes. The coefficient of determination is used to measure the explanatory power of the linear regression line. As previously calculated, the $r^2 = 0.68$. The years of experience of a coder explains 68 percent of the variance in coding time. One application of this regression line is to create personalized workload expectations for each coder based on experience. A performance ratio could then be calculated as the observed coding time divided by the expected coding time for each coder to monitor performance and provide feedback for improvement. A performance ratio greater than one would indicate better than expected performance and a performance ratio less than one would indicate a performance that requires improvement.

Another interesting application of SLR is studying the relationship between charge per inpatient visit and length of stay for inpatient stays. The least squares line may be used to break out the fixed and variable portions of the charges.

Figure 16.9 displays the relationship between patient length of stay and total charges for CHF. The relationship between length of stay and total charge is very strong with an $r^2$ of 0.93. In other words, length of stay explains 93 percent of the variance in total charge. This strong relationship between total charge and length of stay is true for many medical inpatient stays. The relationship between these two variables may be less strong for surgical inpatient stays if the charge for the surgery is a large proportion of the total charge.

Figure 16.8. Example of least squares line

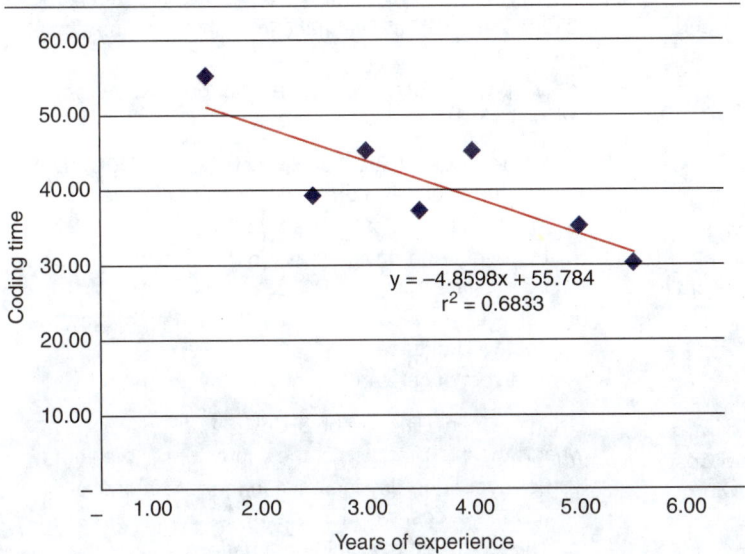

Figure 16.9. Relationship between length of stay and total charge for CHF inpatient stays

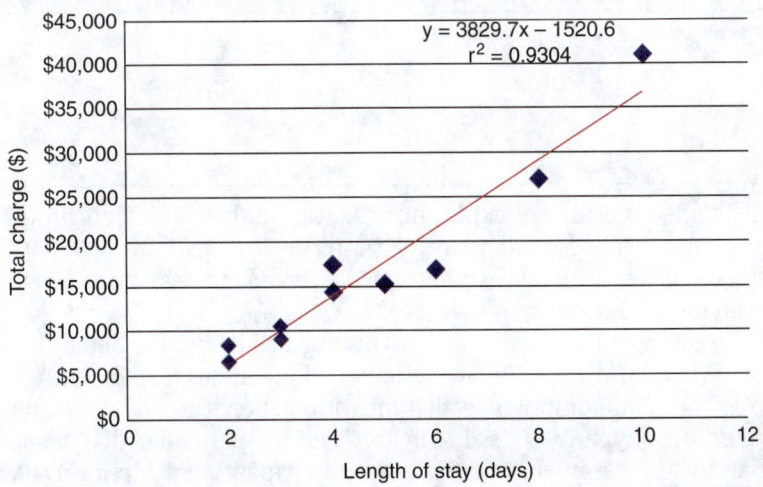

The model in figure 16.9 states that the predicted total charge equals $1,521 + $3,830 × LOS. The intercept of the line, $1,521, represents the fixed charge of a CHF inpatient stay. Fixed charge items are registration, administration, initial laboratory, or radiology workups that are not dependent on how long the patient stays. The slope of the line represents the variable component of the charge. Variable charge items are nursing care, dietary, maintenance medications, and other resources that are used each day of the stay. Breaking the charges into the fixed and variable components facilitates root cause analysis studies into the variation in resources used to treat various types of patients. For instance, the charges for CHF patients are clearly driven more by the variable component than the fixed component. CHF treatment protocols that concentrate on length of stay reduction may be an effective way to ensure proper resources are used to treat these patients. For a joint replacement or other surgical case with significant medical supply costs, it is unlikely that a length of stay study would be very effective.

### Check Your Understanding 16.4

Answer the following questions in a separate document.

1. If the correlation between patient lung volume level and BMI is 0.6, which of the following conclusions is correct?
   a. Patients with low BMI have large lung volume.
   b. Patients with high BMI have large lung volume.
   c. High BMI causes large lung volume.
   d. Large lung volume causes high BMI.

2. Which statistic should a health data analyst recommend to a manager who would like to measure the relationship between length of stay and time to code a medical record?
   a. Slope of the linear regression line
   b. t-Test
   c. Correlation
   d. Intercept of the linear regression line

3. If the coefficient of determination for the SLR model Cost = 2,500 + 450 × LOS is 0.8, then which of the following statements is correct?
   a. 80 percent of the variance in length of stay is explained by cost.
   b. 20 percent of the variance in cost is explained by length of stay.
   c. 80 percent of the variance in cost is explained by length of stay.
   d. 20 percent of the variance in length of stay is explained by cost.

4. Using the model in question 3, Cost = 2,500 + 450 × LOS, what is the interpretation of the slope of the line?
   a. The typical cost of care is $2,500.
   b. For every one-day increase in the length of stay, the cost will decrease by $450.
   c. For every one-day increase in the length of stay, the cost will increase by $450.
   d. The cost of care and length of stay are not related.

5. Using the model in question 3, Cost = 2,500 + 450 × LOS, what is the interpretation of the y-intercept of the line?
   a. For every one-day increase in the length of stay (LOS), the cost will increase by $2,500.
   b. The fixed cost of admitting a patient is $2,500.
   c. For every one-day increase in the LOS, the cost will decrease by $2,500.
   d. The fixed cost of admitting a patient is $450.

## Analytics in Practice

There are numerous practical applications of data analytics in healthcare. Just a few examples include data mining, predictive modeling, analysis of risk-adjusted quality indicators, and real-time analytics.

### Data Mining

The techniques of data analytics may be used to perform data mining. In **data mining**, the analyst performs exploratory data analysis to determine trends and identify patterns in the data set. Data mining is sometimes referred to as knowledge discovery.

In healthcare, data mining may be used to determine if it is cost-effective to expand facilities. An analysis of appointment wait times for patients to see a certain type of specialist or to receive a particular diagnostic test might indicate a need to expand that service. Data mining may also be used to analyze referral patterns of physicians within a particular network.

In traditional data analytics, data are collected for a specific purpose to answer a business or research question. In data mining, data are often used for secondary analysis; that is, the data are used for a purpose that was not the primary reason for collection. Claims data are an excellent data source for mining and finding patterns, but the primary purpose of claims data is for submission to ask for payment and not data mining (White 2021, 2).

In data mining, historical data are analyzed to find trends and patterns. Those trends and patterns are then used in business planning or process improvement. This historical technique may be extended to predict future behavior based on the data via predictive modeling techniques.

## Predictive Modeling

Predictive modeling is another application of data analytics in healthcare. Predictive modeling is a special application of data mining. CMS is using predictive modeling to identify potential fraudulent Medicare claims (White 2011). The pattern of claims submitted by a provider is analyzed to identify unlikely trends, given the claims history of the provider or the patient. For instance, predictive modeling may be used to identify a provider who submits a claim for a service unrelated to their specialty or a high-cost service for which they have not submitted a previous claim. The goal of this technique is to target claims unlikely to be valid and select them for further review.

Predictive modeling applies statistical techniques to determine the likelihood of certain events occurring together (White 2011). Statistical methods are applied to historical data to learn the patterns in the data. These patterns are used to create models of what is most likely to occur. Predictive modeling is used by credit card issuers to determine if transactions are likely fraudulent. Customers who receive a phone call from their credit card company verifying that they authorized a transaction are the subjects of a predictive model.

For example, a customer's typical credit card transaction is $100. The credit card issuer notices that the customer submitted three $5,000 transactions in one day. Given the customer's history and the credit card issuer's historical data regarding fraudulent transactions, those transactions look suspicious. The credit card company may then contact the customer to verify that the customer authorized the suspect transactions. The triggers that tell the credit card company when to suspect a fraud issue are created through predictive modeling techniques.

Predictive modeling techniques use multiple data sources. Data such as the provider's claim history, the patient's demographics and health status, the services included on the claim, and the attributes associated with previously identified fraudulent claims may all be used to develop a statistical model. Statistical techniques used to create the model may include logistic regression, cluster analysis, or decision trees. All these statistical techniques allow the user to combine multivariate (more than one outcome variable) historical data into a model that may be used to assess the probability or likelihood that current claims are fraudulent.

In logistical regression, the likelihood a claim is fraudulent is estimated based on a series of historical data. In cluster analysis, historical data are used to build a model that measures the distance of a claim from the typical claims submitted by that provider or for that type of service. Decision trees use a series of screens or yes or no questions to determine the probability that a claim is valid. The output of each of these methods is the probability of a claim's validity that is expressed as a claim score.

The claim score is typically structured so it is directly related to the probability that a claim is in error. A high score may indicate a high probability that a claim is not legitimate. If the score meets a criterion (either above or below a cutoff value), then it is identified as a potential error. The criteria or cutoff value may be used to tune the model to control the sensitivity and specificity of the model. If the cutoff is too extreme, then the model may not be sensitive enough and will allow fraudulent claims to be paid. If the cutoff is not extreme enough, then the model may not be specific enough and identify many false positives.

In the healthcare setting, the cost of paying fraudulent claims must be weighed against the cost of withholding payment and reviewing the claim prior to payment. For high-cost and low-volume claims, the cutoff may be set lower to ensure no questionable claims are paid. The cost of paying an invalid claim outweighs the cost of reviewing a few false positive claims. The model may be adapted and adjusted as more claims history is aggregated.

Many commercial payers currently use predictive models as one of their fraud prevention tools. The UnitedHealth Group estimated that the use of predictive modeling in the Medicare and Medicaid programs could save the programs $113 billion over the first 10 years of use (UnitedHealth Group 2009).

## Risk-Adjusted Quality Indicators

The values for some quality and outcomes indicators in healthcare are dependent on the mix of patients treated at that facility. For example, the 30-day mortality rate at a major academic medical center cannot be directly compared to the 30-day mortality rate at a rural community hospital without some sort of adjustment for the difference in acuity of the patients. CMS uses a hierarchical regression model to adjust for both individual patient characteristics as well as hospital characteristics. The model calculates an expected 30-day mortality rate for each hospital and then compares the expected rate to the observed rate when reporting statistics on their Hospital Compare website. The method is similar to the observed versus expected productivity ratio presented in the SLR portion of this chapter. The model used to calculate the expected mortality is far more complex, but the interpretation is the same. CMS calculates a risk standardized mortality rate (RSMR) based on the expected mortality rate and the observed mortality rate for each condition and hospital profiled (CMS 2023b). Lower RSMR implies a hospital has better quality as measured by these rates.

Although the details involved in hierarchical regression are beyond the scope of this text, the concept that an observed rate is compared to an expected rate to determine relative performance makes intuitive sense. The exact methodology to derive the expected rate may vary depending on the research question and the data available for modeling.

A more straightforward method for calculating a RSMR is to use **indirect standardization** to derive the expected rate for an outcome variable (White 2020). Indirect standardization is appropriate to use for risk adjustment when the risk variables are categorical and the rate or proportion for the variable of interest is available for the standard or reference group at the level of the risk categories. The expected outcome rate for each risk category is calculated based on the reference group and then weighted by the volume in each risk group at the population to be compared to the standard. Indirect standardization is not useful when trying to compare the outcomes at two facilities but is useful when comparing a facility to a standard.

The example data presented in table 16.4 presents the in-hospital mortality rate for the family of cardiac arrhythmia and conduction disorder MS-DRGs for the US as well as The Hospital. The observed overall in-hospital mortality rate for The Hospital, 1.6 percent, is higher than the national rate, 1.3 percent. The Hospital recorded lower mortality rates for patients assigned to two of the three individual MS-DRGs and had lower mortality rates in MS-DRG 308, which includes patients with MCC. The proportion of the patients in each MS-DRG is not available for the national statistics, and it is not known if The Hospital's mix is more concentrated in the MS-DRGs with MCC.

The national rates for each MS-DRG may be used to estimate the expected mortality rate for The Hospital using indirect standardization.

The first step in indirect standardization is to use the hospital's volume and the national in-hospital mortality rate for each risk category to calculate the expected number of deaths. In this example, the MS-DRGs represent the risk categories. Based on the data in table 16.4, the expected number of deaths for each of the MS-DRGs is as follows:

- MS-DRG 308: $0.049 \times 152 = 7.45$
- MS-DRG 309: $0.008 \times 158 = 1.26$
- MS-DRG 310: $0.002 \times 191 = 0.38$

The three MS-DRG expected deaths are then added together to yield the expected number of deaths at the hospital: $7.45 + 1.26 + 0.38 = 9.09$. The expected in-house mortality rate for the hospital is then $9.09/501 = 1.8$ percent. The observed and expected mortalities may then be used to calculate a standardized mortality ratio (SMR).

$$SMR = \frac{Observed\ Mortality\ Rate}{Expected\ Mortality\ Rate}$$

The SMR for the hospital is 1.6 percent/1.8 percent, or 0.89. An SMR value less than one means the observed mortality rate is lower than expected and an SMR greater than one means the observed mortality rate is higher than expected. The SMR for the hospital is 0.89, indicating that the observed in-hospital mortality rate is lower than expected. Note that the unadjusted observed mortality rate for the hospital was higher than the national rate. Indirect standardization gave the hospital credit for the lower mortality rate in the most resource-intense cases and therefore allowed an apples-to-apples comparison to the national rate.

## Real-Time Analytics

As data analysis tools mature and the granularity of the data available in a healthcare entity increases, real-time analytics and performance dashboards based on key performance indicators (KPIs) are becoming the norm. Once a set of KPIs is identified, data elements to drive those indicators are created in real time and not based on static historical databases. For example, a KPI for an HIM manager at a hospital may be the level of charges in the set of discharged and not final billed (DNFB) charts. If the level of charges goes above a predefined threshold, then an email is sent to the manager to notify him of that fact so action may be taken quickly. Without real-time analytics producing the KPI and alert, the manager may not have been

Table 16.4. MS-DRG 308, 309, 310 mortality rates

| MS-DRG and name | | The Hospital statistics | | | | |
|---|---|---|---|---|---|---|
| | | Estimated US in-hospital mortality rate | The Hospital discharges | Observed in-hospital deaths | Observed mortality rate | Expected deaths |
| 308 | Cardiac arrhythmia and conduction disorders w/mcc | 4.9% | 152 | 6 | 3.9% | 7.45 |
| 309 | Cardiac arrhythmia and conduction disorders w/cc | 0.8% | 158 | 2 | 1.3% | 1.26 |
| 310 | Cardiac arrhythmia and conduction disorders w/o cc/mcc | 0.2% | 191 | 0 | 0.0% | 0.38 |
| Totals | | 1.3% | 501 | 8 | 1.6% | 9.09 |

alerted of the high level of DNFB until a weekly or monthly report was produced.

KPIs included in real-time dashboards may feature both financial and clinical indicators, such as the following:

- Days in accounts receivable
- Charges in DNFB
- Patient census by unit
- Number of patients in ED waiting for inpatient bed
- ED wait time
- Number of patients waiting for discharge
- Time for housekeeping to return a bed to service

KPI dashboards are now used throughout healthcare organizations. Many healthcare IT vendors now include some level of KPI dashboard functionality in their systems. The difficulty in effectively implementing such systems is setting thresholds for the various KPIs that are meaningful and do not identify false positives. Many hospital performance indicators such as volume, length of stay, and ED wait times have a certain amount of typical variability. Setting thresholds that are too sensitive could result in management investigating issues that are not unusual. Combining KPIs with the concepts of analytics, such as confidence intervals and other statistical inference tools, can produce a system of real-time alerts that are both sensitive enough to identify performance issues yet specific enough to avoid false positives.

# Opportunities for Health Information Management Professionals in Healthcare Data Analytics

HIM professionals are uniquely positioned to take on a variety of roles related to healthcare data analytics. Combining the following skills transforms the traditional HIM role into one of a business analyst:

- Understand data structures and coding systems
- Understand available data and methods for integration
- Communicate with both finance and IT staff
- Act as a business analyst—far more valuable than a pure data analyst

For instance, in revenue cycle management, the identification of missed charges is challenging. The traditional approach to identifying missed charges is to perform a charge description master (CDM) review and interview unit staff to ensure charge codes are utilized as designed. The staff may also review departmental order sheets to ensure they include complete and accurate listings of the services available in the department. An HIM professional with strong analytic skills may take a data-driven approach to study this issue.

The charge codes that occur together often may be identified through profiling of historical claims data. Claims with only one of those codes may be selected for focused review. A chart review on that set of records that are most likely to include missed charges may then be completed to understand the root cause of the missing charges. The use of analytics on historical claims may save a significant amount of time in the identification of codes that are particularly problematic. Corrective action may be designed and implemented in a much more efficient manner.

The level of understanding of the relationship between variables analyzed and the complexity of the analytic techniques increase as an HIM professional advances from the entry to senior level. HIM professionals that have a solid grasp of statistical techniques can combine those skills with their knowledge of the clinical application of data to assist with the interpretation and application of the results of analysis projects.

### Check Your Understanding 16.5

Answer the following questions in a separate document.

1. The nurse manager on the internal medicine unit of the hospital noticed that Dr. Smith in the ED admits many patients to the internal medicine unit. The nurse manager is wondering if Dr. Smith admits patients to the hospital from the ED more often than other physicians. What type of analysis should be done to answer the question?
   a. Data warehousing
   b. Data governance
   c. Data mining
   d. Data modeling

2. The business analyst is using claims data to determine the average charges and average length of stay for Medicaid patients to help with setting the budget for next year. What type of data are the claims data in this case?
   a. Secondary data
   b. Primary data
   c. Statistical data
   d. Clinical data

3. What application of data mining is used to identify patients most likely to be readmitted?
   a. Database modeling
   b. Regression analysis
   c. Random sampling
   d. Predictive modeling

4. The coding manager needs a dashboard that shows the discharges pending final billing as it changes throughout the day to plan for staffing. What analysis technique is needed?
   a. Predictive modeling
   b. Indirect standardization
   c. Real-time analytics
   d. Data mining

5. Consider the job responsibilities of a health data analyst. Offer a minimum of five reasons that justify an HIM professional in this role; focus on your own areas of interest in your answer.

# References

Buchner, A., E. Erdfelder, F. Faul, and A. G. Lang. n.d. "G*Power: Statistical Power Analyses for Windows and Mac." https://www.psychologie.hhu.de/arbeitsgruppen/allgemeine-psychologie-und-arbeitspsychologie/gpower.

CMS (Centers for Medicare and Medicaid Services). n.d. "Hospital Compare." https://www.medicare.gov/care-compare/.

CMS (Centers for Medicare and Medicaid Services). n.d. "Program Integrity Manual." https://www.cms.gov/regulations-and-guidance/guidance/manuals/internet-only-manuals-ioms-items/cms019033.

CMS (Centers for Medicare and Medicaid Services). 2009. Roadmap for Implementing Value-Driven Healthcare in the Traditional Medicare Fee-for-Service Program. Technical Report. Baltimore, MD: CMS. http://www.cms.gov/Medicare/Quality-Initiatives-Patient-Assessment-Instruments/QualityInitiativesGenInfo/Downloads/VBPRoadmap_OEA_1-16_508.pdf.

CMS (Centers for Medicare and Medicaid Services). 2023a. "What Are the Value-based Programs?" Baltimore, MD: CMS. https://www.cms.gov/medicare/quality/value-based-programs.

CMS (Centers for Medicare and Medicaid Services). 2023b. "Risk Adjustment and Risk Stratification in Quality Measurement." https://mmshub.cms.gov/sites/default/files/Risk-Adjustment-in-Quality-Measurement.pdf.

CMS (Centers for Medicare and Medicaid Services). n.d. *Important Notes and Considerations for Using these Data: Generating Medicare Physician Quality Performance Measurement Results (GEM) Project*. Accessed June 9, 2024. https://www.cms.gov/Medicare/Quality-Initiatives-Patient-Assessment-Instruments/GEM/downloads/GEMImportantNotes.pdf.

HFMA (Healthcare Financial Management Association). n.d. "HFMA's MAP." Accessed June 9, 2024. http://www.hfma.org/map.

Office of the Inspector General (OIG). 2019. "RAT-STATS Statistical Software." https://oig.hhs.gov/compliance/rat-stats/.

QualityNet. 2023. Specifications Manual for National Hospital Inpatient Quality Measures—Discharges 01-01-24(1Q24) through 06-30-24 (2Q24), Version 5.15a. https://qualitynet.cms.gov/files/6571e06eca7fd3001b35e75f?filename=HIQR_SpecsMan_v5.15a.zip.

UnitedHealth Group. 2009. "Health Care Cost Containment—How Technology Can Cut Red Tape and Simplify Health Care Administration." https://www.unitedhealthgroup.com/content/dam/UHG/PDF/2009/UNH-Working-Paper-2.pdf.

White, S. 2020. *Basic & Clinical Biostatistics*. 5th ed. New York. McGraw Hill.

White, S. 2021. *A Practical Approach to Analyzing Healthcare Data*, 4th ed. Chicago: AHIMA.

White, S. 2011. Predictive modeling 101. *Journal of AHIMA* 82(9): 46–47.

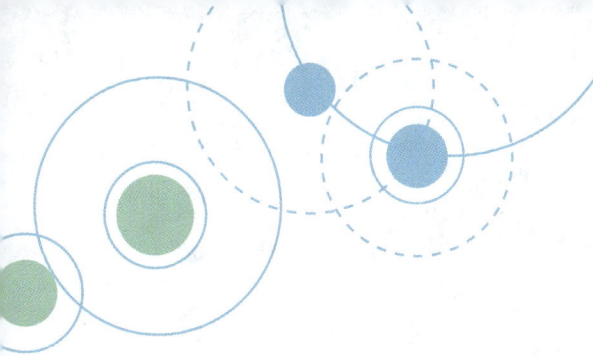

# chapter 17

# Data Visualization

*David T. Marc, PhD, CHDA*

## Learning Objectives

- Defend the role of graphical perception in interpreting a chart
- Propose the most effective method for presenting data
- Differentiate the situations where it is appropriate to use tables versus charts
- Design methods of visualizing data for decision-making
- Construct effective graphical displays of data

## Key Terms

Bar plot
Boxplot
Chart
Dashboard
Data visualization
Dot plot
Graphical perception
Histogram
Information overload
Latency
Line plot
Pie chart
Random oval
Scatterplot
Slicing and dicing
Spatial representation
Symbolic representation
Systematic ovals
Table

In medicine, practitioners and other professionals are faced with almost insurmountable amounts of data pertaining to clinical symptoms, laboratory results, medications, quality reporting, reimbursement and cost data, survey data, and more. This information is ultimately utilized for making decisions. However, given the volume, variety, and complexity of the data, there is the potential for errors in decision-making. In response, methods are being adopted to aid in decision-making processes by presenting information using charts and tables to supplement human information processes to maximize the efficiency of data interpretation while minimizing errors. Charts and tables are powerful tools for data visualization, which is the process of transforming data into graphical forms that can reveal patterns, trends, outliers, and relationships in data. This chapter offers insights and best practices in developing effective visual displays of data using charts and tables. The chapter begins by introducing the basic concept of data visualization as it pertains to graphical perception and decision-making. Next, a comparison on when to use charts and tables as visual displays is provided. The major factors influencing the effectiveness of visual displays are also detailed. The chapter concludes with a case study on developing an effective visual display for a medical scenario involving patient satisfaction and quality of care.

## Data Visualization Related to Perception and Decision-Making

**Data visualization** is a process of formatting data into patterns to support the interpretation of information. A **chart** is a visual display of data that uses symbols on a graph. The purpose of a chart is to display information, and when the chart is viewed by a person, the information is interpreted by the viewer's visual system. A **table** is a display that presents data that are often organized in columns and rows. The purpose of a table is to extract precise values and make decisions based on that value. **Graphical perception** is the term referring to the visual interpretation process and was originally described as the ability to unconsciously extract information from graphics (Cleveland and McGill 1984, 531). The methods selected to present data can have vast implications in healthcare related to presenting information in an abbreviated and easily understood manner. Since the volume of data that health information management (HIM) professionals are held accountable for is vast and continues to grow with technological advancements, including the electronic health record and improved data storage capabilities, there is a need to examine more efficient ways to present information. In addition, new data are constantly being collected in healthcare, which ultimately increases data complexity, thereby offering further considerations for presenting data graphically.

With increasing data complexity, the likelihood for failures in recognizing important findings to guide decision-making rises. The capacity for a human being to process large amounts of information is limited; therefore, new strategies are being explored to improve the presentation of data in order to enhance the efficiency and effectiveness of an interpretation. For example, adopting charts rather than tables for presenting data may support a more efficient interpretation. However, not all charts are created equal. Exploration of the theoretical foundation of graphical presentations allows for a better understanding of the charts that lead to the most effective visualization of data by overcoming human limitations of processing data and making decisions.

Graphical perception research explores human graphical perception and how the interpretation of data is time- and task-dependent. That is, the time of accurately extracting information from visual displays is dependent on the position, length, angle, area, and volume of the chart. Table 17.1 ranks various graphical techniques based on the most accurate presentation methods (Cleveland and McGill 1985, 829; 1984, 532).

When data are presented as a position along a common scale, the information can be extracted faster and with greater accuracy than other methods. By choosing a graphical method that ranks higher on table 17.1 than other methods, one can enhance the accuracy and efficiency of interpreting the data. Various types of charts can be used to present data across the various graphical techniques.

- A **bar plot** is used for presenting data as a position along a common scale. That is, the length of the bar or bars in the plot are referencing the same numeric scale.
- A line chart can also be used for presenting data as a position along a common scale since the line or lines in the plot are referencing the same scale.
- A stacked bar plot is used for presenting data using length along a nonaligned scale. The stacked bar plot includes stacked segments. To obtain the value of each segment, you must calculate the length of the individual segment, which may not be aligned with the scale. The total length of the bar is all the segments added together (see figure 17.4).
- A scatterplot is used to depict direction based on the relationship of two quantitative values.
- A pie chart is used to present data by comparing area based on the percentage of a group relative to the whole.
- A 3D bar plot is used for comparing volume where the height, width, and length of a bar can represent three different numeric values.
- A heat map is used to present data using shading and color saturation where a color scheme is used to represent a range of values.

There are many different types of charts that can be applied along the continuum of the ranked techniques. Notably, the purpose of any type of graphic is to display information to facilitate rapid and accurate interpretation to ultimately guide decisions. Therefore, when designing a chart, it is important to consider using a method that offers greater interpretation efficiency and accuracy.

Early research in behavioral decision-making has observed that when individuals make decisions, they trade the effort required to decide with the accuracy of the outcome (Beach and Mitchell 1978). Research shows that the use of decision aids, such as charts, are used only to reduce effort and not to improve accuracy; however, depending on the task, the use of charts does not extensively compromise the accuracy of the outcome (Speier 2006, 1126). Data literacy and visualization literacy influence a person's ability to interpret and use charts or tables (Franconeri et al. 2021, 111). Literacy is accomplished through repeat exposure to material and learning how to interpret and use the information. Professionals that have experience using a specific type of chart or table may achieve greater literacy using that format and greater success in interpreting data when compared to other display (Franconeri et al. 2021, 126).

A study published in 2022 explored individual differences with interpreting data from charts and found that, depending on user experience, a chart that is ranked lower may have better performance due to past experiences impacting visualization literacy (Davis et al. 2022). For example, a person who has experience interpreting data from a pie chart may make a more accurate and efficient interpretation than what is expected from someone who has less experience using pie charts. Therefore, for individual viewers, an adaptive user interface that meets the specific needs of that individual can be ideal since it accounts for individual differences to maximize interpretation efficiency and accuracy.

When considering the implications of presenting data, one must consider how humans trade accuracy for effort. One example may be when physicians compare changes in laboratory data over time. Rather than taking an approach where the physician must calculate the exact difference in values over time, the physician most likely examines the dimensional differences in the data over time (that is, determines if the value decreases or increases since the previous test). Given this scenario, a graphical display of the laboratory data may be better suited for a dimensional interpretation without compromising on accuracy when compared to the standard approach of presenting laboratory data in a table with only the numbers presented.

**Table 17.1.** Ranking of graphical techniques from most to least accurate

| Rank | Graphical technique | Examples of plots |
|---|---|---|
| 1 | Position along a common scale | Bar plot, line chart |
| 2 | Position along nonaligned scales | Stacked bar plot |
| 3 | Length, direction, angle | Scatterplot |
| 4 | Area | Pie chart |
| 5 | Volume, curvature | 3D bar plot |
| 6 | Shading, color saturation | Heat map |

*Source:* Adapted from Cleveland and McGill 1985, 829; 1984, 532.

## Check Your Understanding 17.1

**Answer the following questions in a separate document.**

1. Prepare an example of a graphical technique that uses length, direction, and angle.
2. Prepare two examples using two different graphical techniques that present data along a common scale.
3. A data analyst is developing a visual display of data to compare the average cost of care over time. What technique should the analyst use to display the data? Explain your rationale.
4. Graphical perception is a term that refers to the visual decoding (interpretation) process and was originally described as the ability to unconsciously extract information from graphics. Determine why principles of graphical perception are important to consider when developing visual displays of healthcare data.

## Charts versus Tables

The most common type of data that is displayed graphically is quantitative data. For example, a child's weight can be tracked over its lifetime. Weight is a quantitative data element. When presenting a child's weight over the period of childhood, the data can be presented in a table where the numeric values for weight are displayed. Alternatively, a chart can be generated, such as a line chart, that displays how weight trends over a period. An example of how these data can be presented using a table or a line chart is shown in figure 17.1. If a user was tasked with identifying the child's exact weight at four years old, the simplest way to complete this task is by referring to the table. To extract the exact weight at four years old from the chart would require more complex perceptual tasks. However, if the task was to identify the trend in weight over time, the simplest way to complete this task is by referring to the chart. The line chart quickly reveals an upward trend in weight for each year. The table would require a user to examine the relationship between the discrete, or specific, numbers for each year to interpret a trend. This example highlights the importance of displaying information with a method that accommodates the desired task.

Charts employ a spatial arrangement of information, whereas tables use a symbolic arrangement (Speier 2006). Charts emphasize a spatially related relationship in data but typically do not present discrete data values. Tables, however, are symbolic since they emphasize discrete data values, but do not present the relationship between the data. **Spatial representations** allow information to be viewed at a glance utilizing perceptual processes without needing to address the individual elements of the information separately or analytically. **Symbolic representations** require analytical processes where information is extracted from specific data values. When considering the advantages and disadvantages of each arrangement, spatial data support a dimensional interpretation, which may decrease effort yet limits the consideration of discrete data points, which may decrease accuracy. Symbolic representations, however, support a holistic interpretation where discrete data points may be determined, allowing for increased accuracy yet requiring increased effort. Simply put, a chart offers the advantage of seeing the general trend of data and comparing differences in data between groups or over time. However, the precise numeric values are more easily discerned when reading a table. Each method has advantages depending on the context of the situation and therefore each can be thought of as task dependent.

The effectiveness of charts to support decision-making can be dependent on the task environment. The task content, task complexity, and task structure can influence the accuracy and efficiency of an interpretation. Charts do not have total superiority over tables and the benefit of charts is task dependent (Davis et al. 2022). In tasks where an accurate interpretation of values is important, especially when a user has experience with tables or tabular presentations, tables are better suited than charts. For tasks that involve viewing the time dependency of large amounts of data, charts are better suited than tables. When the task involves conveying a message from several sets of data on a common subject, presenting subsets of data using both charts and tables is best. Finally, when the task involves large amounts of data and the goal is to recall specific details after the presentation, charts offer better performance than tables. In medicine, data are often presented as both discrete data and time-dependent data depending on the type of data and the context of the situation. Therefore, both tables and charts may be applicable for presenting data depending on the situation.

To expand on the previous explanation, the most suitable situations to provide a chart versus a table depends on the intended use of the information.

**Figure 17.1.** Displaying quantitative data in a table versus a chart

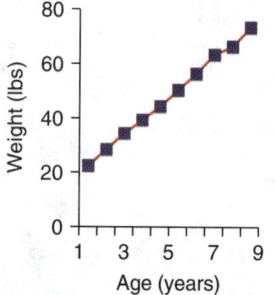

| Age (yrs) | Weight (lbs) |
|---|---|
| 1 | 22 |
| 2 | 28 |
| 3 | 34 |
| 4 | 39 |
| 5 | 44 |
| 6 | 50 |
| 7 | 56 |
| 8 | 63 |
| 9 | 66 |
| 10 | 73 |

The presentation method, whether using charts or tables, must be considered in context to the task at hand knowing each presentation method has advantages in different situations. However, factors other than the context of the task can influence the utility of charts versus tables, such as the experience of the user and the complexity of the data—further explored in this chapter.

---

### Check Your Understanding 17.2

**Answer the following questions in a separate document.**

1. Create a method for presenting data to help a patient identify the trend in their cholesterol levels over the past five years. Consider the merits of a table versus a chart.
2. Create a method for presenting data to help a patient with diabetes identify their latest blood sugar level. Consider the merits of a table versus a chart.
3. Propose an example of when a symbolic representation of data is preferred and explain your rationale.
4. Create a visual display of data that would be effective for interpreting the trend in the monthly number of discharges for heart failure patients.
5. Antoine was asked to assist in the development of an administrative dashboard. In particular, the CEO of the hospital would like to see the trend in the patients that do not show up for appointments and be able to quickly extract discrete values. Develop a prototype of this display and explain why you selected the design features.

---

## Considerations for Adopting Visualization Techniques

Several factors impact the effectiveness of a visual display, including situation context, user experience, chart type, and data complexity. Research has explored the impact these factors have on interpreting visual displays of healthcare data. For example, a prior study in radiology proposed four potential measures to consider recording when designing a visual display: accuracy, which is the measure of correctness; *latency*, which describes the amount of time it takes to answer a question; compactness of the display; and user preference (Starren and Johnson 2000, 16). Although it may not be necessary to explore each of these measures each time a visual display is being designed, the accuracy and latency of interpreting a visual display tend to be the most common measures to consider.

The remainder of the chapter explores how situations with users of varying experience, using different types of charts, and displaying data of varying complexity can influence the adoption and use of visual displays of data.

### Context of the Situation

As described previously, there are certain situations where it may be necessary to present data using numerical values and other situations where a graphical display is ideal. Research has been conducted to compare whether numbers, charts, or a combination of both are best for presenting quantitative data (Feldman-Stewart et al. 2000). One study compared six different display methods including pie charts, vertical bar plots, horizontal bar plots, numbers, systematic ovals, and random ovals. The patients were presented information pertaining to the probabilities of treatment risks and benefits using a combination of methods (figure 17.2). *Systematic ovals* are a graphical technique that displays stacked ovals with the height of the stack corresponding to the maximum of the scale. The ovals are separated into discrete units with each oval corresponding to a specific unit of measurement. The value for the result is summarized by the ovals that are filled in. Figure 17.2 displays an example of systematic ovals where each oval corresponds to one unit. Since the value is 45, there are 45 ovals filled in. A *random oval* display is similar to systematic ovals but it is not as uniform; the ovals are randomly filled in.

The ability to interpret the data presented in figure 17.2 can vary depending on the type of task. If the task required choosing a larger or smaller object, the symbolic representation using vertical bars results in the most accurate and rapid processing, followed by systematic ovals. When the task required an estimate

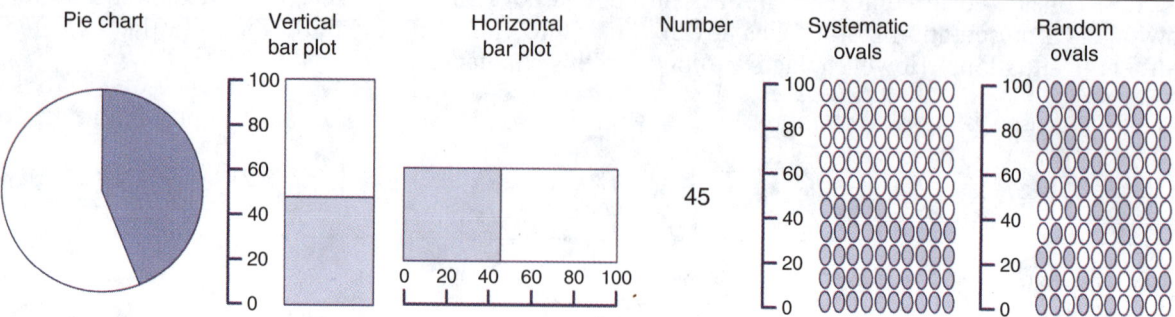

**Figure 17.2.** A comparison of six different graphical presentations of numeric information

*Source:* Adapted from Feldman-Stewart et al. 2000, 238.

of the value, which requires greater precision, numbers resulted in the most accurate estimates, followed by systematic ovals (Feldman-Stewart et al. 2000). These results suggest that quantitative information be presented in one of two ways—either by presenting both vertical bars and numbers or only presenting systematic ovals. Studies such as this demonstrate that the performance of charts to convey quantitative information is highly dependent on the type and complexity of the task at hand, and in some cases the display of both numbers and charts is best.

There are certain characteristics of healthcare data that can be used for determining whether a chart or table is the best method for displaying data. For example, the presentation of a specific number, or set of numbers, is necessary to carry out a task of revealing the last known value for a patient's HbA1c (glycated hemoglobin). The reason the numeric value is the best method is because the task requires an accurate interpretation of a discrete value. Yet when the purpose is to view trends over a period, such as monitoring HbA1c in a diabetic patient over the period of several months, a graphical presentation is more appropriate (see figure 17.3). The reason is that a rapid comparison of several values over time is required for this task. However, to facilitate an accurate and rapid interpretation, one may consider presenting both the specific numbers and a corresponding chart.

### Experience of the User

The ability to interpret data using visual displays is largely dependent on the experience of the person interpreting that display. This is especially relevant in the healthcare setting where health professionals make decisions subconsciously or implicitly and where many tasks are routine and nonreflective when they are in familiar situations, such as in interpreting commonly seen data (Eva 2005, 100). The degree of implicit, nonreflective cognitive processing may be directly related to the experience of the physician (Eva 2005, 101). For example, more experienced health

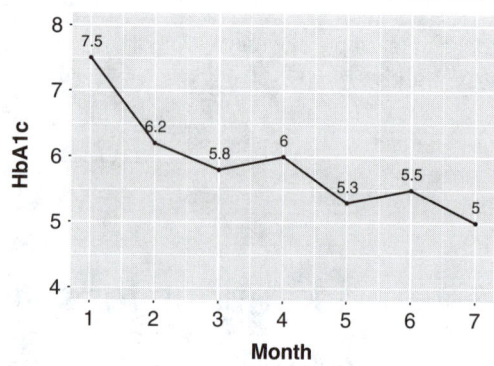

**Figure 17.3.** Displaying HbA1c levels using a chart with numbers

professionals who are trained to look at tabular data (tables) may find a graphical presentation to be a hindrance in effort and accuracy. However, charts may improve the accuracy of interpreting data with less experienced health professionals. Experience must be considered when designing a visual display of data. It is often best to discuss and evaluate the impact that a visual display has on users that vary in terms of their experience in their discipline and experience with specific visualizations.

### Presentation Method

Health professionals often find themselves immersed in data, which can lead to **information overload**, meaning difficulty in making decisions due to the presence of excessive amounts of information. Presentation methods should maximize information retrieval while not causing information overload (Caban and Gotz 2015). Charts can minimize information overload by presenting data in a way that can support an accurate and efficient interpretation of trends without the burden of viewing excessive amounts of information.

In most situations, it is possible to present the same data in more than one way, yet some presentation methods are favored because they can accommodate a more efficient and accurate interpretation method (see table 17.1). For example, consider the graphs displayed in figure 17.4, which compare the average time to code an inpatient chart for three different coders across six months. The graph on the left displays the data using a stacked bar plot while the graph on the right displays the same data using a side-by-side bar plot (figure 17.4). The ability to effectively use the displays is dependent of the intended tasks, which can influence the presentation method selected. If the task was to identify the month that had the lowest average time to code an inpatient chart for each coder, the stacked bar plot is less effective than the side-by-side bar plot. The ability to accurately decide which month has the lowest average time for each coder is very difficult to achieve using the stacked bar plot. The reason is that the side-by-side bar plot offers an advantage because it only requires judgments regarding the position along a common scale, rather than judgments regarding position on identical but nonaligned scales (figure 17.4). The side-by-side bar plot reveals that the lowest average time to code an inpatient chart is April for coder 1, May for coder 2, and April for coder 3. However, when trying to complete this same task using the stacked bar plot, it is very difficult to ascertain which month has the lowest average time to code an inpatient chart for each coder. This exercise demonstrates that even though data can be presented using different graphical methods, certain techniques offer a more accurate and efficient interpretation depending on the task at hand.

The speed and accuracy of interpreting various medical parameters has been researched in depth (Bauer et al. 2010; Lesselroth and Pieczkiewicz 2011; Mielicki et al. 2023; Thomas and Powsner 2005; Tufte 2006; West et al. 2015). In these studies, there were numerous graphical methods that were emphasized as effective ways for presenting data. The methods are largely dependent on the type of data that is available and the type of descriptive summary used (for example, frequency, mean, and median). Table 17.2 displays common graphical methods along with an explanation regarding the most appropriate data to use with each method.

A bar plot is used for two main purposes: (1) for plotting the frequency for one or more groups where the height of each bar represents the count or frequency, or (2) for plotting the mean for one or more groups where the height of each bar represents the average. The bars can be drawn vertically or horizontally. A horizontal bar plot is typically used when presenting data in an ascending or descending order. When a bar plot is used for plotting the mean for one or more groups, the standard deviation or standard error for each level of a group may be added to the plot to show the range of data. When many groups are compared in descending or ascending order on a bar plot, an alternative method for presenting the data is a dot plot.

A **dot plot** presents the frequency or means to compare many groups using dots. The dot plot offers a less cluttered view of the data when there are many groups to compare.

A **pie chart** is used to present the count or proportion of subgroups to the whole. The component parts of a pie chart represent the subgroups of a single factor. If each proportion that is presented in a pie chart is summed, the total should always equal 100 percent.

A **line plot** is used for two main purposes: (1) to present trends or patterns in the number of occurrences between groups, or (2) to present trends or patterns in the mean of a variable between groups. Typically, the change of a variable over time is compared. When more than one group is compared in a line plot, a separate line is drawn for each group.

Figure 17.4. Comparing the stacked bar plot versus side-by-side bar plot

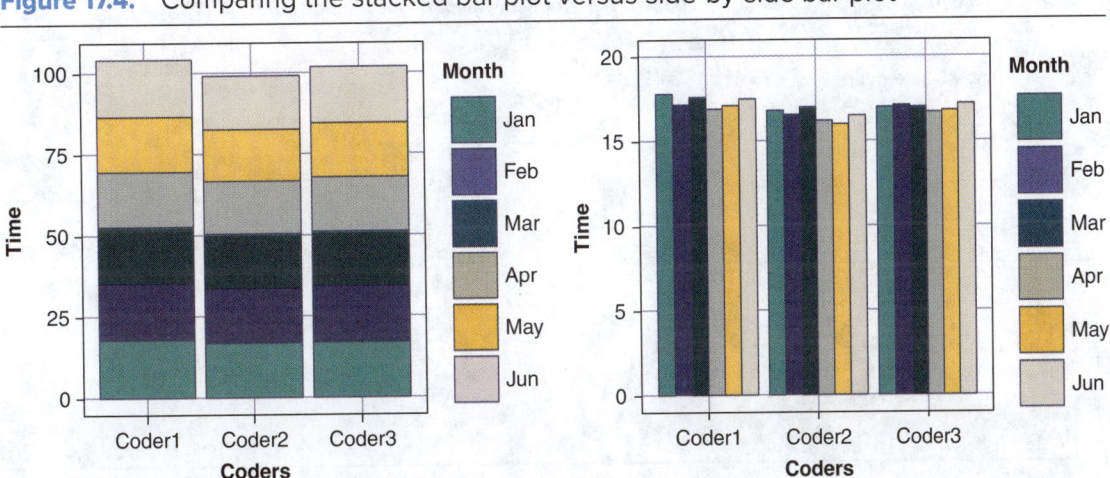

**Table 17.2.** Explanation of the most common graphical methods

**Plotting frequencies**

| Graph type | Definition | Example |
|---|---|---|
| Bar plot | Displays the frequencies for one or more groups. The bars can be drawn vertically or horizontally. | The count of females and males in the selected patient population |
| Pie chart | The count or proportion of subgroups. The component parts of a pie chart represent the subgroups of a single variable. | The count and percentage of females and males in the selected patient population |
| Line plot | Displays trends or patterns in the number of occurrences between groups. Typically, the change of a variable over time is compared. | The number of patient visits for males and females for the years 2021 through 2024. |

*Continued*

Table 17.2. Explanation of the most common graphical methods (continued)

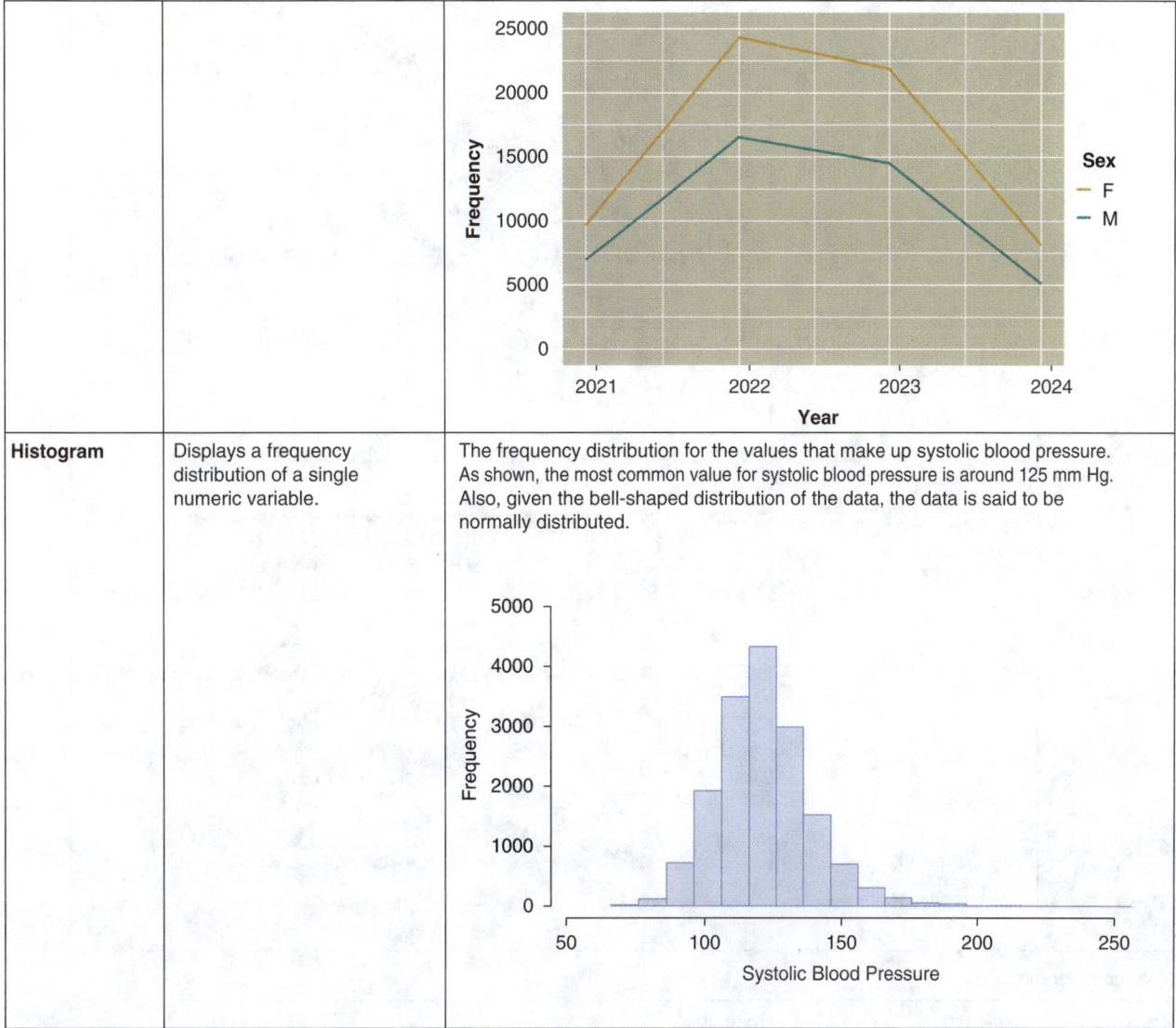

| | | |
|---|---|---|
| Histogram | Displays a frequency distribution of a single numeric variable. | The frequency distribution for the values that make up systolic blood pressure. As shown, the most common value for systolic blood pressure is around 125 mm Hg. Also, given the bell-shaped distribution of the data, the data is said to be normally distributed. |

**Plotting means**

| Graph type | Explanation | Example |
|---|---|---|
| Bar plot | Displays the mean for one or more groups. The bars can be drawn vertically or horizontally. The standard deviation or standard error for each level of a group are typically added to the plot to show the range of data. | The average systolic blood pressure for men and women. The whiskers represent the standard deviation. |

Continued

**Table 17.2.** Explanation of the most common graphical methods (continued)

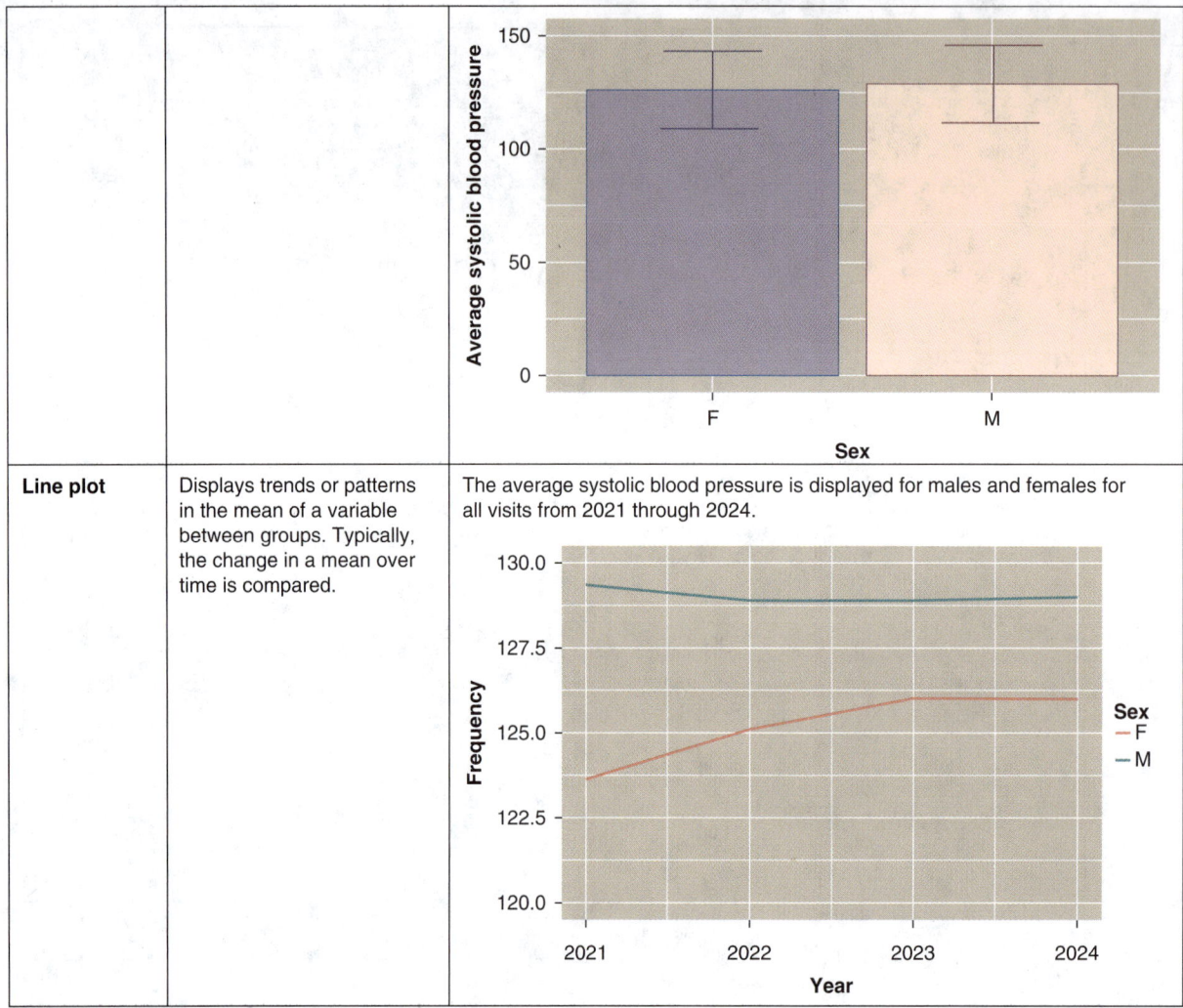

| | | |
|---|---|---|
| | | |
| **Line plot** | Displays trends or patterns in the mean of a variable between groups. Typically, the change in a mean over time is compared. | The average systolic blood pressure is displayed for males and females for all visits from 2021 through 2024. |

**Multimodal graphs**

| Graph type | Explanation | Example |
|---|---|---|
| **Boxplot** | Displays the descriptive statistics of a variable including the minimum, first quartile, medium, third quartile, maximum, and potential outlier values. | Comparing systolic blood pressure in males and females. |

Continued

**Table 17.2.** Explanation of the most common graphical methods (continued)

**Plotting the relationship between variables**

| Graph type | Explanation | Example |
|---|---|---|
| Scatterplot | Displays the relationship between two quantitative variables. | Plot displaying the relationship between systolic blood pressure and body mass index (BMI). |

A **boxplot** displays the descriptive statistics of a continuous variable including the minimum, first quartile, medium, third quartile, maximum, and potential outlier values. The line that makes the bottom of the box represents the value for the first quartile; the first quartile of a data set represents the 25th percentile of numeric data. The number representing the first quartile is interpreted as the value at which 25 percent of the numbers in the data set have a value equal to or less than that value. For example, if ages of a sample of patients were evaluated, and the first quartile is determined to be 15, that would mean 25 percent of the patients in your sample have an age of 15 years or less. The bold line in the center of the boxplot represents the median. The line that serves as the top of the box represents the value for the third quartile; the third quartile is the 75th percentile. The number representing the third quartile is interpreted as a value at which 75 percent of the numbers in the data set have a value equal to or less than that value. If there are dots above and below the boxes, these dots represent potential outliers. An outlier is a value that is distant from other values. For example, if the age of 250 years were present in the data set, this would represent an outlier. Potential outliers are determined on a boxplot when there are values in the data set that are lower than the first quartile value minus $1.5 \times IQR$ and above the third quartile plus $1.5 \times IQR$. IQR stands for interquartile range and is calculated as the value of the third quartile minus the value of the first quartile. When outliers are not present, the whiskers—the lines protruding from the top and bottom of the box—represent the minimum and maximum values.

A **scatterplot** displays the relationship between two quantitative variables. A line is typically drawn through the middle of the points and represents the trend of the data, which is known as the best-fit line. The best-fit line depicts the type of relationship between two quantitative variables. If the line ascends, this is interpreted as a positive association; if the line descends, this is interpreted as a negative association. The slope of the line (that is, the steepness) determines the significance of the relationship between the two quantitative variables. A simple linear regression is the statistical procedure associated with a scatterplot. The simple linear regression offers information related to the significance and strength of an association. The p-value that is calculated from a simple linear regression establishes whether the best-fit line has a slope that is significantly different from zero. A p-value is used for determining significance of a statistical test. The p-value should be compared to a predefined significance level, known as $\alpha$. If the p-value is less than $\alpha$, there is enough evidence to conclude a significant finding. If the p-value is greater than or equal to $\alpha$, there is not enough evidence to conclude significance. Regarding a linear regression, a significant finding means the best-fit line has a slope that is not equal to zero, suggesting that the relationship between the quantitative variables is significant. However, the strength of that relationship is determined based on the distance each point is from the best-fit line. If there are many points scattered far from the best-fit line, the association between the quantitative variables is said to be weak. If the points are close to the best-fit line, the relationship is stronger. The statistic that represents the strength of the relationship is the r² value, which can range from 0 to 1. The strength of the relationship between the two quantitative variables is said to be stronger the closer the r² value is to 1.

A **histogram** displays a frequency or density distribution of a single numeric variable. Categorizing or sorting these numeric variables together is called binning. The numeric variable is broken down into groups based on specific ranges of values to establish the widths of each bar in a histogram. The height of each bar represents the frequency or density of each of the binned groups. The distribution can be described as normally distributed when the pattern follows a bell-shaped pattern. If the histogram has the highest point to the left side of the graph and a right trailing tail, it is referred to as right skewed or positively skewed. If the histogram has the highest point to the right side of the graph and a left leading tail, it is referred to as left skewed or negatively skewed. A bimodal distribution occurs when there is more than one peak in the data. Figure 17.5 displays an example of each of these distribution categories.

**Figure 17.5.** Histogram distribution categories

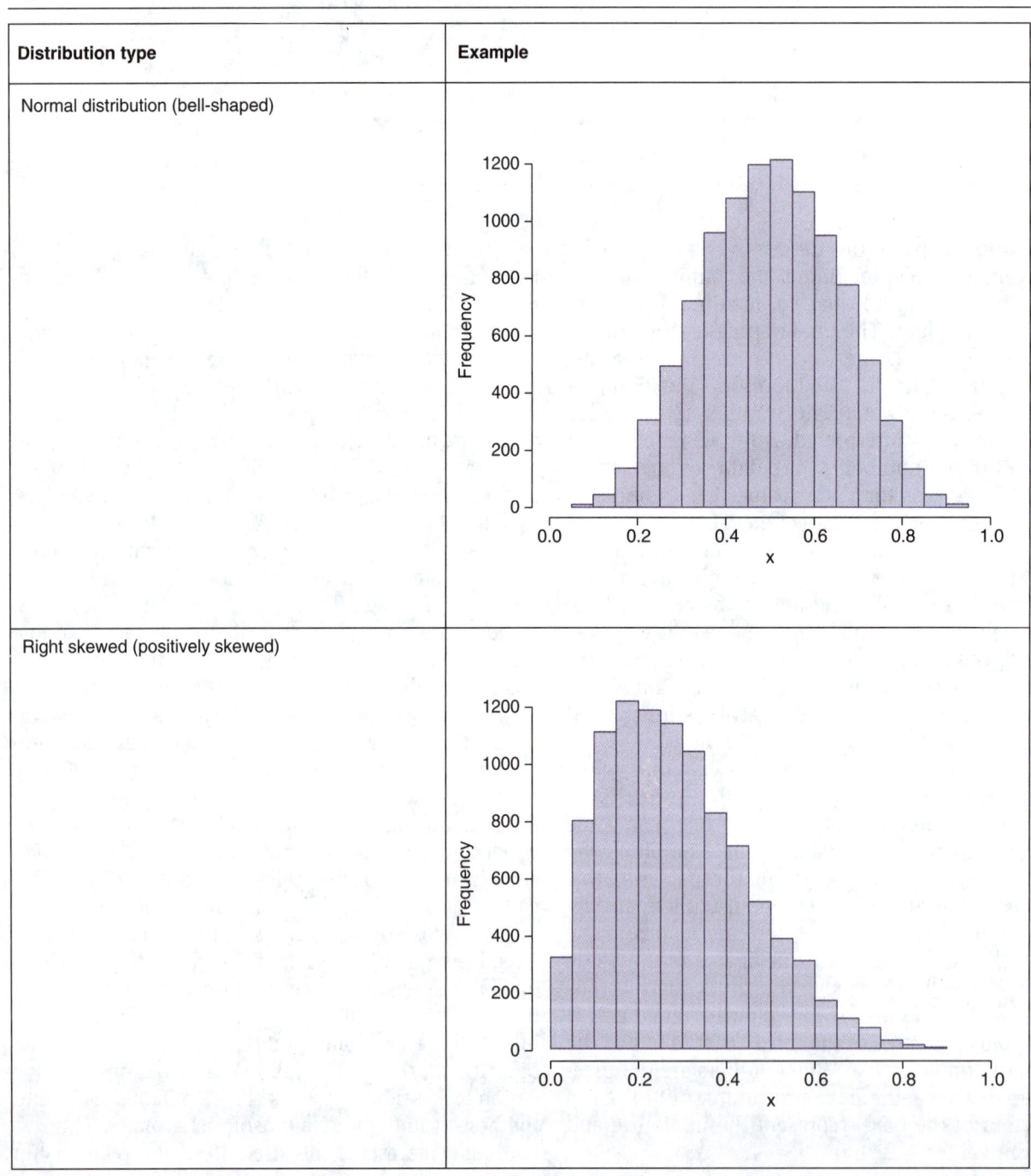

Continued

**Figure 17.5.** Histogram distribution categories (continued)

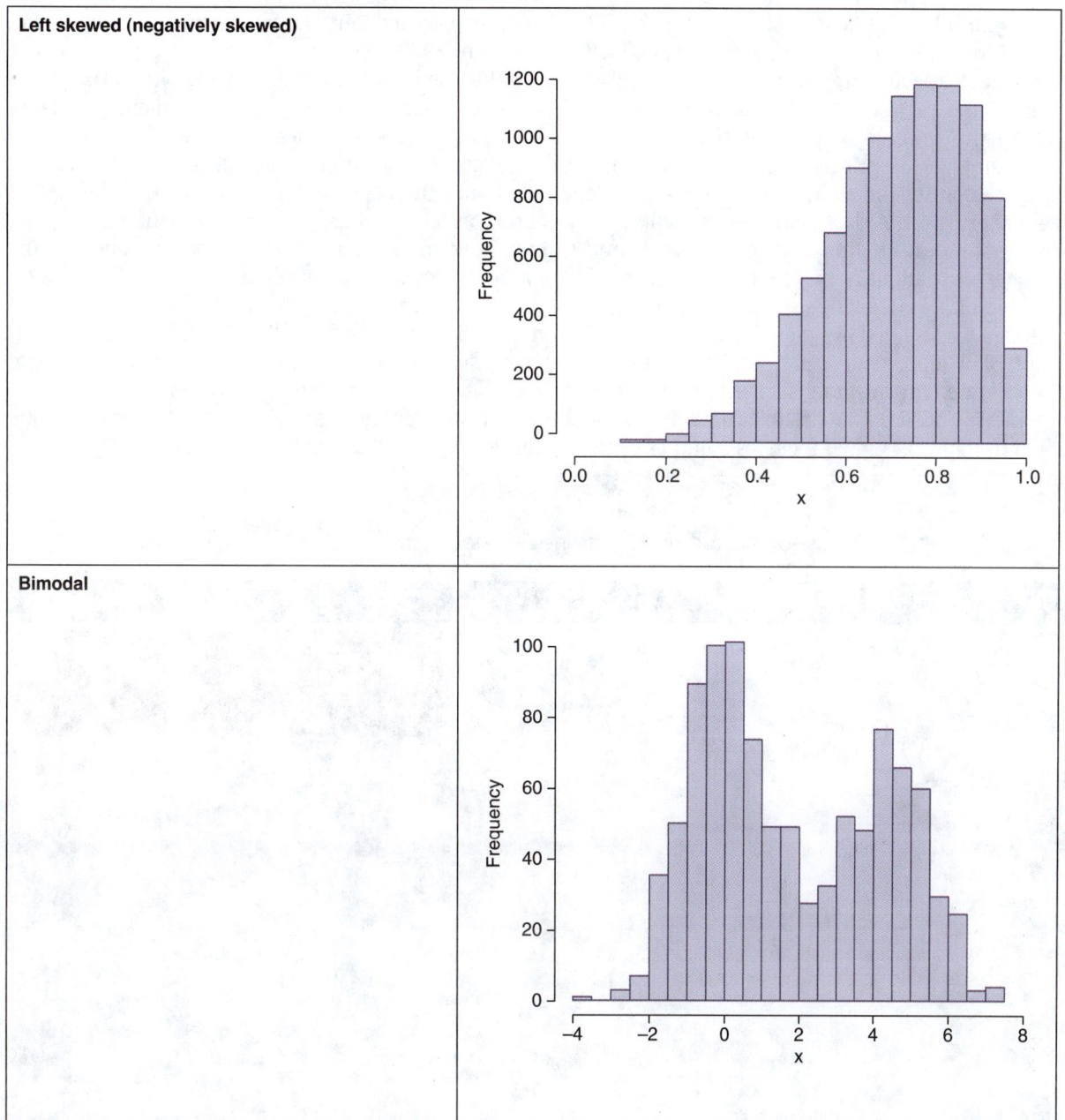

## Complexity of the Data

Data complexity, as it relates to visualization of healthcare data, usually arises when there are multiple parameters that must be viewed simultaneously. When it is necessary to view multiple parameters on one graphical display, difficulties can arise if the data are not standardized (for example, different ranges for each parameter), if the data do not follow a normal distribution, or if a relationship between parameters is meant to be visualized. As healthcare technology expands and more data are collected and utilized, the level of complexity expands even more due to the sheer number of data points meant to be displayed.

A method that has been developed for presenting a variety of data on a single display in an easy-to-read format is called a dashboard. For example, the dashboard in your vehicle presents a variety of data that are important for operating the vehicle. In healthcare, dashboards are used for different purposes, including viewing organization performance data, financial data, and clinical data. The dashboards may use various graphics, including bar plots, pie charts, numbers, textual summaries, and other methods. A dashboard is meant to support a high-level understanding of the data. If additional information is necessary to drill down into more specific findings, a process called slicing and dicing can be adopted. **Slicing and dicing** refers to the process of taking what is known at the highest level of understanding and working downward to identify the underlying causes for the high-level observation. A dashboard helps facilitate a greater understanding of financial, operational, and clinical processes to identify problems and successes.

An example of a dashboard is shown in figure 17.6. This dashboard was created using public data published by the World Bank (2023) and displays worldwide health statistics over time. The death rates for countries across the world are displayed on the dashboard, which is the tab selected in figure 17.6, and includes summaries for the death rates over time, the overall death rate, death rates broken down by continent, and death rates broken down for each country. Users can preview data going back from 1960 until 2022. Interactive tooltips display the values shown through the interactive charts, which consist of a line chart, bar plots, and a digital indicator. For instance, a digital indicator summarizes the overall death rate as the number per one hundred thousand people and the color of the digital indicator is green, yellow, or red depending on the severity of the measure. Upon hovering the cursor over a specific aspect of the plot, an interactive tooltip offers additional information pertaining to the display. For example, when a cursor hovers on a specific dot on the line plot, the year and death rate for that year are displayed in a call out pop-up. Additional tabs can be selected in the dashboard to preview a summary of the worldwide birth rates or life expectancy in addition to the death rates.

**Figure 17.6.** Example of a dashboard for worldwide health statistics

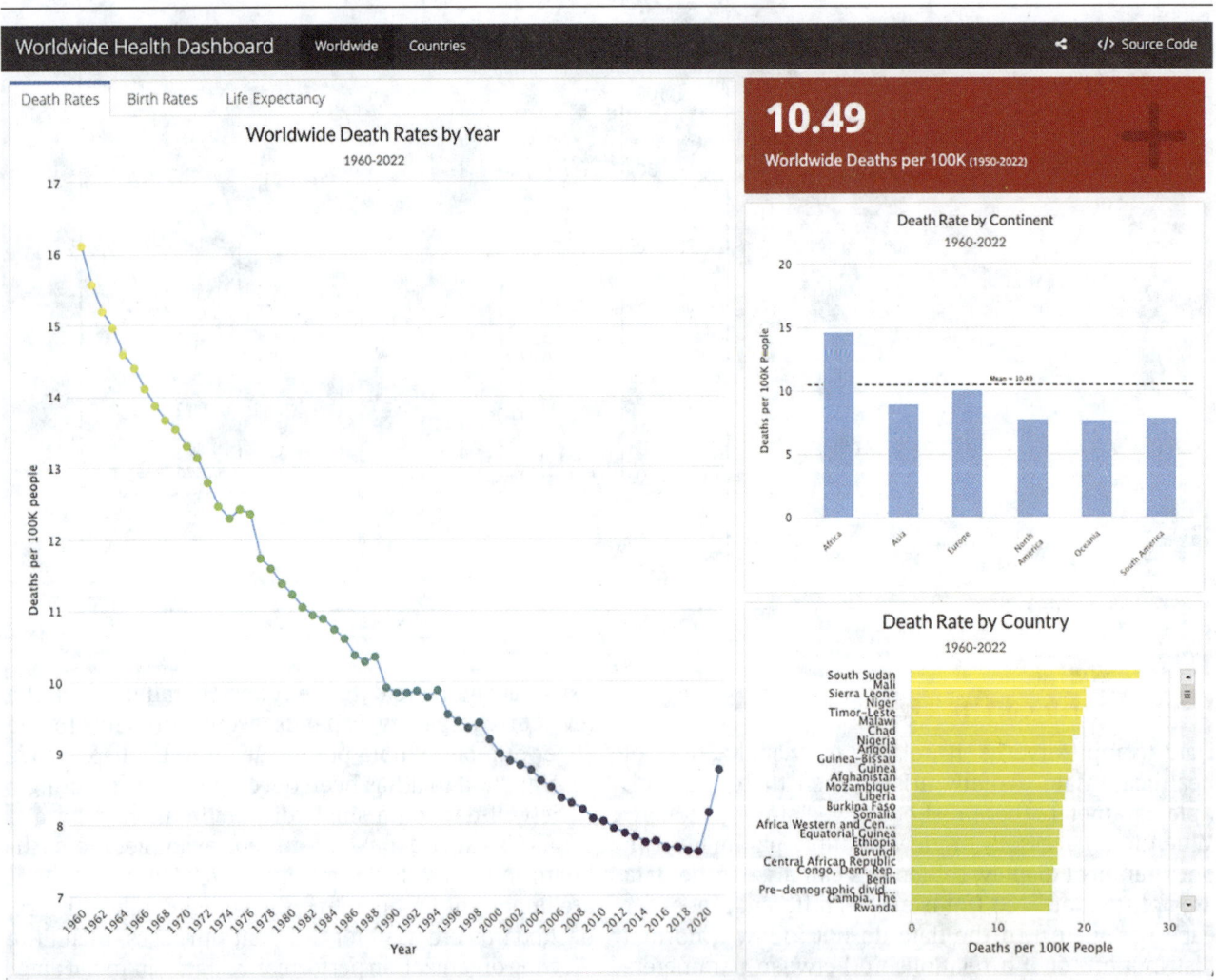

*Source:* Author-created using R Statistical Software with data from World Bank 2023.

# Using Data Visualization to Guide Decisions under the Inpatient Psychiatric Facility Quality Reporting Program

The Centers for Medicare and Medicaid Services (CMS) has initiated the Inpatient Psychiatric Facility Quality Reporting (IPFQR) program. This program's main goal is to provide consumers with information about the quality of care, which can assist them in making informed healthcare decisions. The data provided by this program focuses on quality measures designed to evaluate and promote improvements in the care provided to mental health patients (CMS 2023).

All inpatient psychiatric facilities (IPFs) that receive payments under the inpatient psychiatric facilities prospective payment system (IPF PPS) are required to comply with the IPFQR program's requirements. The IPF PPS is applicable to inpatient psychiatric services provided by psychiatric hospitals or psychiatric units, also known as mental health or behavioral health units, in acute care hospitals (ACHs) or critical access hospitals (CAHs) in the US that participate in Medicare.

The IPFQR program aims to enhance the quality of inpatient psychiatric care by ensuring providers are aware of and report on best practices for their facilities and the care they provide. This is achieved by submitting quality data to CMS on an annual basis. Facilities that are eligible but choose not to participate in the program may face reduced payments from Medicare. Specifically, eligible IPFs that do not participate in the IPFQR program in a fiscal year, or fail to meet all reporting requirements, will experience a two percent reduction in their annual update to their standard federal rate for that year.

Data on the performance of hospitals participating in the IPFQR program is publicly available on the Hospital Compare website. This website provides performance metrics for US hospitals that submit payments to Medicare. Data from Hospital Compare is used in this example to investigate potential geographic differences in IPF clinical outcomes (CMS n.d.). The subsequent analysis revealed that while high-performing hospitals tend to have higher patient satisfaction, there are only moderate improvements in clinical outcomes. This case study, using data visualization techniques, identifies factors that may explain why some hospitals achieve better outcomes than others under the IPFQR program. Table 17.3 displays the IPF quality indicators and the definitions for the data that is published from Hospital Compare.

Hospital Compare was created by CMS and organizations representing consumers, hospitals, doctors, employers, accrediting organizations, and other federal agencies. The Hospital Compare data used in the following analysis are based on IPF quality data from the July 1, 2020, through December 31, 2022, reporting period. The purpose of the analysis is to determine what factors are associated with better quality of care and outcomes when the data is aggregated by state.

The charts in this case study were created using the R Statistical Software package with the ggplot2 package. R is open-source software (available as a free download) that uses a command line language. In this example, each variable was aggregated as the mean for each state. The data dictionary that defines each variable is shown in table 17.3. To identify the variables of interest that have the strongest relationship

**Table 17.3.** IPF quality information from IPFQR program

| Quality Indicator | Definition |
| --- | --- |
| HBIPS-2 | Hours of physical-restraint use |
| HBIPS-3 | Hours of seclusion use |
| HBIPS-5 | Patients discharged on multiple antipsychotic medications with appropriate justification |
| SMD | Screening for metabolic disorders |
| SUB-2 | Alcohol use brief intervention provided or offered |
| SUB-3 | Alcohol and other drug use disorder treatment provided or offered at discharge |
| TOB-2 | Tobacco use treatment provided or offered |
| TOB-3 | Tobacco use treatment provided or offered at discharge |
| TR-1 | Transition record with specified elements received by discharged patients |
| TR-2 | Timely transmission of transition record |
| FUH-30 | Percent of patients receiving follow-up care within 30 days after hospitalization for mental illness |
| FUH-7 | Percent of patients receiving follow-up care within 7 days after hospitalization for mental illness |
| Medcont | Medication continuation following inpatient psychiatric discharge |
| Readmit | Patients readmitted to any hospital within 30 days of discharge from the inpatient psychiatric facility |
| IMM-2 | Influenza immunization |
| COVID | Percentage of healthcare personnel who completed COVID-19 primary vaccination series |

to one another, a correlation matrix was generated. This type of visual display shows the type and strength of the relationship between all variables. (See figure 17.7 for an example.) Several variables are measuring similar phenomenon, causing collinearity. That is, there is a strong correlation only because two variables are measuring something very similar. The strongest relationship appears to exist between medcont and FUH-30 (r-squared = 0.46). The relationship appears to be moderately strong and positive, whereby when one variable is high, the other variable is likely to be high. Past studies have found that around two-thirds of psychiatric inpatients attended a follow-up appointment within 30 days of discharge (Kapoor et al. 2023, 3). Studies explained that some patients did not attend their follow-up visits due to several factors, including lack of trust in the facilities (Shields et al. 2023); the location of the facilities (Hung et al. 2022, 451); their length of stay, the environmental stability, and medication adherence (Warner 2022). Interestingly, the result of our analysis suggests the strongest relationship exists between the probability of having a follow-up visit and medication adherence. Now that we know these variables are related in some way, the next step is to try to understand why they are related.

First, the variance on how each state differs for the variables of interest can be explored using data

**Figure 17.7.** Correlation matrix showing the type and strength of the relationship among all variables

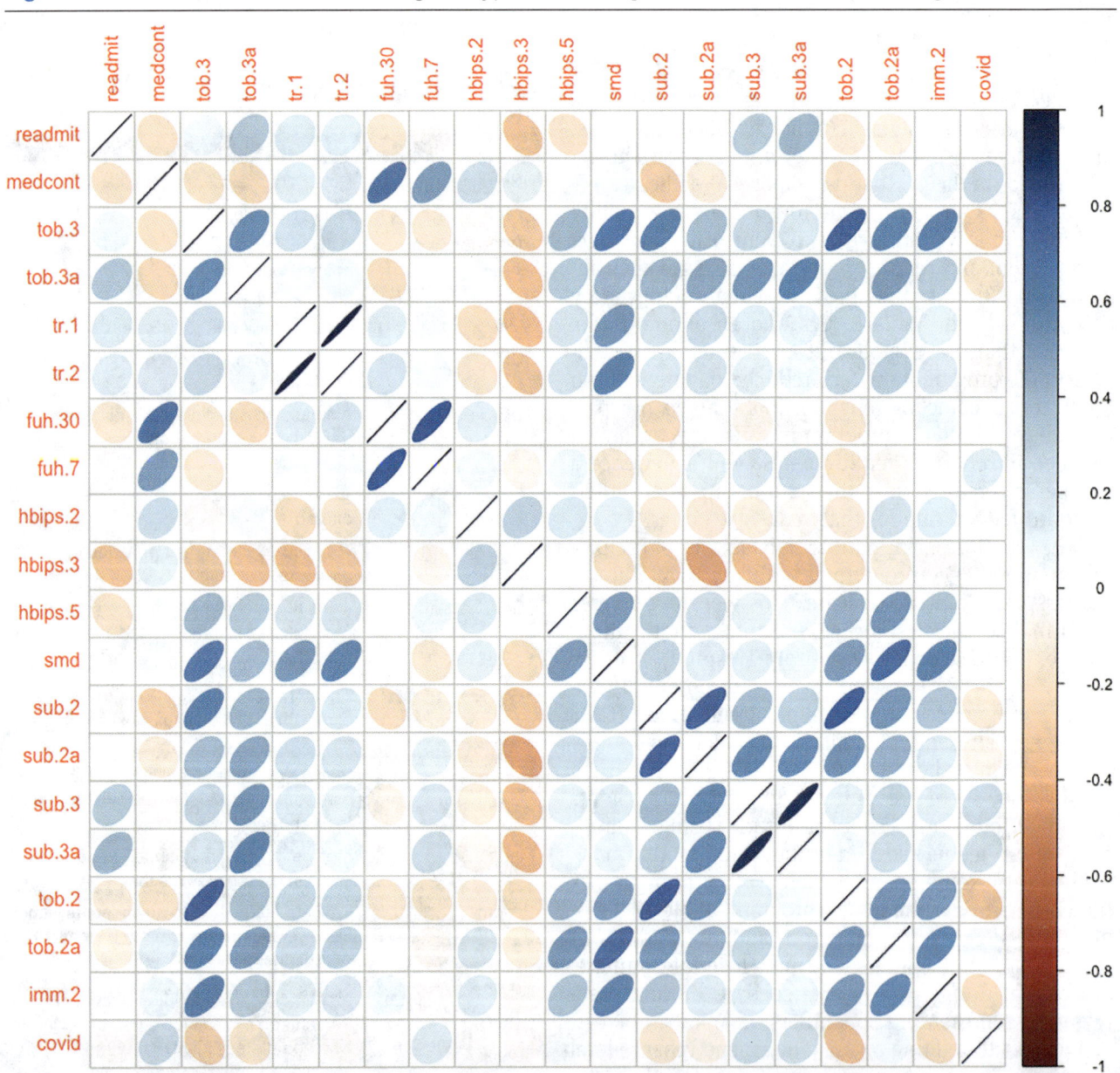

visualization. The first variable that will be explored is medcont, which measures the "patients admitted to an inpatient psychiatric facility for major depressive disorder (MDD), schizophrenia, or bipolar disorder who filled at least one prescription between the 2 days before they were discharged and 30 days after they were discharged from the facility" (CMS 2023). A higher rate is desired as this shows greater patient compliance with treatment. The average of medcont across all states is 73.4 percent. A dot plot was generated to display the mean of the medcont variable for each state and sorted in descending order. Figure 17.8 displays the results of the dot plot which shows Iowa, Minnesota, Wisconsin, and Michigan having the highest rates while Nevada, Alaska, Washington DC, and Florida having the lowest rates. Interestingly, the states with the highest rate are all located in the Midwest.

In comparison, when examining FUH-30, which measures the percentage of patients that received a follow-up within 30 days of an inpatient psychiatric hospitalization, the states with the highest average include Iowa, Montana, New Hampshire, and Minnesota while the lowest include Puerto Rico; Washington, DC; Alaska; and California (figure 17.9). What is interesting is that some of the same states that had the highest or lowest rate for medcont also appear to have the highest or lowest rate for FUH-30. On average

**Figure 17.8.** Average percentage for each state of patients continuing medication after discharge from an inpatient psychiatric facility

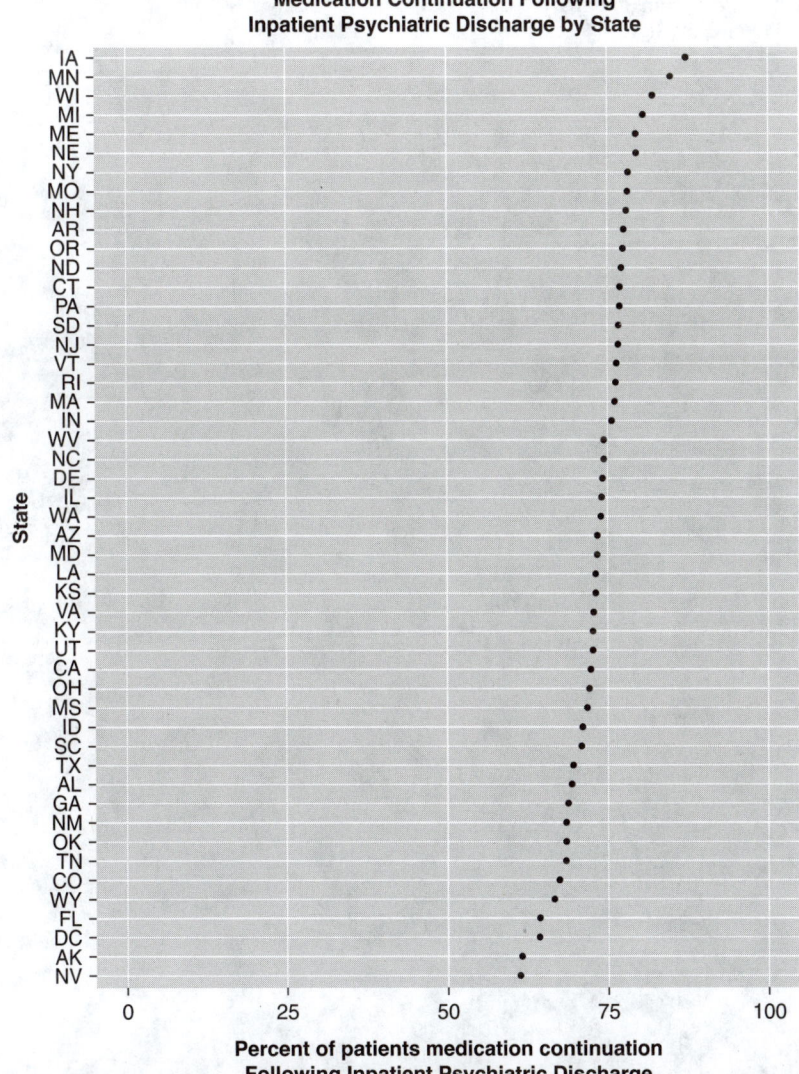

about 52.8 percent of psychiatric inpatients have a follow-up visit within 30 days after discharge. Next, we will want to understand the nature of the relationship between FUH-30 and medcont by conducting a linear regression.

To understand the nature of the relationship between medcont and FUH-30, a linear regression model was created to obtain information about the correlation. As shown in figure 17.10, there is a moderately strong positive correlation. Given the nature of the relationship, an equation of the best fit line can allow the researcher to make a prediction. That is, if the percentage of patients that continue medications is known, a reasonable prediction can be made for the percentage of patients that will comply with a follow-up visit. The equation for the best fit line is determined by knowing the y-intercept and slope. The y-intercept is -18 and the slope of the line is $0.99x$. Therefore, the equation to predict the percentage of patients that have a follow-up visit (denoted by $y$) is $y = -18 + 0.99x$, whereby x is the known percentage of patients that continue to take medications.

The use of data visualization techniques offers a method for examining variables that measure the quality of care received at inpatient psychiatric facilities. Based on the analysis, there is a moderately strong association between the percentage of patients that continue on medications and the percentage of patients that have a follow-up visit after an inpatient psychiatric hospitalization.

**Figure 17.9.** Average the percentage for each state of patients that received a follow-up within 30 days of an inpatient psychiatric hospitalization

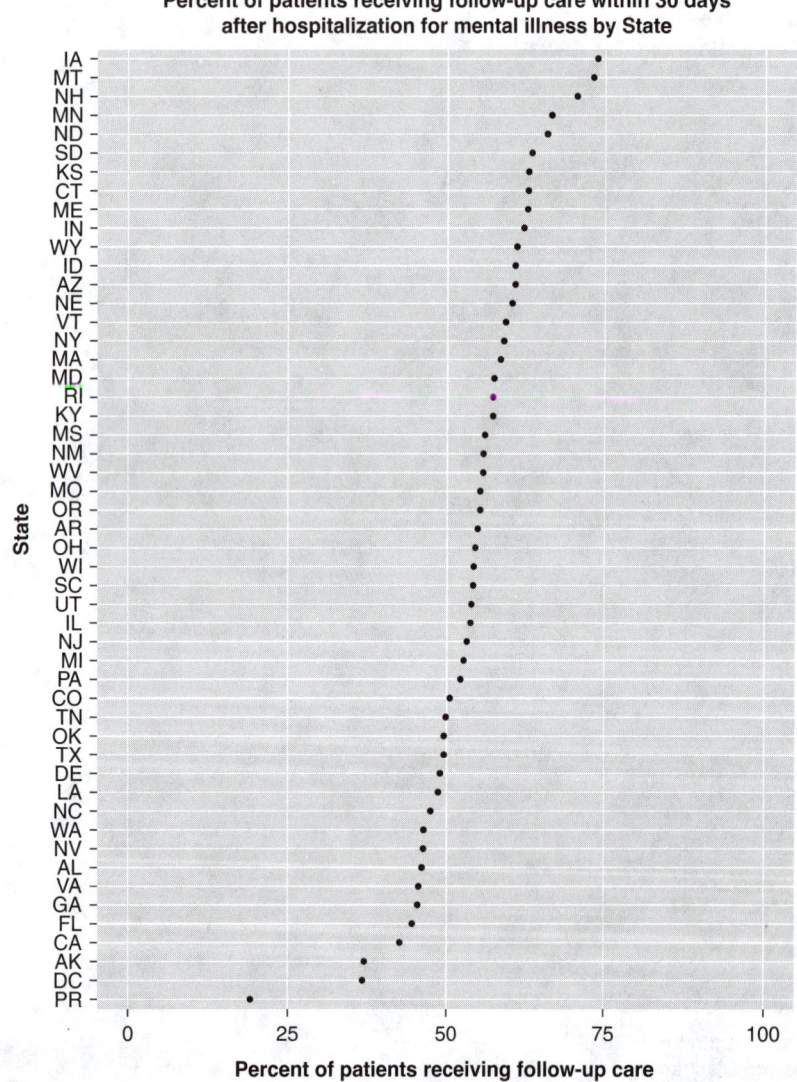

**Figure 17.10.** Relationship between the percentage of patients that will have a follow-up visit and the percentage of patients that continue on medications for each state

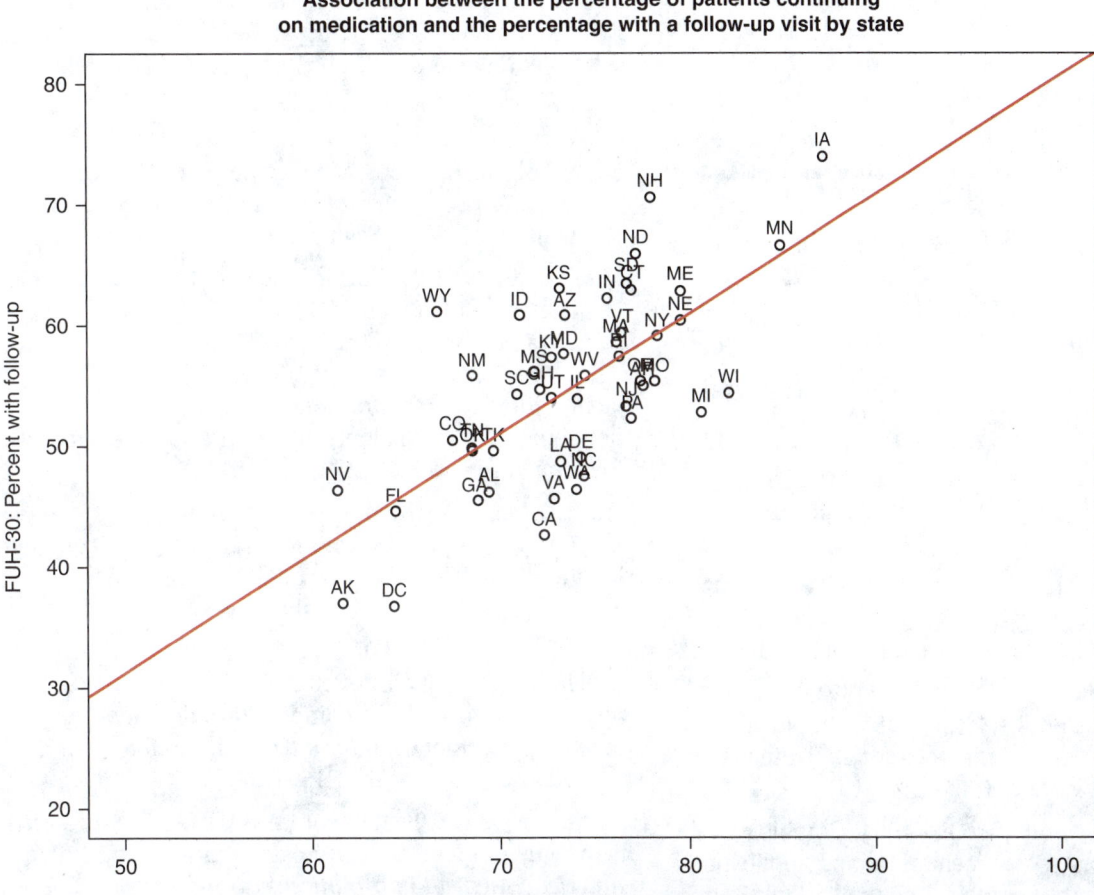

## Check Your Understanding 17.3

**Answer the following questions in a separate document.**

1. If you were tasked with presenting the changes in revenue over the last five years, what graph would you choose? Explain your rationale.

2. Create appropriate scenarios to represent data that would use a line chart and a bar plot. Explain why each plot was used for the respective scenario.

3. Connie was asked to show the median length of stay for the neonatal intensive care unit (NICU). While Connie was evaluating the data, she determined the data are positively skewed and determined that the median was not an appropriate metric to report out. Defend why you agree or disagree with Connie.

4. Your hospital has had staffing challenges over the past year and there are concerns this is affecting patient satisfaction. You were tasked to analyze data to show the relationship between patient satisfaction scores and total RN staffing hours. You were also asked to see if there are differences in the median total RN staffing hours between the surgical, intensive care, and floor nursing units. Create two graphs that would most appropriately display this data.

5. Create a prototype of a financial dashboard that displays the following KPIs for a hospital.
   - Charges and payments by year and month from January 2020–December 2023.
   - Total number of claims by the following insurance carriers: Medicare, Medicaid, BestInsurance, PayerLess, CareB4Cost
   - Average number of days in accounts receivable and the average days to bill against the benchmark
   - Total dollars in accounts receivable by age group of the patient for the following age groups: 0–1, 2–17, 18–44, 45–64, 65–84, 85+

# References

Bauer, D. T., S. Guerlain, P. J. and Brown. 2010. The design and evaluation of a graphical display for laboratory data. *Journal of the American Medical Informatics Association* 17(4):416–424.

Beach, L. R., and T. R. Mitchell. 1978. A contingency model for the selection of decision strategies. *Academy of Management Review* 3:439–449.

Caban, J. J., and D. Gotz. 2015. Visual analytics in healthcare: Opportunities and research challenges. *Journal of the American Medical Informatics Association* 22:260–262.

CMS (Centers for Medicare and Medicaid Services). 2023. "Inpatient Psychiatric Facility Quality Reporting (IPFQR) Program." https://www.cms.gov/medicare/quality/initiatives/hospital-quality-initiative/inpatient-psychiatric-facility-quality-reporting-ipfqr-program.

CMS (Centers for Medicare and Medicaid Services). n.d. "The Total Performance Score Information." https://www.medicare.gov/hospitalcompare/data/total-performance-scores.html.

Cleveland, W. S., and R. McGill. 1985. Graphical perception and graphical methods for analyzing scientific data. *Science* 229:828–833.

Cleveland, W. S., and R. McGill. 1984. Graphical perception: Theory, experimentation, and application to the development of graphical methods. *Journal of the American Statistical Association* 79:531–554.

Davis, R., Pu, X., Ding, Y., Hall, B. D., Bonilla, K., Feng, M., Kay, M. and Harrison, L., 2022. The risks of ranking: Revisiting graphical perception to model individual differences in visualization performance. *IEEE Transactions on Visualization and Computer Graphics*. https://ieeexplore.ieee.org/document/9978718.

Eva, K. W. 2005. What every teacher needs to know about clinical reasoning. *Medical Education* 39:98–106.

Feldman-Stewart, D., N. Kocovski, B. A. McConnell, M. D. Brundage, and W. J. Mackillop. 2000. Perception of quantitative information for treatment decisions. *Medical Decision Making* 20:228–238.

Franconeri, S. L., L. M. Padilla, P. Shah, J. M. Zacks, and J. Hullman. 2021. The science of visual data communication: What works. *Psychological Science in the Public Interest* 22(3):110–161.

Hung, P., J. C. Probst, Y. Shih, R. Ranganathan, M. J. Brown, E. Crouch. and J. M. Eberth. 2023. Rural-urban disparities in quality of inpatient psychiatric care. *Psychiatric Services* 74(5):446–454.

Kapoor, A., P. Ramamurthy, M. Manikandan, and P. Thilakan. 2023. Follow-up attendance of patients with mental disorders and substance use disorders after inpatient treatment in psychiatry ward. *Archives of Mental Health* 25(1):14–18.

Lesselroth, B. J., and D. S. Pieczkiewicz. 2011. *Data Visualization Strategies for the Electronic Health Record*. Hauppage, NY: Nova Science Publishers.

Mielicki, M. K., C. J. Fitzsimmons, L. K. Schiller, D. Scheibe, J. M. Taber, P. G. Sidne, P. G. Matthews, E. A. Waters, K. G. Coifman, and C. A. Thompson. 2023. Number lines can be more effective at facilitating adults' performance on health-related ratio problems than risk ladders and icon arrays. *Journal of Experimental Psychology: Applied* 29(3):529.

Shields, M. C., M. A. Hollander, A. B. Busch, Z. Kantawala, and M. B. Rosenthal. 2023. Patient-centered inpatient psychiatry is associated with outcomes, ownership, and national quality measures. *Health Affairs Scholar* 1(1).

Speier, C. 2006. The influence of information presentation formats on complex task decision-making performance. *International Journal of Human-Computer Studies* 64(11):1115–1131.

Starren, J., and S. B. Johnson. 2000. An object-oriented taxonomy of medical data presentations. *Journal of the American Medical Informatics Association* 7:1–20.

Thomas, P., and S. Powsner. 2005. Data presentation for quality improvement. *AMIA Annual Symposium Proceedings* 2005:1134.

Tufte, E. R. 2006. *Beautiful Evidence*. Cheshire, CT: Graphics Press.

Warner, A. R., L. Lavagnino, S. Glazier, J. E. Hamilton, and S. D. Lane, 2022. Inpatient early intervention for serious mental illnesses is associated with fewer rehospitalizations compared with treatment as usual in a high-volume public psychiatric hospital setting. *Journal of Psychiatric Practice* 28(1). https://journals.lww.com/practicalpsychiatry/abstract/2022/01000/inpatient_early_intervention_for_serious_mental.4.aspx.

West, V. L., D. Borland, and W. E. Hammond. 2015. Innovative information visualization of electronic health record data: A systematic review. *Journal of the American Medical Informatics Association* 22(2):330–339.

World Bank. 2023. "Worldwide Dashboard. World Bank Data." Accessed December 11, 2023. https://databank.worldbank.org/source/world-development-indicators.

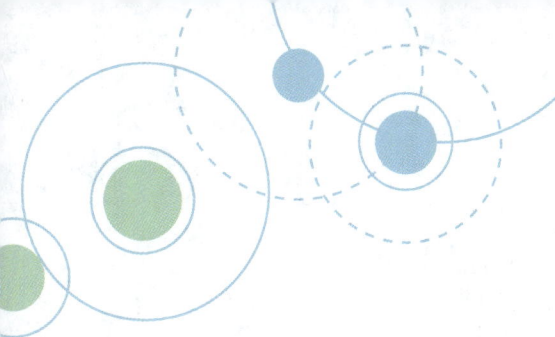

# Research Methods

*Shannon H. Houser, PhD, MPH, RHIA, FAHIMA*

## Learning Objectives

- Articulate a research problem and research questions for topics in health information management
- Use appropriate research process principles in health information management research and practice
- Select appropriate research design approaches and data collection methods
- Conduct research projects using standard and suitable tools and techniques
- Present research findings in formats consistent with recognized standards

## Key Terms

Applied research
Basic research
Bibliographic database
Case study
Causal relationship
Causal-comparative research
Comparative effectiveness research (CER)
Confounding variables
Content analysis
Control group
Correlational research
Deductive reasoning
Dependent variables
Descriptive research
Ethnography
Evaluation research
Experimental (study) group
Experimental research
External validity
Focus group
Generalizability
Grounded theory
Grey literature
Health technology assessment (HTA)
Historical research
Hypothesis
Independent variables
Inductive reasoning
Instrument
Internal validity
Interrater reliability
Interview
Intrarater reliability
Literature review
Likert scale
Living systematic reviews (LSR)
Meta-analysis
Meta-syntheses
Mixed methods research
Naturalistic observation
Needs assessment
Nonparticipant observation
Observational research
Outcome evaluation
Outcomes research
Participant observation
Pilot study
Policy analysis
Primary analysis
Primary source
Problem statement
Process evaluation
Qualitative approach
Quantitative approach
Questionnaire survey

Random sampling
Randomization
Reliability
Research
Research design
Research methods
Research methodology
Research question
Scales
Secondary analysis
Secondary source
Simulation observation
Survey
Systematic review
Treatment
Triangulation
Validity
Variable

**Research** is a systematic process dedicated to discovering or formulating new knowledge about a topic; validating or assessing existing knowledge; or updating antiquated understanding. Knowledge of research and **research methods**—the use of strategies, processes, or techniques to conduct research studies—supports health informatics and health information management (HIM) professionals in their quest to use evidence to address queries or drive decision-making.

Rooted in the combination of business, science, and information technology, HIM research explores the intricate practices of acquiring, analyzing, and protecting digital and traditional medical information—a cornerstone for delivering quality patient care (AHIMA n.d.). As the use of information and technology increases, the relevance and demands placed on HIM Professionals in the research domain have seen a dramatic rise. Professionals across the spectrum of the HIM domain, from coders and data analysts to C-suite executives, collaborate as a cohesive team. By partnering with peers in associated disciplines like medicine, health services administration, health informatics, and information systems [ISs]), they bring diverse insights and data from their respective areas of expertise.

There has been a transformative shift in the understanding and application of research methodologies. This change has been driven by advances in technology, societal and political shifts, pressing environmental concerns, and notably, a global health crisis of unprecedented scale. Collectively, these factors have reshaped how research is conceptualized, carried out, and communicated.

This chapter describes research designs and methodologies for conducting research. Additionally, it showcases exemplary HIM research studies and highlights the connection between research initiatives and the HIM practitioners.

## Research Methodology

**Research methodology** is the science of solving research problems by incorporating a set of procedures or strategies used by researchers to collect, analyze, and present data. A methodology applies tools to guide the research process and outcomes. Generally, there are two types of research: basic research and applied research, and these two types are opposite ends of a continuum, not separate entities. Therefore, the distinction between them is sometimes unclear. However, they can be differentiated as follows.

**Basic research** answers the question "Why?" with the intent of increasing the scientific knowledge base and focuses on the development of fundamental theories and their refinement. Basic research is sometimes called bench science because it often occurs in laboratories, and rarely assists clinical practitioners directly to solve real world practice issues. Although most HIM research is applied in nature, the creation and discovery of the electronic health record (EHR) as a product of technology is an example of basic research. **Applied research** answers the questions "What?" and "How?" and focuses on the implementation of theories into practice. Applied research, particularly clinical applied research, may occur in healthcare settings, such as at the bedside. An example of applied research is identifying the effectiveness of using EHR applications in practice resulting in improvement of healthcare outcomes.

Research methodologists distinguish between two overarching approaches to research: the quantitative approach and the qualitative approach. The **quantitative approach** is the explanation of phenomena by making predictions, collecting and analyzing evidence, testing alternative theories, and choosing the best theory. The goal of this approach is to produce objective knowledge with **generalizability**, meaning it can be applied to other similar situations and populations. As the word *quantitative* implies, the data can often be quantified, and lead to statistical or numerical results. In HIM, an example would be a study that calculates the percentage of a healthcare organization's patients that use its patient portal. The **qualitative approach** is the interpretation of nonnumerical observations and seeking answers of "why" things happened. These nonnumerical observations include words, gestures, activities, time, space, images, and perceptions. These observations are placed in context, which means the specifics of the situation. Context includes time, space, emotional attitude, social situation, and culture. In HIM, an example would be an exploration of the reasons why patients are reluctant and uncomfortable using a healthcare organization's patient portal.

The purpose of the research determines the approach. Research that investigates numerically measurable observations is quantitative; while research that explores reasons or interprets actions is qualitative. Within both approaches, researchers make certain basic assumptions. (See table 18.1.)

**Mixed methods research** is a third approach that combines quantitative and qualitative techniques within a single study or across multiple complementary studies. Mixed methods research is suited to investigations of large topics or complex phenomena, such as in healthcare.

In a series of studies, HIM researchers can use all three approaches. For example, in a quantitative study, researchers might investigate the effectiveness of a community health center's program to educate elders with low incomes on the reliability of health websites. In a qualitative study, researchers may explore the impact of the educational program on elders' application of information from the websites. In a mixed methods study, researchers could investigate factors associated with the implementation of the program, such as the health director's selection of the educational materials and the director's views on barriers and facilitators of the program's implementation.

Researchers use inductive reasoning or deductive reasoning to justify their decisions and conclusions about phenomena. **Inductive reasoning**, or induction, involves drawing conclusions based on a limited number of observations. Inductive reasoning is "bottom up." Researchers employing inductive reasoning begin with observations, detect patterns or clusters of relationships, form and explore tentative hypotheses, and generate provisional conclusions or theories. For example, during the professional practice experience, a student might observe that all coders in the coding department at XYZ hospital had the registered health information technician (RHIT) credential. Thus, one might conclude that all coders have the RHIT credential. **Deductive reasoning**, or deduction, involves drawing conclusions based on generalizations, rules, or principles. Deductive reasoning is "top down." Researchers using deductive reasoning begin with a theory, develop hypotheses to test the theory, observe phenomena related to the hypotheses, and validate or invalidate the theory. For example, the same student might use the generalization to conclude that Jane Doe is a coder, so she must have a RHIT credential because all coders in the department have the RHIT.

As the examples demonstrate, neither induction nor deduction alone is completely satisfactory. Early, exploratory research often takes an inductive approach. Once researchers have generated a theory, they use the deductive approach to test the theory.

**Table 18.1.** Comparison of assumptions in quantitative and qualitative research approaches

| Quantitative | Qualitative |
|---|---|
| Single truth exists | Multiple truths exist simultaneously |
| Single truth applies across time and place | Truths are bound to place and time (contextual) |
| Researchers can adopt neutral, unbiased stances | Neutrality is impossible because researchers choose their topics of investigation |
| Chronological sequence of causes can be identified | Influences interact with one another to color researchers' views of the past, present, and future |

## Check Your Understanding 18.1

**Answer the following questions in a separate document.**

1. When an HIM researcher conducts interviews to evaluate user satisfaction with an EHR system, which research methodology should be utilized, and why?

2. In an investigation of the impact of computer-assisted coding on reimbursement outcomes, an HIM researcher collected data on reimbursement levels and facilitated focus groups to understand the reasons behind any unexpected results. Which research methodology is being implemented in this study and what is the justification for its use?

3. How would an HIM professional categorize a study investigating effective strategies to enhance physician engagement with EHR systems? Provide a rationale for your answer.

4. What type of research approach is used when a researcher analyzes data by using electronic display boards in hospital departments to monitor the number of patients with a list of fall risk factors within 24 hours of admission? Explain your rationale.

5. You are asked to assess the perceptions and user satisfaction of those using mobile phone apps for diet and weight loss. What is the most appropriate research approach to use for conducting this study? Explain your rationale.

## Research Process

The research process identifies the sequential steps a researcher undertakes from the beginning to the end of a study. By adhering to this process, a researcher can pinpoint the problem to be addressed, gather precise and trustworthy data, conduct relevant analyses, and provide credible information. Typically, the research process contains the following steps:

1. Defining the research problem and research question
2. Conducting a literature review
3. Determining the research design
4. Collecting data
5. Analyzing the data
6. Disseminating the results

This six-step process offers a streamlined and effective strategy for conducting a research study. While some researchers might rearrange these steps or modify elements between them, the research process serves as a template. It guides researchers in methodically exploring a research topic and offers a holistic view of the research's progression.

### Defining the Research Problem and Research Question

Research begins with identifying and formulating a research topic from a specific research problem that the researcher aims to address. Subsequently, within that topic, the researcher delineates the research questions they seek to answer. (See figure 18.1 for topic examples.) At this stage, it is critical that the researcher understands the purpose of the research. The researcher's aim should be to address an important question, tackle a pertinent problem, or enrich the existing body of knowledge on the chosen topic. The purpose fundamentally influences choices throughout the various stages of the research process.

A **problem statement** is a concise description of a research problem or an issue that the researcher intends to address or to resolve and explains why the identified study is important. The purpose of a problem statement is to understand the problem and identify the gap between the current problem and intended goal to be achieved. It applies the "five *W*s" (who, what, where, when, and why) to describe and outline the problem. Depending on the complexity of the problem, the length of the statement can vary, but it is usually one or two sentences. An example of a problem statement is "Wide adoption of EHRs is linked with providers' dissatisfaction with the overall system, an overwhelming amount of time to enter data, and an overall decrease in provider productivity."

A **research question** is the central focus of the research and asks about a particular issue within a topic that a researcher wishes to study. It is presented as a question with who, how, what, when, or why. Some may have multiple research questions in one study. An example of a research question related to the first topic in figure 18.1 would be "What is the effect of competitive market forces on the exchange of information among healthcare organizations?" Both the problem statement and research question are important components in the initial and foundational steps in the research process. They establish a direction and outline of which research problem or problems are to be resolved and which research question or questions are to be answered.

The study's purpose guides researchers in formulating their research question(s). In quantitative research, which seeks to produce objective data,

**Figure 18.1.** Examples of topics in health informatics and information management

- Integrated healthcare networks: Understanding the interoperability and seamless information exchange between healthcare institutions, regulatory bodies, accreditation agencies, and other key stakeholders.
- Health information technology (HIT) system analysis: Outcomes and insights from evaluation studies focused on health information systems and emerging technologies.
- IT-driven clinical enhancement: The role of information technology in bolstering clinician efficacy, elevating patient care, and improving health outcomes.
- HIT adoption dynamics: Investigating the determinants and barriers in the uptake and utilization of HIT and platforms.
- Research transparency in health informatics: Establishing robust standards for presenting findings in health informatics and information management studies.
- Consumer digital health landscape: Exploring the accessibility, usage patterns, quality, and variety of e-health initiatives aimed at consumers.
- Health data standardization: Delving into classifications, terminologies, coded datasets, and the creation of structured reporting in healthcare.

questions are crafted with precision. Here, researchers adopt a sequential approach, focusing the question(s) on a topic suitable for investigation. On the other hand, qualitative research, which produces interpretation of nonnumerical data, begins with broad, exploratory research questions. Researchers follow an iterative process, continually refining their question(s) as the study unfolds. Devoting adequate time and energy to developing the research question(s) is crucial. Criteria of a well-constructed research question include the following:

- The question is stated with clarity and precision.
- The question possesses theoretical relevance, practical value, or a combination of both.
- Clear and direct connections exist between the question and an overarching framework, be it a theory or a research model.
- The findings from the research contribute discernibly to the existing body of knowledge.
- The response to the question or the resolution to the issue holds substantive merit. (Aveyard 2023)

Research questions can originate from research models, recommendations of previous researchers, or gaps in the existing body of knowledge.

- *Research models*: These models show the factors and relationships in a theory. Researchers might focus on one or two factors that have previously been highlighted or deemed challenging by other scholars.
- *Recommendations of previous researchers*: In journal articles, theses, and dissertations, researchers specifically make recommendations for additional research based on the results of their own research. For example, researchers may identify unintentional flaws in their own study that future researchers could correct in a replication study.
- *Gaps in the body of knowledge*: Published as journal articles, comprehensive reviews of the literature on a problem or question identify gaps or problematic areas. These review articles can be examined for research questions.

Next, researchers narrow the focus of each question to ensure it is both a manageable and researchable issue. For example, the researcher might initially describe a problem as a broad societal concern and support it with references from popular magazines, journals, and opinion articles. Then, the researcher identifies the impact of this problem or question on health informatics and information management. At this point, researchers draw supporting citations from academic journals, authoritative government reports, or other reputable scientific sources. Finally, the researcher formulates the problem statement.

## Check Your Understanding 18.2

**Answer the following questions in a separate document.**

1. To examine the underuse of patient portals, what steps should a researcher take to craft an initial problem statement based on the methodology outlined in the chapter? Construct a problem statement for the study focusing on the low usage of patient portals.

2. The HIM director is evaluating the privacy and security features of two EHR systems as a part of the purchasing decision for the organization. What is the key driving factor as the HIM director plans this research?

3. Determine and give examples of the components a researcher should consider when designing a research study to assess EHR acceptance by physicians. Include a possible research question.

4. A researcher is investigating the impact of a new telehealth documentation system on the efficiency of patient care coordination among healthcare teams. What type of research methodology would be most appropriate for this study? Provide an example of a research question that might guide the investigation.

5. You are asked to conduct a semistructured interview to assess users' perceived benefits of and barriers to using an EHR and their recommendations on improving the EHR system. What type of research questions would likely be used? Give an example of a research question you created for this study.

## Conducting a Literature Review

After the researcher identifies the topic and develops both a problem statement and research question, the next step is the literature review. A **literature review** is a systematic investigation of all the knowledge available about a topic from sources such as books, journal articles, theses, and dissertations. Literature review has three meanings defined as follows:

- Meaning 1: *Process* of identifying, reading, summarizing, analyzing, and synthesizing the writings of recognized scholars and experts.

- Meaning 2: *Product* that is the introduction to a manuscript or an article in which researchers explain how they arrived at their research question.

- Meaning 3: *Product* in which the introduction of meaning 2 is expanded and refined into an entirely separate, independent, and peer-reviewed article or book chapter. Known as a systematic review or meta-analysis, this literature review is a specialized type of research and is discussed in greater detail in a later section on secondary analysis.

Researchers conduct literature reviews with three main objectives: (1) to acquaint readers with the subject and convince them of the study's relevance, (2) to demonstrate to the reader that the researcher has meticulously examined all aspects of the topic, and (3) to deepen the researcher's understanding of the topic.

The literature review should guide the reader to conclude that the logical and necessary next step is the research proposed by the researchers. The thoroughness of the literature review lends credibility to the study. Researchers come to a complete understanding of the current status of the topic through their literature review.

### Sources for Literature Review

The researcher's first step in a literature review is identifying the relevant sources. Many sources of information are available, such as those shown in appendix B. Many of these sources are available to HIM researchers through educational institutions' libraries or through reciprocal agreements between the researchers' employers and educational institutions. Libraries house many physical and digital resources, including journals (both print and online), e-books, reference handbooks, maps, and multimedia resources like videos and audiotapes. These resources can be located through library catalogs (many of which are available online), bibliographical databases, and specialized databases.

While the bulk of a literature review draws from published works, certain research methodologies might demand alternative information sources, such as multimedia for qualitative studies. It is essential to identify all possible information sources for the review. Published literature includes primary and secondary sources. **Primary sources** are the original works of the researchers who conducted the research study. Research-based articles in *Perspectives in Health Information Management*, *Journal of Medical Internet Research*, or *International Journal of Medical Informatics* are examples of primary sources. **Secondary sources** are summaries of the original works. Encyclopedias and textbooks are examples of secondary sources. For literature reviews, the researcher should predominantly use primary sources.

Additionally, peer-reviewed (refereed) journals have more value than popular (trade) magazines. Peer-reviewed journal articles are scrutinized by subject matter experts before publication to ensure the quality and relevance of the content. Some peer-reviewed journals include the *Perspectives in Health Information Management*, *Journal of the American Medical Informatics Association*, and *Journal of the American Medical Association*. It is worth noting that popular magazines usually do not undergo a peer review process.

For HIM researchers, another important information source is the grey literature. **Grey literature** includes materials that are available in print or digital formats but are not published through traditional commercial publishing channels, including journals (Eden et al. 2011, 98–99). Grey literature is produced by government bodies, like agencies (such as the Institute of Medicine, now the National Academy of Medicine), and private entities such as Deloitte LLP and RAND Corporation. Examples include technical reports, technology assessments, product pamphlets, and technology evaluations. As digital dissemination has grown, repositories and digital libraries have also become crucial sources of both traditional and grey literature. For instance, university researchers increasingly rely on online repositories like institutional digital libraries to access scholarly articles and unpublished theses. These platforms provide not only peer-reviewed research but also grey literature such as technical reports and conference proceedings, which are essential for comprehensive literature reviews and for professionals to stay current in their fields.

### Search of Information Sources

Researchers search and retrieve information sources from knowledge bases, such as bibliographic databases and digital collections. **Bibliographic databases** are databases of published literature such as journals, magazines, newspaper articles, books, book chapters, and other information sources. The databases' scopes vary by type of information source indexed and by academic disciplines covered. For example, some databases index only peer-reviewed journals, while others include conference proceedings and book chapters. Additionally, some focus on specific academic fields like health sciences or computer science, while others cover multiple disciplines. Many databases also offer full texts, not just indices.

Because of its multidisciplinary and wide scope of professions, HIM research is often conducted by searching a variety of databases. Moreover, some of the grey literature is also available through digital collections, such as the resources of the Centers for Medicare and Medicaid Services (CMS) and the Agency for Healthcare Research and Quality (AHRQ). Appendix B lists select databases and digital collections covering business and management, computer science and engineering, health services administration, and medicine and allied health sciences.

For organizing and managing information sources, researchers use various reference management software programs. These software packages allow researchers to do the following:

- Create personal bibliographic databases
- Use the packages' search engines that directly download citations and full-text articles into the researchers' personal bibliographic databases
- Import the contents of databases into word-processing software
- Transform bibliographic entries into the required style of the journal (styles editor)

The literature review is an important part of a research paper. It is used as a foundation to support the new knowledge contribution of this research to a specific field and to identify any differences between the current study and existing literature. The characteristics of a well-developed literature review include the following:

- Balance of comprehensiveness with relevance and focus
- Concise statement of what is known and unknown about a topic
- Logical and succinct summary comprised mainly of primary sources
- Critical analysis and evaluation that includes strengths, weaknesses, limitations, and gaps
- Synthesis

Finally, the literature review concludes with a sentence that specifically links the previous research to the researchers' study. In quantitative studies, the literature review concludes with a clear and explicit **hypothesis**, a statement that describes a research question in measurable terms.

Literature search processes have transformed significantly, reflecting both technological progress and the dynamic nature of research. The surge in preprint servers, open-access journals, and institution-backed digital repositories has diversified the spectrum of sources, ushering in a broader pool of content including grey literature. Advanced search tools now use artificial intelligence (AI) to understand the meaning of words more like humans do, offering another tool for performing literature searches.

## Check Your Understanding 18.3

**Answer the following questions in a separate document.**

1. A researcher is conducting a literature review for the selected research topic of assessing low usage of patient portals. Describe how the literature review will benefit the researcher. Recommend three bibliographic databases or digital resources that may assist the researcher on the topic of patient portal usage and explain why you chose them.

2. An HIM researcher is conducting a qualitative study on user perceptions of mobile health apps for patient care. Compare the three sources of Medline, grey literature, and PubMed, and answer which one of these three sources will be most appropriate, relevant, timely, and useful to this selected topic. Explain the rationale.

3. Conduct a literature review on assessing the association between EHR documentation errors and patient safety issues. Consider the important factors and outline the literature review plan for this topic.

4. How do primary and secondary sources differ in the context of a literature review, and how might they complement each other in research?

5. An HIM researcher is preparing a literature review on the effects of implementing AI technologies in diagnostic processes. The review aims to gather insights from primary sources. Why is it important for the researcher to focus on primary sources, and what type of information should they be looking for?

## Selecting the Research Design

The research design serves as the blueprint for a study, outlining the strategy to achieve the researchers' objectives, whether it is answering a question, addressing a problem, or generating new information. While multiple research designs and methods can be employed to explore the same overarching question or issue, choosing the most suitable design is crucial. This ensures the gathered data is pertinent, of superior quality, and directly correlates with the posed research question or problem.

In selecting a research design, the most important factor that researchers should consider is their purpose as reflected in the problem statement. In addition, researchers should also weigh in other factors, such as the researcher's skill level, time frame for conducting the study, available resources, and potential subjects. The following are specific questions to consider:

- *Skills*: Can the researcher conduct the laboratory experiments, moderate the discussions, or perform the analytical techniques necessary for the research?
- *Time*: Does the researcher have the time to devote to conducting the research, such as in the case of a longitudinal study over a period of 10 years?
- *Money and resources*: Can the researcher afford the equipment and other costs of the research, such as setting up the simulation laboratory as described later in the section on nonparticipant observation?
- *Potential subjects*: Are enough subjects available and are they willing to participate, given their busy schedules? Will people who volunteer to be subjects in the research differ from those who do not volunteer?

There are several prevalent research designs, including historical, descriptive, correlational, evaluation, experimental, and causal-comparative (see table 18.2). The selection of a specific research design is guided by the study's objective and the nature of the research problem.

Preliminary, exploratory research often uses descriptive or correlational designs. As researchers define the investigation, they may opt for causal-comparative and experimental approaches. It is also common for researchers to integrate various designs to cater to specific research questions or challenges. For instance, a study may include both descriptive and correlational elements. The time element, whether retrospective or prospective, and whether cross-sectional or longitudinal, applies to all design types mentioned in this chapter.

### Historical Research Design

Historical research investigates past events to draw associations and develop predictions for present and

Table 18.2. Designs of research, their applications, their associated methods, and examples of HIM studies

| Design | Application | Method | Example of HIM study |
|---|---|---|---|
| Historical | Understand past events | Case study Bibliography | The factors leading to the creation and development of clinical decision support systems in the 1960s and 1970s |
| Descriptive | Describe current status | Survey Observation | A survey of clinicians to determine how and to what degree they use clinical decision support systems |
| Correlational | Determine existence and degree of relationship | Survey Secondary analysis | A study to determine the relationship among individual clinicians' attributes, the health team's characteristics, the setting, and use of clinical decision support systems |
| Evaluation | Evaluate effectiveness | Survey Case study Observation | A study to evaluate the efficacy of the implementation of a clinical decision support system in a specialty clinic in an academic health center |
| Causal-Comparative (Quasi-Experimental) | Detect causal relationship | Cohort study Case-control (retrospective) study | A study to compare the antibiotic prescribing practices for acute respiratory infections of primary care clinician teams using a clinical decision support system versus primary care clinician teams not using a clinical decision support system |
| Experimental | Establish cause and effect | Parallel group trial Cluster trial Randomized, double-blind, controlled trial | A study to evaluate the influence of a clinical decision support system on clinicians' antibiotic prescribing practices for acute respiratory infections with clinicians randomized into an intervention group and a control group |

future events. Researchers focus on studying and analyzing primary and secondary sources as records of past events. Primary sources include wills, charters, hospital patient records, reports, minutes, eyewitness accounts, letters, and email records. Secondary sources are derived from primary sources; secondary sources summarize, critique, or analyze the primary sources. Primary sources are superior to secondary sources. Examining both primary and secondary sources, HIM researchers could explore the origin of standards organizations, the development of transaction standards, and the history of code sets.

## Descriptive Research Design

**Descriptive research** determines and reports the current status of topics and subjects. It provides a clear overview of the situation as it exists. However, descriptive research has limitations, including the lack of standardized questions, the variability of observer training, and sometimes less-than-optimal response rates. HIM researchers have conducted many descriptive studies to keep pace with the dynamic landscape, focusing on areas like the status of the HIM workforce, coding accuracy, the extent of EHR implementation, agreement on the use of specific terms within clinical terminologies, telehealth usage, and obstacles to virtual care implementation.

## Correlational Research Design

**Correlational research** detects the existence, the direction, and the degree of relationships among factors. The factors in correlational research and other research designs are called **variables**. In correlational research, there are at least two measured variables. For example, correlational researchers conducted a study investigating the association between stress and anxiety. They found that the scores for the two variables, stress and anxiety, both moved in the *same* direction—as one increased so did the other. This association is a positive relationship because the variables' scores are moving in the same direction. The researchers also investigated the participants' feelings of personal accomplishment. In this case, the researchers found that the scores for the variables, stress and feelings of personal accomplishment, moved in *opposite* directions—as stress increased, the feelings of personal accomplishment decreased, and vice versa. This association is a negative (inverse) relationship because the variables' scores are moving in opposite directions. However, the design of the researchers' study—correlational—did *not* permit them to state that stress caused anxiety (or vice versa) or that stress decreased feelings of personal accomplishment (or vice versa). Many other factors, such as financial problems, poor coping skills, or low self-confidence, could have been associated with stress, anxiety, and feelings of personal accomplishment.

The degree or strength of the relationship among variables can range from 0.00 to +1.00 (or −1.00), detailed as follows:

- Strength of 0.00 means absolutely no relationship.
- Strength between 0.00 and +1.00 or between 0.00 and −1.00 means that the variables sometimes, but not always, move together.
- Strength of 1.00 or −1.00 means a perfect relationship, with the variables moving exactly in tandem.

The value of correlational research is that it indicates the existence of associations that can be examined and possibly explained using experimental research studies. HIM researchers have conducted various correlational studies to explore the complexities of HIT. These studies focused on examining factors that influence HIT adoption, analyzing the relationship between social media use and perceptions of healthcare laws, exploring the correlation between the severity of drug side effects and mortality rates, and investigating the connection between healthcare professionals' security habits and their individual traits.

## Evaluation Research Design

**Evaluation research** examines the effectiveness of policies, programs, or organizations. Researchers can assess the value of programs, projects, organizations, interventions, policies, technologies, products, and other activities or objects. Criteria to assess these activities or objects can be related to many of their aspects, such as conceptualization, design, components, implementation, effectiveness, efficiency, impact, scalability, and generalizability. Common types of evaluation studies are needs assessments, process evaluations, outcome evaluations, and policy analyses (Shi 2020, 198).

- **Needs assessment**: Collecting and analyzing data about proposed programs, projects, and other activities or objects to determine what is required, lacking, or desired by an employee, group, or organization. The HIM professional could survey patients to determine their preferences and priorities for various features in the healthcare organization's patient portal.
- **Process evaluation**: Monitoring programs, projects, and other activities or objects to check whether their development or implementation is proceeding as planned (also known as

formative evaluation) (Robson 2010, 253). A research team could assess whether the rollout of the new features in the organization's patient portal is occurring per the project's milestones and within budget. Adjustments can be made as needed.

- **Outcome evaluation**: Collecting and analyzing data at the end of an implementation or operating cycle to determine whether the program, project, or other activity or object has achieved its expected or intended impact, product, or other outcome (also known as summative evaluation) (Robson 2010, 253). Researchers could conduct a study comparing the level of patients' interaction with their organization's patient portal to the level of interaction reported by their industry peers. Organizational leaders can use the findings to help decide whether the vendor's contract should be renewed or revised.

- **Policy analysis**: Identifying options to meet goals and estimating the costs and consequences of each option prior to the implementation of any option (Shi 2020, 205). For a federal agency, a research team could identify various ways to increase patient self-management and engagement using HITs and, for each way, analyze its benefits and costs, and predict its consequences.

Other terms are used for the variety of evaluation research depending upon the focus of the research, the researchers' educational background, and the research's funding source.

**Outcomes research** assesses the quality and effectiveness of healthcare as measured by the attainment of a specified result or outcome, improved health, lowered morbidity or mortality, and improvement of abnormal states. An example of outcomes research is a study investigating whether a clinical decision support (CDS) system that links the EHR to treatment protocols, drug information, alerts, and community resources for the care of patients with HIV infection improves a patient's quality of life.

Health services research is conducted about healthcare delivery. This type of research examines organizational structures and systems and the effectiveness and efficiency of healthcare services. The research is usually concerned with relationships among need, demand, supply, use, and outcome of health services. An example of health services research is a study that investigates whether the degree of adoption of HITs affects patient safety.

**Health technology assessment (HTA)** is the evaluation of the usefulness (utility) of a health technology in relation to cost, efficacy, utilization, and other factors in terms of its impact on social, ethical, and legal systems. The purpose of HTA is to inform decision-making to promote an equitable, efficient, and high-quality health system (Chen 2022). Technology, in this context, is broadly defined as the use of scientific knowledge for practical purposes, encompassing methods, techniques, and instrumentation. Health technologies, which include pharmaceuticals, medical devices, procedures, and HITs, aim to enhance health, prevent and treat conditions, or support rehabilitation. For example, the Technology Assessment Program at the AHRQ conducts assessments using primary research, systematic reviews, and meta-analyses to inform national coverage decisions for Medicare (AHRQ 2024).

**Comparative effectiveness research (CER)** is research that generates and synthesizes "evidence that compares the benefits and harms of alternative methods to prevent, diagnose, treat, and monitor a clinical condition, or to improve the delivery of care. The purpose of CER is to assist consumers, clinicians, purchasers, and policy makers to make informed decisions that will improve healthcare at both the individual and population levels" (IOM 2009, 13). Specifically, CER can help determine which intervention, such as a drug or a surgery, may be most effective or beneficial for a given patient. For example, under the Affordable Care Act (ACA) of 2010, the AHRQ is charged to disseminate information gained by federally funded CER. Recent CER information the AHRQ has disseminated includes stroke prevention in atrial fibrillation and treatment of tinnitus (GAO 2015, 280).

### Experimental Research Design

**Experimental research** is a design in which the researcher directly manipulates factors in carefully controlled interventions according to strict protocols (detailed sets of rules and procedures). The purpose of the control in the interventions and protocols is to maintain uniform conditions during the research so that no extraneous factors, known as **confounding variables**, affect the study's outcome. The researchers' goal is to pinpoint the cause of the intervention's effect without any possible, alternative explanations. Thereby, experimental research establishes **causal relationships**—relationships that show cause and effect. For example, smoking (the cause) results in lung cancer (the effect).

Researchers conducting experimental research work with two types of variables. **Independent variables** are antecedent or prior factors that researchers manipulate directly and are the variables used to predict; they are also called treatments or interventions. **Dependent variables** are the measured variables; they depend on the independent variables and are the outcome or variable to be predicted. The dependent variables reflect the results that the researcher theorizes. They occur subsequently or after the independent variables. Therefore, the independent variable causes an effect in the dependent variable.

Experimental researchers design their studies to maximize the likelihood of establishing causal relationships and to minimize any potential effects of confounding variables. To achieve these aims, experimental researchers design the following four key features into their studies:

- *Randomization*: The process begins with **random sampling**—the unbiased selection of subjects from the population of interest. (Random sampling is discussed in greater detail in the section on gathering data.) Then **randomization**, or the arbitrary allocation of subjects between comparison groups, occurs. Of the comparison groups, the **experimental (study) group** comprises the research subjects who receive the study's intervention.

- *Observation*: This is a generic term for the measurements of the dependent variable *before* and *after* the treatment. It could be a pretest and a posttest.

- *Presence of a control group*: Another group, the **control group**, comprises the control subjects who do not receive the intervention.

- *Treatment (intervention)*: In this context, **treatment**, also known as intervention, is defined generically or broadly, beyond its usual meaning of therapy. It is the process in which the researcher manipulates the independent variables. Treatment could mean a physical conditioning program, a computer training program, a particular laboratory medium, or the timing of prophylactic medications (Campbell and Stanley 1963, 13).

As an example of an experimental study, HIM researchers could investigate the effects of an online health promotion program. Adult participants could be randomized between an experimental group and a control group. All participants' baseline data on their consumption of fruits and vegetables could be collected through an online survey prior to the start of the intervention. The intervention could be a multimedia online module containing information and guidance on the benefits of eating fruits and vegetables. Members of the experimental group could be given a link to the program; members of the control group could be told that they were on the wait list and that their access was delayed. Members of the experimental group could access the module from their homes through the link. After three months, all participants could be sent online questionnaires about their consumption of fruits and vegetables. Subsequently, the two groups' data could be analyzed and compared in terms of their initial consumption patterns and their post-intervention patterns.

## Causal-Comparative Research Design

**Causal-comparative research** is a type of quasi-experimental design. *Quasi* means resembling or having some of the characteristics. Therefore, causal-comparative research resembles experimental research by having many, but not all, of its characteristics. Causal-comparative research lacks two characteristics of experimental research: manipulation of treatment and random assignment to a group. Causal-comparative research is also called *ex post facto*, meaning retrospective, because some past variable or phenomenon has already occurred.

Three situations, logistically and ethically, require the causal-comparative design:

- The variables cannot be manipulated (gender, age, race, and birthplace).
- The variables should not be manipulated (accidental death or injury and child abuse).
- The variables represent different conditions that have already occurred (medication error, heart catheterization performed, smoking, and environmental exposure).

These situations prevent people from being assigned randomly into groups. However, by relinquishing manipulation of treatment and randomization, causal-comparative (quasi-experimental) research can only determine the *possibility* of causal relationships.

In an example of a causal-comparative study, HIM researchers may look back in time (retrospective) to investigate the factors associated with inpatient medication errors when a computerized alert system was in place. Identifying inpatient admissions with and without medication errors in the database, researchers could look for patterns in the records associated with errors, such as the patients' diseases, location of care (intensive care unit [ICU] versus regular nursing floor), providers' characteristics, organizational features, and other factors.

As creators of experimental and quasi-experimental research design, Campbell and Stanley formulated the differentiation between these two types of research design, based on the previously described four features (randomization, observation, control group, and treatment) (Campbell and Stanley 1963). Studies having all four key features are classified as experimental (one acceptable omission is the prior observation). Studies totally missing any feature are classified as quasi-experimental.

### Secondary Analysis

In addition to the common types of research design discussed previously, there are additional types of studies focusing on applying secondary data analysis. Researchers distinguish between primary analysis and secondary analysis. **Primary analysis** refers to analysis of original research data by the researchers who collected them. **Secondary analysis** involves using data originally collected by other researchers to address different questions (Wickham 2019). This approach includes techniques like data mining and conducting systematic reviews. Data mining is a technique that uses machine learning, statistics, and database systems to uncover meaningful patterns and hidden relationships in large datasets (Chen et al. 2024). Data mining is considered secondary data analysis because data miners use databases created by others, often for purposes unrelated to research and data mining.

A **systematic review** is a comprehensive review of the evidence on a clearly formulated question that uses systematic and explicit methods to identify, select, and critically appraise relevant published and unpublished research studies; to extract and analyze data from the studies that are included in the review; and to present integrated and synthesized information (Green et al. 2011, 1.2.2). Systematic reviews must meet strict standards to avoid bias.

Systematic reviews are characterized by the following:

- Focusing on a well-defined question
- Using explicit search criteria to identify literature and, if appropriate, grey literature
- Employing inclusion and exclusion criteria to select articles and information sources
- Evaluating evidence in literature against consistent methodological standards
- Including relatively homogeneous (similar) studies with common underlying features

Three other types of systematic reviews exist based on their purpose and on analytical techniques:

- Scoping systematic reviews are exploratory reviews that map the range, extent, and breadth of relevant evidence and literature and other available information resources on a topic.
- Rapid reviews are simplified, less comprehensive reviews that generally conceptualize questions and are conducted when decision makers or policymakers need information within one to six months.
- **Meta-analyses** are a specialized type of systematic review that introduces statistical techniques to combine summary-level information from at least two studies. Meta-analyses estimate the overall, combined effect of several studies' outcomes (effects) for an intervention. This estimate of effect is expressed as an effect size, such as an odds ratio or a Pearson $r$ correlation coefficient. Meta-analyses may also be called overviews or quantitative systematic reviews.

The advantages of systematic reviews are that they integrate and weigh findings from many studies, some of which are contradictory. Researchers synthesize the results from multiple studies to reach overall conclusions.

Systematic reviews have long been a cornerstone in the research community, ensuring rigorous evaluation and synthesis of existing studies on a given topic. However, when new research is produced at a rapid pace, traditional systematic reviews may quickly become outdated. Maintaining currency is addressed by **living systematic reviews (LSR)**, which are dynamic in nature and are continually updated to incorporate new evidence as it emerges (Simmonds 2022). For example, during the COVID-19 pandemic, telehealth platforms rapidly evolved and were adopted in response to the pandemic; thus, new studies on their adoption and efficacy emerged frequently. LSRs in this area ensured healthcare policymakers and providers always had the most current evidence on telehealth best practices, barriers, benefits, and patient outcomes.

While systematic reviews typically focus on quantitative research, qualitative research is increasingly valued for its in-depth, contextual insights. **Meta-syntheses** effectively address the challenge of synthesizing multiple qualitative studies. This approach allows researchers to collate and interpret qualitative findings across studies, leading to deeper theoretical understandings and insights that might not be apparent from individual studies alone. This methodology enhances the depth and richness of data interpretation and contributes to the development of comprehensive conceptual frameworks (Lachal et al. 2017).

For instance, a meta-synthesis of qualitative studies on patient portals might uncover common themes across healthcare settings, patient demographics, or geographical regions regarding the perceived benefits and challenges of using patient portals. This deeper insight could reveal patterns such as the barriers patients face in accessing or navigating these portals, the influence of healthcare provider encouragement on portal utilization, or the concerns patients might have about data privacy and security. Additionally, by synthesizing narratives and experiences, meta-syntheses might identify the role of patient portals in enhancing patient-provider communication, the value patients find in having more direct access to their health information, or potential discrepancies in portal use among different patient populations.

In addition to these advancements, there is a growing emphasis on ensuring the reproducibility of systematic reviews. Transparent reporting and predefined protocols have become essential, ensuring other researchers can replicate the review process and arrive at similar conclusions. Platforms that allow researchers to register their systematic review protocols before beginning the review are instrumental in this regard. By promoting transparency and accountability in the review process, these platforms enhance the trustworthiness and credibility of systematic reviews in the academic community.

---

### Check Your Understanding 18.4

**Answer the following questions in a separate document.**

1. An HIM researcher is conducting a study to evaluate the impact of mobile devices on the accuracy and timeliness of data entry by healthcare providers in emergency departments. Which research design should be used, and why?

2. What is an appropriate research design for a researcher to apply when examining the effect of legislation on the number of hospitals in rural areas in the 1950s and 1960s? Explain your rationale.

3. Develop an experimental research scenario in which you identify and describe the dependent variable and the independent variable.

4. Compare correlational research design with evaluation research design. Recommend which one of these designs is most appropriate for a study to investigate the association between use of EHRs and physician burnout.

5. Consider an evaluation research study for an EHR implementation at either your own workplace or one you researched. Develop five criteria to assess such an implementation.

---

## Collecting Data

High-quality research depends on a carefully conceived plan and flawless execution. Prior to beginning their research study, researchers must write a step-by-step plan that considers every logistical detail from the start of their study to its completion. It is important to document the procedures of and adherence to the plan because the methods section of the study reports the plan's execution in such detail that other researchers can replicate the study.

A data collection method is the strategy that a researcher uses to collect and analyze data. Certain data collection methods are more closely associated with one design than another (see table 18.2). However, considerable overlap exists among methods and designs. For example, researchers can use the survey research method in both descriptive and correlational research designs. Validity and reliability are important concepts in the data collection process and ensure data quality, accuracy and integrity; selection of the proper data collection instrument along with proper procedures helps to ensure valued data.

### Data Collection Methods

Given the evolution of research and advancements in technology, the methods and tools available for data collection have increased and diversified. Traditional methods such as surveys and questionnaires, interviews, focus groups, observations, case studies, and ethnographies remain fundamental. However, the creation of digital platforms and tools has enabled more streamlined, automated, and remote data collection. For instance, digital surveys can be disseminated globally with the potential for real-time analytics. Virtual interviews and focus groups, particularly relevant in the post-pandemic era, circumvent geographic limitations. Wearable devices and health applications are gaining traction for collecting real-time health metrics and behaviors.

The choice of data collection method hinges on several factors, including the study's objective, the nature of the desired information (quantitative versus qualitative), available resources, and the target population's accessibility. For instance, while a digital survey might be appropriate for a broad demographic study, in-depth interviews may be more suitable for understanding nuanced experiences or complex topics. It's not uncommon for researchers to employ multiple methods within a single study to ensure a richer data set, like combining digital health metrics with patient interviews to assess the holistic impact of a health intervention.

Considerations in data collection now also encompass digital ethics, data privacy regulations, and cybersecurity. Ensuring the safe storage and transmission of digital data is paramount, especially with sensitive HIM. Furthermore, acquiring consent, especially in the digital realm, and obtaining Institutional Review Board (IRB) approval remains essential. Digital tools also present opportunities for secondary data analysis and leveraging big data for research purposes, but this comes with ethical and methodological challenges.

**Surveys and Questionnaires** Surveys are a fundamental tool for systematically collecting data from a specific population or a subset of that population. Influenced by remote-working and social-distancing norms, there has been a shift towards using digital platforms for survey distribution, moving away from methods like face-to-face interactions or mailed questionnaires.

Digital surveys offer convenience, rapid response collection, and the capability for real-time data analysis. They can be distributed widely without the constraints of location, eliminating geographical barriers and often leading to higher response rates. QR code-based surveys gained popularity during the pandemic, allowing respondents to quickly scan a code and provide feedback. In healthcare, this approach has been used effectively for patient feedback in clinics and for health screenings at public events, where users can scan a code to access and complete health assessment forms on their mobile devices.

Census surveys are conducted when the population is small. For example, the Health Information Management Association of Australia (HIMAA) conducted a census survey. HIMAA surveyed all its members—approximately 800—to obtain feedback on their views of current challenges facing the profession, challenges facing the profession in the next five to ten years, and other issues (Wissmann 2015, 4). On the other hand, when data from a large population is required, researchers conduct sample surveys. For example, the Health Resources and Services Administration (HRSA) carries out the National Sample Survey of Registered Nurses (NSSRN) to gather data on the US nursing workforce. In the 2022–2023 survey, nearly 50,000 registered nurses provided data (HRSA 2024).

The widespread use of digital tools has greatly streamlined large-scale research initiatives. These online resources enhance the ability to reach vast audiences and improve the efficiency and speed of data collection. For instance, studies such as nursing workforce surveys could greatly benefit from these digital surveying methods, resulting in a more comprehensive and data-rich research process. Questionnaire surveys query members of a population by providing participants a means to record and submit their responses electronically or in print form. Questionnaire studies are efficient because they require less time and money than interview studies do and because they allow the researchers to collect data from many more members of the population.

For example, in the previously discussed investigation on physicians' adoption of patient portals, an earlier phase of the study was an electronic survey (Vydra et al. 2015, 1). Electronic surveys were sent to all 89 primary care physicians affiliated with a university medical center and subject to the departmental patient portal policy. Among the items on the surveys were questions asking the respondents to estimate average amounts of time they spent on various activities associated with the organizational patient portal. Fifty-four physicians (60.6 percent) responded. The results showed that the respondents overestimated the average time they spent on the patient portal's activities (12.5 hours per week) as compared to the institutional log-in records (8.2 hours per week) by approximately 34 percent (Vydra et al. 2015, 14).

As electronic questionnaires become the norm, researchers are integrating them with other digital tools and databases. For example, in the patient portal study, they compare survey responses to actual usage metrics, enhancing data validation and revealing discrepancies between individuals' perceived actions and their actual behaviors.

**Interviews** When a researcher wants to understand a patient's impressions and experiences, interviews can be applied to gain more insight. In interviews, researchers obtain information from individuals through telephone calls or face-to-face interactions. Researchers can conduct a structured interview, controlling the questions and responses, or they can conduct an unstructured interview, allowing a free-flowing conversation. In the structured interview, researchers use a written list of questions called an interview guide. Using an interview guide ensures that all individuals or focus groups are asked the same questions. The structured interview has the advantages of being easier to quantify, tabulate, and analyze than the unstructured interview. However, the unstructured interview is often chosen when the topic is unexplored, poorly understood, or ill-defined. Typically, both types of interviews are recorded and transcribed for later analyses.

For example, a qualitative case study was conducted during an EHR transition at the Department of Veterans Affairs (VA). It involved 122 interviews with 30 clinicians and staff from various disciplines, exploring their perceptions of patient experiences with the portal. This study was part of a larger evaluation of the EHR transition at the initial VA site, conducted before, immediately after, and up to 12 months following the go-live period. Relevant text segments concerning patient experiences and clinician-patient interactions were extracted and analyzed to identify themes (Ball 2024).

**Focus Groups** In a focus group study, researchers and a small number of participants have a group interview on the researchers' topic to uncover information through the participants' discussion of their thoughts and experiences. This method involves engaging 8 to 10 participants in a structured group interview to elicit detailed information. For example, to explore telehealth use in a remote hospital, researchers could conduct a focus group with healthcare professionals. Questions like "What are the main obstacles to implementing telehealth services in remote areas?" and "How can patient information be collected accurately and timely in telehealth practice?" guided the discussion. The purpose was to gather insights into the integration of telehealth, assess its usability, and understand its impact on patient care in remote settings. The session was audio-recorded, transcribed, and analyzed to derive detailed understandings that could inform future telehealth implementations. Focus groups are typically used in health research to explore new issues in depth or to get more detailed views on specific topics, and they often take place in settings familiar to participants to encourage open and honest feedback.

**Observations** In observational research, researchers observe, record, and analyze behaviors and events. Typically, researchers spend prolonged periods in the setting or events under research. However, some research topics, such as behaviors in natural disasters, prevent this prolonged engagement. Observational research is used in multiple research designs but is often classified with the qualitative approach. Highly detailed, observational research provides insight about what subjects do, how they do it, and why they do it. Two common types of observational research discussed in this chapter are nonparticipant observation and participant observation.

In nonparticipant observation, researchers act as neutral observers who neither intentionally interact with nor affect the actions of the population being observed. The researchers record and analyze the observed behaviors and the content of modes of communication, such as documentation, speech, body language, music, television shows, commercials, and movies. There are two common types of nonparticipant observation. In naturalistic observation, researchers record observations that are unprompted and unaffected by their actions. It is difficult to remain unobtrusive in naturalistic observation because the researchers' mere presence can affect people's behavior and other activities. In one naturalistic study, researchers explored how healthcare personnel use personal protective equipment (PPE) across various acute-care hospital settings, including medical and surgical wards, intensive care units, and an emergency department. The study aimed to identify the contextual and behavioral factors that influence PPE usage during patient care under contact and droplet precautions. Observers, comprising research staff, nonintrusively accompanied healthcare personnel and donned PPE to directly experience and observe the procedures. They faced challenges such as distractions during observation, difficulties in documenting in real time, and confusion about proper PPE usage despite having received prior training. This example underscores the effectiveness of naturalistic observation in providing real-time, detailed insights into healthcare practices and the inherent challenges of observing complex clinical environments (Weston 2021).

In simulation observation, researchers stage events rather than allowing them to occur naturally. Researchers can invent their own simulations or use standardized vignettes to stage the events. HIM researchers often employ models of systems or computer applications to replicate their functions in a controlled setting, aiming to analyze and improve performance.

A 2024 study leveraged the simulation observation method to evaluate the effects of a virtual reality (VR) module on stress induction and the potential for stress desensitization through repeated exposure in a simulated environment. Medical students participated in VR simulation modules designed for managing malignant hyperthermia. The participants were divided into two groups: the stress exposure training (SET) group, which was exposed to stressful stimuli during training, and the control group, which was not. Both groups encountered stressful stimuli in a test module. The study assessed both objective and subjective stress indicators following each module. The findings indicated that the VR module successfully induced stress and was positively received by the participants. Notably, members of the SET group reported experiencing less stress and demonstrated greater competence after the test module compared to the control group. These results suggest that repeated exposure to stressors in VR can desensitize individuals to future stress within a simulated context, highlighting the effectiveness of simulation observation in controlled, artificial environments to replicate and study specific conditions or behaviors (Blanchard 2024).

In **participant observation**, researchers are participants in the observed actions, activities, or processes. They can participate overtly (openly) or covertly (secretly). The researchers not only record their observations of other people's daily lives and the contexts of actions, but also record their own experiences and thoughts. Participant observation research is used to investigate groups, processes, cultures, and other phenomena.

For example, one study adopted passive participant observation techniques to evaluate communication practices regarding medication management during annual primary care consultations with elderly patients who have chronic diseases in southern Sweden. Undertaken by two researchers—a male specialist nurse who is also a doctoral student, and a female sociologist with a PhD in applied health informatics—these observations were unbiased, free from any prior involvement with the healthcare professionals or the facilities. Conducted in both Swedish and English to accommodate linguistic needs, the observations ranged in duration from typical to extended consultation times. The researchers used digital recorders to capture verbal communications and detailed field notes to document nonverbal cues, adhering to a specific observation framework. This approach facilitated a comprehensive content analysis that identified key themes and communication barriers within these clinical interactions (Adelsjö 2022).

**Case Studies** A **case study** is used when researchers conduct an in-depth investigation of one or more examples of a phenomenon, such as a trend, occurrence, or incident. The case is a person, event, group, organization, or a set of similar institutions. The researchers identify characteristics of the case with the purpose of understanding similar cases. Case studies are intensive, and researchers amass comprehensive data. Comprehensive data consist of layers of extensive details from multiple sources including administrative records, financial records, policy and procedure manuals, legal documents, government documents, surveys, interviews, and other sources.

In a case study, HIM researchers explored the merging of patient records from two consolidated hospitals into a single Enterprise Master Patient Index (EMPI). The study highlighted the collaboration between the HIM and IT departments, the integration challenges of differing medical record numbers, patient identification systems, and patient name parameters, and the impact and lessons learned from unifying records across different vendor EHR and ancillary systems into hospital's EHR and document imaging system (Crew and Houser 2021).

Case studies are common in evaluation research on HITs and health information systems (HISs). HIM researchers conducted a case study in two hospitals that had used a commercially available computerized physician order entry (CPOE) system or a CDS system for at least two years (Cresswell et al. 2014, e194). These two hospitals were categorized as "early adopters" of technology. The purpose of the case study was to understand the midterm consequences of implementing the systems for early adopters. At both hospitals, the data collected included interviews, nonparticipant observations, and documents of the hospital's system implementation plans (Cresswell et al. 2014, e194).

The researchers used both inductive and deductive reasoning to identify themes in their data. The researchers also analyzed the data from the two hospitals separately. This separation allowed the researchers to subsequently use triangulation to assess the consistency of their evidence. **Triangulation** is the use of multiple sources or perspectives to investigate the same phenomenon. Theses multiple sources or perspectives include data (multiple times, sites, or respondents), investigators (researchers), theories, and methods (Carter et al. 2014, 545). The results or conclusions are validated if the multiple sources or perspectives arrive at the same results or conclusions. The three overarching themes that the researchers found were: (1) impact on individual healthcare professionals, such as greater legibility of prescriptions and, for some, increased workloads; (2) introduction of perceived new safety risks related to accessibility and usability of the systems' hardware and software; and (3) realization of organizational benefits through secondary uses of the hospitals' data, such as reports on adherence to clinical guidelines (Cresswell et al. 2014, e194).

**Ethnography** **Ethnography** is the investigation of a culture by collecting data and making observations while being in the field (naturalistic setting). Ethnographers amass great volumes of detailed data while living or working with the population that they are studying. Coming from anthropology to healthcare, this observational method includes both qualitative and quantitative approaches and both participant and nonparticipant observation.

HIM researchers used an ethnographic study to reveal workarounds that clinicians used to evade security as they accessed the healthcare organization's computer systems in their care of patients (Koppel et al. 2015, 215). To obtain perceptions of computer security rules, the researchers conducted interviews and observations with hundreds of medical personnel (nurses, doctors, line workers, and managers) and with 19 cybersecurity experts, chief information officers, chief medical informatics officers, chief technology officers, and IT personnel. They collected reports from online medical discussion lists and the literature.

The researchers also shadowed many clinicians as they worked to understand the clinicians' motivations and trade-offs for circumvention. The researchers found that to accomplish their essential task of caring for patients, clinicians had invented dozens of ingenious ways to circumvent what they viewed as onerous and irrational computer security rules. For example, the researchers found that "clever clinicians at one hospital defeated proximity-sensor-based timeouts [computer session terminations] by putting Styrofoam cups over the detectors" (Koppel et al. 2015, 217). The researchers pointed out that auditing and analyzing computer access logs would fail to catch these evasions of cybersecurity rules.

## Validity and Reliability

Researchers who fail to plan their study's logistics may violate principles associated with validity and reliability. When study procedures are inconsistent with these principles, the data can be compromised. This not only casts doubt on the findings but also potentially hampers the ability to analyze the data accurately. Ensuring a proper study requires choosing a sample size that represents the target population and supports comprehensive statistical analyses. Adequate sample size is crucial for enhancing result validity and reliability, making the findings more credible and generalizable.

***Validity*** Validity is whether a test or a measurement used in the study achieved what the researcher intended to measure. For example, the researcher used a System Usability Scale (SUS) intending to measure the effectiveness of a mobile phone application with management of diabetes. This intended measurement could be achieved (the study measure is valid), or it actually measured something else, such as efficiency instead of effectiveness (the study measure is invalid).

There are three types of validity—internal validity, external validity, and validity. Internal validity and external validity involve the integrity of the research plan. Validity without a modifier refers to an attribute of instruments (tools or devices that measure or record observations).

Internal validity is an attribute of a study's design that contributes to the accuracy of its findings. Threats to internal validity come from factors outside the study (confounding variables) and are potential sources of error that could contaminate a study's results (Campbell and Stanley 1963, 5). Table 18.3 lists and defines eight common threats to internal validity that researchers attempt to avoid in the design of their research study. If internal validity is breached, researchers cannot state for certain that the independent variable caused the effect.

External validity involves the generalizability of the study's findings to other people or groups, such as patients, hospitals, and countries. Internal validity represents the bare minimum; internal validity combined with external validity is the ideal. For example, a study on the effectiveness of a new EHR system might have high external validity if its results can be applied to a variety of healthcare settings across different regions, demonstrating that the findings are relevant not just to the initial hospital where the study was conducted, but to hospitals nationwide or globally.

An instrument's validity is the extent to which the tool (questionnaire) or device (counter) measures what it is intended to measure. Two important as-

**Table 18.3.** Threats to internal validity

| Type of Threat | Description |
| --- | --- |
| History | Unplanned events occur during the research and affect the results |
| Maturation | Subjects grow or mature during the period of the study |
| Testing | Taking the first test affects subsequent tests; "practice effect" |
| Instrumentation | There is a lack of consistency in data collection |
| Statistical Regression | Subjects are selected because of their extreme scores |
| Differential Selection | Control group and experimental group differ, and the difference could affect the study's findings |
| Experimental Mortality | Loss of subjects occurs during the study |
| Diffusion of Treatment | Members of the control group learn about the treatment of the experimental group |

pects of an instrument's validity are content validity and construct validity, described as follows:

- Content validity concerns whether the instrument's items (content) relate to the topic. For example, a coding test with content validity would have items related to key aspects of coding, such as uses of codes, the appropriate code set to use for healthcare services in various healthcare settings, and sources of guidelines for coding.
- Construct validity is the instrument's ability to measure hypothetical, non-observable traits called constructs. Classic examples of constructs are psychological concepts, such as intelligence, motivation, and anxiety. Although intelligence itself is not visible, its effects are. Therefore, if an instrument is intended to measure patient satisfaction, it should include issues associated with patient satisfaction.

Validity in research has evolved alongside methods and tools. Technological advances such as machine learning and AI raise questions about validity. For example, when textual data is analyzed with AI, researchers must question the validity of these results, especially when compared with conventional human analysis. This is because AI may not fully grasp the nuances of language, context, and cultural subtleties that human analysis can discern, potentially leading to oversimplified or inaccurate interpretations. Additionally, as research spans various cultures, instruments must be culturally sensitive and universally valid. Techniques like translation, back-translation, and pilot testing with diverse groups are essential to ensure validity across different cultural contexts.

**Reliability** Reliability involves the consistency and stability of an instrument's measurements. Over time, a test or observation dependably measures whatever it was intended to measure. Repeated administrations of the instrument will result in reasonably similar findings. Two aspects of reliability are intrarater reliability and interrater reliability. Intrarater reliability means that the same person repeating the test will have reasonably similar findings. Interrater reliability means that different persons completing the test will have reasonably similar findings. Instruments' validity and reliability are often stated in journal articles or can be found in electronic databases of instruments.

### Selecting an Instrument

An instrument is a standardized, uniform way to collect data. Examples of instruments include the previously discussed interview guides and questionnaires, as well as checklists, rating scales, scenarios, and vignettes, among others.

Using a well-designed instrument minimizes bias and maximizes certainty of the variable's (treatment's) effect on the dependent variable (outcome). Researchers can find descriptions of standardized instruments and, often, their validity and reliability listed in electronic databases such as the following:

- Health IT Survey Compendium (AHRQ n.d.)
- HF (Human Factors) Tools (FAA n.d.)
- HaPI (Health and Psychosocial Instruments) (Behavioral Measurement Database Services n.d.)
- Mental Measurements Yearbook with Tests in Print (Buros Center for Testing n.d.)

Researchers can also find standardized instruments during their literature review. Examples of instruments used in HIM research include the System Usability Scale (SUS) (Brooke 1986); the Software Usability Measurement Inventory (SUMI) (Kirukowski and Corbett 1993, 210–212); and the Questionnaire for User Interaction Satisfaction (QUIS) (University of Maryland 2015).

*Factors in Instrument Selection* The most important factor in selecting an instrument is the purpose of the research, so that the data collected are relevant to the research question. Other factors to consider include the following:

- Satisfactory ratings for validity and reliability
- Clarity of language
- Brevity and attractiveness
- Match between the theories underpinning the instrument and the researcher's investigation
- Match between the level of measurement (nominal, ordinal, interval, or ratio scales of data) and the proposed statistical analyses
- Features (see next section)
- Public domain (used for free and can be copied, often with citation) or proprietary (must be purchased and cannot be copied without permission)
- Cost

Researchers should obtain a sample of the instrument (often for free or at a nominal cost) and read it in its entirety to be sure it collects what they want to collect and it operationalizes terms the same way they do. For example, researchers studying workplace social support want to ensure the instrument collects data about social support in the workplace from colleagues rather than social support in the home from family members.

Selecting an existing instrument with established validity and reliability is easier than developing a new instrument. For example, a group of HIM researchers developed a survey to assess telehealth use, the quality of clinical documentation, and challenges during the pandemic. The survey, based on literature and website reviews, included questions validated for clarity, accuracy, and validity. It covered four main categories: health organization demographics, telehealth visit usage, clinical documentation practices for telehealth, and challenges related to telehealth. After refining the survey based on feedback from a pilot test concerning content, technical aspects, and completion time, the final survey was administered through an online platform (Houser et al. 2022).

**Features of Instruments** Researchers consider the following features of instruments in terms of the type of data collected:

- Structure of questions
    - Structured (closed-ended) questions list all the possible responses.
    - Unstructured (open-ended) questions allow free-form responses.
    - Semistructured questions begin with structured questions and then follow with open-ended questions to clarify.

    The advantage of structured questions is that they are easier for the participant to complete and for the researcher to tabulate and analyze than unstructured questions. The advantage of unstructured questions is that they allow in-depth questions and may uncover aspects of a problem unknown to the researcher. Semistructured questions have the advantages of obtaining comparable data for analysis and potentially providing insights.

- Numeric or categorical data
    - Numeric items request the respondent to enter a number in terms of specific unit of measure, such as day, week, or year.
    - Categorical items classify respondents into groupings. The categories must be *all-inclusive* (all respondents fit into a category, even if it is "other"), *mutually exclusive* (no overlapping among categories), *forming meaningful clusters* (logical and understandably different), and *sufficiently narrow or broad* (number of categories may range from two to eight, but respondents should be able to see substantive shades of meaning among the categories).
    - Numeric items are preferable to categorical items when feasible (Alreck and Settle 2004, 113). Numeric items allow for more precise and quantifiable analysis.

- Scaled categorical items. **Scales** are progressive categories such as size, amount, importance, rank, or agreement. (See table 18.4.) Each category is also called a point; a scale with five categories is a five-point scale. A commonly used scale is the **Likert scale**, which allows respondents to record their level of agreement or disagreement along a range. (See table 18.4.) HIM researchers assess the status and quality of clinical documentation in telehealth services using a five-point Likert scale (never, rarely, sometimes, often, always) (Houser et al. 2022). Figure 18.2 shows a Likert scale in a survey. To ascertain perspectives or public relations images, researchers use semantic differential scales that allow respondents to rate products, healthcare organizations, or other services. (See figure 18.3.) The scale places adjectives that are opposites on the ends of the continua. Up to 20 adjective pairs may be used, with half the items beginning with the positive adjective of the pair and the other half beginning with the negative adjective.

- Availability of various formats, such as paper-based, internet, and multiple languages. Prior to using an instrument, researchers should confirm its validity and reliability have been established for the format they intend to use and, in the setting (patient's home, academic health center, and such), of their study.

## Data Collection Procedures

Data collection procedures differ between quantitative and qualitative studies. Quantitative researchers conduct their studies in a linear fashion. They plan their study, collect data, analyze their data, and present their findings. Qualitative researchers conduct their studies in a cyclical, iterative fashion. They plan their study, collect data, analyze the data, revisit and revise their initial questions, create new questions, and collect more data. In collecting more data, they may seek other sources of data and participants and may add alternate techniques for data collection.

**Table 18.4.** Common scales

| Scale | Purpose | Example |
|---|---|---|
| Two-point | Dichotomous question | Yes, no<br>Favor, oppose<br>True, false |
| Three-point | Importance, interest, or satisfaction<br>Satisfaction with amounts | Very, fairly, not at all<br>Too much (many), just (about) right, not enough (too few) |
| Four-point | Generic<br>Measurement of amounts | Excellent, good, fair, poor<br>Very much, quite a bit, some, very little |
| Likert (five-point) | Indication of agreement or disagreement | Strongly agree, agree, neutral, disagree, strongly disagree |
| Verbal frequency (five-point) | Frequency | Always, often, sometimes, rarely (seldom), never |
| Expanded Likert (seven-point) | Extra discrimination desirable | Very strongly agree, strongly agree, agree, neutral, disagree, strongly disagree, very strongly disagree |

**Figure 18.2.** Excerpt from survey

**Survey on Competence**

Rate your level of competence in the following educational subdomains:

|  | Very Weak | Weak | Neutral | Strong | Very Strong |
|---|---|---|---|---|---|
| Classification Systems | | | | | |
| Health Record Content and Documentation | | | | | |
| Data Governance | | | | | |
| Data Management | | | | | |
| Secondary Data Sources | | | | | |

*Source:* Adapted from Sandefer and Karl 2015.

**Figure 18.3.** Example of a semantic differential scale

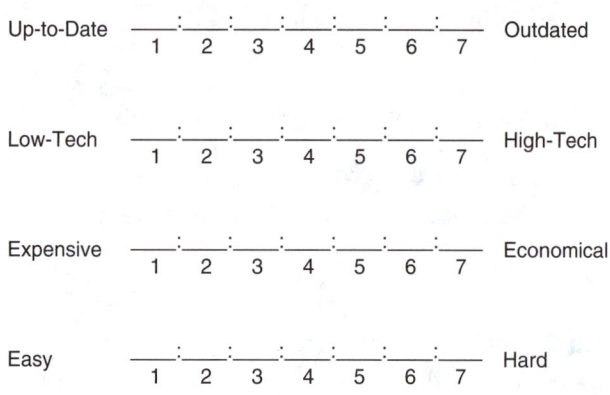

Depending upon the method, issues related to data collection include the following:

- Obtaining approvals of oversight committees
- Listing each data element required to perform the appropriate statistical techniques
- Training for data collection procedures
- Conducting a pilot study
- Considering the response rate
- Assembling and preparing the data for analysis

Prior to conducting studies, researchers must obtain written approvals from the IRB and other oversight entities of their organizations. To obtain approvals, researchers complete the organization's documentation, providing descriptions of their research plan and copies of their informed consent forms. Of note for this chapter on research methods is that researchers must allow sufficient time in their plan for the IRB to review the research, meet, and respond.

Researchers should list each data element required for each statistical analysis they plan to conduct and determine whether their data collection strategies will obtain all these data elements. Therefore, it is advisable to conduct mock statistical analyses on fabricated data and to create tables and figures for the manuscript early in the planning of the research. Running mock statistical analyses also assists researchers in determining their sample size.

Researchers and their assistants may require special training. For example, publishers of some psychological tests require verification of training to administer the tests. The researchers must obtain this verification (or select another instrument). Researchers and their assistants also need training to effectively conduct interviews or to observe vignettes.

A **pilot study** is a trial run that allows researchers to work out the logistical details of their research plan and enhances the likelihood of the research's successful completion. Pilot studies obtain valuable information for researchers, as follows:

- Confirmation of details: volumes of materials or number of study assistants needed, costs, and likely response rates.
- Detection of potential problems: biases in sample selection; flawed performance of equipment, hardware, software, or the website; poorly worded instructions, unclear questionnaire items, and leading questions in interviews; delays in the distribution method; errors in the scoring key; and discrepancies between the order of items on the data collection instrument and the order on the data entry screen.

Ensuring an adequate response rate is of particular concern for surveys. Low response rates jeopardize a study's internal validity. Researchers should carefully review the literature for the response rates of their intended audience, factors affecting response rates, and successful strategies. A study evaluated how different delivery methods—email, regular mail, and a hybrid of the two—affect patient response rates to surveys. Regular mail achieved the highest response rates, followed by the hybrid method and then email. The hybrid method effectively balances high response rates with the convenience of digital (Neve et al. 2021).

Researchers must also be on cautious of response bias, noting that survey participants and responders might differ from nonparticipants and non-responders. It is essential to ensure all groups are representative of the overall population.

Finally, researchers must include a mechanism in the plan for assembling their data and preparing them for analysis. Depending on the research method, procedures should be in place for documenting interviews, data entry, scoring, and quality checks on data entry. In data preparation, missing values and data cleansing must be addressed. Missing values are variables that do not contain values for some cases. Missing values must be resolved before statistical techniques can be applied. Two common rudimentary techniques to resolve missing values are case deletion, in which all cases with a missing value are deleted, and single imputation, in which the missing value is replaced with the average of the available values. The disadvantages of both techniques are the loss of cases and the potential for bias because the missing data may not be random. Multiple imputation avoids these disadvantages by substituting missing values that have been predicted based on producing multiple data sets using existing values, performing statistical analyses on each of them, and combining the results. Data cleaning (also called data cleansing or data scrubbing) is a fundamental step in data preparation. It "is the process of fixing or removing data that's inaccurate, duplicated, or outside the scope of your research question" (NIH 2023). This process involves identifying duplications, such as when a participant returns two questionnaires, verifying internal consistency, for instance, a mismatch between city and zip code, and detecting outliers, like a reported birth weight of 15 pounds in a study on newborn health metrics. Researchers should allocate significant time for this detailed work in their planning.

## Check Your Understanding 18.5

**Answer the following questions in a separate document.**

1. An HIM researcher is assessing the effectiveness of recently introduced telehealth services in a specialty clinic. What data collection methods should the researcher use for this study, and why are these methods chosen?

2. What should researchers consider when selecting data collection instruments for a research study to assess a mobile device usage with weight-loss intervention for diabetes management? Explain your rationale.

3. In a survey evaluating the confidence levels of healthcare professionals in EHR usage within their practice, which measurement scales could an HIM researcher use? Which scale would be most effective?

4. A researcher read a study entitled "EHR use continues to contribute to physician burnout." This study used a new questionnaire to ask physicians about their use of EHR over the years. The researcher decided to examine the strength of this new questionnaire. How does the researcher assess whether the new questionnaire is valid and reliable?

5. Compare and contrast interviews with observations. Recommend your rationale for using the two data collection methods to the researcher who is conducting research to investigate effectiveness of electronic display boards in the hospital.

## Analyzing the Data

In this analytical phase of the research process, researchers try to determine what they have found or what the data reveal. In their plan for the study, the researchers decide which analytical techniques they would use. These techniques are described in the methods section of the manuscript with sufficient detail and clarity so that other researchers can duplicate them.

### Techniques for Qualitative Data Analysis

Qualitative data analysis is a systematic process of working with data to create coherent descriptions and explanations of phenomena (Miles et al. 2014, 10). Qualitative research generates hypotheses and deepens understanding of quantitative data by exploring participants' experiences, perceptions, and behaviors. It focuses on the "hows" and "whys" rather than quantifying "how many" or "how much" (Tenny 2024). Analysis of qualitative data is a cyclical and iterative process with data collection, data analysis, and generation of hypotheses and theories as concurrent, intertwined activities. Although there are many techniques to analyze qualitative data, generally the process is described as having three major activities: data condensation, data display, and conclusion drawing and verification (Miles et al. 2014, 10). Two common qualitative analytical techniques are grounded theory and content analysis.

***Grounded Theory*** Grounded theory refers both to the theories generated using the analytical technique and the technique itself. Researchers, using grounded theory, code (attach meaningful labels), categorize, and compare their data. The term evolved because its early users spoke of their work being "grounded in data." Thus, the term emphasizes that the data generate the theories.

Grounded theory is an iterative or cyclical process. During data collection, researchers using grounded theory record and code their observations (called incidents). However, analysis begins during data collection. From the analysis, the researchers begin creating conceptual categories to fit their data. Both data collection and analysis may uncover gaps or discrepancies that require additional data collection or participants. The grounded theory technique has four stages:

1. Comparing incidents applicable to each category (includes comparing categories' relationships)
2. Integrating categories and their properties (cyclical process)
3. Delimiting theory (reducing and integrating core categories, tying theory to core categories, and achieving higher-level conceptualizations)
4. Writing theory (validating theory by pinpointing data behind it) (Glaser 1965, 439–443)

Development of grounded theory consists of intertwined and concurrent data collection, data coding, categorization, and analysis. Because of the constant analysis and comparisons of categories, the theory and technique are sometimes called *constant comparative method*.

This process results in complex theories that fit the data closely. In grounded theory, researchers seek to develop theories that are unique to groups or settings, unlike quantitative researchers who seek to develop theories that are generalizable.

***Content Analysis*** Content analysis is the systematic and objective analysis of communication to describe and to make inferences about behaviors. Most often, researchers analyze written documentation. However, they may analyze other modes of communication, such as speech, body language, music, television shows, commercials, and movies. Both qualitative and quantitative researchers use content analysis to analyze data.

Content analysis is "essentially a coding operation" (Babbie 2021, 332). Researchers iteratively cycle through a process of coding and categorizing their data until all the meanings of their data have been categorized. Researchers code the text, image, or other means of communication. Coding is the labeling of words or word groups (segments) or images with annotations or scales. These labels are characteristics of the segments. To assess reliability, the agreement between and among coders may be checked. From the coding, researchers identify key terms, characteristics, or other attributes. The coded text (or communication) becomes the data. The data are then categorized into overarching themes. In a quantitative aspect of content analysis, some researchers also tabulate the frequency of coded data. Generally, content analysis is an iterative process characterized by progressively reducing the units of analysis into fewer and fewer categories and, eventually, into themes.

***Qualitative Analytical Software*** Qualitative researchers conduct data analysis, but qualitative analytical software does *not* conduct analysis. Known as computer-aided qualitative data analysis software (CAQDAS), these programs assist researchers in analyzing their data. For example, NVivo, a CAQDAS program, was used in a qualitative study to analyze interview data from postpartum women discussing their pain and depression during pregnancy (Vignato 2022).

Several qualitative analytic software programs exist to aid investigators in their organization, management, collection, coding, and analysis of data. Software may be freeware or proprietary. Table 18.5 describes features of common CAQDAS programs.

**Table 18.5.** Sample of free and proprietary qualitative analytical software

| Qualitative analytical software | Description |
|---|---|
| ATLAS.ti | Codes and analyzes text-based data from open-ended surveys, transcriptions of focus groups, or other sources. ATLAS.ti can be used to code other types of qualitative data, such as photographs. ATLAS.ti allows the retrieval of specific information based on search criteria. ATLAS.ti can also export data as an SPSS data set (ATLAS.ti n.d.). |
| Code-A-Text Integrated System for the Analysis of Interviews and Dialogues (C-I-SAID) | This software facilitates coding and analyzing documents, transcripts, and sound files by allowing investigators to easily label segments with annotations or scales. After coding, the software can analyze the content and generate descriptive statistics, tables and charts. It also supports thematic categorization through content analysis. C-I-SAID is suitable for field notes, open-ended questionnaires, and interviews, and its multimedia version can code video and pictures (LingTranSoft 2019). |
| HyperRESEARCH and HyperTRANSCRIBE | HyperRESEARCH is a cross-platform qualitative analysis software that assists in coding, data retrieval, theory building, and data analysis. The software supports multimedia content including text, graphics, audio, and video sources. HyperTRANSCRIBE assists the transcription of audio or video data into text by allowing keyboard control over playback and looping (Researchware, Inc. n.d.). |
| NVivo | Analyzes unstructured data, aiding in the coding and analysis of text from open-ended surveys, focus group transcriptions, and other sources. NVivo allows investigators to retrieve specific quotes using search criteria to generate tables showing code frequencies. Data can also be exported to quantitative statistical packages (QSR International n.d.). |

## Check Your Understanding 18.6

**Answer the following questions in a separate document.**

1. Why is content analysis crucial in HIM, particularly when evaluating the quality and relevance of EHR data for improving patient care?

2. Differentiate content analysis from grounded theory. Give an example beyond what is in the textbook of when each would be appropriate. The example can be from your own knowledge or experience.

3. Why do some approaches in grounded theory research work better than others, particularly when the focus of the study is hard-to-reach population groups?

4. Differentiate quantitative and qualitative analysis methods. Give an example for each type of analysis method.

5. The quality director has inquired whether NVivo software can be utilized to complete the data analysis and interpretation of your research study. How would you describe NVivo's capabilities in assisting with this task?

## Disseminating Results

The last step of the research process is disseminating, or sharing, the results from the study to intended audiences. HIM researchers provide other HIM professionals with techniques to answer questions and to solve problems in the workplace and with new knowledge. Without presentation and interpretation, the techniques and knowledge would be unavailable to practitioners.

### Reporting the Results

Researchers follow a two-step process when reporting their results. In the first step, they note research findings from their studies with no commentary, explanation, or interpretation. This section of a manuscript is called *research findings*. In the second step, the researchers comment on, explain, and interpret their findings. This section of the manuscript is called *discussion*. Conclusions and recommendations for future research are also included.

In research findings, the researchers describe their results in the past tense; general truths are stated in the present tense. The style of writing for scientific manuscripts is objective, precise, and factual. Maintaining a neutral tone, the researchers record their findings in narrative form. They describe the results for each hypothesis (quantitative study) or research question (qualitative study). Researchers state whether the results support the hypotheses. They also record characteristics about the sample and, depending upon the approach, describe the results of the analyses that investigate whether the sample is similar to or different from the population. Supplemental statistical analyses also are described. Researchers are careful to correctly use the terms *statistical significance* and *significance* (practical or making a difference).

For research findings, researchers generate tables, graphs, and figures to support their narrative reporting of their findings. Researchers present the data in the mode of communication—narrative text, table, or figure—that is most effective for that data element.

In the discussion section, researchers create new knowledge and put their findings in the context of the existing knowledge. This section is not a superficial repetition of the findings section. Researchers compare their findings to the findings in the literature, describing similarities and discrepancies and explaining why their findings were the same or different. In this section, researchers answer the following questions:

- How do their findings answer their research question or address their problem statement?
- What theoretical significance do their findings have?
- What practical significance do their findings have?
- How do their findings explicitly link to the larger body of knowledge?
- How have their findings improved the field's research model?
- How have their findings expanded the body of knowledge?
- What new definitions have they added to the field's area of practice?
- How do their findings support practitioners in the workplace?
- What valid conclusions can the researchers and the readers draw?

In closing their discussion of the findings, researchers state the limitations of their research. A researcher describing a questionnaire survey might state that one limitation is that the data are self-reported. Researchers also make recommendations for future research. In conducting their study, researchers could have seen ways to improve the study or uncovered layers of other questions. These potential improvements and additional questions become the recommendations for further research.

## Presenting the Research

Dissemination makes knowledge public. Knowledge can be disseminated and examined through poster sessions, oral presentations at professional meetings, and publication in journal articles. For the researchers' information to be useful, it must be available and accessible to practitioners and other researchers.

There are two forms of presentation: poster and oral presentation. Poster sessions and oral presentations occur at professional meetings, conferences, and symposia. Months before a professional meeting, professional associations will issue a call for session proposals. In response to the call, researchers submit an abstract with an outline and brief descriptions of their studies to their proposed session. Peer reviewers then review the abstract, and score it in some cases, based on conference presentation criteria and guidelines. The meeting planners determine which proposals or abstracts to accept based on reviewers' scores, if appropriate, the submission's quality, the number of submissions, and relevance of the submission's topic to the theme of the conference.

**Poster Session** Researchers use posters to communicate their work with audiences at scientific or academic meetings. Compared with an oral presentation, posters will do most of the communication through visual materials display. They do so by delivering and conveying the message or research study in a short period of time. Before creating the poster, it is essential to know the target audience, the key message to deliver, and the information audiences would be interested in knowing.

Researchers must conform to the conference's poster guidelines when participating in a poster session. Prior to the event, meeting planners send out the requirements for the poster. Meeting planners will also state the session's time slot on the meeting agenda. During the time slot, the researcher stands near the poster and answers questions from viewers about the research study. Often, researchers have their research abstract or other reference material that expands upon the poster's content available to give to interested people.

Posters typically include the following elements:

- Banner (header): includes title of study, names of researchers, and institutional affiliation. The title of the poster is very important, as this usually is the first thing audiences see. A concise, comprehensive, compelling title can draw audiences' attention and interest.
- Introduction and background: introduces the summary of the study concept, key literature

search on what has been done, and statements about the problems the researcher is trying to solve. Purpose and objectives of the study should also be discussed in this section.

- Methods: explains the study design, samples included in the study, techniques, and procedures used in the research.
- Results: shows key findings of the work and illustrative examples with graphics (such as figures and tables).
- Discussion and conclusions: provides interpretation of the study findings, provides implications and limitations of the study results, indicates further work to be done based on the results of the study, and provides recommendations about how the work could be accomplished.

Institutional printing departments and commercial printing companies provide enhanced poster services, often staffed by artists and designers. Alternatively, online printing websites offer cost-effective solutions with templates for researchers. Over time, traditional paper posters have in many cases been exchanged for a digital format, known as electronic posters or e-posters. Unlike paper posters, which are used in a physical environment, e-posters are hosted online, enabling real-time interaction without the author present. Use of this format has widened the audience from both on-site and online locations.

Poster presentations have evolved significantly with technology, making digital posters a standard feature at many conferences. These posters display dynamically on large screens, incorporate interactive elements such as animations, videos, and real-time data displays. Augmented reality (AR) has further transformed these presentations, allowing researchers to add AR overlays to showcase 3D models and supplementary multimedia content accessible through smartphones or tablets.

Additionally, the power of social media sharing has been utilized to extend the reach of these presentations beyond traditional conference venues, allowing researchers to share their work with academic and non-specialist audiences including the public and policymakers. The broader engagement enhances the societal impact of research, increases public understanding of scientific topics, and can influence policy decisions. The virtual poster sessions allow researchers to present and discuss their work on digital platforms, facilitating global participation and interaction. This modernized approach to poster sessions ensures research dissemination is more engaging, accessible, and in tune with the digital age.

**Oral Presentation** Professional presentations occur during sessions of regional, state, national, and international meetings. As with posters, described previously, researchers submit proposals in response to a call and, if accepted, receive a notice of their time slot. Presenters should be prepared to talk about their research to the audience. Recommendations for delivering an effective presentation advise that presenters do the following:

- Conduct extensive research on the topic, organize material logically, and rehearse multiple times to ensure smooth delivery. Practice the entire presentation to ensure proper timing and pace.
- Know the backgrounds of audience members—whether they are public or technical experts—to tailor the presentation appropriately.
- Focus on delivering a clear "take-home message" that highlights actual findings or implications. Main points should be kept simple and straightforward.
- Use slides, charts, or videos wisely, with each slide generally discussed for about one minute. Visuals should support and not overwhelm the presentation.
- Present information in a logical flow that tells a compelling story. Engage the audience through varying voice tones and interactive elements to keep the narrative dynamic.

The rise of video conferencing platforms has made virtual presentations commonplace, allowing presenters to reach global audiences without travel. These platforms often have interactive features such as polls, breakout rooms, and question and answer sections for dynamic attendee interactions. Additionally, an increasing number of speakers are incorporating multimedia elements such as videos, animations, and interactive demonstrations to enhance engagement, thereby improving audience attention, information retention, and the overall learning experience.

As with poster sessions, AR has found its way into oral presentations, with some speakers using AR tools to showcase 3D models or immersive environments relevant to their topic. Hybrid presentations, which combine both in-person and virtual elements, have also emerged as a flexible format catering to diverse audience needs. These formats also support greater accessibility, ensuring speakers' content is available to those with disabilities by employing features like real-time captioning, screen reader-friendly slides, and sign language interpreters. Additionally, many conferences now offer on-demand replay of presentations, allowing attendees to view content at their convenience, further enhancing accessibility and reach. Coupled with the power of social media, where key insights from talks can be shared instantly with a global audience, the modern oral presentation is more interactive, inclusive, and far-reaching than ever before.

**Publication** Published research may be examined and critically analyzed by practitioners and other researchers. Scientific manuscripts are commonly organized in a prescribed structure. An author's unpublished paper is known as a *manuscript*. A paper published in a journal is known as an *article*.

Editors and researchers have agreed upon reporting guidelines for the content of many types of scientific papers. Using these preexisting guidelines assists authors in producing quality manuscripts. One general guideline for scientific papers is called *IMRAD* (introduction, methods, results, and discussion) (Cooper 2015, 67). The website of EQUATOR: Enhancing the QUAlity and Transparency Of health Research (n.d.) is a source of many reporting guidelines for health research. Examples of specific guidelines include the following:

- Consolidated Standards of Reporting Trials (CONSORT n.d.)
- Consolidated criteria for reporting qualitative research (COREQ) (Tong et al. 2012)
- Preferred Reporting Items for Systematic Reviews and Meta-Analyses (PRISMA) (Moher et al. 2009)

These preexisting guidelines help authors include all key data and information. Table 18.6 serves as a final checklist for the composition and revision of the manuscript.

Publications remain a cornerstone of the academic and research world, serving as a primary means to disseminate findings, innovations, and insights. However, the publication process has shifted significantly over time. One of the most pronounced changes has been the rise of open access (OA) publishing, which allows readers to access articles without a paywall. Funders and institutions are increasingly mandating OA, recognizing its potential to increase the reach and impact of research. Alongside OA, there has been a surge in the popularity of preprint servers like arXiv, bioRxiv, and medRxiv. These platforms allow researchers to share their findings before they undergo peer review, facilitating rapid dissemination of knowledge, especially critical in fields requiring timely updates, such as epidemiology during health crises.

The peer review process itself is undergoing transformation with initiatives like open peer review, where the reviews and sometimes reviewer identities are made public. Technological advancements have also paved the way for interactive publications, integrating multimedia, datasets, and even interactive code within articles, enhancing reader engagement and comprehension. The emergence of altmetrics captures the broader impact of research by tracking mentions in news outlets, blogs, social media, and other nontraditional channels.

As global reach increases, there is a growing emphasis on multilingual publications or at least providing article abstracts in multiple languages (Adema 2023). With concerns about research reproducibility on the rise, journals are increasingly requiring authors to provide data availability statements and, in some cases, the raw data itself, promoting transparency and integrity in the publication process.

**Table 18.6.** Organization of research publications

| Section | Contents |
|---|---|
| Title page | Concise and descriptive title, author, author's affiliation, grant information, disclaimer, corresponding author's address, telephone, fax, and email |
| Abstract | Background, purpose, methods, results, conclusions<br>Context; objective; design, setting, and participants; interventions; main outcome measures; results and conclusions<br>45 to 250 words dependent upon call for papers or journal instructions<br>3 to 10 key words using medical subject headings (MeSH) |
| Introduction | Background; pertinent literature review that provides rationale for research; brief statement of research plan; purpose, objectives, or research question |
| Methods | Protocol with detail for replication<br>Design, setting, and participants<br>Definition of variables<br>Reference to established methods<br>Sampling strategy<br>Collection of data<br>Statement about approval of IRB or other oversight entity<br>Analytical strategy |

*Continued*

**Table 18.6.** Organization of research publications (continued)

| Section | Contents |
|---|---|
| Results | Core<br>Important results followed by less important results<br>Neutral reporting |
| Discussion | Relationship between results and purpose, objectives, or research question<br>Evidence of relationship<br>Similarities to and differences from previous research<br>New knowledge in terms of theoretical framework<br>Limitations<br>Conclusions as related to purpose, objectives, or research question<br>Implications for future research<br>Recommendations as warranted<br>Summary |
| Acknowledgment | Contributors whose level of involvement does not justify authorship |
| References | Citations per format in instructions |
| Tables | Consistent with narrative<br>Expand abbreviations<br>Format per instructions |
| Figures | Consistent with narrative<br>Expand abbreviations<br>Legend<br>Format per instructions |

## Check Your Understanding 18.7

**Answer the following questions in a separate document.**

1. Where should an HIM student search within Dr. Smith's research study to understand the interpretation of the study's results?

2. Differentiate the common approaches used to disseminate research results. Which approach would work best if you wanted your research to be widely available for years to come?

3. The director of HIM will present the results of a study she has done on the utilization of the organization's patient portal in a poster session at the state HIM annual meeting. What would you expect her poster's content and format to be?

4. Differentiate oral presentation and poster presentation. Explain why you select one or the other when presenting at a professional conference.

5. As you prepare to use social media to disseminate the results of your HIM research study, how can multimedia elements improve the effectiveness of your dissemination efforts?

# References

Adelsjö, I., L. Nilsson, A. Hellström, M. Ekstedt, and E. C. Lehnbom. 2022. Communication about medication management during patient–physician consultations in primary care: A participant observation study. *BMJ Open* 2022(12):e062148. doi:10.1136/bmjopen-2022-062148.

Adema, J. 2023 (August 4). "Special Issue on Multilingual Publishing and Scholarship." The Journal of Electronic Publishing [website]. https://journals.publishing.umich.edu/jep/news/71/.

AHRQ (Agency for Healthcare Research and Quality). 2024. "Technology Assessment Program." http://www.ahrq.gov/research/findings/ta/index.html.

AHRQ (Agency for Healthcare Research and Quality). n.d. "Health IT Survey Compendium." Accessed May

10, 2024. http://healthit.ahrq.gov/health-it-tools-and-resources/health-it-survey-compendium.

Alreck, P. L., and R. B. Settle. 2004. *The Survey Research Handbook*, 3rd ed. New York: McGraw-Hill/Irwin.

AHIMA (American Health Information Management Association). n.d. "What Is Health Information?" October 15, 2024. https://www.ahima.org/certification-careers/certifications-overview/career-tools/career-pages/health-information-101/.

ATLAS.ti Qualitative Data Analysis. n.d. Accessed May 14, 2024. https://atlasti.com/.

Aveyard, H. 2023. *Doing a Literature Review in Health and Social Care: A Practical Guide*, 5th ed. Maidenhead, England: McGraw-Hill Education.

Babbie, E. 2021. *The Practice of Social Research*, 15th ed. Boston, MA: Cengage Learning.

Ball, S. L., B. Kim, S. L. Cutrona, B. K. Molloy-Paolillo, E. Ahlness, M. Moldestad, G. Sayre, and S. T. Rinne. 2024. Clinician and staff experiences with frustrated patients during an electronic health record transition: A qualitative case study. *BMC Health Services Research* 24(1):535. doi: 10.1186/s12913-024-10974-5.

Behavioral Measurement Database Services. n.d. "HaPI." Accessed May 14, 2024. http://bmdshapi.com/.

Blanchard, E. E., Z. Trost, M. R. Brown, C. Shum, and M. Mees. 2024. Combining stress inoculation with virtual reality simulation training of malignant hyperthermia. *Advances in Simulation* 9(35). https://doi.org/10.1186/s41077-024-00308-0.

Brooke, J. 1986. "SUS [System Usability Scale]; A Quick and Dirty Usability Scale." https://digital.gov/topics/usability/.

Buros Center for Testing. n.d. "Test Reviews and Information." Accessed September 5, 2024. http://buros.org/.

Campbell, D. T., and J. C. Stanley. 1963. *Experimental and Quasi-Experimental Designs for Research*. Chicago: Rand McNally.

Carter, N., D. Bryant-Lukosius, A. DiCenso, J. Blythe, and A. J. Neville. 2014. The use of triangulation in qualitative research. *Oncology Nursing Forum* 41(5):545–547.

Chen, J., S. Yang, W. Ding, P. Li, A. Liu, H. Zhang, and T. Li. 2024. Incremental high average-utility itemset mining: survey and challenges. *Scientific Reports* 14(1):9924. DOI: 10.1038/s41598-024-60279-0.

Chen, Y. 2022. Health technology assessment and economic evaluation: Is it applicable for the traditional medicine? *Integrative Medicine Research* 11(1). https://doi.org/10.1016/j.imr.2021.100756.

CONSORT. n.d. Accessed September 5, 2024. https://www.consort-spirit.org/.

Cooper, I. D. 2015. How to write an original research paper (and get it published). *Journal of the Medical Library Association* 103(2):67–68.

Cresswell, K. M., D. W. Bates, R. Williams, Z. Morrison, A. Slee, J. Coleman, A. Robertson, and A. Sheikh. 2014. Evaluation of medium-term consequences of implementing commercial computerized physician order entry and clinical decision support prescribing systems in two "early adopter" hospitals. *Journal of the American Medical Informatics Association* 21(e2):e194–e202.

Crew, D., and S. H. Houser. 2021. Overcoming challenges of merging multiple patient identification and matching systems: A case study. *Perspectives in Health Information Management* 18(Winter):1n. https://www.ncbi.nlm.nih.gov/pmc/articles/PMC7883361/.

Eden, J., L. Levit, A. Berg, and S. Morton, eds. 2011. *Finding What Works in Health Care: Standards for Systematic Reviews*. Washington, DC: The National Academies Press.

EQUATOR: Enhancing the QUAlity and Transparency Of Health Research. n.d. Accessed September 5, 2024. http://www.equator-network.org/.

FAA (Federal Aviation Administration). n.d. "Human Factors Tools." Accessed September 5, 2024. https://www.hf.faa.gov/tools.aspx.

GAO-15-280. 2015. "Comparative Effectiveness Research, HHS Needs to Strengthen Dissemination and Data Capacity Building Efforts." Accessed May 14, 2024. https://www.gao.gov/products/gao-15-280.

Glaser, B. G. 1965. The constant comparative method of qualitative analysis. *Social Problems* 12(4):436–445.

Green, S., J. P. T. Higgins, P. Alderson, M. Clarke, C. D. Mulrow, and A. D. Oxman. 2011. What Is a Systematic Review (1.2.2.)? In *Cochrane Handbook for Systematic Reviews of Interventions Version 5.1.0* [Updated March 2011]. Edited by J. P. T. Higgins and S. Green. http://handbook.cochrane.org/.

HRSA (Health Resources and Services Administration). 2024. "National Sample Survey of Registered Nurses (NSSRN)." https://bhw.hrsa.gov/data-research/access-data-tools/national-sample-survey-registered-nurses.

Houser, S. H., C. A. Flite, S. L. Foster, T. J. Hunt, A. Morey, M. N. Palmer, J. Peterson, R. D. Pope, and L. Sorensen. 2022. Patient clinical documentation in telehealth environment: Are we collecting appropriate and sufficient information for best practice? *Mhealth* 2022(8):6. doi: 10.21037/mhealth-21-30.

IOM (Institute of Medicine). 2009. *Initial National Priorities for Comparative Effectiveness Research*. Washington, DC: The National Academies Press.

Kirukowski, J., and M. Corbett. 1993. SUMI: The software usability measurement inventory. *British Journal of Educational Technology* 24(3):210–212.

Koppel, R., S. Smith, J. Blythe, and V. Kothari. 2015. Workarounds to computer access in healthcare organizations: You want my password or a dead patient? *Studies in Health Technology & Informatics* 208:215–220.

Lachal, J., A. Revah-Levy, M. Orri, and M. Moro. 2017. Metasynthesis: An original method to synthesize qualitative literature in psychiatry. *Frontier of Psychiatry*. https://www.frontiersin.org/articles/10.3389/fpsyt.2017.00269/full.

LingTranSoft. 2019. "C-I-Said." http://lingtransoft.info/apps/c-i-said.

Miles, M. B., A. M. Huberman, and J. Saldaña. 2014. *Qualitative Data Analysis: A Methods Sourcebook*, 3rd ed. Thousand Oaks, CA: Sage.

Moher, D., A. Liberati, J. Tetzlaff, D. G. Altman, and the PRISMA Group. 2009. Preferred reporting items for systematic reviews and meta-analyses: The PRISMA statement. *PLoS Medicine/Public Library of Science* 6(7):e1000097.

NIH (National Institutes of Health). 2023. "What Is Data Cleaning?" https://datascience.cancer.gov/training/learn-data-science/clean-data-basics.

Neve, O. M., P. P. G. van Benthem, A. M. Stiggelbout, and E. F. Hensen. 2021. Response rate of patient reported outcomes: The delivery method matters. *BMC Medical Research Methodology* 21(1):220. doi: 10.1186/s12874-021-01419-2.

QSR International. n.d. "NVivo." Accessed September 5, 2024. http://www.qsrinternational.com/product.

Researchware, Inc. n.d. "HyperRESEARCH: What It Is." Accessed September 5, 2024. http://www.researchware.com/.

Robson, C. 2010. Evaluation Research. Chapter 21 in *Research Process in Nursing*, 6th ed. Edited by K. Gerrish and A. Lacey. Chichester, UK: Blackwell Publishing.

Sandefer, R., and E. S. Karl. 2015. Ready or not: HIM is changing—results of the new HIM competencies survey show skill gaps between education levels, students, and working professionals. *Journal of AHIMA* 86(3):24–27.

Shi, L. 2020. *Health Services Research Methods*, 3rd ed. Cengage.

Simmonds, M., J. H. Elliott, A. Synnot, and T. Turner. 2022. Living systematic reviews. *Methods in Molecular Biology* 2345:121–134. doi: 10.1007/978-1-0716-1566-9_7.

Tenny, S., J. M. Brannan, and G. D. Brannan. 2022. Qualitative Study. *StatPearls*. https://www.ncbi.nlm.nih.gov/books/NBK470395/.

Tong, A., K. Flemming, E. McInnes, S. Olive, and J. Craig. 2012. Enhancing transparency in reporting the synthesis of qualitative research: ENTREQ. *BMC Medical Research Methodology* 12:181.

University of Maryland. n.d. "Questionnaire for User Interaction Satisfaction (QUIS™)." Accessed September 5, 2024. https://www.cs.umd.edu/hcil/quis/.

Vignato J., M. Inman, M. Patsais, and V. Conley. 2022. Computer-assisted qualitative data analysis software, phenomenology, and Colaizzi's method. *Western Journal of Nursing. Research* 44(12):1117–1123. doi: 10.1177/01939459211030335.

Wickham, R. J. 2019. Secondary Analysis Research. *Journal of the Advanced Practitioner in Oncology* 10(4):395–400. https://doi.org/10.6004/jadpro.2019.10.4.7.

Wissmann, S. 2015. Addressing challenges to the health information management profession: An Australian perspective. *Perspectives in Health Information Management* International issue:1–10.

Weston, L. E., S. L. Krein, and M. Harrod. 2021. Using observation to better understand the healthcare context. *Qualitative Research in Medicine & Healthcare* 5(3):9821. https://www.pagepressjournals.org/qrmh/article/view/9821/9893.

# Resources

AHRQ (Agency for Healthcare Research and Quality). 2024. "Technology Assessment Program." http://www.ahrq.gov/research/findings/ta/index.html.

AHRQ (Agency for Healthcare Research and Quality). 2022. "AHRQ Data Tools." https://www.ahrq.gov/data/data-tools/index.html.

AHRQ (Agency for Healthcare Research and Quality). 2014a. "Effective Health Care Program Library of Resources." http://www.ahrq.gov/professionals/clinicians-providers/ehclibrary/.

AHRQ (Agency for Healthcare Research and Quality). 2014b. "Results of ARRA-funded CER Dissemination Activities." http://www.ahrq.gov/cpi/about/mission/arra/index.html#s1.

Federation of American Scientists. n.d. "Office of Technology Assessment Archive, Technology Assessment and Congress." Accessed May 11, 2024. http://ota.fas.org/technology_assessment_and_congress/.

Garrard, J. 2020. *Health Sciences Literature Review Made Easy: The Matrix Method*, 6th ed. Sudbury, MA: Jones and Bartlett.

NICHSR (National Information Center on Health Services Research and Health Care Technology) of the National Library of Medicine. 2024. http://www.nlm.nih.gov/hsrinfo/cer.html.

Strunk, W., Jr. and E. B. White. 2000. *The Elements of Style*, 4th ed. New York: Longman.

# chapter 19

# Biomedical and Clinical Research Support

*Shannon H. Houser, PhD, MPH, RHIA, FAHIMA*

## Learning Objectives

- Interpret inferential statistics and statistical data for effective decision-making in research support
- Adhere to Institutional Review Board processes, laws, and regulations to ensure ethical research practices
- Safeguard electronic health information through confidentiality and security measures
- Enhance the role of HIM professionals in research and supportive roles in healthcare research
- Evaluate research designs for conducting comprehensive clinical and biomedical research
- Describe the patient's role in patient-centered outcomes research

## Key Terms

Attributable risk (AR)
Biomedical research
Case-control (retrospective) studies
Clinical research
Clinical trial
Cohort study
Cross-sectional study
Double-blind studies
Epidemiological study
Experimental study
Health Research Extension Act of 1985
Health services research
Human subjects
Incidence
Institutional Review Board (IRB)
Morality
National Committee for Quality Assurance (NCQA)
Observational study
Odds ratio
Office for Human Research Protections (OHRP)
Office of Research Integrity (ORI)
Prevalence
Principal investigator (PI)
Prospective study
Randomized clinical trial (RCT)
Relative risk (RR)
Research protocol
Retrospective study
Single-blind study
Vulnerable subject

**Biomedical research** is the process of systematically investigating subjects related to the functioning of the human body. Its primary aim is to verify the safety and efficacy of innovative drugs, treatments, and medical technologies for patient care. Once these new interventions are made available to healthcare consumers, extensive long-term studies are undertaken to evaluate their outcomes and effectiveness in real-world settings.

**Clinical research** involves direct interaction with human subjects or human-origin materials to explore health and illness, covering areas such as disease mechanisms, therapeutic interventions, and clinical trials, while excluding in vitro studies not linked to living individuals (NIH n.d.). In contrast, biomedical research focuses on understanding biological processes, disease prevention, and various health-related factors (HHS 2022a). The primary differences between clinical and biomedical research lie in their focus, human health versus biological processes; their settings, clinical environments versus laboratories; and their interaction with subjects, direct human involvement versus often using animal models or biochemical assays.

Comparative Effectiveness Research (CER), a subset of clinical research, applies foundational biomedical knowledge to clinical scenarios. While biomedical research focuses on understanding biological processes underlying health and disease and providing critical insights for new interventions, clinical research tests these interventions in human subjects to determine their safety and efficacy.

This chapter explores the various methods by which biomedical and clinical research are conducted. It also examines methods of assessing outcomes and effectiveness, including programs initiated by the Agency for Healthcare Research and Quality (AHRQ), Joint Commission, National Committee for Quality Assurance (NCQA), and the Patient-Centered Outcomes Research Institute (PCORI) in this context. This chapter also highlights the integral role of health information management (HIM) in biomedical research, emphasizing its dependence on the systematic collection, management, and analysis of various types of clinical and nonclinical data.

## Clinical and Biomedical Research

Clinical and biomedical research studies are essential for evaluating disease processes, the safety and efficacy of drugs, and the utility of various diagnostic and preventive measures, such as vaccines and mammography. During the COVID-19 pandemic, these studies were vital for the rapid development and validation of vaccines, drugs, and other treatments to address critical health challenges. The most common examples of these research studies are **clinical trials**, which offer a structured methodology for testing and validating new clinical or biomedical interventions. This systematic approach allows for the careful introduction, thorough evaluation, and ongoing monitoring of new drugs, treatments, and healthcare technologies before widespread implementation.

**Health services research** examines the quality, accessibility, cost, and efficiency of healthcare services to improve the overall patient care standards. *Health Services Research* is a notable journal in this field. It shares findings of studies related to healthcare organizations, technology use, impact of health policy, and research methodologies. The journal frequently publishes research on HIM issues such as use of the electronic health record (EHR) to investigate improvements in patient safety; public perceptions of health information technology (HIT); and analysis of healthcare delivery models, evidenced by studies on hospital report cards, readmission rates, and the efficacy of patient-centered medical homes in reducing emergency department visits (Research and Educational Trust n.d.).

Advancements in artificial intelligence (AI) are transforming clinical and biomedical research. AI enhances the analysis of large datasets in clinical research, speeding up the discovery of insights and advancing personalized medicine. Its algorithms improve research patient recruitment by efficiently identifying suitable participants and predicting potential trial dropouts, increasing trial effectiveness. In drug discovery, AI expedites compound screening and repurposes existing medications. It also improves medical imaging by enhancing diagnostic accuracy and supporting the early detection of diseases. However, it is crucial to address data privacy and concerns of algorithm biases, which occur when algorithm results are unfairly influenced by the data or design. The continuous integration of AI in clinical research makes a new era of advanced medical breakthroughs and improved health outcomes (Senn 2023).

# Ethical Treatment of Human Subjects

In research involving human subjects, researchers must follow ethical principles that guide their behavior and decision-making. Morality includes two separate requirements related to research: recognizing the autonomy of individuals to make their own decisions and providing additional protections for those with decreased autonomy (due to changes in their health capacity) (NIH 1979). This ethical framework is fundamental to responsible research conduct.

Research ethics guide researchers to conscientiously protect human subjects, offering clear boundaries for assessing the benefits and risks involved in studies. In the context of clinical and biomedical research, assessing the benefit versus risk is essential. Benefits can be therapeutic gains for the individual participant or for society. Risks involve understanding both the likelihood and severity of potential harm to the research subject. Stating that 1 out of 100 patients may experience a certain risk suggests likelihood of harm. A rash as a minor effect of the treatment, or liver failure as a major effect of the treatment, suggests severity of harm.

The researcher's dilemma lies in balancing known and unknown risks to subjects against potential benefits, which may be greater for society at large than the individual research participants. However, there are many clinical and biomedical research studies in which the benefits far outweigh the risks to participants. For example, an individual with advanced stage IV pancreatic cancer may only see how the benefits outweigh the risks of participating in a clinical trial that examines the effectiveness of a new medication that could stop the progression of their disease.

The 21st Century Cures Act of 2016, which emphasizes patient empowerment and enhanced data sharing for research, has significant ethical implications for the treatment of human subjects. It advocates for greater access to EHRs and encourages the responsible exchange of data to advance research and innovation. The Act calls for ethical management of health data and sets forth principles like informed, ongoing consent; fostering inclusivity; and upholding consumer trust. These guidelines aim to protect human subjects ethically in a landscape marked by increased data access and interoperability (Durieux et al. 2022).

## The Nuremberg Code and the Declaration of Helsinki

International guidelines also govern the ethical conduct of human research. The Nuremberg Code outlines research ethics that were developed during the trials of Nazi war criminals following World War II. These trials addressed charges that medical experiments were conducted on concentration camp prisoners without their consent. The code was widely adopted as a worldwide standard for protecting human subjects in the 1960s, and beyond. The basic tenet of the Nuremberg Code is that "voluntary consent of the human subject is absolutely essential" (Nuremberg Code 1949, 1). It is the duty and responsibility of the individual initiating, directing, or conducting the experiment to ensure the quality of the informed consent. Additionally, the Nuremberg Code requires that research be based on knowledge from previous animal work, the risks be justified by the anticipated benefits, only qualified scientists conduct the research, and physical and mental suffering be avoided. Research in which death is expected should not be conducted.

The Declaration of Helsinki is a code of ethics for clinical research that was approved by the World Medical Association in 1964. It was a reinterpretation of the Nuremberg Code directed toward medical research with a therapeutic intent. It is a statement of ethical principles that provides guidance to physicians and other participants in medical research involving human subjects, including research on identifiable human material or identifiable data. The document has been revised several times, most recently at the 64th World Medical Association General Assembly in Fortaleza, Brazil, in October 2013 (WMA 2013).

Despite the Nuremberg Code and the Declaration of Helsinki, controversial ethical practices in biomedical research continued to be a problem. In 1966, Dr. Henry K. Beecher, an anesthesiologist, described several examples of research studies with controversial ethics that had been published by prominent researchers in major journals (Beecher 1966). Beecher's article increased public awareness of the ethical problems related to biomedical research, including the following:

- Lack of informed consent
- Coercion of, or undue pressure on, volunteers
- Use of a vulnerable population
- Information being withheld
- Available treatment being withheld
- Information about risks being withheld
- Subjects put at risk
- Risks to subjects that outweigh the benefits
- Deception
- Violation of rights

The work of Beecher enabled others who are doing research or working with researchers to pay attention to these ethical issues and work toward preventing them from occurring during clinical and biomedical research studies.

## The US Public Health Services Syphilis Study

A study conducted in the US that brought ethical issues in research to the forefront was the US Public Health Services Syphilis Study. This study was designed to study the natural history of syphilis in African American men (see figure 19.1). At the time the study began in 1932, there was no treatment for syphilis. However, by the 1940s penicillin had proved to be safe and effective. The men enrolled in the study were denied treatment. They continued to be followed until 1972, when the first public accounts began to appear in the national press. The study resulted in 28 deaths, 100 cases of disability, and 19 cases of congenital syphilis (CDC 2022).

After the press drew attention to the problem, Congress formed an ad hoc panel that determined the study should be stopped immediately and that oversight of human research was inadequate. It was recommended that federal regulations be implemented to protect human research in the future. In 1974, Congress authorized formation of the National Commission for the Protection of Human Subjects in Biomedical and Behavioral Research. The commission was charged with identifying the basic ethical principles that underlie the conduct of human research.

In 1979, the commission published the *Belmont Report: Ethical Principles and Guidelines for the Protection of Human Subjects of Research* (HHS 1979). This report identifies the following three basic ethical principles that underlie all human subject research:

- Respect for persons requires that individuals have the ability to understand and process information and the freedom to volunteer for research without coercion or undue influence from others. Respect for persons requires informed consent and respecting the privacy of research subjects.
- Beneficence is minimizing harms and maximizing benefits.
- Justice requires that people be treated fairly and that benefits and risks be shared equitably among the population. Justice requires that that vulnerable populations or populations of convenience not be exploited. (HHS 1979)

In 1981, the Department of Health and Human Services (HHS) revised its regulations on the protection of human subjects and made them available within the Code of Federal Regulations (CFR) (45 CFR 46). In 1991, subpart A of those regulations was broadened to include 15 other federal departments, creating the Common Rule. Technical amendments, which are amendments that are not substantial and therefore did not require publishing a proposed rule, were made to the Common Rule in 2005. Also, the Office of Management and Budget (OMB) developed a workgroup to examine possible revisions to the Common Rule. Its draft, Advance Notice of Proposed Rulemaking (ANPRM), was circulated for comment, and the ANPRM, titled *Human Subjects Research Protections: Enhancing Protections for Research Subjects and Reducing Burden, Delay, and Ambiguity for Investigators*, was developed (HHS 2011). On September 8, 2015, proposed revisions to the Common Rule were made in a Notice of Proposed Rulemaking (NPRM) published in the *Federal Register* (HHS 2015). Just like the ANPRM, the NPRM seeks comments on this proposed rule. A summary of the changes includes broadening protections for research subjects, such as more focused informed consent documents that are shorter and clearer; and a focus on more oversight for those studies that hold more risk for the research subject and less oversight on those that pose less risk. Public comments were used in the process of developing proposed revisions to the Common Rule. The revised Common Rule went into effect on July 19, 2018 (HHS 2017).

The Office for Human Research Protections (OHRP) is a federal agency that provides leadership and oversight on all matters related to the protection of human subjects participating in research conducted or supported by HHS, as outlined in the regulations.

**Figure 19.1.** Tuskegee Syphilis Study

The Tuskegee Syphilis Study is a notorious chapter in medical research in the United States. From 1932 to 1972, the US Public Health Service conducted research that had the stated purpose of obtaining more information about the clinical course of syphilis. The medical researchers from the US Public Health Service experimented on 399 African American males in Macon County, Alabama. The medical researchers told the men they were being treated for "bad blood." In fact, the researchers were deceiving the men and were denying them treatment for syphilis. Many of the men's wives were infected, and their children were subsequently born with congenital syphilis. The US Public Health Service continued the study despite the advent of penicillin in 1947. The Tuskegee Syphilis Study is a symbol of unethical research.

*Source:* CDC 2022.

OHRP provides clarification and guidance, develops educational programs, maintains regulatory oversight, and provides advice on ethical and regulatory issues in biomedical and behavioral research (HHS 2020). The federal regulations for the protection of human subjects include Title 45 of CFR 46. The Food and Drug Administration (FDA) has a separate set of regulations governing human subjects research (21 CFR 56 IRBs and 21 CFR 50 Protection of Human Subjects). The basic requirements for IRBs and protection of human subjects are similar between the HHS and FDA regulations.

### Check Your Understanding 19.1

Answer the following questions in a separate document.

1. How has the evolution of ethical guidelines for the treatment of human subjects, from the Nuremberg Code to the Declaration of Helsinki and beyond, influenced the integrity and public trust in current medical research practices?

2. Examine the Tuskegee Syphilis Study and identify five ethical concerns as highlighted by Dr. Henry Beecher. Explain how each of these concerns manifested within the study.

3. How would you categorize the major changes to the Common Rule proposed in 2015? What are some potential benefits of the changes?

4. What aspect of the Nuremberg Code is violated in the following scenario? A group of patients with type 2 diabetes were unknowingly included in a study focused on comparing the outcomes related to efficacy of a pharmaceutical. Data related to their use of medications and clinical data related to their disease conditions were used to study drug efficacy.

5. You have been asked to develop an online training on the protection of human subjects participating in research. What resource can assist you in this project?

## Protection of Human Subjects

The ultimate driver for many of the regulations surrounding clinical and biomedical research is protecting the rights, welfare, and well-being of human subjects who participate in research being conducted. The HHS regulations contain three basic provisions for the protection of human subjects (45 CFR 46):

- Institutional assurances of compliance
- Institutional Review Board (IRB) review and approval
- Informed consent

The HHS is only one of the federal agencies that govern and fund human subject research. Others include the US FDA, US Department of Agriculture, US Department of Energy, and US Department of Education, among others.

### Institutional Assurances of Compliance

An institutional assurance of compliance is a commitment of an institution to comply with HHS regulations for the protection of human subjects by documenting this commitment. HHS will support nonexempt research (research that receives a more extensive review by the IRB, such as clinical trials) covered by the regulations only if the organization has an OHRP-approved assurance on file; the research has been reviewed and approved by the organization's IRB; and the IRB will continue to review the research, as necessary (HHS 2016).

Protection of human subjects is required under the HHS CFR. OHRP has formal agreements with more than 10,000 federally funded universities, hospitals, and other clinical and behavioral research institutions in the US and abroad (45 CFR 46). These organizations must agree to abide by the human subject protection regulations found in the CFR. The OHRP's duties include the following:

- Establishing criteria for, and approving assurance of, compliance for the protection of human subjects with institutions engaged in HHS-conducted or HHS-supported human subject research

- Providing clarification and guidance on involving humans in research
- Developing and implementing educational programs and resource materials
- Promoting the development of approaches to enhance human subject protections

The OHRP also evaluates substantive allegations or indications of noncompliance with HHS regulations regarding the conduct of research involving human subjects (45 CFR 46.103). It also provides education and development on the complex ethical and regulatory issues relating to human subjects' protection in clinical and behavioral research. The OHRP helps institutions assess and improve their own procedures for protecting human subjects through a quality improvement program.

## Institutional Review Board

The Institutional Review Board (IRB), one of the basic provisions required by the HHS, is a committee established (within a hospital or university, for example) to protect the rights and welfare of human research subjects involved in research activities. The IRB members are appointed by the specific organization conducting the research.

The IRB determines whether the conducted research is appropriate and protects human subjects as they participate in this research. The primary focus of the IRB is not on whether the type of research is appropriate for the organization to conduct but on whether human subjects are adequately protected (45 CFR 46.111).

The purpose and responsibility of the IRB is to protect the rights and welfare of human subjects as they engage in research activities. The IRB must abide by the regulations as listed in 45 CFR 46.111 and 21 CFR 56.111. The IRB must first determine if research is being conducted and then determine if human subjects are being protected. Research is defined by the Common Rule as "a systematic investigation, including research development, testing and evaluation, designed to develop or contribute to generalizable knowledge" (45 CFR 46.102). Human subjects are defined by the Common Rule as "living individual[s] about whom an investigator (whether professional or student) conducting research obtains (1) data through intervention or interaction with the individual, or (2) identifiable private information" (45 CFR 46.102).

An IRB must review all research activities covered by the HHS regulations and either (1) approve, (2) require changes to approve, or (3) disapprove any research activity. An IRB must perform continuing reviews of ongoing research as often as necessary per degree of risk, but not less than once per year. The IRB has the authority to suspend or terminate approved research that is not conducted in accordance with IRB requirements or that has caused unexpected or serious harm to the subject. If a suspension or termination occurs, the IRB must include a documented statement for the reason and must report this immediately to the investigator, appropriate institutional officials, and the HHS.

The protection of human subjects is a shared responsibility between the institutional officials, the IRB, and the investigator. It should not rest solely with the IRB. The institutional official is responsible for choosing one or more IRBs to review research; providing enough space, staff, and other resources to support the IRB's review and recordkeeping responsibilities; providing education and training for the IRB staff and investigators; providing effective communication and guidance on human subject research; ensuring that investigators carry out their research responsibilities with the utmost respect for human subjects; and serving as the point of contact for OHRP or designating another individual to undertake this responsibility.

The IRB is made up of at least five members with diversified backgrounds per federal regulation, such as including at least one member with a scientific background and at least one member in a nonscientific area. However, most organizations have more than that number. For example, many large universities have 10 IRB members, each functioning as a separate IRB under a central administration and support from the main IRB office. An IRB vice chair and several members with expertise in many diversified areas comprise the IRB committee. Also, the IRB office includes additional staff that reviews exempt or expedited research proposals (University of Pittsburgh 2023).

## Conflict of Interest

No IRB member may participate in the review of a research project in which he or she has a conflict of interest. A conflict of interest may include serving as an IRB committee member to review a research study protocol (a plan or proposal for the study) in which one has a definite interest in the outcome of the specific medical device or medication. If this situation arises, the IRB committee member should resign from the committee (University of Pittsburgh 2020).

Before IRB submissions are reviewed, investigators may be required or encouraged to complete various educational modules, which may include education on research integrity, conflict of interest, use of lab animals in research and education, human embryonic and stem cell research, Health Insurance Portability and Accountability Act (HIPAA) researchers' privacy requirements, blood-borne pathogens, chemical hygiene, responsible literature searching, IRB member education, research with children, and the Good Clinical Practices module (recommended for those investigators involved in FDA-regulated research) (University of Pittsburgh 2021a). Some universities will require students, faculty, and staff to complete Collaborative Institutional Training Institute (CITI) training for all individuals involved in research. Some universities will draw on CITI resources and those from the university to provide research training modules for all individuals involved in research (University of Pittsburgh 2023a).

### Procedures for IRB Submission

The IRB application process varies by institution, but the basic steps outlined in figure 19.2 describe the general sequence from preparing ethical guideline training and study documentation to conducting ongoing reviews and ultimately closing the study.

Exempt, expedited, and full board approval are the three major categories of IRB review for research study proposals. OHRP recommends that clear procedures be developed by organizations so that IRBs can determine whether research is exempt.

Exempt research activities include the involvement of human subjects in one or more of the listed categories according to the HHS Federal Policy regulations (45 CFR 46.101(b)(1–6)). Research that is exempt does not mean the researchers have no ethical obligations to the participants but that the regulatory requirements such as informed consent and yearly renewal from the IRB do not apply to this type of research. The IRB still reviews research protocols to determine their exempt status.

Exempt research activities may include the involvement of human subjects in one or more of the following categories:

- Educational settings (45 CFR 46.101(b)(1)): research conducted in educational settings involving normal educational practices, such as testing different instructional methods (for example, differences in learning outcomes between distance education and traditional classroom)

- Use of educational tests, surveys, interviews, or observation (45 CFR 46.101(b)(2)): research conducted in any setting in which educational tests such as aptitude or achievement tests are conducted unless participants are identified in any way when data are collected

- Use of educational tests, surveys, interviews, or observation (45 CFR 46.101(b)(3)): research conducted that is not exempt under paragraph (b)(2) if (i) the human subjects are elected or appointed public officials or candidates for public office or (ii) federal statute(s) require(s) without exception that the confidentiality of the personally identifiable information be maintained throughout the research and thereafter

- Research involving the collection or study of existing data, documents, records, pathological

**Figure 19.2.** Sample IRB application process

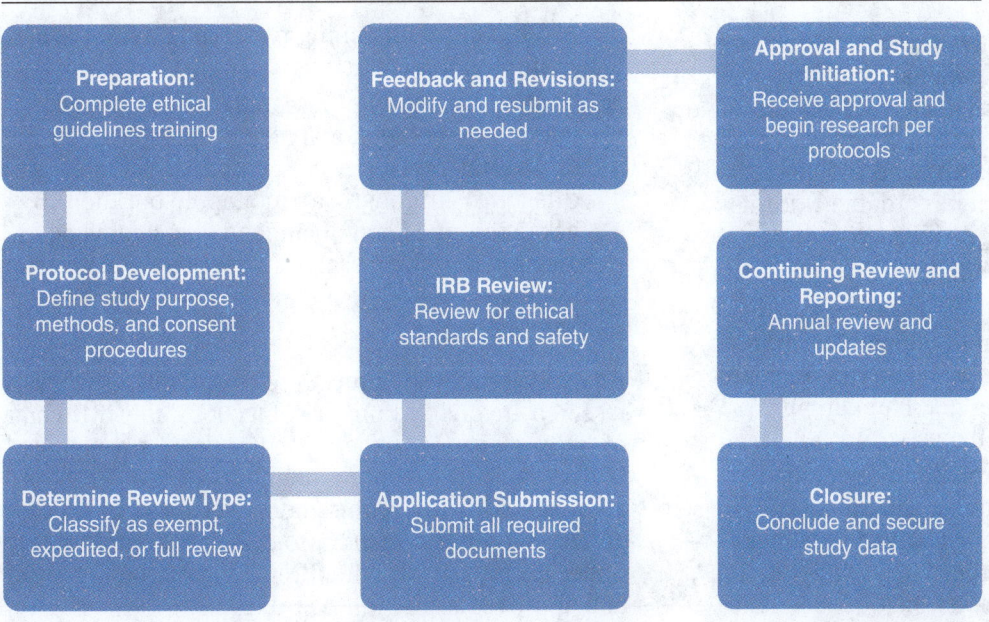

specimens, or diagnostic specimens (45 CFR 46.101(b)(4)): if these sources are publicly available or if the information is recorded by the investigator in such a manner that subjects cannot be identified, directly or through identifiers linked to the subjects

- Research and demonstration projects that are conducted by or subject to the approval of department or agency heads, and are designed to study, evaluate, or otherwise examine (45 CFR 46.101(b)(5)): (i) public benefit or service programs, (ii) procedures for obtaining benefits or services under those programs, (iii) possible changes in or alternatives to those programs or procedures, or (iv) possible changes in methods or levels of payment for benefits or services under those programs

- Taste and food quality evaluation and consumer acceptance studies (45 CFR 46.101 (b)(6)): (i) if wholesome foods without additives are consumed or (ii) if a food is consumed that contains a food ingredient at or below the level and for a use found to be safe, or agricultural chemical or environmental contaminant at or below the level found to be safe, by the FDA or approved by the Environmental Protection Agency or the Food Safety and Inspection Service of the US Department of Agriculture

Expedited research includes those activities that (1) present no more than minimal risk to human subjects, and (2) involve only procedures listed in one or more of the following categories as authorized by 45 CFR 46.110 and 21 CFR 56.110. The categories for expedited IRB review include the following:

1. Clinical studies of drugs and medical devices only when an investigational new drug application or medical device application is not required or when the medical device is cleared or approved for marketing and the medical device is being used in accordance with its cleared or approved labelling
2. Collection of blood samples by finger stick, heel stick, ear stick, or venipuncture
3. Prospective collection of biological specimens for research purposes by noninvasive means. Examples include hair and nail clipping, or placenta removed at delivery.
4. Collection of data through noninvasive procedures (not involving general anesthesia or sedation) routinely employed in clinical practice, excluding procedures involving x-rays or microwaves. Examples include magnetic resonance imaging, electrocardiography, exercise testing, muscle strength testing, and so forth.
5. Research involving materials (data, documents, records, or specimens) that have been collected, or will be collected, solely for non-research purposes (such as medical treatment or diagnosis). (*Note*: Some research in this category may be exempt from the HHS regulations for the protection of human subjects [45 CFR 46.101(b)(4)]. This listing refers only to research that is not exempt.)
6. Collection of data from voice, video, digital, or image recordings made for research purposes.
7. Research on individual or group characteristics or behavior (including, but not limited to, research on perception, cognition, motivation, identity, language, communication, cultural beliefs or practices, and social behavior) or research employing survey, interview, oral history, focus group, program evaluation, human factors evaluation, or quality assurance methodologies. (*Note*: Some research in this category may be exempt from the HHS regulations for the protection of human subjects [45 CFR 46.101(b)(2) and (b)(3)]. This listing refers only to research that is not exempt.)
8. Continuing review of research previously approved by the convened IRB as follows:
   - Where (i) the research is permanently closed to the enrollment of new subjects, (ii) all subjects have completed all research-related interventions, and (iii) the research remains active only for long-term follow-up of subjects; or
   - Where no subjects have been enrolled and no additional risks have been identified; or
   - Where the remaining research activities are limited to data analysis.
9. Continuing review of research, not conducted under an investigational new drug application or investigational device exemption where categories 2 through 8 do not apply but the IRB has determined and documented at a convened meeting that the research involves no greater than minimal risk and no additional risks have been identified

An expedited review procedure consists of a review of research involving human subjects by the IRB chair or by one or more experienced reviewers designated by the chair from among members of the IRB in accordance with the requirements set forth in 45 CFR 46.110. All other research projects that do not qualify under exempt or expedited review must be reviewed and approved at the full board level.

Once the category of submission is determined, the investigator must complete the proper forms for submission to the IRB. The types of forms that must be completed depend upon the level of review. Most IRBs require that research protocols be submitted electronically. An IRB protocol checklist is usually provided so that the investigator can determine what types of documents need to be completed and submitted.

Once the appropriate forms are submitted to the IRB, the investigator awaits a decision from the IRB committee. The decisions from the IRB can include one of the following four categories:

- Full approval
- Approval subject to modifications—protocol is recommended for approval pending inclusion of changes
- Reconsideration—when there are several questions and concerns regarding the protocol and full board review and approval may be necessary once all questions and concerns are addressed
- Disapproval—when major scientific or ethical problems cannot be resolved (University of Pittsburgh 2021a)

## Management of Handling Problems Related to Risk to Human Subjects

Sometimes during the research study protocol, reportable events occur. When this happens, the investigator must notify the IRB and complete an unanticipated problem involving risk to human subjects report. The reportable event report should include the following information:

- Name of principal investigator (PI)
- Title of the study
- IRB study number
- Funding source
- Brief description of the problem
- Severity of the event
- Causality of the event (Was it due to the study protocol or procedure?)
    - Corrective action plan, if necessary
- Whether protocol modification is necessary and, if so, a revised protocol and informed consent must be submitted
- Signature of the PI and date (University of Pittsburgh 2021b)

It is important to document any reportable event that occurs while conducting research. The information listed is critical to protect the safety of future subjects that may participate in the study and for IRB reporting purposes.

## Recordkeeping and Retention

The IRB should prepare and maintain adequate documentation of all IRB activities. This documentation may include the following:

- Copies of all research study protocols reviewed, sample consent forms, progress reports, and reports of injuries to subjects or adverse event reports
- Minutes of IRB committee meetings
- Records of continuing review activities
- Listing of IRB members and their responsibilities
- All written procedures for the IRB
- Statements of significant new findings provided to subjects (45 CFR 46.115)

The records related to this policy should be retained for at least three years, and records relating to research conducted should be retained for at least three years after completion of the research. "All records shall be accessible for inspection and copying by authorized representatives of the department or agency at reasonable times and in a reasonable manner" (45 CFR 46.115).

## Informed Consent

In most cases, clinical and biomedical research requires that subjects give informed consent. Informed consent is a person's voluntary agreement to participate in research or to undergo a diagnostic, therapeutic, or preventive procedure. Informed consent also pertains to a person's voluntary agreement to participate in research; it is based on adequate knowledge and an understanding of relevant information provided by the investigators. In the case of research, it is a thoughtful and respectful explanation of information so that a person can decide whether to participate in a study. The process that encompasses informed consent should educate possible participants in terms they can understand. Informed consent should contain three fundamentals: information, comprehension, and voluntariness. The written presentation of information should document the basis for consent and for the participant's future reference. The consent document should also be revised when necessary to include changes to improve the consent procedure (45 CFR 46.116).

In giving informed consent, subjects do not waive any of their legal rights, nor do they release the investigator, sponsor, or institution from liability for negligence. Federal regulations require that certain information be provided to each human subject. This information includes the following:

- A statement that the study involves research, the purpose of the research, the expected duration of subject participation, a description of the procedures to be followed, and the identification of procedures that are experimental
- A description of reasonably foreseeable risks or discomforts. The description must be accurate and reasonable, and subjects must be informed of previously reported adverse events.
- A description of the benefits to the subject or others who may reasonably benefit from the research
- A disclosure of the appropriate alternative procedures or courses of treatment, if any, that might be advantageous to the subject. When appropriate, a statement that supportive care with no additional disease-specific treatment is an alternative.
- A statement describing the extent to which confidentiality of records identifying the subject will be maintained. The statement should include full disclosure and description of approved agencies, such as the FDA, that may have access to the records.
- For research involving more than minimal risk, an explanation as to whether any compensation or medical treatments are available if injury occurs and, if so, what they consist of or where further information may be obtained. Injury is not limited to physical injury. Research-related injury may include physical, psychological, social, financial, or otherwise.
- An explanation of who to contact for answers to pertinent questions about the research and research subjects' rights and who to contact in the event of a research-related injury to the subject
- A statement that participation is voluntary and that the subject may discontinue participation at any time without penalty or loss of benefits to which he or she is otherwise entitled (45 CFR 46.116)

The federal regulations further require that additional consent information be provided when appropriate (45 CFR 46.116), including the following:

- A statement that the treatment or procedure may involve risks to the subject (or embryo or fetus if the subject is pregnant) that are unforeseeable
- Anticipated circumstances under which the subject's participation may be terminated by the investigator without regard to the subject's consent
- Any additional costs that a subject may incur as a result of participating in the research
- The consequences of a subject's decision to withdraw from the research and procedures for orderly termination of participation by the subject
- A statement that significant new findings developed during the course of the research that may relate to the subject's willingness to continue participation will be provided to the subject
- The approximate number of subjects involved in the study

Federal regulations also require that informed consent be presented in a language the subject understands. If the subject does not understand the language of the consent form, it must be translated appropriately. For subjects who are illiterate, an interpreter must be present to explain the study and translate questions and answers between the subject and the investigator. In institutions where clinical and biomedical research is conducted, consent forms are usually maintained in storage facilities monitored by the PI. The **principal investigator (PI)** is the director of the research project and has full responsibility for all parts of the research conducted. Copies of the consent may or may not be kept in the medical record depending upon organizational policy. Consent forms often contain sensitive information, such as that related to genetic testing. Genetic test results are not to be provided to insurers or other parties, and sometimes not to the subject. To ensure this information is not inadvertently released in the regular course of business related to the release of information process, some organizations choose to maintain these important documents separately. Examples of these documents, which are kept in the research study center files, can be found in figure 19.3.

**Figure 19.3.** Contents of the research study center file

- Investigator's brochure
- Signed protocol
- Revised protocols (if applicable)
- Protocol amendments (if applicable)
- Continuing review documents
- Informed consent form (blank)
- HIPAA consent form (blank)
- Copies of signed consent forms
- Curriculum vitae (resumes) of principal investigator and coinvestigators
- Documentation of IRB or ethical review board (ERB) compliance
- All correspondence between the investigator, IRB or ERB, and study sponsor or contract research organization relating to study conduct
- Copies of safety reports sent to the FDA
- Lab certifications
- Normal laboratory value ranges for tests required by the protocol
- The FDA's Clinical Investigator Information Sheet
- Clinical research associate monitoring log
- Drug invoices
- Study site signature log
- Financial disclosure statement

*Source:* 45 CFR 46.115.

## Vulnerable Subjects

HHS regulations include additional protections for vulnerable or special subject populations as subparts of 45 CFR 46. Federal regulations require that "when some or all of the subjects are likely to be vulnerable to coercion or undue influence, additional safeguards have been included in the study to protect the rights and welfare of these subjects" (45 CFR 46.111; 21 CFR 56.111(b)). When a subject has limited mental capacity or is unable to freely volunteer, the subject is considered a **vulnerable subject**. Examples of vulnerable subjects include the following:

- *Children* may be vulnerable depending on age, maturity, and psychological state. There is potential for control, coercion, undue influence, or manipulation by parents, guardians, or investigators. The risk is greater for particularly young children.
- *Pregnant women, human fetuses, and neonates* may be vulnerable because of the increased potential risk to them. There is potential for interventions or procedures to cause greater risk for both the pregnant woman and the fetus or neonate.
- *Mentally disabled individuals* have problems with capacity. They may not have freedom to volunteer because they may be institutionalized or hospitalized, are economically and educationally disadvantaged, and suffer from chronic diseases.
- *Educationally disadvantaged subjects* may have limitations on understanding the study they will be participating in; some may be illiterate. There is potential for undue influence and manipulation.
- *Economically disadvantaged subjects* may volunteer only because they will benefit economically; that is, because they will receive payment for participating in the research, they may volunteer. They may enroll in research only to receive monetary compensation or medical care they cannot otherwise afford.
- *Individuals with incurable or fatal diseases* may volunteer to participate out of desperation. In many cases, these individuals have failed many treatments and view volunteering in research as their last chance at surviving their illness. Also, because of disease progression or effects of medications, they may not have the mental capacity necessary to make an informed decision. These individuals may accept high risk because they are desperate for a cure, even when there is little or no prospect of direct benefit.
- *Prisoners* have limited autonomy and may not be able to exercise free choice. They may

believe they will receive adverse treatment or be denied certain privileges if they refuse to participate in the research study. In addition, cash payments may be an inducement to participate in research; thus, it could be said that they are not truly volunteering but only participating for the cash benefit. Prisoners represent a population of convenience; that is, they are readily accessible and available. Studies on a contained population can be done more quickly and more cheaply. Lastly, prisoners may not realize benefits from their participation in research because of their incarceration and social and economic status.

## Check Your Understanding 19.2

**Answer the following questions in a separate document.**

1. The researcher aims to investigate the impact of using artificial intelligence (AI) in the anatomy lab on students' unit exam performance. Determine the category of IRB review necessary for this study and justify your reasoning.

2. A researcher plans to conduct a focus group to explore the factors that motivate healthcare workers to adopt new technologies in their professional roles. What level of IRB review is necessary for this study, and what is the rationale?

3. How does IRB approval influence the design and implementation of COVID-19 vaccine trials, and what are some specific examples of ethical considerations addressed by the IRB during the review process?

4. Amanda has been approached to participate in a study using a particular drug to treat her rheumatoid arthritis. She was given a lot of information to read, and her doctor explained the study. She is willing to participate but she really did not understand what her doctor was saying in regard to overall effects. Is this considered proper informed consent?

5. A prisoner agrees to be a subject in a clinical trial assessing the effectiveness of the combination of two cancer agents. Is this legal?

## Role of HIM Professionals in Research

The role of HIM professionals in the research they do can take on two different functions. First, an HIM professional may act as the PI for a research study. The PI is responsible for ensuring the study undergoes the proper IRB review and approval and adheres to all relevant protocols and regulations. This includes following the IRB checklist and completing consent forms that comply with IRB standards. As a PI, the HIM professional must rigorously follow the research protocol approved by the IRB and submit any protocol modifications for re-approval.

In a second function, HIM professionals can provide crucial support to other investigators in healthcare research settings. They offer guidance on the necessary policies and procedures for conducting research, assist in developing research study protocol and consent forms, and help educate investigators on IRB review processes. Moreover, they play a vital role in patient advocacy, informing patients of their rights in research participation. Additionally, HIM professionals may contribute as members or consultants to the IRB, leveraging their expertise in data management, patient privacy, and confidentiality.

### Privacy Considerations in Clinical and Biomedical Research

In response to a congressional mandate in HIPAA, HHS issued regulations entitled Standards for Privacy of Individually Identifiable Health Information. Known as the Privacy Rule, the regulations protect medical records and other individually identifiable health information from being used or disclosed in any form (HHS 2022).

The Privacy Rule establishes a category of protected health information (PHI), "which may be used or disclosed only in certain circumstances or under certain conditions. PHI is a subset of what is termed individually identifiable health information" (NIH 2004a). It includes information in the patient's medical records as well as billing information for services rendered. PHI also includes identifiable health information about subjects of clinical and biomedical research. Deidentification is important in protecting patient privacy and includes removing identifying information such as patient name and zip code.

The Privacy Rule defines how human research subjects are informed about the way their protected medical information will be used or disclosed. It also outlines their rights to access the information. The Privacy Rule protects the privacy of individually identifiable information while ensuring researchers continue to have access to the medical information they need to conduct their research. Investigators are permitted to use and disclose PHI for research with individual authorization or without individual authorization under limited circumstances (HHS 2022).

Individuals must agree to disclose their PHI for research purposes. "A valid Privacy Rule authorization is an individual's signed permission that allows a covered entity to use or disclose the [patient's] PHI for the purpose(s) and to the recipient(s) stated in the authorization" (NIH 2004b). Per the Privacy Rule, when a researcher receives authorization for research purposes, the authorization applies to the specific study for which it was requested and to no other studies. There are certain situations when authorization is not required.

> For some types of research, it is impracticable for researchers to obtain written authorization from research participants. To address this type of situation, the Privacy Rule contains criteria for waiver or alteration of the authorization requirement by an IRB or a privacy board. Under the Privacy Rule, either board may waive or alter, in whole or in part, the Privacy Rule's authorization requirements for the use and disclosure of PHI in connection with a particular research project. (NIH 2004c)

For example, an IRB may partially waive the authorization requirement so the covered entity can provide contact information to investigators, so that they can contact and recruit subjects into their research study (NIH 2004c; HHS 2022b).

It is believed the Privacy Rule will promote participation in clinical trials. Reasons for lack of participation in clinical trials cited most often are concern about health insurance discrimination and loss of privacy should the information be released.

## Oversight of Clinical and Biomedical Research

Because of past abuses of human subjects in the conduct of clinical and biomedical research in the US, Congress began hearings in 1981 to investigate scientific misconduct. Twelve cases of scientific misconduct were reported in the country between 1974 and 1981 (ORI n.d.a). Representative Albert Gore Jr., chairman of the Investigations and Oversight Subcommittee of the House Science and Technology Committee, held the first hearing. Continued abuses were reported throughout the 1980s, which resulted in the creation of the Office of Research Integrity to provide oversight of clinical and biomedical research. Examples of scientific misconduct include researchers falsifying research data, enrolling study subjects who did not qualify for the protocol, disregarding the well-being of vulnerable human subjects, and falsifying personal information in grant applications (ORI n.d.a).

In response to the public outcry over scientific misconduct in clinical and biomedical research, Congress passed the **Health Research Extension Act of 1985** (Public Health Service [PHS] regulation 42 CFR 493). The act requires the secretary of HHS to issue a regulation requiring applicant or awardee institutions to establish "an administrative process to review reports of scientific fraud" and "report to the Secretary any investigation of scientific fraud which appears substantial" (42 CFR 493).

Before 1986, reports of scientific misconduct were received by funding institutes within the PHS. In 1986, the NIH assigned responsibility for receiving and responding to complaints of scientific misconduct to its Institutional Liaison Office. This was the first step in creating a central locus of responsibility for scientific misconduct within the HHS. In March 1989, the PHS created the Office of Scientific Integrity (OSI) and the Office of Scientific Review (OSIR) in the Office of the Assistant Secretary for Health (OASH). In 1992, the OSI and the OSIR were consolidated to form the **Office of Research Integrity (ORI)** in the OASH. The creation of these groups removed responsibility for reviewing complaints of scientific misconduct from the funding agencies.

In 1993, the NIH Revitalization Act established the ORI as an independent agency within HHS. The "role, mission, and structure of the ORI [are] focused on preventing research misconduct and promoting research integrity principally through oversight, education, and review of institutional findings and recommendations" (ORI n.d.a). Responsibilities of the ORI include the following:

- Developing policies, procedures, and regulations related to the detection, investigation, and prevention of research misconduct and the responsible conduct of research
- Reviewing and monitoring research misconduct investigations conducted by applicant and awardee institutions
- Implementing activities and programs to teach the responsible conduct of research, promote research integrity, prevent research misconduct,

and improve the handling of allegations of research misconduct
- Providing technical assistance to institutions that respond to allegations of research misconduct
- Conducting policy analyses, evaluations, and research to build the knowledge base in research misconduct and research integrity (ORI n.d.b)

The ORI within the HHS conducted a study that examined scientists' reports on suspected research misconduct. From this study, it found that investigators believe that the best way to detect and prevent research misconduct is to have the PI supervise research work closely by reviewing data and applying quality control procedures or audits on the data. The ORI also found that more open communication is necessary to detect research misconduct, and that anonymity is necessary for the person reporting the possible misconduct. Policies and an effective training guide with a system for reporting were also found to be important (ORI 2008).

## Types of Clinical and Biomedical Research Designs

Research designs in clinical and biomedical studies vary widely. One frequently used type is the randomized clinical trial, in which individuals are randomly assigned to experimental and control groups to study the effect of interventions, such as an experimental drug. Other common types of designs for research involving human subjects include epidemiological studies, cross-sectional studies, case-control (retrospective) studies, and cohort studies.

### Clinical Trials

Clinical (medical) research is a specialized area of research that primarily investigates the efficacy of preventive, diagnostic, and therapeutic procedures. Efficacy involves both safety and effectiveness. Clinical trials are the specific, individual studies within the field of clinical research. They offer a systematic way to introduce, evaluate, and monitor new drugs, treatments, and devices prior to their dissemination throughout the healthcare system. As a result, they have proved to be effective means of advancing knowledge about medicine and health and, thus, improving the quality of healthcare in the US. Because clinical trials involve patients, they can begin only after the researcher has shown promising results in the laboratory or the results have been well documented in the literature. Clinicaltrials.gov from the NIH is a database of clinical trials that have been or are currently being conducted around the globe. Examples of certain types of clinical trials can be searched in this database to determine if a specific topic or disease has been researched. It is required by the FDA that the researcher post a description of the clinical trial on the database and make the subject aware of this through informed consent (NIH n.d.).

The NIH supports thousands of clinical trials. Private organizations such as drug companies and health maintenance organizations (HMOs) also support them. Trial sites are teaching and community hospitals, physician group practices, or health departments. Many clinical trials are multicentered; that is, several research institutions cooperate in conducting the study. In randomized clinical trials (RCTs), participants are assigned to a treatment or a control group. They may be single-blind studies in which case the subject does not know the treatment or double-blind studies, in which neither the investigator nor the subjects know who is in the treatment or control group until the end of the study.

Researchers conduct clinical trials using protocols. Research protocols are sets of strict procedures that specify the language of informed consent, the types of subjects, the timing of treatments, the period of participation, and the evaluation of efficacy. For example, in RCTs, researchers must follow strict rules in assigning patients to groups. The rules ensure both known and unknown risk factors will occur in approximately equal numbers between the group of patients receiving the treatment and the group of patients not receiving it.

Most clinical trials consist of three phases. For example, in a phase 1 drug trial, studies are performed on 20 to 80 healthy volunteers who are closely monitored (NIH n.d.). The objectives of phase 1 drug trials are to determine the metabolic and pharmacological actions of the drug in humans, to determine the side effects associated with increasing dosages and to gain early evidence of effectiveness. Historically, phase 1 trials are considered the safest and usually involve administering a single dose to healthy volunteers (NIH n.d.). However, they also can pose a high level of unknown risk because this is the first administration of a drug to a human. When the drug is highly toxic, such as a cancer chemotherapy, patients who have the disease the drug would treat (in this example, cancer patients) would be the subjects for phase 1 trials.

In a phase 2 drug trial, the number of participants is usually increased to between 100 and 200 (NIH n.d.). The purposes of this trial are to evaluate the drug's effectiveness for a certain indication in patients with the condition under study and to determine the short-term side effects and risks associated with the drug. Subjects included in phase 2 studies are usually those with the condition the drug is intended to treat. Phase 2 studies are randomized, well controlled, and closely monitored. They may include randomization to treatment and control groups and be double-blinded. Treatment and control groups allow for comparison between subjects who received the drug and those who did not.

Phase 3 drug trials involve the administration of a new drug to a larger number of patients in different clinical settings to determine its safety, effectiveness, and appropriate dosage. The number of subjects involved may range from several hundred to several thousand. Phase 3 trials are conducted only after evidence of effectiveness has been obtained. Phase 3 studies are designed to collect more information on drug effectiveness and safety for evaluating the drug's overall risk benefit.

The FDA, in collaboration with the research study sponsor, may decide to conduct a phase 4 postmarketing study to obtain more information about the drug's risks, benefits, and optimal use. Phase 4 studies may include studying different doses or schedules of administration than what was used in phase 2 studies, the use of the drug in other patient populations or other stages of the disease, or the use of the drug over a longer period. See table 19.1.

During the COVID-19 pandemic, the traditional clinical trial phases underwent a rapid transformation. Strategies were implemented to fast-track the development without compromising on safety and efficacy. This included conducting phase 1 and phase 2 trials concurrently, accelerating regulatory reviews and approvals, bolstering research with unprecedented levels of funding, and fostering international cooperation for data sharing and resource allocation. Adaptive trial designs also played a pivotal role, allowing for real-time adjustments based on initial findings. These collective efforts ensured that despite the accelerated pace, the vaccines met the stringent standards required for widespread public deployment.

## Epidemiological Studies

Epidemiology is the study of health and disease in populations rather than individuals. It examines epidemics as well as chronic diseases. The purpose of an **epidemiological study** is to compare one group or population with the risk factor of interest to one group or population without it. In such studies, the investigator attempts to identify risk factors for diseases, conditions, behaviors, or risks that result from particular causes, such as environmental factors and industrial agents.

The goals are to quantify the association between exposures and outcomes and to test hypotheses about causal relationships. Epidemiological research has several objectives:

- Identify the cause of disease and its associated risk factors
- Determine the extent of disease in a given community
- Study the natural history and prognosis of disease
- Evaluate new preventive and therapeutic measures and new modes of healthcare delivery
- Provide the foundation for public policy and regulatory decisions relating to environmental problems

Epidemiological studies may be observational or experimental. In an **observational study**, the exposure and outcome for individuals in the study is observed. In an **experimental study**, the exposure status for individuals in the study is determined and the individuals are then followed to determine the effects of the exposure.

Observational studies are used to generate hypotheses for later experimental studies. They may consist of clinical observations at a patient's bedside. For example, one researcher observed that every patient he operated on for lung cancer had a history of cigarette

**Table 19.1.** Phases of clinical trials

| Phase | 1 | 2 | 3 | 4 |
|---|---|---|---|---|
| Number of subjects | 20–80 | 100–300 | 1,000–3,000 | Multitudes postmarketing |
| Purpose | Evaluate safety<br>Determine dosage<br>Identify side effects | Evaluate safety<br>Determine effectiveness | Collect more information about safe usage<br>Confirm effectiveness<br>Monitor side effects<br>Compare to alternatives | Collect data on effect on specific groups (population)<br>Monitor long-term side effects |

*Source:* NIH n.d.

smoking (Gordis 1996). If he had wanted to explore the relationship further, he would have compared the smoking histories of a group of his lung cancer patients with a group of his patients without lung cancer. This would be a case-control study. Research designs that are considered observational are cross-sectional studies, prospective cohort studies, retrospective cohort studies, and case-control studies. The element of time frame cuts across all types of designs. There are two pairs of time frames—retrospective versus prospective and cross-sectional versus longitudinal. Retrospective looks back in time to collect data regarding observations that happened, while prospective looks forward to collect data on observations to happen. A longitudinal time frame requires collecting data at multiple points in time. Examples include studies of breast cancer and cardiovascular disease, such as Nurses' Health Study, which has followed the health of more than 238,000 nurses since 1976 (Colditz et al. 1997). Cross-sectional designs involve collecting data during observation at one point in time, versus multiple points in time.

A major purpose of epidemiological studies is to determine risk. In prospective studies, a 2 × 2 table is a tool used to evaluate the association between exposure and disease. (See table 19.2.) The table is a cross-classification of exposure status and disease status. The total number of individuals with the disease is $a + c$, and the total number without disease is $b + d$. The total number exposed is $a + b$, and the total number not exposed is $c + d$.

The number of individuals who had both exposure and the disease, is recorded in cell $a$; the number who had exposure, but no disease, is recorded in cell $b$; the number who had the disease, but no exposure, is recorded in cell $c$; and the number who had neither the disease nor exposure is recorded in cell $d$.

## Cross-Sectional Studies

In a cross-sectional study, both the exposure and the disease outcome are determined at the same time in each subject. A cross-sectional study may also be referred to as a prevalence study because it describes characteristics and health outcomes at a particular point in time. It provides quantitative estimates of the magnitude of a problem. After the population has been defined, the presence or absence of exposure and of disease can be established for everyone in the study. Each subject is then categorized into one of four subgroups that correspond to the 2 × 2 table that appears in table 19.3. An example of a cross-sectional study is determining the prevalence rate of individuals who receive yearly eye exams with type 2 diabetes mellitus.

The prevalence of disease in persons with exposure ($a/a + b$) is compared with persons without exposure ($c/c + d$). Alternatively, the prevalence of exposure in persons with the disease ($a/a + c$) is compared to the prevalence of exposure to persons without the disease ($b/b + d$).

A major advantage of the cross-sectional study is that it is relatively easy to conduct and may produce results in a short period of time. The disadvantage is that because exposure and disease are determined at the same time in each subject, the time relationship between exposure and onset of the disease cannot be established. It describes only what exists at the time of the study.

## Case-Control Studies

Case-control (retrospective) studies are a major component of epidemiological research. In them, persons with a certain condition (cases) and persons without the condition (controls) are studied by looking back in time. The objective is to determine the frequency of the risk factor among the cases and the frequency of the risk factor among the controls to determine possible causes of the disease. In a case-control study, if there is an association between exposure and disease, the prevalence of history of exposure will be higher in persons with the disease (cases) than in those without

**Table 19.2.** 2 × 2 table for classifying disease status and exposure status

|  |  | Disease status | | |
|---|---|---|---|---|
|  |  | Yes | No | Total |
| Exposure status | Yes | a | b | a + b |
|  | No | c | d | c + d |
|  |  | a + c | b + d | a + b + c + d |

**Table 19.3.** 2 × 2 table for cross-sectional studies

|  | Disease | No disease | Totals | Prevalence of disease for exposed/not exposed |
|---|---|---|---|---|
| Exposed | a | b | a + b | a/a + b |
| Not exposed | c | d | c + d | c/c + d |
| Totals | a + c | b + d | a + b + c + d | a + b + c + d |
| Prevalence of exposure for disease/no disease | a/a + c | b/b + d |  |  |

Group a: Persons exposed with the disease
Group b: Persons exposed without the disease
Group c: Persons with the disease, but not exposed
Group d: Persons without disease and without exposure

it (controls). For a case-control study, see the 2 × 2 table in table 19.4. The proportion of cases exposed is $a/a + c$, and the proportion of controls exposed is $b/b + d$. For example, a researcher may be interested in examining the relationship between cell phone use and brain cancer. The researcher selects the cases as those individuals with brain cancer and the controls as those individuals without brain cancer but very much like the cases in all other characteristics. When selecting the controls, the researcher may choose a sibling or friend of the cases, if he or she does not have brain cancer. Then, the researcher may review cell phone records or conduct a person-to-person interview asking them questions about their past cell phone use. After gathering the data, the researcher will determine the odds ratios. The odds ratio is the probability that a certain outcome will occur if an individual is exposed to a certain variable or risk factor. This finding is then compared to the odds that a certain outcome will occur for those individuals not exposed to that variable or risk factor. For example, if the odds ratio is five, the researcher can conclude that those individuals who use cell phones are five times more likely to develop brain cancer than those individuals who do not use cell phones (see Risk Assessment later in the chapter).

The advantages of case-control studies are that they are easy to conduct and cost-effective, with minimal risk to the subjects. Also, existing records may be used to conduct the studies. Case-control studies also allow the researcher to study multiple causes of disease. Although the use of existing health records is advantageous, there are problems associated with using them for retrospective research. One major problem is that the cases are based on hospital admissions. Admissions are based on patient characteristics, severity of illness and associated conditions, and admission policies. These vary from hospital to hospital, making standardization of the study difficult. In addition, there are problems related to poor documentation, illegibility, and missing records. Lack of consistency in diagnostic and clinical services between hospitals also makes comparability difficult. Further, validation of the information can be difficult. An important aspect of epidemiological studies is the identification of risk. In studies using medical records, the population at risk is generally not defined.

## Cohort Studies

A cohort study is a prospective study in which the investigator selects a group of exposed individuals and unexposed individuals who are followed for a period to compare the incidence of disease in the two groups. The length of time for follow-up varies from a few days for acute diseases to several decades for cancer and cardiac diseases. For a cohort study, see the 2 × 2 table in table 19.5. If there is an association between exposure and disease, the incidence of disease is greater in the exposed group ($a/a + b$) than in the unexposed group ($c/c + d$). New cases of the disease are identified as they occur so it can be determined whether a time relationship exists between exposure to disease and development of disease. The time relationship must be established if the exposure is to be considered the cause of the disease.

One of the most famous cohort studies is the Framingham Study, which began in the 1950s (Framingham Heart Study n.d.). The research project was designed to monitor the incidence of coronary artery disease in more than 5,000 residents who were examined every two years for a period of 20 years. This study has provided important data demonstrating the relationship between the development of heart disease and risk factors such as smoking, obesity, diet, and high blood pressure.

Cohort studies offer several advantages. First, the researcher can control the data collection process throughout the study. Also, outcome events can be checked as they occur; and many outcomes can be studied, including those that were not anticipated at the start of the study. The disadvantages of cohort studies include high cost and a long wait for the study

### Table 19.4. 2 × 2 table for case-control studies

|  | Cases (with disease) | Controls (without disease) |
|---|---|---|
| Exposed | a | b |
| Not exposed | c | d |
| Total | a + c | b + d |
| Proportions exposed | a/a + c | b/b + d |

Group a: Persons exposed with the disease
Group b: Persons exposed without the disease
Group c: Persons with the disease, but not exposed
Group d: Persons without disease and without exposure

### Table 19.5. 2 × 2 table for cohort studies

|  | Disease develops | Disease does not develop | Totals | Incidence rates of disease |
|---|---|---|---|---|
| Exposed | a | b | a + b | a/a + b |
| Not exposed | c | d | c + d | c/c + d |

Group a: Persons exposed with the disease
Group b: Persons exposed without the disease
Group c: Persons with the disease, but not exposed
Group d: Persons without disease and without exposure

results. Also, subjects may be lost to death, withdrawal, or lack of follow-up.

One difference between case-control and cohort studies is that the former is a retrospective study, and the latter is a prospective study. A retrospective study is conducted by reviewing records from the past; a prospective study is designed to observe events that occur after the subjects have been identified. The advantages and disadvantages of retrospective and prospective studies are outlined in table 19.6.

Another difference is that in a cohort study, the subjects are individuals with or without the disease and the focus is disease status; in the case-control study, the subjects are individuals who have been exposed or not exposed to the disease and the focus is exposure status.

## Risk Assessment

As stated earlier, one objective of epidemiological studies is to assess risk. Risk is the probability that an individual develops a disease over a specified period, provided that he or she did not die as a result of some other disease process during the same time period. It is usually expressed as relative risk (RR). Before risk can be assessed properly, prevalence and incidence should be defined. Prevalence refers to the number of existing cases of a particular disease. Incidence refers to the number of new cases of a disease. The prevalence rate is therefore the number of existing cases of disease in a particular region during a specific time divided by the number of individuals in the specific region for a specific time. The incidence rate is the number of new cases of disease in a particular region during a specific time divided by the number of individuals in the specific region for a specific time. RR is calculated from cohort studies and compares the risk of some disease in two groups differentiated by some demographic variable such as sex or race. The group of interest is referred to as the exposed group and the comparison group is the unexposed group. The risk ratio is calculated as:

$$\frac{\text{Risk for exposed group or the incidence rate of the exposed group}}{\text{Risk for unexposed group or the incidence rate of the unexposed group}}$$

An RR of 1.0 indicates that there is identical risk in both groups. An RR that is greater than 1.0 indicates an increased risk for the exposed group; an RR of less than 1.0 indicates a decreased risk for the exposed group.

### Odds Ratio

In a case-control study, the primary aim is to identify differences in exposure frequency associated with one group having the disease under study and the other group not having it. The incidence of disease in the exposed and unexposed populations is not known because persons with the disease (cases) and without the disease (controls) are identified at the onset of the study. Thus, RR cannot be calculated directly. So, the question becomes, what are the odds that an exposed person will develop the disease? Or, put another way, what are the odds that a nonexposed person will develop the disease?

In a case-control study, the odds ratio compares the odds that the cases were exposed to the disease with the odds that the controls were exposed. Using the 2 × 2 table in table 19.4 as a reference, the odds ratio is calculated as:

**Table 19.6.** Advantages and disadvantages of study designs

| Retrospective study (e.g., case-control study) | |
|---|---|
| **Advantages** | **Disadvantages** |
| Short study time | Control group subject to bias in selection |
| Relatively inexpensive | Biased recall possible |
| Suitable for rare diseases | Cannot determine incidence rate |
| Ethical problems minimal | Relative risk is approximate |
| Hospital medical record may be used | |
| Potential large sample of subjects | |
| No attrition problems | |
| **Prospective study (e.g., cohort study)** | |
| Control group less susceptible to bias | Requires more time |
| No recall necessary | Costly |
| Incidence rate can be determined | Relatively common diseases only |
| Relative risk is accurate | Ethical problems may be considerable and influence study design |
| | Volunteers needed |
| | Results may not be generalizable to a larger population |
| | Requires many subjects |
| | Problems with attrition |

$$\frac{(a/a+c)}{(b/b+d)}$$
or
$$\frac{(ad)}{(bc)}$$

The odds ratio measures the odds of exposure of a given disease. For example, an odds ratio of 1.0 indicates that the incidence of disease is equal in each group; thus, the exposure may not be a risk factor for the disease of interest. An odds ratio of 2.0 indicates that the cases were twice as likely to be exposed as the controls. This implies that the exposure is associated with twice the risk of disease.

### Attributable Risk

The **attributable risk (AR)** is a measure of the public health impact of a causative factor on a population. In this measure, the assumption is that the occurrence of a disease in an unexposed group is the baseline or expected risk for that disease. Any risk above that level in the exposed group is attributed to exposure to the risk factor. It is assumed that some individuals will acquire a disease, such as lung cancer, whether they were exposed to a risk factor, such as smoking, or not. The AR measures the additional risk of illness resulting from an individual's exposure to a risk factor. The AR is calculated as risk for the exposed group minus the risk for the unexposed group. AR percent is calculated as follows:

$$\frac{(\text{Risk for exposed group}) - AR = (\text{Risk for unexposed group})}{\text{Risk for exposed group}} \times 100$$

## Check Your Understanding 19.3

**Answer the following questions in a separate document.**

1. A researcher conducting a study related to exposure to certain environmental factors and the odds of disease prevalence finds that individuals who were exposed to these factors have an odds ratio of 3.7. How would you interpret this finding?

2. In the second quarter of 2024, City D reported 1,800 new cases of COVID-19. What epidemiological measure does this represent, and why is it important for public health monitoring and response?

3. Construct a 2 × 2 table for a case-control study involving individuals with and without a diagnosis of hypertension and whether each group eats fast food >2 times per week. Conduct the odds ratio based on the odds of exposure in each group.

4. How would you interpret an RR of 2.5?

5. How is the Privacy Rule being violated in the following scenario?

   A researcher at Hospital A has been investigating the impact of prescribed supplements on anxiety disorders for the past three years. The researcher has obtained IRB approval and obtained signed authorizations from a group of patients to use their medical records for the purpose of the study. Since the conclusion of anxiety-related research project, the researcher has started using the medical record data to explore the relationship of prescribed supplements on sleep apnea.

## Use of Comparative Data in Outcomes Research

Healthcare organizations such as the **National Committee for Quality Assurance (NCQA)** and the Joint Commission have developed measures for evaluating the effectiveness of healthcare providers. The NCQA is a "private, not-for-profit organization dedicated to improving healthcare quality. Since its founding in 1990, NCQA has been a central figure in driving improvement throughout the healthcare system, helping to elevate the issue of healthcare quality to the top of the national agenda" (NCQA n.d.). The purpose of the measures developed by the NCQA is to provide purchasers of healthcare, primarily employers, with information about the cost and effectiveness of organizations with which they contract for services.

The Joint Commission measures are designed primarily to encourage organizations to improve their own performance and to provide a comprehensive picture of the care provided within the organization.

## Comparative Effectiveness Research

It is increasingly accepted within healthcare that what works best in the care and treatment of one patient or group of patients may not work best with another individual or group. One research approach that is used to understand these variances and determine evidence-based best practices is comparative effectiveness research (CER). This type of research is typically performed in real-world clinical settings versus being research based on theoretical frameworks. The purpose of CER is the "generation and synthesis of evidence that compares the benefits and harms of alternative methods to prevent, diagnose, treat, and monitor a clinical condition or to improve the delivery of care. CER is meant to help consumers, clinicians, purchasers, and policy makers make informed decisions that will improve healthcare at both the individual and population levels" (IOM 2009). Findings from CER can not only inform the risks and benefits of treatment options, as examples, but can also illustrate the costs of such options.

In recent years, there has been debate about the risks of cesarean section versus vaginal delivery of newborns, and there is a growing body of knowledge on the subject. Hospitals and obstetricians, as well as patients and others, have a stake in this topic because issues addressed in these debates include patient safety, quality of care, reimbursement rates, autonomy in patient decision-making, and provider decision-making. In one CER study about the benefits and risks of vaginal versus cesarean births researchers from the Department of Obstetrics and Gynecology at the Johns Hopkins School of Medicine found that cesarean section births are associated with higher instances of respiratory distress and Apgar scores of 7 or less in newborns (Werner et al. 2013).

## Patient-Centered Outcomes Research Institute (PCORI)

CER has gained attention in recent years because of the Patient-Centered Outcomes Research Institute (PCORI). PCORI is an entity funded through the Patient-Centered Research Trust Fund and was established by the Patient Protection and Affordable Care Act (ACA) of 2010 (ACA 2010).

PCORI was established to provide evidence that assists patients and healthcare providers in making informed decisions about prevention and treatment options, based on research and comparative evidence that supports these choices. The major difference in this type of research is patients playing a major role in the types of research conducted and receiving clear and easy to understand information and research results. These studies compare medications, medical devices, assistive technologies, surgeries, and such to determine the best ways to provide healthcare to patients. The National Strategy for Quality Improvement of Healthcare (2016) was developed by the HHS as part of the ACA. It sets priorities and a strategic plan for quality improvement of healthcare in the US. The Hospital Consumer Assessment of Healthcare Providers and Systems (HCAHPS), under Medicare, now requires all hospitals to publicly report standardized information on the perspectives of all patients to include the patient experience and patient satisfaction in the quality reporting. The AHRQ has established a patient-centered care improvement guide. It provides best practices to assist hospitals in moving toward patient-centered care. It also provides evidence behind these best practices and examines barriers to establishing patient-centered care.

A major part of patient-centered research is developing questions important to patients and providers of care. Such questions include the following:

- Given my personal characteristics, conditions, and preferences, what should I expect will happen to me?
- What are my options, and what are the benefits and harms of those options?
- What can I do to improve the outcomes that are most important to me?
- How can the healthcare system improve my chances of achieving the outcomes I prefer?

To answer these questions, PCORI will do the following:

1. Assess benefits and harms to inform decision-making, highlighting comparisons that matter to people
2. Focus on outcomes that people notice and care about
3. Incorporate a wide variety of settings and diversity of participants (PCORI n.d.)

A patient-centered research question should include the following elements:

1. Population of patients and research participants
2. Intervention(s) relevant to patients in target population
3. Comparator(s) (usual care or no specific intervention) relevant to patients in target population

4. Outcomes meaningful to patients in target population
5. Timing: outcomes and length of follow-up
6. Setting and providers (PCORI n.d.)

PCORI explains that people sometimes care about outcomes that are different than the outcomes of interest to investigators (PCORI n.d.). They care about things they notice such as pain and fatigue levels even though these elements may be more difficult to measure. For example, when measuring the outcomes related to a new drug for cancer, investigators may measure the difference in blood markers, while patients will focus on the end result of nausea.

The role and goal of PCORI is to redirect research investigations so they include patient-centered outcomes such as nausea, pain, and functional status, and other scientific elements that may be important. PCORI strives to engage the end users to help shape the research so the outcomes matter to them—survival, function, symptoms, and health-related quality of life, versus biomarkers, chemistry panels, and cost of end-of-life care.

A priority of the National Quality Strategy in Person and Family-Centered Care is to increase the use of EHRs that capture the voice of the patient by integrating patient-generated data in EHRs and routinely measuring patient engagement, self-management, shared decision-making, and patient-reported outcomes. One of its indicators for doing this is to collect the percentage of patients asked for feedback. This is an example of how the EHR will be used to demonstrate at what rate the patient is involved in his or her care, and patient-centered outcomes research will be a major component in this data analysis.

Therefore, the HIM professional will play a vital role in making effective decisions about how to incorporate patient- and family-centered data within the EHR so research in this area can be continued and needed outcomes generated.

### Check Your Understanding 19.4

**Answer the following questions in a separate document.**

1. As Blue Cross initiates contract negotiations with a local healthcare organization, which set of measures are they likely to prioritize, NCQA or Joint Commission, and for what reason?
2. How does Comparative Effectiveness Research (CER) contribute to improving patient outcomes, and what are some challenges faced in conducting CER studies?
3. How does the National Quality Strategy in Person and Family-Centered Care plan to increase the use of the EHR in patient-centered care?
4. What is the major focus of PCORI? Why do you think this is important to patients?
5. How is patient-centered outcomes research different than research historically performed by investigators?

## References

ACA (Patient Protection and Affordable Care Act). 2010. http://housedocs.house.gov/energycommerce/ppacacon.pdf.

Beecher, H. K. 1966. Consent in clinical experimentation: Myth and reality. *Journal of the American Medical Association* 195(1):34–35. http://www.ncbi.nlm.nih.gov/pubmed/5951827.

CDC (Centers for Disease Control and Prevention). 2022. "US Public Health Service Syphilis Study at Tuskegee—The Tuskegee Timeline." http://www.cdc.gov/tuskegee/timeline.htm.

Colditz, G. A., J. E. Manson, and S. E. Hankinson. 1997. "The Nurses' Health Study: 20-year contribution to the understanding of health among women." *Journal of Women's Health* 6(1):49–62.

Durieux. B. N., M. DeCamp, and C. Lindvall. 2022. 21st Century Cures Act: Ethical recommendations for new patient-facing products. *Journal of the American Medical Informatics Association* 29(10):1818–1822. https://pubmed.ncbi.nlm.nih.gov/35876830/.

Framingham Heart Study. n.d. Accessed June 8, 2024. http://www.framinghamheartstudy.org.

HHS (Department of Health and Human Services). 2022. "HHS Instruction 42-3: Senior Biomedical Research and Biomedical Product Assessment Service." https://www.hhs.gov/about/agencies/asa/ohr/hr-library/42-3-sbrbpas/index.html.

HHS (Department of Health and Human Services). 2022. "Summary of the HIPAA Privacy Rule." Office for Civil Rights, Health Information Privacy. https://www.hhs.gov/hipaa/for-professionals/privacy/laws-regulations/index.html.

HHS (Department of Health and Human Services). 2020. "History." Office of Human Research Protections. https://www.hhs.gov/ohrp/about-ohrp/history/index.html.

HHS (Department of Health and Human Services). 2016. "Organization." Office of Human Research Protections. https://www.hhs.gov/ohrp/about-ohrp/organization/index.html.

HHS (Department of Health and Human Services). 2017. "Revised Common Rule." https://www.hhs.gov/ohrp/regulations-and-policy/regulations/finalized-revisions-common-rule/index.html.

HHS (Department of Health and Human Services). 2015. Federal policy for the protection of human subjects. *Federal Register* 80(173). https://www.govinfo.gov/content/pkg/FR-2015-09-08/pdf/2015-21756.pdf.

HHS (Department of Health and Humans Services). 2011. Human subjects research protections: Enhancing protections for research subjects and reducing burden, delay and ambiguity for investigators. *Federal Register* 76(143). http://www.gpo.gov/fdsys/pkg/FR-2011-07-26/pdf/2011-18792.pdf.

HHS (Department of Health and Human Services). 1979. *The Belmont Report: Ethical Principles and Guidelines for the Protection of Human Subjects of Research*. https://www.hhs.gov/ohrp/regulations-and-policy/belmont-report/index.html.

IOM (Institute of Medicine). 2009. *Initial National Priorities for Comparative Effectiveness Research*. Washington, DC: National Academies Press.

NCQA (National Committee for Quality Assurance). n.d. "About NCQA." Accessed June 8, 2024. http://www.ncqa.org/about-ncqa.

NIH (National Institutes of Health). 2004a. "Clinical Research and the HIPAA Privacy Rule." https://privacyruleandresearch.nih.gov/clin_research.asp.

NIH (National Institutes of Health). 2004b. "HIPAA Authorization for Research." NIH Pub. No. 04-5529. http://privacyruleandresearch.nih.gov/authorization.asp.

NIH (National Institute of Health). 2004c. "Institutional Review Boards and the HIPAA Privacy Rule." NIH Pub. No. 03-5428. http://privacyruleandresearch.nih.gov/irbandprivacyrule.asp.

NIH (National Institutes of Health). n.d. Accessed May 14, 2024. http://clinicaltrials.gov.

NIH (National Institutes of Health). n.d. "NIH Inclusion Outreach Toolkit: How to Engage, Recruit, and Retain Women in Clinical Research: NIH Definitions." Accessed May 14, 2024. https://orwh.od.nih.gov/toolkit/nih-policies-inclusion/definitions.

National Strategy for Quality Improvement in Healthcare. 2016. https://archive.ahrq.gov/workingforquality/reports/2016_ahrq-agencyspecificplan.pdf.

Nuremberg Code. 1949. Reprinted in *Trials of War Criminals before the Nuremberg Military Tribunals under Control Council Law* no. *10 Nuernberg, October 1946–April 1949*. Washington, DC: US Government Printing Office. https://www.loc.gov/item/2011525364/.

ORI (Office of Research Integrity). 2008. "Final Report: Observing and Reporting Suspected Misconduct in Biomedical Research." https://ori.hhs.gov/sites/default/files/gallup_finalreport.pdf.

ORI (Office of Research Integrity). n.d.a. "Historical Background." Accessed September 5, 2024. http://ori.hhs.gov/historical-background.

ORI (Office of Research Integrity). n.d.b. "About ORI." Accessed September 5, 2024. http://ori.hhs.gov/about-ori.

PCORI (Patient-Centered Outcomes Research Institute). n.d. "About PCORI." Accessed November 14, 2023. https://www.pcori.org/about/about-pcori.

Research and Educational Trust. n.d. "Health Services Research." Accessed September 5, 2024. https://www.hsr.org/hsr-journal.

Senn, C. 2023 (October 17). Revolutionizing clinical research: The profound impact of AI. *Clinical Researcher* 37(5). https://acrpnet.org/2023/10/revolutionizing-clinical-research-the-profound-impact-of-ai/.

University of Pittsburgh. 2023a. "Welcome University of Pittsburgh and UPMC Researchers." https://www.citi.pitt.edu/.

University of Pittsburgh. 2023b. "Chapter 7: IRB Committee Membership." *Human Research Protection Office, Policies and Procedures*. https://www.hrpo.pitt.edu/policies-and-procedures/chapter-7-irb-committee-membership.

University of Pittsburgh. 2020. "Chapter 20: Conflict of Interest." *Human Research Protection Office, Policies and Procedures*. https://www.hrpo.pitt.edu/policies-and-procedures/chapter-20-conflict-interest.

University of Pittsburgh. 2021. "Chapter 22: Education and Training." *Human Research Protection Office, Policies and Procedures*. https://www.hrpo.pitt.edu/policies-and-procedures/chapter-22-education-and-training.

University of Pittsburgh. 2021a. "Chapter 17: Reportable New Information." *Human Research Protection Office, Policies and Procedures*. https://www.hrpo.pitt.edu/policies-and-procedures/chapter-17-reportable-new-information.

Werner, E., C. Han, D. Savitz, M. Goldshore, and H. Lipkind. 2013. Health outcomes for vaginal compared with cesarean delivery of appropriately grown preterm neonates. *Obstetrics and Genecology* 121(6). https://www.ncbi.nlm.nih.gov/pubmed/23812452.

WMA (World Medical Association). 2013. "Declaration of Helsinki Ethical Principles for Medical Research Involving Human Subjects." https://www.wma.net/policies-post/wma-declaration-of-helsinki-ethical-principles-for-medical-research-involving-human-subjects/.

21 CFR 56: IRBs. 2015.

21 CFR 50: Protection of human subjects. 2015.

21 CFR 56.110: Expedited review procedures for certain kinds of research involving no more than minimal risk, and for minor changes in approved research. 2015 (April 1).

21 CFR 56.111(b): IRB. 2015 (April 1).

42 CFR 493: Public Health Service Act laboratory requirements. 1990 (March 14).

45 CFR 46: Protection of human subjects. 2009 (July 14).

45 CFR 46.101(b)(1–6): To what does this policy apply? 2009 (July 14).

45 CFR 46.102: Definitions. 2009 (July 14).

45 CFR 46.103: Assuring compliance with this policy–research conducted or supported by any federal department or agency. 2009 (July 14).

45 CFR 46.110: Expedited Review Procedures for certain kinds of research involving no more than minimal risk and for minor changes in approved research. 2009 (July 14).

45 CFR 46.111: Criteria for IRB approval of research. 2009 (July 14).

45 CFR 46.115: IRB records. 2009 (July 14).

45 CFR 46.116: General requirements for informed consent. 2009 (July 14).

# PART IV

# Organizational Management and Leadership

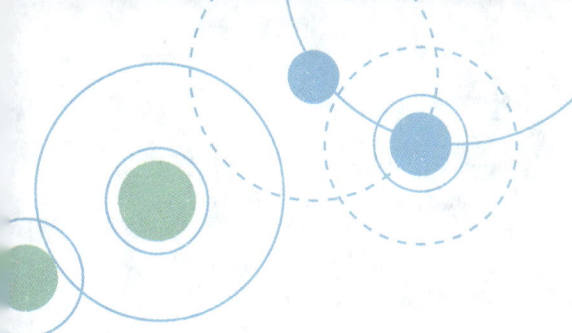

# Chapter 20

# Leadership and Management Theories and Strategies

*Pamela K. Oachs, MA, RHIA, CHDA, FAHIMA, and Amy Watters, EdD, RHIA, FAHIMA*

## Learning Objectives

- Synthesize how the evolution of management theory has formed the management discipline
- Apply situation-based approach to management and leadership
- Evaluate the relationship between skills needed for each level of management and key management functions
- Create a plan for introducing change to staff addressing the impact of the change at various stages
- Differentiate between the actions of managers versus leaders within an organization
- Assess the key ideas of prominent leadership theories

## Key Terms

Administrative management theory
Autocratic leadership
Bureaucracy
Business process reengineering (BPR)
Champion
Change agent
Change driver
Cognitive complexity
Complex adaptive system
Conceptual skills
Controlling
Critic
Democratic leadership
Discipline
Early adopter
Early majority
85/15 rule
Emotional intelligence (EI)
Esprit de corps
Evidence-based management
Exchange relationship
Executive dashboard
Expectancy theory of motivation
Goal
Great person theory
Hawthorne effect
In-group
Innovator
Interpersonal skills
Inventor
Laggard
Late majority
Leader–member exchange (LMX)
Line authority
Management by objectives (MBO)
Maslow's Hierarchy of Needs
Mission statement
Operations management
Organization development (OD)
Organizational chart
Organizing
Out-group
Path–goal theory
Piece-rate incentive
Role
Role theory
Scalar chain
Scientific management
Servant leadership
Situational theory of leadership
Socioeconomic approach to management (SEAM)
Span of control
Sponsor
Staff authority
Systems thinking

Technical skills
Theory X
Theory Y
Theory Z
Time and motion studies
Total quality management (TQM)
Trait approach
Unity of command
Values statement
Values-based leadership
Vertical dyad linkage (VDL)
Vision statement
Worker immaturity–maturity

Management theories are ways of describing how managers think about the way organizations work, which in turn influence their decisions and direct their efforts and behavior. The theories described in this chapter reflect the development of management theories from the early 1900s to the present, including newer, developing approaches. Many elements of even the early theories are still practiced widely. By identifying working theories, managers may evaluate how appropriate these theories are for the setting and how they can be revised to work better.

A key idea is that management theories and practices grow out of the unique intersection of forces or **change drivers** that operate at the time. Change drivers are large-scale forces such as demographic, social, political, economic, technical, and more recently, global and informational factors that require organizations of all sizes to revise how they operate. Management theories assist leaders to more effectively and efficiently allocate resources to respond to these changes.

In this first section of the chapter, some of the key historical and theoretical developments in management are summarized, many of which are still used in organizations today. The functions, skills, and roles of managers are identified, along with trends in management theory. Leadership of the organization will be examined through the evolution of leadership theories and how the transition can be facilitated during organization change.

## Landmarks in Management as a Discipline

Management is a **discipline**, a field of study characterized by a knowledge base and perspective that are distinctive from other fields of study. The knowledge base and perspective, principles and practices, and code of conduct form a foundation for the field. Over time, changing social conditions and growing technological innovations have contributed to the way the management discipline has evolved and management theories are framed (see figure 20.1).

### Scientific Management (1880–1920)

The late 19th and early 20th centuries marked the emergence of scientific management concepts. **Scientific management** was an early effort to apply scientific principles and practices to business processes. The concepts of bureaucracy, efficiency, and project management were developed during this period and are still relevant today.

#### Bureaucracy

Management theory emerged with the onset of the Industrial Revolution in the mid-19th century and initially took the form of scientific management. During this period, political economist Max Weber recognized the variability in production standards that lead to inefficiencies and proposed that organizations be structured as **bureaucracy**. Clear hierarchies of roles, relationships, rules, and regulations to standardize behavior, and the use of trained specialists for jobs typified this form of organization. Consequently, the subjective judgment and favoritism bias of earlier organizations could be eliminated, and planning could be based on the position and task rather than the person and personal preferences. Large organizations are often structured as bureaucracies in which authority is hierarchically organized—with a rigid division of labor, rigid rules and regulations, and impersonal culture. In the modern marketplace, including the healthcare market, where competitive advantage is maintained through innovation, such bureaucracy has come more often to refer to slow decision-making, unresponsiveness, lack of appreciation for the uniqueness of individuals, a culture which discourages innovation, and rules without reasons.

#### Efficiency

Around the same time ideas about bureaucracy were being formed, Frederick W. Taylor discovered that his company and most others had tremendous unused potential. Pay and working conditions were poor, waste and inefficiency were prevalent, and management decision-making was unsystematic and not based on research of any sort. Taylor proposed that organizations

**Figure 20.1.** Foundations of management timeline

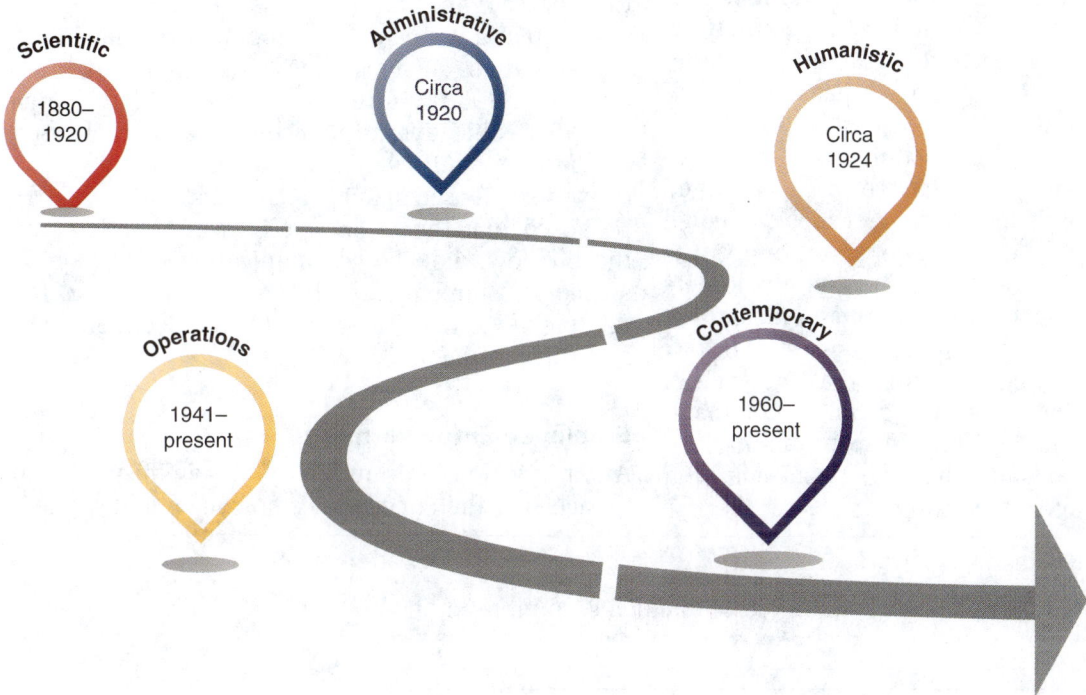

observe and study how jobs were performed and then streamline the actions to be more efficient. He conducted **time and motion studies** in which tasks were subdivided into their most basic movements. Detailed motions were timed to determine the most efficient way of carrying them out. After the "one best way" was found, the best worker match for the job was hired, tools and procedures were standardized, instruction cards were written to guide workers, and breaks were instituted to reduce fatigue. Taylor also developed a **piece-rate incentive** system in which workers received additional pay when they exceeded the standard output level for their task. In addition to task analysis and specialization which are still relevant today, Taylorism also established an awareness that organizational layers and professions must communicate more efficiently across departments and specialties to avoid silos and fragmentation of work.

In the early 1900s, when time and motion studies became popular, Frank and Lillian Gilbreth developed many of the early ideas of ergonomics—the study of people working efficiently—and their work identified how unnecessary or inefficient motions could be reduced. This resulted in higher productivity, less fatigue, and better planning.

### Project Management

As productivity increased in the early 1900s, managing more complex projects, maintaining time schedules, and coordinating multiple tasks became essential. A tool still used today, the Gantt chart, was developed by Henry Gantt in 1915. This task-by-time chart is used for project management and healthcare operations management to show how the components of a task are scheduled over time (Langabeer and Helton 2020). See figure 20.2 for an example of a basic Gantt chart showing an initial electronic health record (EHR) implementation timeline.

## Administrative Management (Circa 1920s)

Attempting to compensate for the theory of scientific management's exclusion of senior management, the **administrative management theory** proposed a rational approach to designing organizations, with formal structure, clear division of labor, and use of delegation. It argued that management was a profession and could be learned. This theory gave rise to identifying the key functions of management, clarification of the executive role, and employee empowerment.

### Key Functions of Management

Henri Fayol was a French mining engineer whose major contribution includes a description of the key functions of management and 14 principles for organizational design and administration.

Fayol's management functions have persisted with some variation into modern organizations, including healthcare, and identify key functions that define the manager's role. Fayol's managerial functions include planning, organizing, leading, and controlling.

Like his four managerial functions, most of Fayol's 14 principles of management have been incorporated into modern organizations and are widely accepted today (see figure 20.3). For example, authority was proposed as the right of an executive to give orders and expect obedience. **Unity of command** meant that each employee reports to only one boss. The **scalar chain**, or line of authority, ensured that everyone in the organization appears in the chain of command and reports to someone. **Esprit de corps** emphasized the work climate in which harmony, cohesion, and high morale promoted good work.

### The Executive Role

Chester Barnard, an American business executive and public administrator, elaborated on the role of top executives in his classic book, *Functions of the Executive* (1938). He emphasized formulating organizational objectives, establishing a system of essential services, and even envisioning an early version of evidence-based management (Barnard 1938). He proposed that the leader receives information from those below, that the communication system be designed and implemented by the executive, and that the role of middle management is to implement plans and solve problems.

### Employee Empowerment

Another major contribution to the administrative approach was the concept of employee empowerment.

**Figure 20.2.** Gantt chart showing sequence of initial EHR implementation timeline

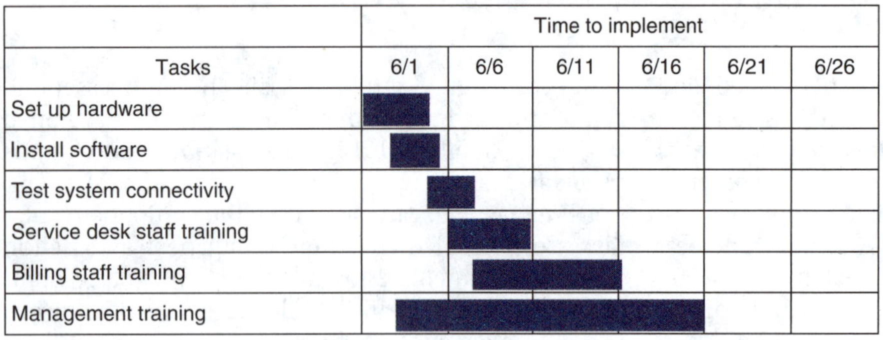

| Tasks | Time to implement | | | | | |
|---|---|---|---|---|---|---|
|  | 6/1 | 6/6 | 6/11 | 6/16 | 6/21 | 6/26 |
| Set up hardware | ■ |  |  |  |  |  |
| Install software |  | ■ |  |  |  |  |
| Test system connectivity |  | ■ |  |  |  |  |
| Service desk staff training |  | ■ ■ |  |  |  |  |
| Billing staff training |  |  | ■ ■ |  |  |  |
| Management training |  | ■ ■ ■ ■ |  |  |  |  |

**Figure 20.3.** Fayol's 14 principles

1. *Specialization of labor:* Work allocation and specialization allow concentrated activities, deeper understanding, and better efficiency.
2. *Authority:* The person to whom responsibilities are given has the right to give direction and expect obedience.
3. *Discipline:* The smooth operation of a business requires standards, rules, and values for consistency of action.
4. *Unity of command:* Every employee receives direction and instructions from only one boss.
5. *Unity of direction:* All workers are aligned in their efforts toward a single outcome.
6. *Subordination of individual interests:* Accomplishing shared values and organizational goals take priority over individual agendas.
7. *Remuneration:* Employees should receive fair pay for work.
8. *Centralization:* Decisions are made at the top.
9. *Scalar chain:* Everyone is clearly included in the chain of command and line of authority from top to bottom of the organization.
10. *Order:* People should clearly understand where they fit in the organization, and all people and material have a place.
11. *Equity:* People are treated fairly, and a sense of justice should pervade the organization.
12. *Tenure:* Turnover is undesirable, and loyalty to the organization is sought.
13. *Initiative:* Personal initiative should be encouraged.
14. *Esprit de corps:* Harmony, cohesion, teamwork, and good interpersonal relationships should be encouraged.

*Source:* Fayol 1917.

In contrast to what was often considered a mechanistic view of workers by Frederick Taylor, Mary Parker Follett (1868–1933), one of the first women pioneers in management theory, was interested in broader social ideas and championed the role of relationships and conflict in organizations. Although she drew mixed attention in the late 1920s, she foresaw the development of a systems view of business, the role of empowered employees in organization development (OD), and the use of workgroups to implement solutions. Follett promoted using teamwork and creative group effort, involving people in OD, and integrating the organization, which involved many elements of systems management theory (Parker 1984).

## Humanistic Management (Circa 1924)

Although the US has always touted itself as the home of democracy, the equity of power in the workplace has not always existed. By the early 1900s, there were growing social pressures to treat workers in a more enlightened and respectful manner. Barnard's and Follett's ideas that people should be treated fairly and that effective controls come from individual workers, formed the basis for a shift in management thought. Concepts such as the Hawthorne effect, the hierarchy of needs, and theories X and Y illustrate this shift.

### The Hawthorne Studies

Between 1927 and 1932, Elton Mayo, Franz Roethlisberger, and others from Harvard University conducted a series of experiments at the Western Electric Hawthorne Works in Chicago. The studies originally were designed to explore how fatigue and monotony affected job productivity and how these might be mitigated by breaks, variable work hours, temperature, humidity, and lighting. Although performance increased when desirable conditions were increased, unexpectedly, performance also improved when these conditions were reduced. The researchers concluded that human factors made the difference: receiving attention during the study, freedom to participate, and feeling important by being singled out for participation in the project—the so-called Hawthorne effect (Landsberger 1958). This popularized study gave strong impetus to the consideration of social factors at work. In healthcare, the Hawthorne effect (also called the observer effect) is based on the principle that what gets attention and measured is what gets improved, and that is a key concern to increasing patient satisfaction (Gandolf n.d.).

### Human Resources Management

In the 1950s, the psychology field in the US was just coming to prominence, as were theories of motivation. Observing that many problems were derived from an inability to meet needs, Abraham Maslow (1908–1970) suggested that an understanding of employees' psychological needs might help to explain behavior and provide guidance for managers on how to better motivate workers. Maslow's Hierarchy of Needs began with physiological existence needs and progressed through safety, social belongingness, self-esteem, and finally self-actualization or creativity needs. This developmental view of needs meant that to motivate people, lower-order needs should be satisfied before higher-order needs could serve as motivators (Maslow 1943).

### Theory X and Theory Y

This era marked the shift in conceptual models from assumptions that workers were incapable of independent action to beliefs in their potential and high performance. Douglas McGregor (1906–1964), a Sloan Management Professor at MIT, formulated these contrasting views as Theory X and Theory Y (McGregor 1960). Theory X presumed that workers inherently disliked work and would avoid it, had little ambition, and mostly wanted security; therefore, managerial direction and control were necessary. Theory Y took a more enlightened view and assumed that work was as natural as play, that motivation could be both internally and externally driven, and that under the right conditions people would seek responsibility and be creative. Theory X found more application in situations where workers were typically immature, less skilled or educated, or uninterested in the work, while Theory Y found more applications in situations where workers were more mature, educated, motivated, and creative.

## Operations Management (1941–Present)

Operations management, developed after World War II, applies statistical, mathematical, and quantitative methods to decision-making in the business setting to better understand how products and services could be manufactured and delivered. Techniques such as forecasting, linear programming, break-even analysis, queuing theory, logistics, and, more recently, data mining emerged from this emphasis on statistical control, especially with the growing capacity of computers.

## Contemporary Management (1960–Present)

Although many aspects of older theories of management are still widely practiced in organizations, research and practical experience have led to many refinements and new developments in the field. More contemporary approaches to management include management by objectives (MBO), total quality management (TQM), theory Z, an emphasis on excellence in quality and performance, and the socio-economic approach to management (SEAM). Each of these has improved understanding of how effective management works.

## Management by Objectives

Peter Drucker (1909–2005) revolutionized the role of business strategy by wresting it from the hands of top management and making it everyone's job, helping workers understand how mission, strategy, goals, and performance were related. Because strategy was action-oriented, starting in the 1950s, Drucker elaborated on the technique of **management by objectives (MBO)**, in which clear target objectives could be stated and measured and could direct behavior (Drucker 1986). Drucker's MBO approach was further developed by his promotion of the ideas that workers should be considered assets rather than liabilities, the corporation is an interpersonal community, and business is customer-centered (Byrne 2005).

## Total Quality Management

The **total quality management (TQM)** approach sought to overcome the limitations of MBO, criticizing the use of quotas because workers often spent too much time trying to look good or protect themselves by seeking short-term objectives and ignoring long-term and critical outcomes. TQM offered a way to build in high performance by maximizing employee potential and continuous improvement of process. The **85/15 rule** of TQM proposes that 85 percent of problems encountered are the result of faulty systems and only 15 percent are due to unconscientious or unproductive employees. The manager's job, then, becomes one of anticipating and removing barriers to high employee performance.

From the late 1970s to the mid-1980s, the US was beset with a series of economic setbacks. Serious recessions, a growing trade deficit, government deregulation, and huge operating losses led to the downsizing of hundreds of thousands of workers. Quality became the focus as a means of increasing competitive position, and much of the idea was derived from W. Edwards Deming (1900–1993), an American statistician. Deming's 14 points of TQM are illustrated in figure 20.4. (Deming 1986).

**Figure 20.4.** Deming's 14 principles

1. Create a constancy of purpose toward continual improvement of products and services, with the objectives to stay in business, be competitive, and provide jobs.
2. Adopt the new philosophy for a new economic age by correcting superstitious learning, calling for a major change, and looking at the customer rather than competition.
3. Cease dependence on inspection to achieve quality by eliminating emphasis on mass inspection and building quality in from the beginning.
4. Do not award business based on price tag alone, and minimize total costs by developing trusting and loyal long-term relationships with single suppliers.
5. Constantly and continually improve production and service systems and thereby improve quality and decrease costs.
6. Institute training on the job, where barriers to good work are removed and managers provide a setting that promotes worker success.
7. Institute leadership with the aim of revising supervision to better help people, machines, and processes do a better job.
8. Drive out fear so everyone can work effectively toward company goals.
9. Break down barriers between departments so various departments can work as a team and anticipate problems of production or use of a product or service.
10. Avoid asking for new levels of productivity and zero defects through slogans and targets because most problems of low productivity lie with the system rather than the worker.
11. Replace work standards such as quotas, numerical goals, and MBO with good leadership.
12. Remove barriers that rob people at all levels of their pride of workmanship; shift from numbers to quality.
13. Institute a program of education and self-improvement by emphasizing lifelong learning and employment.
14. Transformation of the workplace occurs through everyone's action.

*Source:* Deming 1986.

TQM principles continue to be a popular and effective application to change management and have been widely used in healthcare. However, TQM is not a one-size-fits-all approach. In healthcare it should be customized to the needs of the organization, including their unique environment, structures, cultures, and processes (Mosadeghrad 2016).

## Theory Z

Responding to the growing efficiency of Japanese production in the 1980s, William Ouchi, a Japanese American management professor, proposed an extension of McGregor's Theory Y and Deming's TQM in his **Theory Z** (Ouchi 1981). This approach is based on the values of long-term employment, employee engagement and participation, and consensual decision-making. It is different from McGregor's employer-employee relationship in its focus on the broader structure and culture of the organization.

## Business Process Reengineering

In the mid-1990s, there was a growing frustration with the status quo and encouragement to reinvent organizations. While TQM focused on incremental changes and gradual progress, the emerging emphasis on reengineering organizations focused on more disruptive change strategies. Fostered by Michael Hammer and James Champy's book, *Reengineering the Corporation* (1993), **business process reengineering (BPR)** (also known as business transformation and process change management) became popular. It proposed the radical redesign of the organization and its business processes to reduce costs, streamline operations, and improve quality of service. BPR responds to a need in the business environment to rapidly adapt to changing situations brought about by technology in the workplace. In some ways harkening back to Taylor's best way, BPR attempts to find the best work processes to maximally improve cost, quality, service, and speed. Like TQM, it emphasizes ongoing improvement and use of IT to provide real-time information about customers, competition, and change. However, in contrast to TQM's incremental and top-down approach, BPR has been adopted in healthcare emphasizing extensive redesign and empowering individuals and teams to be involved in developing the change (Bhaskar 2015).

## The Search for Excellence

Although elements of most major theories can be found within successful managers' practices, developments and refinements in thinking have continued to become part of management practice and history. In 1982, Tom Peters and Robert Waterman published *In Search of Excellence*. Based on a sample of highly successful business firms, they described the management practices that led to their success. Eight characteristics were described that became the rage in management circles for a time, with managers hoping to reproduce in their own organizations what top firms had done (Peters and Waterman 1982) (see figure 20.5).

The lesson from the excellence studies highlights some important principles, including the following:

- Whether you succeed or fail, try to understand what brought about that result.
- When you succeed, recognize that the success factors are not static but, rather, are continually changing.
- Do not let past success strategies keep you from discovering new ones for the future.
- What may contribute to the success of one type of organization or competitive setting may not be as useful to other types and settings or at other stages of OD.

Researchers continue to search for the essential ingredients that will make firms most successful. Dynamic

**Figure 20.5.** Characteristics of highly successful firms

1. *A bias for action:* They establish a value for action and implementation rather than overanalyzing and delaying with endless committees.
2. *Close to the customer:* They listen and respond to customers to satisfy their needs.
3. *Autonomy and entrepreneurship:* They empower people and encourage innovation and risk taking.
4. *Productivity through people:* They increase employees' awareness that everyone's contributions lead to shared success.
5. *Hands on, value driven:* Their managers should be visible, involved, and know what is going on.
6. *Stick to the knitting:* They stay with the core business, what they do well, and avoid wide diversification.
7. *Simple form, lean staff:* They have fewer administrative layers and keep the structure simple.
8. *Simultaneous loose–tight properties:* They maintain dedication to core principles but encourage flexibility and experimentation in reaching goals.

*Source:* Adapted from Peters and Waterman 1982.

and diverse work environments increase the complexity and challenge as this search continues.

## Socioeconomic Approach to Management

The **socioeconomic approach to management (SEAM)** is a method of organizational change that originated in Lyon, France in 1973 by Henri Savall. This approach emphasizes the importance of both the human side and the economic side of successful management. The socioeconomic focus suggests that investing in human potential enriches an organization's profit. SEAM is contrary to early management models which indicate employees are a commodity, when in times of financial shortfall should be disposed of. Instead, it promotes the thought that one of the ways to increase organizational effectiveness is to increase collaboration, cohesion, and participation in the workplace. When there is a problem, staff do not look for someone to blame; they look for a collaborative solution. In a socioeconomic model, respect for each individual goes together with the effort to increase profits. In an organization using SEAM, managers are trained to be effective at meeting strategic goals, and dysfunctions and hidden costs are exposed. Like the TQM model, the SEAM model suggests that most dysfunctions are due to systems, not people (Conbere and Heorhiadi 2018).

The history of management reflects significant development in our understanding of how people work and how that work can be more effectively organized. From Taylor's and Fayol's early efforts to create structured work systems to more contemporary views on the importance of integrating human factors with work conditions, management theories continue to evolve and tend to focus on adapting to and leading organization change (see figure 20.1).

### Check Your Understanding 20.1

Answer the following questions in a separate document.

1. Give an example of a situation or job in which the Theory X approach to management would be appropriate. Explain your rationale.
2. How have management theories changed over the years and what are some factors that have contributed to such change?
3. In what ways do you feel the SEAM model may affect the productivity of an organization's staff. Explain your rationale.
4. Using the example of the Gilbreths' time and motion research, identify a complex activity you engage in (such as packing for a trip, dressing in the morning, or such) and streamline the sequence to become more efficient.
5. Think of a small project you must complete, such as writing a paper. Draw a Gantt chart, breaking down each step of writing a paper and plot each step over time to completion.

## Functions and Principles of Management

As theories of management began to be refined, so did the formal nature of the manager's role. As organizations increased in diversity, complexity, and size, managers often shifted their expertise from expert knowledge in doing a task to expert knowledge in managing other people. Mary Parker Follett reputedly said, "Management is the art of getting things done through people" (Peek 2023). Specific functions and principles of management were an extension of the work done by historical practitioners, as were a range of skills and roles that contribute to successful problem solving, depending on the level of management.

### Managerial Functions

Fayol identified the key functions of management as planning, organizing, directing and leading, and controlling and evaluating. These functions vary in emphasis according to the level of management within an organization from frontline supervisors to middle managers to top management. Within each managerial level, there are certain categories of skills that are needed to carry out the functions.

## Planning

Planning is the first step in management and involves determining what should be accomplished and how. Although planning occurs at all levels, top-level or strategic planning is most critical in formulating the mission and providing direction for change. When these strategies are defined, they can be implemented at the lower levels of the organization. High-quality planning and implementation capability provide competitive advantage over those who minimize the importance of planning (Dunn 2021).

Plans are usually organized hierarchically into planning levels, with a **mission statement** driving the enterprise by defining exactly the purpose of existence for the organization. The mission statement is a written statement that sets forth the core purpose and philosophies of an organization or group. The mission may also incorporate or be accompanied by a **values statement** that reflects the social and cultural beliefs an organization wishes to support among its members. A **vision statement** describes the ideal and desired future state toward which an organization is directed, in contrast to the mission statement, which is current and realistic. The strategic plan follows from the mission. It is formulated by top management, sets the priorities and positioning of the organization for a time period, and is based on the internal strengths and weaknesses and external opportunities and threats (often identified using the SWOT acronym). These are translated through the lower levels of the organization by middle management in formulating tactical plans, which are strategic plans for the organization's major divisions. At the lower departmental levels, these finally become operational plans implemented as daily activities (see figure 20.6).

Plans are usually expressed in terms of goals. **Goals** are statements of intended outcomes that provide a source of direction and motivation as well as a guideline for performance, decision-making, and evaluation. Good goals should cover key result areas of the strategy and have the characteristics of being SMART goals—specific, measurable, achievable, realistic, and time-bound.

## Organizing

After the goals have been specified, the task changes to deciding how resources can be allocated to achieve them. **Organizing** is the way in which the organization is designed and operated to attain the desired goals. It involves the way that tasks are grouped into

**Figure 20.6.** Planning levels

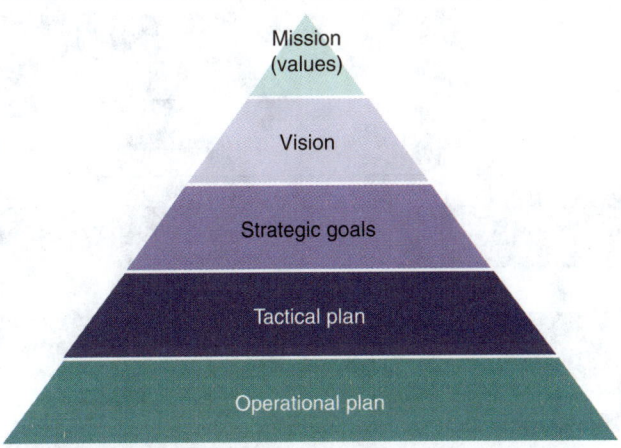

departments and resources are distributed to them. Traditionally, division of labor has been used to divide work into separate jobs. This specialization allows for development of greater expertise and standardization of tasks and for clear selection and training criteria. However, too narrow or specialized a task, such as data entry or scanning and indexing, may produce boredom or fatigue from routine, affecting productivity.

Jobs are most often organized by positions, and the positions are arranged hierarchically by an organizational chart. (An example of a typical hospital organizational chart is shown in figure 20.7.) The **organizational chart** graphically represents the formal structure of an entity, often includes departmental subdivisions, and follows the scalar chain (everyone from top to bottom knows who they report to and is clearly included in the chain of command) and unity of command (every employee receives direction and instructions from one boss). The vertical structure refers to the formal design of positions within departments and divisions of the organization, the lines of authority and responsibility, and the allocation of resources to them. Two kinds of authority are found in organizations. **Line authority** is the right of managers to direct the activities of employees under their immediate control; **staff authority** is related to the expert knowledge of specialists in the organization and involves their ability or right to advise and recommend courses of action.

Each supervisor oversees a certain number of people, which is referred to as the span of management or the **span of control**. There are several factors to consider in optimally balancing the span of control. In general, the span of control is larger when work is routine and homogeneous, workers have similar tasks, rules and guidelines are available, people are well trained and motivated, workers are located together, and task durations are short (Dunn 2021).

**Figure 20.7.** Sample hospital organizational chart

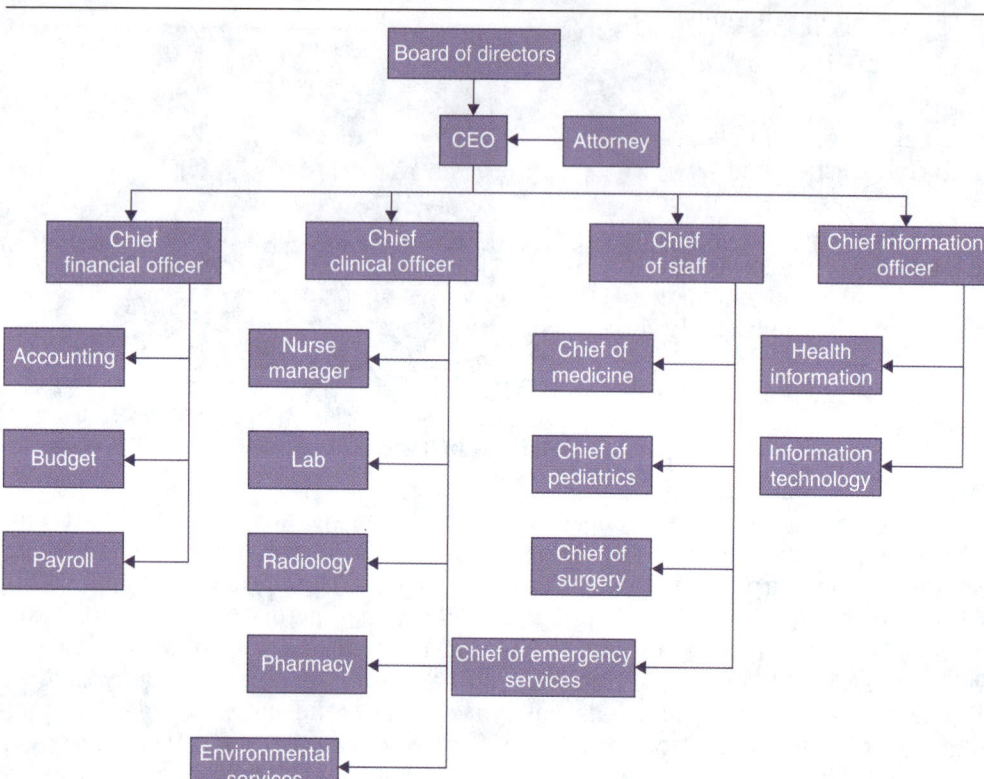

Span of control factors include the number of managers and supervisors, departmental fragmentation, and layers of management (Advisory Board 2015). Organizational charts help visualize span of control considerations.

## Directing and Leading

The third managerial function of directing and leading accomplishes goals by influencing behavior and by inspiring people to high performance. Leading motivating, creating shared culture and values, and communicating with all levels of the organization with the intent to influence behavior to perform well.

Power—the ability to influence—is central to leadership. It derives from several sources, including the following:

- *Authority* or legitimate power comes from the right of the position in the organization to direct the activities of employees (French and Raven 1959).
- *Reward power* is based on the leader's ability to withhold or provide rewards for performance (French and Raven 1959).
- *Coercive power* maintains control over punishments (French and Raven 1959).
- *Referent power* exists when the leader possesses personal characteristics that are appealing to the constituency, and the constituency follows out of admiration, charismatic impact, or the desire to be like the leader (French and Raven 1959).
- *Expert power* occurs when the leader has knowledge or expertise that is of value (French and Raven 1959).
- *Information power* is based on being able to provide information to decision makers (Raven 1993).

A large part of the directing and leading function of management relates to motivating people to perform at their best. Motivating employees should be a top priority for managers. There are two categories of motivational theory a leader should consider: content theory and process theory. Content theory focuses on factors individuals need to feel energized and the motives that drive people to behave in a certain way. These needs vary for each person. Process theory focuses on an individual's feeling of equity in regard to how they are treated and compensated and whether or not they feel they are rewarded for their effort in the way they expected (Dunn 2021).

Leadership behaviors and most models of leadership are categorized as task-oriented behaviors and social or group-oriented behaviors. Task-oriented behaviors are directed toward defining tasks, creating structure and rules, ensuring production, and placing emphasis on quality and speed of output. Social orientation focuses on interpersonal behaviors that develop and maintain harmonious work relationships, encourage morale, reduce stress and conflict, and build worker satisfaction. For much of the history of management, an autocratic and centralized view of leadership was considered appropriate. As humanistic views have prevailed over more recent decades, leadership has become decentralized and distributed throughout the organization.

### Controlling and Evaluating

The final managerial function of controlling refers to monitoring performance and using feedback to ensure that efforts toward achieving the prescribed goals are on target, and making course corrections as needed. The controlling function includes employee performance evaluations, budget reports, and quality and productivity monitoring. It is sometimes referred to as "evaluating." Managers are obligated to ensure progress is made toward achieving goals.

While some organizations allow experienced and responsible employees to self-monitor, technology has enabled remote monitoring of performance. With so many tasks requiring computer input, it is possible to analyze many aspects of performance, such as rate of entry, number of patients seen, or tasks completed. The employee can view personal performance compared to required levels or to a standard, and high and low performers may come to the attention of a manager. The function of controlling includes regular performance evaluations for all employees to ensure personal and organizational goals are met. This method of evaluation can also serve to motivate employees and can be a tool for the leading function discussed previously.

Significant breakthroughs in control have occurred with the development of the executive dashboard and balanced scorecard (BSC) introduced in 1992 (Kaplan and Norton 1996). The executive dashboard is an information management system providing decision makers with regularly updated information on an organization's key strategic measures. The dashboard typically contains regularly updated information on key strategic measures such as forecasts, patient satisfaction, billings, profit, and so on.

The BSC is an extension of strategic planning in which key performance indicators (KPIs) are measured at all levels of the organization. The BSC shows progress related to meeting the KPIs and offers workers and management ongoing feedback. Categories of feedback usually include financial information, customer satisfaction, internal processes (for example, quality or response time), and learning and growth.

### Levels of Management

The four functions of management vary in emphasis according to the level of management involved (see figure 20.8). In general, as one moves from frontline (supervisory) to middle management to top managers, planning increases, organizing increases, directing decreases, and controlling stays about the same (Jones and George 2021; McConnell 2018).

Larger organizations often have three levels of management—supervisors, middle managers, and executives; in addition, they have a board of directors. These different levels of management within organizations also have different levels of leadership functions.

Supervisory managers are hands-on managers of daily operations over a unit or division or within a department. They ensure staff meet preestablished standards of performance, policy, and procedures. They often have high-level technical skills but may have limited hiring and financial authority.

Middle managers have a broader scope of responsibility than supervisory managers, often overseeing all functions in a department, such as the health information management (HIM) department, the admission and registration department, and others. They can facilitate the work of positions above and below them, both supervisory and executive. More specifically, their responsibilities often include the following:

- Developing, implementing, and revising the policies and procedures of the organization under direction by the executive level
- Carrying out organizational plans developed at the executive and board level
- Communicating operational information to executives so they can continue ongoing planning

**Figure 20.8.** Relative degree of managerial function by level in the organization

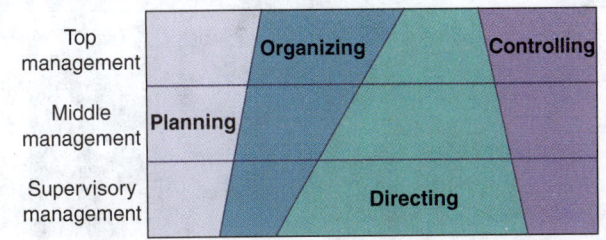

In an HIM department, middle managers can modify department-level policies and procedures as needed and analyze information to get at a root cause of a problem and use discretion in dealing with it. They may also track quality of clinical databases, oversee compliance programs, participate on interdisciplinary committees, and conduct risk and quality audits. Middle managers typically report to an executive manager, who could be the chief operations officer (COO), chief information officer (CIO), chief financial officer (CFO), or chief executive officer (CEO).

At the highest level of the organization are executive managers and the governing board. Executives are mostly responsible for formulating the strategic plan, ensuring consistency in the direction of the organization with its vision and mission, and allocating assets and resources toward that end. They establish policies and lead the organization toward quality improvement and compliance. In the typical "C-suite" of a large healthcare organization, there is commonly a COO, a CFO, a chief nursing officer (CNO), a CIO, and a chief medical officer (CMO), all of whom report to the CEO. The CEO reports directly to the board of directors, also called the board of trustees or governing board.

Governing boards are legislated to be responsible for the operation of the entire organization. They are the final authority when it comes to the approval of the strategic plan and mission, vision, ethics, and values statements, and are accountable for quality and finances. In healthcare, a board is usually made up of a chairperson and internal directors, and board members who bring legal, insurance, business, and other expertise (Price 2018).

## Managerial Skills

The categories of skills required to perform the four management functions are conceptual, interpersonal, and technical (Katz 1974). As management has become increasingly complex, the requisite skills for carrying out the four managerial functions also vary by level in the organization, as shown in figure 20.9. Technical skills are most pertinent for frontline management while conceptual skills are most relevant for top management. Interpersonal skills are used largely in middle management.

### Conceptual Skills

The need for conceptual skills has increased significantly over the years. Where it was once important only to have effective technical skills, a successful manager must now understand diverse fields and deal with complex situations. Conceptual skills, especially at the higher levels of the organization, include such competencies as visioning, planning, decision-making, problem solving, creativity, and conceptualizing the connections among parts of a complex organizational system, or systems thinking. Cognitive complexity—the ability to see the many parts of a problem, process conflicting information, and integrate that diversity into a coherent picture—is very important for top managers (Houghton et al. 2018). For example, EHRs involve high levels of information complexity, and inattention to the demands this places on providers can lead to higher patient care risks (Roberson et al. 2014; Stephenson and Schwartz 2014). Conceptual skills are needed to consider the results of making a change. In another example, computerized provider order entry reduces variation in orders, thereby reducing risks (Connelly and Korvek 2023). In this example, conceptual skills have been used to develop solutions to the existing issue of variation.

### Interpersonal Skills

Interpersonal skills involve the ability to work with and through others to accomplish goals. Depending on the nature of the work and the level of interaction needed among individuals, interpersonal skills may or may not be critical for employee success. However, managers need to cultivate impeccable interpersonal skills in their interactions with employees and with each other.

Interpersonal competency is based on self-awareness and understanding; effective managers are those who can articulate both their strengths and weaknesses. Consistently high performers also demonstrate self-monitoring, referring to the ability to observe the reactions that one's behavior has on others and then adjust one's behavior to improve the relationship and quality of care (Lei et al. 2023). Other important interpersonal skills include communicating, motivating and influencing, managing conflict, and complementing different ways of interacting.

Emotional intelligence (EI), the sensitivity and ability to monitor and revise one's behavior based on the needs and responses of others, is an important and relevant topic in management and healthcare. Advocates of EI believe awareness and use of feelings

**Figure 20.9.** Relative degree of functional skills by level

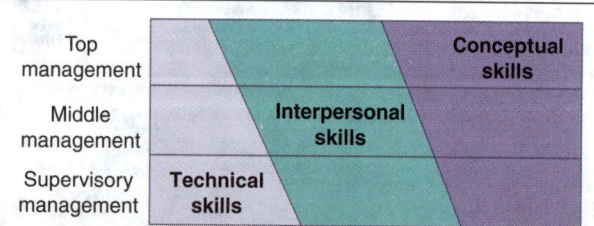

complement rational intelligence and experience. The combination of these is key to more effective care (Karmi et al. 2021) (see figure 20.10).

### Technical Skills

Understanding and mastering the technical information, methods, and equipment involved in a discipline constitutes **technical skills**. Examples of these include data collection, scanning and indexing, analysis and reporting, and other task-specific responsibilities. Although most important at the staff level of the organization, technical skills are still required of upper management for a comprehensive understanding of the workings of the organization. However, conceptual and interpersonal skills are more useful in obtaining promotion in most organizations because, at higher levels in organizations, these types of skills are used more often than technical skills. Conceptual skills are more useful in leading and planning functions because they involve understanding how the organization should be viewed as a complex system of interconnecting parts and processes. For example, as healthcare information systems continue to shift from decentralized to more centralized operations, HIM managers need to effectively collaborate with IT and other departments to ensure information consistency and quality of care (Crew et al. 2021). The ability to understand complex connections, recognize gaps in continuity of information, and anticipate unintended consequences does much to reduce errors.

### Managerial Activities

Managerial and leadership activities are typically organized around several roles. A **role** refers to a set of expectations about how a person is to behave from the perspective of oneself, peers, managers, staff, consumers (patients), and others (such as legislators). **Role theory** has been a prominent framework for examining behavior in the field of medical sociology for decades, and it has been applied in management to clarify the wide range of responsibilities.

Managers often complete a great deal of work at an unrelenting pace, but the activities are characterized by variety, fragmentation, and brevity. Information overload and multitasking pose continuing challenges. A study showed that executives spend about 72 percent of their time in meetings, 62 percent of non-face-to-face communications are electronic, and only 3 percent of the time is spent with customers (Porter and Nohria 2018).

Henry Mintzberg's research with managers showed that their activities could usually be described by 10 roles organized into three categories (see table 20.1):

- *Interpersonal activity* arises from the manager's formal authority in the organization and is supportive of the informational and decisional activities. It includes the roles of figurehead for ceremonial and formal occasions, of leader for motivating and using power, and of liaison to link and network for information and support.

- *Informational activity* includes the roles of monitor of performance information, disseminator of values and information, and spokesperson for the organization with outside groups.

- *Decisional activity* includes the roles of entrepreneur, to promote improvement and change; disturbance handler, to deal with disruptions; resource allocator, for overseeing resources and setting priorities; and negotiator, for making arrangements with other organizations. (Mintzberg 1992)

These roles are intricately intertwined and cannot easily be separated, especially when responsibilities are often distributed among team members. However, they provide a realistic portrayal of the wide range of skilled behaviors required of effective managers.

**Figure 20.10.** Attributes of emotional intelligence

- *Self-awareness:* The ability to monitor, notice, and label one's feelings as they occur. This allows one to be more certain about feelings and to identify early vague feelings.
- *Self-regulation:* The ability to manage one's emotions and impulses. A person with this skill is often viewed as being reflective, comfortable with change and ambiguity, and able to control impulsiveness.
- *Motivation:* Being highly motivated is essential for focusing attention, mastering situations, showing creativity, and being productive and successful.
- *Empathy:* The ability to recognize emotions in others. This is important for teamwork as well as for helping adjust one's behavior to the emerging reactions of others.
- *Social skills:* The ability to handle relationships with others is central to being perceived as popular, effective with others, and having the qualities of a leader.

*Source:* Adapted from Goleman 1998.

In healthcare, as well as other fields of management, decisions tend to be based more often on political and value considerations than on empirical sources. For example, the increased interest in alternative approaches to healthcare (for example, acupuncture and nutrition) and to healthcare delivery is driven by the desire to reduce errors, decrease costs, improve outcomes of care, and reduce liabilities. Such diverse and in some cases controversial practices are leading to an emphasis on **evidence-based management**, or information-based management, in which more informed decisions are made based on the best clinical and research evidence that such proposed practices are valid.

## Trends in Management Theory

As change drivers impact the healthcare marketplace, organizations must adapt to survive and thrive. Management theories become a guide for thinking about the structure and processes by which business is revised and conducted. As the marketplace changes, old theories may lose their explanatory power and be replaced with more relevant theories and principles for managing the organization. In general, there has been a shift in paradigm from more traditional hierarchical, centralized, and uniform approaches to more flexible and adaptive ones that utilize the advantages of technology. Table 20.2 differentiates the factors in a traditional management paradigm with the factors in the modern management paradigm. At the same time, as managers become accustomed to, and develop expertise with, a certain viewpoint, they may become biased in its use and fail to see exceptions to it. A requisite skill for managers is to know when to use a particular framework and when to change it.

Although managers at the turn of the 20th century faced a host of changes, the unrelenting pace of change is even more constant for managers today. The successful manager must be able to see patterns of change and prepare others to respond to them.

**Table 20.1.** Mintzberg's managerial roles

| Managerial activity | Related roles |
|---|---|
| Interpersonal | • *Figurehead:* The manager represents the organization and is a symbol for ceremonial, social, legal, and inspirational duties.<br>• *Liaison:* The manager maintains networks of relationships outside his or her organizational unit to gather information and favors.<br>• *Leader:* The manager directs, guides, motivates, and develops subordinates. |
| Informational | • *Monitor:* The manager oversees internal and external information sources.<br>• *Disseminator:* The manager communicates facts and values to others in the organization.<br>• *Spokesperson:* The manager communicates with others outside the organization. |
| Decisional | • *Entrepreneur:* The manager promotes development and planned change in the organization.<br>• *Disturbance handler:* The manager resolves crises and unexpected problems.<br>• *Resource allocator:* The manager uses authority to allocate budget, personnel, equipment, services, and facilities.<br>• *Negotiator:* The manager resolves dilemmas and disputes and determines the use of resources. |

*Source:* Mintzberg 1989.

**Table 20.2.** Trend shift in management

| Traditional management approach | Modern management approach |
|---|---|
| Multilevel hierarchical organization | Flatter, distributed organization |
| Centralized decision-making | Decentralized decision-making |
| Status measured by amount of turf controlled | Status measured by success in achieving outcomes |
| Funding inputs and intentions | Funding outcomes |
| Face-to-face interaction | Telecommunication and virtual interaction |
| Homogenous staffing | Workforce diversity |
| Job description | Skill portfolio |
| Annual strategic plan | Learning organization |
| Financial bottom line | Triple bottom line; social, environmental, and financial aspects |
| Efficiency and stability | Ongoing innovation, digital management |
| Mass services | Market segmentation |
| Work at central office | Remote work |

### Check Your Understanding 20.2

**Answer the following questions in a separate document.**

1. Consider a job description for a position you have held or are working toward. What is the distribution of conceptual, interpersonal, and technical skills required?
2. Draw an organizational chart of your college, a hospital, or some other organization with which you are familiar. Be sure to designate both line and staff positions. Can you identify any issues with the structure?
3. Discuss reasons for the four management functions changing in emphasis over the three levels of management. Why do you think leadership functions, usually reserved for the top, are now emphasized more for supervisory managers?
4. Analyze the three categories of roles in the Mintzberg model and give an example of a situation that fits in each category.
5. Using table 20.2 and your own perspective, evaluate your current employer, the college you attend, or your academic department against each paradigm. Choose three paradigms from the list and describe if your organization uses the traditional management or the modern management approach and why you have made that determination.

## Trends in Leadership Theory

A theory guides examination of a phenomenon, such as leadership. The theory labels important features, then uses them to describe, explain, and help predict what might happen if certain actions were pursued. The idea that leadership makes a difference is undisputed, but exactly how and why it makes a difference needs further examination.

Leadership theories suggest that consistency between leadership behaviors exhibited by leaders and those expected by their followers can increase employee satisfaction and performance (Tsai and Qiao 2023). Leadership impacts productivity and profitability, as well as the level of quality and integration of care for both patients and professionals (Sfantou et al. 2017). Without effective leadership organizational performance suffers and growth of employee engagement declines. Gallup has found that 70 percent of the variance in team engagement is determined solely by the manager (Pitonyak and Desimone 2024). In 2023 only 30 percent of US employees were found to be engaged at work (13 percent worldwide), leading organizations to focus more on manager engagement to ensure lasting growth (Harter 2024).

Leaders had to respond to the changes the COVID-19 pandemic brought to the workplace, particularly related to the increase in remote work. Today, the proportion of hybrid and fully remote workers has stabilized, with 29 percent of employees reporting they are working fully remotely and 52 percent working a blend of in the office and at home. However, it is crucial that leaders are equipped to respond to this new-normal. In 2023, there was an increase of employees in the US who felt more detached from their employers, with less clear expectations, lower satisfaction levels with their organization, and less connection to its mission, than they did four years ago (Harter 2024). Gallup found the most fundamental element for employee engagement is knowing what is expected of you, and that there are strong links between this element and organizational performance including productivity, employee wellbeing and retention, safety, and customer engagement (Harter 2024). The decrease in clarity of expectations may be due to post-pandemic layoffs, budgets cuts, or staffing challenges. Managers may also have no formal training on how to lead a hybrid or remote group of employees. To succeed in this new work environment leaders must find new ways to engage with their employees in a meaningful way.

Trends in leadership theory have shifted from classical approaches focused on a defined use of authority to behavioral approaches, which allowed for movement to a variety of leadership styles including those contingent on a particular situation and those based on values and core beliefs.

### Classical Approaches to Leadership Theory

Classical leadership theories tended to focus on the principled and effective use of authority. This emphasis began to change with the many social changes emerging in the early to mid-1900s. Inventions and innovations in manufacturing and technology increased competition, which made managers more open to new ideas. Workers became increasingly better educated and skilled, thereby requiring managers with authoritative styles to adopt more democratic approaches. The workforce also became increasingly diverse, much like today, and this required a broader understanding of different cultures and motivational approaches. The classical models evolved from great person theory to trait theory to the autocratic-democratic continuum.

### Great Person Theory

The course of human history is marked with the contributions of great people. Great person theory is based on the belief that outstanding individuals originally led to the conception of leadership as an inborn ability, sometimes passed down through family, position, or social tradition, as in the cases of royal families in many parts of the world. The problem with the great person theory is that some of those who took positions of such greatness were terribly lacking, as in the cases of Caligula in ancient Rome or Stalin in Russia. In the US, there were people who were leaders in one aspect but who failed in others. For example, Ulysses S. Grant excelled as a general, which got him elected president—a role in which he did not perform well (Waugh 2009).

### Trait Approach

The trait approach gradually replaced the great person model and proposed that leaders possessed a collection of traits or personal behaviors and attributes that distinguished them from non-leaders. In research during the 1930s and 1940s, leadership traits were often grouped into categories related to physical needs, values, intellect, personality, and skill characteristics. Some researchers have organized traits on the three leadership requirements of conceptual, interpersonal, and technical skills. Others add a fourth category—administrative skills—which includes the four managerial functions of planning, organizing, directing, and controlling (Yukl 2006).

Unfortunately, in much of the early research, only a weak relationship was discovered between traits and individuals who would emerge as leaders, and many leaders did not share all the traits in common. During later studies in which traits and skills were correlated with leader effectiveness rather than leader emergence, stronger connections appeared. Some of the more important traits included adaptability, social alertness, ambition, assertiveness, cooperativeness, decisiveness, dominance, energy, stress tolerance, and confidence. Skills included intelligence and conceptual abilities, creativity, tact, verbal fluency, work knowledge, organization, and persuasion (Stogdill 1974). Despite this extensive work, it appears that no single traits are absolutely required for leadership. Certain traits and skills may be more helpful in some situations and may lead to greater effectiveness.

### Autocratic versus Democratic Leadership

America's reaction to World War II and the Cold War with Russia contributed to research that attempted to distinguish the benefits of democratic over autocratic values. This also found expression in management theories of Douglas McGregor, Robert Lippit and Ronald White, and Robert Tannenbaum and Warren Schmidt. McGregor's formulation of Theory X and Y identified two types of work environments and leaders that corresponded to autocratic and democratic behaviors (McGregor 1960). White and Lippitt (1960) conducted studies on democratic and autocratic leaders. They found that groups under autocratic leadership, where the manager made decisions without others' input and gave very specific direction, performed well if they were closely supervised; however, levels of member satisfaction were low. In contrast, democratic leadership that involved members in decision-making led members to perform well whether the leader was present or absent, and members were more satisfied. This kind of research led to the emphasis on participative management in many organizations. The autocratic–democratic dimension was useful for understanding a range of managerial behavior that could be applied across different settings.

Based on the autocratic–democratic dimension, Tannenbaum and Schmidt (1973) designed a continuum that described seven degrees of leader involvement in decision-making (see figure 20.11). At one end (autocratic) of the continuum, the leader makes a decision alone and announces it. At the other end (democratic), the leader encourages his or her employees to make their own decisions within prescribed limits. This model was new in that it reflected a shift from looking at the leader in isolation or in terms of a rigid or permanent style and suggested a person had a range of available behaviors depending on the situation. But what behaviors made leaders successful?

## Behavioral or Task-Relationship Theories of Leadership

While most earlier theories focused on what leaders *should* do and what was expected of them, emerging behavioral theories describe what managers *actually* do. The emerging theories clearly emphasize a leader's orientation toward both tasks and people and enable leaders to describe a variety of styles rather than just the one "right" style.

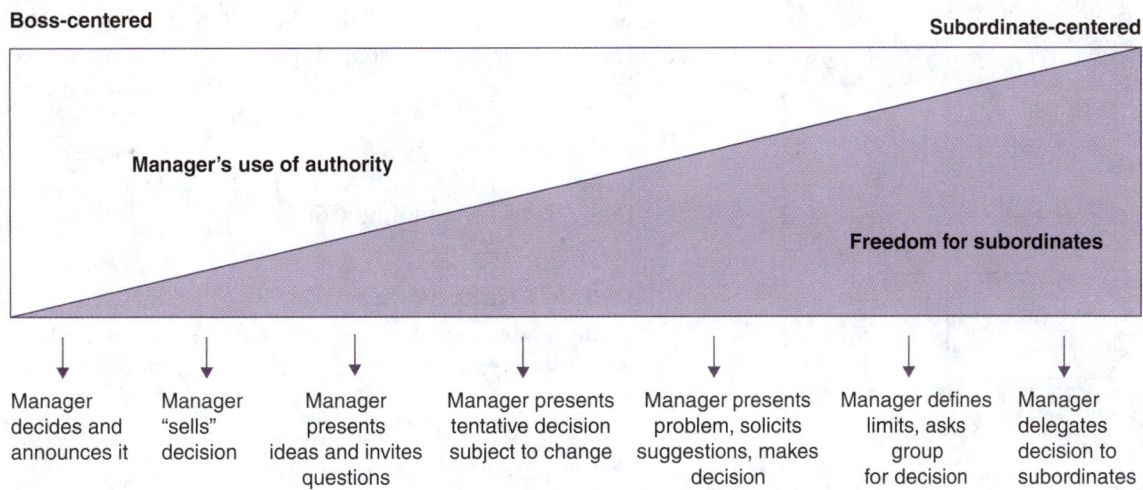

Figure 20.11. Tannenbaum and Schmidt's leadership continuum

Source: Tannenbaum and Schmidt 1973.

During the 1950s and 1960s, researchers at Ohio State University examined the behavior of leaders in several hundred studies and reduced them to two categories: consideration or relationship orientation and initiating structure or task orientation (Shartle 1979). Consideration (as defined in the study) refers to attention to the interpersonal aspects of work, including respecting the staff's ideas and feelings, maintaining harmonious work relationships, collaborating in teamwork, and showing concern for the staff's welfare. Initiating structure is a leadership skill that is task-focused and centered on giving direction, setting goals and limits, and planning and scheduling activities. During the same period, researchers at the University of Michigan developed a similar model. Comparing effective and ineffective managers, they found that a key difference was that the effective employee-centered managers focused more on the human needs of their staff whereas their less effective task-oriented managers emphasized only goal attainment (Likert 1979). This distinction led to the development of several assessment tools or inventories that helped identify a manager's preference or managerial style.

Building on the Ohio State and Michigan studies, Robert Blake and Jane Srygley Mouton (1976) at the University of Texas identified the same two dimensions: concern for people (consideration) and concern for production (initiating structure). Their leadership grid marked off degrees of emphasis a leader may have toward people or production using a nine-point scale and finally separated the grid into five styles of management based on the combined people and production emphasis. Although this model has been considered a key theory, and it clearly presents a collaborative or team management approach as the ideal, subsequent contingency theories show that there are situations in which other emphases may be as effective. (see figure 20.12 for an example of a leadership grid).

## Contingency and Situational Theories of Leadership

Most of these early theories of leadership have emphasized identifying a cluster of traits or a single style or orientation for leadership. As research in leadership has continued, it has become apparent that successful leadership does not depend on style or skills alone but, also, on matching a leader's style with the changing demands or contingencies of a specific situation.

### Hersey and Blanchard's Situational Theory

One of the more popular leadership models still widely used for training, and one that has attempted to integrate other ideas from management, is Paul Hersey and Kenneth Blanchard's situational theory of leadership (Hersey et al. 1996). Situational leadership is based on the relationship between leaders and followers and provides a framework to analyze each situation based on task behavior (the amount of guidance and direction given by a leader) and relationship behavior (the amount of socioemotional support a leader provides) (The Center for Leadership Studies 2017). In addition, worker immaturity–maturity is a concept that suggests that job maturity (work-related ability) and psychological maturity (motivation related to work) of employees also influence

**Figure 20.12.** Leadership matrix models

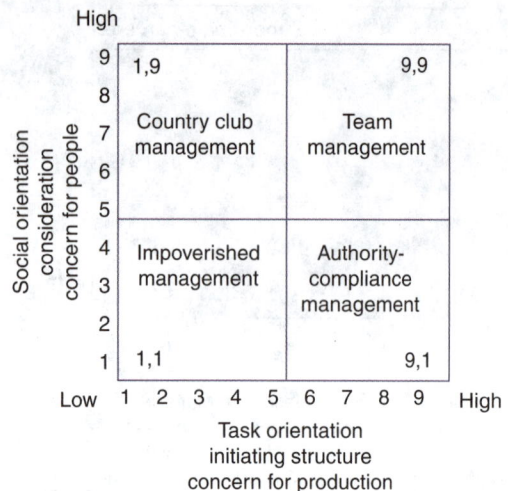

*Source:* Blake and Mouton 1976.

the selection and effectiveness of the leadership style (Argyris 1957). Situational theory refers to the idea that the leader's style should be adjusted to different situations and employees encountered.

## Path–Goal Theory

Another model of leadership, initially introduced by Robert House in 1971 and revised in 1996, is path–goal theory. While some theories have focused on the motivation of the leader, the path–goal theory (House 1996) examines the motives and needs of the staff and how the leader can respond to them. This theory was based on the **expectancy theory of motivation**, which proposes that one's degree of effort is influenced by the expectation that the effort will result in the attainment of desired goals and meaningful rewards. **Path–goal theory** states that a person's ability to perform certain tasks is related to the direction and clarity available that lead to organizational goals. For example, if a worker is unclear about what a task involves and what should be done, performance will be improved when clear instructions are given. The role of leaders, then, is to facilitate progress on the path toward the goal by removing barriers to performance.

Path–goal theory identifies four different situations, each requiring a different facilitative response from leadership (see figure 20.13). When staff lack self-confidence, leaders provide support by being friendly, approachable, concerned about needs, and equitable. This increases the staff's confidence to achieve the work outcome. When the staff has an ambiguous job, the leader is more forthright in providing the worker with direction, schedules, rules, and regulations that clarify the path. When staff do not have sufficient job challenge, the leader uses an achievement approach by setting challenging goals, continually seeking improvement, and expecting high performance. Finally, when the reward is mismatched with staff needs, the leader takes a more consultative or participative role in which workers share work problems, make suggestions, and are included in decision-making to ensure more appropriate rewards. All four strategies result in improved task performance and satisfaction—again, the task and social dimensions.

## Dyadic Relationship Theory

Some leadership theories are macro theories and attempt to explain leadership across large domains, but there also are micro theories that focus on a specific context for leadership. Leader–member exchange (LMX) (Graen and Skandura 1987) and closely related vertical dyad linkage (VDL) represent micro theories that focus on dyadic relationships, or those between two people or between a leader and a small group. More specifically, they explain how in-group and out-group relationships form with a leader or mentor and how delegation may occur.

**Vertical dyad linkage (VDL)** was first formulated in 1975 to describe the single-person mentoring relationships that occur in organizations (Dansereau et al. 1975). It was later supplemented by **leader–member exchange (LMX)** theory, which applied the same idea to the leader's relations with groups. In these situations, leaders look for employees with high-performance and leadership potential that distinguishes them from employees with less potential. The best predictors of being selected for in-group, in addition to competence, include compatibility of the employee with the leader, interpersonal liking for each other, and being extroverted. Once identified, the leader and employee form an **exchange relationship**, in which a leader offers greater opportunities and privileges to an employee in exchange for loyalty, commitment, and assistance. The leader may delegate special responsibilities, offer interesting and desirable tasks, give opportunities for highly visible or skill-building projects, and provide mentoring.

Those employees who form a group around the leader are referred to as the **in-group**; those employees not included form the **out-group**. Being in the in-group may sound attractive, but it involves performance beyond the call of duty. In-group members may work longer hours, work during off-hours, and take on more difficult tasks compared to members in the out-group. The out-group expects to be treated fairly by the leader, and if the exchanges are viewed as fair, there is little or no conflict between the in- and out-groups; they can remain fairly stable over

**Figure 20.13.** Path–goal theory

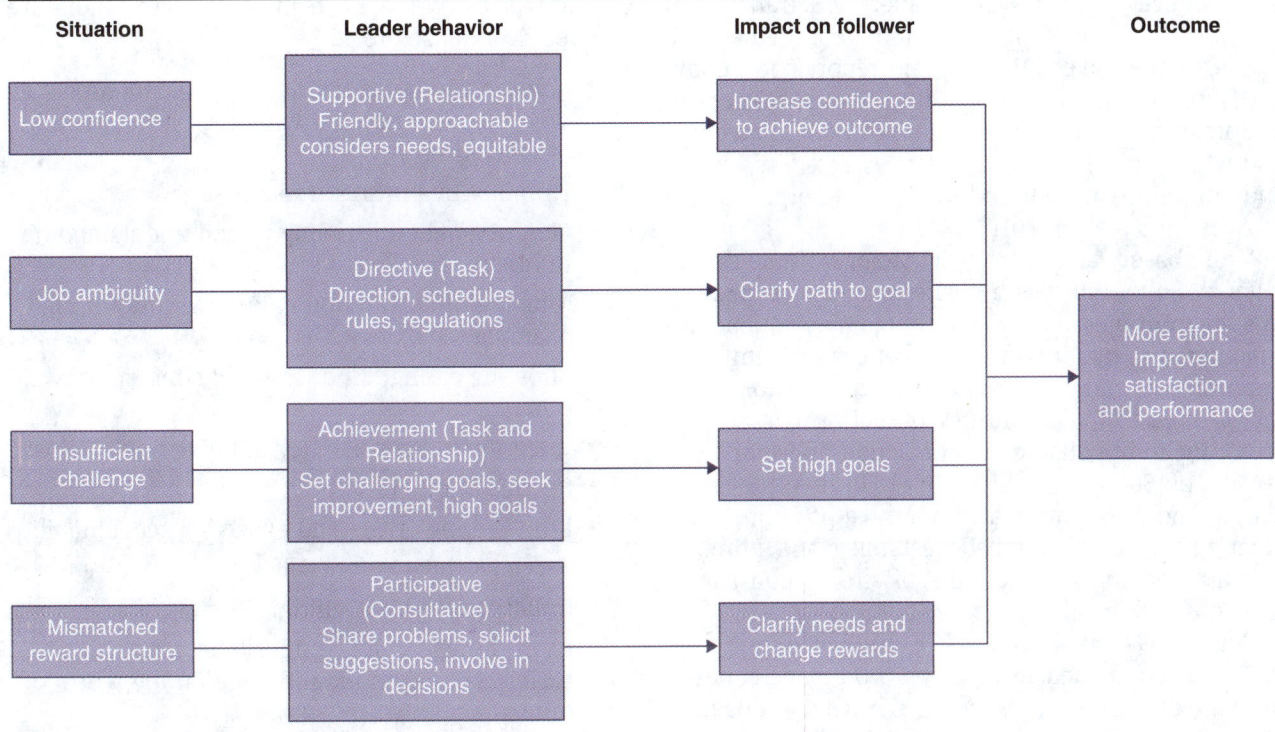

*Source:* Adapted from House 1996.

time. However, when the out-group perceives that the in-group is receiving greater privileges for doing the same work as the out-group, the latter can feel resentment, alienation, and hostility and show lower performance. The leader must ensure fair treatment and clear expectations for both groups. In addition, leaders can promote high-quality relationships with all employees by speaking with people personally, using active listening, not imposing the leader's view on issues discussed, and sharing expectations about the job and working relationship. A 2008 study of the theory supported its key hypothesis that when there was variance in employees' perceptions of equity and fairness, this negatively affected job satisfaction and feelings of well-being (Hooper and Martin 2008).

LMX theory is somewhat different from other leadership theories in that it emphasizes the interaction and quality of the relationship between leader and follower rather than just leadership behavior alone or the same approach applied to everyone. In a review of LMX literature related to HIM, favorable benefits to both leaders and followers were found. These included enhanced group performance, self-efficacy, more initiative, reasonable risk taking, lower turnover, job satisfaction, higher trust levels with supervisors, and career advancement (Hunt 2014).

## Values-Based Leadership

Values are core beliefs that guide and motivate attitudes and actions and both form and express an organization's culture. Values make a difference to most people, and ethical leaders tend to promote more trust and loyalty among their employees and increase efficiency and productivity (Fox et al. 2018; Verbos et al. 2007). Values-based leadership refers to leadership behaviors that emphasize moral, authentic, and ethical orientations to how the organization and employees function (Copeland 2014). The values-based leadership theories are like James McGregor Burns' transformational leadership in which an inspired and enthusiastic leader engages employees to strive toward higher vision for the organization and ethical performance for themselves (Burns 1978). This is also like other contingency theories such as path-goal leadership in which the leader's role is to empower and facilitate employee satisfaction and productivity.

### Role of Values and Ethics

"Everything a leader does sets a tone," especially regarding ethics, according to a National Business Ethics Survey (Ethics Resource Center 2014). Both top leaders as well as direct supervisors were found to have an important role in modeling and supporting ethical behavior and corporate values. Employees who believe managers and leaders are transparent and honest in their communication are more likely to conduct themselves ethically and report bad behavior. However, one of the significant consequences of the organization and its leaders not being perceived as highly ethical is that employees feel less loyalty and commitment and tend to leave the organization (Trevino and Nelson 2011).

Value-based healthcare is replacing volume-driven organizations, but it is a challenging transformation to shift from fee-for-service to outcomes, patient satisfaction, and quality—and perceptions of culture are important for morale and quality. Organizations with the strongest ethical cultures outperform in several areas, including customer satisfaction and employee loyalty, by 50 percent (LRN 2024). To retain talented people and to maintain a competitive position, organizational leadership must reestablish and promote ethical behavior and a culture of strong, consistent, and compatible values.

Since 1994, the Ethics & Compliance Initiative (ECI) has conducted research on workplace conduct from the employee's perspective. The Global Business Ethics Survey focuses on four major ethics outcomes:

- Pressure in the workplace to compromise ethical standards
- Observations of misconduct by employees in their daily work
- The reporting of misconduct when observed
- Any retaliation perceived by employees after reporting misconduct (Ethics Resource Center 2023)

Establishing an ethical culture in an organization affects performance and reduces the risk of employee misconduct or unethical behavior. In 2022, only 14 percent of US respondents felt they worked in a strong ethical culture, 19 percent felt pressure to compromise standards, 53 percent observed misconduct, 62 percent reported misconduct when observed, and 50 percent perceived retaliation after reporting misconduct (Ethics Resource Center 2023). To remedy problems in ethical leadership, commitment to and reinforcement of ethical practices at all levels of management are required so these practices become embedded in the organization's culture.

### Servant Leadership

A prominent values-based approach is **servant leadership**, in which the leader's role is viewed as serving others (Greenleaf Center for Servant Leadership n.d.). To Robert Greenleaf, the concept's founder, servant leaders put the needs, interests, and aspirations of others above their own. A review of more than 100 characteristics of servant leadership in the literature has been condensed to 12 key values:

- Valuing and being committed to people for who they are, not just what they bring to the organization
- Humility by putting others first
- Nonjudgmental listening to and understanding of others
- Trusting others and being trustworthy through example
- Showing caring, kindness, and concern for others
- Integrity and consistency in living one's values
- Service to others
- Empowering others and expecting accountability
- Serving others before self
- Collaboration and building community
- Love (for example, composite of acceptance, caring, appreciation, and belief in the worth of others)
- Continuous learning and personal growth (Focht and Ponton 2015)

The popularity of servant leadership has spread worldwide and to many of the best companies in the US. It has also been explored in healthcare. Servant leadership has been found to positively impact the quality of relationship between healthcare leader and employees (Hanse et al. 2015), job satisfaction (Farrington and Riyaadh 2019), teamwork and patient outcomes (Trastek et al. 2014), customer satisfaction, and financial performance (Jones 2012).

## Complexity Leadership and Systems Thinking

Management guru Peter Drucker states that healthcare workplaces are "the most complex human organization(s) ever devised" (Drucker 2002). Healthcare organizations can be thought of as **complex adaptive systems**, which refers to the complexity of structures and processes involved in healthcare, and the ongoing changes and rearrangements of these structures and processes. Such systems tend to have diverse values, individuals, and rules; and the parts and relationships reorganize as they continually learn about demands that impact them. An example might be a health system comprised of many hospitals and clinics, pharmacies, long-term care facilities, online resources, and social networking (Martinez-Garcia and Hernandez-Lemus 2013). The interconnections among these entities and how they influence behavior and decision-making can be complex and a source of unexpected consequences. Healthcare leaders must be able to tolerate the ambiguity that accompanies such dynamic change, collaborate with diverse thinkers to help conceptualize and plan services, and identify feedback loops that can be used to anticipate change.

The significance of broad criteria used to measure success such as customer focus, cost, and staff development underline the focus required for change leadership. Change strategies must not only include sound financial reasoning to reduce costs, but also create patient satisfaction and employee development, produce evidence-based outcomes, and demonstrate concern for impact on the environment.

Decision makers often focus on the immediate problem as defined and seek to find a single solution to that problem without trying to understand the broader system that has enabled the problem to emerge in the first place. In addition, many problems are considered only in the context or department in which they occur, though the stream of events that led to the problem may have occurred elsewhere. Furthermore, a solution may work within that department but may cause more or worse problems downstream in other departments. Correcting this issue involves viewing more than the cause-and-effect relationship between problem and solution, and it also needs to go further than just considering the immediate context or situation.

**Systems thinking** is based on understanding that a system refers to the interconnections among many components that make up a whole. In healthcare, systems thinking can involve many levels of people and actions involved in a single event, or it can involve an evolving series of connections over time. Not taking time to understand the systemic connections can lead to neglecting factors that may be critical to patient care. For example, medication errors can be mitigated by electronic prescribing, but new errors can also be generated. Inconsistencies between the structured input fields of dose and frequency of administration and the instructions entered in the free-text field can result in delays and potential adverse events (Coiera et al. 2017; Turchin et al. 2011).

One of the important concepts in systems thinking is that of feedback loops or causal loop diagrams (Maccoby et al. 2014). While we typically think of events as a linear series of actions, in many cases each action can have nonlinear spin-off events or lead back to the previous action adding to the complexity and uncertainty in the outcome. A somewhat complex situation is shown in a causal loop diagram in figure 20.14.

**Figure 20.14.** A systems view of overtime effects

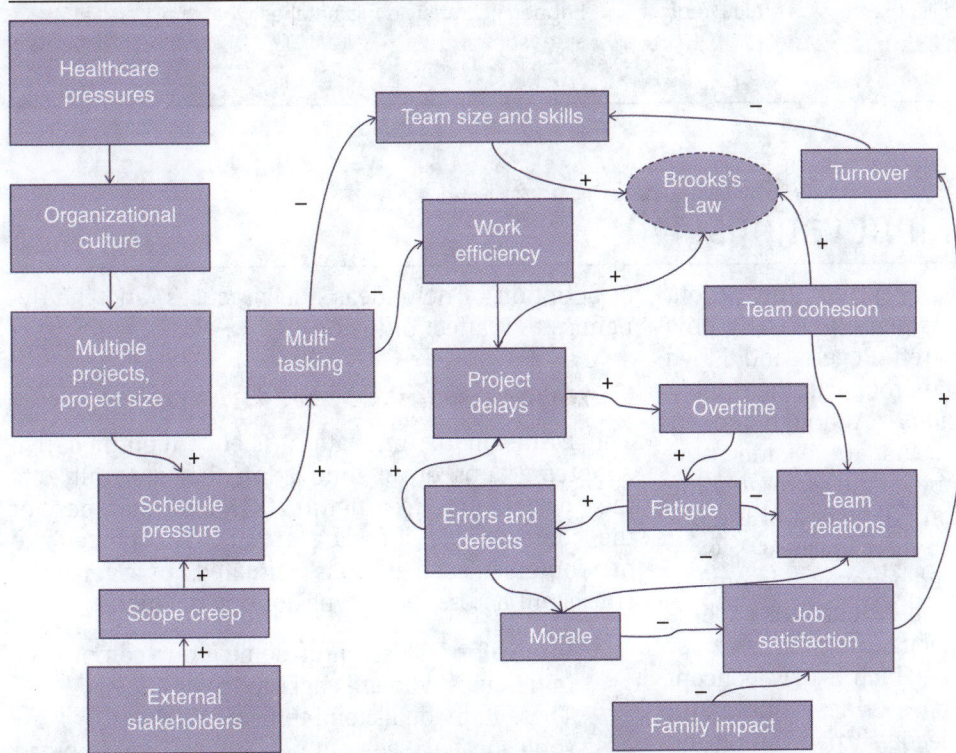

*Note:* Plus signs indicate the next task is increased, while a minus sign indicates a decrease.
*Source:* Swenson 2014.

Unintentional consequences are a relatively common outcome resulting from approaching complex problems with a simple solution mindset. Systems thinking is requisite for healthcare leaders that should be a cornerstone of strategic thinking and a shared skill among all leadership in the organization (de Savigny and Adam 2009; Trbovich 2014).

> **Check Your Understanding 20.3**
>
> Answer the following questions in a separate document.
>
> 1. Make a list of your traits and skills. Then, describe two separate leadership situations you may experience; these could be at work, at school, on a sports team, as a volunteer, and such. Rank your traits and skills in order of how effective they would make you as a leader in each leadership situation you identified. Which skills give you an advantage and which ones might be a disadvantage? Explain your rationale.
> 2. Imagine you have been asked to be a consultant to an aspiring political or managerial figure. You are asked to recommend how this person should appear to others to increase his or her chances for election or promotion. What behaviors would you advise for and against and why? What ethical issues are involved in this type of image building?
> 3. Think of situations where you have noticed effective and ineffective leaders. What makes them different from each other? Consider their personalities, limitations in skills or adaptability, aspects of the situation, as well as what is required of them, and list the traits as effective or ineffective.
> 4. What are some work situations in which an autocratic style might be effective and appropriate?
> 5. The HIS manager would like to streamline the work processes in the release of information (ROI) area so that staff can be scheduled only during business hours, Monday through Friday, 8 a.m. to 4:30 p.m., instead of seven days a week from 7 a.m. to 7 p.m. To show the value of the staff's input, the manager tasked the ROI team to analyze the process, identify inefficiencies, and propose a new process that worked well in the identified work hours. Considering the concept of systems thinking, what might be some unintended consequences in this scenario?
> 6. Think of people with whom you have worked and rank them along the continuum of stages of worker maturity. What are the behaviors that led you to place them at those positions of the immaturity–maturity continuum? What leadership behaviors would you use with them as a supervisor given their maturity levels? Explain what might happen if your style mismatches what they need at these stages.

## Diffusion of Innovations

Innovations have occurred throughout history, but little attention was given to exactly how they were adopted until Everett Rogers and Floyd Shoemaker (1971) clarified the process in their book, *Communication of Innovations*. Although Rogers and Shoemaker were not the first to consider how ideas were diffused and adopted, their presentation of the categories of innovation adopters and the diffusion curve came at a time when businesses were eager to understand consumer behavior. As organization change is considered and innovations such as the EHR are introduced, understanding diffusion, or the way and rate of speed in which a new concept spreads in the market, becomes critical. Successful innovation is dependent on leaders appreciating the way segments of adopters differ, the stages and rates of adoption of new ideas and practices, and the dynamics that affect diffusion.

### Categories of Adopter Groups

The Diffusion of Innovation Theory identified five adopter groups of an innovation that generally fits the normal curve (see figure 20.15 for a summary of the characteristics of each group). The percentage of adopters in each group is estimated but is generally consistent across many types of organizations.

- **Innovators**: This venturesome group comprises individuals who are eager to try new ideas. These individuals tend to be worldly and sophisticated, seek out new information in broad networks, and are more willing to take risks.

- **Early adopters**: The individuals in this group have a high degree of opinion leadership. They are more localized than worldly, and often look to the innovators for advice and information. These are the leaders and respected role models in the organization, and their adoption of an idea or practice does much to initiate change.
- **Early majority**: Although usually not leaders, the individuals in this group represent the backbone of the organization, are deliberate in thinking about and accepting an idea, and serve as a natural bridge between early and late adopters.
- **Late majority**: This skeptical group usually adopt innovations only after social or financial pressure to do so.
- **Laggards**: The traditional members of this group are usually the last ones to respond to innovation. The laggards are often characterized as isolated, uninformed, and mistrustful of change and promoters of change, but they may serve a function by keeping the organization from changing too quickly. (Rogers 2003)

When planning a change, each of these groups should be considered as an internal market segment whose needs must be responded to by leaders.

**Figure 20.15.** Characteristics of innovation stakeholders

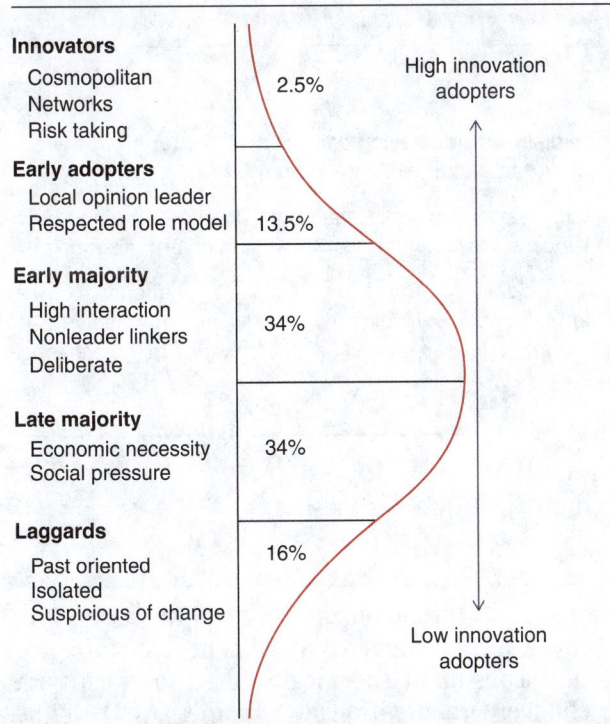

*Source:* Adapted from Shoemaker 2010.

## Dynamics Affecting Innovation Diffusion

Innovations are often difficult for people to adopt, but they can be made more attractive when they meet certain conditions. In general, people are more responsive when a change is presented with consideration to the following factors:

- **Relative advantage.** Innovations are defined as having some advantage over what a person is already doing, and identifying improvements and advantages to work can help a person or an organization accept a change. For example, with a new technology, is it more secure, mobile, or easy to use over current technology? For an adopter, does the EHR provide an advantage over paper records or other legacy information systems?
- **Compatibility.** This refers to how well the innovation matches or fits in with the adopter's needs, work pattern and style, personality, values, and other personal requirements.
- **Simplicity.** Some innovations are too complex and easily overwhelm people, and EHRs are no exception. If they can first be presented simply and with fewer choices, they can be expanded to greater complexity later.
- **Trialability.** Being able to try or experiment with an innovation can reduce the anxiety of making an initial commitment. Working with smaller parts of an innovation or implementing in stages can enable people to become more comfortable with the change.
- **Observability.** If the advantages of an innovation are readily observable to oneself and others, it is more likely to be adopted. Unfortunately, many EHR implementations are not particularly eventful, but satisfaction and successes should be shared among users.
- **Communication channels.** Identifying the pathways used by opinion leaders to influence adoption can improve the diffusion.
- **Homogeneous groups.** Innovations tend to spread faster among groups who share similar characteristics, as opposed to heterogeneous groups who may differ in important ways.
- **Pace of innovation or reinvention.** Some innovations are relatively stable over time, while others are more dynamic and may be changed by adopters as they are used.

- Norms, roles, and social networks. The culture, climate, norms, and social rules tend to shape and modify innovations to fit that system. Culture usually wins out over strategy.
- Opinion leaders. The pace of diffusion can be affected by the influence of leaders and other respected and key persons.
- Infrastructure. Adoption can be further influenced by the support structures available, such as technologies related to the innovation (Cain and Mittman 2002; Shoemaker 2010).

The more these factors can be identified and used to plan, communicate, and execute change, the greater the likelihood there will be fewer barriers, more acceptance, and more successful outcomes. Diffusion theory also accounts for why some innovations are accepted rapidly while others are delayed regardless of substantial evidence supporting their benefits (Sanson-Fisher 2004).

### Innovator Roles

In the late 1960s and early 1970s, the literature reflected a new interest in the roles of organizational innovators who become gatekeepers or nodes for the flow of information (Allen and Cohen 1969). Four roles have been identified for the successful implementation of an innovation:

- **Inventor** (innovator): The individual who develops a new idea or practice in the organization. However, it is not sufficient to merely originate and understand the new idea. Rather, the idea must be facilitated by several other roles in the organization before it is adopted or brought to market.
- **Champion**: Someone in the organization who believes in the idea, acknowledges the practical problems of financing and political support, and assists in overcoming barriers.
- **Sponsor**: Usually a high-level manager who approves and protects the idea, expedites testing and approval, and removes barriers within the organization.
- **Critic**: A crucial but sometimes overlooked role. This role is essential in challenging the innovation for shortcomings, presenting strong criteria, and, in essence, providing a reality test for the new idea. (Daft 2012; Roberts 2007)

In an innovative environment, all these roles are important and exemplary of how role responsibilities are distributed in an organization.

### Check Your Understanding 20.4

Answer the following questions in a separate document.

1. Why are all four innovator roles important for establishing innovations?
2. Think of an innovation you have adopted in your personal life—a technical device, appliance, clothing, or the like. What were the factors that influenced your adoption (for example, trialability, advantage, compatibility, simplicity, and such)?
3. Explain why identifying each of the adopter groups is important during an innovation.
4. Laggards tend to resist change and slow down the innovation process. How can this be valuable in an organization?
5. The release of information (ROI) manager intends to implement a new ROI software. Describe three actions the manager can take to gain acceptance for this change.

## Change Management

A more global role for practitioners of organization change is often referred to as the change agent. The **change agent** is a specialist in organization development who facilitates the change brought about by the innovation. He or she may be internal or external to the organization, as in the case of an employee on a change management task force, or business consultant specifically hired to assist with the change. **Organization development (OD)** is the process in which an organization reflects on its own processes and consequently revises them for improved performance. OD is "an effort planned, organization-wide, and managed from the top, to increase organization effectiveness and health through planned interventions in the organization's processes, using behavioral-science knowledge" (Beckhard 1969, 9).

## Differences between Leaders and Managers

Traditionally, the terms *manager* and *leader* are often used interchangeably (Schyve 2009), but technically they refer to different role functions in the organization. Managers tend to focus on the present situation, maintain efficiency of the status quo, direct others to follow the rules, control risks, carry out requirements to reach the vision through others, and focus within the organization. In contrast, leaders focus on distant opportunities, challenge the status quo, make and break rules by doing things right, inspire, and focus more externally (see table 20.3). These roles tend to become blurred as organizations become flatter, decisions are driven downward, employees are more empowered, and initiative is encouraged. However, since organizations differ in culture, the roles should be explicitly clarified for those new to the position.

Leaders involved in implementing change are most active at three critical points: during the initial stage of change when they explain the reasons for change and offer the vision; during transition when people struggle and need encouragement; and, finally, as the change becomes accepted, success is acknowledged, and the changes need to be stabilized. Managers work closely with people to reduce errors and ensure understanding, provide encouragement and support during transition, and reward behavior that reinforces the new status quo. In some ways, the roles of managers and leaders have become blurred as have the stages since there is rarely a plateau when change is not occurring in modern organizations, and change seems continuous. It is during these long transitions that expert facilitators, from inside or outside the organization, can be of great assistance.

## Organization Development Change Agent Functions

The concept of an agent for change has moved from the narrow specialty of OD, to permeate most professions, including healthcare. Although managers may perform change agent functions, generally managers are viewed as helping maintain efficiency and the status quo. Change agents are more like leaders in that they encourage and facilitate change by thinking about what can be better. OD change agents perform a range of five functions with management:

- *Acceptant function* uses counseling skills to help the manager sort out emotions to gain a more objective perspective of the organization
- *Catalytic function* helps collect and interpret data about the organization
- *Confrontation function* challenges the manager's thinking processes and assumptions
- *Prescriptive function* tells the manager what to do to correct a given situation
- *Theory and principle function* involves helping the client system internalize alternate explanations of what is occurring in the organization (Blake and Mouton 1976)

These functions are essential for HIM professionals who are leading change in healthcare, such as facilitating the transition from the *International Classification of Diseases, Tenth Revision* (ICD-10) to the *International Classification of Diseases, Eleventh Revision* (ICD-11).

## Internal and External Change Agents

Change happens on its own but is usually most desirable when it is intentionally directed toward the benefit of the organization and its members. The role of the change agent is to facilitate this change process by utilizing reflective learning: drawing attention to important processes, helping people understand what the processes mean, and considering and implementing plans of action. Exactly who performs this role can be critical (Lunenberg 2010; Weick and Quinn

Table 20.3. Differences between managers and leaders

| Manager | Leader |
|---|---|
| Administers | Innovates |
| Reproduces/replicates | Originates |
| Maintains | Revises |
| Plans short view | Plans long term |
| Bottom line | Horizon |
| Works with the status quo | Challenges the status quo |
| Does things right | Does the right thing |
| Limited focus | Systemic focus |
| Directs | Inspires |
| Follows the vision | Delivers the vision |
| Controls risks | Seeks opportunities |
| Focuses on "what" | Focuses on "why" |
| Rules oriented | Outcome oriented |
| Transactional | Transformational |

1995). There are advantages and disadvantages to using change agents from within the organization as well as from outside the organization (see table 20.4).

Choosing a change agent can be difficult, and the wrong decision can delay the change process or discourage participants from the effort. When an organization plans to use internal or external change agents, it should consider several questions, including the following:

- How confidential and proprietary is the information involved? Would either type of agent present a disclosure or confidentiality risk?
- Are there conflicts of interest? Is the external agent working with any competitor or internal agent loyal to conflicting parties?
- What level of commitment and availability is required? What is the potential effect of an external agent with many other clients or an internal agent with other work obligations?
- What skills are required for a successful change effort? What constellation of experiences and skills do the external and internal agents offer?
- How important is it that stakeholders view the agent as being objective, fair, and neutral? Which type of agent would best be viewed this way?
- To what extent does the culture of the organization require changing? Which type of agent is better positioned to influence the change?

There are many factors to consider when deciding to use an internal or external change agent. This decision is critical for gaining acceptance and cooperation to work toward an effective change in the organization.

## Stages of Change

People and organizations move through stages of transition in response to change, and as they do, they have different needs and require different skills from the leader. Change is difficult for most people even when parts of the change are desirable, and resistance should be expected as a normal response to doing things differently. Understanding the reasons for resistance to change and the various stages of change can help change agents facilitate this process.

### Resistance to Change

Kurt Lewin, one of the founders of OD, said, "If you wish to understand something, try changing it" (Lewin 1951). When one attempts to change a system, the mechanisms that maintain it spring to its defense. Change does not come easily to most people, and in organizations, "resistance to change is experienced at almost every step" (DeWine 1994, 281). The first step for leaders who are trying to reduce resistance to change is to understand its source and function in the system.

Resistance to change occurs for several reasons, including self-interest and anxiety about the unknown, different perceptions, suspiciousness, and conservatism.

**Table 20.4.** Advantages and disadvantages of internal and external change agents

|   | Internal change agent | External change agent |
|---|---|---|
| Advantages | 1. **Familiarity:** Knows and can maintain the environment, culture, people, issues, and hidden agendas | 1. **Objectivity:** Provides fresh, outside, objective perspective |
|   | 2. **Development of internal staff:** Develops and keeps expertise and resources internal | 2. **New skills:** Brings skills and techniques not available from within organization |
|   | 3. **Personal investment:** Has strong personal investment in success | 3. **Outside perspective:** Brings diverse organizational experiences, benchmarks, comparisons; may have more legitimacy to insiders by not taking sides |
|   | 4. **Trust:** May already have trust and respect of others | 4. **Willingness to challenge:** Is willing to assert, challenge, and question norms |
| Disadvantages | 1. **Bias:** May be biased; has already taken sides, or may be disliked or mistrusted by some stakeholders | 1. **Lack of commitment:** May or may not be available when needed by the organization; may split time and commitments with other clients |
|   | 2. **History:** May have previous relationships that contribute to subgrouping or fragmentation; may be enculturated and is part of the problem or does not see it | 2. **Expense:** Incurs high expense |
|   | 3. **Coverage:** Takes agent away from other duties | 3. **Lack of history:** Takes time to become familiar with the system |
|   | 4. **Internal pressure:** Is subject to organizational sanctions and pressures as an employee | 4. **Co-dependency:** May create co-dependency or may abandon the system |

When confronted with change, the first thing many workers want to know is how it will affect them and their jobs (Quast 2012). Because the turbulence of the marketplace makes many changes uncertain, workers may not receive satisfactory answers to their questions. Those who have attained expertise and status from their positions now may face new job descriptions or expanded or new duties. For example, managers in downsized organizations may have been reassigned as coaches to newly formed teams. This new role raises questions about their authority, status, and responsibility.

Other workers may resist change simply because they perceive the situation differently and believe the proposed change is unjustified. Ongoing change makes many people uneasy about, and even mistrustful of, any innovation. Some people view all change as just another fad based on the whim of management rather than a survival strategy for the organization. Finally, some people are very conservative in their beliefs, are isolated in their social networks and information, and dislike the inconvenience of change.

Resistance can distract workers from their tasks, preoccupy them with gossiping, and contribute to stress and workplace violence. To confident change leaders, indications of resistance can be viewed as useful information about what stakeholders need before the transition can continue. When change is resisted, continued efforts to implement the change are often presented as "overcoming" resistance to change. However, this way of thinking about change implies an adversarial approach rather than collaborative one. Early on in change theory, Lewin (1951) recognized the importance of understanding resistance as a way of reducing it, and offered a tool called the force field analysis as a way of describing the opposing forces and how they could be reconciled. Change efforts are described as an interaction between driving forces for change and those that resist or restrain change. These can be represented as opposing arrows that maintain a status quo, each arrow having an estimated magnitude representing how much it is perceived as driving or resisting change. Rather than increase the driving forces that often result in eliciting a counterreaction and even greater resistance from the restraining forces, Lewin suggested understanding the restraining forces and finding ways to reduce them. When they are reduced, change can occur without as much adversity or conflict.

For example, a hospital is planning to implement a BSC to track KPIs, and the administration suspects it may not be easily accepted. They bring in a consultant to help identify issues on the topic and discover that while there are several driving forces, there are also several resistances that would complicate, delay, or perhaps defeat the effort (see figure 20.16). On the driving side there is administrative support, incentives, vendor support, consumer demands, and legislative requirements. These vary in strength and are opposed by several resistors including a climate of mistrust, fatigue from too many changes, unwillingness to learn new skills, union support for resistance, and frequent miscommunication. Trying to push the change without appreciating the resistance factors would be problematic. Instead, strategic change would involve asking staff more about their resistances and listening and understanding their reasoning. Once staff feels understood, leaders may be able to find ways to reduce each of the objections. More transparency and involvement of representative staff in the planned change may reduce mistrust and miscommunication. Training periods and pay for training might reduce anxiety about new skills or time pressures. While there is no guarantee that all forces against change can be reduced, this broad view can at least identify factors that are more responsive.

### Facilitation of Change

The purpose of transition management is to make the potential upheaval and chaos posed by both planned and unexpected changes less disruptive to the people and processes of healthcare. It is helpful to think of a transition as a series of stages through which people move as they adjust to changes. Each stage has its own set of challenges and tasks to master, the successful completion of which forms the foundation for moving on to the next stage.

The understanding of how change happens and how it affects people has developed considerably

**Figure 20.16.** Force field analysis of forces for and against implementing the balanced scorecard

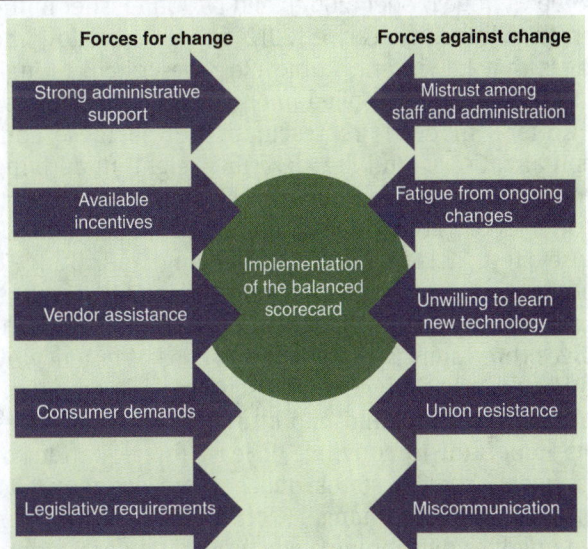

since the original work by Kurt Lewin in the 1940s. Each subsequent generation of management theorists seems to present it with even more detailed distinctions in stages of transition. Lewin initially described how it was important for organizations to "unfreeze" or disrupt the status quo of an organization to mobilize and prepare people for change. The unfreezing could be done by showing discrepancies between expectancies and actual performance, challenging values and attitudes, and proposing a more compelling future. The second stage of change is often awkward and uncertain but involves putting into practice a deliberate plan for transition and implementing new behaviors. Finally, Lewin suggested that as new behaviors become normalized, the change becomes "refrozen" as the new and more effective status quo.

Deming's recognition that as market forces change, organizations correspondingly need to review and revise their operations for continuous change was not widely accepted until the turbulent markets of the late 1970s and early 1980s. By the 1990s, it was apparent that the real focus of organization change was not just the revision of structure and procedures but the engagement and facilitation of the people who were involved in making the transition. William Bridges' book *Managing Transitions* emphasized the distinction between *change* and *transition*: while change referred to a shift in the structure and processes, transition involved the psychological adjustment of people as they adapt to and internalize those changes (Bridges 1991).

Another trend in conceptualizing transition was the description of how people make that psychological adjustment across the stages of change. A seminal work in healthcare by Elizabeth Kubler-Ross is her detailed description of how people deal with grief and loss (Kubler-Ross 1969). This theme was built on by Bridges in his *Transitions* book, by John Kotter in the 8-Step Change Model (2007), and by John Fisher in the Personal Transition Curve (2012). These all follow the stages that Lewin and Kubler-Ross described, though in more detail and applied in organizational settings.

Kotter's model is representative of all these conceptualizations, and he describes eight underlying process steps related to success in transformation (Kotter 2007; 2014). See figure 20.17 for a visual of these steps. Like Lewin's unfreezing and Bridge's ending stage, Kotter proposes phase one for developing a climate for the change process to occur. This involves three steps starting with a sense of urgency by noticing market drivers and discussing related potential crises, threats, and opportunities. Kotter believes it is important to convince at least three-quarters of managers that the status quo is more dangerous to survival than the change (Kotter 2007; 2014). Step two involves developing a coalition of power vendors

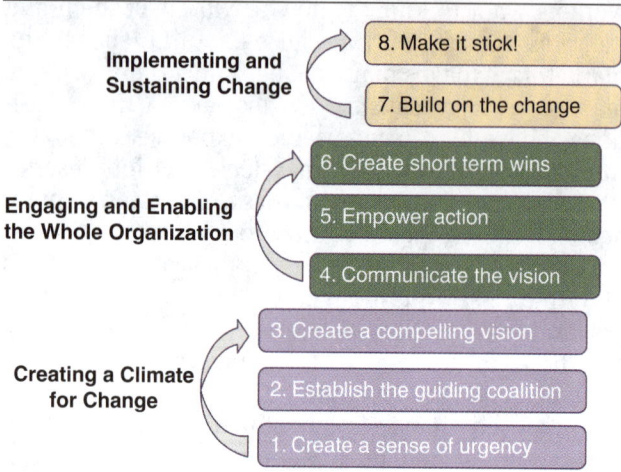

Figure 20.17. Kotter's Phases of Change

who can work together and lead the change efforts. Creating a compelling vision of the future is step three that helps formulate strategies for directing and achieving the change effort.

Phase two engages and enables the organization to participate in and drive the change. Step four involves using multiple vehicles to communicate the new vision and use the coalition to role-model new behaviors. Some consultants recommend overcommunicating by delivering the message seven times to make the change clear (Eligible 2016). Step five empowers others to act by removing obstacles, changing structures and systems that undermine the vision, and encouraging risk taking and innovative ideas and actions. Step six plans and creates short-term wins that are visible, demonstrate improvements, and reward employees for improvements.

Phase three consists of ways to implement and sustain the change. Step seven consolidates what has been improved already and encourages more change. This is accomplished by using earned credibility to change systems not yet compliant with the vision, mobilizing employees who implement the vision, and reinvigorating the process by introducing new themes, projects, and change agents. Step eight integrates the changes into the newly emerging culture by showing connections between behaviors and success and ensuring leadership development and succession throughout the organization.

The more carefully and thoroughly an organization proceeds through these stages, the greater the chances for success, while mistakes at any stage can jeopardize the transition. Over half of the organizations Kotter has consulted with have failed during phase one (Kotter 2007). This has often been due to leaders underestimating the difficulty of creating urgency, overestimating the ease of success, lacking patience for what will likely take years, or becoming paralyzed with the complexity of the situation. Kotter's model has been promoted for use during the implementation of the EHR and provides a detailed and unique approach (Neumeier 2013).

Vision is the centerpiece of Kotter's and others' change strategy, but "vision" is not just an imagined favorable view of the possible future. The current strategic situation for an organization is a resolution of multiple forces and change drivers operating in the environment. Although it is unlikely that any imagining of the future can be completely accurate, especially during turbulent change, any envisioning should be framed around projections of how change drivers will shape the business environment of the future. Vision for the organization becomes more accurate the more that leaders have a sound understanding of trends and patterns among the change drivers that shape the current and emergent environment.

## Leading through Cultural Change

A significant trend in healthcare is the pressure for mergers and acquisitions among healthcare systems, pharmaceutical firms, and health insurance companies (Sanborn 2018). A merger is the combining of two or more companies to form a new one, while an acquisition is where one company purchases another, absorbing it into the parent company. The pace of these has increased substantially, in part due to the pressures resulting from the Affordable Care Act (Singer 2019). Proponents argued that combining resources enables healthcare organizations to benefit from consolidating leadership, organizational structure, and reducing unnecessary duplication in skills. Merging separate entities' cultures can be a major issue—like trying to merge two different personalities (Plank and Cervantes 2015).

Culture- and people-related problems following the merger are two of the leading issues affecting success (Schroeder 2015). Mergers between healthcare systems, facilities, and even departments require a well-thought-out and agreed-on alignment that covers several areas of operations (Chesley 2020). Governing boards must be blended, and they may have different styles of decision-making and doing business. The executive committee and full board may also have difficulty balancing the authority between them. There are often different approaches for alignment with medical staff members and failing to find the best combination of physicians can suboptimize operations, clinical services, and market potentials. Finally, leaders should have a candid discussion of the integration of visions for the unified system.

Merged organizations need to commit time and effort to rebuilding a new culture from the merged organizations. The stages of culture change are very similar to the stages of transition already considered. However, the initial stages for defining the emerging desired culture are worth detailing. Stage one typically involves a culture task force or other designated group that starts by describing the pre-existing cultures from which the organization originated. This shows respect for the previous cultures and clarifies differences and similarities to consider. Both positive and negative perceptions of the two cultures are also openly identified and discussed to surface potential conflicts and establish a norm of openness (Trimnell et al. 2015).

The resulting data from stage one is organized during stage two into a meaningful conceptual framework comprised of seven attributes:

- Physical environment—décor, symbols, artifacts, design
- Beliefs and values—recognitions, ceremonies, stories, traditions
- Communication process and styles—language, blogs, newsletters, memos
- Social environment—events, interactions, ceremonies, rewards
- Work attributes—attendance, punctuality, work ethic, retention
- Management attributes—leadership styles, opportunities for advancement
- Emotional environment—humor, conflict resolution styles, climate (Trimnell et al. 2015)

In stage three, the change team generates a list of desirable culture characteristics to carry into the new culture, and those to leave behind. Stage four takes the list, makes brief definitions or descriptive phrases of each, and then reduces it to the top 10 most desirable culture characteristics. Discussion then focuses on the enablers and constraints that operate on the top 10 in preparation for the implementation plan.

Stage five prepares a synthesis of the top 10 most desirable characteristics into a draft of the culture and recommendations on how they can be implemented. Development of the statement by a widely representative team and sanctioned by top leadership ensures more widespread ownership. It is important that the higher-level culture descriptors are translated down to individual behavior where people are engaged and accountable.

## Response to Change

As much as individuals differ in their responses to change, it should not be surprising that various departments, units, professions, and other stakeholders can vary in their responses. The level of perceived impact on organizational and unit culture and the effect on work styles and turf can dramatically affect responses. For example, in some departments where there is little direct impact, staff may experience minor disruption of daily work and status quo. On the other hand, those who are more affected may show a decline in productivity, have lower morale, and express more complaints. Those who feel violated may actively defy the change or seek employment elsewhere, resulting in job gaps and loss of important knowledge and expertise. The more such reactions can be anticipated and people from all levels engaged in transition planning, the less the adverse impact on individuals, departments, and the organization as a whole. As shown in figure 20.18, different departments may react differently depending on how they perceive the impact of change. Their reactions may also have different trajectories, increasing and decreasing over time.

One should think of these theories as lenses through which organization change and innovations can be viewed. Each organization is different, and change agents may need to customize the transition management model they are using. Nonetheless, the frameworks presented in this chapter are a helpful toolkit for leaders in the turbulent environment of healthcare.

**Figure 20.18.** Variable impact of change on different stakeholders

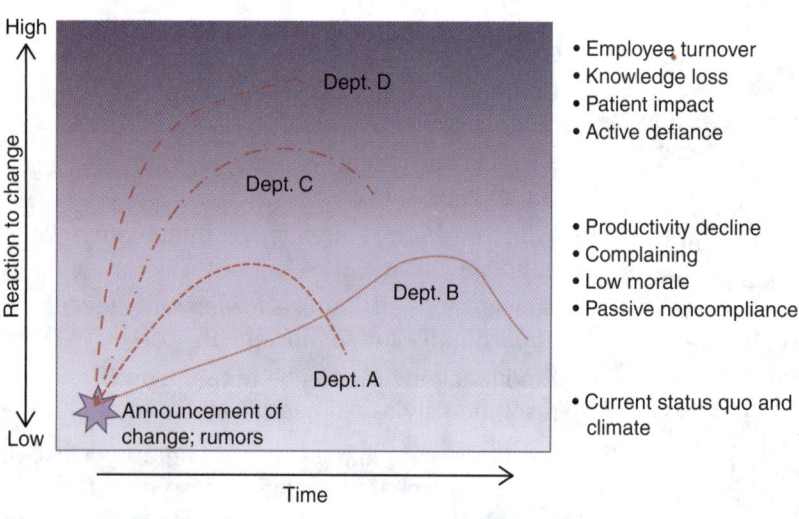

*Source:* Adapted from Creasey 2022.

## Check Your Understanding 20.5

**Answer the following questions in a separate document.**

1. Make a list of reasons that people resist change. For each reason, suggest a way to reduce resistance.

2. Stages of change are a prominent feature of change theories. Explain why the idea of stages is important and how they can be used by a change agent to reduce stress on the people affected by transition.

3. If you were informed that your position was being eliminated due to reorganization but that you could apply for a new position, how would you react? What would you expect from management to help cope with the stress of this change?

4. An external change agent was just hired to facilitate an important organizational change. What are some of the issues that an executive team needs to know before going through a transition? What should they expect and how should they respond?

5. Describe the work cultures of two different departments in an organization with which you are familiar. What are the implications of these differences, and how they could be merged if necessary? What common core do they share (for example, values, outcomes, and such)?

6. Administration has mandated that all departmental policy and procedure manuals need to be updated before the upcoming Joint Commission survey. Differentiate how a manager would approach this request versus how a leader would approach this request.

# References

Allen, T. J., and S. I. Cohen. 1969. Information flow in two R&D laboratories. *Administrative Science Quarterly* 14(1):12–19.

Argyris, C. 1957. *Personality and Organization*. New York: Harper and Row.

Barnard, C. 1938. *The Functions of the Executive*. Cambridge, MA: Harvard University Press.

Beckhard, R. 1969. *Organization Development: Strategies and Models*. Reading, MA: Addison-Wesley.

Bhaskar, H. L. 2015 (June). A comparative analysis of business process reengineering and total quality management. *Global Journal of Business Management* 9(1):11–28.

Blake, R. R. and J. S. Mouton. 1976. *Consultation*. Reading, MA: Addison-Wesley.

Bridges, W. 1991. *Managing Transitions: Making the Most of Change*. Reading, MA: Addison-Wesley.

Burns, J. M. 1978. *Leadership*. New York: Free Press.

Byrne, J. A. 2005. The man who invented management. *Business Week*, November 28, 97–106.

Cain, M., and R. Mittman. 2002. Diffusion of Innovation in Healthcare. Prepared by Institute of the Future for the California HealthCare Foundation. https://www.chcf.org/wp-content/uploads/2017/12/PDF-DiffusionofInnovation.pdf.

Chesley, C.G. (2020). Merging cultures: Organizational culture and leadership in a health system merger. *Journal of Healthcare Management* 65(2):135–150.

Coiera, E., J. Ash, and M. Berg. 2017. The unintended consequences of health information technology revisited. *Yearbook of Medical Information* 2016(1):163–169.

Conbere, J., and Heorhiadi, A. 2018. *The Socio-Economic Approach to Management: Steering Organizations into the Future*. New Jersey: World Scientific.

Connelly, T., and S. Korvek. 2023. *Computer Provider Order Entry*. https://www.ncbi.nlm.nih.gov/books/NBK470273/.

Copeland, M. K. 2014. The emerging significance of values-based leadership: A literature review. *International Journal of Leadership Studies* 8(2):105–135.

Creasey, T. 2022 (November 9). "Understanding Resistance—Prosci's Flight and Risk Model." Accessed February 7, 2024. https://www.prosci.com/blog/understanding-resistance-to-change.

Crew, D., P. Furlow, and S. Houser. 2020. Overcoming challenges of merging multiple patient identification and matching systems: A case study. *Perspectives in Health Information Management* 18(Winter). https://www.ncbi.nlm.nih.gov/pmc/articles/PMC7883361/.

Daft, R. L. 2012. *Management*. Mason, OH: Southwestern.

Dansereau, F., G. Graen, and W. Haga. 1975. A vertical dyad linkage approach to leadership within formal organizations: A longitudinal investigation of the role-making process. *Organizational Behavior and Human Performance* 13:46–78.

Deming, W. E. 1986. *Out of the Crisis*. Cambridge: Massachusetts Institute of Technology, Center for Advanced Engineering Study.

de Savigny, D., and T. Adam. 2009. *Systems Thinking for Health Systems Strengthening*. Alliance for Health Systems Policy and Research, World Health Organization. https://iris.who.int/bitstream/handle/10665/44204/9789241563895_eng.pdf?sequence=1&isAllowed=y.

DeWine, S. 1994. *The Consultant's Craft: Improving Organizational Communication*. New York: St. Martin's Press.

Drucker, P. 2002. *Managing in the Next Society*. New York: St. Martin's Griffin.

Drucker, P. 1986. The appraisal of managerial performance. *Management Decision* 24(4):67–78.

Dunn, R.T. 2021. *Dunn and Haimann's Healthcare Management*, 11th ed. Chicago: HAP.

Eligible. 2016. "Multichannel Marketing for Healthcare." https://eligible.com/community/multichannel-marketing-healthcare/.

Epstein, R. M., C. Hassed, and C-A. Moulton. 2012. *Promoting Self-Monitoring as a Core Competency*. San Francisco: Association of American Colleges Conference.

Epstein, R. M., D. J, Siegel, and J. Silberman. 2008. Self-monitoring in clinical practice: A challenge for medical educators. *Journal of Continuing Health Professions* 28(1):5–13.

Ethics Resource Center. 2023. "Global Business Ethics Survey (GBES): Interactive Dashboard." https://www.ethics.org/gbes-database/dashboard/.

Ethics Resource Center. 2014. *Ethical Leadership*. https://www.ethics.org/wp-content/uploads/2014-ECI-WP-Ethical-Leadership-Every-Leader-Sets-Tone.pdf.

Farrington, S. M., and L. Riyaadh. 2019. "Servant Leadership and Job Satisfaction within Private Healthcare Practices." https://emeraldinsight.com/doi/abs/10.1108/LHS-09-2017-0056?af=R.

Fayol, H. 1917. *Administration Industrielle et Générale; Prévoyance, Organisation, Commandement, Coordination, Controle*. Paris: H. Dunod et E. Pinat.

Fisher, J. 2012. "Process of Personal Transition." www.businessball.com/personalchangeprocess.htm.

Focht, A., and M. Ponton. 2015. Identifying primary characteristics of servant leadership: Delphi study. *International Journal of Leadership Studies* 9(1):44–61.

Fox, E., B. J. Crigger, M. Bottrell, and P. Bauck. 2018. Ethical leadership: Fostering an ethical environment and culture. Integrated Ethics: Improving ethics quality in healthcare. https://www.ethics.va.gov/elprimer.pdf.

French, J. R. P. and B. Raven. 1959. "The Bases of Social Power." In *Studies in Social Power*. Edited by D. Cartwright. Ann Arbor, MI: Institute for Social Research.

Gandolf, S. n.d. "What the Heck is the Hawthorne Effect and How Can It help Hospital and Healthcare Marketing?" Accessed August 8, 2023. *Healthcare Success* (blog). http://www.healthcaresuccess.com/blog/healthcare-marketing/hawthorne-effect.html.

Goleman, D. 1998. What makes a leader? *Harvard Business Review* 74(6):92–102.

Graen, G., and T. A. Skandura. 1987. Toward a psychology of dyadic organizing. *Research in Organizational Behavior* 9:175–209.

Greenleaf Center for Servant Leadership. n.d. "What is Servant Leadership?" Accessed October 14, 2024. https://www.greenleaf.org/what-is-servant-leadership/.

Hammer, M., and J. Champy. 1993. *Reengineering the Corporation*. New York: Harper.

Hanse, J. J., U. Harlin, C. Ulin, and J. Winkel. 2015. The impact of servant leadership dimensions on leader-member exchange among health care professionals. *Journal of Nursing Management*. https://pubmed.ncbi.nlm.nih.gov/25879275/.

Harter, J. 2024 (January 23). "In New Workplace, U.S. Employee Engagement Stagnates." https://www.gallup.com/workplace/608675/new-workplace-employee-engagement-stagnates.aspx.

Hersey, P., K. H. Blanchard, and D. E. Johnson. 1996. *Management of Organizational Behavior: Utilizing Human Resources*, 7th ed. Upper Saddle River, NJ: Prentice-Hall.

Hooper, D. T., and R. Martin. 2008. Beyond personal leader-member exchange (LMX) quality: The effects of perceived LMX variability on employee reactions. *Leadership Quarterly* 19(1):20–30.

Horsky, J., D. R. Kaufman, M. I. Oppenheim, and V. L. Patel. 2003. A framework for analyzing the cognitive complexity of computer-assisted clinical ordering. *Journal of Biomedical Informatics* 36(1–2):4–22.

Houghton, S. M., A. C. Stewart, and P. S. Barr. 2018 (February). Cognitive complexity of the top management team: The impact of team differentiation and integration processes on firm performance: Organizational Behavior, Performance, and Effectiveness *Current Topics in Management* 14:95–118.

House, R. 1996. Path-goal theory of leadership: Lessons, legacy, and reformulated theory. *Leadership Quarterly* 7(3):323–352.

Hunt, T. J. 2014. Leader-member exchange relationships in health information management. *Perspectives in Health Information Management* 11(Spring):1–8.

Jones, D. 2012. Servant leadership's impact on profit, employee satisfaction and empowerment within the framework of a participative culture in business. *Business Studies Journal* 4(1):35–49.

Jones, G. R., and J. M. George. 2021. *Contemporary Management*, 12th ed. New York: McGraw-Hill Irwin.

Kaplan, R. S., and D. P. Norton. 1996. *The Balanced Scorecard*. Boston: Harvard Business School Press.

Karimi, L., S. Leggat, T. Bartram, L. Afshari, S. Sarkeshik, and T. Verulava. 2021. Emotional intelligence: Predictor of employees' wellbeing, quality of patient care, and psychological empowerment. *BMC Psychology* 9(1):93. https://www.ncbi.nlm.nih.gov/pmc/articles/PMC8176682/.

Katz, R. L. 1974. Skills of an effective administrator. *Harvard Business Review* 52:90–102.

Kotter, J. P. 2014. *Accelerate: Building Strategic Agility for a Faster Moving World*. New York: Harvard Business Review Press.

Kotter, J. P. 2007. Leading change: Why transformation efforts fail. *Harvard Business Review* 85(1): 96–103.

Kubler-Ross, E. 1969. *On Death and Dying*. New York: Simon and Schuster/Touchstone.

Landsberger, H. A. 1958. *Hawthorne Revisited*. Ithaca, NY: The New York State School of Industrial and Labor Relations.

Langabeer, J. R., and J. Helton. 2020. *Health Care Operations Management: A Systems Perspective*, 3rd ed. Burlington, MA: Jones and Bartlett.

Lei, L., C. Wang, and J. Pinto. 2023. Do chameleons lead better? A meta-analysis of the self-monitoring and leadership relationship. *Personality and Social Psychology Bulletin.* https://doi.org/10.1177/01461672231210778.

Lewin, K. 1951. *Field Theory in Social Science.* New York: Harper and Brothers.

Likert, R. 1979. From production- and employee-centeredness to systems 1–4. *Journal of Management* 5:628–641.

LRN. Benchmark of Ethical Culture 2024 Report. 2024. https://chat.lrn.com/2024-benchmark-ethical-culture-report?submissionGuid=5ae37544-36de-407f-8015-7677974d3398.

Lunenberg, F. C. 2010. Managing change: The role of the change agent. *International Journal of Management, Business, and Administration* 13(1):1–6.

Maccoby, M., C. Norman, C. Norman, and R. Margolies. 2014. *Transforming Healthcare Leadership: A Systems Guide to Improve Patient Care Decrease Costs and Improve Population Health.* New York: John Wiley and Sons.

Martinez-Garcia, M., and E. Hernandez-Lemus. 2013. Health systems as complex systems. *American Journal of Operations Research* 3:113–126.

Maslow, A. H. 1943. A theory of human motivation. *Psychological Review* 54:370–396.

McConnell, C. R. 2018. *The Effective Healthcare Supervisor*, 9th ed. Burlington, MA: Jones and Bartlett.

McGregor, D. 1960. *The Human Side of Enterprise.* New York: McGraw Hill.

Meyer, R. M. 2008. Span of management: Concept analysis. *Journal of Advanced Nursing* 63(1):104–112.

Mintzberg, H. 1992. The Manager's Job: Folklore and Fact. In *Managing People and Organizations.* Edited by J. J. Gabarro. Boston: Harvard Business School.

Mintzberg, H. 1989. *Mintzberg on Management: Inside Our Strange World of Organizations.* New York: Free Press.

Mosadeghrad, A. M. 2016. Total Quality Management in Healthcare. In *Management Innovations for Healthcare Organizations: Adopt, Abandon or Adapt?* Edited by A. Örtenblad, C. A. Löfström, and R. Shaeff. Routledge.

Neumeier, M. 2013. Using Kotter's change management theory and innovation diffusion theory in implementing the electronic health record. *Canadian Journal of Nursing Informatics* 8(1–2). http://cjni.net/journal/?p=2880.

Ouchi, W. 1981. *Theory Z: How American Business Can Meet the Japanese Challenge.* New York, NY: Avon.

Parker, L. D. 1984. Control in organizational life: The contribution of Mary Parker Follett. *Academy of Management Review* 9:736–745.

Peek, S. 2023 (February 21). "The Management Theory of Mary Parker Follett." https://www.business.com/articles/management-theory-of-mary-parker-follett/.

Peters, T. J. and R. H. Waterman. 1982. *In Search of Excellence: Lessons from America's Best-Run Companies.* New York: Harper and Row.

Pitonyak, J., and R. Desimone. 2024. "How to Engage Frontline Managers." https://www.gallup.com/workplace/395210/engage-frontline-managers.aspx.

Plank, W. and A. Cervantes. 2015 (September 9). What's driving merger and acquisition activity? *Wall Street Journal.* http://www.wsj.com/articles/whats-driving-merger-and-acquisition-activity-1441846542.

Porter, M. E., and N. Nohria. 2018. How CEOs manage time. *Harvard Business Review* 96(4):42–51.

Price, N. 2018 (July 31). The roles and responsibilities of a board of directors of a hospital. BoardEffect. https://www.boardeffect.com/blog/roles-responsibilities-board-directors-hospital/.

Quast, L. 2012. Overcome the five main reasons people resist change. *Forbes.* http://www.forbes.com/sites/lisaquast/2012/11/26/overcome-the-5-main-reasons-people-resist-change/.

Raven, B. H. 1993. The bases of power: Origins and recent developments. *Journal of Social Issues* 49(4):227–251.

Roberson, D., S. M. Connell, K. Dillis, R. Gauvreau, E. Gore, K. Heagerty, L. Jenkins, A. Ma, A. Maurer, J. Stephenson, and M. Schwartz. 2014. Cognitive complexity of the medical record is a risk factor for major adverse events. *The Permante Journal* 18(1):4–8.

Roberts, E. B. 2007 (January–February). Managing invention and innovation. *Research Technology Management* 50(1):35–54.

Rogers, E. M. 2003. *Diffusion of Innovations*, 5th ed. New York: Free Press.

Rogers, E., and F. F. Shoemaker. 1971. *Communication of Innovations: A Cross-Cultural Approach.* New York: Free Press.

Sanborn, B. J. 2018 (March 29). Merger and acquisition activity has record-breaking first quarter in 2018. *Healthcare Finance News.* https://www.healthcarefinancenews.com/news/merger-and-acquisition-activity-has-record-breaking-first-quarter-2018.

Sanson-Fisher, R. W. 2004. Diffusion of innovation theory for clinical change. *The Medical Journal of Australia* 180(6 suppl):s55.

Schroeder, H. 2015. "The Art and Science of Post-Merger Integration." Association for Corporate Growth. https://www.schroeder-inc.com/2016/03/23/the-art-and-science-of-post-merger-integration/.

Schyve, P. M. 2009. *Leadership in Healthcare Organizations: A Guide to Joint Commission Leadership Standards*. San Diego, CA: The Governance Institute.

Sfantou, D. F., A. Laliotis, A. E. Patelarou, D. Sifaki-Pistola, M. Matalliotakis, and E. Patelarou. 2017. Importance of leadership style in quality of care measures in healthcare settings: A systematic review. *Healthcare* 5(4):73. https://www.ncbi.nlm.nih.gov/pmc/articles/PMC5746707/.

Shartle, C. L. 1979. Early years of the Ohio State University leadership studies. *Journal of Management* 5:126–134.

Shoemaker, E. M. 2010. *Diffusion of Innovations*, 4th ed. New York: Simon and Schuster.

Singer, L. E. 2019. Considering the ACA's impact on hospital and physician consolidation. *The Journal of Law, Medicine, and Ethics* 46(4):913–917.

Stephenson, J., and M. Schwartz. 2014. Cognitive complexity of the medical record is a major risk factor for adverse events. *Permanente Journal* 18(1):4–8.

Stogdill, R. M. 1974. *Handbook of Leadership: A Guide to Understanding Managerial Work*. Englewood Cliffs, NJ: Prentice-Hall.

Tannenbaum, T., and W. Schmidt. 1973 (May–June). How to choose a leadership pattern. *Harvard Business Review*. No. 73311. First published in 1958 by *Harvard Business Review* 36:95–101.

The Center for Leadership Studies. 2017. *Situational Leadership: Relevant Then, Relevant Now*. https://www.situational.com/content/uploads/2017/10/FINAL_CLS_History_CaseStudy_Digital.pdf.

Trastek, V. F., N. W. Hamilton, and E. E. Niles. 2014. Leadership models in healthcare—A case for servant leadership. *Mayo Clinic Proceedings* 89(3):374–381.

Trbovich, P. 2014. Five ways to incorporate systems thinking into healthcare organizations. *Horizons* 48(s2):31–36.

Trevino, L. K., and K. A. Nelson. 2011. *Managing Business Ethics*. New York: John Wiley & Sons.

Trimnell, J., D. Butterill, W. Skinner, G. Golyea, L. Yue-Chan, and D. MacFarlane. 2015. Rebuilding organizational culture in the wake of a merger. *Healthcare Management Forum* 14(3):11–23e.

Tsai, C., and K. Qiao. 2023. A cross-cultural examination of the fit between expected and observed leadership behaviors and employee satisfaction: An empirical study of the expectations and satisfaction of Chinese employees toward the leadership behaviors of their expatriate supervisors. *International Studies of Management & Organization* 53(1), 19–39.

Turchin, A., M. Shubina, and S. Goldberg. 2011. Unexpected effects of unintended consequences: EMR prescription discrepancies and hemorrhage in patients on warfarin. *AMIA Annual Symposium Proceedings* 2011:1412–1417.

Verbos, A. K., J. A. Gerard, P. R. Forshey, C. S. Harding, and J. S. Miller. 2007. The positive ethical organization: Enacting a living code of ethics and ethical organization identity. *Journal of Business Ethics* 76(1):17–33.

Waugh, J. 2009. *U. S. Grant: American Hero, American Myth*. Chapel Hill, NC: University of North Carolina Press.

Weick, K. E., and R. E. Quinn. 1995. Organizational change and development. *Annual Review of Psychology* 50:361–386.

White, R. K., and R. Lippitt. 1960. *Autocracy and Democracy: An Experimental Inquiry*. New York: Harper.

Yukl, G. 2006. *Leadership in Organizations*, 6th ed. Upper Saddle River, NJ: Prentice-Hall.

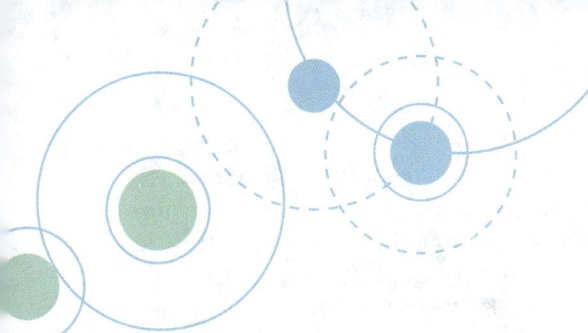

# chapter 21

# Strategic Management

*Ryan H. Sandefer, PhD*

## Learning Objectives

- Lead a strategic planning process leveraging innovative thinking to identify initiatives within a changing and complex healthcare environment
- Conduct and communicate the results of external and internal assessments
- Establish strategies, implementation plans, and evaluations that include measurement for organizational success
- Develop and apply leadership, ethical management, and interpersonal skills to effectively impact change in an organizational setting

## Key Terms

Areas of excellence
Balanced scorecard
Mission statement
Process innovation
Scenarios
Service innovation

Stakeholder
Strategic goals
Strategic management
Strategic objectives
Strategic planning
Strategic profile

Strategic thinking
Strategy
Strategy map
SWOT analysis
Vision
Vision statement

Traditional strategic and business planning techniques are no longer effective in this quickly changing healthcare landscape. An updated and innovative leadership approach to assess the environment; understand risks and opportunities; and plan, manage, and monitor strategic plans is needed. Organizations achieve *sustained* success if their leaders, including managers, (1) have an astute, timely strategic plan for running their department, division, or company; (2) include managers, staff, customers, medical staff, and community leaders in the development of the plan; and (3) implement and execute the plan with proficiency.

Setting strategy has often been viewed as the work of senior managers and boards of trustees. Strategy is often thought of as being mandated from senior leaders, handed down from planning departments and consultants, embodied in slogans, and not very relevant to the day-to-day work of most employees in the organization. The ability to develop effective strategies and plans at the department or division level and contribute significantly at an organizational level is a key attribute and skill of successful HIM managers and leaders today.

Simply stated, **strategy** is the art and science of planning and marshaling resources for their most efficient and effective use to intentionally position and focus your organization for the future. **Strategic management** is the process a leader and his or her leadership team uses for assessing a changing environment to create a vision of the future; determining how the organization fits into the future environment based on its mission and vision and gaining knowledge of its strengths, weaknesses, opportunities, and threats; and then setting in motion a strategic plan of action to position the organization accordingly.

**Strategic planning** is a management tool used to develop a formalized roadmap that spells out where an organization is going over the next one to five years and describes how the company can focus on its continuing mission and execute the chosen vision and strategy. A **vision** gives a short description of an organization's ideal future state. A **mission statement** is a statement that sets forth the core purpose and philosophies of an organization or group; it defines the organization or group's general purpose for existing. The mission stays static, but the vision may change, as it depicts a future strategy. Management theories about the importance of strategy and how to set strategy are changing. This reconsideration reflects the speed of change in every facet of contemporary life, including healthcare. One of the key components seen as missing or poorly done in current strategic planning processes is strategic thinking.

**Strategic thinking** is the thought process of an organization's leaders that helps them determine the vision for some point in the future and identify a strategy to achieve this vision. Strategic thinking is the framework for the strategic and operational improvement plans. Game-changing strategies come from a connection between different ways of thinking strategically, inspired to invent new ways of doing business (Brandenburger 2019, 58).

This chapter explores the importance of strategic thinking and planning to effective strategic management, describes approaches to making and communicating strategic choices, provides approaches for maximizing organizational learning, and illustrates how HIM professionals can use strategy to shape and influence change in their department and organization.

## From Strategic Planning to Strategic Management and Thinking

Strategic planning was first described in management literature in the 1940s and continued to grow as a prominent and highly touted organizational function in the decades that followed. Strategic planning was developed to prevent organizations from crisis planning. Competitors were outpacing them in innovation and they quickly had to develop reactive strategies to maintain a competitive advantage. Early applications were characterized by rigorous and formal analysis of data to determine a desired future and the steps to achieve a three-to-five-year plan. In large corporations, departments of planners prepared forecasts with the aid of computer analysis. The complex reports were delivered to senior leaders, who made decisions with little or no involvement from managers or employees in the process.

These approaches have fallen out of favor for several key reasons. First, forecasting the future, particularly in such rapidly changing times, is difficult. Second, by the time a complex multi-year plan is finalized and delivered to its managers and employees, it is undoubtedly out of date. If customers, employees, and all levels of managers are involved in strategy development, the plan is likely to be seen as relevant and likely to be implemented. Third, for strategic planning to really be more than an operations improvement plan, the plan must include a clear vision for the future and innovative strategies that not only help the organization redefine its existing products and services but also create new products and services that strategically move the organization forward toward its vision.

For an organization to stay strong and viable, HIM professionals must understand the organizational vision. They must engage the best thinking of everyone in and outside their area, consider where the organization is today and where it needs to be in the future, and then design the path for their area to assist the organization in achieving the new vision as a team. When departmental and organizational strategic plans are reviewed and updated at least annually, the effort will result in plans that cause transformative organizational change.

No one phrase is the accepted label for this type of comprehensive strategic planning and thinking. Today's managers and directors in many organizations are likely to still hear the activity referred to as *strategic planning*. However, it can embody many concepts that encapsulate strategic management and strategic thinking:

- It is framed by the organization's vision, mission, and values.
- It considers possible future scenarios rather than trying to forecast only one future.
- It is the work of all levels of management and involves key **stakeholders**, defined as individuals within the company who have an interest in, or are affected by, the results of a project.
- It is action-oriented and measurable, with a commitment to bringing about change.
- It results in organizational innovation, change, and learning.

Strategic thinking is a way of introducing innovation and creativity into decision-making and engaging others in the change process. The competencies that distinguish a strategic thinker include the following:

- An ability to plan (consensus building) and formulate strategy (leadership)
- Flexibility and creativity
- Comfort with uncertainty and risk
- A sense of urgency and vision of how to move change forward positively
- An understanding of how to gain a powerful core of organizational supporters and customers
- An ability to communicate the vision and plans

Strategic thinking should be viewed as a component of each of the four functions of management namely planning, organizing, directing, and controlling. Every aspect of management involves a strategic component, as described here. With organizational learning as a centerpiece, the approach described in this chapter unifies change management, strategy development, and leadership. In all three areas of organizational learning, managers learn by observing and reflecting on the results of their experiences. To undertake deliberate change, individuals use their experiences to find new ways of looking at the patterns and trends that they did not previously perceive. Innovative thinking is considered important when testing and applying new ways of what can and should be, along with continuous improvement and evaluation.

## Skills of Strategic Managers

The definition of strategy is straightforward, but the skills for setting and executing strategy are far from simple. HIM professionals must take advantage of opportunities to learn and develop skills for strategic management, including the following:

- Monitoring industry trends in healthcare and information management
- Reflecting on how industry trends can affect existing and new products and services
- Considering how changes in one area can affect others in the organization
- Considering how a strategic course for change is set for their organizations and how to apply it to the department level
- Helping others visualize the need for change and recruiting them as partners in moving a change agenda forward
- Implementing and measuring strategic plans effectively
- Questioning the status quo on a continuing basis
- Leading innovative change
- Being self-reflective and lifelong learners

Strategy is no longer a management domain reserved for senior managers. Today, all managers must develop skills and competencies that enable them to think and act strategically. Strategic managers watch for changes in the larger environment beyond the healthcare industry, including political, economic, social, and technological changes. Such changes may involve staff attitudes, public policy, ethics, or inventions and innovations within the healthcare industry or externally. Managers must consider how these changes are affecting—or might affect—healthcare and the organizations in which they work. For example, shifts in public attitudes regarding the value placed on personal privacy and security of health information have implications for health information policies and practices regarding patients who are electronically requesting copies of their health records.

Strategic managers develop skills reflecting the implications and opportunities afforded by trends. Whether reading a journal or discussing new ideas with others, strategic managers are always testing new ideas, identifying those that have merit, and discarding those that do not. They are creating links between the trends and the value-adding actions they can take. For example, federal programs to adjust provider reimbursement based on certain quality parameters suggest a need to elevate organizational health information standards for data integrity so pay-for-performance determinations are accurate and fair.

Effective strategic managers and thinkers are creative in how they make associations among trends, ideas, and new opportunities. These associations are not always direct, as in the examples about privacy and public policy or data quality and pay for performance. Making strategy choices may be the result of drawing lessons from analogous situations. Managers should realize the benefit of connecting with and learning strategy from other colleagues and other industries. For example, faced with a shortage of trained coders, the HIM director institutes a coder training program in partnership with human resources looking to retrain other employees or with a local community college, modeled after a similar program used to address the shortage of nurses in the community.

Strategic managers also continually look for opportunities to improve on the status quo. They do not accept the adage, "If it's not broken, don't fix it." They always look for ways to make things better and are willing to take calculated risks and evaluate new approaches through trial and error. They understand that taking no action may be less tolerable than trying something even if it does not fully succeed. For example, the quality of coded data for inpatient services is at 94 percent and the data quality manager thinks that adjusting staff assignments may make better use of staff skills and improve performance even further. This change must be monitored closely and adjusted appropriately.

New managers may lack the confidence to initiate change and may have few analogous experiences to draw on. Still, they should guard against accepting or perpetuating artificial barriers to creativity characterized by common statements, such as, "We've never done that before," "We have always done it that way," or "That's not my job." Confidence comes from experience, and experience requires asking focused questions, action, and thoughtful reflection on what did and did not work. It is important to use the information from this reflection to move forward strategically.

Finally, strategic managers learn to help their organization contribute to innovative thinking, which leads to new ideas. They know that the best solutions represent the best thinking of all key stakeholders. Thus, strategic managers learn techniques to bring out the greatest thinking of their staff, superiors, colleagues, and customers for their change agenda. For example, in pursuit of decreasing the number of electronic records physicians printed, the health information manager knew that support from nursing and other staff in the patient care units was essential for success. The health information manager oversaw implementation of a multifaceted plan to reduce the rate of printing on the units and shared credit with the nurses and clinicians when the print rate began to decline.

The science and art of leadership required to become a strategic manager can be learned. Learning begins by recognizing the importance of strategy for being a successful manager.

## Elements of Strategic Planning

As shown in figure 21.1, strategic thinking and strategic management are logical processes that comprise several steps in strategic planning that may be explicit or implicit. The four phases are as follows:

- Phase I: Environmental Assessment
- Phase II: Identifying Organizational Direction
- Phase III: Strategy Formulation
- Phase IV: Implementation

**Figure 21.1.** Elements of strategic planning

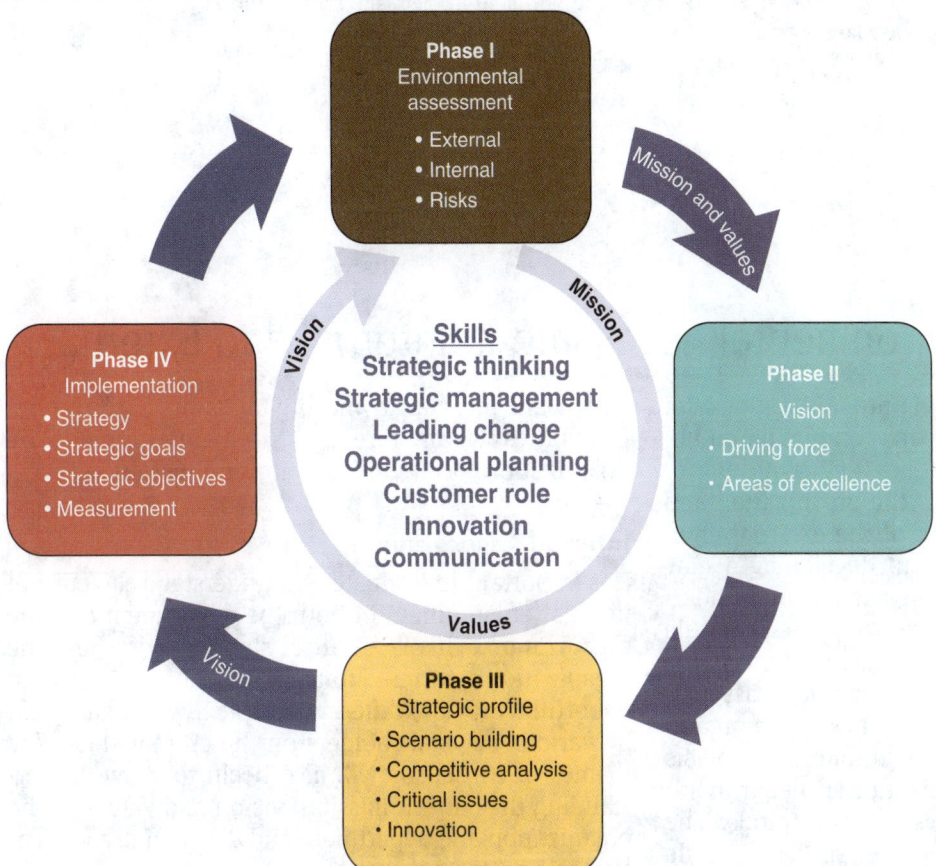

The strategic planning process is depicted as circular because overall strategic management is a never-ending process and often requires revisiting steps as more information is discovered. The best strategies may emerge from trial and error, but an effective strategy will not emerge without a clear idea of where the leaders want to move the organization and a realistic assessment of the environmental issues to overcome. Moreover, strategic management cannot happen in isolation. Stakeholders—whether staff, customers, caregivers, patients, or managers—must be engaged in each phase of the strategic planning process.

Each step involves learning, which in turn enables plans to be improved upon, therefore making subsequent efforts more effective. Thus, experience sharpens and clarifies understanding of the issues, allowing managers to be more precise in setting goals. Strategies and tactics are continually modified with experience. Strategic management is a process that leads to organizational learning and improvement over time.

In contrast to traditional strategic planning, where all steps are neatly outlined before implementation is begun, strategic management requires a willingness to learn and change as the leaders guide an organization through the process. In a fast-paced, changing healthcare environment, constant review of strategy, goals, and objectives is required, as well as new skills focused on strategic thinking, planning, and management.

## Check Your Understanding 21.1

**Answer the following questions in a separate document.**

1. Give an example of when it is strategic to choose not to move forward with an initiative. Justify your reasoning.
2. How does strategic thinking differ from strategic planning? Share a specific example of strategic thinking that you have or might apply to a department, organization, or college.
3. Identify three key stakeholders in your strategic thinking example above. Evaluate what the role of each key stakeholder group might be and explain why.

4. The organization has just developed a new strategic plan that creates a vision of preparing the organization for value-based care. What are three key skills a strategic thinker needs to assist the organization in achieving its vision?

5. How would you explain the distinctions between each of the four strategic planning phases?

6. How would you encapsulate the important concepts of strategic management?

# Phase I: Environmental Assessment: Internal and External

The strategic planning process begins with phase I, with the leadership team conducting an environmental assessment, including a current description and internal assessment of the organization and department and an assessment of the external environment. The beginning stage in developing a new or updated strategic plan is to develop a solid understanding of the organization's current strategic profile through the internal and external assessment of the organization or department. This approach assesses the current mission, vision, and values of the organization or department; completes an internal analysis of the trends within the organization or department; and conducts an external assessment of trends. The final step in completing the current strategic profile is to assess the potential impact of the uncertainties and risks in the internal and external environment on the organization's strategic plan. Based on all the information and intelligence gathered throughout this profiling process, the strategic thinking tools and techniques described here are then utilized to develop a strategic future profile.

## Understand Environmental Assessment Trends

Knowledge of the current internal and external environment is essential to vision and strategy formulation. A comprehensive environmental assessment is conducted, which is defined as a thorough review of the internal and external conditions in which an organization operates. This data-intensive process is the continuous process of gathering and analyzing current information and intelligence about trends that are—or may be—affecting the industry, the healthcare organization, and HIM. It is both internally focused on HIM and the healthcare organization and externally focused on related industries, market, and environmental trends. A **SWOT analysis** tool is commonly used in this step. A SWOT analysis outlines the organization's strengths (S) and weaknesses (W), which are internal to the organization, and the opportunities (O) and threats (T) that are external to the organization. See figure 21.2 for an illustration.

### Internal Assessment

It is important to evaluate and understand the current internal environment of both the department and the organization. This is a critical step to understand the organization's current strategic direction. It is also an opportunity to gain differing perspectives that are held by various key stakeholders on the current state. Key themes of consensus will also begin to show. Understanding the current mission, vision and values of the organization and department and developing a current strategic profile are part of the internal assessment.

***Assess the Current Mission, Vision, and Values*** It is important to review the current mission, vision, and values of the organization and department. The mission is a statement of the core purpose and philosophy while the vision is a description of the desired future that sets the direction and rationale for change; the mission stays static, and the vision is the picture of the future. It is also important to understand the organizational values used to describe the basic philosophy, principles, or ideals of the organizational culture and behavioral expectations. Any strategic plan must be developed in accordance with the mission, vision, and values of the organization to help drive change supported by staff and senior leaders.

***Develop a Current Strategic Profile*** The organizational description needs to include a current **strategic profile** that identifies the existing key services or products of the department or organization, nature of its customers and users, nature of its industry and market segments, and nature of its geographic markets (Robert 2006, 53–54). Another critical step in the assessment process is to conduct a SWOT (strengths,

**Figure 21.2.** Illustration of a SWOT analysis

## SWOT ANALYSIS

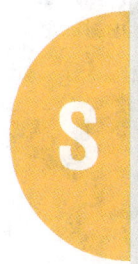

**STRENGTHS**

Internal characteristics of the organization that give an advantage over others

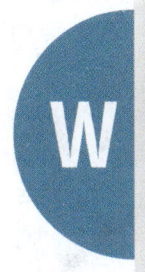

**WEAKNESSES**

Internal characteristics that put the organization at a disadvantage relative to others

**OPPORTUNITIES**

External factors that the organization can capitalize on to improve its performance.

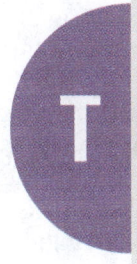

**THREATS**

External factors that have the potential to harm the organization's performance

weaknesses, opportunities, and threats) analysis of the department and organization. A SWOT analysis

> evaluates the internal organization based on its *strengths* compared with regional competitors and community needs and demands, *weaknesses* compared with competitors or patient and staff perceptions of the internal functions, *opportunities* for advancing ahead of competitors or serving a patient population not served well currently, and *threats* from external or internal competitors or agents that could limit the organization's success. (Dunn 2021, 214)

This process should involve multiple key stakeholders (for example, students, faculty, staff, and alumni at a college or university; or providers, patients, and coders in a healthcare setting) and will be an opportunity to begin consensus building about the current internal strengths and weaknesses, along with the external view of opportunities and threats (SWOT analysis) related to your plan. At this point in the process, planning assumptions, data analysis, and identification of potential risks and uncertainties should be finalized.

The internal environmental assessment includes analysis of the following:

- *Role statements and organizational framework*: Organization-wide strategy and priorities; evaluating whether the organization is meeting its mission, vision, and value statements, and whether its structure and processes are designed to achieve business aims; includes an assessment of program development, governance, and management
- *Performance indicators*: Patient experience, quality, patient access to care, human capital, operating margin, budgeted staff, key statistics, educational resources, competencies, and organizational culture; information management strategy, information systems plans and priorities, compliance programs, products and services, and business processes
- *Primary market research*: Information on the organization and its marketplace, staff and customer experience feedback
- *Financial performance and position*: Budget targets and results, financials, performance, and productivity measures (Harris 2018, 35–39)

When the internal assessment is complete, there should be a comprehensive view of the organization's past and current performance and strategy. Developing a comprehensive SWOT analysis and current strategic profile should clearly identify the organization's advantages and disadvantages in the internal and external environment and key planning issues. This information will be useful in the next steps of the strategic planning process, developing an external assessment. Involving employees, leaders, and all key stakeholders in each step of the process is critical.

### External Assessment

The external environmental assessment is conducted to understand the organization's performance as it relates to its marketplace and includes the following:

- *Review forces of the healthcare industry*: Demographic, economic, political, health status, social, technological, and educational factors that may affect the organization
- *Conduct primary market research*: Comparative information on the organization and its competitors and other likely key external factors including the community
- *Assess market forecasts and implications*: Healthcare reimbursement systems, patient and customer engagement trends, and regulatory trends
- *Analyze competitors*: Collect competitor data rigorously using multiple sources
- *Identify potential collaborators*: Current and potential collaborators and partners
- *Assess market trends*: A review of the state of the healthcare industry and other related industries and organizations (Harris 2018, 116–119)

Other key pieces of information needed for the external assessment phase can be used as appropriate.

An HIM manager who focuses exclusively on his or her own area of responsibility, whether managing a department, a service, or a project, will have a difficult time succeeding as a strategic manager. Understanding the external environment provides the context for the tough decisions involved in setting direction, designing strategy, and leading change.

The internal and external environment should be assessed together and summarized with succinct graphs and tables. After reviewing the information gathered during this phase, the organization's strengths, weaknesses, opportunities, and threats should be evident. The assumption about the future environment should now be identified. The product of this phase in the process should be a list of critical issues to be addressed and resolved in the next phase of the strategic planning process (Harris 2018, 129–132).

## Assess and Manage Risk and Uncertainty

Analyzing the changing environment and envisioning the future is an analytic and a highly creative activity. Understanding internal and external trends and forces of risks and uncertainties requires analysis of the following:

- Relationships between trends
- Sequence of events
- Causes and effects
- Priority among items

As a strategic thinker, the ability to consider the internal and external environment is a critical skill requiring an understanding that there is risk and uncertainty as an organization begins to predict possible future trends and design strategies to manage them. It also gives the manager an opportunity to find ways for developing strategies to avoid possible pitfalls or counteract external and internal forces. Examples of key risks and uncertainties to review include the following:

- Market demand—market and industry trends affecting the demand for the service or the organization
- Supply factors—access to trained employees, physicians, or supplies needed by the service or organization
- Competitors—information technology (IT), outsourcing, mergers, and acquisitions
- Macroeconomic shifts—payers, employers, and customer trends
- Policy and Regulation—federal or state government regulatory, policy, and legal changes
- Time (immediately, six months, one year, or several years)—when the forces of risk and uncertainty described earlier are predicted to potentially change or not change (Jennings 2000, 7–14)

Another helpful aspect in reviewing key external forces that may bring risk and uncertainty is understanding they can be categorized into three levels of uncertainty. Categorization helps evaluate how to mitigate risks. A clear trend (CT) is one known to be happening with certainty. An "unknown that is knowable" (UK) is a force or trend where current facts or information may not be known but can be researched and become known. A residual uncertainty (RU) would be defined as a level of uncertainty unable to be determined as the information is not knowable during the needed time frame, even though assumptions about its level of risk must be made. Part of the strategic process must evaluate each of the identified risks and uncertainties by these three categories (Jennings 2000, 10–13). Within HIM, examples of these categories of forces are as follows:

- CT—the move from a paper medical record to the electronic health record (EHR)
- UK—consumer preferences of the electronic patient portal
- RU—fate of IT vendors that develop and support EHRs

When assessing the levels of risk and uncertainty, it is important to understand that there may be elements the leaders will not understand or that may become clearer over time. Organizations must decide whether it is important to continue tracking each of the risks or uncertainties or if they continue to have a high level of importance. The levels of risk and uncertainty that seem important will be helpful to include in the next phase, which focuses on tools for strategic thinking—especially the scenario-building exercise.

The last step in the environmental assessment process is to determine the strategic critical issues facing the organization. This list should serve as an important step in understanding what operational and strategic matters may need to be addressed by strategy development. The review of critical issues can assist in prioritizing critical success factors as key issues to the organization's future, not just current operations.

### Check Your Understanding 21.2

**Answer the following questions in a separate document.**

1. Describe four key types of information that should be collected during the external environmental assessment phase and provide an example of each type as it applies to your organization, department, or college.
2. Explain why is it important to review trends in other industries when conducting the internal and external assessment phase?
3. Summarize the three categories used to assess the possible levels of sources of uncertainty and apply them to at least three identified sources of uncertainty in your organization, department, or college.
4. The current and future strategic profile requires a description of four key aspects of the organization (or department). List these four key elements and describe how the future strategic profile may differ from the current one.
5. Formulate reasons why the SWOT analysis tool is helpful for both the internal and external environmental assessment of an organization during phase I. Generate an example of an internal strength and a weakness and identify an external opportunity and a threat for an organization, department, or college you are familiar with.
6. What is the purpose of an external environmental assessment in relationship to strategic planning?

## Phase II: Identifying Organizational Direction from Vision to Strategy

As defined earlier, a strategy is an action or the set of actions that moves the organization toward its vision. Strategic management is about identifying organizational direction and pursuing a new set of activities or prioritizing ways of carrying out current activities that move the organization toward its vision. It may take the form of new or redesigned programs or services. It may involve implementing new systems, outsourcing certain operations, or merging functions with another organizational entity. It also may entail phasing out an outdated program or adopting new technologies. Finally, it may be aimed at bringing an organization into compliance with new regulations or finding new ways to reduce operating costs.

It is important to remember that strategic management is not the same as operations management improvement. Operations improvement is ongoing and internally focused and if aligned with the strategic plan, will assist in bringing the organization toward its goals. Strategic management seeks to improve the position of the organization for the future and in the broader marketplace in which it operates. The vision statement may require review and alignment of the organization's mission and values.

## Create a Commitment to Change with the Vision

The organization's vision sets the broad future direction for the new strategy, leaving the details to be worked out. An effective, bold organizational **vision statement**, or picture of the desired future state of the organization, has the following characteristics:

- Conveys a memorable and simple picture of what the future will look like
- Evokes strong emotion and creates a strong sense of urgency
- Is clear enough to provide guidance in decision-making
- Is flexible so that alternative strategies are possible as conditions change
- Is easy to describe and communicate (Kotter 2012a, 72)

A vision states the direction of what the organization aspires to become and helps motivate people to act. The AHIMA Board of Directors developed the AHIMA vision, "A world where trusted information transforms health and healthcare by connecting people, systems, and ideas" (AHIMA n.d.). This vision led to the need to develop an updated strategic plan that included both short- and long-term priorities. This is evidence of AHIMA using its vision to strategically lead its members in the advancement and use of health data and information management for the delivery of quality healthcare worldwide.

A vision must be worth pursuing. Designing a compelling vision requires a solid understanding of the internal and external environmental assessment. It also requires the ability to break free of the current paradigms, which are philosophical or theoretical frameworks within which a discipline formulates its theories and makes generalizations, and to think creatively about a new reality for the future.

The following are examples of effective and ineffective vision statements within HIM organizations. A director of HIM services for a health system envisions services that make full use of staff and technology to provide high-quality, cost-effective information to authorized users. The director expresses this idealized vision as follows:

*Utilizing state-of-the-art information technology and evidence-based practices, we will deliver accurate electronic information to support patient care and healthcare operations.*

This is an example of an effective vision that lays out a substantial challenge, yet it provides focus. First, the overarching vision is to be able to deliver all information electronically to all users of HIM services. It acknowledges that technology is only as effective as the enabling processes; therefore, it promises use of evidence-based or research-proven practices, which are practices substantiated by applied research that demonstrate their validity. The vision statement acknowledges that achieving this vision will require new ways of working. First, success will require gaining a deeper understanding of the needs of those working in patient care and healthcare operations, who rely on the information and whose collaboration is needed to achieve the vision. Second, it will require effective teamwork among HIM staff, who must become more comfortable with both change and risk taking.

In another example, an HIM consultant for a long-term care system was having difficulty gaining support for a vision of what an EHR could contribute to the residents, staff, and overall organization. The consultant developed the following description of the vision:

*All members of the care team have immediate access to complete and accurate information for each resident. This information recaps care delivered, and presents the status of all health, social, activity of daily living (ADL), and other resident-specific issues being managed. Information needs to be entered just once and is available for a variety of patient care, quality improvement, and administrative uses. Summary reports are used as the basis for shift change briefings and for periodic care conferences. The information system prompts caregivers to actions that need to be taken and alerts them to changes in status that require special vigilance. Data entered in the system summarizing observations, care given, orders, and activities produce a record of care that meets licensing and other external requirements. The system also automatically accumulates the information needed for care and operations management and for external reporting.*

This vision is ineffective because it highlights the difficulty many have in creating a brief, compelling vision, since it includes too many specific objectives. The vision could be simplified and revised as follows:

*All members of the care team and management will have immediate access to complete and accurate information for each resident to improve patient care, quality, and timeliness.*

This brief but compelling vision statement serves as a starting point for creating a more detailed set of specifications and evaluating potential EHR system vendors.

Visions can be created to narrow focus on a particular project. For example, a data quality manager for a multispecialty group practice clinic prepared the following vision statement to help the physicians and coding staff rally around a proposed project to improve the timeliness and accuracy of billing processes by using computer-assisted coding tools:

*During each patient visit, the physician will document using an electronic tablet. This will assist the practice in achieving 90 percent of visits billed within one business day, 95 percent within three business days, and the balance within five business days.*

This vision statement has three major elements. It sets aggressive, measurable goals of billing 90 percent of visits on the day of service, 95 percent within three business days, and the balance within five business days. To do so, physicians must initiate the process using an electronic tool to eliminate time-consuming handling of handwritten information. It also requires physician coding specialists with advanced data quality and compliance management skills to do concurrent coding.

These vision statements relate to HIM challenges. However, it is important that the HIM vision complements the organization's overall vision and mission. For example, the organization's vision is to be known for its advanced clinical services in cardiac and oncology care. To achieve this vision, the organization is pursuing a strategy of attracting clinical talent with national reputations and expanding clinical research programs. This overall organization vision and strategy should be accounted for when crafting the HIM- or department-level vision and strategies.

Strategic managers must understand the overall organizational vision, strategy, and goals and take them into account when crafting their own plans. They seek ways to support and further the overall strategy of the organization through the priorities they set for their areas of responsibility. Advancing the organization's goals through synergistic efforts is the mark of a successful strategic manager.

## Define Areas of Excellence

Understanding and developing clear current and future areas of excellence is another key concept of strategic thinking. The concept of **areas of excellence** refers to describable skills, competencies, or capabilities that a department or company cultivates to a level of proficiency greater than anything else it does (Robert 2006, 62–63). To determine a strategic direction, the leader must develop a clear understanding of current key areas of excellence in the organization and what future areas of excellence are needed to achieve the new vision. Over time, the strategy of an organization, like a person, can become stronger and healthier or it can grow weaker and sicker. What determines the future success of the strategy are the areas of excellence a department or an organization deliberately cultivates to keep the strategy strong and healthy (Robert 2006, 62). For an HIM director, understanding special capabilities—such as managing the collection of patient and clinical quality data to improve quality of patient care or obtain value-based payment incentives—can be an important area of excellence. It becomes much easier to make difficult choices involving resources and time allocation if it is clear which strategies and current and future areas of excellence are pursued.

## Formulate Key Strategies

The next step in strategic planning is to formulate and refine key strategies aligned with the driving force for the future and areas of excellence needed to achieve the identified vision. The strategies need to address the critical issues identified earlier in the internal and external assessment process. For example, implementing the strategy, "Acquire and implement electronic signature software" requires researching the company's areas of excellence, developing requests for proposals, evaluating technology vendors that offer software compatible with the clinical data systems and clinical processes, and designing staff training plans.

Building a strategy grounded in a vision provides a context in which one can continually assess whether the organization is on track and if it is making progress. The AHIMA Board of Directors identified five key strategies in its future visioning sessions and a deep understanding of the external environment. They were cast as focused aims for the Association, reflecting the key changes AHIMA must lead over the next decade:

- Build brand and increase influence
- Elevate and broaden the profession
- Demonstrate exceptional financial stewardship
- Embed culture and values into our daily work
- Commit to innovation and performance excellence (AHIMA 2024)

It is important to look at the range of strategies being pursued to be clear about priorities, recognize opportunities for synergy and integration, and identify strategies to remove that no longer add value. When formulating strategies, question whether the leaders are getting too involved in how the strategy will be implemented.

### Check Your Understanding 21.3

**Answer the following questions in a separate document.**

1. Create a vision statement for your organization, department, or college and evaluate it using three of the characteristics of an effective vision statement.
2. Justify why a vision statement for a department or division should or should not be aligned with the organization's vision.
3. Summarize what areas of excellence are and why they are important in moving a strategic plan forward.
4. Why might it be important for AHIMA to build and update its strategy to achieve its vision?
5. What is the relationship between strategic management and an organization's vision.

## Phase III: Strategy Formulation

The third phase in the strategic planning process requires using the information and strategy development from phases I and II, along with tools for strategic thinking to build possible future scenarios, assess the competition, and then develop the future strategic profile and innovations. If all these aspects are done correctly, strategic thinking is ensured. The final strategies and future strategic profile can then be confirmed before moving into the implementation phase (phase IV).

### Use Techniques and Tools for Strategic Thinking

To bring out the best strategic thinking of a team or workgroup, it is often helpful to use techniques that help participants consider factors from different perspectives. Several group process techniques such as brainstorming, storytelling, scenario building, nominal group technique, and other techniques help unleash each individual's strategic thinking. The following section reviews how storytelling and scenario-building techniques may be used in the strategic planning process.

Storytelling is a powerful group process technique. Stories are defined as one way to transmit an organization's truths, insights, and commitments. Using compelling stories is a powerful way to persuade people by uniting an idea with an emotion. Essentially, a story can connect the organization to its audiences on an emotional level (Kemp et al. 2023). Telling stories about possible futures suggested by the external and internal assessment of trends has a few advantages, including capturing an understandable and emotional story that builds long-lasting value for a business. Stories are memorable, making it easier to remember essential points, and they generate excitement.

One storytelling technique used in more sophisticated strategic planning is scenario planning. The word *scenario* means a script of a play or story, or a projected sequence of events. **Scenarios** are stories describing the current and feasible future states of the business environment. They are plausible stories about how the future might unfold. They are not meant to predict but, rather, simply to interpret and clarify how internal and external environmental trends may influence the organization's strategy and how it might play out. As healthcare has become more complex, the scenario planning tool has become more widely used in strategic planning. It is helpful in dealing with complex new factors (Coates 2016, 99).

Scenario planning is based on analysis and interaction of environmental variables. Environmental assessment, along with assessing risks and uncertainties, is an important preparatory step in scenario development. Based on the study of the environment, two to four scenario themes are developed, reflecting alternate possible futures using differing potentials around the key forces or risks and uncertainties described earlier. Scenarios are constructed that describe possible ways in which each of these themes might be played out. These scenarios or stories are refined through input and further study until they reflect the decision maker's best thinking about what futures might be in store for the organization under various circumstances. Productive scenarios meet four tests: they are relevant, are internally consistent, describe clearly different futures, and are long term in perspective (Schoemaker 1995, 25–41). Other approaches that promote strategic thinking include contingency planning, sensitivity analysis, simulation, decision analysis and game theory, and blue ocean strategy (Harris 2018, 91–96). The following section is a brief overview of how these other approaches might be used:

- Contingency planning to address a single uncertainty in each situation or to develop plans to address multiple possible outcomes in the future
- Sensitivity analysis to examine the effect of a change in one variable while other variables all remain constant
- Simulation to analyze the effects of simultaneous change in multiple variables
- Decision analysis and game theory to address future uncertainties creatively
- Blue ocean strategy to create uncontested market space and to expand the current boundaries of an organization's market or create entirely new market space (the blue ocean) (Harris 2018, 91–96)

Strategic planning efforts study environmental trends, consult with subject matter experts, review open positions in the marketplace, and develop bold new scenarios, each highlighting a slightly different, but plausible, future environment. The impact of rapidly evolving technology, such as EHRs, digitized health information, and computerized coding requires a change in HIM professionals' education and preparation. Strategic managers can develop plans focused on the key strategic variables that shape the education and professional roles in this future vision.

## Determine Impact of Competition

Developing ways to understand the department's and organization's competitors is also valuable during the strategic planning process. Innovations or changes are always being planned by the competition. During the strategic planning process, leaders take the time to understand the current and potential strengths and weaknesses of the organization's key competitors. The organization's strategies should be developed to have the most influence on increasing its market share. Once the organization has selected a strategic direction, it should take time to evaluate and anticipate any impact that competitors, current or future, might have on the strategy. As the industry has matured, more and more secondary industry providers such as insurance, technology, biomedical, pharmaceutical, and retail organizations are revising their strategies for healthcare. This is an example of how stealthy or unusual competitors need to be considered and may have a significant impact on an organization's plan. The mergers and consolidation of organizations within healthcare are dramatically changing the landscape and competition. Understanding the impact of these market changes on the proposed future strategy may significantly affect the future strategic profile.

## Identify a Future Strategic Profile

Based on the findings and conclusions from the internal and external assessment, a new or updated vision statement and strategies are identified. It is critical to review the current strategic profile to determine if a new or updated future strategic profile of the organization needs to be developed. The future strategic profile serves as a filter to determine the following:

- What products or services the organization will offer in the future
- What markets it should geographically be in
- What customers and users will be served
- The industry and market segments to be emphasized more and less in the future (Robert 2006, 54)

At this time, the organization reevaluates what it focuses on and where it will be geographically located in the future. This future strategic profile serves to determine a more optimal way to allocate resources of staff, time, and money.

For example, an updated vision for a managed care health plan might be to fully engage members with chronic diseases who are focused on maintaining their health as partners with the health plan. The health plan's new future strategic profile may now emphasize patient portal use and chronic disease management with an accountable care organization as its key products, rather than traditional types of insurance plans for its members. It may choose to partner with specific market segments within healthcare that provide better outcomes for patients with chronic diseases (a change in its future customers and market segments). This new future strategic profile will be helpful in allocation of resources, determining if new market opportunities should be pursued, and ensuring strategic thinking is included in the plan.

## Create a Platform for Strategic Innovation

Techniques such as scenario development and environmental and competitive assessment are useful in formulating strategy because they include a focus on both the internal and external environments. However, one should not expect to identify exciting new strategies by only looking at the past, looking inward, or looking within the healthcare industry. As a critical part of this process, time should be taken to seek information by looking outside the organization and the healthcare industry, and looking to the future in formulating innovative strategy. New or innovative services or products come from identifying potential new needs based on determining the possible future scenarios that might occur. Organizations should seek to find or develop innovations that will differentiate their services or products from competitors'. Strategic product or service innovations are often overlooked when finalizing key organizational strategies.

> Product or *service innovations* create new market opportunities, and in many industries are the driving force behind growth and profitability. *Process innovations* enable firms to produce existing products or services more efficiently. As such, process and service innovations are one of the main determinants of productivity growth [emphasis added]. (Robert 2006, 118–119)

Strategic innovation requires an understanding of the department's and organization's strategic capabilities, anticipation of future needs by reviewing and predicting future trends, a willingness to take risks and think strategically. Many healthcare innovations came from unexpected industry stress, research and development, and a willingness to test new services or products with the ultimate goal of improving the health of a population. The strategic plan needs to include time for thoughtful development of product, service, and process innovations.

An important part of strategic planning, often overlooked yet vital to developing effective strategy, is the customer's role. Traditional ways of collecting customer information include consumer focus groups and patient surveys along with more innovative methods, such as patient advisory boards. If designed correctly, these tools can be effective in gathering patient engagement information within the proper context of strategic planning. Unfortunately, the strategic planning process often ignores customers, users, and suppliers or involves them too late to provide effective feedback. Strategic planning should involve patients and their families in the design of the strategies, strategic goals and objectives, and implementation plans for new patient-focused tools. By using a tool such as a consumer advisory board, the organization might begin to understand needs and expectations from the customers' perspective, making it easier to develop ways to provide a truly innovative product and service. These customers are often readily available, whether it involves using volunteers, staff members, or their family members who are customers. Clinicians and office staff who get calls from patients on a regular basis are well versed in understanding what their customers want and need and should be included on the board.

## Develop Final Strategic Findings and Conclusions

After reviewing all the information from both internal and external assessments, a shared list of strategic findings is developed with the strategic planning team. Based on these findings, the leader should determine if there are further informational needs or data points that will be important for developing the final set of strategic findings and conclusions. Strategic findings and conclusions help solidify the new vision, areas of excellence, future strategic profile, and key strategies for achieving the vision.

The essence of strategy is deciding what to do and what not to do. Managers are urged to rethink the meaning of strategy as making choices necessary to distinguish an organization in meeting customers' needs and focusing on improving value for patients (Porter and Lee 2015, 1681–1682). Major strategic change will impact current activities and may require their modification or even elimination as no organization has the resources to take on major new programs without considering their impact on current programs. Letting go of even a marginal program may produce a backlash, but making trade-offs, no matter how difficult, is essential for leaders and managers to create effective strategy. After completing all aspects of the first three phases of strategic planning, the leaders will now need to put a strategic "stake in the ground" to move forward with implementing the selected key strategies.

## Check Your Understanding 21.4

**Answer the following questions in a separate document.**

1. Describe two important tools often used for strategic thinking and how they could be incorporated in the strategic planning process of a department, organization, or college.
2. Describe the four tests that scenarios must meet to be effective for the strategic planning process; additionally, describe how these tests can be applied.
3. A current strategic profile is first identified by describing the products or services offered, what customers and users will be served, what markets it is geographically located in, and the industry and market segments that are emphasized. Compare and contrast through examples of how the current strategic profile might differ when developing the future strategic profiles in these four key areas.
4. Strategic service or product innovations are often overlooked when finalizing key organizational strategies. Generate two strategic innovations for one of your current services or products.
5. Why are strategic findings and conclusions critical to the project's success?

# Phase IV: Implementation

Determining how to accomplish each strategy by further defining strategic goals and objectives is the critical phase in creating an effective implementation plan. Unless strategy is implemented, it is of no value. The Balanced Scorecard Collaborative estimates that 90 percent of all companies fail to execute their strategies (Butler 2022). The reasons companies fail to execute include (1) loss of energy and focus for the plan; (2) lack of managing the implementation; (3) disconnecting the strategy from operations; and (4) a lack of resources to support implementing the strategy (Harris 2018, 231–232). Resources must be reallocated to programs that enable the organization to operate at a new level of innovative strategy. The final phase in strategic planning will outline the role of using strategic goals and objectives to accomplish each strategy. The use of an implementation planning tool is also helpful.

## Roles of Strategic Goals and Strategic Objectives

The next step in iterative strategic planning is to develop strategic goals and objectives to advance each identified key strategy to achieve the described future vision. It is important to select key strategies based on resolving the identified critical issues and future strategic profile needed for the future vision to be realized. Strategies are the high-level focus areas to pursue to achieve the vision. These strategies must be clearly identified and understood. To achieve a strategy, managers should develop a set of strategic goals and objectives that define a series of more precise key action steps that are needed to achieve each strategy.

### Defining Strategic Goals

Strategic goals should not be confused with annual operational goals. Often strategic plans are written as operational goals or objectives rather than at a strategic level. A **strategic goal** is a high-level set of key activities describing the actions needed to carry out each of the newly selected organizational strategies. For example, if the strategy is to meet the 95th percentile performance on timely billing to payers, the strategic goal might be to reduce the accounts receivable days attributable to coding backlogs by moving to computer-assisted coding (CAC), and strategic objectives may include selecting a new CAC software, training contract coders for concurrent review, and redesigning the medical record completion processes.

### Defining Strategic Objectives

**Strategic objectives** are detailed steps to achieve the identified strategic goal and include specific timelines, resource allocation needs, and assignment of responsibility to the person(s) accountable for implementation of each strategic goal. Continuing with the timely billing example, the strategic objectives should state (in more detail than the strategic goal) the person(s) responsible and the detailed action steps of how to authorize more overtime, who will and how to hire the contract coding professionals, and who will and how to redesign the record completion process. Another example is for the strategic objective of hiring contract coding professionals. The objective should state with whom the organization will be contracting, how many contract coding professionals are needed, the potential additional costs, the timelines for implementation, and who is responsible for making it happen.

The next step is to take each strategic goal and identify the strategic objectives or short-term specific and detailed action plans needed to accomplish each strategic goal. For a strategic goal focused on wellness, the organization can format incentives for members to engage in wellness activities and use their electronic patient portals to improve health. The objectives are as follows:

- Develop insurance premium rebates of $20 per month for key wellness activities of which a patient can show evidence. These could include gym membership, coaching sessions, and nutrition education sessions attended. The participation goal is 30 percent of members.
- Monitor members' electronic patient portal use to schedule physician annual visits and preventive care visits with the goal of increasing it by 20 percent.
- Develop an incentives system for members to upload their daily walking steps into their patient portal directly from the health-monitoring device with the goal of increasing member participation by 50 percent.

The vision describes where the organization wants to go, and the strategies are broad directional frameworks for how the organization intends to pursue its vision. The strategic goals describe specific action plans to be implemented to achieve each strategy. Within each of these strategic goals are even more detailed strategic objectives that need to be identified to accomplish each of these strategic goals.

## Importance of Implementation Plans

For any strategic plan to become effective and to ensure a successful implementation plan, detailed strategic goals and objectives must be written out and supported by those responsible for the implementation. This requires involvement in the design of and understanding the rationale for and the outline of detailed responsibilities and expectations required of all leaders and staff in the department or organization. The strategic goals and objectives need to be clearly outlined, with assignments for who will be accountable, timelines, allocation of resources, and measurements used to ensure success of implementation. When a detailed implementation plan includes all these elements laid out clearly, the likelihood of strategic success increases significantly (see table 21.1). The measurement of these detailed implementation plans must be done on a regular basis, more often than annually or periodically, because what is measured becomes a priority of leaders and employees in the organization.

### Check Your Understanding 21.5

**Answer the following questions in a separate document.**

1. Identify the four key aspects of a detailed implementation plan. Why is it important for healthcare organizations to have such a detailed plan? Give a brief description for each of the four aspects noted.
2. Identify two differences between a strategic goal and a strategic objective.
3. Based on the following AHIMA vision statement, "A world where trusted information transforms health and healthcare by connecting people, systems, and ideas," do the following:
   a. Create one strategy to achieve this vision (please do not copy a current identified AHIMA strategy; use your own unique strategy).
   b. Create one strategic goal to achieve the above strategy.
   c. Create one strategic objective related to how to achieve the strategic goal noted above (remember to include who's responsible, timelines, and resources needed).
4. What are some reasons companies fail to execute their developed plans?

**Table 21.1.** Detailed implementation plan

| Strategy #1: Increase utilization of the patient portal within ABC Health System ||||
|---|---|---|---|
| **Strategic goal** | **Strategic objectives** | **Implementation plan** | **Measurements** |
| A. Develop a Patient Portal Consumer Advisory Board | 1. Develop and gain approval for a patient portal consumer advisory board charter within the organization's patient experience structure. | **Timeline:** Gain charter approval by first quarter | Increased use of Health System patient portal achieved: |
| | 2. Identify and contact active health system consumers who are willing to serve on the patient portal advisory board. | Select membership and complete orientation by second quarter | By Q3 = 27% |
| | 3. Design a detailed patient portal orientation program for new members, establish board leadership, and set annual objectives. | Begin holding quarterly meetings by third quarter | By Q4 = 50% |
| | | **Who is responsible:** | Consumer Rating of patient portal: |
| | | HIM director and patient experience director | Score 4.0–5 = 70% |
| | | **Resource needs:** | Score 3.5–3.99 = 20% |
| | | Operating budget support $2,000 for food and 0.1 FTE staff time | Score 3.0–3.49 = 10% |
| B. Develop a Patient Portal Clinician Advisory Board | 1. Develop and gain approval for a patient portal clinician advisory board charter within the Health System's information governance board | **Timeline:** | Increased use of Health System patient portal achieved: |
| | 2. Identify and contact active health system clinicians who are willing to serve on the patient portal advisory board. | Gain charter approval | By Q3 = 27% |
| | 3. Design a detailed patient portal orientation program for new members, establish board leadership, and set annual objectives. | by first quarter | By Q4 = 50% |
| | | Select membership and complete orientation by second quarter | Consumer Rating of patient portal: |
| | | Begin holding quarterly meetings by third quarter | Score 4.0–5 = 70% |
| | | **Who is responsible:** | Score 3.5–3.99 = 20% |
| | | HIM patient portal manager; departmental reps from hospital, clinics and radiology. | |
| | | **Resource needs:** | Score 3.0–3.49 = 10% |
| | | ($1,000) for food and staff time for meetings. | |

## Support for the Change Program

Sound change strategies and tactics alone do not ensure success. Success depends on great execution, including securing support for the needed organizational change efforts. Healthcare organizations are highly complex with many competing priorities. Gaining approval, even for the best-designed efforts, may be difficult. Developing a systems approach, creating a sense of urgency and a structure to support change efforts, and developing a plan to navigate the politics and communication needs are critical to success.

### Take a Systems Approach

There are five activities related to creating an effective strategic plan, including motivating change, creating a vision, developing political support, managing the transition, and sustaining momentum (Cummings and Worley 2019). As a part of creating a vision and strategic plans, it is important to include all levels of staff in the organization by asking them to be involved in the strategic planning and visioning process. This assists in motivating change within the organization, as people tend to support what they help create. Understanding the influence political systems have on the distribution of power and influence within the organization may give insight during the process (for example, the authority of the medical staff and the approval and decision-making processes of the board of directors within an organization).

Organizations may move quickly into chaos as existing health systems are experiencing significant changes. This is a time of great vulnerability, and leaders must be vigilant, watching for and thoughtfully managing transitions and attending to unintended effects that make achieving realignment difficult. Leaders must be sensitive to the emotional relationships among individuals in a group and how change will affect relationships between individuals and between the manager and others. Times of change are times of high stress and anxiety. This may play out in several ways. For example, in times of major change, employees may be more inclined to look for other employment opportunities as it is threatening and unsettling to go through change. Some turnover in staff may be an acceptable and unavoidable result, but the leader should be attentive and sensitive so that turnover does not derail the ability to carry out the project.

The organization's systems are highly interdependent, and any change will have intended and unintended impact on all systems. For example, when implementing new technology such as EHRs or other major systems, the focus is often on features and functions of the system. Securing the right champions for system implementation planning and understanding how it affects the workflow, procedures, and formal and informal interactions of staff, are more challenging and important to successful implementation than all the features and functions. The successful strategic manager leading wide-scale technology change is the one who excels at helping people get behind and involved in the change. The manager who focuses only or primarily on installing the hardware and software will not succeed. Managers should not let these challenges of change keep them from pursuing the strategies their organization needs. However, success will depend on how well change is managed from a systems perspective. The manager must attend to system aspects throughout the implementation process. He or she also should be aware that implementation is not complete until all systems are back in a new alignment after the changes are in place.

### Create the Structure for Change

Organizational structure is an important element to ensure success of the change process. Once a new vision and strategies are determined, the current structure should be reviewed, and focus placed on how to best restructure (if needed) to achieve the new vision. Structure is an organizational function often overlooked and yet important to successful implementation. As strategic goals and objectives are identified in the implementation plan, they are assigned to a leader. Another important aspect of consideration regarding structure is where the department is positioned within the structure of the organization. This placement in the structure and strategy is important to understanding how allocation of resources and capital will be made. The importance of structure for accomplishing an organization's strategic goals and objectives should not be underestimated.

### Manage the Politics of Change

Organizational change can be a political process. Change leadership requires the courage to persevere even in the face of criticism; however, charging ahead without considering the political implications may be ineffective. While strategic planning has traditionally been a top-down process, many organizations are realizing the power of senior leaders creating a framework and having strategic planning from the bottom up. This change in focusing the planning process within the business units allows strategic planning to be with the "real" action and closer to the customer (Harris 2018, 51). Political savvy entails skill in mediating and shaping inevitable conflicts when people are being offered multiple choices with significant consequences. Deliberately enlist the support of thought and opinion leaders. Engage those who may be most threatened by the proposed change; do not wait for them to come to you. Early engagement may turn potential resisters into supporters. At the very least, it will help change leaders build their arguments and communication plan to address the concerns of those who oppose the change.

Collaboration is one technique for managing the political dimensions of change. Change may threaten to shift the balance of power, and employees or coworkers who feel threatened may react by joining together to increase their own power to influence the course of events. The use of collaborations is essential for positive change.

The first step in building a collaboration is to honestly assess subgroups in terms of how they will view the proposed change. Before embarking on a major change, the following questions should be considered carefully:

- Who will be most affected by the change?
- What benefits (for example, power) might these individuals perceive they will lose?
- Are their fears real? If so, what options are available to help overcome their fears?
- Does the change have the potential to create new benefits for these individuals?
- Can a negative reaction be avoided by engaging individuals or groups in the process?
- If the leader is not successful in getting them on board, is their influence likely to be strong enough to derail the change plan?

Even when a leader is not successful in getting resisters on board, he or she will have better information about the strength of their feelings and their resolve to oppose change. At the same time, leaders are always working to diffuse potential resistance and to focus on building support for the change.

## Create a Sense of Urgency

When trying to change organizations and move forward strategically in tumultuous times, developing a sense of urgency to change is important (Kotter 2012a, 37). Leaders may overestimate the extent to which they can force or drive change in the organization. To increase the sense of urgency, leaders must remove or minimize the sources of complacency. With this rapid change in the healthcare industry, dynamic strategic planning has replaced static planning. Some examples of how this might be done include the following:

- Engage employees, customers, and coworkers in a dialogue about change through a series of input meetings (namely, having them participate in the SWOT analysis)
- Convene a guiding coalition (GC) committee with opinion leaders and representatives from major stakeholder groups
- Develop inspiring and stretching vision statements and strategies
- Present believable stories and scenarios that illustrate the potential futures using both head and heart that may occur if action is not taken
- Identify revolutionary goals, encourage strategic thinking, and drive decision-making down to all levels
- Create new effective vehicles for communication, such as a project website or newsletter

The need for strategic planning has changed with the fast-paced environment. After the initial longer-term strategies are developed, strategic planning must be a continuous process. It is important to engage everyone in the strategic plan to ensure it is not just reviewed once a year but integrated into the organization. "Sufficient urgency around a strategically rational and emotionally exciting opportunity is the bedrock upon which all else is built" (Kotter 2012b, 54). The need to build a sense of urgency among the employees in the organization is required for successful implementation. Creating a culture that emotionally engages employees and leaders will ensure strategic change is a priority.

## Engage with Communication

Communication is key to engaging others in the vision and change process. A benchmarking study of how companies have successfully communicated change showed that communication is critical at three stages of the change process: as it is being planned, throughout implementation, and after it is complete. Communication must be two-way to ensure open dialogue among all members of the organization throughout the process. Long term, the interests of key stakeholders and those of the organization need to be served if the organization is to continue to operate successfully. Furthermore, a core element of strategic communication is research that informs and influences an organization in relation to public expectations, concerns, interests, and needs (McNamara 2012). All strategic communication needs to allow for two-way, honest interactions.

At the planning stage, leaders should communicate the need for change and the vision. Remember, if followers do not accept the vision, the rest of the change process is likely to be very rocky. Communicating results, even when they are incomplete, is an important reinforcement. It makes the change real and maintains the necessary momentum.

Communication is most effective if the message is tailored to the recipient. The leader identifies needs and opportunities to customize the organization's message to subgroups that have a particular set of issues. For example, the message to the medical staff will be different from the message to staff in health information services. Before implementing the use of report templates to expedite document creation, the manager may design a tactical plan that details all the elements of the communication plan for each of the constituent groups affected by, or with an interest in, the project.

The communication plan must offer groups the opportunity to discuss issues with leadership and share their opinions. This may mean that feedback could indicate that the proposed vision and new course is not moving the organization in the right direction. However, it is worth reconsidering and reworking the vision and strategic plans to ensure they are moving the organization in a direction that the employees believe in and will follow (Kotter 2012a, 128). The importance of open communication and developing a culture of transparency within an organization cannot be underestimated.

Communication is a critical element to engaging all stakeholders in strategic planning. Communication comes in two forms—words and actions—and the most effective communication is characterized by deeds. Behavior from important people that is inconsistent with the vision overwhelms other forms of communication (Kotter 2012a, 90). As leaders are beacons for change, others will watch the leaders' actions for signals of commitment to the course of action and rightly insist on their integrity. Therefore, leaders' actions are closely scrutinized, and their motives may be suspect.

Ethics and integrity must be front and center all the time, but particularly during times of important change. At these times, the political, cultural, and technical systems are out of alignment. There is opportunity for events to take unexpected turns.

## Implement Strategic Change

Once the vision and strategies are agreed upon, the change management team is in place, and the guiding coalitions are organized, the hard work of implementation begins. Reviewing multiple studies of executives, 90 percent fail to successfully implement strategy (Gibson 2023). Implementation requires all the managerial skills including planning, budgeting, monitoring, and producing results.

### Create and Communicate Short-Term Wins

Major change takes time. The organization's vision may be compelling and its strategies right on target, but if short-term results cannot be demonstrated, the leaders may lose support, and the momentum for change may begin to erode. The best way to sustain change efforts is to sequence the implementation plan through strategic objectives and goals in such a way that short-term successes are clearly demonstrated and celebrated. For example, in implementing a new coding and billing compliance plan, the data quality manager for a group practice reported statistics to the chairs of clinical services or related executives showing the monthly claims rejection rate. As this rate began to decline, the manager organized special events such as a recognition event for office managers and staff at each improvement milestone. The consistent measurement reporting and recognition touches garnered attention and maintained momentum for the project.

The implementation plan can be deliberately seeded with several short-term objectives and goals with a high likelihood of success. This tactic enables the implementation team to work together to assess how much effort and how many resources will be required for later phases. It demonstrates that the program of planned change is real and not just talk. Moreover, it strengthens the courage and commitment of the leaders and the GCs.

New programs can be launched quickly by using techniques such as rapid prototyping, demonstration projects, or pilot tests. The details do not always need to be fully worked out to create visible demonstrations. The leader may not need to secure approval for full implementation, as testing an approach to see its value is often accepted as a pilot. In test mode, all operational details do not need to be worked out before go-live. The leader need not anticipate all the intricacies up front but should just begin the journey and adjust while implementing the pilot stage. Prototyping and pilot tests also offer a way to show others how redesigned processes or new technology might work when fully implemented.

## Pace and Refine Change Plans

Implementation requires managing interdependent projects at various stages of design, development, and deployment. A difficult implementation challenge is deciding what strategies should be advanced first and how fast or slow to move through them. Sequencing and pacing change require thorough knowledge of the organization and its capacity for change, again considering all organizational components—cultural, political, and technical—and the available financial and managerial resources.

The higher the stakes, the more likely it is that a proposed change will be controversial. If the only viable approach is likely to be met with resistance, more time and effort are needed up front to gain acceptance before the approach is implemented. The importance of two-way communication and involvement of staff and management throughout the process cannot be overemphasized.

The timing of change is critical. Change leaders can cite examples of projects that moved too quickly and projects that moved too slowly. In rapidly evolving environments, there is a need to increase the speed of business cycles and bring innovation to market in order to respond quickly to unanticipated changes.

Implementation is critical to the success of the plan being realized. If the strategic plan is not implemented, all may be lost in moving an organization toward its best future. Implementation, as a process, will guide, show when adjustments are necessary, and find ways to improve as the plan moves forward. Implementing change is a highly iterative process. Leaders should expect their plans and tactics will need to be modified as they gain experience. They should create strategies, strategic goals and objectives, budgets, and timetables that permit frequent course corrections. The organizations that can act quickly will see immediate and long-term success. Those who lag will suffer, if they survive at all (Kotter 2012b, 58).

## Maintain Momentum and Stay the Course

Because leading change is a process of learning and adjusting, change leaders must learn to tolerate—and even enjoy—uncertainty. Change sponsors are eager to see their well-crafted strategies take hold and inevitably feel discouraged by a lengthy process. In addition to celebrating short-term wins, other ways to maintain momentum and keep moving include the following:

- Work quickly to resolve the difficult issues.
- Reiterate what will happen if change either does not occur or is watered down by compromise. If possible, focus on the consequences due to external trends.
- Stay focused on the prize. Put every action in context. Regularly revisit the vision, strategies, goals, and objectives to regenerate a sense of purpose. Help others by making the goals as tangible as possible.
- Remember that resistance to change is natural. Do not take it personally.
- Rethink the tactics, sequence, and pace regularly to keep from getting bogged down. If momentum slows, institute actions that produce short-term gains. Keep moving forward.
- Maintain the sense of urgency. Although it is important to celebrate short-term wins, do not let these celebrations mitigate the sense of urgency the organization has created. Also, do not let intermediate gains be mistaken for the bigger goals.

For maximum and sustained impact, the change being introduced must become part of the fabric of the organization. It must become the way the organization operates, thinks, and behaves. At some point, it must become part of the culture. Even after change is implemented, there often continues to be a move backward toward the old reality. So strong is the effect of culture that leaders should be on the lookout for signs of slippage and for opportunities to reinforce the value of the new reality. To ensure change is lasting and to prepare the organization for more change, leaders should quantify the impact, benefits, and value of the changes and use data to identify the direction for future change. As noted previously, continue intensive communication on issues facing HIM and the organization. The leaders will need to integrate change competencies and behaviors into performance appraisal and management development programs. Finally, due to the rapidly changing times, leaders must approach strategy, change, and organizational development as an ongoing process.

## Measure Your Results

Environmental assessment was shown to be an important prerequisite to launching major change. It is also the way to measure the impact of change and determine what further change is needed. Any time strategic change is undertaken, the measures by which its success will be judged should be made part of the performance measures data set. A systematic and ongoing environmental assessment, both internal and external, must become a core competency of the organization and part of its routine work. It must include information on performance, health system–related trends, customer and employee attitudes, and satisfaction.

Once the key strategies are identified, a strategy map is designed that begins with a brief description of the current state and the desired future state. A strategy map is a visual representation of the cause-and-effect relationships among the components of an organization's strategy. Depicting strategies as a road map is a useful way to help others understand the next steps of implementation, which focuses on developing strategic goals and objectives to lead to the needed strategy change.

The balanced scorecard is a framework for measuring organizational performance across the following four perspectives (Kaplan and Norton 2004, 31):

- *Customer perspective*: To achieve the vision, how should the organization appear to internal and external customers?
- *Financial perspective*: How must the organization be held financially accountable?
- *Internal process perspective*: To satisfy customers, in which operational processes must the organization excel?
- *Learning and growth perspective*: How will the organization enhance its ability to change and improve?

A strategy map enables examination of the cause-and-effect relationships among the preceding perspectives. Figure 21.3 shows a sample balanced scorecard using these four perspectives which becomes the basis of a strategy map for improving the real and perceived value of HIM services. The purpose of using the balanced scorecard methodology is to improve implementation and demonstrate how a strategy is more clearly defined and tied into operations using a strategic goal, strategic objectives, detailed implementation plans, and measurements. Each department or division can model their strategy maps and balanced scorecards to reflect the overall organization's strategy maps and balanced scorecard.

**Figure 21.3.** Balanced scorecard with strategy map

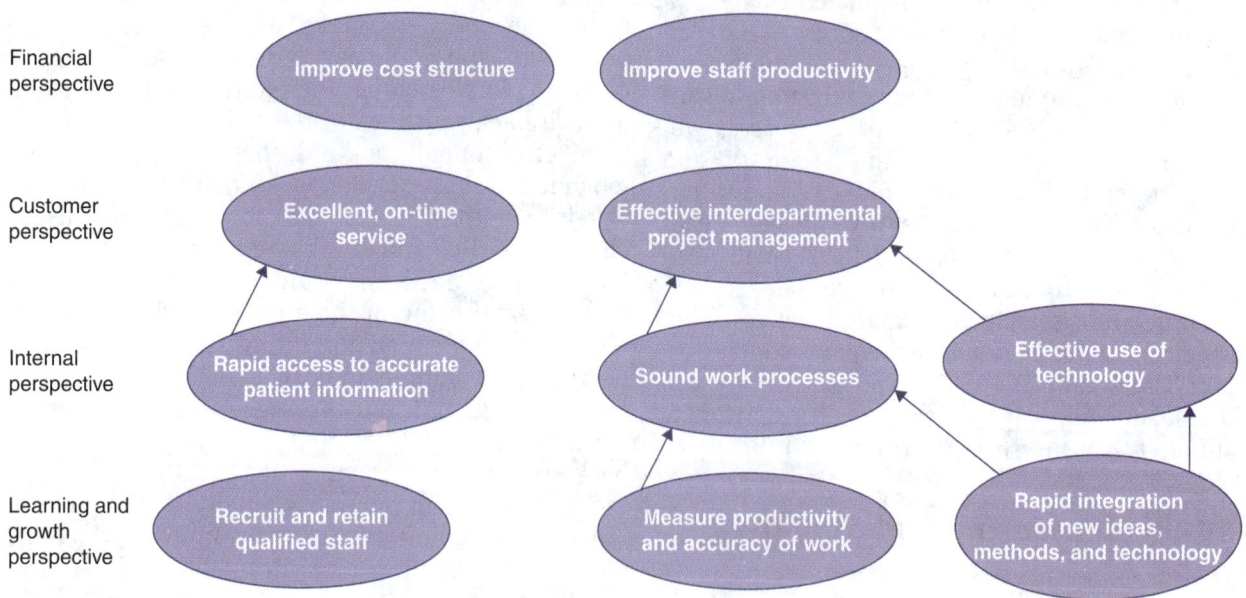

## Check Your Understanding 21.6

**Answer the following questions in a separate document.**

1. Differentiate between change management and collaboration, and examine how they can improve strategic planning outcomes.
2. What is one of the most important skills required of a leader that is engaging other employees and key stakeholders in conducting strategic planning?
3. What are the four perspectives typically found when using the balanced scorecard methodology? Give an example of each perspective for your organization, department, or college.
4. Based on the AHIMA vision and using the four perspectives of customer, financial, internal processes, and learning and growth, develop a strategy goal and measure for each of the perspectives for AHIMA.
5. The best practice in the process of who to involve in strategic planning of an organization on an annual or periodic basis is to include which of the following?
   a. Only the executive team and board of directors
   b. Only the directors, executive team, and board of directors
   c. The staff, managers, directors, executive team, board of directors, patients, and community stakeholders
   d. Only patients and community stakeholders
6. Why is it useful to utilize a strategy map for assessment purposes?

# References

AHIMA (American Health Information Management Association). n.d. "About Us." Accessed June 12, 2024. https://www.ahima.org/who-we-are/about-us/.

AHIMA (American Health Information Management Association). 2024. "2024–2027 AHIMA Strategic Plan." https://ahima.org/media/023o4jwl/ahima-2024-2027-strategic-plan.pdf.

Brandenburger, A. 2019. Strategy needs creativity. *Harvard Business Review* 97(2):58–65.

Butler, J.. "90 Percent of Organizations Fail to Execute Their Strategies Successfully: A White Paper to Help You Avoid Being a Statistic." 2022. https://www.intellibridge.us/90-percent-of-organizations-fail-to-execute-their-strategies-successfully.

Coates, J. F. 2016. Technological forecasting and social change. *Journal of Business Strategy* 113(A):99–102.

Cummings, T., and C. Worley. 2019. *Organization Development and Change*, 11th ed. Stamford, CT: Cengage Learning.

Dunn, R. T. 2021. *Haimann's Healthcare Management*, 11th ed. Chicago: Health Administration Press.

Gibson, K. 2023. 5 reasons strategy execution fails. Harvard Business School. https://online.hbs.edu/blog/post/why-do-strategic-plans-fail.

Harris, J. M. 2018. *Healthcare Strategic Planning*, 4th ed. Chicago: Health Administration Press.

Herskovitz, S., and M. Crystal. 2010. The essential brand persona: storytelling and branding. *Journal of Business Strategy* 31(3):21–28. https://doi.org/10.1108/02756661011036673.

Jennings, M. C. 2000. *Health Care Strategy for Uncertain Times*. San Francisco: Jossey-Bass.

Kaplan, R. S., and D. P. Norton. 2004. *Strategy Maps: Converting Intangible Assets into Tangible Outcomes*. Boston: Harvard Business School Press.

Kemp, A., R. Gravois, H. Syrdal, and E. McDougal. 2023. Storytelling is not just for marketing: Cultivating a storytelling culture throughout the organization. *Business Horizons* 66(3): 313–324. https://doi.org/10.1016/j.bushor.2023.01.008.

Kotter, J. P. 2012a. *Leading Change: Why Transformation Efforts Fail*. Boston: Harvard Business Review Press.

Kotter, J. P. 2012b. The big idea: Accelerate! *Harvard Business Review* 90(11):44–58.

Porter, M. E., and T. H. Lee. 2015. Why strategy matters now. *New England Journal of Medicine* 372:1681–1684 DOI: 10.1045/NEJMp1502419.

Robert, M. 2006. *The New Strategic Thinking: Pure and Simple*. New York: McGraw-Hill.

Schoemaker, P. J. H. 1995. Scenario planning: A tool for strategic thinking. *Sloan Management Review* 36(2):25–41.

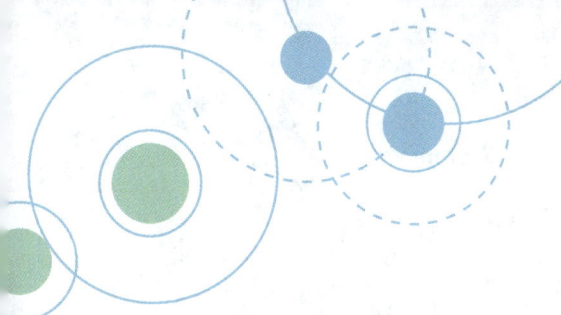

# chapter 22

# Human Resources Management

*Madonna M. LeBlanc, MA, RHIA, FAHIMA*

## Learning Objectives

- Map key federal legislation to human resources (HR) functions.
- Design position descriptions for use in HR planning and management
- Utilize best practices to acquire and retain staff
- Determine the key steps a manager should take in performance counseling and disciplinary action, adjusting them appropriately to each situation
- Evaluate the impact of workforce trends on the organization's HR management activities

## Key Terms

Age Discrimination in Employment Act (ADEA) of 1967
Americans with Disabilities Act (ADA) of 1990
Arbitration
Authority
Behavioral description interview
Civil Rights Act of 1964, Title VII
Civil Rights Act of 1991
Compensable factors
Compromise
Conflict management
Constructive confrontation
Control
Delegation
Discrimination
Employment-at-will
Empowerment
Equal Employment Opportunity Act of 1972
Equal Employment Opportunity Commission (EEOC)
Equal Pay Act (EPA) of 1963
Exempt employees
Exit interview
Factor comparison method
Fair Labor Standards Act (FLSA) of 1938
Family and Medical Leave Act (FMLA) of 1993
Genetic Information Nondiscrimination Act (GINA) of 2008
Grievance
Grievance procedures
Harassment
Hay method of job evaluation
Job classification method
Job evaluation
Job ranking
Job specification
Labor-Management Relations Act (Taft-Hartley Act) of 1947
Labor-Management Reporting and Disclosure Act (Landrum-Griffin Act) of 1959
Labor relations
Layoffs
Mediation
National Labor Relations Act (Wagner Act) of 1935
Nonexempt employees
Occupational Safety and Health Act (OSHA) of 1970
Orientation
Panel interview
Performance review
Policy
Point method
Position (job) description
Pregnancy Discrimination Act of 1978

| | | |
|---|---|---|
| Procedure | Structured interview | Reemployment Rights Act (USERRA) of 1994 |
| Progressive discipline | Team building | |
| Recruitment | Termination | Union |
| Reference check | 360-degree evaluation | Workers' Adjustment Retraining and Notification (WARN) Act of 1988 |
| Responsibility | Uniformed Services | |
| Retention | Employment and | |

Healthcare organizations are extremely complex. They must operate as effective and efficient businesses in a very tight financial environment. They must also employ a variety of well-educated technical specialists and professional employees to provide or support increasingly sophisticated healthcare services. Contemporary healthcare managers work in a unique environment characterized by the need to control costs and, at the same time, meet the needs of healthcare consumers and healthcare workers.

Managers work at many levels within healthcare organizations—as supervisors of functional units, as middle managers of departmental units or service lines, and as executive managers of multiple departmental units or service lines. At each level of management, the practice of managing the human resources (HR) within the prescribed scope of authority and responsibility is critical to the manager's success and the success of the entire organization.

Managing HR is both an art and a science. Managers can learn much in this arena by partnering with HR management specialists, observing experienced colleagues, reflecting regularly on their own experiences, and continuing to develop their competencies throughout their careers.

This chapter is not meant to provide a comprehensive background in HR management but to present a general introduction to the subject of managing HR within the context of health information management (HIM) operations. The chapter begins with a brief overview of the principles and nature of organizations and a discussion of the roles of the various levels of management. Its primary focus is the interrelationship of HIM managers and HR professionals and the roles the supervisor and middle manager play in implementing HR policies and practices in healthcare organizations.

## Role of the Human Resources Department

Payroll and benefits consume most healthcare organizations' financial resources (Dunn 2021). Therefore, adequate time and attention must be paid to HR management. Effective HR management is also important for reasons beyond financial impact. HR management factors affect the attitudes and morale of employees and, therefore, affect their ability to perform their work effectively. Employee morale becomes important when the work involves caring for patients directly or indirectly supporting those who provide hands-on care.

Entities such as hospitals, large physician groups, and integrated health systems commonly have a dedicated HR department that supports managers at all levels. However, every manager must understand the principles of HR management to implement them effectively within the manager's scope of authority and responsibility. Every manager must also know how to appropriately and effectively work with the organization's HR department.

The HR department is responsible for several types of interrelated activities. HR management is a set of closely related activities focused on contributing to an organization's success by enhancing its productivity, quality, and service. Each of these interrelated activities is shown in figure 22.1, which illustrates the extensive factors involved in creating a desirable, functioning employee environment. Performing HR activities with the organization's unique mission, culture, size, and structure in mind, as well as the greater social, political, legal, economic, technological, and cultural environment in which it operates, is also important (Mathis and Jackson 2016).

### Human Resources Planning and Analysis

HR planning and analysis ensure the long-term health of the organization's human assets. Internal trends such as a shortage of employees in the workforce or the changing nature of the skill mix required to handle the organization's evolving product lines must be addressed.

As one of the 25 largest healthcare occupations, 30.1 percent of the medical records specialists are 55 years and older and closer to leaving the workforce

**Figure 22.1.** HR management activities

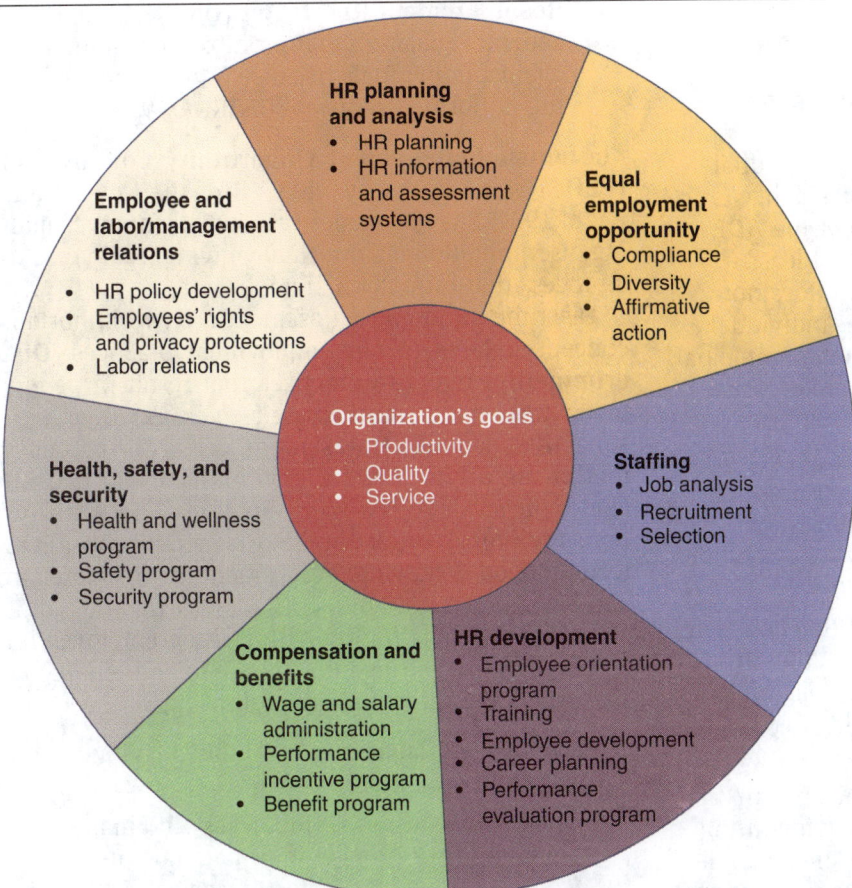

*Source:* Adapted from Mathis and Jackson 2016.

(Bureau of Labor Statistics 2022). The COVID-19 pandemic led to unprecedented understaffing and, in combination with residual employee burnout, complicated recruitment. These workforce challenges, among others, requires healthcare employers to evaluate current HR policies and practices to determine if they are effectively retaining their existing staff, creating job opportunities for new employees, and planning for potential workforce shortages (AHIMA 2023).

In addition to planning for a change in workforce numbers, the skills needed in healthcare are also shifting. As healthcare becomes more complex and sophisticated, the need for highly skilled professionals also increases. Further, the growth of information technology within healthcare necessitates continuing education for current HIM and other healthcare professionals as processes undergo dramatic change with more technology solutions, requirements, and regulations to manage.

The HIM profession has experienced and will continue to experience rapid and significant change driven by the increased use of healthcare technology and the many government programs and regulations that affect the delivery of healthcare and the creation, use, and maintenance of health records. These changes will drive the HIM workforce to require more advanced technical skills, more advanced conceptual and analytical skills, and greater communication skills (AHIMA 2023). HR professionals and HIM managers need to collaborate to ensure intentional employee retention strategies, continuing education programs, and strong recruitment plans meet both the short-term and long-term workforce needs.

## Equal Employment Opportunity Practices

The HR department takes the lead in ensuring the various laws and regulations associated with equal employment opportunity (EEO), affirmative action, and the US Department of Labor (DOL) are scrupulously applied in the organization's hiring and promotion practices. Federally enacted DOL and EEO legislation includes the following:

- **Age Discrimination in Employment Act (ADEA) of 1967**: The federal act that states it is unlawful for an employer to discriminate against an individual in any aspect of employment because that individual is 40 years old or older, unless one of the statutory exceptions applies, such as the capacity to safely perform the job at a particular age. Favoring an older individual over a younger individual because of age is not unlawful discrimination under the ADEA, even if the younger individual is at least 40 years old. However, the ADEA does not require employers to prefer older individuals and does not affect applicable state, municipal, or local laws that prohibit such preferences (ADA 1990; Library of Congress 2007).

- **Americans with Disabilities Act (ADA) of 1990**: Federal legislation that ensures equal opportunity for and elimination of discrimination against persons with disabilities (ADA Amendments Act 2008)
- **Civil Rights Act of 1964, Title VII**: The federal legislation that prohibits discrimination in employment on the basis of race, religion, color, sex, or national origin (Civil Rights Act 1964)
- **Civil Rights Act of 1991**: The federal legislation that focuses on establishing an employer's responsibility for justifying hiring practices that seem to adversely affect people because of race, color, religion, sex, or national origin (Civil Rights Act 1991)
- **Equal Employment Opportunity Act of 1972**: The amendment to the Civil Rights Act of 1964 prohibiting discrimination in the workplace on the basis of age, gender, race, color, religion, sex, or national origin (EEOC 1972)
- **Family and Medical Leave Act (FMLA) of 1993**: The federal legislation that allows full-time employees time off from work (up to 12 weeks) to care for themselves or their family members with the assurance of an equivalent position upon return to work (FMLA 1993)
- **Genetic Information Nondiscrimination Act (GINA) of 2008**: Legislation which prohibits genetic information discrimination against employees or applicants (GINA 2008)
- **Pregnancy Discrimination Act of 1978**: The federal legislation that prohibits discrimination against women affected by pregnancy, childbirth, or related medical conditions by requiring that affected women be treated the same as all other employees for employment-related purposes, including benefits (Pregnancy Discrimination Act 1978)
- **Uniformed Services Employment and Reemployment Rights Act (USERRA) of 1994**: Federal legislation that prohibits discrimination against individuals because of their service in the uniformed services (USERRA 1993)

The **Equal Employment Opportunity Commission (EEOC)** was created by Title VII of the Civil Rights Act of 1964. It is the agency responsible for investigating discrimination claims, finally giving legal voice to a process that formally had none.

Discrimination and harassment are two important concepts related to fair employment practices. **Discrimination** refers to practices that result in people being treated differently based solely on their personal distinctions. **Harassment** refers to practices that create a hostile work environment that can include physical, verbal, or emotional harassment. Both are illegal under the EEO laws, and the EEOC recommends following best practices to create an anti-harassment environment: adopt a rigorous anti-harassment policy, routinely train each employee on its contents, and stringently adhere to and enforce it. The policy should include the following:

- "A clear explanation of prohibited conduct, including examples;
- Clear assurance that employees who make complaints or provide information related to complaints will be protected against retaliation;
- A clearly described complaint process that provides multiple, accessible avenues of complaint;
- Assurance that the employer will protect the confidentiality of harassment complaints to the extent possible;
- A complaint process that provides a prompt, thorough, and impartial investigation; and
- Assurance that the employer will take immediate and appropriate corrective action when it determines that harassment has occurred" (EEOC n.d.a)

It is important for both managers and employees to know these policies so that employers can ensure a safe work environment free of discrimination and harassment and so that employees are not fearful to report when these issues occur.

## Rights of Employees and Employers

Although many of the basic rights of employees are defined in law, others are expectations that may be debated within organizations. For example, **employment-at-will** is a well-established concept—either an employer or an employee can terminate an employment relationship without providing either notice or reason. Other issues are less clear. What are the privacy rights of employees? Can an employer monitor employees' emails and voicemails? Organizations are well advised to address the rights of employees and the rights of the employer in an employee handbook to clarify expectations for employees and supervisors. A well-developed employee handbook also improves the organization's legal position should the organization be called on to defend its actions in a court proceeding.

## Staffing

The HR department also helps managers define staffing needs; develop job descriptions; and recruit, screen, and select staff. After an employee is brought into the organization, the HR department plays a significant role, in partnership with the employee's direct supervisor, by spearheading the employee's immediate orientation to the organization's policies, practices, and procedures. The HR department is also active in addressing the employee's ongoing training and development requirements; for the HIM department, that could include ongoing education regarding new technology, new software programs, or annual code and coding guideline updates.

## Compensation and Benefits Program

An organization's compensation and benefits program is the most prominent activity associated with HR management because it is directly connected to the employee's financial status. This activity involves the establishment of basic definitions of employment and compensation status for the organization (for example, full-time versus part-time, temporary versus permanent, independent contractor versus employee, wage versus salary). The Fair Labor Standards Act (FLSA) of 1938, which federally enacted minimum wage and overtime payment regulations, and the Equal Pay Act (EPA) of 1963, which requires equal pay for men and women performing substantially the same work, serve as fundamental legislative mandates in this area. Social Security, unemployment and disability insurance, leave benefits, and workers' compensation are benefits organizations are required to offer by law (SBA n.d.). Other common benefits voluntarily offered to employees by the organization are health insurance, retirement plans, wellness programs, holidays (time off with pay), vacation time, and employee assistance programs. The HR department also leads the development and administration of the organization's job evaluation and classification systems, wage and salary systems, and incentive pay systems.

## Health and Safety Program

The HR department is also involved in activities designed to protect the health, safety, and security of the workforce. Healthcare organizations have given substantial attention to safety management since the enactment of the Occupational Safety and Health Act (OSHA) of 1970. Its intended purpose is "to ensure safe and healthful working conditions for workers by setting and enforcing standards and providing training, outreach, education and assistance" (OSHA n.d.). This act established a national reporting system for accidents and injuries on the job and led to the development of specific safety management programs in most businesses. Safety concerns such as chemical exposure, injury related to repetitive motion, and workplace violence continue to receive special attention by HR professionals (Dunn 2021). For the HIM manager, concerns may include ventilation, workstation ergonomics, lighting, and fire hazards.

The use of artificial intelligence (AI) presents a particular trio of related technologies that offer to improve workplace safety: natural language processing, computer vision technology and, predictive and prescriptive analytics. Natural language processing (NLP) provides the capacity for HR to manage data collection across multiple software platforms for analytical trending of safety reports. Computer vision technology capitalizes on workplace camera placement to analyze safety practice compliance, such as confirming personal protective equipment use. Predictive and prescriptive analytics engine use provides the potential for strategizing mitigation practices should safety incidences occur. While new technologies may be cost-prohibitive, a return on investment (ROI) analysis may illustrate the benefits such use can afford. Transparency of using these tools with employees is pivotal to their buy-in and understanding of importance in improving workplace safety (Zielinski 2023).

## Labor Relations

Employee, labor, and management relations are established through the day-to-day interactions between employees and their managers. However, the organization's managers and employees often seek leadership and support from the HR department. The HR department sets the stage for developing and sustaining the quality of these critical relationships by establishing and communicating to both managers and employees the contracts, policies, practices, and rules that constitute the organization's expectations of its employees.

HR management activities associated with unions and collective bargaining are referred to as **labor relations**. Labor organizations known as **unions** enter negotiations with employers on behalf of groups of employees who have elected to join a union. The negotiations relate to compensation and safety and health concerns. In a unionized environment, three laws came into existence over a period of 25 years (1935 through 1960) and constitute a code of practice for unions and management. HR departments pay strict attention to these three acts:

- **National Labor Relations Act (Wagner Act) of 1935**: Federal pro-union legislation that provides, among other things, procedures for union representation and prohibits unfair labor practices by unions, such as coercing non-striking employees, and by employers, such as interference with the union selection process and discrimination against employees who support a union (NLRA 1935)

- **Labor-Management Relations Act (Taft-Hartley Act) of 1947**: Federal legislation passed in 1947 that imposed certain restrictions on unions while upholding their right to organize and bargain collectively (Labor-Management Relations Act 1947)

- **Labor-Management Reporting and Disclosure Act (Landrum-Griffin Act) of 1959**: Federal legislation passed in 1959 to ensure union members' interests were properly represented by union leadership; it also created, among other things, a bill of rights for union members (Labor-Management Reporting and Disclosure Act 1959

For the manager who oversees a group of employees covered by a union contract, these laws represent the basic rules for their interactions with employees in the areas of pay, benefits, safety, health, and performance evaluation. (See table 22.1 for a list of prominent employment laws.) Grievance management is referred to later in the chapter as part of performance management.

## Check Your Understanding 22.1

**Answer the following questions in a separate document.**

1. What are some specific examples of internal and external environmental trends in the HIM field that are factors in HR planning and analysis?

2. An HIM manager is interviewing applicants for a scanning and indexing specialist. Required qualifications include a high school diploma, two years of work experience, and one year of experience in healthcare. Applicant 1 has a high school diploma and has one year of work experience in healthcare. Applicant 2 has a high school diploma and three years of healthcare experience but is in a wheelchair due to multiple sclerosis. The manager is concerned about the applicant's physical ability to do the job. Identify and describe the legislation available to the manager to help make the best hiring decision. Using this information, which applicant should be hired?

3. Ashley manages the transcription staff and notices the newest employee, Eva, is struggling to adjust to her workstation. Eva is very petite, and her chair and keyboard appear oversized for her stature. Her discomfort may be impacting her potential productivity. Who should Ashley contact to have Eva's equipment assessed for appropriate sizing?

4. Troy just started working as a registration supervisor and will soon be hiring a new registration specialist. Troy's staff is unionized. What resources are available to Troy as he begins his new job and the process of hiring new staff?

5. Larry is the coding manager and one of his best coders just informed him that she has been diagnosed with breast cancer and treatments will begin next week. She is very concerned she will lose her job. What legislation should Larry investigate and share with his employee?

## Role of the HIM Manager in Human Resources

Because the day-to-day management of an organization's HR is the responsibility of supervisory, middle, and executive managers, every manager is responsible for many of the same HR activities as the HR professionals. In an HIM department, for example, the supervisor of coding services would be

**Table 22.1.** Federal labor legislation

| Legislation | Concern or content | Administrative or enforcement agency |
|---|---|---|
| National Labor Relations Act of 1935 (Wagner Act) | Encouraged collective bargaining | National Labor Relations Board (NLRB) |
| Fair Labor Standards Act (FLSA) of 1938 | Addressed the need for minimum wage, overtime pay, and record keeping | US Department of Labor (DOL) |
| Fair Employment Act of 1941 | Prohibited discrimination against race, creed, color, or national origin | Committee on Fair Employment Practices |
| Labor Management Relations Act of 1947 (Taft-Hartley Act) | Amended provisions of the Wagner Act; restricted activities and power of labor union | NLRB |
| Labor-Management Reporting and Disclosure Act of 1959 (Landrum-Griffin Act) | Required financial disclosures of labor organizations | DOL |
| Equal Pay Act (EPA) of 1963 | Discouraged compensation relative to the sex of a worker | Equal Employment Opportunity Commission (EEOC) |
| Title VII of the Civil Rights Act of 1964 | Removed bias related to sex, color, race, religion, and national origin | EEOC |
| Age Discrimination in Employment Act of 1967 (amended in 1978, 1986) | Prohibited discrimination due to age (protection for those 40 and older) | EEOC |
| Occupational Safety and Health Act (OSHA) of 1970 | Established regulation around workplace safety | Occupational Safety and Health Administration |
| Equal Employment Opportunity (EEO) Act of 1972 | Promoted equal employment opportunities for all Americans | EEOC |
| Rehabilitation Act of 1973 | Prohibited discrimination against people with disabilities; specific to federal programs | DOL |
| Employee Retirement Income Security Act (ERISA) of 1974 | Established pension and healthcare plan rules | DOL |
| Pregnancy Discrimination Act of 1978 (amendment to Title VII of the Civil Rights Act of 1964) | Prohibited discrimination due to pregnancy, childbirth, or related medical conditions | EEOC |
| Immigration Reform and Control Act of 1986 | Established employment eligibility verification | DOL |
| Employee Polygraph Protection Act of 1988 | Prohibited use of polygraphs by most private employers | Secretary of Labor |
| Americans with Disabilities Act (ADA) of 1990 | Prohibited discrimination against people with disabilities, specific to private sector; much based on Sec. 504 of the Rehabilitation Act of 1973 | EEOC |
| Civil Rights Act of 1991 | Established provisions for damages for intentional employment discriminations | EEOC |
| Uniformed Services Employment and Reemployment Rights Act (USERRA) of 1994 | Protected veterans' civilian jobs | DOL |
| Family Medical Leave Act (FMLA) of 1993 | Permitted unpaid leave for certain healthcare reasons related to family or self | Employment Standards Administration |
| Health Insurance Portability and Accountability Act (HIPAA) of 1996 | Established regulation around securing health insurance coverage | DOL |
| Nursing Relief Disadvantaged Areas Act of 1999 | Permitted temporary employment of alien or foreign RNs | DOL |
| Genetic Information Nondiscrimination Act (GINA) 2008 | Prohibits genetic information discrimination against employees or applicants | EEOC |

*Source:* Adapted from Dunn 2021; DOL n.d.a.; EEOC n.d.b.

responsible for the day-to-day management of clinical coding specialists. Managers at all levels can use any of a variety of HR tools and processes to handle these responsibilities efficiently and effectively.

## Human Resources Planning

Several tools may be used to plan and manage staff resources. Position descriptions, for example, outline the work and qualifications needed to perform a job. Position descriptions should be aligned with the mission and goals of the organization. Policies and procedures are tools allowing for consistent and transparent communication of information to staff how best to accomplish their work.

### Position Descriptions

A **position (job) description** outlines the work to be performed by a specific employee or group of employees with the same responsibilities. Position descriptions generally consist of three parts: a summary of the position's requirements and purpose, its functions, and the qualifications needed to perform the job. Position descriptions also include the official title of the job and to whom (the position) the employee will directly report. While working and collaborating with a variety of positions, it is essential to define the person ultimately responsible for the employee. For example, a scanning and indexing clerk reports to the clerical supervisor. It is critical the employee have one person to whom they report and the reporting relationship is very clear, ensuring no confusion about from whom the employee should take direction. See figure 22.2 for a job description template that demonstrates important components of the job description.

A **job specification** is a document (or a section of the job description document) focused on the knowledge, skills, abilities, and characteristics required of an individual to perform the job. These specifications may include education and training, professional certifications, and experience (Dunn 2021, 21).

Position descriptions, including the job specification, are used during the recruitment process to explain the work to prospective candidates. They also enable managers and HR staff to set appropriate salaries and wages for various positions. In addition, they may be used to evaluate job performance, either during probationary periods or annually, and to resolve performance problems. For this reason, it is essential that position descriptions are written in a criteria-based language that correlates directly to the established job functions. The manager can use the position description to clarify the tasks the employee is expected to perform.

**Figure 22.2.** Job description template

---

Job title:                                              Department:

Reports to:                                             Cost center:

Job category:                                           Salary (exempt) or hourly (nonexempt)

Job type: Full-time or part-time

Job summary:

Description of the job:

**Required employment qualifications**: Knowledge, skills, abilities, mental capacity, education, experience, and licensure or credentials required for the job.

**Preferred employment qualifications**: Knowledge, skills, abilities, mental capacity, education, experience, and licensure or credentials preferred but not required for the job.

**Physical demands/safety requirements/working conditions**: Lifting, standing, sitting, walking, and reaching requirements; keyboarding and use of computer monitor, noise, smells, use of chemicals, and any other physical demands and safety considerations that are part of the working conditions.

**Job responsibilities and functions/competencies**: All required job functions and responsibilities, can include the weight of each job function.

**Mission/values/behavioral expectations**: Mission and stated values of the organization including behavioral expectations for this job.

**Decision-making authority**: Decision-making authority required of this job role, if any.

**Supervisory and/or budget responsibilities (if applicable)**: Supervisory responsibilities or budget responsibilities, if any.

**Date Reviewed**: Last date job description was reviewed for accuracy and relevance.

Generally, new or revised job descriptions are needed in the following circumstances:

- When an entirely new kind of work is required
- When a job changes and the old description no longer reflects the work
- When a change in technology or processes dramatically affects the work to be accomplished

Sometimes top performers outgrow their job descriptions. They may find more efficient ways of doing part of their assigned tasks and want more interesting or meaningful work. The job description may need to be updated to better reflect additional assigned responsibilities to support an increase in salary and benefits or a change in title.

When writing new position descriptions, managers may use existing descriptions of other, related jobs or interview staff who are currently performing some of the tasks intended for the new job. They also may assign staff members a work measurement technique to record how they spend their time on the job for a period that reflects a comprehensive cycle of their work. Staff with more repetitive daily activities may only need to record their activities for a short period of time (for example, a week). In contrast, staff with more diverse tasks may need more time, perhaps a month, to document the scope of their duties.

### Policies and Procedures

Policies and procedures are critical tools that may be used to ensure consistent quality performance. A **policy** is a directive statement that describes how a specific situation or process should be handled and reflects the organization's values and mission. For example, a policy might state that patients are allowed to review their health records under certain conditions, such as when a clinical professional is present or in the HIM department. Policies should be clearly stated and comprehensive. They must be developed in accordance with applicable laws, and they must reflect actual practice. Because they may be used as documentation of intended practice in a lawsuit, policies should be developed very carefully. Organization and departmental policies are often found on the organization's internal network or intranet. A **procedure** describes how work is to be done and how policies are to be carried out. Procedures are instructions that ensure high-quality, consistent outcomes for tasks done, especially when more than one person is involved. One of the benefits of developing a procedure is that time is taken to analyze the best possible method for completing a process. A detailed procedure is also useful in training new staff or in providing instructions to anyone needing to perform a task in the regular employee's absence.

## Recruitment and Retention

Armed with a position description, the manager is ready to begin recruiting candidates for a new or open position. **Recruitment** is the process of finding, soliciting, and attracting new employees. However, the manager should be sure to understand the organization's recruitment and hiring policies and to seek the assistance of the HR department before the vacancy is publicized. This preparation ensures the organization's legal obligations and policies and procedures are followed throughout the recruitment, selection, and hiring process.

### Recruitment

The first thing to consider in recruiting candidates to fill a staff opening is whether to promote someone from inside the organization or to look for candidates outside the organization. The advantage of promoting from within is that the practice often motivates employees to perform well, learn new skills, and work toward advancement. To advertise a vacancy internally, the organization might post it on facility bulletin boards or list it in the organization's newsletter or intranet. The department manager may announce an opening at a routine staff meeting or use any other communication channels available. Initial communication of job opportunities internally suggests that internal candidates are considered first whenever possible.

When the position cannot be filled from within, however, there are several ways to advertise externally. For example, the organization might place an ad in a newspaper or professional journal, post the job on the organization's employment site or on external internet recruitment sites, announce the opportunity at professional meetings, contact people who have previously applied or expressed interest in working at the organization, or work through a professional recruiter.

In most cases, the approach used depends on the nature of the open position. For example, the facility might run an ad for a clerical position in a local newspaper or on an internet recruitment site, but not in a professional journal because the market for entry-level positions is often locally strong. Alternately, the facility might turn to a professional recruiter when trying to fill a department director or experienced coding position because the number of qualified candidates for these positions is more limited.

As in every industry, job seekers looking for professional-level healthcare positions submit detailed resumes. A resume describes the candidate's educational background and work experience and usually includes information on personal and professional achievements. Candidates often submit a cover letter describing the type of position in which they are interested along with their resume. Today, it is common for candidates to submit, and organizations to accept, application letters and resumes through electronic systems, including email and employer websites.

Applications are formal documentation that job seekers complete to give prospective employers their chronological work history, current employment status, and the specifics of their skill sets. People seeking entry-level positions may be asked to complete an application rather than submit a resume. In many cases, completion of applications can be done online. It is imperative that job descriptions used in the job postings are comprehensive and up to date, so the most qualified candidates are not excluded. It is equally important that applicants are as specific as possible in their applications while highlighting their skill sets so, in turn, they are not excluded by an electronic HR management system that uses keyword matches to determine eligible applicants. These systems are designed to compare key skills and knowledge from the job description requirements to those identified skills and knowledge included in the employee application or resume; when the terms match between the two, that person becomes a candidate for the position.

## Selection

When a sufficient pool of applicants has been recruited, the selection process can begin. The goal of the selection process is to identify the candidate most qualified to fill the position. Testing and interviewing applicants are the two basic tools employed in the selection process. Employment testing is commonly conducted during the applicant's first visit to the facility. Reliability of a test refers to the consistency with which a test measures an attribute. Validity refers to a test's ability to accurately and consistently measure what it purports to measure. Testing practices are under increasing legal scrutiny, which places a special burden on organizations to ensure tests used are clearly job related. Use of tests as a selection procedure violates federal anti-discrimination laws if used to exclude people based on race, color, sex, national origin, disability, religion, or age (EEOC 2007). HR professionals are generally familiar with a variety of ability (achievement) tests that assess applicants' current skills, aptitude tests, mental ability (cognitive) tests that assess applicants' reasoning capabilities, personality tests, and honesty (integrity) tests that are designed to evaluate honesty via a series of hypothetical questions that are suitable for use in the organization (EEOC 2007). Many healthcare organizations also perform routine drug testing on candidates for employment to create a drug-free work environment.

The interview is generally considered the most important phase of the selection process, and there are three effective interview formats:

- **Structured interview** uses a set of standardized questions that are asked of all applicants. It ensures that the same questions based on predetermined selection criteria are asked of and evaluated for each applicant.

- **Behavioral description interview** requires applicants to give specific examples of how they have performed a specific procedure or handled a specific problem in the past. The worksheet in figure 22.3 also allows a space for documenting specific information from the applicant for each criterion.

- **Panel interview** includes a team of people who interview applicants at one time. (Mathis and Jackson 2016)

Interviewing is one of the most important skills managers need for selecting new staff. Unfortunately, many managers receive little formal training in interviewing techniques or have little practical experience. This shortcoming can be overcome through self-education, mentoring by more experienced managers, or instructional sessions with HR professionals in the organization.

Failure to adequately prepare for conducting the interview has very serious consequences for the organization and the applicant. Reviewing the position description, reading the applicant's resume and application form, and preparing appropriate and relevant questions are important steps to take before beginning an interview.

The interview itself has four basic purposes:

- Obtain information from the applicant about his or her past work history and future goals
- Give information to the applicant about the organization's mission and goals and the nature of the employment opportunity
- Evaluate the applicant's work experience and alignment with the organization
- Give the applicant an opportunity to evaluate the organization as a potential fit for his or her current and future employment goals

EEO regulations dictate the types of questions that may be asked during interviews and on employment applications. For example, questions pertaining to

**Figure 22.3.** Interviewing and selection worksheet

| Selection criteria | Information on [applicant name] | Score rate 1–10 | Information on [applicant name] | Score rate 1–10 | Information on [applicant name] | Score rate 1–10 |
|---|---|---|---|---|---|---|
| | | | | | | |
| | | | | | | |
| | | | | | | |
| | | | | | | |
| | | | | | | |
| | | | | | | |

age, religious affiliation, and marital status should be avoided (EEOC n.d.b). These regulations apply during all activities associated with the interview, including during formal interview sessions and during less formal lunches, dinners, or hallway and elevator small talk, when it is very easy to inadvertently lapse into discussions on these topics. Managers should always seek the advice of HR professionals when they are uncertain about which questions to ask.

Employers must be certain to conduct careful background checks of potential employees. The Centers for Medicare and Medicaid Services (CMS 2010), as well as many states, mandate that healthcare organizations must conduct comprehensive background checks and fingerprinting (ACA 2010) for employees who have direct vulnerable patient contact in long-term care environments. Managers or HR professionals also check the references of candidates and communicate with the past employers of candidates by telephone or through correspondence. **Reference checks** are background investigations conducted by the employer specifically to assess the applicants' compatibility with the position and to validate the accuracy of information the applicants provide on their application, resume, and during the interview.

## Hiring

After all the internal and external interviews, tests, and reference and background checks are complete, the hiring manager usually has enough information to make a hiring decision. A tool that can assist with making a hiring decision is the decision matrix in figure 22.4. In this figure, the decision analysis matrix is designed for hiring an inpatient coder. The MUST criteria are the criteria required for the applicant; these criteria must be present to the hiring manager's satisfaction for them to be met. The WANT criteria are desired criteria. These criteria would not be considered if all the MUST criteria are not met. The WANT criteria have a weight of importance noted in parentheses after each criterion. If the criteria are met to the hiring manager's satisfaction, that weight is assigned to the criteria for the applicant. If not, a zero is given. This is an all-or-nothing scoring. A manager may decide to use a range between zero and the weighted score as another methodology. The total at the bottom of the matrix is the total of the WANT or desired criteria for each applicant.

In some organizations, the manager shares the hiring decision with key department staff, HR staff, and executive staff, depending on the level of the

**Figure 22.4.** Decision analysis matrix

| DECISION: | Applicant to select for inpatient coder position. | | | |
|---|---|---|---|---|
| Evaluate each applicant (A, B, and C) based on the criteria specified in the job description by applying the decision analysis technique. | | | | |
| Criteria | | A | B | C |
| MUST (required) | | | | |
| Place an X across from each MUST criteria the applicant meets. All MUST criteria must be met before evaluating the WANT criteria. | | | | |
| 1. Two years inpatient coding experience | | ___ | ___ | ___ |
| 2. Coding credential (CCS, CPC, CIC) | | ___ | ___ | ___ |
| 3. Experience using an encoder | | ___ | ___ | ___ |
| 4. Ability to communicate clearly | | ___ | ___ | ___ |
| WANT (desired) | | | | |
| Each WANT criterion is weighted with the number in parentheses after it. If the applicant meets the criteria and expectations fully, assign that weight as noted. If not, give them a 0. Only rate the WANT criteria if all the MUST (required) criteria are met. | | | | |
| 1. Responsible, dependable (5) | | ___ | ___ | ___ |
| 2. Neat appearance (3) | | ___ | ___ | ___ |
| 3. Experience with CAC (2) | | ___ | ___ | ___ |
| 4. RHIA credential (3) | | ___ | ___ | ___ |
| Total Points | | ___ | ___ | ___ |
| Comments: | | | | |

position. When the details of the job offer have been approved by the HR department, a formal job offer should be made. The HR department should prepare a letter that describes the duties and responsibilities of the position, states the employment start date, and explains the salary and benefits package. In addition, the hiring manager may choose to communicate the offer to the candidate through a personal telephone contact, which is subsequently confirmed by an official letter (Anthony et al. 2010).

## Workforce Retention

According to the Bureau of Labor Statistics, a certain level of staff turnover is expected; variable rates for healthcare are typically in the 3.0 percent range (BLS 2024). Employees move, retire, or seek other careers. A manager can do little to prevent turnover resulting from changes in the personal lives of employees. However, the actions of managers and the policies of the organization can have an impact, either positive or negative, on staff retention. **Retention** is the ability to keep valuable employees from seeking employment elsewhere.

The following questions should be considered when assessing employee retention:

- Is there a comprehensive new employee orientation and training program giving the employee the resources needed to be successful?
- Does the organization support continued education either financially or through flexible work schedules?
- Do employees have opportunities to advance their careers within the organization?
- Are salaries and benefits competitive with similar organizations?
- Do working conditions provide a comfortable and safe environment as well as hybrid or remote options?
- Does the manager treat employees fairly and follow employment regulations and guidelines?
- Is there frequent and clear communication between management and employees?

Although individual managers may have limited influence on some of these factors, they must always be aware of the impact that broader organizational HR policies and practices have on employees. Gone unnoticed or left unaddressed, concerns in these areas are often what make employees look for other jobs. For example, employees become dissatisfied when they feel they are being treated unfairly or that HR practices are needlessly rigid. In some cases, employees become dissatisfied simply because they do not know the rationale for a particular HR policy or because a concern they have voiced about an unsafe condition in their work area is not acted on by the manager. The challenge to the manager is to communicate frequently, be informed as soon as possible when employees express an HR-related concern, and encourage an open door policy.

Staff turnover is expensive in terms of both lost productivity and recruitment and training costs. To ensure effective management, turnover should be monitored across time and benchmarked with the rest of the organization and other organizations in the community or geographic area. Routine employee satisfaction surveys provide information about how employees feel about their jobs and insights into how the facility might improve working conditions. An HR representative and the direct supervisor often conduct exit interviews with employees who leave the organization as another way to obtain information on how employees feel about their jobs and what issues cause them to leave. By using a checklist format, employers can consistently gather information from the departing employee and feed that back to the department for consideration and correction as appropriate.

## Effective Communication

Maintaining regular and effective communication with staff is one of the ongoing challenges in managing HR. Communication is important because it contributes significantly to staff morale and their ability to contribute to the department's operations. To address this challenge, a manager should establish a communication plan that includes routine and timely opportunities for both verbal and written information sharing within the department or workgroup. The plan should include, as appropriate, the following types of communication:

- Daily personal contact with every employee to maintain a sense of connectedness and, as necessary, to create opportunities for casual discussions of emerging work-related changes or issues
- Intranet-based or traditional bulletin boards located in an area convenient to staff to publicize official announcements, permissible personal news, written status updates, and written highlights from departmental meetings
- Weekly status meetings with the staff for each functional unit in the department in larger organizations or the entire department in smaller organizations
- Monthly departmental meetings with highlights recorded for posting, including the topics, discussions, actions to be taken, who is responsible to complete the action, and the timeframe
- Quarterly performance discussions with individual employees
- Ad hoc verbal or electronic (email) status updates, as appropriate, to alert staff to information of interest from organizational meetings
- Written departmental communications to disseminate a change in policy, new procedure, or special notification

On a day-to-day basis, when problems emerge that require resolution within the department or when decisions are made that affect the employees in the department, the management team is responsible for establishing a unique communication plan that conforms to the situation. Such a plan identifies all employees affected by the problem or the decision and defines the specific approach that managers will take to engage or inform each person appropriately.

In general, keeping staff well informed is a key factor in developing and sustaining a healthy level of trust in the relationship between employees and managers. Communication plans are simple tools that managers can use to ensure that this critical aspect of their responsibilities is handled with the level of routine and regular attentiveness it requires.

## Employee Empowerment

Creating an environment that encourages employees to use and develop their problem-solving and decision-making competencies is an established HR management practice that has many benefits. It increases the manager's capacity and productivity, improves the quality and timeliness of decision-making, enhances employee morale, and contributes to improved employee retention. Through effective team-building and appropriate delegation of duties, the manager empowers employees to grow in capability and confidence.

### Empowerment

Empowerment is the concept of providing employees with the tools and resources to solve problems themselves. In other words, employees obtain power over their work situation by assuming responsibility. Empowered employees have the freedom to contribute ideas and perform their jobs in the best possible way.

Healthcare organizations that empower their employees believe all employees can perform—and truly want to perform—to their highest potential when given the proper resources and environment. Because they perform jobs on a regular basis, they are intimately familiar with the specific steps required in their daily work responsibilities. What the employees may lack are skills in analysis and problem solving that may help them become more effective performers. Training sessions in skills such as data analysis, use of control charts, or flowcharting will help employees to identify problems, develop alternatives, and recommend solutions.

To perform effectively, employees also need to be given responsibility, authority, and the trust to make decisions and act independently within their area of expertise. Figure 22.5 offers suggestions on how managers can empower their employees. Empowered employees are less likely to complain or feel helpless or frustrated when they cannot resolve a problem on their own. Moreover, they are more likely to feel a sense of accomplishment and to be more receptive to solutions they develop themselves. In addition, they tend to demonstrate commitment and self-confidence and produce high-quality work.

One disadvantage frequently mentioned by managers is that empowerment involves too much time for meetings and discussion and takes employees away from their "real work." It is much more efficient to take the time necessary to prevent problems than to solve them after they occur. In the long run, empowered employees work more efficiently and productively.

Indeed, some managers are afraid to share power. They feel they have worked hard to gain the power they have and are reluctant to give it up. But the manager who empowers others usually increases his or her own power because a high performing unit reflects the manager's expertise.

An example of empowerment in the HIM department is training ROI employees to solve a slow turnaround issue. The employees are probably more aware than the supervisor of problems that prevent them from filling requests for information (such as missing documents, insufficient fees, and incomplete records). With proper training in brainstorming and flowcharting, and a supportive environment, the employees may be able to develop a procedure that can be performed differently to prevent delays.

### Team Building

Today, people need to work collaboratively with others; thus, the need for **team building**—the process of organizing and acquainting team members to enhance the outcomes of collaborative work. The team may consist of people who perform the same function within the same department—a coding team, for example. The team may bring together people who perform different functions within the same department to solve a shared problem or people from across the organization with different expertise to implement a new computer system or to study an issue that would affect the overall organization (for example, improvements in the employee evaluation system).

At their best, teams increase the creativity and improve the quality of problem solving. Often team-based decisions are more widely accepted than managerial decisions because team members enlist support for the decisions from their peers and coworkers. In addition, teams can use their collective energy to produce more work than individuals can. Moreover, teamwork establishes strong relationships among

**Figure 22.5.** Ten steps that empower

1. Know what each of your employees does and how well the tasks are done.
2. Decide what additional authority they can handle right now.
3. Ascertain what preparation each of your employees needs to achieve the competencies and mental toughness that empower them.
4. Reduce micromanaging and match the level of supervision with the ability, maturity, and motivation of each employee.
5. Ensure that workers know the purpose (mission) of their jobs.
6. Delegate activities that involve decision-making and problem solving.
7. Review your education and training program; design a cross-training and job rotation program so that people become more flexible.
8. Make tasks more challenging; assign complete rather than fragmented tasks.
9. Provide sufficient resources, time, and psychological support.
10. Emphasize commitment rather than conformity.

*Source*: Adapted from McConnell 2018, 435–436.

employees. Teamwork can enrich jobs and provide variety in work assignments as well. Finally, teams can develop new leaders and expose employees to issues that would not be within the usual scope of their jobs.

One thing that binds team members together is having a common purpose. The purpose for an ongoing work team, for example, might be to ensure cross-training, improve procedures, and monitor quality and productivity. In other cases, teams are created for a specific purpose. Some teams exist for long periods of time because they have an ongoing reason to exist. Other teams function for limited periods of time and disband after their purpose has been fulfilled.

However, having a common purpose is only one element of an effective team. The team also must have an effective leader. This individual must be able to create agendas and organize meetings, lead discussions, and ensure the work moves forward. The team may either appoint or elect its leader, depending on its purpose and the experience and expertise of its members.

In addition, effective teams set ground rules. For instance, team members might decide that all meetings will start on time, minutes will be recorded, decisions will be reached by consensus, and everyone will participate in discussions. The early establishment of rules can reduce conflict as the team moves forward. Team strength lies in engaging the collective brainpower of all members, and so the team leader should use techniques that effectively engage every member of the team.

Not all teams are effective, and the causes for problems vary. A team without a clear purpose could create a product that does not accomplish the work it was designed to accomplish; for example, a request to improve the release of information process without knowing the issues or problems will likely lead to the team not meeting the expected goal. A leader who dominates the team could reduce its effectiveness and frustrate its members. Members who do not participate, have insufficient expertise, or are unconcerned with the team's success could cause the team to fail. Members who work outside the team or do not support its decisions can create dissension and reduce support for the outcome. Contrarily, having a highly cohesive team that consistently thinks alike may make a poor decision because of a lack of varying perspectives.

Managing staff teams is an important aspect of every manager's assorted responsibilities. Careful consideration should be given to developing the team's purpose and composition. Team members must feel their work is important and their contributions make a difference. A well-run team can be an effective and productive force. A poorly run team can waste time and frustrate and demoralize its members.

## Delegation

Managers have specific responsibilities and the authority to act within the scope of that responsibility. Delegation of this authority expands the manager's capacity, improves the timeliness of decisions, and develops the competencies of other staff members. **Delegation** is the process by which managers distribute work to others along with the authority to make decisions and take action. To be effective, delegation should correspond with authority and responsibility. A manager must assign **responsibility**, which is an expectation that another person will perform tasks. At the same time, **authority**—or the right to act in ways necessary to carry out assigned tasks—must be granted. An employee cannot be expected to perform a job for which he or she is not given authority to obtain resources. Authority should equal responsibility when work is delegated. Finally, there must be accountability, which is the requirement to answer to a supervisor for specific results. Successful delegation includes assigning responsibility, granting authority, and creating accountability (Schermerhorn and Bachrach 2023).

Guidelines for delegating are presented in figure 22.6. As an employee development tool, delegation can give employees the opportunity to try new tasks previously performed by someone in a higher position. It can lead to empowerment because employees contribute ideas and fully utilize their skills. At the same time, the manager should remain available to aid and support.

Sometimes managers have difficulty delegating because they feel that only *they* can do the job correctly. In other cases, they feel threatened by the idea that another employee can do their tasks and perhaps do them better. This thinking can induce poor morale and result in talented employees leaving the organization. In addition, it can lead to managers

**Figure 22.6.** Ground rules for effective delegation

- Carefully choose the right task and right person to whom you delegate
- Define the responsibility; make the assignment clear
- Agree on performance objectives and standards
- Agree on an action plan and set checkpoints
- Give authority; allow the other person to act independently
- Show trust in the other person
- Provide adequate training so the delegate has competence to succeed
- Give performance feedback
- Monitor, recognize, and reinforce progress
- Help when things go wrong
- Do not forget your accountability for performance results

*Source:* Adapted from McConnell 2018, 430–434.

being overburdened with work doable by others and to employees being denied opportunities to learn new skills.

In some situations, employees may be unwilling to accept delegated responsibilities when they feel that they are unqualified to do the tasks or are being dumped on. Dumping can involve assigning an employee unpleasant or unpopular work that seems to have little value or asking an employee to take on work in addition to an already demanding workload. This results in resentment or anger. Employees may feel this way when they have a poor working relationship with their supervisor, know that others have refused the same task, or have been taken advantage of in the past. To avoid these problems, employees who are either competent to perform the tasks or willing to undergo the necessary training should be delegated to.

People are more willing to accept tasks that they understand and have a choice in doing, in addition to those they recognize as adding value to the organization and their personal growth. Managers should set checkpoints, monitor how the delegate is doing, and allow the opportunity for questions and feedback.

Delegation is a skill that matches the right employee with the right task. It requires communication, support, and an environment that fosters risk taking. It is essential to identify and develop successors and is important if a manager wishes to provide a path to advance in the organization. Effective delegation leads to a more efficient and productive department overall and mutually benefits the manager, employee, and institution.

### Check Your Understanding 22.2

Answer the following questions in a separate document.

1. Consider a job you have had or someone you know has had. Develop a job description for it.
2. You are the HIM director and are hiring a new administrative assistant. Develop three criteria for the job that you will use to rate each candidate.
3. You just completed the job description for a new business analyst and can now proceed with hiring someone. Map the process you will use from this point until you have chosen a candidate.
4. You manage a relatively limited HIM staff in a 42-bed rural hospital. While employee performance is adequate, the department climate is lackluster of late. You plan a one-day team building retreat and you need to justify the expense to administration. Create a rationale you would use to qualify your funding request.
5. Construct three questions that would be unlawful to ask a candidate. State why each would be considered unlawful.

## Compensation Systems

Employee compensation systems reward employees equitably for their service to the organization. Organizations also use compensation systems to enhance employee loyalty and encourage greater productivity. The FLSA, the EPA, and several of the EEO laws (for example, Title VII of the Civil Rights Act, Age Discrimination in Employment Act, and the ADA) all have provisions that affect compensation systems. Provisions of the FLSA, for example, cover minimum wage, overtime pay, child labor restrictions, and equal pay for equal work regardless of sex (DOL 2023). Federal regulations specify exemptions from some or all the FLSA provisions for a number of groups of employees (Myers 2011). These groups are referred to as **exempt employees** and are paid a salary per pay period. Covered groups are referred to as **nonexempt employees** and are paid an hourly wage.

Managers who control employee work schedules and process employee timecards at the close of each pay period become quite familiar with the provisions of the FLSA that relate to overtime pay. In general, the FLSA requires that employers pay one and a half times the employee's regular rate for all hours that a covered (nonexempt) employee works in excess of 40 per week (DOL 2023). Some organizations institute overtime pay for all worked hours in excess of eight hours per day and others when employees work in excess of 40 hours per week or 80 hours per two-week pay period. In calculations of worked hours, the FLSA specifies that rest periods of up to 20 minutes each be counted as worked time, but meal periods of 30 minutes or more are not counted as worked time (DOL 2023). Time spent in mandated job-related training is considered worked time, and significant travel time (beyond the usual time required to commute to and from work) associated with a work-related event is counted as worked time (DOL 2008). Compensatory time, taken in lieu of overtime pay, may be used when it is part of the organization's compensation plan (Myers 2011). Because of the complexities and sensitivities associated with compensation issues, HR professionals are a manager's best advisor when questions related to compensation regulations and practices arise.

## Compensation Surveys

The HR department routinely consults compensation surveys published by government agencies and professional and trade associations to ensure that pay for the organization's employees is fair, equitable, and aligned with other organizations. This is important for effective employee recruitment and retention. In some cases, an HR department may choose to conduct an independent survey to obtain data more specific to the organization's needs. Often consultants experienced with survey design and data analysis are employed by the organization to either assist in or do the survey project to ensure a successful outcome from this costly activity. Compensation surveys provide benchmark data that the organization can use to evaluate or establish its compensation system for unique jobs within the organization or for jobs throughout the organization (Dunn 2021).

## Job Evaluations

Job evaluation projects are undertaken by an organization to determine the relative worth of jobs as a first step toward establishing an equitable internal compensation system. **Job evaluation** is the process of applying predefined compensable factors to jobs to determine their relative worth. A **compensable factor** is "a characteristic used to compare the worth of jobs" and "the EPA [Equal Pay Act of 1963] requires employers to consider [several] compensable factors in setting pay for similar work performed by both females and males" (Myers 2011, 691). These factors include skill, effort (mental and physical exertion required to perform job-related tasks), responsibility, and working conditions.

Four job evaluation methods are commonly used:

- **Job ranking** is the simplest and the most subjective method of job evaluation. It involves placing jobs in order from highest to lowest in value to the organization.
- **Job classification method** involves matching a job's written position description with a description of a classification grade. Jobs in the federal government are graded on the basis of this method of job evaluation.
- **Point method** is a commonly used system that places weight (points) on each of the compensable factors in a job. The total points associated with a job establish its relative worth. Jobs that fall within a specific range of points fall into a grade associated with a specific wage or salary.
- **Factor comparison method** is a complex quantitative method that combines elements of both the ranking and point methods. Factor comparison results indicate the degree to which different compensable factors vary by job, making it possible to translate each factor value more easily into a monetary wage. (Mathis et al. 2016)

The Hay method of job evaluation is another system used. The **Hay method of job evaluation** is a modification of the point method that numerically measures the levels of three major compensable factors: the knowledge, problem-solving, and accountability requirements of each job (Mathis et al. 2016).

In addition, most healthcare organizations establish some type of job classification system that combines jobs with similar levels of responsibility and qualifications into job grades that determine salary ranges and benefit packages. For instance, all supervisory-level managers might be classified into one salary and benefit category, but each would have a unique job description. Job classifications also may determine whether an employee belongs to a union or is a candidate for unionization at the time a union attempts to organize the workforce, as may be the case if clerical staff is organized.

# Performance Management

Most organizations use some form of **performance review** system to evaluate the performance of individual employees. Figure 22.7 offers an example of a performance appraisal form illustrating the appraisal ratings, criteria for evaluation, strengths, areas for improvement, and goals. This type of format supports a uniform approach to assessing each employee. Although performance reviews should be

**Figure 22.7.** Performance appraisal form

| PERFORMANCE APPRAISAL | |
|---|---|
| Employee name: _____ | Date: _____ |
| | Title: _____ |
| Department: _____ CC: _____ Emp. No: _____ | DOH: _____ |
| Appraisal period: _____ to _____ | |

Instructions: Carefully evaluate employee's work performance in relation to current job requirements. Check rating box to indicate the employee's performance. Indicate N/A if not applicable.

**DEFINITION OF APPRAISAL RATINGS:**

Exemplary (E): Performance is exceptional in all areas and is recognizable as being superior to others.
Proficient (P): Results clearly meet most position requirements. Performance is of high quality and is achieved consistently.
Novice (N): Competent and dependable level of performance. Meets performance expectations of the job.
Unsatisfactory (U): Results are generally unacceptable and require immediate improvement.
N/A: Not applicable to this person's job.

| APPRAISAL FACTOR | RATING |
|---|---|
| Applies past experiences to new problems | |
| Retains information; does not repeatedly ask the same questions or make the same mistakes | |
| Follows instructions and takes notes when necessary | |
| Has gained the skills necessary to navigate the computer system for the functions for which he or she is responsible | |
| Takes care of equipment | |
| Uses supplies wisely; exercises apparent stewardship | |
| Follows department procedures | |
| Completes assigned work accurately | |
| Completes volume required | |
| Makes efficient use of time | |
| Meets accuracy requirements | |
| Completes assigned work with little or no dependence upon others | |
| Handwriting is legible | |
| Does not transpose numbers | |
| Willing to work with overtime | |
| Requires minimum supervision | |
| Improved in all areas that were marked "improvement needed" or "unsatisfactory" in last evaluation | |
| Achieved goals outlined in last evaluation | |
| Maintained strengths in same areas as last evaluation | |
| Days of absence | |
| Tardies | |

Area(s) for improvement:
Strengths:
Goals:
1.
Target Date: _____ Employee's initials: _____
2.
Target Date: _____ Employee's initials: _____
Employee Comments:
Employee's initials: _____
Employee's Signature: _____ Date: _____
Supervisor's Signature: _____ Date: _____
Manager's Signature: _____ Date: _____

a part of regular communications between managers and employees, formal performance review discussions are routinely held on an annual or biannual basis. The functions of performance reviews include the following:

- Assessment of the employee's performance compared to performance standards or previously set performance goals
- Development of performance goals for the future year
- Development of a plan for professional development

Performance reviews also may include employee self-assessments. In some organizations, other employees may contribute information to the reviews of colleagues and coworkers. In the case of a supervisory manager, his or her staff may participate in the evaluation. This form of evaluation to which managers, peers, and staff contribute is called a **360-degree evaluation**.

Many organizations' base pay increases on the results of annual performance reviews. Whether or not the evaluation affects salary, the annual review is an opportunity to formally discuss past accomplishments, career development, and expectations for future performance.

Performance management is an ongoing challenge, and performance issues, as well as measurable successes, should be addressed in real time, not harbored until the annual review. Information about performance should be collected regularly and shared with employees, whether their jobs involve coding clinical records or directing a department. Good performance results should be shared to encourage and reward ongoing success. Performance issues are rarely resolved by ignoring them. Understanding the causes of problems and working with employees to resolve them are important management tasks. Actions that can be taken to improve performance include retraining, streamlining responsibilities, reestablishing expectations, and monitoring progress.

## Performance Counseling and Disciplinary Action

When actions taken to improve performance are unsuccessful, more formal counseling and even disciplinary action may be required, such as suspension without pay, demotion, or less pay. Most organizations have formal processes in place to ensure all staff are treated fairly and that employment laws are followed. Managers should consult with the HR department to ensure any disciplinary actions comply with approved procedures. Refer to table 22.1 for references to common employment law.

The steps described in establishing performance standards, hiring and training employees, and conducting routine performance reviews are all necessary before doing performance counseling or taking disciplinary action. Moreover, steps to improve performance should be taken in all cases.

Performance counseling usually begins with informal counseling or a verbal warning. No record of these actions is typically required in the employee's official file. However, a manager may choose to include it. The **progressive discipline** process begins with a verbal warning that may or may not be a part of the employee's file depending on organization policy and the severity and frequency of the offense. When the next offense occurs, the process progresses to a written reprimand with formal documentation of the problem and delineation of the steps needed to correct it. This, and any further related action, is typically a part of the employee's official HR file. Employees may be required to submit a step-by-step action plan to resolve issues and improve their performance. The next offense often results in suspension, with further related infractions resulting in termination.

In some environments, disciplinary actions include suspension from employment without pay or demotion to a job with lower expectations and less pay. In some cases, more than one of these actions may be taken. Generally, however, suspension and demotion are less popular than the use of binding performance improvement plans because suspension and demotion create a punitive atmosphere. Such punitive actions also affect the morale of other employees and staff. Empowering employees to create a plan of action places the responsibility for performance improvement in their own hands.

Regardless of the counseling and disciplinary actions mandated by the organization, managers should take some key steps of their own, including the following:

- Discussing performance problems and consequences for poor performance with the employee in a clear and direct manner as soon as possible after the performance problem is discovered
- Supporting the employee's efforts to improve performance or resolve performance issues
- Documenting the steps taken to improve performance
- Carefully following the organization's HR policies
- Consulting HR professionals before acting
- Keeping performance issues confidential
- Following the same process for all employees

By following these steps in a timely, impartial, and considerate manner, managers will construct a consistent disciplinary message and hopefully coach the employee to job performance improvement. Documentation of the steps taken in the progressive discipline process is critical if performance does not improve, necessitating advanced actions up to suspension or termination. This documentation may be critical in the event of employee denial, grievance, or litigation.

## Termination and Layoff

One of the most difficult duties of a manager is delivering the notification of **termination** (ending of a job) to an employee. The HR department is a vital resource for advising and supporting the manager through this process to ensure accepted HR practices as established by the organization are adhered to. The general guidelines to use when terminating an employee are as follows:

- Determine the most appropriate location to hold the discussion privately.
- Review the employee file and the progressive discipline process that has occurred.
- State position quickly and concisely and end the discussion.
- Be sensitive to appropriate timing for the discussion.
- Be prepared with all of the appropriate severance information.
- Treat the employee with dignity and respect. (Delpo n.d.)

**Layoffs** are like terminations except they are essentially unpaid leaves of absence initiated by the employer as a strategy for downsizing staff in response to a change in the organization's status (for example, an unexpected or a seasonal downturn in business volume). In many cases, unlike termination, employees are called back to work at some future date.

The **Workers' Adjustment Retraining and Notification (WARN) Act of 1988** requires that organizations employing more than 100 people give the employees and the community a 60-day notice of its intent to close the business or to lay off 50 or more members of its workforce (DOL n.d.b). The intent of the act is to provide time for employees and their families to adjust to an impending unemployment event and seek new skills to be competitive in the current job market. Managers must understand this requirement so they can plan accordingly for that time, should they be in a position where employee layoffs are imminent. It is important to plan for a potential downturn in employee morale and productivity during this time.

## Conflict Management

Sometimes problems arise because of conflicts among employees. It is common for people to disagree, and sometimes a difference of opinion can increase creativity. However, too much conflict can also waste time, reduce productivity, and decrease morale. When taken to the extreme, it can threaten the safety of employees and cause damage to property. **Conflict management** focuses on working with the individuals involved in a disagreement to find a mutually acceptable solution. There are three ways to address conflict:

- **Compromise**: In this method, both parties must be willing to lose or give up a piece of their position. One scenario in which this approach may be well served is job sharing where one position (FTE) is split between two employees. If only one set of benefits apply to a position, the employees will need to determine who will enjoy the insurance benefits and who receives the paid time off (PTO). The outcome of this decision will require each employee to give up something for the job-sharing arrangement to work.
- **Control**: In this method, interaction may be prohibited until the employees' emotions are under control. The manager also may structure their interactions. For example, the manager can set ground rules for communicating or dealing with specific issues. Another form of control is personal counseling. Personal counseling focuses on how people deal with conflict rather than on the cause of specific disagreements.
- **Constructive confrontation**: In this method, both parties meet with an objective third party to explore their perceptions and feelings. The desired outcome is to produce a mutual understanding of the issues and to create a win-win situation. For example, there are two registry abstracters sharing a desk space on their respective back-to-back shifts that are at odds, each perceiving that their method of organization is most beneficial. The opposing methods of processing are creating tension reported to be exacerbating their anger with each other, rather than being resolved during attempted one-on-one encounters. With appropriate moderating between the two employees and a third party, often the parties

at odds can receive a new understanding of a coworker's perspective.

Conflict is an expected part of working with others, but managing and resolving conflict is crucial to an effective work unit.

### Grievance Management

Employees have the right to disagree with management and can express their opinions or complaints in a variety of ways. They should be encouraged to bring problems and concerns directly to their manager. When they do not achieve satisfaction at that level, the manager should explain other options to the employee. For example, dissatisfied employees should understand that they can either take their issues to the next management level or discuss them with HR staff.

Organizations establish **grievance procedures** that define the steps an employee can follow to seek resolution of a disagreement they have with management on a job-related issue. A complaint becomes a **grievance** when it has been documented in writing and brought to the attention of management or union representatives. At that point, the formal grievance procedure is set in motion. Depending on organizational policy or a union contract, the grievance procedure may vary.

Employees who belong to a union should follow the grievance procedures set by their union. Union contracts usually specify the types of actions employees can take and the time frames for filing grievances and define the formal process for elevating the consideration or resolution of a grievance. Grievances taken to the highest levels will likely have to be resolved through mediation or arbitration. **Mediation** is when a dispute is taken to an objective third party to facilitate agreement between the disputing parties. **Arbitration** is when an objective third party is brought in to make a binding decision in a case where the parties cannot come to agreement. Each of these steps takes time and can cost money. Therefore, managers should try to avoid grievances by maintaining open and effective communication with their staff.

## Maintenance of Employee Records

Official documentation about an employee's job performance must be maintained under the control of the HR department. Any employee records maintained under the control of the manager must be kept secure at all times.

Federal legislation such as Title VII of the Civil Rights Act of 1964, the Age Discrimination in Employment Act, the Immigration Reform and Control Act, and the FLSA place numerous recordkeeping and reporting requirements on the HR department. The Environmental Protection Agency and the OSHA also have recordkeeping requirements. Several of these additional recordkeeping obligations are as follows:

- Employers must protect the confidentiality of personnel records and files.
- Employers must protect the health records of employees.
- Employers must avoid intruding into the personal lives of employees, such as their other associations, alcohol use, spending habits, and financial obligations, unless there are valid job-related reasons for making such intrusions.
- Employers must prevent the public disclosure of personal information that may be embarrassing to an employee.
- Employers must protect the results of employment-related tests, including written tests used in making selection decisions, and the results of both pre-employment and random drug testing. (Myers 2011, 125–126)

Employers must have consistent and stringent recordkeeping processes to protect the privacy of employees. This is a legal and ethical obligation.

## Human Resources Trends and Practices

Human resource management and practice are directly impacted by the trending labor force composition and must keep apprised of those trends to be best positioned. The following workforce trends in employment are likely to affect the labor market in the US during the first decades of the 21st century:

- Women will constitute a greater proportion of the labor force than in the past, with 56.2

percent of all US women in the workforce in 2016. In the healthcare industry, women are more than 70 percent of the workforce. Approximately 71 percent of the women in the workforce have children under the age of 18, and 47.6 percent of women in the workforce hold college degrees. This trend indicates a need for daycare availability, which is an example of how an organization may need to position itself as a desired employer (BLS 2023).

- Minority racial and ethnic groups will account for a growing percentage of the overall labor force. Immigrants will expand this growth. Organizations can facilitate that transition with diversity training for all employees.
- The average age of the US population will increase, and more workers who retire from full-time jobs will work part-time. As a result of these and other shifts, employers in a variety of industries will face shortages of qualified workers (EEOC n.d.c).

From this information, employers must be prepared to function with an increasingly diverse workforce in terms of gender, age, health status, race, and ethnicity. In general, the management of an increasingly diverse workforce is receiving considerable attention in the HR literature, and some organizations have initiated diversity training programs. Three content areas that are often included in diversity training programs include the following:

- *Legal awareness:* Federal and state laws and regulations on EEO and the consequences of violating these laws and regulations
- *Cultural awareness:* Attempts to deal with stereotypes, typically through discussions and exercises
- *Sensitivity training:* Attempts to sensitize people to the differences among them and how their words and behaviors are perceived by others (Mathis et al. 2016)

There is still work to be done within healthcare organizations and HIM departments to prepare for the anticipated growth in the multicultural profile of human assets over the coming decade.

The DOL data also indicate that employees will increasingly seek ways to gain more control over their time (BLS 2017). The time pressure associated with trying to balance work and personal lives (especially when both parents are working outside the family home), coupled with the time pressure associated with increasingly long commutes, appear to be driving this concern to the surface in HR management. Flextime, job sharing, and home-based (telecommuting) staffing options have emerged as viable solutions to the workforce retention issue. Within work units in HIM, flextime and home-based staffing options are being implemented to address the labor shortages already affecting departmental operations. The advancement of technology is playing a key role in the increased availability of staffing options and growing opportunities for work and personal life balance.

Effective management of HR begins with attention given to the adoption of appropriate policies, procedures, and practices in each of the HR activity areas: HR planning and analysis; EEO; staffing; HR development; compensation and benefits; health, safety, and security; and employee and labor management relations. HIM professionals working in close partnership with the organization's HR department hire and retain qualified employees by following these employment guidelines and fostering effective working relationships between employees and management.

Effective recruitment, selection, and hiring practices involve the consistent use of the tools designed to identify the best-qualified candidates for each position. Once hired, ensuring employees are well-oriented and trained is the critical first step toward a successful long-term outcome. Subsequently, maintaining open and meaningful communications with employees, setting realistic performance expectations for employees, engaging employees in ways that give them appropriate control of their work schedule and environment, delegating appropriate levels of decision-making authority, and providing them with opportunities for ongoing staff development all serve to enhance employee morale and increase job satisfaction.

Managing HR is both a science and an art. As such, it is learned through a combination of study and observation. Published HR management resources are readily available to provide the knowledge foundation associated with this field. In the workplace, HR professionals are available to serve as advisors to HIM managers who want to handle this complex aspect of their management responsibilities knowledgably and artfully.

## Check Your Understanding 22.3

**Answer the following questions in a separate document.**

1. Trauma registrars Mitch and Tom have been increasingly at odds. They are going as far as attempting to win co-workers to their side of their perceived issues. Aside from affecting the department's morale, you notice their productivity is also nearing subpar. Explain which conflict management approach would best apply to address their issues.

2. Jill is a record analyst; she is an hourly employee whose overtime is defined as time over eight hours per day. Her supervisor needs her to occasionally assist a physician with documentation, which would require her to work beyond her eight-hour workday. Overtime pay is not currently allowed due to budget constraints. How could the supervisor handle this situation?

3. Tom has just completed his third month as a coder. Quality standards for new coders are that they will be at 80 percent accuracy in the first month, 85 percent in the second month, 90 percent in the third month, and 95 percent by fourth month. Tom achieved a 75 percent accuracy rate in his first month and 82 percent in the second month. The supervisor will conduct his three-month probationary performance review tomorrow, and Tom has reached 89 percent accuracy. How should the supervisor use the progressive discipline process to approach Tom?

4. The registration area has consistently been understaffed during the morning shift. Registrars are not able to easily step away for breaks and sometimes even miss lunch. Despite efforts with talking to the supervisor to get more staff scheduled, the issue continues. The supervisor feels that the busy times are sporadic and does not want to schedule another person. The issue is escalated to the union by registration staff. Determine how this situation is most easily resolved at this point.

5. Bernice is a reliable employee who typically does good work. She has had strong performance reviews consistently. Her coworkers have told the supervisor that Bernice has been out drinking at least two to three times per week and they are surprised that she even makes it to work. What should the supervisor do?

# References

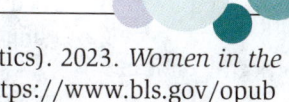

AHIMA (American Health Information Management Association). 2023. *Health Information Workforce: Survey Results on Workforce Challenges and the Role of Emerging Technologies*. https://www.norc.org/content/dam/norc-org/pdf2023/AHIMA-Workforce-Survey-Report-Final-2023.pdf.

Age Discrimination in Employment Act (ADEA) of 1967, Public Law 101-336. https://www.eeoc.gov/statutes/age-discrimination-employment-act-1967.

Americans with Disabilities Act (ADA) of 1990. Public Law 101-336. https://www.govinfo.gov/content/pkg/STATUTE-104/pdf/STATUTE-104-Pg327.pdf.

Americans with Disabilities Act (ADA) Amendments Act of 2008. Public Law 110-325. https://www.congress.gov/110/plaws/publ325/PLAW-110publ325.pdf.

Anthony, W. P., P. L. Perrewe, and K. M. Kacmar. 2010. *Human Resource Management: A Strategic Approach*, 6th ed. Boston: Cengage Learning.

BLS (Bureau of Labor Statistics). 2024 (February). "Job Openings and Labor Turnover." https://www.bls.gov/news.release/jolts.htm.

BLS (Bureau of Labor Statistics). 2023. *Women in the Labor Force: A Databook*. https://www.bls.gov/opub/reports/womens-databook/2022/home.htm.

BLS (Bureau of Labor Statistics). 2022 (June). "Spotlight on Statistics: Healthcare Occupations." https://www.bls.gov/spotlight/2023/healthcare-occupations-in-2022/home.htm.

BLS (Bureau of Labor Statistics). 2017 (March). "BLS Spotlight on Statistics: Women at Work." https://www.bls.gov/spotlight/2017/women-at-work/home.htm.

CMS (Centers for Medicare and Medicaid Services). 2010. Advance notification of upcoming national criminal background check federal matching grants solicitation under section 6201 of the Affordable Care Act. *CMCS Informational Bulletin*. https://www.medicaid.gov/Federal-Policy-Guidance/downloads/06-01-2010-Criminal-Background-Checks.pdf.

Civil Rights Act of 1964. Public Law 88-354. https://www.govinfo.gov/content/pkg/STATUTE-78/pdf/STATUTE-78-Pg241.pdf.

Civil Rights Act of 1991. Public Law 102-166. https://www.govinfo.gov/content/pkg/COMPS-344/pdf/COMPS-344.pdf

Delpo, A. n.d. "What to Say When You Fire an Employee." Accessed May 28, 2024. http://www.nolo.com/legal-encyclopedia/what-to-say-fire-employee-36140.html.

DOL (US Department of Labor). 2023. "Handy Reference Guide to the Fair Labor Standards Act." https://www.dol.gov/sites/dolgov/files/WHD/legacy/files/Digital_Reference_Guide_FLSA.pdf.

DOL (US Department of Labor). 2008. "Fact Sheet #22: Hours Worked Under the Fair Labor Standards Act (FLSA)." https://www.dol.gov/agencies/whd/fact-sheets/22-flsa-hours-worked.

DOL (US Department of Labor). n.d.a. "Summary of the Major Laws of the Department of Labor." Accessed May 28, 2024. https://www.dol.gov/general/aboutdol/majorlaws.

DOL (Department of Labor). n.d.b. "The Worker Adjustment and Retraining Notification Act (WARN)." Accessed May 28, 2024. https://www.dol.gov/general/topic/termination/plantclosings.

Dunn, R. T. 2021. *Dunn and Haimann's Healthcare Management*, 11th ed. Chicago: AUPHA.

Equal Employment Opportunity Act of 1972. Public Law 92-261. https://www.govinfo.gov/content/pkg/STATUTE-86/pdf/STATUTE-86-Pg103.pdf.

EEOC (Equal Employment Opportunity Commission). 2007. "Employment Tests and Selection Procedures." http://www.eeoc.gov/policy/docs/factemployment_procedures.html.

EEOC (Equal Employment Opportunity Commission). n.d.a. "Best Practices for Employers and Human Resources." Accessed May 28, 2024. http://www.eeoc.gov/eeoc/initiatives/e-race/bestpractices-employers.cfm.

EEOC (Equal Employment Opportunity Commission). n.d.b. "Laws Enforced by EEOC." Accessed May 28, 2024. http://www.eeoc.gov/laws/statutes/index.cfm.

EEOC (Equal Employment Opportunity Commission). n.d.c. "Prohibited Employment Policies/Practices." Accessed May 28, 2024. https://www.eeoc.gov/prohibited-employment-policiespractices.

FMLA (Family and Medical Leave Act) of 1993. Public Law 103-3. https://www.govinfo.gov/content/pkg/COMPS-1832/pdf/COMPS-1832.pdf.

GINA (Genetic Information Nondiscrimination Act) of 2008. Public Law 110-233. https://www.govinfo.gov/content/pkg/PLAW-110publ233/pdf/PLAW-110publ233.pdf.

Labor-Management Relations Act (Taft-Hartley Act) of 1947. Public Law 104-320. https://www.govinfo.gov/content/pkg/COMPS-8190/pdf/COMPS-8190.pdf.

Labor-Management Reporting and Disclosure Act (Landrum-Griffin Act) of 1959. Public Law 86-257. https://www.govinfo.gov/content/pkg/COMPS-1511/pdf/COMPS-1511.pdf.

Library of Congress. 2007. Online registration of claims to copyright. *Federal Register* 72(129):36883–36889.

Mathis, R. L., J. H. Jackson, and S. R. Valentine. 2016. *Human Resource Management: Essential Perspectives*, 7th ed. Boston: Cengage Learning.

McConnell, C. 2018. *Umiker's Management Skills for the New Health Care Supervisor*, 7th ed. Sudbury, MA: Jones and Bartlett.

National Labor Relations Act (Wagner Act) of 1935. Public Law 98-620. https://www.govinfo.gov/content/pkg/COMPS-8189/pdf/COMPS-8189.pdf.

OSHA (Occupational Safety and Health Administration). n.d. "About OSHA." Accessed December 27, 2023. https://www.osha.gov/aboutosha.

DOL (US Department of Labor). n.d.a. "Summary of the Major Laws of the Department of Labor." Accessed May 28, 2024. https://www.dol.gov/general/aboutdol/majorlaws.

Patient Protection and Affordable Care Act of 2010. Public Law 111-148. https://www.congress.gov/111/plaws/publ148/PLAW-111publ148.pdf.

Pregnancy Discrimination Act of 1978. Public Law 95-555. https://www.govinfo.gov/content/pkg/STATUTE-92/pdf/STATUTE-92-Pg2076.pdf.

Schermerhorn, J. and D. Bachrach. 2023. *Management*, 15th ed. New York: John Wiley & Sons.

SBA (Small Business Administration). n.d. "Required Employee Benefits." Accessed May 28, 2024. https://www.sba.gov/business-guide/manage-your-business/hire-manage-employees#id-plan-to-offer-employee-benefits.

USERRA (Uniformed Services Employment and Reemployment Act) of 1994. Public Law 103-353. https://www.opm.gov/retirement-center/publications-forms/benefits-administration-letters/1995/95-101.pdf.

Zielinski, D. 2023 (September 24). "Companies Turn to AI to Improve Workplace Safety." Society of Human Resource Management. https://www.shrm.org/topics-tools/news/technology/companies-turn-to-ai-to-improve-workplace-safety.

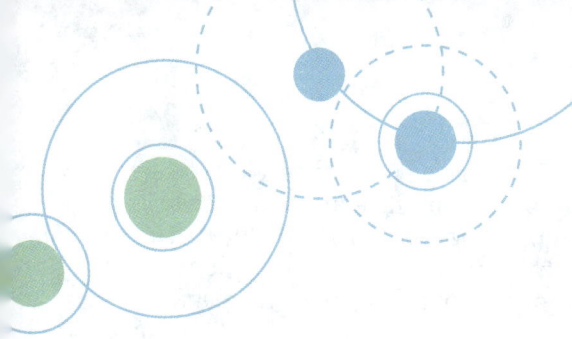

# chapter 23

# Employee Training and Development

*Barbara A. Glondys, MA, RHIA, CHPS*

## Learning Objectives

- Implement an employee training and development program
- Develop training using delivery methods to meet the needs of adult learners and various learning styles
- Evaluate the effectiveness of employee training and development programs
- Facilitate professional development and continuing education

## Key Terms

- ADDIE model
- Asynchronous
- Avatars
- Blended learning
- Blog
- Career plan
- Coaching
- Computer-based training (CBT)
- Continuing education (CE)
- Cross-training
- Curriculum
- Development
- Diversity training
- E-learning
- Employee handbook
- Group discussion
- Incentive pay
- In-service education
- Job rotation
- Just-in-time training
- Learning
- Learning content management system (LCMS)
- Learning curve
- Learning management systems (LMSs)
- Massed training
- Mentor
- M-learning
- Motivation
- Multiuser virtual environment (MUVE)
- Needs assessment
- Onboarding
- One-on-one training
- On-the-job training
- Programmed learning module
- Promotion
- Reinforcement
- Reverse mentoring
- Role playing
- Simulation
- Socialization
- Soft skills
- Spaced training
- Succession planning
- Synchronous
- Task analysis
- Team building
- Train-the-trainer
- Training
- Videoconferencing
- Webinar
- Wiki

As a service industry, healthcare relies on the availability of competent workers. The growth of new technologies, the increasing amount of big data (data sets so large and complex that new tools for analysis are required), the introduction of new and revised laws and standards, the application of new vocabulary and processes, and the decreasing numbers of employees with adequate skills to respond to this new environment mean that healthcare organizations must frequently assume responsibility for preparing and developing their own labor pool, unless they choose to outsource domestically or overseas. Providing the necessary training to workers is costly in terms of both money and time. Using overseas workers creates its own training needs. Moreover, organizations must do what they can to protect their investment by retaining a capable and motivated workforce.

In addition, health information management (HIM) professionals must keep up with the rapidly changing healthcare environment. Principle number nine of the AHIMA *Code of Ethics* directs the HIM professional to: "Advance health information management knowledge and practice through continuing education, research, publications, and presentations" (AHIMA 2019). This reflects the critical importance of both educating others and continually pursuing ongoing personal professional development. See online appendix C for the complete AHIMA *Code of Ethics*.

This chapter focuses on training and professional development of employees in the healthcare organization. It describes the orientation process and methods for training new employees as well as developing current employees for more advanced job responsibilities. It discusses adult learning strategies, techniques for delivering employee training including e-learning methods, and ways that training and development programs can enhance job satisfaction, personal career growth, and the discovery of one's own leadership style. Special training issues, such as diversity, soft skills, and preparation for future e-HIM roles, are addressed. Finally, the chapter describes how to implement a departmental employee training and development plan.

## Training Program Development

Traditional management theory differentiated between **training**, or providing entry-level skills required to begin a job for technical employees, and **development**—maintaining or upgrading competencies for management staff who needed to improve skills such as decision-making and interpersonal communication. Today, the terms *training* and *development* are often used interchangeably with the primary goal of improving knowledge, skills, abilities, attitudes, and social behavior of workers at all levels. As employees who make up the organization grow, so does the organization.

Training programs should accommodate all employees. Examples of accommodation include providing instructions in another language for employees who are non-English speakers or making equipment and locations accessible to those with disabilities. In addition, the organization should develop diversity training programs. **Diversity training** facilitates an environment that fosters inclusion and appreciation of individual differences within the organization's workforce.

Investment in training programs helps the organization to accomplish goals on an individual, group, and organizational level. Other important reasons for providing employee training and development include the following:

- Introducing new employees to the organization
- Providing a path for employee promotion and retention
- Improving employee performance and productivity
- Updating skills for employees in new or restructured positions resulting from organizational or technological change
- Reducing organizational problems caused by absenteeism, turnover, poor morale, or substandard quality
- Delivering high-quality healthcare within budgetary constraints

One way to view training and development needs is as a progression through orientation, on-the-job training, staff development through internal in-service education programs, staff development through external and professional continuing education (CE) programs, and personal career development beyond the current job. This chapter covers each of these steps in depth.

Investment in employee development does not end with training. Organizations need to find ways to gain the commitment of employees so they remain productive. Retaining good employees and developing their potential is an area of great importance, particularly in an industry that has a shortage of qualified workers.

# Departmental Employee Training and Development Plan

Every healthcare organization and every HIM department have unique training needs. The level of education and experience of the employees, the tasks they perform, and the resources available directs the focus of training efforts. The content, objectives, and frequency of a training program are all dependent on the specific situation that exists in an organization.

## Training and Development Model

Several models for designing training and development programs have been developed. Each organization needs to review their needs using a systematic approach to instructional systems design. A model frequently used is the **ADDIE model**: **A**nalyze, **D**esign, **D**evelop, **I**mplement, **E**valuate (Sampson and Fried 2023, 211). This method emphasizes the how, what, why, where, who, and when of training. Begin with an analysis or needs assessment that identifies what training is required. Next, design the training program by defining the objectives and methods to be used. In the third step, the program is developed and pilot tested. Then, the program is rolled out with the support of the management for successful delivery. After the program is delivered, it is important to evaluate whether the program achieved the objectives identified in the needs assessment. Figure 23.1 displays this model.

The following is a step-by-step training and development plan that expands upon the ADDIE model and can be applied on various levels to help an organization's HR department, or a health information manager, identify and fulfill the training and development

**Figure 23.1.** ADDIE model

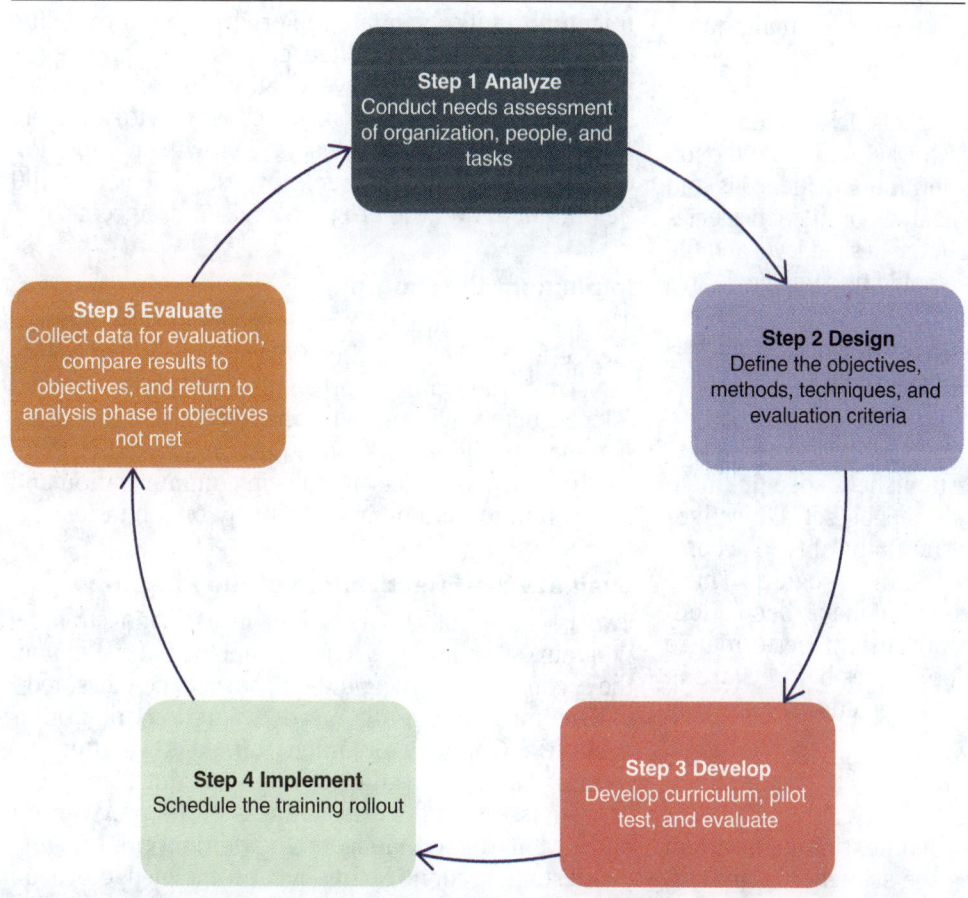

*Source:* Adapted from Sampson and Fried 2023, 211.

needs of an employee group. The plan includes the following steps:

1. Perform a needs assessment.
2. Set training objectives.
3. Design the curriculum.
4. Determine the location and method of delivery.
5. Pilot the program.
6. Implement the program.
7. Evaluate the effectiveness of the program.
8. Make changes as needed.
9. Provide feedback to interested groups.

The plan should be approved and supported by upper management. Implementing a training program requires a substantial investment of time, money, and personnel. Developing a curriculum based on a systematic evaluation of needs is a much wiser investment than creating a program around the latest hot topic.

### Perform a Departmental Training Needs Assessment

The needs assessment is critical to the design of the plan. This approach typically focuses on three levels: the organization, the specific job tasks, and the individual employee. The outcome of the needs assessment is an understanding of where training is needed in the organization (entry-level, remedial, or management development), based on the firm's strategic mission and goals. In addition, a list of the tasks to be learned at each level (based on the job description, job specification, and the specific skills and knowledge required), and an analysis of the deficiencies in knowledge and skills between the desired level and the current level of each employee, should be completed. This information is obtained through observation, employee and manager interviews, surveys, tests, and task analysis of the job descriptions and job specifications.

### Set Training Objectives

After the needs have been established, specific, measurable training objectives should be set. Objectives stipulate what the employee should be able to accomplish upon completion of the training program. These are based on the deficiencies that have been identified between the desired and current performance levels. It is important to set objectives before starting the program so the results can be evaluated following completion of training.

### Design the Curriculum

The curriculum is the subject content of the program that will be taught, including the sequence, activities, and materials. The curriculum designer should prepare a budget that identifies costs and available resources. Examples of training resources include face-to-face trainers, computer-based modules either purchased or developed in-house, books, training manuals and web-based learning management systems (LMSs). LMSs assist the trainer by tracking grades and student access, presenting the content in a user-friendly manner, and collating statistics on use. After these decisions are made, the curriculum must be organized into a program that supports adult learning and the stated objectives. All program elements must be carefully prepared to ensure quality and effectiveness.

### Determine the Location and Method of Delivery

Where and when the program should be delivered is an important part of the training plan. When space is available and the instructor and materials are available internally, a classroom setting might be suitable. On the other hand, when employees work over several shifts and days or in remote locations, computer-based courses and web-based delivery might permit the employee to more readily achieve the training objectives.

### Pilot the Program

It is important to validate the program by introducing it to a test audience. When computer technology is part of the program delivery, all computer programs should be tested to make sure they work with a variety of hardware and web browsers. Following completion of the program by a few employees, feedback should be obtained, and the program revised, if necessary.

### Implement the Program

The tested program can now be given to the entire audience for which it has been developed. When necessary, train-the-trainer workshops should be conducted for instructors who may not have formal training experience. In these workshops the trainer—either manager or employee—learns skills in communication and instruction to train others effectively on job tasks.

### Evaluate the Effectiveness of the Program

Two issues should be addressed in evaluating training programs. The first is selecting the method of evaluation; the second is identifying the outcomes to be measured.

The most frequently used evaluation method is a survey. Opinions obtained immediately after the training, and again after a period of time, are valuable in assessing the effectiveness of the program for both trainees and managers. In addition, pretests and posttests help identify the level of knowledge or skill that has been learned.

Four outcomes can be measured in evaluating effective training programs:

- *Reaction:* What is the reaction of the trainees immediately after the program? Are they excited about what they learned?
- *Learning:* What have the trainees actually learned? Can they now use a new software program?
- *Behavior:* Have supervisors noticed a change in employee behavior? Has morale improved?
- *Results:* How does the actual level of performance compare with the established objectives? Can the employees assign codes more accurately? (Dessler 2019, 225)

Evaluating these outcomes determines whether the training has been successful, connecting back to the gaps identified in the initial needs analysis, or whether modifications to the training program are required.

### Make Changes as Needed

When the results of the evaluation show less-than-expected results, it is important to determine where changes may be helpful. This may include a change in the materials, location or time of program delivery, or subject content. In any case, it is important to adjust if needed. A program not meeting the desired objectives is costly.

### Provide Feedback to Interested Groups

After tallying the results of the evaluations and making any needed adjustments, it is important to provide feedback to the course developers, managers and supervisors of the involved departments, and trainees. Communication is vital to maintaining interest in and support for the training program. Feedback demonstrates a desire to respond to the needs of everyone involved in this important activity.

---

### Check Your Understanding 23.1

**Answer the following questions in a separate document.**

1. John has been hired as an outpatient coder. He indicated in his interview he would like to advance to an inpatient coder position and that he was even interested in leadership. Propose a two-to-three-year plan for John to achieve his goal to be in a lead inpatient coder role at some point in the future using each concept of employee development progression.

2. Susan is the supervisor of the registration department. She recently created an employee training and development plan for her area and began by setting objectives. Next, she developed training materials, reserved a room for training, and notified the employees of the date, time, and place. She arranged for another supervisor to provide coverage so the employees could concentrate on the training. Susan tested the program prior to full implementation to ensure it was appropriate, then implemented the program. After the conclusion of the training, the employees completed a posttest and evaluation form. Susan was disappointed that the employees performed poorly on the posttest and gave unfavorable comments on the evaluation. Susan is now planning to make changes, but wondered why she did not accomplish her objectives. Did Susan follow the ADDIE model? Explain your answer and suggest what she should do differently.

3. To ensure Susan's training plan is successful, examine and justify key considerations to address at the beginning of the initiative.

4. What is the relationship between setting objectives and evaluating a training program? Give an example. Why is this important?

5. Angela is the supervisor of the release of information (ROI) function in the HIM department. For each of the four outcomes of effective learning, give a specific example of how Angela could determine the effectiveness of an organization-wide training session she held on HIPAA requirements.

---

## Elements of Workforce Training

The goal of any institution's training program is to provide employees with the skills they need to perform their jobs. Because employees are at different stages in their career development, the training program must be flexible and adaptable to meet many needs. At any given time, new employees will need to know basic information about the organization and their specific job function, and long-term employees will want to improve their ability to contribute at higher levels within the organizational structure through developing new proficiencies. Today's workforce needs both technical skills and soft skills, such as critical thinking and team building—the process of organizing and acquainting team members to enhance the outcomes of collaborative work.

## New Employee Orientation and Training

One of the key ingredients in employee satisfaction is the feeling of being knowledgeable about the organization and competent in the job. This feeling begins with an effective orientation and training program for new employees. Just as a manager prepares for the interview and selection of a new employee, he or she must plan how the new employee will learn about the organization, department, and job.

Most large organizations have a formal new employee orientation, or onboarding process. This process, which includes a series of activities designed to acclimate the new employee to the organization and job, may involve a one-on-one session with an advisor from the HR department, group training with new employees from across the organization, or some form of individual computer-based training (CBT) which provides electronic training that individual learners can complete at their own pace. In addition to the basic skills needed to do the job, the employee needs to experience a period of socialization in which he or she learns the values, behavior patterns, and expectations of the organization.

In a large facility, new employee orientation is usually presented on-site and coordinated by the HR department; in a small facility, it may be performed entirely by the employee's supervisor. The orientation may consist of a brief and informal presentation, or it may be a formal program that takes place over several days on a regularly scheduled basis. The requirements of an orientation program may be expressed on three levels: organizational, departmental, and individual. An effective tool, which reflects all three levels of orientation and can be used in familiarizing new workers, is the orientation checklist (figure 23.2). This checklist helps the employer know that the employee is receiving the information he or she needs to begin the job and serves as an agenda for presenting the information in a logical manner. Rather than presenting everything the new employee needs to know all at once, it is helpful to spread the orientation over several days.

### Orientation to the Organization

Formal orientation programs typically begin with presentations by HR and other department heads, such as the privacy officer and the director of safety and security, before the new employee is introduced to his or her immediate supervisor. The program usually addresses organization-specific information, such as the organization's mission and vision, goals, policies, and structure; employee relations practices; and employee-centered information such as compensation and benefits.

At the organizational level, the orientation program provides the information that every employee who works for the organization needs to know. This information typically includes the following:

- A brief review of the organization along with explanation of its mission and its vision
- The institution's ownership form, mode of governance, and administrative structure
- An overview of the various departments and services
- A review of specific employee policies:
  - Drug, alcohol and substance abuse considerations
  - Sexual harassment
  - Nondiscrimination issues
  - Conflict of interest prohibitions and gifts
  - Dress codes
  - Use of computers, accessing the Internet, using electronic mail (email)
  - Computer security and passwords
  - Privacy and confidentiality of all aspects of patient care
  - Security, fire and safety
  - Infection control
  - Review of the organization's disaster plan including modified operations schedule in emergencies (Liebler and McConnell 2021, 194)

In addition, it is helpful to present policies and requirements all employees must know—employee benefits such as paid time off, insurance programs, payroll requirements, the performance appraisal process and personnel policies—in an employee handbook given to new employees during the orientation. The handbook provides a convenient reference after the immediate orientation period has ended. Often, a tour of the facility is given to familiarize new employees with locations such as the cafeteria, elevator banks and offices such as the human resources department.

**Figure 23.2.** Sample orientation checklist

Employee Name_____
Department_____
Supervisor Name_____ Date of Hire_____
Date of Orientation_____

Instructions: Supervisor or person responsible for completing task should initial and date each item as completed

**Prior to first day**
_____Send welcome packet and orientation information
_____Prepare employee's workspace
_____Inform other employees

**First day**
**Morning: Review organization-specific information**
_____Overview of the organization's history, mission, organizational structure
_____Safety policies and procedures
_____Anti-harassment and discrimination policy, diversity awareness
_____Confidentiality and privacy policies and procedures
_____Emergency fire and other safety procedures, disaster plan
_____Disciplinary policies and procedures
_____Active shooter training

End with tour of the facility

**Lunch**

**Afternoon: Review employee-centered information**
_____Photo ID badge, computer username and password
_____Federal and state tax forms
_____Benefits and deadlines—insurance
_____Educational assistance programs
_____Time reporting, sick leave, vacation and holiday policies
_____Performance reviews
_____Employee handbook

At the end, the department supervisor will escort employee from orientation meeting to department

**Department information**
_____Introduce to department co-workers
_____Introduce to a buddy and/or mentor
_____Provide tour of department, workspace, keys
_____Confirm work hours, attendance requirements
_____Department dress code

**Second day**
_____Ask employee how the first day went and if they have any questions
_____Provide overview of job duties
_____Review computer, phone, copy, and fax machine use
_____Provide job description and department organization chart
_____Begin on-the-job training

**Third day**
_____Ask employee if they have any questions
_____Review department sick leave and vacation policy, procedures
_____Review compensation and performance evaluation process
_____Continue on-the-job-training

**Fourth day**
_____Ask employee if they have any questions
_____Ask how employee is feeling about job, coworkers
_____Review department quality and quantity standards

*Continued*

**Figure 23.2.** Sample orientation checklist (continued)

```
_____ Describe department emergency procedures, disaster plan
_____ Discuss email, internet, social media policies
_____ Continue on-the-job training

Fifth day
_____ Ask employee if they have questions
_____ Provide oversight as employee works independently for the morning
_____ Take employee to lunch
_____ Provide competency assessment for employee to complete
_____ Provide feedback on results of assessment and suggestions for improvement as needed
_____ Allow employee to complete orientation evaluation form

Orientation completed
Employee signature_____ Date_____
Supervisor signature_____ Date_____
```

## Orientation to the Department

The employee's supervisor then continues the orientation process within the employee's assigned department. The employee is introduced to the department and team, given a tour of the department, shown their workstation, and introduced to the specific job responsibilities. A "buddy" who has the same position as the new employee could be assigned. In addition to providing guidance to the new person, the experience serving as a buddy offers an opportunity for further development of the experienced employee as well (Liebler and McConnell 2021, 195).

At the departmental level, orientation information typically includes the following:

- Departmental policies and procedures
- Email and internet usage policies
- Introduction to other employees
- Tour of department
- Work hours, schedule, and time and absence reporting
- Reporting incidents and emergencies
- Training in operation of equipment (for example, telephone, photocopying machines, or computers)
- Fire and safety regulations specific to the department (Liebler and McConnell 2021, 199)

## Individual Orientation

As with all training programs, the orientation must be customized to the employee through a needs assessment. A needs assessment determines whether gaps exist between the employee's actual and desired knowledge and skill level at the organization, department, and work unit level (Sampson and Fried 2023, 206).

To develop an individualized orientation program, it is helpful to begin with a **task analysis** to determine the specific skills required for the job. The job description and job specification are excellent sources for this part of the process. The job tasks should, at a minimum, include specific, measurable objectives for productivity and performance and the supervisor's explanation of each job task, followed by a demonstration and an opportunity for the employee to demonstrate the task (Dessler 2019, 202). The new employee's individual orientation in the department is usually the longest portion of the orientation program. It is an ongoing process that lasts as long as it takes for the new employee to feel comfortable in the job and proficient performing the job functions.

The individual portion of the orientation should continue as described in the suggested schedule with some portion of each day devoted to job training and work rules so the new employee can gradually understand the requirements of the job and become acclimated to the work environment. As the new employee is trained and tested in each important aspect of the job, the supervisor should document the employee's demonstrated competency. This documentation helps the organization comply with the standards of various accrediting bodies.

## Assessment of the New Employee Orientation and Training Program

After the orientation process, all new employees should be asked for feedback. HR should develop a form to be completed by the new employee.

Figure 23.3 presents an example of a form for evaluating the general portion of the orientation program. Typical questions include the following:

- Was the program relevant to your job and needs?
- What part of the program was most useful to you?
- What part of the program was least useful to you?

After the new employee completes the form, supervisors should be asked to evaluate the effectiveness of the orientation process. For example, they should be asked for feedback on the employee's ability to apply his or her newly acquired job skills and for an assessment of the employee's comfort level with the department.

## On-the-Job Training

Preparing staff to carry out the tasks and functions of their jobs should continue beyond orientation for both new and experienced employees. A variety of methods are available to employers. Effective training programs are matched to the specific education, experience and skill level of employees and can include an appropriate combination of methods, media, content, and activities.

**Figure 23.3.** Sample orientation evaluation form

---

**Employee orientation program evaluation form**

Date:

Job title:

1. Please rate each of the following items to indicate your reaction to the session. If ranking is less than *agree*, please comment below.

| Item | Strongly disagree | Disagree | Agree | Strongly agree |
|---|---|---|---|---|
| Objective 1: The program explained my job responsibilities. | ___ | ___ | ___ | ___ |
| Objective 2: I was able to practice using technology needed to perform my job. | ___ | ___ | ___ | ___ |
| Objective 3: I was able to interact with other participants. | ___ | ___ | ___ | ___ |
| Objective 4: The program length was appropriate for the content. | ___ | ___ | ___ | ___ |

Comments:

2. Describe the part of the program that was most useful for you.
3. Describe the part of the program that was least useful to you.

4. Please use the following scale to comment on the instructor's ability to lead the program, wherein:
1 = Needs improvement  2 = Adequate  3 = Good  4 = Excellent

| Item | Instructor rating |
|---|---|
| Organization and preparation of content | 1  2  3  4 |
| Presentation of content | 1  2  3  4 |
| Clarity of instructions | 1  2  3  4 |
| Appropriate use of time | 1  2  3  4 |
| Connected content to your job functions | 1  2  3  4 |
| Stimulated interaction with other participants | 1  2  3  4 |

5. How would you rate your level of skill/knowledge:

   a. Before the program?      1  2  3  4
   b. After the program?     1  2  3  4

6. What changes do you recommend to the program?
7. Other comments:

*Source:* Adapted from Dessler 2017, 268.

## Definition of On-the-Job Training

**On-the-job training** is a method of training in which the employee learns a task by performing it. Along with teaching basic skills, on-the-job training gives employees and supervisors opportunities to discuss specific problem areas and initiates socialization among the new employees and their coworkers. On-the-job training offers several advantages, including its relatively low cost compared to outside training programs, the ability to tailor it specifically to the department's policies and procedures, and the fact that work is still in progress while the employee is being trained. Training may be performed by either a supervisor or a coworker with particular expertise. The selection of an appropriate trainer, both skilled in the job and willing to teach, is critical to the success of this method.

## Needs Assessment and Job Requirements

The training program should begin by reviewing the job description and the job specifications. Job descriptions and specifications should include a list of tasks performed; the skills, ability, and knowledge required; and the expected standards of performance for quality and quantity. Next, a needs assessment should be completed to assess the gap between expected performance and the employee's current performance level. What the employee does not know or cannot do becomes the basis for additional training. The requirements may include any of the following:

- Physical skills (for example, operation of equipment)
- Academic knowledge (for example, medical terminology or English spelling and grammar)
- Knowledge of institutional policies (for example, safety regulations)
- Technical skills, which may include both physical and mental skills (for example, use of computer software)

After the specific requirements for training are identified, the appropriate delivery methods for training can be matched to the topic.

## Components of On-the-Job Training

On-the-job training methods can be used individually or in combination and should be adapted to each learner. On-the-job training offers a variety of delivery options, including one-on-one training by a supervisor or an experienced peer, job rotation, CBT, coaching or mentoring, and informal learning during meetings or discussions with supervisors and peers.

**One-on-one training** is the technique used most often. In this type of training, the employee learns by first observing a demonstration and then performing the task under supervision. One-on-one training by the supervisor gives the supervisor an opportunity to observe how the trainee is doing and to adjust the process to meet the employee's skill level.

In **job rotation**, the employee moves from job to job at planned intervals, usually three to six months. This method is most useful for supervisory positions, where the employee needs to learn a variety of tasks performed by several different employees, as well as their interrelationships. In **cross-training**, the employee learns to perform the jobs of many team members. Cross-training provides opportunity for competent employees to experience greater task variety in their jobs and affords flexibility in shifting resources for workload or attendance fluctuation. This method is most useful when work teams are involved.

CBT, including web-based training, provides an opportunity to individual learners to supplement job task instruction with electronic training at their own pace. It is effective in situations where repetition aids learning; for example, with medical terminology and tasks that cannot be duplicated entirely in the practice session, such as role playing with different cases where employees are requested to release patient information. **Role playing** is an activity where learners are presented with a hypothetical situation they may encounter on the job, and they act out the response.

After the trainee has demonstrated the ability to do the job, **coaching** should continue by the supervisor or an expert peer on a continuous basis. The experienced worker observes or reviews the work of the employee in a nonthreatening manner, offering advice and suggestions for revising techniques to improve productivity and efficient work performance. In a formalized arrangement in which a specific person is assigned to follow up on a regular basis, the coach is referred to as a **mentor**. In this scenario, the mentor meets with the trainee on a regular basis and often gives advice on personal career growth and development within the organization. In **reverse mentoring**, the new employee mentors a senior person on subjects in which he or she may have more expertise, such as use of social media or digital technologies. This provides an opportunity for the newer employee to gain an important sense of belonging and contribution (Schermerhorn and Bachrach 2021, 219).

## Assessment of On-the-Job Training Programs

By its nature, on-the-job training provides an opportunity for immediate assessment of its effectiveness. The trainer can observe the employee's skills and can question the employee regarding knowledge of policies, procedures, and other academic knowledge that may be required. If the assessment reveals areas of weakness, the training can be adjusted to reinforce knowledge or repeat steps performed incorrectly.

When the employee is working independently, the supervisor should check the quantity and quality of the employee's work against performance standards as appropriate for the job and level of employee expertise. It could be daily for an entry-level employee to weekly or monthly or more for a more experienced employee. If the employee's performance is below standard, the training can be repeated before poor performance becomes a habit.

Finally, the employee should be encouraged to ask questions both during and after the training and should receive positive and constructive negative feedback as appropriate. Following the training program, the employee should be asked for feedback on the training program and any changes that may be helpful.

## Staff Development through In-Service Education

The healthcare industry grows and changes constantly. Whether it is a new law passed by the state or the federal government, new reimbursement regulations, updates to *International Classification of Diseases* (ICD) or Current Procedural Terminology (CPT) codes, new or revised accreditation standards, or future HIM roles, change is a permanent factor. Preparing workers for such changes requires continuous training and retraining.

### Definition of In-Service Education

In-service education is the third step in employee development, which is a continuous process that builds on the basic skills learned through new employee orientation and on-the-job training. In-service education is concerned with teaching employees the specific skills and behaviors required to maintain job performance or to retrain workers whose jobs have changed. In-service education may include external programs or may be delivered at the worksite or through CBT.

### Needs Assessment for In-Service Education

The need for in-service education may be triggered by many events, including the following:

- A restructuring of the department or organization
- Updates to coding or reimbursement requirements
- Implementation of electronic health records (EHRs)
- A decline in productivity or morale or an increase in absenteeism
- A new organizational policy or procedure
- An external requirement imposed by accreditation or licensing organizations, such as an annual renewal of CPR certification or retraining in infectious disease precautions or safety procedures
- Regulatory changes, such as required by HIPAA or Health Information Technology for Economic and Clinical Health (HITECH) legislation (McConnell 2018, 416)

The amount of in-service education needed varies with the event and the education and experience of the employee. Downsizing or reorganizing structure often causes changes in an individual employee's job responsibilities. Employees may need to learn other job functions within the workgroup or may even be placed in a new department. This can require a series of formal training sessions, including on-the-job training.

Renewal of training required by external organizations may be subject to defined content and duration, often including a test or demonstration of the employee's competence. On the other hand, implementation of a new policy or procedure may simply include distributing the information accompanied by a short meeting.

The department manager needs to determine the appropriate format of the in-service education based on the topic and experience and education level of the employees. The following types of questions may help with the determination of format.

- Should the instruction be given as massed training (training in one highly concentrated session) or as spaced training, which occurs in several shorter sessions?
- Should the task be broken down into parts or be taught as a single unit?
- How will competence be assessed? Is the topic a skill that needs to be demonstrated by the learner, or is it a level of knowledge that should be tested with a written assessment?

As with other training categories, periodic analysis of actual versus desired job performance will create a list of topics that should be addressed with in-service education.

## Requirements for an In-Service Education Program

Unlike orientation programs, which are delivered primarily at one point in time, in-service education programs need to be available on an ongoing basis. Depending on the size of the organization, some programs (such as a refresher on the response to the institution's disaster plan) may be offered monthly. The HR department may coordinate programs on topics that affect the organization. Programs specific to HIM, such as a coding update, are more likely to be developed by a supervisor or manager in the HIM department.

Finally, some topics serve the needs of more than one department. For example, a program on *International Classification of Diseases, Tenth Revision, Clinical Modification* (ICD-10-CM) coding may be given by the coding supervisor to employees from the HIM, patient accounting, and physician billing departments. This type of program would probably take place in a more formal setting and require coordination with other department managers.

Examples of in-service education topics and the individuals within the organization who are likely to have responsibility for them are shown in figure 23.4.

## Steps in Conducting In-Service Education

Presenting an effective in-service program requires planning. The time frame depends on the complexity of the material and the number of participants but should include enough time to prepare materials and publicize the event. Generally, a formal in-service program should follow these steps:

1. *Set objectives*. Is the purpose of the program to teach a new job task to an individual or to improve morale within the department?
2. *Understand the audience*. Is the training intended for one employee or 50 employees? Are the participants from the same department or from several departments? Are they in the same location or dispersed?
3. *Decide whether the content should be delivered as a unit or in parts (massed or spaced)*. This may be resolved by the availability of the employee as well as the topic.
4. *Determine the best method of delivery*. The education and experience of the audience, time available, and cost of preparing and delivering the instruction should all be taken into consideration. Is there a qualified expert in-house? Are software or cloud-based resources available? Is space available to train a large group at one time? (See the discussions of adult learning strategies and delivery methods later in this chapter.)
5. *Prepare a budget*. If a specific amount has been allocated, the plan should be compared to the predetermined budget and revised, if necessary. Approval should be obtained if the proposal is a new one. In addition, the proposal should include the costs of developing printed materials, speaker fees, and training resources.
6. *Publicize the program*. Flyers, posters, or electronic notices should announce the program and should include the date, time, length, location, topic, and a summary of the content. When it is important to know the number of attendees in advance, the notice should include a method for RSVP.
7. *If appropriate, prepare handout materials*. Handouts would include materials to be used for instruction as well as documents to reference following the program. At a minimum, an agenda of the topics and a schedule should be developed.
8. *Practice, practice, practice!* The person presenting the program should be adequately prepared and comfortable with the content. Also, a training room should be scheduled ahead of time and any needed equipment should be checked to ensure it is available and in good working order. Anyone planning to use a computer or a projector should know how to operate it.
9. *Use a variety of methods and be alert to your audience*. In addition to the lecture, the presenter should engage the audience through interactive questioning and activities. People learn by doing. Opportunities should be provided from time to time for questions and periodic breaks when the program lasts more than two hours.
10. *Obtain feedback from the audience*. It is important to give the participants an opportunity to document their reactions to the training. To that end, an evaluation form should be created and distributed.

A sample in-service education evaluation form is shown in figure 23.5.

## Assessment of In-Service Education

Because some amount of cost, in terms of both time and resources, is usually involved with in-service training, it is important to determine whether its objectives have been met. The organization's administrative staff will want evidence that the training was cost-effective and there was return on investment in terms of increased productivity and employee development. Methods for assessing the impact of in-service education are as follows:

- *Pretests and posttests*. Administer a short questionnaire, with the same questions, before and after the in-service program to measure the level of improved understanding of the content presented.
- *Completion of an evaluation form at the conclusion of the program*. Immediate feedback provides an assessment of the effectiveness of the delivery methods (Refer to figure 23.5 as an example.)
- *Formal or informal feedback from the employee's supervisor*. Within a few days of the program, the supervisor should be contacted to determine whether the learner has applied the new skills and knowledge on the job.
- *Follow up with the employee later*. Thirty days after the in-service program, the attendees should be asked to validate the value of the program. Are they able to perform their job better? Is there something they feel they did not learn that should have been included?

Feedback from learners and instructors should be incorporated to improve in-service content and delivery methods to best meet the purpose of the educational programs.

**Figure 23.4.** Examples of responsibility for in-service education

**Organization-wide:** The human resources department typically assumes responsibility for the following topics and may include staff from other departments in the planning and presentation:
- Fire and safety awareness
- Disaster plan implementation
- Infectious disease/universal precautions
- Diversity training
- Team building
- HIPAA training

**Multiple departments:** The health information manager may work with managers of several departments to coordinate presentation of the following topics:
- ICD or CPT annual updates
- Medical terminology training
- Use of office productivity software for employee productivity measurement
- Clinical documentation integrity
- Quality improvement

**Health information management department:** The health information manager may develop in-service training within the department for the following topics:
- Release of information
- Fire and safety procedures
- Record security in the event of disaster
- EHR implementation
- Data analysis

## Figure 23.5. Sample in-service education evaluation form

**In-service education evaluation form**

To help us improve the quality of future programs, please complete the following evaluation of today's session. Please use the following scale to answer questions 1 through 6:

1 = Needs improvement  2 = Satisfactory  3 = Excellent

1. How satisfied were you with the content of the presentation?   1  2  3
2. How would you rate the organization of the presentation?   1  2  3
3. How would you rate the effectiveness of visual media used in the presentation?   1  2  3
4. How would you rate the delivery of the presentation?   1  2  3
5. How well did the presenter meet the learning goals of the program?   1  2  3
6. How satisfied were you with the following aspects of the program?
    a. Meeting location   1  2  3
    b. Parking   1  2  3
    c. Accessibility   1  2  3
    d. Registration process   1  2  3
    e. Meeting room setup and seating   1  2  3
    f. Handout materials   1  2  3
7. What is one thing you learned that you did not know prior to attending?
8. What would you like to have learned more about?
9. Please provide any additional comments that could improve future programs.

## Check Your Understanding 23.2

**Answer the following questions in a separate document.**

1. Propose a general structure for the levels of a formal employee orientation program. Why does an orientation program promote employee retention?

2. Sandra is the HIM operations supervisor. As summer approaches, she will need to accommodate for staff vacations. How do you recommend she approach this issue through training with her staff?

3. Identify the elements of an orientation that are similar to an in-service education program. Identify the elements that are different.

4. Midwest Hospital has recently merged with Southern Hospital, and all HIM staff are reporting to a corporate director. Coding staff jobs are being reorganized, and coders may encounter patient conditions with which they are unfamiliar. The director is proposing an in-service refresher of ICD-10-CM coding skills. Assess whether in-service education is the best approach and include in your answer what else should be done to address this situation.

# Adult Learning Strategies

Training refers to the process of providing individuals with the educational content and activities they need to function in the workplace. **Learning** is the acquisition of knowledge or skills through experience, study, or by being taught. In the healthcare work environment, learning translates into achieving the goals of the institution through improved job performance. To accomplish this objective, it is important to understand how employees learn and the factors affecting the learning environment.

## Characteristics of Adult Learners

One of the most difficult tasks faced by employees is achieving balance. Ideally, people shift their time between the demands of work, the demands of home, and their own needs and desires to accomplish more with fewer and fewer hours. Too much stress can lead to burnout. Therefore, training must be viewed as an integral part of the work environment and not as an additional requirement. The individuals responsible for training need to understand that time is a very valuable resource.

Because time is scarce, employees need to see relevance in the activities that consume their time. They will be more willing to accept tasks that can be accomplished quickly and that provide satisfaction or tangible benefits. Three fundamental concepts in helping adults learn are motivation, reinforcement, and knowledge of results.

### Motivation

Motivation is the inner drive to accomplish a task. At different stages in life, adults are motivated by specific needs. Understanding that employees differ in the relative importance of these needs at any given time is important in designing a training program.

Employees will be more motivated when they perceive a need for the training. The trainer should call attention to the important aspects of the job and help employees understand how to perform these tasks efficiently and effectively. The manager should help the employee know the answer to the question, "What's in it for me?" (Lang 2020). Moreover, employees should see a direct connection between the knowledge learned and the work goal. It is helpful when the trainer explains the reason for performing a task in a certain order and relates policies to objectives.

### Reinforcement

Reinforcement is a condition following a response that results in an increase in the strength of that response. For example, additional pay after an employee attends a training course that requires extra work hours would serve as a positive reinforcement for the new health information technician. Reinforcement is most effective when it occurs immediately after a preferred response. This connects the reinforcement with the response and is more likely to result in the desired effect.

Incentive pay is a form of positive reinforcement. The higher the quality and quantity of work, the better the pay increase given. For example, coders might be compensated based on the number and quality of cases coded rather than an hourly rate.

### Knowledge of Results

Many adults appreciate feedback on their performance. It is important to understand the concept of the learning curve. As shown in figure 23.6, when a new task is learned, productivity may decrease while a great deal of material is being learned. Later, there is little new learning, but productivity may increase significantly. Either situation can be frustrating, so guidance and feedback are important to help employees understand what they have accomplished. It is

**Figure 23.6.** Learning curve

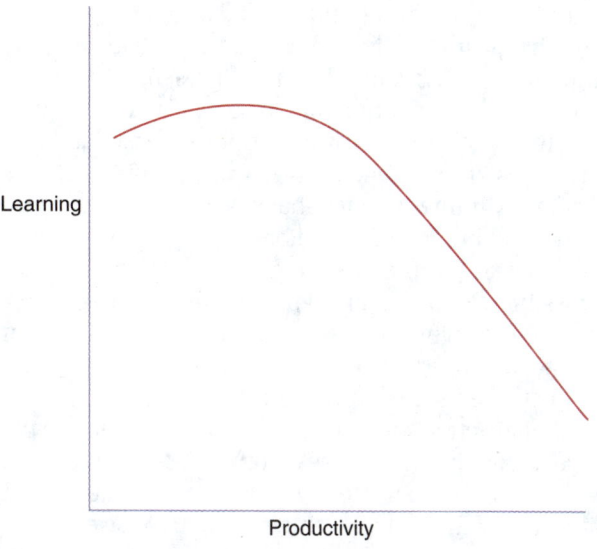

important to provide encouragement when new tasks are mastered, even though the quantity of work may not be at the level desired. In addition, it is important to explain that the employee may reach a plateau where improvement slows or levels off, and that this is normal.

### Education of Adult Learners

When an organization wants its workers to improve their work habits, it must demonstrate that it values the effort behind the improvements. The organizational climate must support the continued learning and growth of its employees. Some actions the administration might take to indicate this commitment include:

- Providing training during work hours rather than outside the employees' regular work schedules
- Conducting the training off-site to avoid interruptions from day-to-day activities
- Compensating voluntary education with incentives such as bonuses and promotions

Adults tend to remember and understand material that is relevant and has value to them. Therefore, it is important to present an overall picture along with the objectives they are expected to accomplish. Performance standards should be realistic and attainable. Setting artificially high standards reduces motivation and results in feelings of frustration, anxiety, and stress. Employees should feel challenged, but not overwhelmed.

Consideration should be given to the importance of motivation, reinforcement, and knowledge of results. Establishing individual goals that challenge employees and satisfy their personal motivators is the ideal. Training methods that allow for the design of individualized programs, such as CBT or print-based programmed learning modules, should be considered. **Programmed learning modules** lead learners through subject material that is presented in short sections, followed immediately by a series of questions that require a written response based on the section just presented. Answers are provided in the module for immediate feedback.

Learning is accomplished best by doing. Therefore, it is important to provide as many hands-on activities as possible. People recall 10 percent of what they read, 20 percent of what they see and hear, and 75 percent of what they practice doing (Beskar 2022). Therefore, the most effective training includes a combination of verbal instruction, demonstration, and hands-on experience, using multiple senses. Correct responses should be reinforced immediately. Recognition by the trainer or feedback about achievement may be just as effective as monetary rewards in providing reinforcement.

Adults want to know why it is important to learn something. In addition, they want to be in control of the situation and learn at their own pace. Where possible, training should be delivered with spaced repetition, which is the same material repeated after a lapse in time and presented in varying formats. The employee who learns quickly can move forward, whereas the slower learner can devote more time to a specific activity.

## Learning Styles

Just as there are varying types of personalities, there are several different ways in which people learn. The most effective trainers use a variety of styles to meet the needs of all participants. If relevancy, meaning, and emotion are attached to the material taught, the learner will learn. Learners tend to progress only as far as they need to achieve their goal. Therefore, the best time to learn is when doing so is viewed as useful, which has made **just-in-time training** popular. Content is taught in small, relevant portions where and when the learner can use it most readily. The learner can then put the newly learned information to practice quickly.

Although an individual may have a preferred learning style, other approaches may sometimes be used. Learning styles are influenced by factors such as the physical environment of the learning space, age, maturity, energy level, education, ability, and experience, and they may change over time. Following are various models for categorizing learning styles:

- *Feelers:* Feelers focus on emotions and people. They favor a learning environment where they can share experiences and opinions and enjoy working in groups.
- *Observers:* Observers take their time before participating and like to watch and listen.
- *Thinkers:* Thinkers enjoy activities that require them to analyze and evaluate. They rely on logic and reason and prefer to work independently, questioning the relevance of simulations and role play activities.
- *Doers:* Doers like to take charge and tend to dominate discussions. They prefer opportunities to practice and apply what they have learned to the real world. (Lawson 2016, 32)

In addition to differences in learning styles, effective training recognizes six modalities that describe how learners process information:

- *Visual:* Learning through the eyes (videos, slides, demonstrations)
- *Print:* Learning through the written word (text, paper and pencil exercises)
- *Aural:* Learning through the ears (lecture, audio recordings)
- *Interactive:* Learning through exchange of ideas with others (group discussions)
- *Tactile:* Learning through hands-on (model building)
- *Kinesthetic:* Learning through movement (role play, games) (Lawson 2016, 33)

Good training creates a multisensory learning environment, using a variety of activities to ensure all participants' needs are addressed.

Various teaching techniques may be used to address different learning styles. These include the following:

- Individual tasks (reading, answering questions)
- Working with a partner (exchanging ideas, problem solving)
- Lecturing to a group (keep to a minimum for key learning points)
- Working in groups (role playing, simulations)

In general, effective training results when the participants do most of the work, and content is distributed incrementally and using a variety of activities. Easy-to-follow materials should be distributed for use during and after the training.

## Special Considerations for Staff Development

Several factors should be considered when delivering all levels of training programs, from orientation to staff development. Employees bring differing cultural norms, experiences, skills, abilities, and expectations to the workplace and the employer must help these individuals coexist and succeed. Trainers should consider diversity, language, and disabilities when preparing training programs. Just as it is important to match the teaching technique to the learning style, it is important to accommodate differences in culture, language, skill level and abilities. Doing so will enhance the value an employee brings to the workplace by maximizing their potential, and it may be required by law. In addition to appreciating diversity, team-building exercises can enhance the productivity of the work unit and prepare them for evolving roles in HIM.

## Diversity

Awareness of the impact of culture and human differences on the workforce has become an increasingly important issue. Organizations find it is important to learn about issues such as the effect of culture on communication and learning styles and the impact of these differences on training and expectations.

Diversity training attempts to develop sensitivity among employees about the unique challenges facing diverse groups and strives to create a more harmonious working environment. It is important to help all employees from diverse backgrounds feel included and respected as part of the team, remain committed and productive, and understand how to respond appropriately to other employees, customers, or patients. The emphasis should be on learning from each other's viewpoints. Training should be provided for the entire organization with additional, specific training for management staff.

A suggested training course might begin with a review of various cultures from a social studies perspective (that is, location of the country, climate, customs, or food preferences). Other topics to include later would be cultural norms, such as communication styles (strong eye contact or standing close when conversing), use of first versus formal names, or tolerance of jokes. Behavior that may be offensive or inappropriate in one culture but not another should be discussed, and acceptable alternatives should be presented. Additional guidelines to consider when providing diversity training include support from top management, periodic repeating of the program and presenters who are culturally neutral (Liebler and McConnell 2021, 207).

## English as Second Language

In addition to considering cultural diversity issues when creating training programs, many healthcare institutions include employees whose primary language may not be English, either in the US or overseas. This may also be true if the department is responsible for orienting or training employees of outsourced services. When the demand for health information technicians in functions such as transcription or coding exceeds the current US supply, healthcare providers may move some of their work to overseas vendors (often referred to as offshoring). Although most of the employees are in countries where English is frequently spoken, outsourcing has resulted in some unique requirements for training. In addition to the requirements for orientation of all new employees, orientation training for overseas workers may include English proficiency, American etiquette, and cultural differences. If the number of such employees is significant, thought should be given to obtaining materials written in their primary language.

## Disabilities

In general, employers are required to make reasonable accommodation for workers with disabilities. This may include altering training materials, modifying equipment, and making existing facilities accessible and usable. For example, employees in the HIM department may require adaptations to computer equipment.

The US Department of Education has established minimum requirements for developers of electronic and information technology to ensure accessibility for those with or without disabilities (2001). When designing training programs for use on computers, keep in mind that adjustments may need to be made so that users with disabilities can use the program if it requires a keyboard and monitor. Some programs may be developed using voice recognition software or screen readers. Web design should be compliant with requirements of the Americans with Disabilities Act of 1990 (ADA). If graphics, audio, or video are to be used, a text alternative should accompany them to be accessible with a screen reader. Options for the user to control animation, flashing or blinking objects, or color contrast should be provided, as well as an option to extend time available on timed responses.

### Check Your Understanding 23.3

Answer the following questions in a separate document.

1. Develop topics for diversity training programs; include in your answer case examples that you may have encountered in your own work or personal experiences.

2. Department director Cindy is planning a series of workshops on data analysis using spreadsheets for her health information technicians. Develop four different learning activities that would correspond to each of the four categories of learning styles.

3. Lori recently assumed the position of chief privacy officer at a large academic medical center. She has completed a needs assessment and decided to offer a training program on new HIPAA law updates and open it to all employees and medical staff. To not impact regular work hours too much she has scheduled the training program to begin at 6 a.m., taking place for two hours every Monday through Friday for two weeks, plus a final eight-hour day on Saturday. She has set up a website for registration, but 48 hours prior to the start date, only three people have signed up. In your opinion, why is there no motivation among employees to register for this important training program? What can Lori change to get a better response?

4. Develop a checklist for orienting the employees of an outsourced transcription company with employees in another country.

5. Sarah is a coding supervisor and wants to develop a workshop on confidentiality for her coders who work remotely. Design the instructional program using methods that will help learners retain the most content.

6. Sam recently hired a disabled veteran, Susan, as an ROI supervisor in his department. Susan has arrived for her first day on the job and is required to attend an orientation program. The program is being held in a room that is only accessible by a partial staircase from a main hallway. When Susan mentioned she will have difficulty accessing the room (she is in a wheelchair), Sam said, "Well, you need to figure it out—this is an old building and we have many programs in that room." Examine what might be wrong with Sam's response, and propose adaptations to accommodate diversity and disability issues in training.

# Delivery Methods

There are many techniques for delivering training, just as there are many purposes for training. Factors that influence selection of a training method include the following:

- Purpose of the training
- Level of education and experience of the trainees
- Preference for instructor-directed or self-paced
- Amount of space, equipment, and media available for training
- Number of trainees and their location
- Cost of the method in comparison to desired results
- Need for special accommodation due to disability or cultural differences among the trainees

When the purpose of training is to increase the level of knowledge or to introduce new policies, a different method is appropriate than when the goal is to teach a hands-on skill. Training that requires a lot of room and equipment located near the employees' work area will require a different method than training that needs to be delivered across a distance. Some subjects, such as demonstration of a new fire safety procedure, are best taught to a group of learners at the same time and place; for example, in a traditional classroom setting. In-person training would also be preferred when hands-on practice of new equipment or processes is desired—for example, cardiopulmonary resuscitation (CPR) training. Other subjects, such as use of computer software, may be taught at a time and place more effective for employees to learn, like a computer lab or remotely.

**Blended learning** uses several delivery methods, thereby gaining the advantages and reducing the disadvantages of each method alone. Common examples are classroom lecture plus online discussion, or a combination of asynchronous discussion with synchronous webinars. Various delivery methods are categorized here as either instructor-directed or self-paced.

## Delivery Methods: Instructor-Directed

Instructor-directed training and development programs, delivered in a face-to-face environment, allow for personal interaction among instructors and students. Questions can be immediately addressed, and examples given to supplement and clarify the content being delivered. Examples of instructor-directed delivery methods include classroom learning, group discussions, seminars and workshops, intensive study courses, and coaching and mentoring.

### Classroom Learning

Classroom learning takes place in a physical classroom, where learners are present in-person with their teachers and peers. The classroom provides a structured environment, which helps learners stay on task, focus on their work, and receive immediate feedback from the teacher (Oreed 2023). In-person training allows the instructor to convey practical experience and broadcast corporate culture, makes communication occur in real time, and allows information to flow in two ways. It enables immediate feedback and can improve communication skills. The class itself may be recorded and used to deliver the same material to other shifts or workers unable to attend the class.

To supplement content or add interest to both lectures and computer-based training, videos are useful for presenting events or demonstrations such as scenarios on interpersonal communication, conflict resolution, viewing surgical procedures, or product presentations.

### Group Discussions

Other techniques are frequently used in combination with the large classroom setting. **Group discussion** is effective following a lecture. Learners form smaller groups to generate ideas through interactive sharing of ideas. Role playing is useful for practicing tasks such as interviewing, grievance handling, team problem solving, conflict resolution, or communication difficulties.

### Seminars and Workshops

Seminars and workshops offer training over the course of one or more days and usually consist of several sessions on specific topics related to an overall theme. Some sessions are large, general classes and others are small, breakout classes on topics of limited interest. The cost of workshops and seminars, especially when they are held outside the workplace, is usually high because of the costs of materials, room rental, refreshments, and speaker fees. This training is typically conducted by experts on a subject and may be held in-house or offered by professional organizations, public or private colleges, or vocational schools. It is often used to develop new skills or to retrain employees whose jobs have been affected by changes in the organization, external requirements, or new policies or procedures.

### Intensive Study Courses

Intensive study courses allow a great deal of material to be compressed into a short time frame. A common example is the weekend college, where learners attend 10 to 12 hours per day on Saturday and Sunday. These courses are usually delivered on a college campus or at a hotel setting and require an overnight stay. This training method is suited for teaching special skills that can best be learned in a setting away from day-to-day operations. Examples of courses include cultural awareness, training in teamwork and empowerment, and management development.

### Coaching and Mentoring

Both new employees and experienced employees who may be ready for a change can benefit from coaching or mentoring (Schermerhorn and Bachrach 2021, 193). As discussed earlier in this chapter, coaching is an ongoing process in which an experienced person offers performance advice to a less experienced person. However, coaching goes beyond teaching. A good coach is also a counselor, a resource person, a troubleshooter, and a cheerleader. Coaches deal with improving attitudes and morale, correcting performance problems, and encouraging career development, in addition to giving instruction in specific tasks.

Effective coaches are dedicated leaders who display a high level of competence and can push or pull employees to their highest level of performance. They are role models who set a good example; show workers what is expected and how to get the job done well; provide praise or constructive feedback where appropriate; and are ready to help with routine work alongside the employee, if necessary. Department managers are well positioned to share their knowledge and expertise of the job they manage.

Coaching starts with orientation of the new employee and continues throughout his or her time with the organization. The more time the coach spends observing and listening to employees, the more opportunities there will be to support, praise, and offer advice. Helping employees should be done in a manner that encourages self-sufficiency. For example, when an employee comes forward with a problem, a good coach does not simply give the answer but, rather, asks the employee for suggestions. In other words, the coach's response should be, "What do you think?" rather than, "Here's what you should do."

Mentoring is a form of coaching. A mentor is an experienced employee who works with other employees early in their careers, giving them advice on developing skills and career options. Several employees may be assigned as protégés to the mentor, but contact is usually one-on-one. Through the mentoring relationship, employees have an advisor with whom they can solve problems, analyze and learn from mistakes, and celebrate successes. Successful mentoring depends on effective interaction between mentor and protégé. Mentors who enjoy passing on their experience and knowledge to others must be chosen.

## Delivery Methods: Self-Paced

There are numerous methods available for independent learning. Depending on the learner's situation and preferences, self-paced learning is an effective option. Computer-based training, webinars, simulations training, e-learning, videoconferencing, web-based courses, social networking, and m-learning allow individuals to learn at their own pace, often asynchronously, and remotely.

### Computer-based Training

CBT is a method designed to provide individual learners with electronic training at their own pace (Dessler 2019, 211). Learners must use a computer to access the program as content is delivered locally by access to a vendor's web server. Similar to text-based programmed learning, the explanatory material is presented and followed by a series of questions. The content is accompanied by sound or images to maintain interest and to present the material in a creative way. After each question is answered, there is an immediate response or reinforcement. In most systems, students can repeat sections of the material until they have mastered it. Students can work on different topics, at varying speeds, and in several languages. The cost of developing CBT courses may be higher than classroom instruction or printed instructional material; but once developed, the cost of delivery is less because the course can be used multiple times. It is especially useful for content that does not change frequently, such as basic medical terminology or general ROI policies.

The advantages of CBT include lower training costs, reduction in travel or time away from work for workshops, and better learning retention than with traditional classroom teaching. In addition, interactive technology has been demonstrated to reduce learning time by an average of 50 percent (Dessler 2019, 211). Disadvantages are that initially it may require a cost investment, and some students prefer a live setting and instructor for interaction.

### Webinars

Webinars are seminars delivered through a web browser, either in real time or as a recorded broadcast. This medium reduces training costs as presenters and trainees can sit in their own offices in different locations, avoiding the need for travel. Webinars can be very interactive using such tools as polling, chat box, and audio, and can add quick accessibility to responses and enhance a webinar (Sampson and Fried 2023, 216).

### Simulation Training

Simulation training is a form of education through an application that mimics work-related situations and imparts knowledge and skills as the user progresses (Fonarov 2021). A typical simulation provides the learner with a fictional scenario of a problem, and the learner decides what action to take next, as if it were a real experience. Simulations have been found to be a highly effective means to facilitate learning of complex skills (Chernikova et al. 2020).

The online realm brings another dimension to learning. A multiuser virtual environment (MUVE) is a computer-based virtual environment that can be accessed by multiple users simultaneously. MUVEs are accessed over the internet and can be used to simulate a work environment. MUVEs "are structured with three-dimensional objects, in which users can actively navigate their avatars to different areas of the immersive environment" (Doğan et al. 2018). Users create representations of themselves (avatars) and interact with other users (Doğan et al. 2018). Healthcare organizations can use a MUVE in a variety of soft skills training exercises, such as interpersonal communication, decision-making, and leadership. Individuals can role play to practice skills, try real-world experiences, and learn from their mistakes. Team-building scenarios can be developed where avatars, working together as a team, might put together a puzzle or solve a problem. Cultural diversity sensitivity may be explored simulating scenarios that present potentially controversial situations.

### E-learning

E-learning refers to training courses delivered in a variety of electronic formats. Although most often used to designate web-based training, e-learning may also refer to self-directed CBT and videoconferencing. There is increased demand for online training because traditional methods lack the flexibility and broad-based delivery necessary to meet the rising demand for updated skills in many areas of healthcare.

Electronic training works best when:

- There are many employees to train
- Employees are geographically dispersed at several sites and work varied schedules
- Just-in-time training is required
- The purpose is to gain knowledge or learn applications
- There is a blend of solid instructional design, instructor creativity, and proven technology (Kibbee and Gerzon 2008)

Advantages of e-learning include flexibility of class time and place, consistency of delivery, reduced time and cost of training, the ability to be combined with other training delivery methods, and the ability to reuse and easily maintain content. Drawbacks include technical problems, such as connectivity or availability for large blocks of time, and learner issues with motivation or distraction. Additionally, e-learning does not work well for teambuilding and does not motivate social interaction. Trainers may not be available for some time, and therefore a lag may occur between the time a problem arises and the time it can be solved. As mobile devices increase in usage, it is anticipated that the frequency of web-based training will increase. Table 23.1 shows classroom versus e-learning advantages and disadvantages.

## Videoconferencing

With **videoconferencing**, a computer monitor equipped with speakers, or a monitor and telephone, is required. This enables learners to listen and respond to the same material presented by an instructor located at another site. Interactive videoconferencing offers one- or two-way video together with two-way audio. With one-way video, students receive the image of the instructor and demonstrations and can both see and hear the presenter, but the instructor cannot see the students. Two-way video permits both parties to see each other and interact. Improved technology is enhancing the quality as well as reducing the cost of this delivery method.

Videoconferencing permits additional flexibility in delivering courses that may be enhanced through visual and audio presentation, such as those that include demonstrations or simulation exercises. It is useful for training employees in organizations with multiple sites, such as integrated delivery networks with inpatient and outpatient facilities. The disadvantage is the high cost, but the expense is justified for large organizations that do extensive training.

## Web-Based Courses

The most frequent mode of e-learning is the web-based course. Internet-based training is delivered through a universally available medium and is relatively low cost. It permits on-demand training, removing both time and space barriers. The medium is familiar to individuals and requires a minimum of instruction in the specific courseware used to deliver the course. This method provides instruction at a place, time, and

**Table 23.1.** Classroom versus e-learning advantages and disadvantages

|  | Classroom | Asynchronous web-based | Synchronous web-based |
|---|---|---|---|
| Advantages | • Learners can interact with instructors and other learners<br>• Real-time two-way communication<br>• High-quality, personal delivery<br>• Immediate answers to questions<br>• All students get same info at the same time<br>• Allows instructor to convey personal experience and broadcast corporate culture | • Just-in-time training<br>• Self-paced learning<br>• Consistency<br>• Content is reusable<br>• Training materials easy to update<br>• Flexible time and place<br>• Cost-effective<br>• Measurable—test scores can be used for evaluation | • High-quality delivery<br>• Flexibility of asynchronous learning and effectiveness of real-time support<br>• Enables extensive collaboration<br>• Immediate answers to questions<br>• Rapid, low-cost content |
| Disadvantages | • Expensive<br>• Not scalable<br>• Training too soon or too late<br>• Scheduling can be difficult<br>• Requires time off work<br>• Effectiveness is dependent on professionalism and personality of the lecturer | • Motivation can be difficult<br>• Lack of classroom collaboration<br>• No real-time interaction<br>• Delay in trainer response<br>• Not effective for teaching interpersonal skills<br>• Reduced cultural and social interaction<br>• Requires technical expertise | • Higher cost per student than asynchronous<br>• Instructor and students must be available at same time |
| Best for | • Multiple students with similar skills<br>• Training in single location<br>• Interpersonal skills<br>• Discussion is needed | • Basic training<br>• Large number of students in multiple locations<br>• Students are self-motivated | • Basic training<br>• Students in multiple locations that need to convene<br>• Highly interactive knowledge sharing<br>• Technical support is available |
| Worst for | • Students of varying skill levels<br>• Consistency across learner groups | • Observing interpersonal skills and feedback<br>• Real-time knowledge sharing<br>• Complex content | • Students of varying skill levels<br>• Observing interpersonal skills and feedback |

*Source:* Adapted from Kibbee and Gerzon 2008.

pace suited to each learner. The instruction can be delivered in several forms.

Web-based courses can be delivered **synchronously**, which means in real time with employees and trainers interacting via chat rooms, whiteboards, or application sharing at a predetermined time with review of materials. This closely mimics a traditional classroom setting. Another option is **asynchronous** delivery, where learners and instructors interact through email or discussion forums. It is not necessary to be online at the same time and is therefore more convenient than synchronous delivery. The discussion board format is the most frequently used, where learners post comments and then review and respond at different times. Materials also can be posted for review at the learner's convenience.

Software can be distributed simultaneously to learners by download from a website. Learners can interact with other learners and the instructor through a variety of communication tools. A common form of delivery today is to access courses developed by training organizations or universities through a website. Widely available course-authoring tools permit trainers to develop e-learning courses easily and quickly without professional course developers. Most rapid e-learning tools also incorporate search tools, bookmarking, and data tracking. Employees are issued a username and password to access the course. Material can be presented using a variety of methods, including text, audio, or video. Relevant material can be accessed through hypertext links embedded on the website that learners can access with the click of a mouse.

Software for delivering web-based courses is developed as LMSs and **learning content management systems (LCMSs)**. While LMSs manage the instructional activities, LCMSs provide a technical framework to develop the content and permit sharing and reusing content. Most courseware used by colleges and universities has both components. Rapid e-learning tools can be linked to LMSs to facilitate course development.

### Social Networks

The popularity of social networking websites provides another opportunity for e-learning. These sites provide an online community where participants can share information including file attachments, website bookmarks, or multimedia files. **Blogs** provide a web page where users can post text, images, and links to other websites. While blogs originally started as a type of online personal diary, they are now used for a variety of purposes, including communication within organizations, and can be helpful for distributing training materials. **Wikis** are a collection of user-modified web pages that together form a collaborative website. Healthcare organizations may use wikis as a tool where trainers or supervisors can post material, and employees can respond and discuss questions. Social networking websites and apps enable users to interact with each other, and may provide easily accessible tools to post documents and reminders for employee groups and provide platforms for asking questions.

### M-Learning

**M-learning**, or mobile learning, is an electronic learning mode in which content is typically delivered through the internet to computers, smartphones, or tablets, thereby expanding accessibility to a true anytime, anyplace level. Content is easy to access and delivery permits viewing on the learner's schedule. As with any form of e-learning, effective instructional design is important. M-learning is not appropriate for very long courses with a great deal of material but is good for delivering key points and short updates. It is an effective way to quickly deliver multimedia information to many people (Al-Amri 2020).

## Artificial Intelligence in Training and Development

The term artificial intelligence (AI) means a machine-based system that can, for a given set of human-defined objectives, make predictions, recommendations, or decisions influencing real or virtual environments. AI systems use machine and human-based inputs to:

**(A)** perceive real and virtual environments;

**(B)** abstract such perceptions into models through analysis in an automated manner; and

**(C)** use model inference to formulate options for information or action. (H.R.6216 National Artificial Intelligence Initiative Act of 2020)

AI technology enables computers and machines to simulate human intelligence and problem-solving capabilities. It is a tool that can deliver and enhance education and training by tailoring educational content to meet individual students' needs and preferences. Personalized learning provides relevant content suggestions and recommendations based on an employee's job title, interests, and the content they have already learned.

As healthcare progresses from human-powered effort to increasing use of AI and health information technologies, healthcare professionals will perform with more autonomy and on ever-changing tasks. This will require continuous learning to prepare for and adapt to continuous transformations in their workplaces (Hopper 2024).

---

### Check Your Understanding 23.4

**Answer the following questions in a separate document.**

1. As corporate director of HIM for a large healthcare system recently formed through merger of six smaller hospitals, you are tasked with developing a team-building program for your staff who are in areas several miles apart. Propose the best training method for this situation, and explain factors you considered in your decision.
2. Bringing all the employees in question 1 together for training will result in a large amount of travel expenses. Propose two options that would reduce costs.
3. Assess types of training appropriate for delivery on mobile devices such as smartphones and tablet computers.
4. Larry is comparing synchronous and asynchronous web-based training using an LMS as a training method for data analysts in his department. The staff members are familiar with the basics of spreadsheet programs, but he wants to teach them more advanced functions. What would you recommend to Larry?
5. Janice has hired a new coding supervisor. There is an open position in the coding section, and Janice wants to train her new supervisor on interviewing skills. What would you recommend as the best training methods for this situation. State your reasons.
6. Linda has recently revised the department's policy and procedure for ROI on emancipated minors. Evaluate the use of the organization's intranet to deliver this training. What other method could you suggest?
7. Explain the difference between mentoring and coaching.
8. Provide a scenario that would be appropriate to use MUVEs for training.

---

## Positioning Employees for Career Development

Developing strong healthcare leaders in an increasingly competitive market is a growing need. Successful organizations have a formal process in place for leadership development. Creating an environment that encourages and allows employees to use and develop their problem-solving and decision-making competencies is an established HR management practice with many benefits. It is critical for organizations to prepare HIM staff for emerging roles. In addition, encouraging continuing education, promoting soft skill development, sharing opportunities for promotion and succession planning, encouraging the development of a personal career plan, and ensuring a strong awareness for and development of employment law and regulation training is imperative for sustaining a strong organization.

### Preparing the HIM Staff for Future Roles

HIM professionals must continuously transform their knowledge, skills, and abilities to keep pace with the competencies needed for new roles. A study on workforce challenges and the role of emerging technologies identified next steps for health information professionals to prepare for these roles. Competencies are needed in the areas of data quality and analytics, consumer health information, revenue cycle, and privacy, risk and compliance (NORC and AHIMA 2023).

In addition, HIM professionals must become skilled in the use of AI to ensure its implementation in healthcare does not compromise patient safety, decrease care quality, or violate health data privacy. "Professionals in HI will require upskilling and training to build capacity to oversee technology use and develop innovative ways of utilizing these tools to support healthcare operations and improvement" (NORC and AHIMA 2023, 18).

### Continuing Education

**Continuing education (CE)** is a requirement for most credentialled professionals, including those in HIM. It usually requires a person to complete a certain number of hours of education within a given period to maintain a credential or license status. As the HIM field is changing rapidly, it is important that credentialed professionals remain current in their knowledge of the profession so they can provide high-quality skills to the organizations for which they work.

CE programs for HIM are most often provided by external organizations such as AHIMA or its component state associations. Career development, by contrast, usually includes a combination of internal methods, such as job rotation through progressively increasing job responsibilities in-house and externally taught formal classes and workshops.

As part of the formal performance appraisal process, CE goals should be set for all employees. Management should support the individual's achievement by such activities as providing time off to attend workshops, flexible scheduling for formal classes offered at educational institutions, and financial reimbursement.

## Soft Skills

The technical skills required to perform a job, acquired through education, experience and training, are known as "hard" skills. While these are integral to employee success, skills that are more difficult to define are those intangible factors, or **"soft" skills** that contribute to an employee's career advancement and recognition beyond job knowledge (Lavender 2019). Soft skills include the following:

- Oral and written communication
- Critical Thinking
- Organization
- Teamwork
- Work ethic
- Flexibility
- Attention to detail
- Empathy
- Self-confidence
- Positive attitude
- Leadership
- Time management
- Problem solving

Soft skills training refers to the formal programs and activities that help employees develop key nontechnical competencies. Training can be delivered in many of the ways that have been discussed in this chapter. In addition, employees can research self-help resources and participate in informal activities outside the workplace to strengthen their skills.

## Promotion and Succession Planning

Promotion may be another tool to encourage employee development and commitment. When tied to training programs, it can become a powerful incentive. **Promotion** usually refers to the upward progression of an employee in both job and salary. However, it also can mean a lateral move to a different position with similar job skills or a change within the same job because of completing higher education or credentialing requirements. To attract, retain, and motivate employees, organizations should provide a career development system that promotes from within. When tied to promotion, career development programs offer an incentive to ambitious employees. Goals can be incorporated into the performance review process

**Succession planning** is a specific type of promotional plan in which senior-level position openings are anticipated and candidates are identified from within the organization. The candidates are given training through formal education, job rotation, and mentoring so that they can eventually assume these positions. It should be considered an essential part of every manager's job to identify and develop potential successors.

## Developing a Personal Career Plan

While an organization can use the methods discussed to assist employees with career advancement, the major responsibility still falls on employees themselves. Employers no longer have the sole responsibility to identify career paths and offer promotional or growth opportunities. After careful self-examination of strengths and weaknesses as well as professional interests and career opportunities, a career plan can be developed.

A **career plan** is a strategic plan for an individual, providing direction, goals, and an action plan to reach those goals. It includes the individual's own strengths, weaknesses, personal values, and interests, all of which should be used to model a personal leadership style that can be developed during the career plan. A solid career plan will identify the skill sets and resources needed to reach one's goals, and how to better align them with those of the organization (Broscio and Scherer 2014, 62). When an opportunity for a lateral or advanced opportunity presents itself, an individual with a career plan will have developed the necessary skills, such as project management, data analytics, or leadership, and will be ready to act when called upon. A career plan must be flexible and updated regularly. See figure 23.7 for the key components of a career plan.

AHIMA has created tools to assist HIM professionals with personal career development. The *AHIMA*

**Figure 23.7.** The key components of a career plan

A strategic career plan should have these core components:
- Statement of one's personal values set and short- and long-term goals, clearly outlined but flexible based on the iterative process of building a plan to meet the needs of the individual, employer, and market
- Answers to the following questions:
  - What do I require for fulfillment in my work and life?
  - What does my current or future employer contribute that meets my requirements for fulfillment?
  - What is required of me to be successful by my current or future employer?
  - What do I contribute to my current or a future employer's success?
  - What am I doing well (and not so well) to meet my current or potential employer's needs, and what is my current or potential employer doing well (or not so well) to meet my needs?
- Analysis of gaps between one's own needs and aspirations and the current situation and market requirements
- Your value proposition today, what it should be in the future, and how this positions you to reach your goals
- Action steps to close the gaps and achieve your goals, including:
  - Market research: to stay informed
  - Learning plan: to stay relevant
  - Personal marketing: to build relationships
  - Managing risk: to eliminate career barriers
  - Identifying sources of support: to determine the need for a coach or mentor
- Process to monitor progress, gain feedback, and update the plan on an ongoing basis

**Source:** Broscio and Scherer 2014. What's your plan? *Healthcare Executive* 29(6):60–62. Used with permission.

*Career Prep Workbook* prompts new and practicing HIM professionals to compare their own skills and knowledge to what is required to pursue future career opportunities (AHIMA n.d.a). The Health Information Career Map illustrates jobs and career paths for HIM professionals (AHIMA n.d.b.). One can select a particular HIM job title at a given educational level, view job responsibilities, and see promotional paths to other positions (AHIMA n.d.a).

## Employment Laws and Regulations Impacting Training

In developing training programs, healthcare organizations must recognize that special accommodations may be required to address the needs of both a culturally diverse workforce and employees with disabilities. Employers need to understand the requirements affecting training included under Title VII of the 1964 Civil Rights Act, the 1991 Civil Rights Act, and the ADA. If completion of a training program is part of the selection process for a particular job, the organization must be able to demonstrate that the requirements for training are valid and do not discriminate against, or have a negative impact on, women, minorities, or disabled individuals. For example, the vocabulary in written documents used for training should match the level required for the job, and training equipment and locations should be accessible to individuals with mobility disabilities.

For employers to avoid liability for harassment and discrimination acts of and by their employees, they must not only implement anti-discrimination policies but also provide training to ensure employees understand their rights and responsibilities. The courts interpret this as exercising reasonable care to prevent harassment. The training should cover all types of harassment, be provided for all employees shortly after they are hired and periodically thereafter, be of substantial length, and permit the employee to repeat as necessary until competence is demonstrated. Inadequate training exposes employers to potential liability for negligent training if an employee harms a third party (McConnell 2018, 330).

The Occupational Safety and Health Act of 1970 (OSHA) was established by the federal government to ensure safe working conditions. Among its many requirements is training to reduce unsafe acts. Hospitals are required to train employees in fire safety and other job-related safety measures. If necessary, the training must be provided in the worker's native language (other than English), and the worker must demonstrate proficiency following the training.

The ADA requires employers to provide reasonable accommodations for physical or mental limitations regarding many employment-related functions, including training (ADA 1990). For example, this would require that accommodations be made to CBT to provide accessibility through voice recognition or screen readers, if necessary. The World Wide Web

Consortium's Web Accessibility Initiative publishes information about ADA compliance for websites (WWW Consortium n.d.). Section 508 of the Rehabilitation Act of 1973 provides accessibility standards for electronic and information technology. Finally, accrediting organizations such as the Joint Commission require staff orientation and CE to meet requirements of a particular position and define several topics for training, including cultural diversity sensitivity (Joint Commission 2024).

### Check Your Understanding 23.5

Answer the following questions in a separate document.

1. David has worked as a cancer registrar for two years in his current position. Recently, the layout of one of the screens he uses for abstracting was changed by the software company. David mentions to Beth, his supervisor, that he has ideas for reorganizing the fields on the screen to make his job easier. Propose how Beth could use this situation to empower David.

2. Evaluate the HIM profession and the needs of the future workforce. Provide examples of the top skills required for the future HIM workforce. Assess your skills and propose what skill sets are your strengths, and those you'd like to develop further.

3. Julie has worked in her coding position for about three weeks. A backlog of records to code that are more advanced than her skill level exists due to a senior coder being on vacation. Julie has reviewed her pathophysiology textbook to try to come up with the correct code for a complex cardiac patient but remains unsure. She asks John, her supervisor, for help, but he simply says, "Here, let me do it, I don't have time to explain!" Recommend a better response for John that would incorporate coaching into the situation.

4. Julie has worked in her position for one year. Her supervisor recognizes she clearly has increased the quality and quantity of her work. She earned her certified coding specialist (CCS) credential and maintains CE requirements. When a supervisory position opened, Julie applied for it. However, another employee, who Julie knows does not perform as well and is not credentialed, was given the position, as she has more seniority and has threatened to resign if not given the promotion. Examine how this situation was handled and what should be done differently to make promotion in this department useful as a motivational tool.

5. You were promoted to the position of supervisor of the cancer registry at your facility and asked to review the current employee orientation and training program to be sure it is compliant with laws and regulations. Provide three examples of topics that may be affected and reference the applicable law.

6. Identify three soft skills and give a specific example of how each one can contribute to an HIM employee's professionalism.

# References

Al-Amri, S., Noor, N. F. B. M., Hamid, S. B., and Gani, A. B. (2020). Designing mobile training content: challenges and open issues. *IEEE Access*, 8, 122314–122331. https://doi.org/10.1109/ACCESS.2020.3006712. https://proxy.cc.uic.edu/login?url=https://doi.org/10.1109/ACCESS.2020.3006712.

AHIMA (American Health Information Management Association). 2019. "AHIMA Code of Ethics." https://bok.ahima.org/doc?oid=105098.

AHIMA (American Health Information Management Association). n.d.a. *Career Prep Workbook*. Accessed May 29, 2024. https://www.ahima.org/media/o0dl1qdo/ahima_career_prep_workbook_fillable.pdf.

AHIMA (American Health Information Management Association). n.d.b. "Career Map." Accessed May 29, 2024. https://www.ahima.org/career-mapping/career-map/.

Americans with Disability Act of 1990. Public Law 101-336.

Beskar, D. 2022 (January 13). "Understanding the Learning Pyramid." https://davidbeskar.org/understanding-the-learning-pyramid/.

Broscio, M. A., and J. E. Scherer. 2014. What's your plan? *Healthcare Executive* 29(6):60–62.

Chernikova, O., N. Heitzmann, M. Stadler, D. Holzberger, T. Seidel, and F. Fischer. 2020.

Simulation-based learning in higher education: A meta-analysis. *Review of Educational Research* 90(4):499–541.

Dessler, G. 2019. *Fundamentals of Human Resources Management*, 5th ed. Upper Saddle River, NJ: Pearson Education.

Dessler, G. 2017. *Human Resources Management*, 15th ed. Upper Saddle River, NJ: Pearson Prentice-Hall.

Doğan, D., M. Cnar, and H. Tuzun. 2018. "Multi-user Virtual Environments for Education." In *Encyclopedia of Computer Graphics and Games*, edited by N. LeeSpringer https://doi.org/10.1007/978-3-319-08234-9_172-1.

Fonarov, O. 2021 (July 26). "The Basics of Employee Training Through Simulation." https://www.forbes.com/sites/forbestechcouncil/2021/07/26/the-basics-of-employee-training-through-simulation/?sh=54b0429d1422.

Hopper, A. M. 2024. *Preparing Healthcare Workers for an AI-Driven Workplace*. Auerbach Publications. New York. https://doi.org/10.1201/9781003175841.

House Rule 6216—National Artificial Intelligence Initiative Act of 2020. 116th Congress (2019–2020)

Lang, D. 2020. "Three Ways to Reinforce Training–What's In It For Me?" Langevin Learning Services, Ogdensburg, NY. https://langevin.com/3-ways-to-reinforce-training-whats-in-it-for-me/.

Lavender, J. 2019. "Soft skills for hard jobs." *Journal of Continuing Education Topics and Issues* 21(2):48–52.

Lawson, K. 2016. *The Trainer's Handbook*, 4th ed. Hoboken, NJ: John Wiley & Sons.

Liebler, J., and C. McConnell. 2021. *Management Principles for Health Professionals*, 8th ed. Burlington, MA: Jones and Bartlett Learning.

McConnell, C. 2018. *Umiker's Management Skills for the New Health Care Supervisor*, 7th ed. Sudbury, MA: Jones and Bartlett.

NORC and AHIMA. 2023. *Health Information Workforce: Survey Results on Workforce Challenges and the Role of Emerging Technologies.* https://www.norc.org/content/dam/norc-org/pdf2023/AHIMA-Workforce-Survey-Report-Final-2023.pdf.

Oreed. 2023 (March 28). "The Seven Biggest Differences Between Online and Classroom Learning." https://oreed.org/en/article/the-7-biggest-differences-between-online-learning-vs-classroom-learning.

Sampson, C., and B. Fried. 2021. *Human Resources in Healthcare: Managing for Success*, 5th ed. Chicago: Health Administration Press.

Schermerhorn, J., and D. Bachrach. 2021. *Exploring Management*, 7th ed. New York: John Wiley & Sons, Inc.

Title VII of the Civil Rights Act of 1964. Public Law 88–352.

WWW Consortium. n.d. "Web Accessibility Initiative." Accessed January 6, 2019. http://www.w3c.org/WAI.

# chapter 24

# Work Design and Process Improvement

*Pamela K. Oachs, MA, RHIA, CHDA, FAHIMA*

## Learning Objectives

- Evaluate the functionality of a work environment
- Determine alternate methods for distributing work assignments and scheduling staff
- Develop job procedures to support employees in delivering effective and efficient services
- Differentiate the methods of standard setting
- Construct performance management measures
- Select the appropriate tool(s) for use in different types of improvement efforts

## Key Terms

Affinity diagram
Benchmarking
Brainstorming
Business process
Business process redesign (BPR)
Check sheet
Closed system
Common cause variation
Compressed workweek
Continuous quality improvement (CQI)
Control chart
Cybernetic system
Cyclical staffing
DMAIC
Employee self-logging
Ergonomics
External customer
Feedback control
Fishbone diagram

Flextime
Float employee
Flowchart
Force-field analysis
Goal
Histogram
Internal customer
Job procedure
Job sharing
Key indicator
Lean
Multivoting technique
Narrative
Nominal group technique (NGT)
Objective
Offshoring
Open system
Outsourcing
Parallel work division
Pareto chart

Performance improvement
Performance measurement
Playscript
Preventive control
Procedure manual
Process improvement
Productivity
Qualitative standard
Quantitative standard
Run chart
Scatter diagram
Serial work division
Service level agreement (SLA)
Shift differential
Shift rotation
Six Sigma
Spaghetti diagram
Special cause variation
Standard
Swimlane diagram

Telecommuting
Total Quality Management (TQM)
Unit work division
Use case analysis
Volume log
Work distribution analysis
Work distribution chart
Work measurement
Work sampling

Management is the art of getting work done through and with people (Peek 2023). It is an art because effective management depends on the use of sound judgment, intuition, communication, and interpersonal skills. It is also a science because it is based on theory and principles that have been—and continue to be—tested and explored. Managers engage in specific functions, including planning, organizing, directing, and controlling, to create and facilitate effective work processes so the desired outcome can be achieved in a cost-efficient manner.

Management of human resources is one of the most challenging and critical functions in a healthcare organization. Whether a lead staff person, supervisor, manager, or department director, one's ability to successfully achieve organizational goals is impacted by people and performance management skills. Performance management does not occur by accident. Careful consideration of the availability, organization, and performance of staff resources is fundamental to delivering effective and efficient services related to health information management (HIM).

This chapter introduces key concepts, tools, and techniques associated with evaluating, designing, redesigning, and implementing effective and efficient work processes within an organization. It includes discussion of various methods of work division and work scheduling; management of work procedures; components of the work environment; elements of a performance management program, including methods for establishing performance standards; and various process improvement methodologies to continuously improve or reengineer workflow, work processes, and staff performance to accommodate changes in service requirements and fiscal limitations.

## Functional Work Environment

Considering the amount of time the average full-time employee spends in the work environment, it is prudent for management to create a workplace infrastructure and ambience that evokes comfort and productivity. Whether creating new space or evaluating current space for the remote or on-site employee, developing the work environment involves consideration of these fundamental elements: workflow, space and equipment, aesthetics, and ergonomics.

### Departmental Workflow

The workflow in a departmental setting is the established path along which tasks are sequentially completed by any number of staff to accomplish a function. Well-designed workflow is critical to achieving optimal efficiency when a function requires the coordinated activity of a group of employees. Spatial relationships among a group of people who perform tasks and the equipment required to perform them are critical factors in planning efficient workflow. In such situations, creating a workflow diagram such as a spaghetti diagram (see figure 24.1) helps the manager to visualize the flow of people, products, and process documents in a defined work area (Hessing n.d.).

### Space and Equipment

Workspace design can influence the department culture, including employee morale, productivity, quality, and job satisfaction. The design of efficient workspace involves several considerations, including the number of employees, physical activity of employees, communication requirements among employees and customers, workflow, equipment used, the type of environment (paper or electronic), job functions, and the need for privacy. Even in a highly electronic environment, there may still be an abundance of paper to manage, equipment to place, and workflow to design. For example, whether health records are scanned or physically stored, there needs to be a plan for their location throughout the record processing functions that keeps them safe and secure while still being available to the employees.

Space is considered a precious and costly commodity in healthcare facilities and must be used efficiently. Department managers should understand basic facility planning techniques and know who their facility planning resources are in the organization. They must be able to consider the facility's master plan when reviewing their department or work unit needs to collaboratively develop a design for the work area.

Figure 24.1. Spaghetti diagram: Inefficient (top) and efficient (bottom)

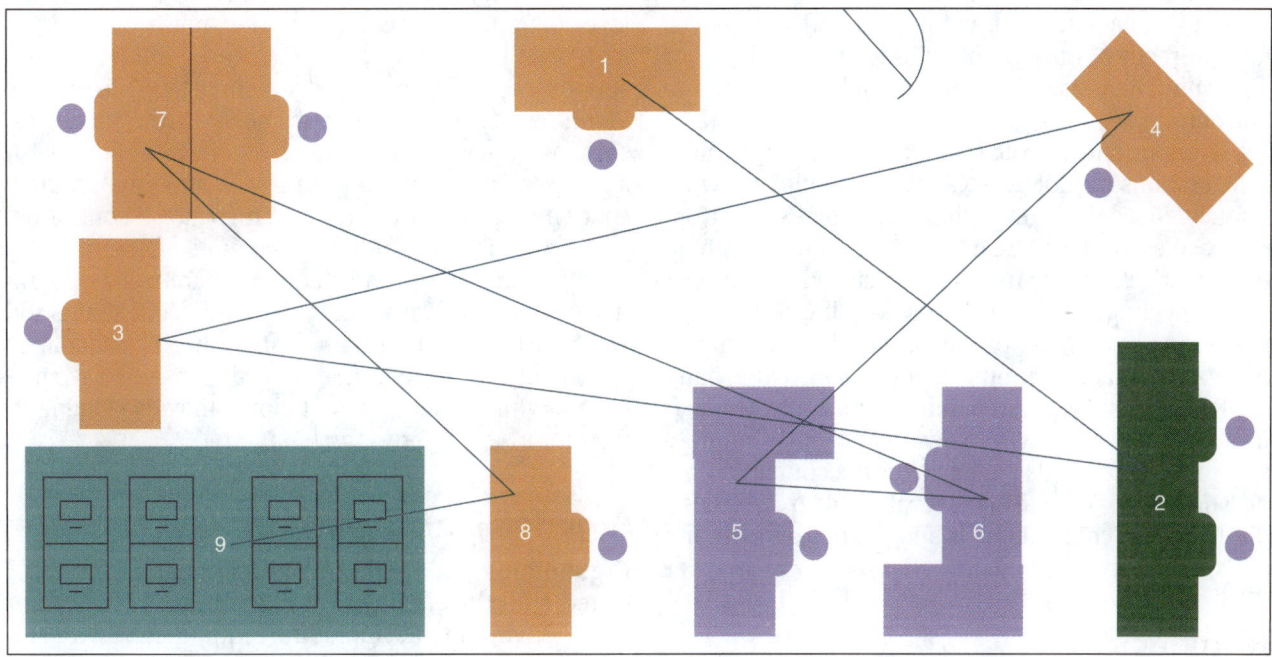

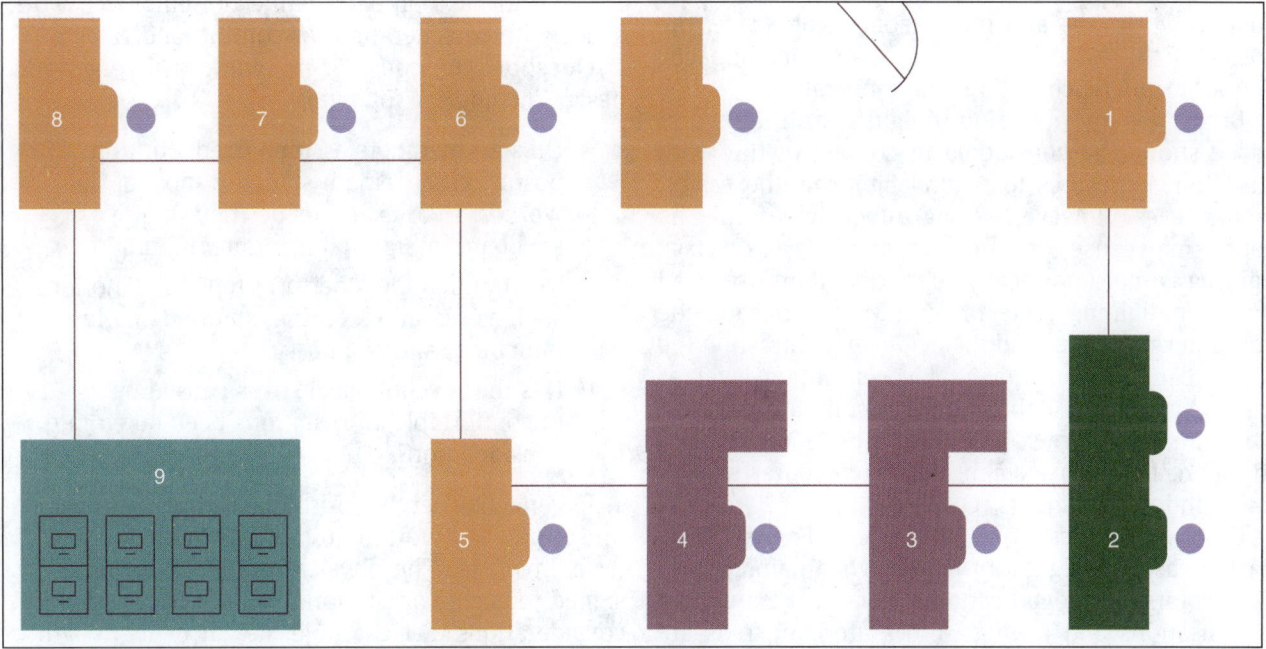

Reorganization of a department because of changes in workforce numbers, telecommuting efforts, a shift in workforce functions, or acquisition of new functions constitutes a space planning process. Departmental reorganization in response to changes in methods or functions, such as a move to remote coding or implementation of an electronic health record (EHR), can trigger the need for revised space planning. Sometimes the basic need to improve workflow and the appearance of a department can be a pivotal reason for space planning.

Another space consideration is personal space, or the area of privacy surrounding an employee. Depending on the employee's job role, confidentiality may be a concern. If the employee is in a mentoring or leadership role, privacy may be necessary when offering feedback to other employees. If the employee works directly with patients either on the phone or in person, there are also confidentiality concerns to consider.

It is important to realize that space and equipment considerations do not go away when employees work remotely. Telecommuting will require redesign of on-site space as workers begin to vacate work areas, temporary workspace may need to be designed for required on-site meetings, and employees working from home also need to have their home offices properly equipped.

Effective space planning contributes to the quality of the work, employee satisfaction, and the services the department provides; and it minimizes costs too. Space needs change over the course of time and should be periodically reevaluated to determine whether these characteristics and the department and staff's needs are still being met.

## Aesthetics

Aesthetics of the workplace are the physical surroundings of the employees' workspace. They have physiological as well as psychological effects on employees. Aesthetic elements include the lighting of both the general work area and the personal workspace, the colors of the walls and furniture, auditory impacts, and atmospheric condition and temperature.

Brightness and diffusion of light within the workspace should be considered in context of the work situation. Exposures to natural light may be easiest on the eyes. However, strong direct light from any source may cause eye strain and fatigue. Desk or task lighting is more physically supportive than overhead florescent lighting alone. Many HIM functions include computer monitors, and the degree of contrast on the screen can influence the employee's comfort level, as can the glare from light sources or computer screens. There are several ways to address these issues, including glare filters, placement of the computer screen, and window treatments (OSHA n.d.a).

Color influences how people feel. For example, dark areas feel brighter or lighter when painted with light colors. Moreover, certain colors evoke a variety of sensations and feelings. Blues are cool, reds are warm, greens evoke luxury, neutral colors can have a calming effect, and so on (Cherry 2019). When choosing color schemes, it is important to consider the area, the function of the area, and who will occupy it.

Music and sound may be incorporated to improve working conditions and relieve both mental and visual fatigue. Certain kinds of music can reduce tension and make employees generally feel better. Sound conditioning and soundproofing are important considerations because a noisy office may not be efficient. A certain level of routine office background noise is expected and, usually, is not irritating. However, loud or abrupt sounds can be alarming, distracting, and disruptive. Planning separate space for noisy work processes, such as copying and printing, is effective because it addresses the source of the noise. Carpeting, window coverings, and partitioning can offer noise control because they absorb significant amounts of sound.

Air conditioning and ventilation impact temperature, circulation, and moisture content. Air that is too warm or too cold is equally distracting, and a balance can be difficult to maintain. Dry air can cause eye irritation, while a lack of circulation can cause stagnant, uncomfortable conditions (OSHA n.d.a).

## Ergonomics

Ergonomics is a discipline of functional design associated with the employee in relationship to his or her work environment, including equipment, workstation, and office furniture adaptation to accommodate the employee's unique physical requirements with a goal to facilitate effectiveness of work functions. It is considered "fitting the job to the person" (OSHA n.d.b) and has helped redefine the employee workspace with consideration for comfort and safety.

Questions to consider in workspace ergonomic design include the following:

- Do staff members assume fixed working postures that remain static for most of the workday? For example, do they sit at a keyboard or stand at a counter all day?
- Do staff members perform repetitive motions such as scanning, typing, stamping, hole punching, and so on?
- Has the psychological stress caused by uncomfortable workstations been taken into consideration?

In effective ergonomic planning, the designer must know the work requirements of the job and the tasks involved. The physical traits of the worker assigned to each workstation also influence ergonomic considerations. For example, height or leg length or back or waist length will determine specific needs. Another consideration is whether an individual or multiple persons share one workstation. Finally, one must consider what equipment is currently available at the workstation and what equipment must be purchased to create an ergonomically correct work environment. Often, organizations employ ergonomic specialists to perform assessments on employees and their work environment. These specialists may be employees of the organization, possibly physical or occupational therapists; or they may be consultants to the organization brought in on an as-needed basis. Managers must collaborate with these professionals to ensure the employees' needs and work functions are understood, allowing the ergonomic specialist to perform a proper evaluation and make appropriate recommendations.

When the work environment is not ergonomically sound, issues such as back and neck strain, carpal tunnel syndrome, tension headaches, and eyestrain can occur. Preventive, proactive ergonomic management includes educating staff on how to care for themselves to reduce potential ergonomic injuries or discomfort. Careful consideration and professional assessment of individual employees' work environment needs will help reduce or eliminate physical barriers to employee comfort and productivity. Preemptive, ergonomically correct practices markedly reduce employee absence and workers' compensation usage due to workplace injury (OSHA n.d.c).

### Check Your Understanding 24.1

**Answer the following questions in a separate document.**

1. John is the HIM manager at ABC Health System. He manages a total of 20 scanning and indexing, deficiency analysis, coding, document audit, and release of information (ROI) staff. The organization implemented an EHR one year ago and John realizes at least half of his staff could work remotely. Recommend ways in which John could approach the redesign of the department space if the appropriate staff began to work remotely.

2. Using the scenario in question 1, how can John justify this change in physical work environment to his boss?

3. Construct a spaghetti diagram of your existing work, classroom, or home environment. You can evaluate a restaurant or business if you like. Look for inefficiencies in the way people move about in this environment and develop an improved spaghetti diagram.

4. Peter has been having neck and back pain and headaches for the last couple of weeks. As his supervisor, what would you recommend?

5. Considering the impact that aesthetic elements, such as lighting, the colors of the walls and furniture, noise, and temperature have on employees, state your position on the feasibility and effectiveness of remote work.

## Methods of Organizing Work

Staffing involves the determination of which types of employees, how many of each type, and what kind of work schedule are needed. The types of employees needed depend on the skills, experience, and education required for the specific work that must be done. The number of employees needed depends on the volume of work and the pattern of work division selected for the work setting. Work scheduling is based on when employees are needed to provide the services they are responsible for delivering within the organization.

### Work Division Patterns

The method to dividing work among employees used in a process-oriented department depends in large part on the nature of the work to be performed and the number of employees available to perform it. Three basic types of work division patterns are serial, parallel, and unit work division.

### Serial Work Division

The sequential handling of tasks is called **serial work division**. Often referred to as a production line, serial work division tends to create task specialists. The example in figure 24.2 illustrates an ROI process using serial work division. In this staffing model, each type of employee sequentially handles a step in the total ROI work process.

### Parallel Work Division

The concurrent handling of tasks is called **parallel work division**. Multiple employees do identical types of tasks and basically see the process through from beginning to end. The example in figure 24.3 illustrates an ROI process using parallel work division. In this staffing model, all ROI specialists are expected to perform all of the tasks that comprise the ROI work process independent from the others.

**Figure 24.2.** Serial work division of release of information process

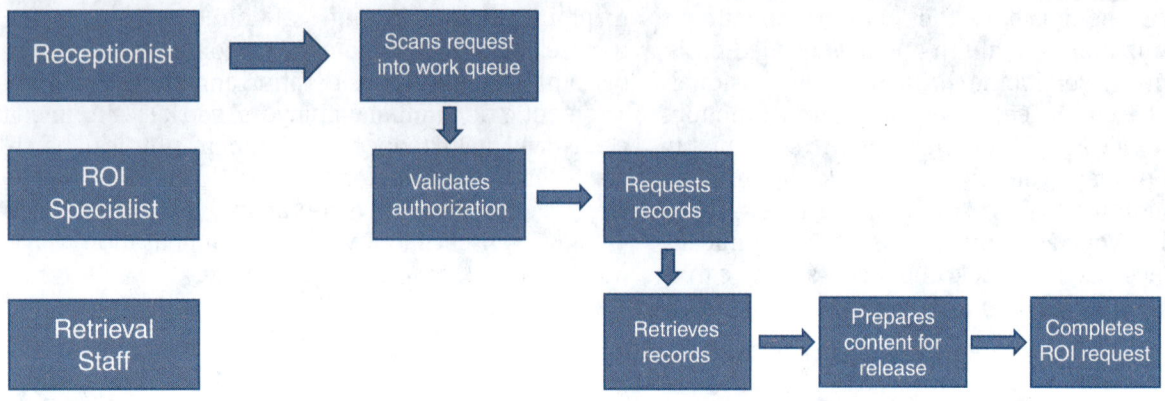

**Figure 24.3.** Parallel work division of release of information process

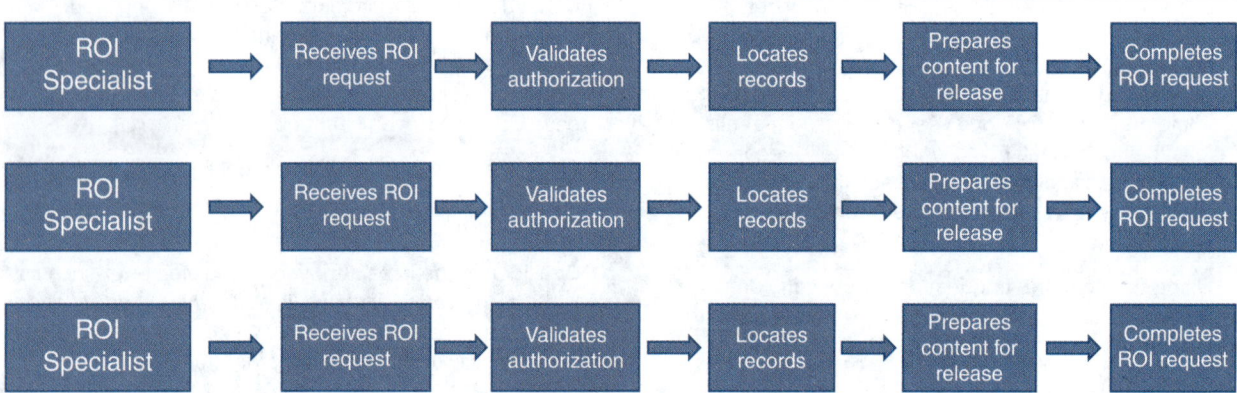

### Unit Work Division

When different specialized tasks are performed at the same time, it is called **unit work division**. The tasks are all related to the same product but are not dependent on each other. The work is specialized, but the sequence of tasks is not fixed. For example, the coding professional codes records, the patient access staff registers patients, and the records staff scans and indexes reports. All tasks relate to the creation of a patient's medical record but occur independently.

## Work Distribution Analysis

**Work distribution analysis** is a process for evaluating the types of work functions performed in a department, the amount of time given to those functions, who is performing each function, and the way work is distributed among the employees. It is used to document and describe the major functions of a work unit, determine whether a department's current work assignments and job content are appropriate, and identify process variation. Making time to perform this analysis can lead to one or more of the following observations:

- Large amounts of time are being dedicated to functions of minor importance.
- Small amounts of time are being dedicated to functions of key importance.
- There is too much or too little job function specialization.
- There is duplication of efforts or functions.
- Some employees are overloaded with work assignments.
- Some employees do not have enough work to keep busy.
- Staff are performing tasks inappropriate to their positions.

Work distribution analysis can be helpful in determining whether adequate time is available and appropriate for each task and whether employees are overburdened or have time for additional responsibilities. In addition, it can help the manager assess whether the work is organized and distributed appropriately.

Some basic work distribution data can be collected through work queues or work volume dashboards. Other data may best be collected in a **work distribution chart** initially completed by each employee and includes all responsible task content as well as hours or parts of hours spent on tasks gathered over a designated period. Work distribution charts can be formulated in a variety of ways but frequently are tables, with work tasks forming the row headings and a double column of employee names and hours spent on tasks forming the column headings. (See table 24.1.) Actual data collection time and methods varies depending on what is needed to get a representative sample of activities and times. When adequate data have been collected, the manager compiles them, clusters similar job tasks together, and completes the chart.

In table 24.1, four HIM department employees have identified how much time they have spent on each of the identified tasks in a 40-hour workweek. Task content should come directly from the employee's current job description. In addition to task content, each employee tracks each task's start time, end time, and volume or productivity within a typical workweek. In the example in table 24.1, the work distribution chart shows that the supervisor spends just over half of the time doing administrative work (often in meetings), yet there is a rather large amount of time given to ROI, particularly in giving depositions. The admissions clerk spends most of the time receiving visitors and performing data entry. The discharge clerk spends the same amount of time on ROI as analysis. The scanning and indexing clerk spends most work time on prepping, scanning, and indexing records. Analysis using this chart may indicate that an unusual amount of time is spent by the supervisor in the ROI function and that there is little time left for supervising duties; or possibly the discharge clerk is distracted by a large amount of ROI activity. This information can be used to investigate these questions further to determine if a change should be made.

The results of a work distribution analysis can lead a department to redefine the job descriptions of some employees, redesign the office space, or establish new or revised procedures for some department functions to gain improvements in staff productivity or service quality.

## Work Scheduling

After management has determined the appropriate work distribution within a department and adjusts accordingly, a work-scheduling system can be developed. Determining the work schedule for departmental staff involves more than simply assigning the correct number of work hours to each employee. Effective scheduling results in the following:

- A core of employees always on duty when services must be provided
- Enough employee hours scheduled to meet the required volume of work to be done per established performance standards
- A pattern of hours (shifts) to be worked and days off that employees can be reasonably sure will not change except in extreme emergencies
- Fair and just treatment of all employees regarding hours assigned
- A committed workforce with high morale and a strong rate of retention

**Table 24.1.** Work distribution chart

| Position/employee | Supervisor/J. Johnson | | Admissions clerk/A. Jones | | Discharge clerk/B. Olson | | Scanning/indexing clerk/R. Smith | |
|---|---|---|---|---|---|---|---|---|
| Activity | Task | # of Hours | Task | # of Hours | Task | # of Hours | Task | # of Hours |
| Release of information | Post requests; give depositions | 2 / 10 | Photocopy/scan | 8 | Certify content | 15 | Retrieve records | 4 |
| Analysis | Determine completion | 2 | Place in queue | 3 | Tag for incomplete | 15 | Collect records | 5 |
| Scanning / indexing | Audit scanned records | 2 | — | — | Check for scanned record for MDs | 4 | Prep records; scan/index records | 30 |
| Administrative overhead | Attend meetings; supervise employees | 12 / 10 | Receive visitors; data entry | 14 / 14 | Generate MD letters | 5 | — | — |
| Training | Read literature | 2 | Attend software training | 1 | Attend computer training | 1 | Attend computer training | 1 |
| Totals | 40 hours/40 hours | | 40 hours/40 hours | | 40 hours/40 hours | | 40 hours/40 hours | |

Several staffing concerns should be considered when devising an effective staff schedule. Answers to the following questions will help determine the department's or work unit's course of action:

- How is the workweek defined by policy? The workweek is generally established to begin on Sunday, but organizational policy may dictate otherwise.
- What days of the week is the department open? How many and what hours and days are covered?
- What functions must be performed each day and within what time frame?
- How many full-time equivalents (FTEs) are needed to handle the work volume?

HIM departments often are on a standard Monday through Friday, eight-hour-day pattern but, depending on the services the department provides, may need evening or weekend coverage to handle specific functions that must be provided 24 hours per day, seven days a week. The emergency department registration function is one where 24-hour coverage may be necessary. Understanding the type and volume of work that needs to be done during specific time frames, along with knowing the number and type of staff available, is critical to effective scheduling.

### Shift Rotation and Shift Differential

Employee schedules may involve **shift rotation** and shift differential depending on departmental needs. Rotation among morning, afternoon, and evening shifts is not the ideal scheduling situation but is often necessary when coverage is needed, and personnel have not been specifically hired to work afternoons or evenings on a regular basis. Specific start and end times should be determined for every shift, and a reasonable amount of time should elapse between the time an individual ends one shift and begins another. An employer should allow adequate time off between shifts to avoid employee fatigue; however, there is no state or federal law requiring a minimum amount of time off between shifts (Stone 2019). Time spent on the more undesirable shifts should not exceed time spent on the preferred shift. It may be prudent to adopt **cyclical staffing**, which is the rotation of work schedule for a group of employees to allow for a fair distribution of day, evening, and weekend shifts for each person within the group. **Float employees**, staff that are cross-trained in several departmental functions, may be used to enable this scheduling.

In situations where weekend coverage is an issue, employees should have at least alternate weekends off. Many employers pay a slightly higher hourly wage to employees who work less desirable shifts (evening, night, or weekend). This is referred to as a **shift differential**. Under the Fair Labor Standards Act, an employer is not required to pay a shift differential (DOL n.d.), but it may be beneficial for employee morale and retention.

Mandatory work functions and the minimal staff needed to cover them should be defined by the manager when determining weekend or holiday coverage. All employees should participate in holiday and weekend rotation. Employees may be required to provide their own holiday or weekend replacements but should not be responsible for providing replacements when their absence is due to illness.

### Vacation and Absentee Coverage

To keep productivity optimal, the HIM manager must plan appropriately for vacation staffing and absentee coverage. Temporary staff hired to cover for vacationing employees, the use of cross-trained or float staff, or extra hours for existing staff may be options but are not always financially feasible. Moreover, some positions are too complex to be filled with temporary employees. For example, due to the complexity of the role, it is unlikely that a temporary assistant director could be hired to fill in for an assistant director on a two-week vacation. In such a case, key tasks that must be performed should be identified and distributed appropriately among staff who will handle them while the employee is on vacation. Generally, lengthy staff absences can add undue stress on the remaining employees and adversely affect department service levels. Thus, it is advisable to ensure there is a plan for when a lengthy absence is expected.

### Alternate Work Schedules

Today's work environment has not only accepted but also seeks work scheduling alternatives to the regular 40-hour workweek when possible; the following are examples:

- **Compressed workweek**: A week in which more hours are combined within fewer days (for example, four 10-hour days, three 12-hour days, seven 10-hour days with seven days off [seven on/seven off], and so on).
- **Flextime**: Employees choose their arrival and departure times around a fixed core work time. For example, if management feels full coverage is essential between 10 a.m. and 2 p.m., employees could start as early as 5:30 a.m. or end as late as 6:30 p.m. and still provide the department with core coverage.
- **Job sharing**: Divides one job between two part-time employees, each with partial benefits (as they apply). Job sharing may work well in some

cases, but it also can be problematic depending on the compatibility of the two individuals involved. And should one person terminate employment, finding a compatible new job-sharing partner could present a challenge.

In general, the benefits to employers of alternative work schedules include easier staff recruitment and better retention, increased morale, decreased absence and tardiness, and some productivity improvements. For employees, the benefits can include less home stress, reduced commuting time, and a perception of greater autonomy in the workplace.

### Telecommuting

With a **telecommuting** option, employees work full- or part-time in their own homes. The first employees in HIM departments to take advantage of telecommuting were transcriptionists; they were soon followed by coding professionals. The EHR has enabled even more employees to work remotely including employees performing discharge analysis, abstracting, auditing, and reporting. The advantages of this type of work scheduling are that it saves space in the department, reduces long commutes to the workplace, retains employees who prefer to be home, and offers work opportunities to the physically challenged. On the other hand, employers may feel a loss of control when employees telecommute. And some employees in alternative work situations, such as telecommuters, need contact with other employees to avoid feeling disconnected from the department.

### Outsourcing

In some cases, flexible job arrangements may not be an option or solve a staffing issue. A potential solution to the problem of a shortage of qualified staff is **outsourcing**. In this arrangement, the organization contracts with an independent company with expertise in a specific job function. The outside company then assumes full responsibility for performing the function rather than just supplying staff. Outsourcing (domestic and offshore) provides access to staff as needed, even in a tight labor market; frees up internal resources for other things; eliminates some process or service headaches; provides access to the newest technologies quickly; offers lower labor cost; and may accelerate change. **Offshoring** is a type of outsourcing where a company's workforce is based overseas. Jobs most suitable for offshoring have the following characteristics:

- No face-to-face customer service requirements
- Work is easily documented with written rules and procedures
- High wage differential with workers in the destination country
- Low social networking requirement
- No need to understand the customer's culture (Lee and Mather 2008)

The challenges with outsourcing for the health information manager include less immediate control over the quantity and quality of the work, the need to know negotiation techniques and contract language, reliance on the vendor, and the need to understand protections for both patient and employee data. The Health Insurance Portability and Accountability Act (HIPAA) requires special arrangements regarding security and confidentiality for outsourcing contractors (covered entities) (HHS 2003). In an outsourced environment, the health information manager's responsibility shifts from supervising employees to managing a vendor relationship.

Outsourcing occurs in any number of health information functions including transcription, ROI, document imaging, coding, and registries. The outsourcing company may perform the functions either at the facility or partially or completely off-site. Advances in secure communication and EHRs have resulted in many remote workers being employed by such independent companies.

When healthcare organizations decide to use outsourcing, a manager is challenged to select the most appropriate vendor to provide the services desired. Specific key factors to consider when selecting a vendor or partner include a commitment to quality, high level of collaboration, advanced technology, outsourcing experience, strong staff training, reasonable and clear cost, positive references and reputation, common goals, flexible contract terms, and effective employee policies.

Senior executive support is a requisite for achieving success when adopting an outsourcing vendor or contracted service. The administration's confidence in the process is essential to creating the seamlessness necessary for continued, smooth, functional operation. Administrative support can best be engaged when the manager understands the organization's goals for each outsourcing or contracted service effort being planned. Selecting the right vendor is a definite variable for successful outsourcing.

Suggestions for successful outsourcing arrangements include the following:

- Seeking assistance from someone skilled in negotiation when developing the contract with the vendor
- Engaging legal counsel to review the language of the contract to ensure it complies with HIPAA and other regulatory requirements

- Requiring competitive bidding for each outsourced service at regular intervals
- Establishing quality expectations and key performance indicators for contractors
- Monitoring compliance with performance indicators
- Performing periodic customer surveys to assess satisfaction with the service

Effective management of the relationship between the healthcare organization and the outsourcing partner includes properly constructed contracts, open communication and collaboration among partners, and careful attention to personnel issues. Careful review and evaluation of the functions and performance of the outsourced staff regarding contract requirements is critical to a successful outsourcing arrangement.

As in any outsourcing arrangement, quality control and compliance with privacy and security standards for both patient and employee information are important issues to be addressed in contracts and performance monitoring.

### Contracting for Services

While outsourcing seeks a vendor to assume full responsibility for performing a function, contracting for services seeks an arrangement to supply staff to only assist with maintaining or enhancing a function. The organization maintains responsibility for that function. When a manager is planning to contract for staffing typically in a transitional or temporary situation, various types of arrangements can be considered, including the following:

- *Full service:* Contracting for enough staff to handle a complete function within the department; for example, the ROI function
- *Project-based:* Contracting for staff to focus on completion of a specific project; for example, a master patient index (MPI) cleanup in which duplicate records are resolved
- *Temporary:* Contracting for staff to cover for a temporary situation to keep productivity in line; for example, a coding backlog due to staff vacancy, vacations, or a learning curve on a new system or technology

Clear definitions of the work or services needed as well as the performance expectations are crucial to a successful contract for services. **Service level agreements (SLAs)** provide this detail in writing, plus price and payment terms, the reporting chain of command, terms for termination of the relationship, and privacy, security, and confidentiality expectations of the contracted staff.

## Work Procedures

Management has the responsibility to develop procedures for employees that fully aid them in effectively and efficiently carrying out their job functions. A **job procedure** is a structured, action-oriented list of sequential steps involved in carrying out a specific job or solving a problem.

### Procedure Writing Guidelines

To be effective, procedure writing requires considerable attention to detail. The following criteria facilitate the development of well-written procedures:

- Display the title of the procedure accurately and clearly.
- Number each step of the procedure for easy reference.
- Begin each activity with an action verb.
- Keep sentences short and concise.
- Include only procedures, not policies. Policy manuals should be maintained as separate documents, though it is appropriate to include references to related policies or a policy statement within the procedure so the employee can easily locate the policy as may be necessary or desired.
- Identify logical beginning and end points to simplify directions.
- Consider the audience and construct the procedure to be of most help to that audience. For example, new staff, temporary staff, or cross-trained staff who perform these procedures only occasionally need a basic, simplified version to ensure completion of a new or seldom-performed task.

In addition, the written procedure should provide completed samples of forms used during the procedure.

It is effective to have an experienced employee who does the job write (or at least draft) the procedure because he or she knows it best. Supervisory personnel should collect all the written procedures and determine whether they are complete and follow a consistent format. Supervisory personnel are also responsible for ensuring procedures are reviewed at least annually and updated in a timely way when the procedure is modified.

### Procedure Formats

When determining the appropriate format for a procedure, the HIM manager needs to consider the audience and the complexity of the task. The following are formats that can be followed for procedural documentation:

- **Narrative**: Narrative formats are the most common for procedure writing. The author details the processes of the procedure in a step-by-step descriptive method.
- **Playscript**: This format describes each player in the procedure, the action of the player, and the player's responsibility regarding the process from the start to completion of a specific task within the procedure.
- **Flowchart**: A flowchart is a visual illustration of the procedure using standard flowcharting symbols. These symbols are provided in various software programs to depict the steps associated with a procedure.

Sometimes a combination of formats is used. However, whatever format is chosen, all procedures should be available to employees at any time.

### Procedure Manuals

A **procedure manual** is a compilation of all of the procedures used in a specific unit, department, or organization. Procedure manuals may be kept as hard copies that have been printed and bound together in a book or binder, or they may be maintained on an organization's secure website or intranet. The valuable aspects associated with procedure manuals include promoting teamwork, promoting consistency in employee work, reducing training time, establishing guidance on work unit standards, documenting expectations, and answering employee questions.

The manual's content and format are relatively straightforward. Procedure manuals should include the following elements:

- *Titles:* Name of the facility, name of the manual, name of the department, and date
- *Foreword:* Paragraph form, purpose of manual, suggestion for use by employees
- *Table of contents:* List of all procedures in the manual referenced to page number
- *Job procedures:* Step-by-step job procedures and the forms used in each procedure, including completed forms together with explanations to ensure accurate use of forms
- *General rules and regulations:* Information that includes department- or unit-specific details often influenced by state or federal law and regulatory agencies
- *Index:* Alphabetical list of topics covered in the manual (optional)

Procedure manuals are particularly important for work units with a variety of duties or staff who may not routinely do the same tasks. An updated, organized procedure manual readily available and in a standardized format saves employees time and ensures accurate results.

---

### Check Your Understanding 24.2

**Answer the following questions in a separate document.**

1. ABC Hospital has recently had a shortage of coding staff due to one person being out on a maternity leave and two open positions posted for over a month with no experienced applicants at this time. The coding manager is determining whether she should temporarily outsource until staffing is back to the expected level, permanently outsource some of the coding volume, or continue to recruit and offer extra hours to existing staff. Evaluate the pros and cons of each option in this scenario and present your recommendation along with rationale.

2. Differentiate the three procedure formats. If you were a new ROI specialist, which procedure format would you prefer? Explain why.

3. The HIM operations manager, Angela, has noticed productivity is dropping, yet employees seem to be very busy. What do you suggest Angela do to address the situation?

4. Differentiate flextime, job sharing, and the compressed workweek as three unique alternatives to the regular 40-hour staffing schedule. Identify a scenario in the HIM profession or from your own experience where you think each would work well as an alternative schedule.

5. As the registration manager, you have been asked to staff the new urgent care clinic with your registration staff working at the family practice clinic. The registration staff currently works Monday through Friday from 7 a.m. to 5 p.m. You will now need to incorporate evenings and weekends into their schedule. What scheduling considerations will you use for staffing the new urgent care clinic?

## Performance and Work Measurement Standards

Work is the task to be performed; performance is the execution of the task. Effective management involves discerning what work is to be done, what performance standards are achievable and appropriate, how performance can be measured in terms of efficiency and effectiveness, and how performance can be monitored for variances from the standards set. Employees want to know for which tasks they are responsible, what is expected of them, and how they are performing relative to that expectation. Through performance standard setting and measurement processes, managers can confirm the level of success of a work unit or identify opportunities for improvement.

A standard may be defined as a performance criterion established by custom or authority for the purpose of assessing factors such as quality, productivity, and performance. Managers are responsible for controlling all the resources available to them, including human resources (staff), materials (supplies), machines (equipment), methods (procedures), and money (budget). Thus, managers are expected to set standards for each of these resources and then use them as ways to assess the quality, productivity, and performance of those resources. Performance standards should be aligned with the mission and goals of the organization.

### Criteria for Setting Effective Standards

To create viable, significant standards, it is important to be aware of the criteria commonly considered as the foundation for developing effective standard setting. Effective standards are as follows:

- *Understandable:* The person(s) affected by the standard knows what it means, and it makes sense to him or her.
- *Attainable:* It is reasonable to expect that the person(s) affected by the standard can achieve it.
- *Equitable:* If more than one person is affected by the standard, all are held accountable for it.
- *Significant:* Meeting the standard is important to the goals of the work unit or organization; the effort it takes to meet the standard is worth it.
- *Legitimate:* The standard has been formally accepted within the organization and is documented in appropriate places and ways.
- *Economical:* The standard can be met and monitored without incurring costs that are beyond the value of that which is gained by having it. In other words, achieving the standard must be worth the expense associated with achieving it.

### Types of Standards

Standards are worded differently at various levels within the organization depending on whether they reflect a goal or an objective. A goal is a generalized statement of a unit, department, or organization standard. An objective is a statement of the result in measurable terms with time and cost limits, as applicable. The development of specific objectives can bring goals to a practical, working level (Dunn 2021). For example, the HIM department might have a general standard (often called a *goal*) for its document creation function to support patient care through accurate and timely auditing of medical reports. The standard may then be stated in objective form to make it more specific and measurable; for example, to audit routine history and physical, operative, and consultation reports within eight hours of creation. Note that this objective is related directly to the timeliness aspect of the preceding goal statement.

#### Qualitative and Quantitative Standards

Objective-level standards are commonly characterized in two ways—as quantitative standards and qualitative standards.

Qualitative standards specify the level of service expected from a function, such as the following:

- *Accuracy rate:* For example, assignment of diagnostic and procedure codes for inpatient records is at least 98 percent accurate.
- *Error rate:* For example, mistakes in the assignment of diagnostic and procedure codes occur in no more than two percent of inpatient records coded.
- *Turnaround time:* For example, dictation must be transcribed within 12 hours.
- *Response time:* For example, requests for information are responded to within three working days of receipt.

**Quantitative standards** specify the level of measurable work, or **productivity**, expected for a specific function, such as the following:

- *Number of units of work per specified period:* For example, 70 records audited per full-time employee per day
- *Amount of time allotted per unit of work:* For example, no more than 15 minutes to code one inpatient record

Quantity standards (also called productivity standards) and quality standards (also known as service standards) are generally used by managers to monitor individual employee performance and the performance of a functional unit or the department. They are also used for planning, staffing, and budgeting purposes. To properly communicate performance standards, managers need to make the distinction between quantitative and qualitative standards and identify examples of each for the HIM functions.

### Key Indicators

**Key indicators** are current measurement thresholds that alert a department or work unit to its existing level of service. Common key indicator examples include the following:

- Transcription turnaround time
- Days outstanding in accounts receivable (A/R)
- ROI turnaround time
- Percentage of incomplete records

The following red flag indicators are examples that would move a department manager to take corrective action:

- The number and severity of complaints increase. When the number or severity of complaints increases, the circumstances surrounding the complaints must be assessed immediately so corrections to the process or personnel involved can be made.
- Compliance surveys to assess performance on accreditation, legal, or regulatory standards indicate that the organization has failed to comply in one or more areas. When this occurs, the organization needs to correct the variance(s) as soon as possible and return to compliance.

Key indicators allow managers to monitor critical service standards on a current and ongoing basis so they can make timely staffing or process adjustments to ensure that department service performance remains as expected.

## Methods of Communicating Standards

After standards have been created, they must be communicated to staff. All the given types of standards can be provided to staff in several ways:

- Written specifications: In job descriptions, performance evaluation forms, equipment specification sheets, and forms design guidelines
- Documented rules, regulations, or policies: In policy manuals, regulations or accreditation manuals, and employee handbooks
- Demonstration models: In samples, videos, and computer-based learning modules
- Verbal confirmations: In departmental or work unit meetings or individual employee counseling sessions

Whatever the method of communication deemed most appropriate, it is critical that employees are aware of departmental standards so they can be successful in meeting them.

## Methods of Developing Standards

Several methods can be employed to develop performance standards in a work unit. Two approaches are commonly used: benchmarking comparable performance and measuring actual performance.

### Benchmarking Comparable Performance

**Benchmarking** is the systematic comparison of the products, services, and outcomes of one organization with those of a similar organization, or the systematic comparison of one organization's outcomes with regional or national standards such as professional associations and standard-setting organizations. Internal benchmarking may also be performed. Benchmarking against a prior period within a department or function, or benchmarking against a higher-performing but similar department, unit, or service line can be effective. To engage in a benchmarking effort, the manager should first select key functions of the department to benchmark (for example, coding, documentation creation, or ROI). Relating benchmarks to the specific process is critical. Thought must be given to the type of performance measure(s) desired as indicators (for example, for coding, dollars remaining in A/R due to uncoded records and dollars remaining in A/R due to coding disputes; for documentation creation, turnaround time [creation to audit] for consultations, operative reports, history, and physicals).

When the key functional areas have been selected and the types of indicators identified, the research for benchmarks (preferably) available through published sources can begin. Investigation of benchmark standards gathered through this research must also involve a critical assessment of their relevance to the department's specific situation; then, the standard can be successfully sold to the rest of the entity. Benchmarking involves the following steps:

1. Identifying peer organizations and departments that have achieved outstanding performance based on some key indicator (for example, 98 percent of health records coded within two days post discharge)
2. Studying the best practices within these organizations that make it possible to achieve that performance level
3. Acting to implement those best practices in one's own organization to achieve a similar performance

Before officially adopting a benchmark standard, a manager should routinely gather performance data in the department to compare actual performance against the benchmark and then evaluate factors in department processes that must be changed to eventually move actual performance into the benchmark range.

## Measuring Actual Performance

**Work measurement** is the process of studying the amount of work accomplished and the amount of time it takes to accomplish it. It involves the collection of data relevant to the work, such as the amount of work accomplished per unit of time. Its purpose is to define and monitor productivity.

Work measurement can support a manager in many activities, including the following:

- Setting production standards
- Determining staffing requirements
- Establishing incentive pay systems
- Determining direct costs by function
- Comparing performance to standards
- Identifying activities for process and methods improvement

Gathering the information available through work measurement efforts will be invaluable to the manager in making administrative decisions. When selecting the work measurement technique that best suits the department or work unit, the manager should consider the following factors:

- Amount of financial resources available
- Availability of qualified personnel to take part in the study
- Amount of time available to devote to study
- Attitudes of employees toward participation in a study

Work measurement can be accomplished through various techniques. Analysis of historical or past performance data generally uses work volume (direct or estimated) and hours paid from past records to establish the standard. When using historical data, managers are cautioned to keep in mind that volume figures are not adjusted for the level of quality, and the number of hours paid is different from the number of hours worked.

**Employee self-logging** is a form of self-reporting in which the employees track their tasks, volume of work units, and hours worked. **Volume logs** are sometimes used to document information about the volume of work units received and processed in a day by keeping track of the number of products produced or activities done. (See table 24.2.)

The scientific methods of work measurement include time studies and the use of preestablished time and unit standards. For example, time studies use a stopwatch to record and document the time required to accomplish a specified task.

**Work sampling** is a technique of work measurement that involves using statistical probability (determined through random sample observations) to characterize the performance of the department and its functional work units.

Each of the work measurement techniques offers calculations of employee productivity in either unit per measure of time or time per unit.

**Table 24.2.** Sample volume log

| Task | Number of worked hours | Number of units |
|---|---|---|
| Coding | 40 | 120 records |
| ROI | 36 | 85 requests |

The coding standard calculates at three records per worked hour for this employee (120 records/40 hours) and an ROI standard of 2.4 requests per worked hour (85 requests/36 hours). It does not capture any interruptions or unworked time in the eight-hour day, but is a simple way to arrive at a ballpark figure.

## Check Your Understanding 24.3

Answer the following questions in a separate document.

1. Sarah is using benchmarking to develop coding standards for her hospital coders. In her research within the geographic region, she learns there is not a common standard. Explain why one hospital may have different productivity standards for coders than another hospital.
2. Analyze the following standard and determine if it is qualitative or quantitative. Give your rationale. "Answer all phone calls by the third ring."
3. Develop one quantitative and one qualitative standard that is not already used as an example in the chapter. Consider your own work experience or experience as a student.
4. The outpatient coding manager wants to know the amount of work being done in her department for future planning. She needs the information by the end of the week. Her staff tends to react negatively when they are asked about their productivity. What work measurement technique would you suggest she use? Why?
5. Why would the coding staff ask their manager to perform a work measurement study in their work unit? Describe how you would feel if a work measurement study was being done in your work unit.

# Performance Measurement

**Performance measurement** is the process of comparing the outcomes of an organization, work unit, or employee to preestablished performance standards. Performance measurement is used to assess quality and productivity in clinical services and in administrative services. Examples of performance measures maintained by acute-care hospitals in clinical services include the rate of nosocomial infection, the percentage of surgical complications, the average length of stay, and the ratio of live births to stillbirths. Examples of performance measures maintained by an administrative service such as the HIM department include lines transcribed, turnaround time for ROI requests, and days in A/R due to uncoded patient discharges.

Performance measurement is a fundamental management activity that supports two of the basic functions of management—planning and controlling. The planning function is concerned with defining the expectations of performance (standards or objectives), the processes required for achieving those expectations (procedures), and the desired outcomes of performance (goals). The goals, objectives, standards, and processes established during the planning process become the criteria used in the control process to evaluate actual performance.

## Performance Controls

In the control process, specific monitors, or controls, are established for the purpose of identifying undesirable circumstances occurring in a work process that could lead to an undesirable outcome; the intent is to introduce appropriate intervention into the process.

The characteristics of effective performance controls include the following:

- Flexibility refers to the fact that controls must be adaptable to real changes in the requirements of a process. For example, a budget is a control on the use of money. Money budgeted in one category (equipment) may need to be spent in another category (travel) because of a change in a program or a new law or regulation.
- Simplicity refers to the fact that those involved in the process must find the controls understandable and reasonable. For example, ROI specialists agree that responding to requests for information within 48 hours of receipt is a clear and achievable expectation.
- Economy implies that controls should not cost more than they are worth. The time and money spent to implement a control should be in line with the level of risk (loss) involved if the process fails to meet performance expectations. For example, potential loss of a life calls for a significant investment in controls; potential criminal liability calls for significant investment in controls; while the potential for having to pay for a day of overtime to correct clerical errors calls for a minimal investment in controls.
- Timeliness suggests that controls should be implemented to detect potential variances within a time frame that allows for corrective

action before any adverse effect has occurred. For example, the accuracy of a health record number assignment should be confirmed at the time of registration or the coding checked before a bill is transmitted to avoid the adverse effects associated with errors that are then transmitted to other areas of the organization or outside the organization.

- Focus on exceptions demands controls be targeted at those aspects of a process that are most likely to vary significantly from expectations. For example, a new registration specialist who is likely to make more errors that could do damage to customer service ratings is generally monitored (controlled) more closely and more frequently than one who is experienced and has performed well for the past year.

There are two general types of controls—preventive (self-correcting) and feedback (non-self-correcting). **Preventive controls** are front-end processes that guide work in such a way that input and process variations are minimized. Simple things such as standard operating procedures, edits on data entered in computer-based systems, calendar notifications, use of work queues, and training processes are ways to reduce the potential for error by using preventive controls.

**Feedback controls** are back-end processes that monitor and measure output and then compare it to expectations and identify variations. Variations must be analyzed so corrective action plans can be developed and implemented. Some may be self-regulating (such as thermostatic systems or pacemakers), but most are non-self-regulating, meaning they require intervention by an oversight agent (a supervisor, manager, or auditor) to identify the variance and take action to correct it. A customer survey or routine performance reviews are examples of this type of control.

## Variance Analysis

In the context of performance measurement, when variations are identified (that is, actual performance does not meet or significantly exceeds expectations), further analysis is needed. Analysis of the resources involved in the work (people, procedures, supplies, equipment, and money) is conducted to help determine what, if any, changes should be made. Changes may involve activities such as additional staff training, modifications in procedures, adjustments in workflow, revision of policies, or purchases of updated equipment. As a result, the analysis and the changes to address findings may also lead to revisions in performance criteria and expectations.

## Assessment of Departmental Performance

When establishing a performance assessment program, the steps in the control (evaluation) process include the following:

1. Monitoring and measuring outcomes through established performance indicators
2. Comparing performance against established goals
3. Identifying variances between the actual performance and the target goals
4. Determining potential causes for variance
5. Developing an action plan to address the variance
6. Implementing the action plan
7. Continuing to monitor and measure outcomes to assess whether the action plan has resulted in improved performance

It is not enough to measure and compare the measurements to goals and target measures; it is also important to identify and evaluate any variances, develop and implement action plans, and measure again to see if positive changes have been made. If not, the causes for variance must again be assessed and further action taken until performance indicators are met.

### Monitoring and Measuring Performance

Monitoring and measuring performance involve taking an aggregate look at performance over a period of time. Options include operating with an employee self-reporting method such as self-logging, using computerized monitoring to audit productivity, manually auditing work samples, or relying on customer feedback to measure performance.

Effective outcomes performance monitoring depends on both employee performance measurement and management execution. The focus of the effort is on service indicators such as turnaround time, cost and revenue reports, and customer feedback. Consider this practical application of department outcomes performance monitoring. Assume that one established expectation of the department is that routine response to an authorized ROI request occurs within five working days of receipt of the request in the department.

The first step in controlling this function would be to set up data collection and reporting to obtain information that can be used to monitor the time it takes the department to respond to a routine ROI. (See table 24.3.)

**Table 24.3.** ROI variance report

| On June 6, 20XX, total routine ROI requests in processing: 130 | | | | | |
|---|---|---|---|---|---|
| Days since receipt | 6–10 days | 11–15 days | 16–20 days | >20 days | Summary |
| Number of total requests | 12<br>9% | 15<br>12% | 2<br>2% | 1<br>1% | 30<br>24% |
| **Reasons** | | | | | |
| Unable to locate record | 0 | 2 | 0 | 1 | 3<br>10% |
| Incomplete record | 12 | 12 | 2 | 0 | 26<br>87% |
| Issue with authorization | 0 | 0 | 0 | 0 | 0 |
| Unavailable record | 0 | 1 | 0 | 0 | 1<br>3% |
| Other | 0 | 0 | 0 | 0 | 0 |

Next, the department should determine the kinds of controls it wants to establish. The department wants to monitor routine requests, but how are routine requests defined? A routine request may be any request that is not urgent (that is, it does not have to be handled within minutes, hours, or some stipulated amount of time under five working days). For example, a subpoena for a record that must be handled within three days or a request for a record needed for an appointment in a clinic the next morning would not be considered a routine request.

The line related to ROI turnaround time (TAT) in the middle of the performance report shown in table 24.4 indicates the average number of days it took the HIM department to respond to routine ROI requests in January (3), February (3), March (6), and April (5). This report may also be electronically displayed as an easy-to-read dashboard.

The average turnaround time is calculated by dividing the total response days attributed to the volume of routine requests responded to within the reporting period by the volume of routine requests responded to. For example, if the department responded to 300 routine requests in the month of May and 100 were responded to in six days, 100 in two days, and 100 in four days, the average turnaround time in May would be four days:

$$\frac{(600 \text{ days} + 200 \text{ days} + 400 \text{ days})}{300 \text{ requests}}$$
$$= 4 \text{ days (average)}$$

Having the information monthly to include as part of the regular performance reporting within the department allows the manager to review monthly trends and identify potential focus areas for future process improvement activities.

The underlying data indicate that a considerable number of requests are not responded to within the five-working-days standard set by management (for example, 100 [or 33 percent] were responded to in six working days). In this case, the direct supervisor of the ROI function would likely want access to data of this

**Table 24.4.** Sample health information services performance report

| Indicator | January 20XX | February 20XX | March 20XX | April 20XX |
|---|---|---|---|---|
| Discharge equivalents | 5,000 | 5,400 | 5,360 | 5,500 |
| Labor cost per discharge equivalent (DCE): <$10.00 | $10.00 | 9.25 | 9.33 | 9.90 |
| FTE budgeted at 50 | 50 | 50 | 50 | 48 |
| Coding: Days in A/R due to uncoded records <5 days | 3 | 5 | 4 | 5 |
| Document Creation: TAT for History & Physicals (H & Ps) <24 hours | 12 | 16 | 18 | 26 |
| ROI requests received | 200 | 245 | 300 | 260 |
| Release of info: TAT ≤5 days | 3 | 3 | 6 | 5 |
| Resignations: <1% | 0 | 0 | 0 | 2/50 = 4% |

nature more often than once a month. For example, a weekly report showing the number of routine requests in the system for five days or more that have not yet been answered would allow the supervisor or ROI clerk to identify problem requests and take corrective actions over the course of the following week.

## Comparing Performance to Established Goals and Standards

The next step in monitoring and measuring outcome performance is to compare current performance against established goals (standards). Continuing with the example in the preceding section, when comparing performance against the standard performance indicator of responding to routine ROIs within five days, the data in table 24.4 show an upward trend in March and April.

When comparisons are done, the manager should evaluate any variances and develop an action plan specific to each. Action plans can be additional staff training, modifications in procedures, adjustments in workflow, revision of policies, purchase of updated equipment, and others. For example, in an evaluation of the performance variance in responding to routine ROI requests, the direct supervisor would likely begin to collect data that will provide the following types of information to uncover the factors that triggered the variances (see table 24.3):

- How many open ROI requests exist with a date of receipt of more than five working days?
- What is the aging profile of those open ROI requests; that is, how many are 6 to 10 working days, 10 to 15 working days, 16 to 20 working days, or more than 20 days?
- What are the reasons the requests are still open?
- In what time increments since receipt of the requests has the requesting party been notified of the delay and the reason for the delay?

After the variances have been evaluated, an action plan can be formulated to address areas for performance improvement:

- Establish a procedure to ensure weekly contact with the requestor to determine continuing need for the information and to update the status of the request.
- Flag the incomplete record with ROI REQUEST PENDING to ensure it is routed to ROI immediately when required documentation is complete.
- Hold a staff in-service to ensure all employees understand the policies and procedures impacting the turnaround time requirements.

The supervisor, working with the ROI staff, will take the actions put forth in the plan and then continue to monitor the ROI function to determine if the actions taken are effective in resolving the identified performance variance.

## Check Your Understanding 24.4

Answer the following questions in a separate document.

1. Differentiate between preventive controls and feedback controls. Develop one preventive control and one feedback control related to your school or your personal life.
2. Develop one preventive control and one feedback control for ensuring an accurate MPI.
3. Describe which functions of management are evident in performance management and the rationale for your answer.
4. Anne is the ROI supervisor. As a part of her role, she noticed when reviewing performance measures that the turnaround time for requests was about 24 hours higher than the established goal last month. She looked at the schedule for the month and realized one of the staff members was on vacation that month. She noted that as the variance justification and filed her report.
Evaluate Anne's process. Will the turnaround time meet the established goals next month? Why or why not?
5. Recommend changes or actions a manager might take to address performance issues revealed when he or she completes an analysis of performance variances in the department.

# Performance Improvement

**Performance improvement** is the continuous study and adaptation of a healthcare organization's functions and processes to increase the likelihood of achieving desired outcomes. The reason managers set performance standards and routinely measure departmental performance against those standards is to ensure the department is serving its internal and external customers in ways that meet their needs and expectations. A natural outcome of any performance measurement system is the identification of variances from performance expectations and thus the opportunity to engage in performance improvement activities to bring performance back into line.

Performance improvement requires an appreciation and knowledge of how systems and processes work together. Whether improvement is a result of incremental or radical changes, a thoughtful approach to assessing existing and designing new workflows is important.

## The Role of Customer Service

All performance improvement efforts today focus on the customer and work to create a true customer orientation within the work environment by listening and responding to customers, thinking about their needs, and using that information to improve.

To focus on customer orientation, management and staff should do the following:

- Identify the key processes in the department or organization.
- Identify the customers of those processes.
- Define quality and expectations from a customer perspective.
- Develop and collect quality measures to meet expectations for the identified key processes.
- Evaluate and continuously monitor performance measures to ensure expectations are being met.

Customers are the people, external and internal, who receive and are affected by the work of the organization or department. They have names and needs and are the reason(s) for the collective work of the organization.

**Internal customers** are located within the organization. They may be anyone within the work unit who is affected by the HIM functions. Physicians and clinical staff need high-quality, expedient patient health information to deliver high-quality patient care. Administrative staff members are customers of the information harvested from collective databases for use in planning facilities and services. The HIM department staff are customers who work in each of the functional areas and rely on each other in various ways to get their work done.

**External customers** reside outside the organization. Patients seen by providers are considered external customers, as are payers who need information so they can reimburse their enrollees in a timely manner. Regulatory agencies look to HIM for data on conditions of accreditation or participation. Vendors assist HIM, with the department's direct input, in making optimal selections of products. Public health agencies look to HIM for information and data on the health status of the community population to earmark services the population needs to maintain a healthy existence.

## Identification of Performance Improvement Opportunities

In a department that employs performance standards and engages in routine performance measurement, opportunities for improvement present themselves as a natural outcome of that effort. Even when a department is lacking a formal performance measurement program, the following can be seen as symptoms of performance problems:

- Inaccuracies and errors in work
- Complaints from customers
- Delays in getting things done or lots of interruptions
- Low employee morale or high rates of absenteeism or turnover
- Poor safety records and on-the-job injuries

When any of these issues are observed, they indicate performance is not meeting expectations and there are opportunities for improvement. An investigation of underlying cause(s) is required, and appropriate actions must be taken so the performance issues can be resolved. Issues related to workflow or process, ineffective procedures, inadequate training, faulty equipment, or a poor work environment may all need to be reviewed.

Collecting meaningful performance data, being alert, and observing and listening to customers and key staff are all ways to identify improvement opportunities. It is a continuous improvement culture that has no tolerance for complacency. Excellence is not an accident; it is an intended outcome that requires a manager's commitment and continuous attention.

## Principles of Performance Improvement

The concepts of performance improvement, work improvement, process improvement, and methods improvement all relate to a management philosophy that is, at its core, systems oriented. It views the work processes in an organization as being systematic in nature and seeks to constantly improve them by adjusting various components of the system.

Process improvement consists of a series of actions taken to identify, analyze, and improve existing processes. It includes methodologies that inform and further the goal of performance improvement.

A system is a set of related components that work together to achieve a common purpose and the desired outcomes. Systems come in manual, automated, and hybrid forms. A system is made up of the following components:

- *Input*: Resources available to the system, namely human resources (staff), materials (supplies), machines (equipment), methods (procedures), and money (budget).
- *Process:* The transformation of the inputs. What is done to or with the inputs that result in something being accomplished?
- *Output*: The finished product or the result of the process, such as an educated student, a transcribed report, a coded record, and such.
- *Controls and standards*: The expectations of what the output should be and the mechanisms in place to monitor, track, and observe how well actual performance measures up to expectations.
- *Feedback*: Information reported when output is compared to the standards to identify how well actual output met standards (desired output). Feedback sometimes comes in the form of customer complaints, and certainly feedback can and should come in the form of compliments to staff as well, when performance expectations are met.
- *External environment*: Anything outside the system that affects how the system functions (for example, laws or regulations set by the local, state, or federal government). In HIM departments, examples of external factors that affect its systems include the following:
  - The HIPAA regulations related to patient information confidentiality and security
  - Joint Commission or other accrediting body requirements related to patient care and documentation
  - Medicare severity diagnosis-related groups (MS-DRGs) and Present on Admission (POA) regulations that impact coding and reimbursement systems in hospitals
  - A tight labor market, which makes it difficult to hire well-qualified employees for specialized jobs

Open systems are those systems affected by what is going on around them and must adjust as the environment changes. These are systems that cannot function in isolation; they must consider influences outside of the system itself. For example, the healthcare system is an open system; it must adjust to external influences such as HIPAA regulations, Joint Commission standards, economic status, and patient needs. They also can be considered cybernetic systems because they have standards, controls, and feedback mechanisms built into them. On the other hand, a closed system operates in a self-contained environment; that is, it is not affected by outside factors. A mechanical system (engines, motors, and such) is the best example of a closed system.

The aim of all performance, work, method, or process improvement efforts is to increase the effectiveness, efficiency, or the adaptability of the systems that are operating within an organization. These three goals of improvement efforts are described as follows:

- *Effectiveness:* How closely the output of a system matches what is expected of it. If a department is effective, it is getting done what it is supposed to get done.
- *Efficiency:* How well the department is using its resources; that is, is the department getting the most bang for its buck, or is it wasting staff time, money, or other resources?
- *Adaptability:* The ease with which the system can adjust when circumstances require it to change to meet new demands or expectations. Adaptable systems respond appropriately to changing needs.

Organizations need to accomplish their goals with the fewest number of resources while being able to adjust as needed. This is the intent of improvement efforts.

## Check Your Understanding 24.5

**Answer the following questions in a separate document.**

1. Sam has just taken a supervisory position in the HIM department and her first assignment is to develop a departmental performance improvement program. First, she identified the key processes in the department, then she set some performance expectations for each area and measured how the staff was doing against those expectations. She continually monitors and measures performance to ensure the staff is meeting the established expectations, yet she is still hearing complaints from others in the organization. What is Sam missing?

2. Construct a diagram that illustrates the components of a system.

3. Using the diagram constructed in question 2, evaluate the components of the ROI function and apply them to your diagram.

4. Amber works in registration. Several times per day she has an urgent admission who needs to be assigned a bed. The bed placement process requires her to call the appropriate nursing unit based on the patient's diagnosis to request a bed assignment. Amber hates to call the cardiology unit because every time she does, the health unit coordinator is abrupt and tells Amber she must call back later because she is busy with her patients and that "they are her customers." Amber then must call back again, hoping to get results. What is the main issue in this scenario related to improving performance? Name any secondary issues as well.

5. Identify an external customer and an internal customer to a healthcare organization that has not already been named in the chapter. Explain why they would be considered customers.

## Continuous Quality Improvement

**Continuous quality improvement (CQI)** is a management philosophy that emphasizes the importance of knowing and meeting customer expectations, reducing variation within processes, and relying on data to build knowledge for process improvement. Its focus is on improving the quality of services provided to customers, whether internal or external. The approach is to make efforts to meet or exceed customer expectations by conducting small tests of change aimed at improving the quality of services. It can be applied to individuals as well as entities. CQI does not seek to blame problems on individuals but, instead, suggests systems or processes may have inherent flaws that contribute to problems.

CQI seeks to improve the system through small, incremental changes with the expectation that over time the changes will continually improve the quality of care. CQI never stops; it is a way of doing business in which processes are continually improved. To achieve this, CQI relies on the collection and analysis of data that can be used to make informed decisions. Several principles are incorporated into the CQI philosophy. They include constancy of variation, importance of data, vision and support of executive leadership, focus on customers, investment in people, and importance of teams.

Systems will always produce some normal variation in their output; the manager's job is to reduce the amount of variation as much as possible so the process can become more stable and produce a more reliable output. Managers should not assume any variation is a defect but, rather, should monitor and measure data over time to ensure any variation is, in fact, caused inherently by the system. This type of variation is **common cause variation**. A greater-than-expected variation is a **special cause variation**. An example of variation in HIM departments might be found in the coding of records. A coding professional may complete 20 records one day but only 18 the next. The variation is not due to the coding professional's lack of productivity but perhaps to the size of the records that day. In other words, the change is attributed to common cause variation. A significant drop in coding might indicate a special cause is in effect. Perhaps the coding professional was assigned duties in addition to coding that day.

Far too often, decisions for improvement are based on faulty assumptions. CQI recognizes the importance of collecting sufficient data to make informed decisions. An entity must continually collect and analyze data related to performance measures to improve decision-making accuracy, gain consensus when making and implementing decisions, and allow the ability to predict further (ASQ 2023a).

Acceptance of the CQI philosophy must funnel down from the top to truly permeate the organization's culture. Executive leadership must communicate a clear vision and mission statement that every employee can understand and share. To be successful, the entity must know and understand what its customers need and want. One way to obtain customer feedback is to administer satisfaction surveys on a regular basis. Any identified needs should be addressed.

The CQI philosophy assumes people want to do their jobs well. However, some employees may need training on how they can more adequately serve their customers. Management can empower employees by giving them opportunities to learn and grow and feel more competent in performing their jobs. Because CQI seeks to improve processes that may extend beyond the boundaries of individual departments, the people directly involved with the processes must work together. Teams should include individuals with different expertise and from different levels of the organization. Team members should be knowledgeable about portions of the process and able to contribute to the improvement effort. Having members from different areas on the team brings fresh perspectives and opens communication. A good team can also communicate its purpose and activities to other parts of the organization.

CQI attempts to involve people in the examination and improvement of existing systems. Commonly used methods of continuous improvement, such as total quality management, Lean, Six Sigma, and Lean Six Sigma, promote employee involvement and teamwork, work to measure and systematize processes, and reduce variation, defects, and cycle times (ASQ 2023c).

### Total Quality Management (TQM)

**Total quality management (TQM)** offers a way to build in high performance by maximizing employee potential and continuous improvement of process. It uses data, strategy, and effective communications to build a culture of quality. There are eight principles of TQM:

1. Customer-focused: The customer determines the level of quality.
2. Total employee involvement: All employees work toward common goals.
3. Process-centered: There is a focus on process thinking.
4. Integrated system: Differing processes are interconnected.
5. Strategic and system approach: The strategic plan incorporates quality as a key component.
6. Continual improvement: Continual improvement drives the overall entity.
7. Fact-based decision making: Data is continually collected and analyzed to improve decision-making.
8. Communications: Effective communications maintain morale and motivate employees. (ASQ 2023a)

When planning and implementing a quality management system, there is no one solution for every situation or workplace. Each entity is unique in terms of the culture, management practices, and the processes used to create and deliver its products and services (ASQ 2023d).

### Lean

**Lean** is a management strategy in which the core idea is to maximize value while minimizing waste, basically creating more value with fewer resources (Lean Enterprise Institute n.d.). Lean is known for its focus on the reduction of waste and is based on the Japanese success story of Toyota. Toyota's steady growth from a small company to one of the largest automobile companies in the world using Lean principles has made Lean a hot topic in management science in the 21st century.

Lean implementation focuses on eliminating waste and creating a smooth workflow. Through analysis of the process versus a prime focus on the end goal, quality problems are exposed, and waste reduction occurs naturally. The goals of the entity remain the same; the approach toward achieving the goals differs in the Lean methodology. Lean works to eliminate non-value-added work, or waste, brought about by a lack of error detection, confused responsibilities, unnecessary work, disconnects, and workarounds. Waste can be defined as "any action or step in a process that does not add value to the customer" (Skhmot 2017). Lean is about creating a continually improving system that achieves more while using less.

Lean has been applied in many industries, not just manufacturing. It has been used in healthcare with significant improvements in quality and efficiency. The principles of removing activities that do not add value can be applied anywhere. Value in a hospital setting may be described as patient comfort, competent caregivers, or patient discharge after achieving the desired outcomes. Anything that helps treat the patient is value-added; everything else is waste. There are eight areas of waste: waiting, extra-processing, inventory, transportation, motion, overproduction, defects, and unused talent (Skhmot 2017). Examples of how these areas of waste may relate to healthcare are found in table 24.5.

There are several Lean tools and techniques used in manufacturing that have a strong application to

Table 24.5. Eight areas of waste related to healthcare

| Area of waste | Healthcare examples |
|---|---|
| Waiting | Waiting for discharge order, waiting for a report holding up surgery, waiting for long term care placement |
| Extra-processing | Multiple requests for patient demographic information, duplicate lab tests, multiple patient signatures |
| Inventory | Outdated forms kept on hand, excess supplies |
| Transportation | Transporting patients, retrieving health records, transporting medication |
| Motion | Searching for records in various locations, seeking physicians for documentation queries, providers giving care in different locations |
| Overproduction | Creating paperwork for potential surgery patients, preparing extra patient meal trays in case of overflow |
| Defects | Medication errors, assignment of duplicate health record numbers, equipment malfunctions |
| Unused Talent | RNs transporting patient to car following discharge, supervisor covering for data entry staff breaks |

*Source:* Adapted from Skhmot 2017.

the healthcare industry. Following are just a few Lean tools. When they are used, they can uncover large amounts of waste.

- *Root Cause Analysis:* In this technique, the focus is to resolve the underlying problem. The five whys are often used. Simply ask "why" in every situation until you discover the root cause of the problem. Usually, this process takes approximately five tries before the root cause is identified.
- *The five Ss:* The five Ss are *sort, straighten, scrub, standardize,* and *sustain.* This method focuses on cleaning, decluttering and organizing the workstation to minimize waste.
  - Sort—Remove everything that is not used or expected to be used.
  - Straighten—Organize what is kept, have a place for everything.
  - Scrub/Shine—Clean the area.
  - Standardize—Establish procedures to keep the area organized.
  - Sustain—Maintain the gains and avoid backsliding.
- *Visual controls:* The visual controls tool is used to create a workplace where all that is needed is displayed and immediately available.
- *Value stream mapping:* This is a visual method of documenting both material and information flows of a process. It shows both the current and future state of processes to highlight opportunities for improvement.
- *Pull system (Kanban):* This is a method of controlling the flow of resources by replacing only what the customer has consumed. Pull systems consist of production based on actual consumption, small volumes, low inventories, management by sight, and better communication. To create value, services must coincide with demand. (Vorne Industries n.d.)

Identifying the value streams, mapping and understanding each action in the value stream, and identifying and implementing immediate and future improvements using Lean tools and techniques are all a part of building a culture of continuous improvement in the organization.

## Six Sigma

**Six Sigma** is a data-driven methodology for removing defects in any process. Some industry experts doubted that Six Sigma could be applied to the healthcare industry because of the human variability of patients. However, the 2000 Institute of Medicine report highlighting the alarming statistic of up to 98,000 deaths linked to medical errors soon resulted in a movement to review statistical data in the healthcare industry (IOM 2000). Both industry and healthcare are customer driven and rely on feedback regarding success and failure in relevant data. Healthcare leaders became invested in enlisting this philosophy of excellence, reducing costs, lowering lengths of stay, and raising the bar for high-quality healthcare.

Six Sigma uses a scientific methodology that involves the following steps: define, measure, analyze, improve, and control (**DMAIC**).

- Define the problem, improvement opportunity, goals, and customer requirements
- Measure performance
- Analyze the process to determine root causes of variations or poor performance

- Improve the process by addressing the root causes
- Control the improved process and future performance (ASQ 2023b)

The DMAIC process is used in a variety of quality improvement initiatives, not just Six Sigma.

Six Sigma employs many of the same tools used by other quality management systems. In addition, Six Sigma uses soft tools that are not mathematically based. Rather they have a subjective quality to them. Examples of basic soft tools are a set of ground rules, a team agenda, a parking lot to track ideas not immediately pertinent, and activity or progress reports.

Six Sigma focuses on improving management and clinical processes. Statistical analysis is used to find the most defective part of a process, and rigorous control procedures are used to ensure sustained improvement. To achieve Six Sigma, a process must not produce more than 3.4 defects per million opportunities (Feldman 2022).

Six Sigma provides a systematic approach to validate data and focuses on the most meaningful improvements. Successful implementation of Six Sigma in healthcare organizations has produced benefits such as increased productivity, effectiveness, and efficiency; improved quality of products and services, organizational communication and employee engagement, and customer satisfaction; and reduced operating costs, waste, and variation. (Feldman 2022).

As in other quality management concepts, the customer defines acceptable performance with the focus on delivery, quality, and cost. This parallels with the Triple Aim from the Institute for Healthcare Improvement (IHI), consisting of "improving the patient experience of care (including quality and satisfaction), improving the health of populations, and reducing the per capita cost of healthcare" (IHI n.d.).

### Lean Six Sigma

The uses of Lean methods along with Six Sigma techniques have been successful. Despite numerous debates over which methodology is best, it may be that the two methods work quite well together. Lean provides tools to identify and implement value-added activities designed to streamline processes and improve efficiency because of waste reduction. Six Sigma focuses on reducing variation through statistical analysis, validation of data, and measuring improvements. Lean and Six Sigma complement each other with goals aimed toward overall improvement, organizational buy-in, and a culture change that promotes continuous improvement through a structured methodology and identified tools and techniques.

### Basic Continuous Improvement Tools

A number of tools and techniques are frequently used with process improvement initiatives. Some of them are used to facilitate communication among employees; others are used to assist people in determining the root causes of problems. Some tools show areas of agreement or consensus among team members; others permit the display of data for easier analysis. The following section presents a brief description of the tools and techniques commonly used by improvement teams.

***Brainstorming*** Brainstorming is a technique used to generate many creative ideas free of criticism and judgment. It encourages team members to think outside the box and offer ideas. There are some variations in using the technique—one can use an unstructured method for brainstorming or a structured method. The unstructured method involves having a free flow of ideas about a situation. The team leader writes down each idea as it is offered so all can see. There should be no evaluative discussion about the worthiness of the idea because nothing should inhibit the flow of ideas. Each idea is captured and written for the team to consider at a later point (Brassard and Ritter 2020).

Structured brainstorming uses a more formal approach. The team leader asks each person to generate a list of ideas for themselves and then, the team leader proceeds around the room eliciting a new idea, one by one, from each member. The process may take several rounds. As team members run out of new ideas, they pass, and the next person offers an idea until no one can produce any fresh ideas (Brassard and Ritter 2020). Brainstorming is highly effective for identifying several potential processes that may benefit from improvement efforts and for generating solutions to particular problems. It helps people think in new ways, involves them in the process, and facilitates open communication.

***Affinity Diagram*** An affinity diagram allows the team to organize and group similar ideas together. Ideas that are generated in a brainstorming session may be written on sticky notes and arranged on a table or posted on a board. Without talking to each other, each team member is asked to walk around the table or board, look at the ideas, and place them in groupings that seem related or connected to each other. Each member is empowered to move the ideas in a way that makes the most sense. As a team member moves the ideas back or places them in other groupings, the other team members consider the merits of the placement and decide if further action is needed. The goal is to have the team eventually feel comfortable with the arrangement. The natural groupings that emerge are then labeled with a category. This tool brings focus to the many ideas generated. (See figure 24.4.)

***Nominal Group Technique*** Nominal group technique (NGT) is a process designed to reach consensus about an issue or an idea that the team considers most important. In NGT, each team member ranks each idea according to its importance. For example, if there were six ideas, the idea that is most important would be given the number 6. The second most important idea would be given the number 5. The least important idea would have the number 1. After each team member has individually ranked the list of ideas, the numbers are totaled. The ideas deemed most important are clearly visible to all. Those ideas that people did not think were as important are also made known by their low scores. NGT demonstrates where the team's priorities lie.

***Multivoting Technique*** The multivoting technique is a variation of NGT and has the same purpose, to narrow and prioritize a group of ideas. Team members are asked to rate the issue using a distribution of points. For example, a team member may be asked to distribute 25 points among 10 total issues. Thus, one issue of particular importance may receive 12 of the team member's points, four others may receive some variation of the remaining 12 points, and five others may receive no points. After the vote, the numbers are added, and the team can see which issue has emerged as particularly important to its members.

This process also can be done with colored dots. For example, if there are eight items on a chart, team members may be given four dots to distribute on the four items they find most important. This method particularly enables team members to quickly visualize where consensus lies and what issue the team deems most important.

***Fishbone Diagram*** When a team first identifies a problem, it may use a fishbone diagram, also known as a cause-and-effect diagram, to help determine the root causes of the problem. (See figure 24.5.) The problem is placed in a box on the right side of the paper. A horizontal line is drawn (somewhat like a backbone), with diagonal bones, like ribs, pointing to the boxes above and below the backbone. Each box contains a category. The categories may be names that represent broad classifications of problem areas (for example, people, methods, equipment, materials, policies and procedures, environment, measurement, and so on). The team determines how many categories it needs to classify all the sources of problems. Usually, there are about four. After constructing the diagram, the team brainstorms possible causes of the problem. These are then placed on horizontal lines extending from the diagonal category line. The brainstorming of potential causes continues among team members until all ideas are exhausted. The purpose of this tool is to permit a team to explore, identify, and graphically display all the potential root causes of a problem.

After identifying several causes of a problem, the team must identify the root causes and work on eliminating those. If the root cause is not eliminated, then the problems will continue to occur. CQI involves continually making efforts to improve processes. Techniques such as multivoting and NGT can help bring consensus among the team about what to work on first.

**Figure 24.4.** Affinity diagram

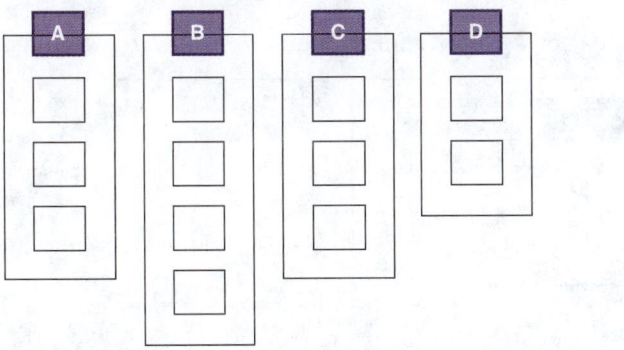

**Figure 24.5.** Fishbone diagram

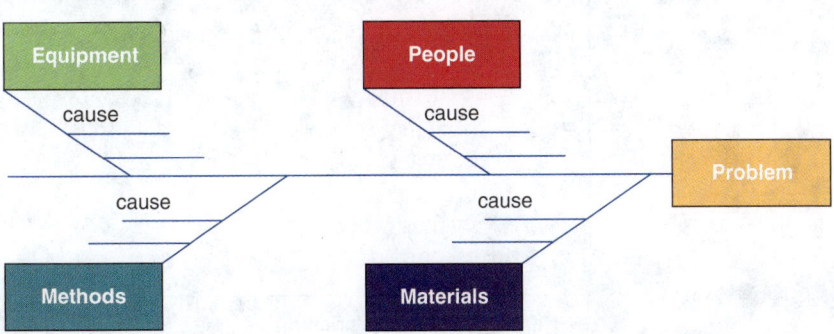

***Pareto Chart*** When a team decides to use multivoting or NGT, each team member places a number or mark next to an item indicating his or her opinion about the item's importance. When the numbers are tallied, the items can be ranked according to importance. This ranking can then be visually displayed in a Pareto chart (see figure 24.6). A Pareto chart looks like a bar chart except that the highest-ranking item is listed first, followed by the second highest, down to the lowest-ranked item. Thus, the Pareto chart is a descending bar chart. This visualization of how the problems were ranked allows team members to focus on those few that have the greatest potential for improving the process. The Pareto chart is based on the Pareto principle, which states that 20 percent of the sources of the problem are responsible for 80 percent of the actual problem (Brassard and Ritter 2020).

***Force-Field Analysis*** A force-field analysis also visually displays data generated through brainstorming. The team leader draws a large T formation on a board. (See figure 24.7.) Above the crossbar and on the left side of the T is a title related to positive drivers, such as benefits or forces for change; and above the bar and written on the right side of the T is a title related to negative drivers, such as barriers or forces against change. Team members are then asked to brainstorm and list on the chart under the crossbar the reasons or factors that would support a change for improvement and those reasons or factors that can create barriers. Thus, the force field enables team members to identify factors that support or work against a proposed solution. Often the next step in this activity is to work on ways to either eliminate barriers or reinforce drivers.

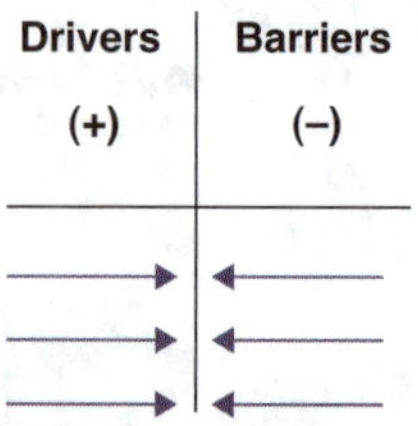

***Check Sheet*** A check sheet is a data collection tool that permits observations or occurrences to be recorded and compiled. It consists of a simple list of categories, issues, or observations on the left side of the chart and a place on the right for individuals to record marks next to the item when it is observed or counted (see figure 24.8). After a period of time, the checkmarks are counted, and the patterns or trends can be revealed.

A check sheet is a simple tool that allows a clear picture of the facts to emerge. After data are collected, several tools can be used to display the data and help the team more easily analyze them.

***Scatter Diagram*** A scatter diagram is a data analysis tool used to plot points of two variables suspected of being related to each other in some way. For example, to see whether age and blood pressure are related, one variable (age) would be plotted on one line of the graph, and the other variable (blood pressure) would be plotted on the other line. After several people's blood pressures are plotted along with their ages, a pattern might emerge. If the diagram indicates that blood pressure increases with age, the data could be interpreted as revealing a positive relationship between age and blood pressure. (See figure 24.9.)

**Figure 24.8.** Check sheet

|   | 1 | 2 | Total |
|---|---|---|---|
| A | ₩₩ | /// | 8 |
| B | //// | //// | 8 |
| C | // | / | 3 |

**Figure 24.6.** Pareto chart

**Figure 24.7.** Force-field analysis

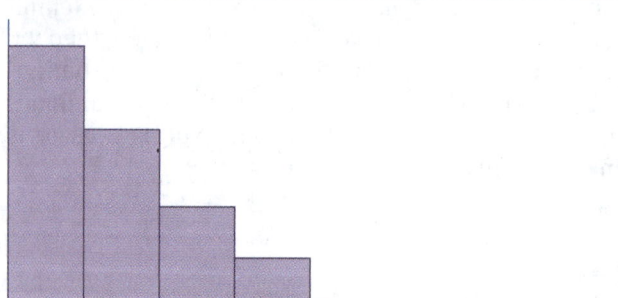

**Figure 24.9.** Scatter diagram

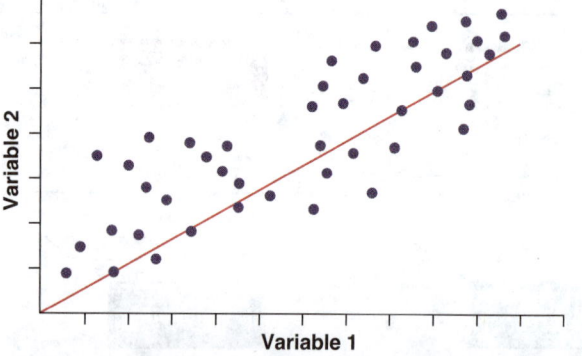

In some cases, a negative relationship might exist, as with variables such as number of hours of training and number of mistakes made. Whenever a scatter diagram indicates the points are moving together in one direction or another, conclusions can be drawn about the variables' relationship, either positive or negative. In other cases, however, the scatter diagram may indicate no linear relationship between the variables because the points are scattered haphazardly, and no pattern emerges. In this case, the conclusion would have to be that the two variables have no apparent relationship.

*Histogram* A histogram is a data analysis tool used to display frequencies of response. It offers an easier way to summarize and analyze data than having them displayed in a table of numbers. A histogram displays continuous data values that have been grouped into categories. The bars on the histogram reveal how the data are distributed. For example, an HIM administrator may want to show the number of minutes it takes to respond to patient requests for information. Minutes may be categorized into four groups—for example, 1 to 30 minutes, 31 to 60 minutes, 61 to 90 minutes, and more than 90 minutes. Checkmarks may be recorded indicating the category of minutes taken to respond to the request. After some time, the checkmarks are added and the histogram is plotted with the frequencies shown on the vertical axis, or *y*-axis, and the minute intervals shown on the horizontal axis, or *x*-axis.

A histogram such as one in figure 24.10 indicates the different intervals in which patients had to wait for their requests to be filled. A histogram can give an excellent idea of how well a process is performing; it can show how frequently data values occur among the various intervals, how centered or skewed the distribution of data is, and what the likelihood of future occurrences is.

*Run Chart* A run chart displays data points over time (see figure 24.11). Measured points of a process are plotted on a graph at regular time intervals to help team members see whether there are substantial changes in the numbers over time. For example, suppose an HIM manager wanted to reduce the number of incomplete records in the HIM department. The manager might first plot on a graph the number of incomplete records each month for the past six months and then enact a change in the processing of records designed to improve the process. Following the improvement effort, data on the number of incomplete records would continue to be collected and plotted on the graph. If the run chart shows that the number of incomplete records has decreased, the HIM manager could attribute the decrease to the improvement effort.

A run chart is an excellent tool for providing visual verification of how a process is performing and whether an improvement effort appears to have worked.

*Control Chart* A control chart looks like a run chart except that it has a line displayed at the top, called an upper control limit (UCL), and a line displayed at the bottom, called a lower control limit (LCL). (See figure 24.12.) These lines have been statistically calculated from the data generated in the process and represent two standard deviations above and below the mean (Shaw and Carter 2019, 89).

Like the run chart, the SPC chart plots points over time to demonstrate how a process is performing. However, the two control limit lines enable the interpreter to determine whether the process is stable, or predictable, or whether it is out of control. Remembering

**Figure 24.11.** Run chart

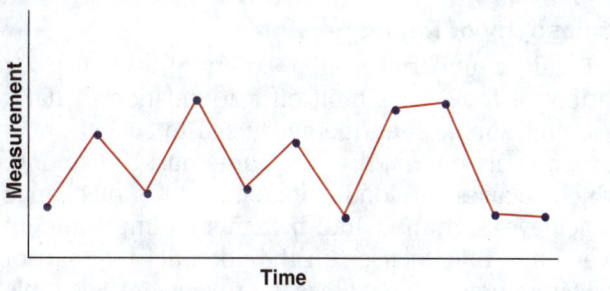

**Figure 24.10.** Histogram

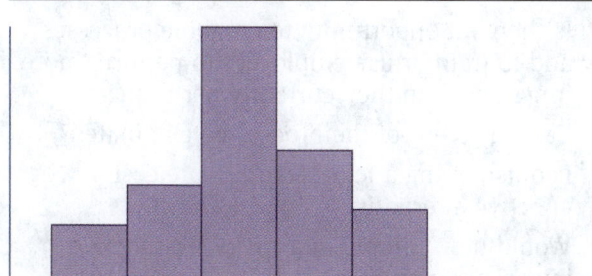

**Figure 24.12.** Statistical process control chart

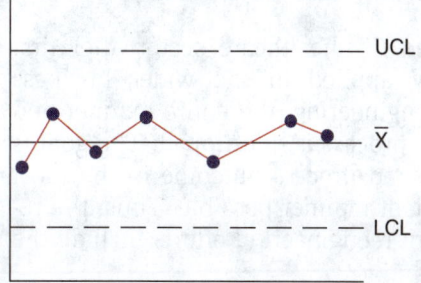

the constancy of variation principle, it is easy to see the purpose of the control chart. The control chart indicates whether the variation occurring within the process is a common cause variation or a special cause variation. It indicates whether it is necessary to try and reduce the ordinary variation occurring through common cause or to seek out a special cause of the variation and try to eliminate it.

## Business Process Reengineering

Business process reengineering has been met with resistance in the healthcare sector because of the fear it has evoked among healthcare workers. The term *reengineering* may be confused with reorganizing or downsizing, which can result in the loss of jobs. Because salaries comprise up to 70 percent of a healthcare facility's operating expenses, a drop in personnel can have a significant impact on reducing expenditures (BLS 2023). Due to negative connotations related to downsizing, restructuring, and outsourcing, the perception of reengineering went from a strategy an organization does to something that is done to the organization. Although the term *reengineering* itself is not always favorable in organizations today, **business process redesign (BPR)** is still a focus strategy for rethinking and drastically improving and sustaining overall performance, not a strategy for cutting costs (Dunn 2021). A **business process** can be defined as a collection of interrelated work tasks initiated in response to an event that achieves a specific result for a customer of the process (Sharp and McDermott 2009).

### Philosophy of Reengineering

BPR can be undertaken in a variety of ways using a variety of tools; it is built on a foundation of data. The philosophies and methods used to collect, measure, and act on that data are numerous. Unlike CQI, which focuses on conducting small tests of change to achieve continuous but incremental improvement over time, BPR focuses on the potential redesign of the entire process to achieve improvement. (See table 24.6 for a comparison of reengineering and quality management.) Reengineering implies making massive changes to the way a facility delivers healthcare services.

BPR has entered the healthcare sector after first being successfully applied in the wider business community. In reengineering, the entire manner and purpose of a work process is questioned. The goal is to achieve the desired process outcome in the most effective and efficient manner possible. Thus, the results expected from reengineering efforts include the following:

- Increased productivity
- Decreased costs
- Improved quality
- Maximized revenue
- More satisfied customers

The goal of reengineering is to develop sustained improvements and efficiencies over the long term, not just a quick fix.

### Process of Reengineering

When an organization decides to use reengineering as an improvement strategy, it commits itself to looking at selected processes within the organization in fine detail. Processes are selected for reengineering based on several criteria, including the following:

- Frequency and severity of problems created by the process, such as slow turnaround time or excessive waiting time
- Impact on customer satisfaction
- Complex processes involving multiple departments, procedures, and employees
- The feasibility of creating improvement (McConnell 2016)

Selecting a process for reengineering raises several questions:

- What is the intended purpose of the process? Is that purpose being accomplished efficiently?
- Is the process necessary? Could any redundancies or non-value-added activities be eliminated?
- Which employees are involved in the process, and which ones are needed? In other words, what are the minimum qualifications and minimum number of employees needed to do the job?
- Is the process as efficient as it could be, or are there more efficient means for accomplishing the goal?
- Is the process contributing to the efficiency of other processes that may be affected by its results?
- Is there an opportunity to combine processes and to train or use employees to perform more functions than they currently perform?
- Can any steps of the process be eliminated?
- Is outsourcing a feasible and more cost-effective alternative?
- Would new equipment or new technologies improve the process?

Table 24.6. Reengineering compared to quality management

| Reengineering | | Quality management | |
|---|---|---|---|
| Rethinking and radical redesign | Focus | Incremental improvements | Focus |
| Rethink | Think creatively | Quality planning | Focus on the customer |
| Redesign | Think both process and outcome | Quality control | Measure and monitor performance |
| Retool | Use technology to control and define work processes | Quality improvement | Use data, eliminate boundaries, and empower work |

Many of the tools and techniques used in systems analysis and CQI are also used in reengineering. In reengineering, it is essential to thoroughly understand how the process contributes to how the organization functions and to determine whether a better method exists. Therefore, observation of processes, customer input, interviews with employees, and the use of cross-functional teams to discuss the current steps of the process are frequently used methods for obtaining data. Data must be collected for a sufficient time to reflect the effectiveness of the process.

In addition, the data must be appropriately analyzed, and the analysis should include the input of individuals qualified to interpret the findings. Thus, a team composed of individuals involved in various aspects of the process should be permitted access to the data and should give input about alternative strategies. Moreover, the team can investigate the acceptability of new technologies that might allow for greater efficiency. Before new technologies are adopted, however, the team should thoroughly analyze the potential benefits, costs, and feasibility of using them in the organization.

After a reengineered process has emerged, new policies and procedures must be written and distributed to the people involved in the process. In addition, employees should be given adequate time to be trained in and master the redesigned process. Managers play an important role in reengineering through their support, encouragement, and commitment to the process.

### Factors for Success in Reengineering Efforts

One critical factor for the success of the reengineering effort is the visible and persistent commitment of senior administration. A second critical factor is management's commitment to excellence. Managers must demonstrate a can-do attitude in working through the change. In addition, the fact that change is needed to address an unacceptable problem must be effectively communicated throughout the organization. Having everyone, or almost everyone, acknowledge a problem exists creates a great deal of buy-in. Employees, including physicians, should be encouraged to overcome any reluctance to participate in the change process due to fears about restructuring. Many healthcare organizations make the mistake of not including their physicians in critical decision-making. The likelihood of a successful reengineering effort increases when every stakeholder is involved in the process.

Reengineering takes time. The organization should realize that change cannot be achieved overnight and should avoid trying to change too many processes at one time. Instead, it should focus its efforts on a few processes at a time. A great deal of planning, information gathering, and analysis must occur before an actual redesign can be implemented. When the planning phase has been completed, the organization should revise or develop policies and procedures accordingly and distribute them throughout the organization.

Finally, implementation of the redesigned processes requires patience. Glitches may occur with any new system, but reengineering can produce significant performance improvement with careful monitoring and persistent adjusting.

## Workflow Analysis and Process Redesign

Whatever the methodology or strategy used, workflow analysis and process redesign are necessary components of overall organizational improvement. The study of workflow as "who does what when" has become a critical part of process analysis and design methodologies.

### Process and Workflow Theory

The delivery of healthcare is increasingly complex. Therefore, the related workflows are also increasingly complex. As the use of technology becomes critical in all aspects of patient care, understanding how the work flows within and between processes is critical. The success of information technology (IT) projects is not solely dependent on the technology, but also on the people and the process. A process must remain customer focused and redundancy, delay, and error must be avoided. The goal of workflow analysis is BPR.

Workflow analysis should be done any time work involves multiple departments or functions and prior to identifying an IT solution. It is important to ensure all the stakeholders are a part of the analysis, the entire process is considered when making improvements, the business process is accurately identified, and the team does not get stalled in over-analysis of the current process. HIM professionals are well suited for workflow analysis because they can see the big picture of the overall healthcare process. They understand how healthcare professionals work together toward quality patient care, and they understand information flow and the users of the information. It is also important to understand the organizational structure and how to manage change. An essential, necessary distinction in workflow analysis is the difference between a process and a function. A process, as stated earlier, is a collection of interrelated work tasks done in response to an event that achieves a specific result for a customer. For example, the coding process requires multiple skill sets and is interdepartmental, including registration, clinical documentation, charge entry, qualitative analysis, coding, and billing. A function is an occupation or a department that focuses on related activities and similar skills. For example, the coding function is intradepartmental using one skill set primarily. The coder selects a case from the work queue, reviews clinical documentation and charges, determines the adequacy of the information, applies coding rules and selects or audits codes, and verifies codes for billing and reporting (AHIMA 2006). If a function is identified erroneously as a process for analysis, work methods will be defined for the benefit of the individual function, not to optimize the manner in which work flows through the function and through other areas of the organization as a whole. Focusing on functions and not business process perpetuates the development of functional silos. This should be avoided in process redesign.

Once a process is identified, the subsequent steps in workflow analysis are to frame the process, understand the current (as-is) process, design the new (to-be) process, and develop use case scenarios (Sharp and McDermott 2009). Framing that process is crucial in establishing and documenting the process boundaries. This will clarify the scope of the process—what is both within and outside of the scope. Documenting all the pertinent information about the process is called developing the process frame. In the process frame, one must do the following:

- Describe the process triggers, steps, results, and stakeholders.
- Understand the environment, including the mission, vision, goals, and culture.
- State the case for analysis.

The purpose of analysis is to understand processes to identify bottlenecks, sources of delay, rework due to errors, role ambiguity, duplication, unnecessary steps, and handoffs. This understanding of the current (as-is) process will lead to a redesigned future (to-be) process that can then be tested through a use case analysis.

## Tools and Techniques

There are several process mapping tools that can assist with workflow analysis and process redesign. Process mapping shows the activities of the process, including the sequence and flow of the work. Tool selection will depend on the level of precision needed and the nature of the process being mapped. Tools may be simple or complex, paper-based, automated, or web-based. Some of these tools are considered CQI tools, such as the workflow diagram for illustrating the movement of information (see figure 24.1) and the process flowchart for illustrating each step in a process and the sequence of steps (see figure 24.3). Other process mapping tools include the top-down process map, the swimlane diagram, and process simulation software.

***Spaghetti Diagram*** A spaghetti diagram is a visual depiction of the layout of the workspace with all the furniture, equipment, doorways, and so on sketched in. Superimposed on the layout are the movements of either individuals or things (for example, documents, files, and such). This diagram can be used to evaluate the workflow and to redesign one that is more efficient. An inefficient workflow is depicted in figure 24.1 (top), showing long distances between connected points in the workflow, crisscrossing paths, and paths that backtrack in the workspace. A redesigned diagram in figure 24.1 (bottom) depicts a smoother workflow resulting in improved efficiency.

***Flowchart*** Whenever a team examines a process with the intention of making improvements, it must first thoroughly understand the process. Each team member comes to the team with a unique perspective and significant insight about how a portion of the process works. To help all members understand the process, a team will develop a flowchart (see figure 24.13). This work allows the team to thoroughly understand every step in the process and the sequence of steps. It depicts each decision point and each event to complete. It readily points out places where there is redundancy and complex and problematic areas.

***Top-Down Process Map*** The top-down process map identifies the least number of steps necessary in a process. The main steps are worded broadly and simply,

**Figure 24.13.** Release of information flowchart

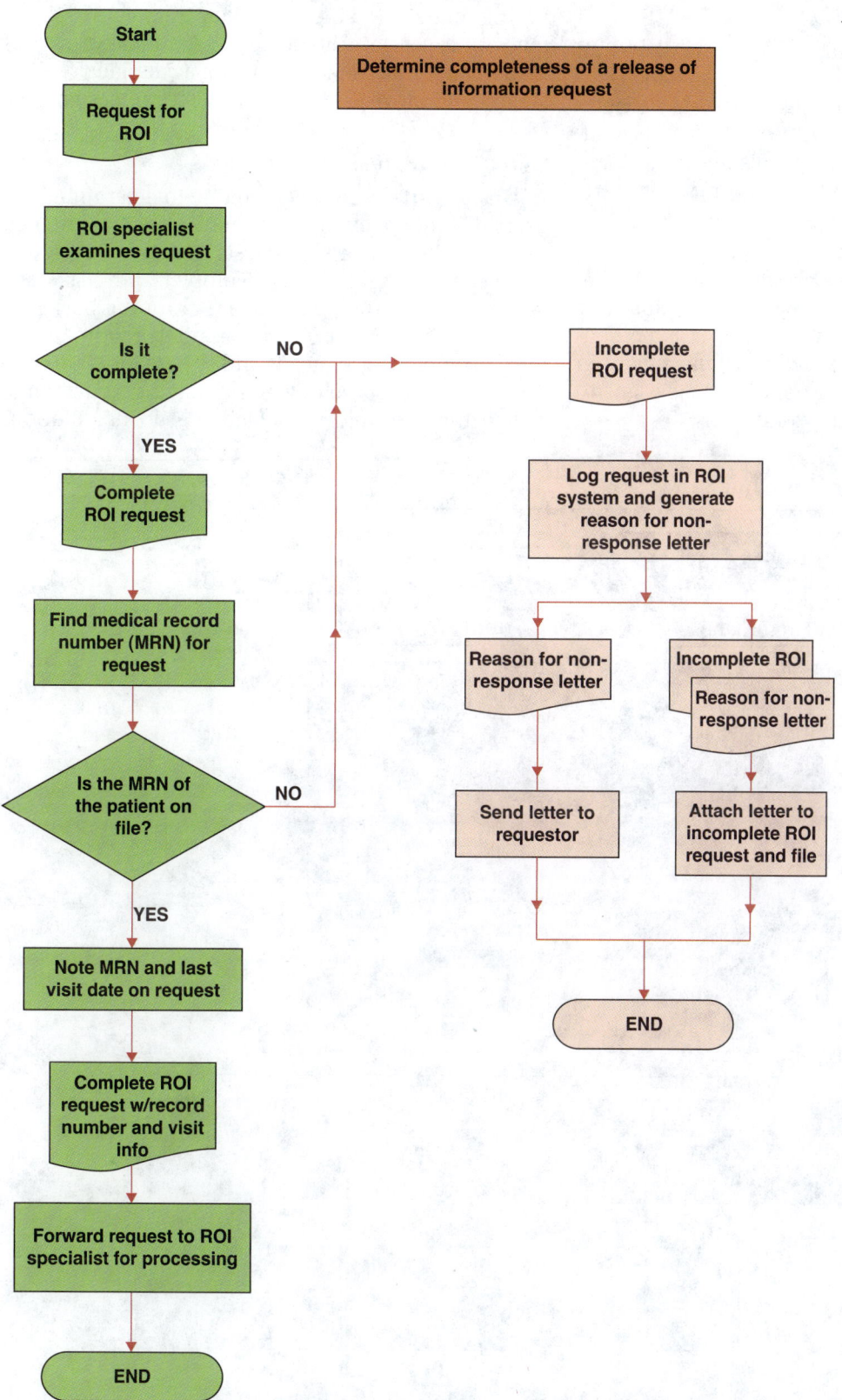

with each step showing only three to four subtasks in more detail (see figure 24.14).

**Swimlane Diagram** A swimlane diagram shows an entire business process from beginning to end and is especially popular because it highlights relevant variables (who, what, and when) while requiring little or no training to use and understand. The swimlane diagram is often used to identify the current (as-is) process as well as to design the new (to-be) process (see figure 24.15).

**Process Simulation Software** Process simulation software can show the flow of work, individuals, or movement of information in existing or hypothetical situations. This software can show movement in existing situations and various alternative designs to identify the most appropriate workflow.

These tools and techniques assist in analyzing current workflows to focus on facts rather than opinions, to truly understand the existing process, and to document all aspects of the process. Additionally, process maps can bring stakeholders to a common understanding to move forward with process redesign.

## Use Case Analysis

A use case analysis is a technique to determine how users will interact with a system. It uses the designed future (to-be) process and describes how a user will interact with the system to complete process steps and how the system will behave from the user perspective. The purpose of use case analysis is to bridge the gap between user needs and system functionality. A use case analysis helps identify system requirements, design the user interface, facilitate documentation,

**Figure 24.14.** Top-down process map

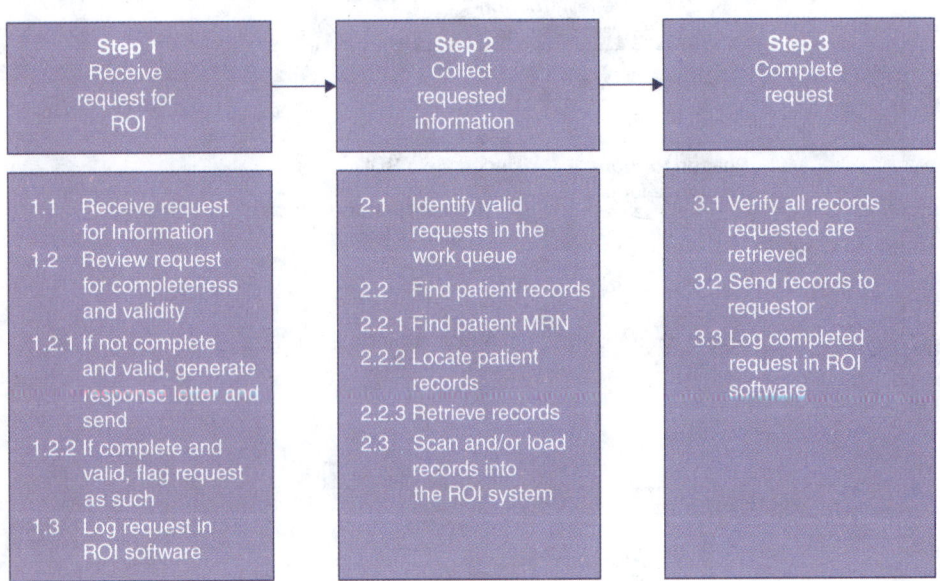

**Figure 24.15.** Sample swimlane diagram

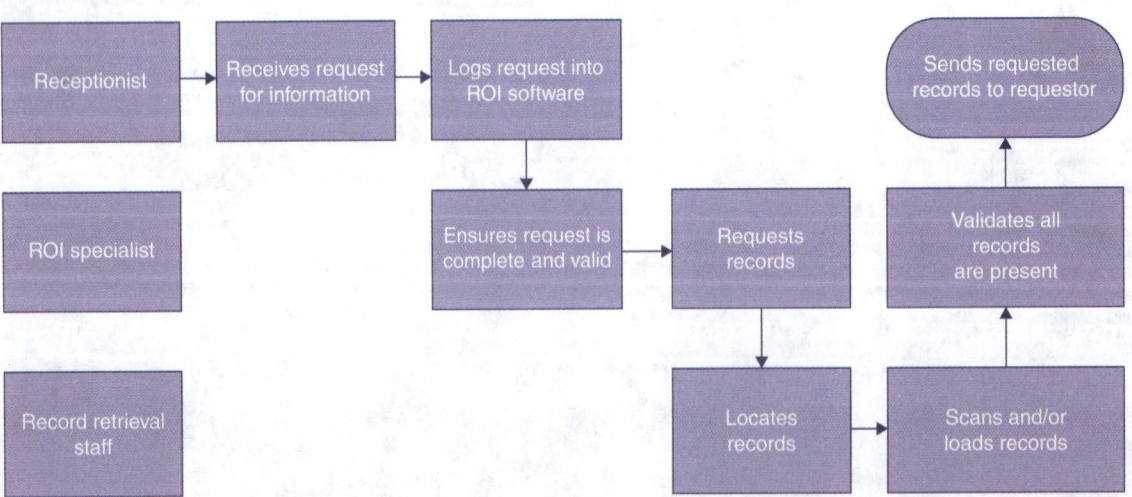

create test plans, and develop training and support plans. It is critical to list all use case scenarios that impact every user so that no case is overlooked. Priority should go to developing use case scenarios focusing on areas with the most impact on the success of the project, such as those affecting multiple users' workflows (Sharp and McDermott 2009).

Identifying all potential use cases is valuable to ensure nothing is overlooked and all users are involved.

More value emerges when each use case is not only identified but also described. Basic elements of a use case description are the use case name, a description of the use case, the users of the system for that use case, preconditions that must be in place before the use case can be tested, the normal sequence of steps, the post conditions or results expected, any alternate steps as needed, and any variations or issues known to that particular use case that are important to know. (See example in figure 24.16.)

**Figure 24.16.** Use case description

**Use case name**
Provider orders lab work for inpatient.

**Description**
When a provider determines a need for lab work for an inpatient, he or she will complete the ordering process for lab.

**Actor(s)**
Care provider

**Preconditions**
- The patient must currently be admitted in the hospital.
- The provider has active privileges at the hospital.
- The computerized provider order entry system is functioning properly.

**Normal sequence of steps**

1. Provider signs on to the system using a password.
   System validates the password and displays the patient search screen.
2. Provider enters the patient's health record number.
   System verifies the health record number and displays the patient's electronic health record.
3. Provider selects the lab module.
   System verifies the user is allowed access to the module and displays the lab module.
4. Provider selects the lab test from drop-down list.
   System verifies the lab test name.
5. Provider enters the lab test.
   System verifies the test.
6. Provider submits the lab order by selecting the Submit button.
   System sends lab order.

**Postconditions**
- The order is submitted to the laboratory information system.
- The lab receives electronic notification of pending order.
- A pending order is recorded in the patient's electronic health record.

**Alternative sequence of steps**
- If the provider does not have the health record number, he or she may enter the patient's last name and the first name. The system will then provide a list of patient names that the physician may choose from.
- An additional free-text field may be provided to the physician to record any additional notes or messages in relation to the lab being ordered.

**Comments, issues, and design notes**
- When searching for a patient's electronic health record, it may be necessary to also be able to search by patient date of birth.
- For the lab test fields, it may be necessary to create drop-down lists that can be selected from, instead of allowing free text. This will allow more control of the data entry and reduce data entry errors.

*Source:* Adapted from Sharp and McDermott 2009.

## Check Your Understanding 24.6

**Answer the following questions in a separate document.**

1. Brian has been asked to lead a process improvement project for a vocal and varied team of laboratory system users. They really want their ideas heard. What tool(s) would you recommend to Brian in this situation?

2. The process improvement team working on reducing registration errors has tried many fixes with no results. They are committed to identifying exactly what the issue is that will lead to a process improvement. What tool(s) would you recommend?

3. As the ROI supervisor, you need to ensure the staff understand the procedure for processing requests. It is important that the staff know each step of the procedure and who does what. What tool would be best to quickly and effectively illustrate this procedure?

4. The use case analysis is a technique that shows how users will interact with a system and helps with designing a user interface that is user-friendly. Using figure 24.16 as a guide, develop a use case description for registering for a class at your educational institution.

5. Computer-assisted coding will be implemented on June 1. Staff have been trained but will have a learning curve once the system is live. As the coding manager, you want to monitor the success of the project regarding productivity and quality while maintaining morale and motivation among the coding staff. What tools would you use in your weekly staff meetings to maintain the momentum of this new technology?

# References

AHIMA (American Health Information Management Association). 2006. *Optimizing Investment in the EHR: Workflow Analysis as the Foundation for Success* [Workshop resource book]. Chicago: AHIMA.

ASQ (American Society for Quality). 2023a. "Total Quality Management (TQM)." https://asq.org/quality-resources/total-quality-management.

ASQ (American Society for Quality). 2023b. "The Define Measure Analyze Improve Control (DMAIC) Process." https://asq.org/quality-resources/dmaic.

ASQ (American Society for Quality). 2023c. "Continuous Improvement." https://asq.org/quality-resources/continuous-improvement.

ASQ (American Society for Quality). 2023d. "What Is a Quality Management System (QMS)?" https://asq.org/quality-resources/quality-management-system.

BLS (Bureau of Labor Statistics). 2023 (September 12). "Employer Costs for Employee Compensation–June 2023." https://www.bls.gov/news.release/pdf/ecec.pdf.

Brassard, M., and D. Ritter. 2020. *The Memory Jogger II*, 2nd ed. Salem, NH: GOAL/QPC.

Cherry, K. 2019. "Color Psychology: How Colors Impact Moods, Behaviors, and Feelings." http://psychology.about.com/od/sensationandperception/a/colorpsych.htm.

DOL (US Department of Labor). n.d. "Night Work and Shift Work." Accessed December 14, 2023. https://www.dol.gov/general/topic/workhours/nightwork.

Dunn, R. T. 2021. *Dunn & Haimann's Healthcare Management*, 11th Ed. Chicago: HAP.

Feldman, K. 2022 (June 14). "What Is Six Sigma?" https://www.isixsigma.com/getting-started/what-six-sigma/.

Hessing, T. n.d. "Spaghetti Diagram." Accessed December 14, 2023. https://sixsigmastudyguide.com/spaghetti-diagram/.

HHS (US Department of Health and Human Services). 2003. "Business Associates." http://www.hhs.gov/hipaa/for-professionals/privacy/guidance/business-associates/index.html.

IHI (Institute for Healthcare Improvement). n.d. "Triple Aim and Population Health." Accessed December 13, 2023. https://www.ihi.org/improvement-areas/triple-aim-population-health.

IOM (Institute of Medicine). 2000. *To Err Is Human*. Washington, DC: National Academies Press.

Lean Enterprise Institute. n.d. "What is Lean?" https://www.lean.org/explore-lean/what-is-lean/.

Lee, M., and Mather, M. 2008 (June 22). U.S. labor force trends. *Population Bulletin* 63(2). https://www.prb.org/resources/u-s-labor-force-trends/.

McConnell, C. R. 2016. *Umiker's Management Skills for the New Health Care Supervisor*. Burlington, MA: Jones and Bartlett.

OSHA (Occupational Safety and Health Administration). n.d.a. "Computer Workstations eTool." Accessed December 10, 2023. https://www.osha.gov/etools/computer-workstations.

OSHA (Occupational Safety and Health Administration). n.d.b. "Ergonomics." Accessed December 10, 2023. https://www.osha.gov/ergonomics.

OSHA (Occupational Safety and Health Administration). n.d.c "Business Case for Safety and Health." Accessed December 10, 2023. https://www.osha.gov/businesscase.

Peek, S. 2023 (February 21). The management theory of Mary Parker Follett. https://www.business.com/articles/management-theory-of-mary-parker-follett/.

Roberts, J. G., J. G. Henderson, L. A. Olive, and D. Obaka. 2013. A review of outsourcing services in health care organizations. *Journal of Outsourcing and Organizational Information Management* 2013(1). https://ibimapublishing.com/articles/JOOIM/2013/985197/985197.pdf.

Sharp, A., and P. McDermott. 2009. *Workflow Modeling: Tools for Process Improvement and Application Development*, 2nd ed. Norwood, MA: Arctech House.

Shaw, P. L., and D. Carter. 2019. *Quality and Performance Improvement in Healthcare*, 7th ed. Chicago: AHIMA.

Skhmot, N. 2017 (August 5). "The 8 Wastes of Lean." https://theleanway.net/The-8-Wastes-of-Lean.

Stone, J. 2019. "Labor Law on Time Between Shifts." https://smallbusiness.chron.com/night-shift-day-shift-labor-laws-76454.html.

Vorne Industries. n.d. "Top 25 Lean Tools & Techniques." Accessed December 13, 2023. https://www.leanproduction.com/top-25-lean-tools/.

# Financial Management

*Rick Revoir, EdD, MBA, CPA*

## Learning Objectives

- Determine appropriate financial structure for a healthcare organization
- Justify the importance of financial stewardship
- Apply accounting concepts and principles
- Analyze and interpret financial statements
- Calculate and interpret basic financial ratio results in terms of organizational impact
- Assess the importance of internal controls and their role in financial management

## Key Terms

Accounting
Accounting rate of return (ARR)
Accounts payable
Accounts receivable
Accrue
Activity-based budget
Asset
Balance sheet
Capital budget
Conservatism
Consistency
Corporation
Cost accounting
Current ratio
Days in accounts receivable
Debt ratio
Debt service
Detective control
Depreciation
Direct cost

Equity
Expense
Favorable variance
Financial Accounting Standards Board (FASB)
Fiscal year
Fixed budget
Fixed cost
Flexible budget
For-profit organization
General ledger
Generally accepted accounting principles (GAAP)
Going concern
Income statement
Indirect cost
Internal rate of return (IRR)
Internal Revenue Service (IRS)
Liabilities
Liquidity

Managerial accounting
Matching
Materiality
Net assets
Net income
Net loss
Net present value (NPV)
Not-for-profit organization
Operational budget
Partnership
Payback period
Preventive control
Profitability
Public Company Accounting Oversight Board (PCAOB)
Return on investment (ROI)
Revenue
Revenue Principle
Securities and Exchange Commission (SEC)

Sole proprietorship
Statement of cash flow
Statement of retained earnings
Statement of stockholder's equity
Total margin ratio
Variable cost
Variance
Zero-based budget

A physician treats a patient. A hospital admits a woman in labor. A professional association offers continuing education (CE) for its members. These scenarios are examples of organizations providing services for which they receive compensation. How organizations arrange to provide those services, determine compensation, and handle the flow of funds that these activities both require and generate is guided by financial management.

This chapter focuses on the concepts and tools associated with planning and controlling the financial resources required to operate a department or a work unit. It presents operations, labor, and capital budgeting processes and techniques; reviews organizational and departmental financial performance measures; and explores techniques for improving financial performance at the departmental level. Finally, the chapter acquaints readers with the language of financial and managerial accounting to enhance their understanding of the role of the health information management (HIM) professional as a manager.

## Healthcare Financial Management

The process of financial management involves various players within the organization's financial arena. Table 25.1 lists and describes the roles of the financial personnel who work in health systems. However, healthcare financial management also involves several players outside the financial arena. For example, HIM professionals are involved with reimbursement through the coding function. Record retention and release of information activities help support claims auditing and claims denial appeals. HIM professionals play an important role in clinical documentation integrity (CDI) activities, including clinical training to support medical necessity and reimbursement. Figure 25.1 illustrates a potential organizational structure of personnel in a health system.

HIM professionals are familiar with financial data as one component of a health record, or the data related to payers and billing. To financial managers, financial data are the individual elements of organizational financial transactions. (The term *financial* refers to money and, as is discussed later, money is the measurement of financial transactions.) A financial transaction is the exchange of goods or services for payment or the promise of payment. Financial data are compiled into informational reports for users. The degree of detail that users require depends on their needs and is largely influenced by the relationship of the user to the originator of the transaction.

Table 25.1. Financial personnel and their roles in a hospital

| Position | Typical or minimum background | Financial roles |
|---|---|---|
| Board of directors or trustees | Depends on the needs of the facility | Ultimate responsibility for the fiscal integrity of the organization |
| Chief executive officer (CEO) | Master's degree prepared in public administration, hospital administration, or business administration; occasionally, clinical background | Overall responsibility for administration of the organization |
| Chief information officer (CIO) | Bachelor's degree and often a master's degree in information technology or a Master of Business Administration | Overall responsibility for information systems (ISs) and HIM |
| Chief financial officer (CFO) | Bachelor's degree and certified public accountant (CPA) or certified management accountant (CMA) | Overall responsibility for related departments, including patient accounts, accounting, decision support, and internal auditing |
| Controller or accounting manager | Bachelor's degree and CPA | Oversees accounting and cash disbursement, including payroll |
| Patient accounts manager | Bachelor's degree | Oversees claims processing |

**Figure 25.1.** Organization of the nonphysician side of the health system

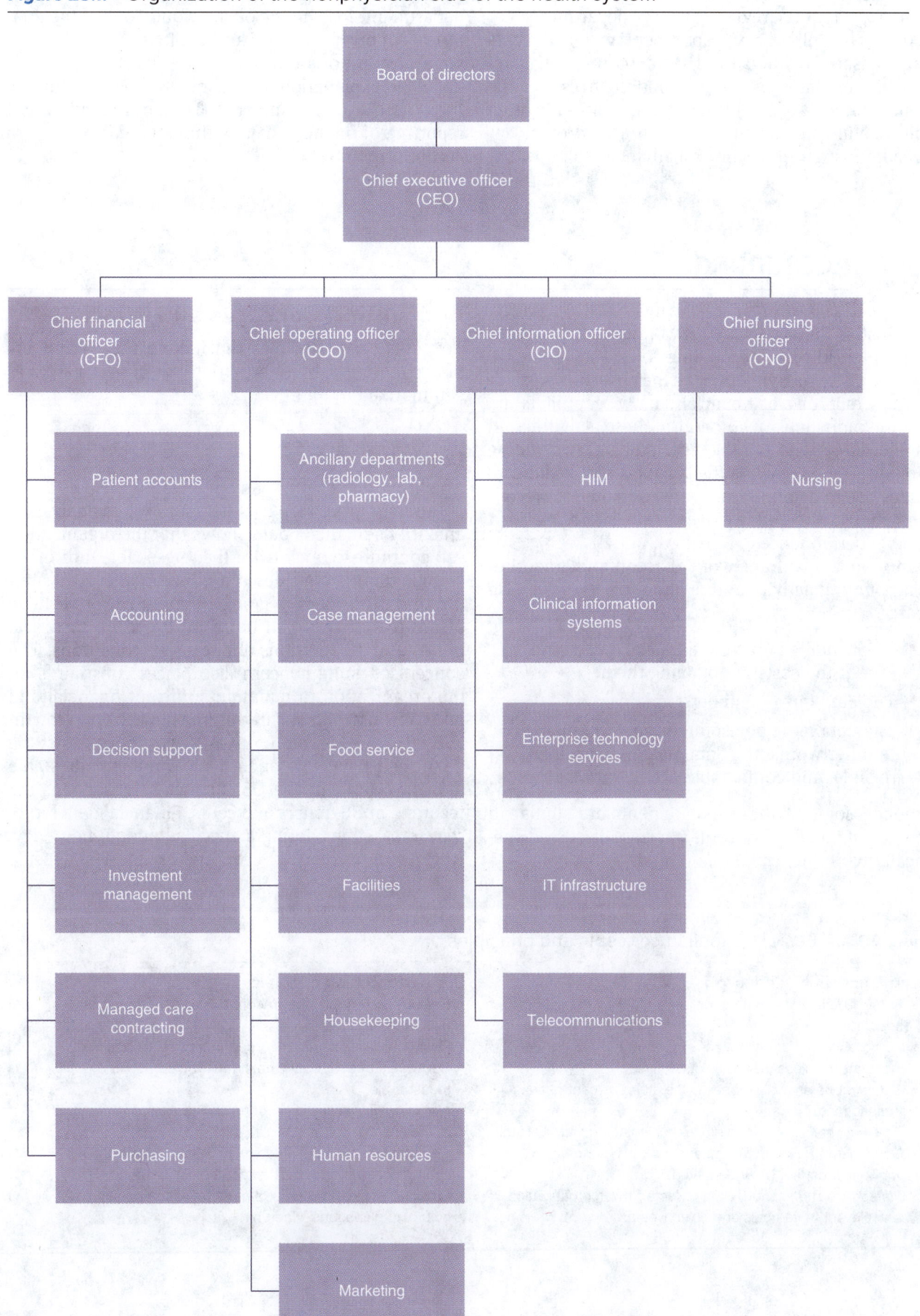

Financial transactions that originate at the department level require review by that department. For example, the pharmacy department will review its drug transactions, and the HIM department will review its purchases of supplies and services. On the administrative level, informative summaries are often more useful than detail. For example, an organization administrator does not usually need to know the number of cases of copier paper purchased in each department. Instead, he or she would look at the total office supply purchases and evaluate whether they were at appropriate and expected levels. Additional detail or explanation would not be required unless the purchases were unusual. The accumulation and reporting of financial data within an organization are accounting functions.

## Accounting

**Accounting** is an activity as well as a profession. Just as there are many HIM roles and functions, so are there diverse accounting roles and functions. The accounting activity involves the collection, recording, and reporting of financial data. Accountants are both the individuals who perform these activities and many of those who use the reported data. Accounting is important because it is the language that healthcare entities use to communicate with each other to record transactions, determine investment strategies, and evaluate performance.

The conceptual framework of accounting underlies all accounting activity and is based on the following ideas:

- The benefits of having financial data should exceed the costs of obtaining them.
- The data must be understandable.
- The data must be useful for decision-making. In other words, the data must be relevant, reliable, and comparable.

Although some of these requirements are similar to general data quality concerns, they are discussed specifically with financial data in mind.

### Accounting Concepts and Principles

Concepts and principles that define the parameters of accounting activity are briefly discussed here and summarized in figure 25.2.

### Concepts

An entity is a person or an organization such as a corporation or professional association. When analysis of an entity's financial data shows that the organization can continue to operate for the foreseeable future, the organization is considered a **going concern**. Assuming that a business is going to continue, projections of future activities can be made based on historical trends and assumptions about future conditions. The concept of going concern also places constraints on the organization to maintain sufficient financial and other resources to ensure future stability and growth.

Every one of an entity's transactions must be quantified using a standard measurement or stable monetary unit. In the US, financial transactions are recorded in US dollars and cents. Financial data represent transactions during a specified period: hour, day, week, month, quarter, year, and so on. The specific

**Figure 25.2.** Basic accounting concepts and principles

| Basic accounting concepts | Basic accounting principles |
|---|---|
| • *Entity:* The financial data of different entities are kept separate.<br>• *Going concern:* Organizations are assumed to continue indefinitely, unless otherwise stated.<br>• *Stable monetary unit:* Money is the measurement of financial transactions.<br>• *Time period:* Financial data represent a specified period of time.<br>• *Conservatism:* Resources must not be overstated, and liabilities must not be understated.<br>• *Materiality:* The financial data collected by an organization are relevant to its goals and objectives. | • *Reliability:* Amounts represent the transactions that occurred.<br>• *Cost:* Transactions are recorded at historical cost.<br>• *Revenue:* To record revenue, it must be earned and measurable.<br>• *Matching:* Expenses are recorded in the same period as the related revenue.<br>• *Consistency:* When an accounting rule is followed, all subsequent periods must reflect the same rule.<br>• *Disclosure:* Financial reports must be accompanied by helpful explanations, when necessary. |

period depends on the use of the data. The fiscal year (also called the financial year) is defined by the tax year. Individuals generally have a tax year that coincides with the calendar year. Organizations, on the other hand, use fiscal years that correspond to their business needs, usually their business cycle, representing the total activities of the organization. Many not-for-profit healthcare organizations have a fiscal year end of June 30.

For financial reporting purposes, a fiscal year is divided into quarters (three-month periods) and months. Because the months generally end on the last calendar day, the quarters can be of slightly different duration. For example, the first quarter of a fiscal year that begins April 1 includes April, May, and June: 91 days. The second quarter of that same fiscal year includes July, August, and September: 92 days. Over time, it is common to compare similar quarters from year to year.

Not all financial data represent completed transactions within the period represented. Sometimes estimates are involved, or transactions are completed between periods. When amounts are estimated, efforts must be made to ensure their use does not misrepresent the actual financial transaction. Therefore, financial data must comply with conservatism, meaning they fairly represent the financial results of the period and do not overstate or understate information in a significant (material) way.

Materiality refers to the thresholds below which items are not considered significant for reporting purposes. These thresholds may be a dollar value or a percentage of a dollar value. For example, if an organization made a $10,000 error in estimating bad debt expense, this error would be material for a company that has $100,000 in expenses, but the error would be immaterial to an organization that has $1 billion in expenses. An item is material when it could affect the decision-making of anyone using the financial statements. This issue arises when determining the significance of errors, potential liabilities, and the necessity for disclosures.

## Principles

Accounting principles support the quality of financial data. Financial data must possess the same data quality characteristics, such as timeliness and validity, as any other type of data. In financial data, reliability refers to whether the data represent what occurred and are free of material error both in the current period and over time. Transactions are recorded at their historical cost measured at the time of the transaction. For some transactions, such as the purchase of equipment or investment in marketable securities, such as stock or shares in a company, there may be a change in the actual or perceived value of the underlying asset or liability. In those cases, adjustments or disclosures are made when reporting the financial data. Revenue consists of earned, known amounts. It is the compensation that has been earned by providing goods and services to the client or patient as well as amounts received or earned from other sources. The Revenue Principle states that earnings resulting from activities and investments may only be recognized when they have been earned, can be measured, and have a reasonable expectation of being collected. For an organization to generate revenue, it must incur expenses. For example, payroll, rent, travel, and raw materials. Expenses represent the utilization of resources by the organization to generate revenue. Whenever possible, expenses are recorded in the same period as the associated revenue, thereby matching the expenses and revenues. The principle of consistency requires that the method not change over the life of the asset. Thus, the financial data are prepared in the same way from one period to the next. In fact, organizations sometimes change their choices. Consistency then requires that financial data be restated to show the effect of the change applied to previous periods. Sometimes the financial data alone do not provide enough information for data users to make informed decisions. The impact of a building fire, a potential or ongoing lawsuit, or an expiring collective bargaining agreement cannot be reflected in the financial data when no financial transaction has occurred. Therefore, notes or disclosures that help the user to make informed decisions must accompany all financial reports.

## Authorities

Just as clinical data are organized and reported in predetermined formats for ease of communication, financial data also are organized and reported in specific ways. Theoretically, organizations can design their own accounting systems and reporting mechanisms. Internally, this is often the case, as will be seen with budgeting. However, organizations that want to borrow funds or attract investors must follow generally accepted rules that apply to their industry and accounting in general. Five major sources of accounting and reporting rules apply to healthcare organizations. These sources will be discussed in the sections that follow.

### Financial Accounting Standards Board

The Financial Accounting Standards Board (FASB) is an independent organization that sets accounting standards for businesses in the private sector. Its counterpart, the Government Accounting Standards Board (GASB), sets standards for accounting for government entities. The FASB makes the rules by which financial data are compiled, reported, reviewed, and audited publicly known. These rules, which include the conceptual framework, are referred to as **generally accepted accounting principles (GAAP)** and generally accepted auditing standards (GAAS).

### Securities and Exchange Commission

The **Securities and Exchange Commission (SEC)** is a federal agency that regulates public and some private transactions involving the ownership and debt of organizations. The SEC sets standards regarding reporting financial data, disclosures, timing, marketing, and execution of these transactions. Public transactions take place through an exchange, such as the New York Stock Exchange (NYSE) or the National Association of Securities Dealers Automated Quotation System (NASDAQ). Organizations whose ownership interests (stocks) are traded on these exchanges are called public companies.

### Internal Revenue Service

The tax status of an organization influences its administration. The **Internal Revenue Service (IRS)** regulates and collects federal taxes. Healthcare organizations fall into one of two major tax categories: for-profit and not-for-profit. The primary differences between for-profit and not-for-profit organizations are related to the level of accountability and the distribution of profits. Within these categories are several legal structures, such as sole proprietorship, partnership, and corporation. A summary of legal structures is provided in table 25.2.

### Public Company Accounting Oversight Board

Historically, the accounting profession has been largely self-regulated. The FASB and GASB, although technically independent, have strong ties to the profession. Although IRS and SEC standards and regulations constrained the specific representation of financial activities, the accounting profession was free to accomplish its reporting and other activities without government intervention. However, that changed in 2002. The federal government responded to the collapse of ENRON, WorldCom, and others with the Sarbanes-Oxley Act of 2002, which restricted the professional services of independent auditors of public companies and, among other things, created the **Public Company Accounting Oversight Board (PCAOB)**, which oversees the audits of companies that are publicly traded. Sarbanes-Oxley had a significant impact on the degree of scrutiny and testing of internal controls, financial reporting, and governance of organizations.

### Centers for Medicare and Medicaid Services

CMS is the federal agency that administers the Medicare program and the federal portion of the Medicaid program. The federal government is the largest single payer of healthcare expenses in the US. Although CMS does not set accounting rules, it enforces the federal regulations regarding the reimbursement for Medicare and the federal portion of the Medicaid program and sets standards for the documentation and reporting of transactions related to such reimbursement. Since CMS requires significant reporting from participant organizations, its influence on financial activities and data collection should not be underestimated.

## Financial Organization

The way an entity organizes itself depends on its financing, leadership, and tax status. The three basic forms of business organization are the sole proprietorship, the partnership, and the corporation (see table 25.2). Other organizational entities, such as

Table 25.2. Common legal structures of nongovernmental organizations

| Structure | Description | Healthcare examples |
|---|---|---|
| Sole proprietorship (for-profit only) | One owner; all profits are owner's personal income | Solo practitioners |
| Partnership (for-profit only) | Two or more owners; all profits are owners' personal income | Physician group practices |
| Corporation | One or many owners; profits may be either retained or distributed as dividends. May be public or private. "Owners" may be individuals, other organizations, or an interest group. Not-for-profits are often understood to be owned by the communities they serve. | Hospitals, insurance companies |

trusts and variations like limited liability corporations (LLCs), are beyond the scope of this discussion.

**Sole proprietorship** is a venture with one owner in which all profits are considered the owner's personal income. For example, an independent coding consultant who operates from home and has no employees may choose to operate as a sole proprietor. The owner, or proprietor, is the leader of the organization and is responsible for all aspects of the business. Income from the business flows through the owner's individual tax return. If the consultant's business expands, employees or subcontractors can be added without changing the organizational structure. Some physicians are solo practitioners and therefore sole proprietors.

Two or more consultants who want to be in business together may choose a partnership structure. In a **partnership,** partners share in the responsibility for the business, and income still flows through the individuals' tax returns. Partners do not need to share equally in the financial or other business responsibilities. A partnership agreement details the contractual arrangement. Because a partnership is a separate legal and accounting entity from the individuals, a tax identification number is required for the partnership, and the partnership may be required to file its own tax returns detailing the income allocated to each partner. Partnerships survive as entities only so long as the partners remain together. A change in ownership dissolves the original partnership and a new one must be created.

A **corporation** is a legal entity that exists separately from its owner(s). Corporations pay their own taxes and have their own legal rights and responsibilities. In fact, the owner(s) of the corporation may have nothing to do with its leadership or day-to-day operations. A corporation is typically governed by a board of directors or trustees, and the day-to-day operations are led by one or more administrators who report to the board. The corporation's income after taxes may be kept, to invest in its growth, or it may be distributed in whole or in part to the owner(s). This after-tax distribution is a dividend and is taxable income to the owner(s). This two-tiered taxation, on the corporation and then again on the distributed dividend, is referred to as double taxation and may make this structure less attractive to individuals.

The purpose of the organization drives another consideration in the financial organization of the business. Is the purpose of the business to generate income for the owners, or is there a more altruistic foundation? The answer to this question helps to define the tax status the organization can obtain.

### For-Profit Organizations

**For-profit organizations** may be sole proprietorships, partnerships, or corporations. In this context, profits are the funds remaining after all current obligations have been met, including taxes. Inherently, the underlying goal of for-profit organizations is to increase the wealth of the owners. Increase in wealth can be accomplished through the generation of profits to be distributed to the owners or by increasing the value of the organization so that the owners' investment is more valuable. The leadership of the organization may distribute the profits to the owners or otherwise invest them as they see fit. For-profit organizations may be privately or publicly owned.

Private ownership may be by an individual, a group of individuals, or an organization. Physician practices, urgent care centers, and freestanding ancillary care organizations are often privately owned. The distribution of profits from a privately owned organization is at the discretion of the owners or as defined by contract among owners.

Public ownership means the ownership interest in the organization may be bought and sold in the financial marketplace. For example, Tenet Healthcare Corporation (THC) is a publicly held organization with hospitals in numerous states. Its stock is traded on the NYSE under the symbol *THC*. A publicly held organization's board of directors determines the distribution of profits. Boards are constrained in these determinations by contractual obligations such as mortgage contracts and preferred stock obligations, stockholder expectations, and strategic organizational goals.

### Not-for-Profit Organizations

**Not-for-profit organizations** are not owned but, instead, are held in trust for the benefit of the communities they serve. Many hospitals fall into this tax category. Other not-for-profit organizations include professional associations such as the American Health Information Management Association (AHIMA) and charitable organizations such as the American Red Cross. The IRS defines numerous types of not-for-profit organizations. The two categories of not-for-profit organizations discussed here are 501(c)(6) and 501(c)(3).

***501(c)(6)*** Most professional associations are organized under 501(c)(6), which gives them some federal tax benefits and the freedom to engage in activities unrelated to their organizational purpose. For example, organizations under 501(c)(6) may lobby and sell goods and services but are largely involved in activities that benefit their major interest group, which may be defined as paid membership. Such organizations may be subject to state sales tax, both as purchaser and seller. AHIMA and most of its component state associations (CSAs) are 501(c)(6) organizations.

**501(c)(3)** On the other hand, 501(c)(3) organizations are largely exempt from federal taxes, but must confine their activities to the public benefit. Donations to 501(c)(3) organizations are generally tax deductible (for the donor) to the extent that no goods or services have been received in return. For that reason, charities are generally 501(c)(3) organizations, and many 501(c)(6) organizations have charitable components that are separately incorporated. Organizations classified as 501(c)(3) may also be exempt from state sales tax under certain circumstances.

### Tax Status Issues

It is important to understand the underlying tax status of an organization because tax status affects the organization's business decisions and long-term strategies. Undistributed profits from a for-profit organization may stay in the business and be available for investment or future distribution. There is no need to identify the future use of these funds, although stockholders may ultimately press for distribution when undistributed profits appear excessive. Occasionally, portions of undistributed profits are held in reserve for specific uses.

On the other hand, profits from a not-for-profit organization stay in the business. Because all such profits must be used for the benefit of the community the organization serves, the future use of these profits should be clearly defined. Excessive unrelated business income or high unrestricted reserves (effectively, too much savings) may result in the loss of not-for-profit status. For further information about tax exemptions of organizations, see IRS Publication 557 (IRS 2023).

## Sources of Financial Data

Just as a health record is constructed from the data collected, financial records are also composed of data. Health records are built from medical decision-making; financial records originate with financial decision-making, the smallest component of which is the transaction.

### Transactions

Virtually every financial transaction consists of three fundamental steps:

1. Goods or services are provided.
2. A transaction is recorded.
3. Compensation is exchanged.

Each step may require a few additional steps, depending on the service and the industry. In addition, the steps are not always performed in the same order. Independent contractors that perform hospital coding represent a simple example. The contractor codes the records, submits an invoice, and receives payment from the hospital. In this case, four specific steps may be needed to support the transaction: keeping a log to track the records that have been coded, preparing an invoice to bill the hospital, keeping a list of the invoices sent, and checking the invoices off when they are paid.

In a hospital, multiple individuals and departments perform services and provide administrative support for financial transactions. Four areas are of particular concern in the context of this discussion: clinical services, patient accounts, HIM, and administration.

***Clinical Services*** Just as contract coders keep track of the records they have coded, clinical or patient care services providers also keep track of the services they perform. The documents of original entry or source documents enable the healthcare facility to verify the services were provided and communicate to supporting departments that a transaction has been initiated. The source document includes two elements—the clinical documentation and the billing documentation.

Clinical documentation is a record of who has seen the patient, which tests or treatments were performed, and why these tests and treatment were administered; in other words, everything clinically relevant that happened to the patient during his or her interaction with the organization. The documentation must include a proper clinician order and medical necessity to ensure the cost of treatment is covered.

Along with the recording of clinical documentation is the capture of the associated billing information. Regardless of the reimbursement system, the organization must capture the billable event in such a way that the financial transaction can be completed. Therefore, when a medication is administered to a patient, the clinical record reflects the medication; dosage; time, date, and route of administration; and the clinical personnel who administered it. At the same time, the charge for the drug must be communicated to patient accounts. This detailed tracking of billable events also supports the cost accounting function, which is discussed later in this chapter.

***Patient Accounts*** The patient accounts department is responsible for collecting recorded transactions, billing the payer (generating the claim), and ensuring the correct receipt of reimbursement. This department depends on the reliable recording of services. This means the capture of billing information must be timely and accurate to efficiently complete the financial transaction. In addition to the clinical support staff and departments, the patient accounts department relies on the HIM professionals for coded data.

*Health Information Management* HIM professionals are responsible for identifying and recording the appropriate clinical codes to describe the patient's interaction with the organization. The coding supports billing which drives the reimbursement to the facility. In addition to the coding activity, HIM professionals are responsible for aggregating and maintaining the documentation that supports the reimbursement.

*Administration* Financial transactions occur throughout the facility. Employees are paid, equipment and supplies are purchased, and departments perform services for each other. The finance department accumulates and analyzes all the financial data. Ultimately, the entire management team participates in the review and analysis of financial data.

## Uses of Financial Data

Financial data are generated virtually everywhere in a healthcare facility. Managerial and supervisory personnel use these data for four key purposes—tracking reimbursement, controlling costs, planning future activities, and forecasting results.

### Reimbursement

Healthcare facilities are service organizations that derive almost all their income from clinical activities. Therefore, a key use of financial data is to track reimbursement and ensure the desired amount of profit is generated. In the current industry environment where payers often dictate the amount of reimbursement, the provider is increasingly unable to control pricing as a method of managing desired profit. Therefore, the cost of providing services has become the controllable factor.

### Control

Controlling costs is best done at the department level. For example, the chief executive officer (CEO) of a hospital does not shop around for the best price on copier paper, and the chief financial officer (CFO) does not monitor employee productivity in the food services department. Each department is charged with responsibility for ensuring prudent management of financial and other resources. Departments are given this charge through the budget process, which is one of the outcomes of administrative planning.

### Planning

Administrative planning reflects the organization's mission. From that mission, goals and objectives are derived that help move the organization toward achieving its mission. Financial data are used to analyze trends, develop budgets, and plan. Planning cannot be accomplished by using historical data alone because the industry changes, sometimes rapidly. Therefore, the administration must forecast future scenarios.

### Forecasting

Forecasting is the prediction of future behavior based on historical data and environmental scans. It can be as simple as predicting the profits of an organization according to anticipated changes in reimbursement. It also can involve complicated predictions of consumer behavior based on market research and news reports.

## Check Your Understanding 25.1

**Answer the following questions in a separate document.**

1. If an insurance company representative contacted the HIM department about a claims audit, to which financial personnel should he or she be directed and why?
2. Three physicians plan to create a community clinic that will offer low-cost and free charity care. The purpose of the clinic is to improve the health of the community and provide charity care. The clinic will solicit donations to support the operations. Any earnings from the clinic will be reinvested back into the clinic to serve the community. Evaluate the situation and determine which type of organization status would be appropriate for this clinic.
3. Big Medical Center earned a lot more revenue than expected this year but does not expect to earn as much next year. To make the financial reports more consistent,

a junior accountant suggests that the hospital record some of next year's expenses this year. Would you agree or disagree that this is a good strategy? Why?

4. St. Sara's Surgical Center is forecasting and budgeting surgery cases for their next fiscal year. Marketing manager Ryan believes surgery cases are going to increase 30 percent next year because of a new marketing campaign. CFO Sophia is budgeting a one percent increase in surgical cases based on analyzing the actual number of cases over the past three years. Which staff member's recommendation best reflects the concept of conservatism and why?

5. Analyze the two following scenarios and determine which situation would meet the materiality criteria. Clinic A is a large multispecialty clinic with $3 billion in revenue, and an accountant discovers a $10,000 mistake in one of the revenue accounts. Clinic B is a small clinic with $80,000 in revenue. It discovers a $10,000 mistake in a revenue account. Which clinic would consider this to be a material error? Explain your answer.

## Basic Financial Accounting

A basic understanding of the mechanics of financial accounting helps department managers to understand the impact of their financial transactions on the overall organization. The system of recording financial transactions is based on balancing the *purpose* of the transactions with their impact on the organization. For example, a facility purchases drugs with the purpose of ensuring sufficient and appropriate drugs are on hand to treat patients. The purchase of the drugs increases the facility's pharmaceutical inventory. The impact of that purchase is the outlay of cash. After the cash is spent on drugs, it cannot be spent on something else. Recording both the increase in inventory and the outlay of cash enables the organization to understand and communicate information about its activities. Fundamental to this communication is an understanding of the components of financial data and their relationship to each other.

### Assets

Assets are things that are owned or due to be received. In a transaction, the compensation that has been earned by providing goods or services becomes an asset as soon as it has been earned. Examples of assets include cash, inventory, accounts receivable, buildings, and equipment.

### Cash

Cash consists of monetary instruments, including those instruments that can be converted into cash quickly. Those that can be converted to cash—for example Treasury bills—are often referred to as cash equivalents. Included in cash are funds maintained in bank accounts. It is important to remember that currency and bank accounts are both considered cash, for accounting purposes. At the point of sale, such as purchasing lunch in the cafeteria, currency may be tendered. CMS, on the other hand, does not deliver reimbursement to a hospital in truckloads of currency. Instead, it electronically transfers funds between financial institutions. Both are considered cash to the hospital. Cash is only recorded, and becomes an asset, when it has been received.

### Inventory

An organization has inventory if it maintains goods on hand it intends to sell to a client. Drugs are part of a hospital's pharmaceutical inventory because they are effectively on hand to be sold to patients. It is important to distinguish between goods that are available for sale and goods that the organization uses in other ways. Photocopy paper is inventory to the office supply store. To the hospital HIM department, it is used for general business purposes and is considered a supply. In this case, the hospital is the client (the consumer of the goods). Because hospitals are primarily service organizations, and the provision of goods is incidental to the services provided, hospitals tend not to have a great deal of inventory other than supplies.

### Accounts Receivable

When an organization has delivered goods or services, payment is expected. Remember that the second step in a transaction is to record the transaction. Because the revenue has been earned upon delivery or a provision of the goods and services, the organization must have some way to keep track of what is owed as a result. Accounts receivable then is merely a list of the amounts due from various customers (in this case, patients). Payment on the individual amounts is expected within a specified period. A schedule of those expected amounts is prepared to track and follow up on payments that are overdue (late). Figure 25.3 shows one way to prepare a simple aged accounts receivables report. One can use this report to prioritize follow-up efforts on the accounts that are most delayed (for example, those greater than 120 days overdue) or those accounts that are the highest dollar amount despite the aging (for example, accounts over $250 such as the two accounts noted under the 31 to 60 days column). This report could be sorted by discharge date and the amounts subtotaled.

### Building

Many organizations own the buildings in which they reside. These buildings are assets to the organization because they are part of its physical plant, its infrastructure. Buildings are considered long-term assets because they are typically owned for many years.

### Equipment

Equipment is another long-term asset. Hospitals include CT scanners, hospital beds, and surgical robots in this category. Each organization decides what items are relevant to this category, depending on industry conventions and materiality. For example, a large hospital would rarely consider a $500 personal computer to be equipment, whereas an independent coding consultant might view it as a significant, long-term investment.

**Purchase Price** In acquiring a piece of equipment (and certain other assets), the transaction is recorded at the purchase price. For example, the hospital purchases digital mammography equipment for $200,000. The hospital then would have a $200,000 asset in equipment. However, the equipment gradually wears out from use over time. That $200,000 asset is not worth $200,000 four years after it was purchased. To provide better information about the financial value of its equipment, the organization provides an estimate of this decrease in value, called **depreciation**, every year.

**Depreciation** Depreciation is an example of a contra-account. This estimate of the cumulative decrease in value of an asset actually reduces the cost of

**Figure 25.3.** Aged accounts receivable

| A/C # | D/C | SER | 0–30 days | 31–60 days | 61–90 days | 91–120 days | >120 days | Total A/R |
|---|---|---|---|---|---|---|---|---|
| 46153153 | 04/15/24 | OR | | | | | 149 | |
| 46160492 | 07/06/24 | ED | | | | 25 | | |
| 46162518 | 07/31/24 | ED | | | 10 | | | |
| 46162874 | 08/31/24 | ED | | | 30 | | | |
| 46163484 | 08/07/24 | ORTHO | | | | | 165 | |
| 46162580 | 07/30/24 | OB | | | | 114 | | |
| 46125122 | 06/19/24 | OP | | | | | 16 | |
| 46160520 | 07/06/24 | OP | | | | 50 | | |
| 46169245 | 10/09/24 | OP | 175 | | | | | |
| 46165628 | 09/30/24 | OB | | 266 | | | | |
| 46163713 | 08/12/24 | OP | | | 52 | | | |
| 46166048 | 09/04/24 | ORTHO | | 380 | | | | |
| 46161964 | 07/23/24 | OP | | | 94 | | | |
| 46162506 | 07/30/24 | OP | | | 104 | | | |
| 46164953 | 08/25/24 | OP | | | 152 | | | |
| 46169231 | 10/09/24 | ED | 125 | | | | | |
| 46157104 | 05/30/24 | OB | | | | | 50 | |
| 46124651 | 06/15/24 | OB | | | | | 84 | |
| 46126673 | 07/09/24 | ED | | | | | 148 | |
| 46122160 | 05/20/24 | OP | | | | | 227 | |
| Total amounts | | | $300 | $646 | $244 | $387 | $839 | $2,416 |
| Total number of accounts | | | 2 | 2 | 4 | 5 | 7 | 20 |

the underlying asset. Thus, the mammography equipment purchased for $200,000 may have an accumulated depreciation of $75,000 after two years. At that point, its remaining book value to the organization is $125,000. The following shows this illustration:

| | |
|---|---|
| Mammograph | $200,000 |
| Accumulated depreciation | $75,000 |
| Book value | $125,000 |

## Liabilities

Liabilities are debts. They are amounts that are owed, often due to the acquisition of an asset. Examples of liabilities include accounts payable, loans payable, and mortgages.

### Accounts Payable

Accounts payable is a liability that is created when the organization has received goods or services but has not yet remitted the compensation (that is, paid for the goods or services). Referring to the accounts receivable discussion, the provider of the goods and services records a receivable when payment is not received at the point of the sale. On the other side of that transaction is the organization for which the goods and services were provided. When the recipient of the goods and services does not intend to pay immediately, the amount is recorded by the recipient as an account payable. The recipient also records either the acquisition of an asset or the recognition of an expense (discussed later in this chapter).

### Loans Payable

A loan is an amount an organization has borrowed that will be repaid over a specified period. The creation of the loan may be associated with the purchase of goods or services, and the material goods may be guaranteed by the value of specific assets (collateral). For example, the organization may need $50,000 more than it has on hand to purchase a CT scanner. It might take a two-year loan from the bank (or the vendor), using the scanner as collateral, meaning that if the organization does not pay the loan back on a timely basis, the lender is entitled by contract to take possession of the scanner.

### Mortgage

A mortgage is a liability that is created when the organization borrows money and uses a physical asset, such as a building, as collateral. Organizations may use a mortgage to finance the construction of a clinic or building. Individuals obtain a mortgage to finance the purchase of a home.

## Equity or Net Assets

All financial accounting is based on an equation that pictures the organization holistically, balancing what is owned against what is owed: assets versus liabilities. Equity (or owner's equity) is the arithmetic difference between assets and liabilities. In a not-for-profit environment, the difference between assets and liabilities is referred to as net assets. These relationships can be expressed in the following equation:

$$\text{Assets} - \text{liabilities} = \text{net assets (equity)}$$

The purchase of a building illustrates this equation. The purchase of a house typically involves a deposit of cash and an assumption of a mortgage. The building is an asset whose value is, historically, the price paid at the time of the purchase. The mortgage is a liability. As mortgage payments are made, the amount of the mortgage owed declines. The deposit of cash is the owner's equity in the building. As mortgage payments are made, the amount of owner's equity in the building increases. For example, Dr. James purchases an office building for $200,000. She makes a down payment (or deposit) of $50,000 and assumes a mortgage of $150,000. As the mortgage is paid over 30 years, the historical value of the house remains the same, the amount of the mortgage decreases, and the owner's equity in the property increases. When the mortgage is completely paid, the owner's equity in the house equals the historical value of the house, as shown here:

| | Assets | | Liabilities | | Equity |
|---|---|---|---|---|---|
| At purchase | $200,000 | − | $150,000 | = | $50,000 |
| After 10 years | $200,000 | − | $100,000 | = | $100,000 |
| After 20 years | $200,000 | − | $50,000 | = | $150,000 |
| After 30 years | $200,000 | − | —0— | = | $200,000 |

Earlier, it was stated that an equation balances what is owned and what is owed. Therefore, another way to look at the accounting equation is as follows:

$$\text{Assets} = \text{liabilities} + \text{net assets (equity)}$$

Using the previous mortgage example, the second version of the equation proves useful. At every step in the following calculation, the equations balance.

An increase in assets increases equity. A decrease in assets decreases equity. An increase in assets with an equal increase in liabilities has no impact on equity. Notice that increasing a liability reduces equity in the same manner that decreasing an asset does.

|  | Assets |  | Liabilities |  | Equity |
|---|---|---|---|---|---|
| At purchase | $200,000 | = | $150,000 | + | $50,000 |
| After 10 years | $200,000 | = | $100,000 | + | $100,000 |
| After 20 years | $200,000 | = | $50,000 | + | $150,000 |
| After 30 years | $200,000 | = | —0— | + | $200,000 |

Assets, liabilities, and equity are the components of the balance sheet (discussed later in this chapter). First, it is important to understand the revenue and expense components of financial information.

## Revenue

Revenue can be broken down by sources. For example, hospitals generate revenue from patient care and nonpatient care. Revenue is also categorized as operating revenue which includes patient care and nonoperating revenue, which includes nonpatient care and investment revenue.

### Sources of Revenue

Patient services is the main source of revenue for a healthcare facility. Depending on the nature of the facility, patient services may be its only source of revenue. Examples of nonclinical services that are a source of revenue include employee food services, monetary donations, and gift shop.

### Categories of Revenue

How an organization describes its revenue depends on industry convention, materiality, and whether the revenue is recurring or unusual. Revenue from any source increases equity. A coding consultant works for a week at a client hospital and earns $1,500. He receives a check from the hospital and deposits it in his bank account. This increases his cash asset by the amount of the deposit: $1,500. The increase in the asset, absent an associated liability, increases equity by the same amount. Most organizations can group their revenue sources into at least two categories—operating and nonoperating.

**Operating Revenue** A hospital considers patient services revenue to be operating revenue. Because the hospital is in the business of serving patients, patient services is its main source of revenue and thus falls under the heading of operating revenue. Consider food services. Inpatients must be fed, so food services are a patient service and thus an operating expense. The employee cafeteria also generates revenue, but the revenue it generates is unrelated to patient services. In the HIM department, small revenue streams may be generated through release of information activities or through contracting services out to other facilities. Since the pricing of these activities is generally cost based, it is more appropriately thought of as an offset or quasi-reimbursement of the underlying cost.

**Nonoperating Revenue** A hospital with a large endowment that generates significant income may want to highlight this investment revenue in a separate category. Investment income is one example of nonoperating income. Other examples include gift shop sales and unrestricted monetary donations.

## Expenses

It is unlikely that revenue is generated without any reduction of cash or liability being incurred. The coding consultant in the previous example must purchase coding software, travel from home to the client and back, and engage in CE. Expenses, then, represent the organization's use of resources to generate revenue. The consultant coder uses cash to purchase coding software. The software helps to generate revenue for one year, at which time it expires. Therefore, the price of the software is an expense to the coder.

The simple example that follows in table 25.3 illustrates the impact on the accounting equation of the financial transactions discussed thus far. The chart shows how one's financial transactions affect one's equity; as liabilities are subtracted from one's assets, equity or net assets is calculated. This individual began with a balance in assets of $1,500; after purchase of coding resources, payment of health insurance, attendance at a CE session, and purchase of a computer with $200 cash down, total assets equal $4,520. Subtracting $800 on credit for the computer (liability), this person has net assets or equity of $3,720.

### Purchasing

As previously stated, healthcare organizations typically cannot affect revenue by raising prices, so they must attempt to control expenses as much as possible. One way to do this is through the purchasing function. Individuals responsible for purchasing activities must adhere to their facility's policies and procedures, which may vary somewhat from the basic descriptions in this section.

**Table 25.3.** Impact on accounting equation

| | October activity | | | | |
| --- | --- | --- | --- | --- | --- |
| | Assets | − | Liabilities | = | Equity |
| Beginning balance | $1,500 | − | —0— | = | $1,500 |
| Purchase coding resources | <100> | − | | = | <100> |
| Pay health insurance | <100> | − | | = | <100> |
| Receive payment from client | $1,200 | − | | = | $1,200 |
| Purchase computer (on credit) | 1,000–200 | − | 800 | = | 0 |
| Receive payment from client | $1,300 | − | | = | $1,300 |
| Attend CE session | <80> | − | | = | <80> |
| Ending balance | $4,520 | − | 800 | = | $3,720 |

Organizations handle the purchasing function differently depending on their size and needs. Large organizations tend to maintain a central purchasing and distribution department that is responsible for the acquisition of supplies and equipment.

Significant savings can be obtained by purchasing supplies in bulk and distributing them as needed to departments. Central purchasing also has the benefit of minimizing the space required for storage of items on hand. Central purchasing systems should be designed to minimize the risk of loss due to misappropriation of stored items. The periodic comparison, by counting, of items on hand with the items recorded and the itemized distribution of stored items can assist in this process.

To obtain the benefits of purchasing in large quantities, some facilities combine their purchasing efforts. Healthcare systems, for example, may offer coordinated purchasing on behalf of multiple facilities. Nevertheless, the control over the use of the items remains with the department.

Maintaining a central purchasing and distribution department results in direct administrative costs to the organization (for example, salary, facility maintenance, and administrative processing). Therefore, the control benefits of centralized purchasing must be weighed against the cost of such operations. Savings also can be obtained by limiting the source of supplies to one or two key vendors who offer discounts to the organization. In this scenario, department managers would order items as needed, but only from approved vendors.

Finally, an organization may choose to allow individual departments to make purchases independently. Although this can result in additional supply and equipment costs, there may be overall savings in not maintaining a central purchasing department. The major disadvantages of independent or decentralized purchasing are the need for supply storage space in the ordering department and the allocation of managerial resources to purchasing.

Regardless of the purchasing system used, controls must be in place to ensure the efficient execution of approved transactions. Purchase orders, shipping and receiving documents, and invoices are the key controls over the purchasing process.

**Purchase Orders** The purchase order system ensures that purchases have been properly authorized prior to ordering. Authorization is often tied to dollar limits or the budget process. Purchase orders are numbered sequentially so all orders can be verified. A purchase order is typically a template the user fills out with details of the intended purchase. Purchase orders for routine, budgeted items often require only the authorization of a supervisor or manager. For large-dollar items, as specified in the organization's policy and procedure manual, additional authorization may be required.

The purchase order shows the appropriate individual with the appropriate authorization ordered the specific items. The order is then forwarded to the vendor. The originator of the order has an electronic copy, and notification is sent to the accounts payable department. When there is a central receiving department, that department also has access to the details of the purchase order which are verified when goods are received.

**Shipping and Receiving Documents** Items received from a vendor contain a packing slip, also known as a shipping and receiving document. This document lists the quantities and descriptions of the items sent from the vendor, but not usually the price. The recipient of the items must verify the items received match the ones that were ordered. The verified shipping and receiving document is forwarded to accounts payable.

**Invoices** The vendor sends an invoice (bill or request for payment) directly to accounts payable. The accounts payable department matches the invoice to the shipping and receiving document and the purchase order on file. When all the documents match, the invoice can be processed, and payment scheduled. Invoices generally have terms: for example, payable upon receipt or within 30 days. Some vendors offer discounts for early payment, such as "2/10, net 30," which means the seller will grant a 2 percent discount for payment within 10 days; otherwise, the full amount is due within 30 days. Other terms may include interest charges for late payment. The facility's accounting department must balance expected payments (receivables) with obligations (payables). Departments often receive invoices directly. It is important to forward all invoices to the accounting department immediately upon receipt and verification so accounting has the information it needs to make appropriate and timely decisions about payment.

**Statements** A statement is a list of outstanding invoices the vendor has sent but for which no payment has been received. Some companies send statements that include all activity for the period, including payment. The statement is one way the vendor lets the customer know that payments are late. Statements are not payable without supporting documentation. When there is no purchase order, receiving document, and invoice, accounts payable will not remit payment.

Statements received for which there is no underlying documentation should be treated as suspicious. Purchases may have been made without proper authorization. Additionally, there are fraudsters that send statements when no transaction has taken place in the hope the receiving organization's controls are lax, and payment will be made. This is particularly true of fraudulent subscriptions and advertising schemes.

**Inventory Slips** The purchase of large quantities of supplies is called *supplies inventory* and may be recorded as an asset at the time of purchase. Items are then removed from assets and recorded as expenses as they are used. This same system may be used to track pharmacy inventory (by patient rather than department). In a centralized purchasing system, some mechanism must be in place to track the distribution of items to other departments. The financial transaction consists of moving the responsibility for the expense of the items from the purchasing department to the requesting department.

## Recording Transactions

As previously discussed, financial transactions begin with the documents of original entry or source documents. Whether the organization's transactions are recorded on paper or through a computer, there must be a way to determine the origination of the transaction. The originating document details the parties involved in the transaction, the amount of the transaction, the type of financial impact involved (revenue or expense, asset or liability), and the individual responsible for the transaction. Table 25.4 shows some common accounts and what they represent.

**Table 25.4.** Common accounts

| Account | Example |
|---|---|
| Assets | Cash |
| | Accounts receivable |
| | Inventory |
| | Equipment |
| | Land |
| | Buildings |
| | Prepaid rent |
| | Prepaid insurance |
| Liabilities | Accounts payable |
| | Loans payable |
| | Mortgage payable |
| **Equity or Net Assets** | |
| Revenue | Patient services revenue |
| | Parking revenue |
| | Food service revenue |
| | Interest earned |
| Expenses | Salaries/wages |
| | Utilities |
| | Rent |
| | Supplies |
| | Insurance |
| | Repairs |

## Double-Entry Bookkeeping

All financial transactions are recorded with the accounting equation in mind: assets = liabilities + net assets (equity). To simplify the recording of transactions, accountants use special terminology to reflect the maintenance of a balanced equation.

***Debits and Credits*** Visually, transactions have two sides—left and right. Debits are shown on the left; credits are shown on the right. Each account has two sides—increase and decrease. In asset accounts, the left-hand debit side represents the natural balance of the account and debits increase the account. Conversely, credits decrease an asset account. For the accounting equation to balance, the opposite is true of liability and equity accounts. The right-hand credit side of liability and equity accounts represents the natural balance, and credits increase the accounts. Instead of using minus signs or brackets to represent the increases and decreases, debits and credits provide an additional safeguard against clerical error because every transaction must balance.

Look at the coding consultant example again in table 25.5, using debits and credits. It is shown that as assets increase with payments from clients, that amount is placed on the left side of the asset account (debited). As the asset decreases due to purchases, that amount is placed on the right side of the asset account (credited). As previously noted, for the accounting equation to balance, the opposite is true of liability and equity accounts; the credit side of the equity account increases when accounts payables are increased. As liabilities and equities decrease (for example, when accounts payables are paid off), the liability account is debited.

***Impact on Individual Accounts*** Assets involve multiple accounts, as described previously: cash, accounts receivable, and building. Similarly, liabilities have their own accounts. Revenues and expenses fall into the equity section. This system of debits and credits enables us to understand immediately whether a transaction increases or decreases a particular account. Individual accounts increase and decrease in value; however, the overall equation always remains in balance.

## Transaction Tracking

Financial transactions are recorded, or posted, to the accounts described earlier, according to a system of journal entries.

***Journal Entry*** Each journal entry contains at least one debit and one credit. For every transaction, the sum of the debits must equal the sum of the credits. Ensuring that the debits and credits equal is one aspect of ensuring the accuracy of financial data. Other aspects include posting to the correct accounts and in the correct period. Table 25.6 shows the purchase of supplies on credit. The supplies are delivered on February 24, and the supplier's invoice is paid on March 15. Note that no financial transaction is recorded until the supplies are received.

The accounts payable amount is eliminated when the invoice is paid. It is common business practice to record, or **accrue**, liabilities as they are incurred. This accrual basis of accounting enables organizations to understand their total liabilities continuously and to match expenses with the associated revenue. Some organizations, such as small professional associations and sole proprietorships, only record transactions when the cash is paid or received. This cash basis of accounting is analogous to the way individuals handle their private transactions.

In the preceding tabulation, the supplies expense entry is a debit to increase that account. Expenses are temporary equity accounts that close annually. Revenue increases net income; expenses reduce net income. Therefore, revenue accounts have a natural credit balance and expenses have a natural debit balance.

It should be noted that all the financial accounting examples in this chapter relate to corporate and not-for-profit accounting. Government accounting activity, although a system of debits and credits, is significantly different in some respects. For example, a supply purchase would be recorded (encumbered) at the time the supplies were budgeted and then reduced at the time they were ordered. Government accounting is outside the scope of this discussion.

***General Ledger*** In a paper-based accounting system, journal entries are recorded chronologically in a general journal and their component debits and credits are posted to the individual accounts. The list of all the individual accounts is referred to as the **general ledger**. In a computer-based environment, only the original journal entry is posted. The computer stores the entries and generates summaries of the individual accounts on request.

The example in figure 25.4 is based on this chapter's original description of a financial transaction. The result of this completed transaction is an increase in cash and an increase in equity (revenue). Note that the amount in accounts receivable is eliminated when the reimbursement is received.

Nonfinancial managers are rarely required to make actual journal entries to record financial transactions. However, they do initiate the transactions and receive reports that detail them. Often the reports only show the department's side of the transaction. For example,

**Table 25.5.** Debits and credits

| October activity | Assets | | − | Liabilities | | = | Equity | |
|---|---|---|---|---|---|---|---|---|
| | Debit | Credit | | Debit | Credit | | Debit | Credit |
| Beginning balance | $1,500 | | − | —0— | | = | | $1,500 |
| Purchase coding resources | | 100 | − | | | = | 100 | |
| Pay health insurance | | 100 | − | | | = | 100 | |
| Receive payment from client | $1,200 | | − | | | = | | $1,200 |
| Purchase computer (on credit) | $1,000 | 200 | − | | 800 | = | 0 | |
| Receive payment from client | $1,300 | | − | | | = | | $1,300 |
| Attend CE session | | 80 | − | | | = | 80 | |
| Ending balance | $4,520 | | − | | 800 | = | | $3,720 |

**Table 25.6.** Journal entry for purchase of supplies

| Date | Description | Debit | Credit |
|---|---|---|---|
| 2/24 | Supplies expense | $300 | |
| | Accounts payable | | $300 |
| | Purchase office supplies | | |
| 3/15 | Accounts payable | $300 | |
| | Cash | | $300 |
| | Pay 2/24 office supply invoice | | |

**Figure 25.4.** Example of a financial transaction

**Service provided:**
Physician sees a new patient, whose chief complaint is an itchy rash.

**Transaction recorded:**
Clinical record: History and physical or progress note reflect examination of rash and notation that the patient encountered poison ivy while weeding his garden. Over-the-counter (OTC) topical ointment prescribed.
Billing record: Encounter form—office visit recorded

Journal entry:

| | Debit | Credit |
|---|---|---|
| Accounts receivable—Patient X | 60 | |
| Patient service revenue | | 60 |

**Reimbursement received:**
Journal entry:

| | Debit | Credit |
|---|---|---|
| Cash | 60 | |
| Accounts receivable—Patient X | | 60 |

a purchase of supplies would appear to the manager on a list of expenses and be added to a summary of all supply expenses on another report. The cash and accounts payable portions of the transaction would not show because they are controlled by the accounting department. Another example is the discharged, not final billed (DNFB) report (discussed later in this chapter). The DNFB lists individual patient accounts, which are accounts receivable to the organization.

## Financial Statements

At the departmental level, individual financial transactions are reviewed for data quality and compliance with policies and procedures. On an administrative level, the overall impact of transactions is generally of more interest than the individual transactions; therefore, summary reports are prepared. These summaries also are used to communicate with lending institutions, potential investors, and regulatory agencies. A variety of summaries are useful for analyzing an organization's financial activities. The three key reports are the income statement, statement of retained earnings, and balance sheet.

### Income Statement

The **income statement** summarizes the organization's revenue and expense transactions during the fiscal year. The income statement can be prepared at any point in time and reflects results up to that point. The income statement contains only revenue and expense accounts and reflects only the activity for the current fiscal year.

The arithmetic difference between total revenue and total expenses is **net income** in a for-profit organization or excess of revenue over expense in a not-for-profit organization. When total expenses exceed total revenue, net income is a negative number, or a **net loss**. Net income increases equity; net loss decreases equity.

At the end of the fiscal year, all income statement accounts are closed, and the net results are added to, or subtracted from, the appropriate equity account (net asset). For the purposes of periodic reporting, net assets are adjusted in this manner every time this report is prepared. However, at the end of the fiscal year, the income and expense accounts are closed so the new fiscal year begins at zero.

### Retained Earnings or Change in Net Assets

The statement of retained earnings expresses the change in retained earnings from the beginning of the balance sheet period to the end in a for-profit organization, while a statement of change in net assets is prepared in a not-for-profit organization. Retained earnings are affected, for example, by net income and loss, distribution of stock dividends, and payment of long-term debt. Net income and loss are carried forward from the income statement. When the income statement accounts are closed, the net income and loss are transferred to equity. The mechanics of this transaction are to take the balance in each revenue and expense account and record the opposite amount so that all the income statement accounts have a zero balance. The net dollar amount of the debits and credits is recorded to equity. The statement of changes in retained earnings highlights this transaction. The ending balance in retained earnings is then reported on the balance sheet.

### Balance Sheet

The balance sheet is a snapshot of the accounting equation at a point in time. Because every financial transaction affects the equation, theoretically, the balance sheet will look different after every transaction. To ensure a meaningful evaluation, the balance sheet is typically reviewed on a periodic basis (monthly, quarterly, semiannually, and annually). It is often compared to balance sheets from previous fiscal years to analyze changes in the organization.

The balance sheet lists the major account categories grouped under their equation headings: assets, liabilities, and equity and fund balance. Figure 25.5 shows a set of simple statements. The dollar amount shown next to each account category is the total in each category on the ending date listed at the top of the report. This figure also shows the relationship among the income statement, statement of retained earnings, and balance sheet.

### Analysis Statements

Several other types of summary statements are required by users to analyze an organization's financial activity and position. Depending on the organization and its use of the analysis statements, the additional financial statements may be required by GAAP as part of a complete financial summary report. Figure 25.6 shows a two-year, side-by-side comparative balance sheet and three simple examples of statements to help explain the changes from one year to the next. These statements are included for completeness of discussion and are not statements that HIM professionals usually need to analyze.

The statement of cash flow details the reasons that cash changed from one balance sheet period to another. It shows the analyst whether cash was used to purchase equipment or to pay down debt and whether any unusually large transactions took place. The statement of stockholder's equity (also called the statement of net assets) details the reasons for changes in each of the stockholder's equity accounts, including retained earnings.

## Ratio Analysis

After the financial statements have been prepared, they are ready for ratio analysis. Financial analysts can use financial statements, particularly the balance sheet, to determine whether an organization is using its resources similarly to or differently from other organizations in the same industry. For example, hospitals compare their days in accounts receivable ratio to peer hospitals and industry averages. In any industry, one of the most common reasons to analyze financial statements is to lend money to the organization or to invest in it. Thus, the organization's use of assets compared to its liabilities is extremely important. Changes in an organization's ratios are of particular interest.

Ratios, as a comparative tool, are only meaningful within the context of the organization's industry. It is not useful to compare a ratio for a hospital against a ratio for an automobile manufacturer, except to state that one would expect the ratios to be different. Whether an organization's particular ratio is inherently good or bad depends on expected ratios for similar organizations in that industry.

### Liquidity and Debt Service

A key issue to lenders and investors is the organization's ability to repay its financial obligations. Liquidity refers to the ease with which assets can be turned into cash. This is important because payroll, loan payments, and other financial obligations are typically paid in cash. Debt service is the extent to which those financial obligations are loans.

***Current Ratio*** An organization's ability to pay current liabilities with current assets is important to lenders. Current assets include cash, short-term investments, accounts receivable, and inventory. Current assets implicitly will be (or could be) converted to cash at some point

**Figure 25.5.** Financial statements and relationship among the income statement, net assets, and balance sheet

**Sample hospital income statement**

| | 12/31/24 (000) |
|---|---|
| **Revenue** | |
| Net patient service revenue | $650 |
| Unrestricted gifts | 40 |
| Other | 95 |
| Total revenue | $785 |
| **Expenses** | |
| Salaries and wages | $430 |
| Fringe benefits | 95 |
| Supplies | 175 |
| Total expenses | $700 |
| Income from operations | $85 |
| **Nonoperating gains** | |
| Unrestricted gifts | $15 |
| Excess of revenues over expenses | $100 |

**Sample hospital statement of changes in net assets**

| | 2024 (000) |
|---|---|
| Beginning balance January 1 | $900 |
| Excess of revenues over expenses | 100 |
| Ending balance December 31 | $1,000 |

**Sample hospital balance sheet**

| | 12/31/24 (000) |
|---|---|
| **Assets** | |
| Cash | $500 |
| Accounts receivable | 600 |
| Inventory | 400 |
| Building | 2,500 |
| Total assets | $4,000 |
| **Liabilities** | |
| Accounts payable | 600 |
| Mortgage | 2,000 |
| Total liabilities | $2,600 |
| **Net Assets** | |
| Restricted net assets | 400 |
| Unrestricted net assets | $1,000 |
| Total fund balance | $1,400 |
| Total liabilities and net assets | $4,000 |

*Source:* Adapted from Davis and Revoir 2013, 778.

within a year, through collections, sales, or other business activity. Current liabilities include accounts payable and the current portion of loan obligations. Again, the term *current* implies that the liability will be discharged within a year. The **current ratio** compares total current assets with total current liabilities:

$$\frac{\text{Total current assets}}{\text{Total current liabilities}}$$

From the balance sheet in figure 25.6, one can take the current assets (cash plus accounts receivable plus inventory) and divide them by the current liabilities (accounts payable) to determine the current ratio:

$$\frac{1,500,000}{600,000} = \frac{15}{6} = 2.5$$

The current ratio indicates that for every dollar of current liability, $2.50 of current assets could be used to discharge the liability. A higher current ratio is more favorable than a lower current ratio. In this example, the current ratio is 2.5, which is more favorable than another organization that has a current ratio of 1.0.

**Figure 25.6.** Two-year comparative balance sheet with analytical statements

**Sample hospital income Statement**

|  | 12/31/24 (000) | 12/31/23 (000) |
|---|---|---|
| **Revenue** | | |
| Net patient service revenue | $650 | $500 |
| Unrestricted gifts | 40 | 30 |
| Other | 95 | 70 |
| Total revenue | $785 | $600 |
| | | |
| **Expenses** | | |
| Salaries and wages | $430 | $290 |
| Fringe benefits | 95 | 90 |
| Supplies | 175 | 180 |
| Total expenses | $700 | $560 |
| | | |
| Income from operations | $85 | $40 |
| | | |
| **Nonoperating gains** | | |
| Unrestricted gifts | $15 | $10 |
| Excess of revenues over expenses | $100 | $50 |

**Sample hospital statement of revenues and expenses**

|  | 2024 (000) | 2023 (000) |
|---|---|---|
| Beginning balance January 1 | $900 | $850 |
| Excess of revenues over expenses | 100 | 50 |
| Ending balance December 31 | $1,000 | $900 |

**Sample hospital balance sheet**

|  | 12/31/24 (000) | 12/31/23 (000) |
|---|---|---|
| **Assets** | | |
| Cash | $500 | $650 |
| Accounts receivable | 600 | 750 |
| Inventory | 400 | 350 |
| Building | 2,500 | 2,150 |
| | | |
| Total assets | $4,000 | $3,900 |
| | | |
| **Liabilities** | | |
| Accounts payable | 600 | 500 |
| Mortgage | 2,000 | 2,100 |
| | | |
| Total liabilities | $2,600 | $2,600 |
| | | |
| **Net Assets** | | |
| Unrestricted net assets | 400 | 400 |
| Restricted net assets | 1,000 | 900 |
| | | |
| Total net assets | $1,400 | $1,300 |
| | | |
| Total liabilities and net assets | $4,000 | $3,900 |

*Source:* Adapted from Davis and Revoir 2013, 779.

**Days in Accounts Receivable Ratio** A key measure for healthcare organizations to track is the **days in accounts receivable** ratio that reflects how long it takes for an organization to collect its accounts receivable. A lower ratio is preferable, and it means an organization is collecting its receivables more quickly and results in more available cash. The days in accounts receivable divides net accounts receivable by average daily net patient service revenue:

$$\frac{\text{Net accounts receivable}}{(\text{Net patient service revenue} / 365)}$$

For example, if a hospital had net accounts receivable of 90,000 and net patient service revenue for the year of 650,000, the ratio is calculated as follows:

$$\frac{90,000}{(650,000 / 356 \text{ days})} = 50.5 \text{ days in accounts receivable}$$

In this example, patients and payers are, on average, paying their bills within 50.5 days. A lower ratio is preferable and indicates the hospital is efficiently collecting its accounts receivable. A lower ratio provides organizations with more liquidity or access to cash.

**Debt Ratio** Looking back to the mortgage example, the organization's building asset was purchased using 10 percent cash and 90 percent mortgage. Ninety percent of that asset was financed with debt. Looking at all the liabilities and all the assets together gives the analyst an overall picture of how the assets were acquired. The **debt ratio**, therefore, is total liabilities divided by total assets. Using the balance sheet in figure 25.6, the debt ratio is as follows:

$$\frac{2,600,000}{4,000,000} = 65\% \text{ or } 65.0$$

It is important to remember that all ratio analysis is industry specific and varies somewhat depending on the economic environment. Therefore, ratio analysis can be used to compare similar organizations at a specific point in time or the same organization at different points in time. However, a hospital ratio would never be compared with a professional association ratio.

### Profitability

The preceding examples illustrate how organizations can evaluate their ability to pay their bills. Another measure of an organization's health is its profitability. **Profitability** refers to an organization's ability to increase in value: How well does it invest its assets? As with other ratios, profitability measures are only meaningful as benchmarks against like organizations or in trending a single organization over time.

**Return on Investment** Return on investment (ROI) measures the increase in the value of an asset. In a savings account, this increase is measured as the amount of interest received in a period. The beginning balance in the account is the measurement of the asset. Interest received in the period is the return; therefore, the following is true:

$$\text{ROI} = \frac{\text{Interest earned in the period}}{\text{Asset value at the beginning of the period}}$$

Return on individual investments can be calculated in this manner. For an entire organization, interest earned is replaced by earnings, usually after taxes. Asset value is replaced by total assets:

$$\text{ROI} = \frac{\text{Earnings (after taxes)}}{\text{Total assets}}$$

To illustrate ROI, examine the acquisition of technology to generate income:

$$\text{Purchase} : \$100,000 \begin{pmatrix} \text{invest in document} \\ \text{imaging system} \end{pmatrix}$$

$$\text{Liability} : \$90,000 \, (\text{long-term loan from bank})$$

$$\text{Net income} : \$30,000 \, (\text{after taxes})$$

$$\text{ROI} = \frac{\$30,000}{\$100,000} = 30\%$$

In this example, a $100,000 investment generated an ROI of $30,000 or 30 percent. When analyzing new investments, organizations will often identify a benchmark ROI that all new investments must meet or exceed. Additional measures of return are discussed later in the section on capital projects.

**Total Margin Ratio** Overall profitability of an organization is measured by the **total margin ratio**, which compares excess of revenue over expense by total revenue. The ratio is calculated as follows:

$$\frac{\text{Excess of revenue over expense}}{\text{Total revenue}}$$

From the income statement in figure 25.5, the total margin ratio is as follows:

$$\frac{100,000}{785,000} = 0.127 \quad \text{or} \quad 12.7\% \quad \text{or} \quad 12.7$$

The total margin ratio indicates that for every dollar of revenue, the organization earned a profit of 0.12 cents. A higher total margin ratio is preferable because it demonstrates an organization's profitability. It is critical for an organization to maintain profitability to continue to invest in new programs and facilities.

### Check Your Understanding 25.2

Answer the following questions in a separate document.

1. Calculate the total margin ratio for 12/31/23 and 12/31/24 using the income statement in figure 25.6. Interpret the results of the calculation. Is the 12/31/24 ratio more or less favorable than 12/31/23?

2. Evaluate the balance sheet in figure 25.5 and calculate the accounting equation.

3. Discuss the components of the three key financial statements and the relationship among them.

4. Accountant Harriet is analyzing the days in accounts receivable ratio for St. Ava's health system and it increased from 50 days last year to 60 days this year. Is this a favorable or unfavorable trend? Explain your answer.

5. A lender wants to know how quickly a borrower would be able to repay a debt. What is the best ratio to use for this analysis? Why?

## Basic Management Accounting

To obtain appropriate compensation for goods and services provided, the organization must understand and measure the resources used to manufacture, acquire, or otherwise produce those goods and services. The measurement of those resources is monetary and is referred to as their cost. In manufacturing and other goods-oriented businesses, sales are compared to the cost of goods sold, which are composed of raw materials and other manufacturing costs. Calculation of the manufacturing cost of goods sold, byproducts, salvage, and waste is outside the scope of this discussion. In a service industry, the underlying costs consist largely of human resources, supplies, and the tools of the trade.

Management accounting focuses on the internal communication of accounting and financial data for the purpose of facility-based decision-making. Management accountants use the same transaction data that are summarized in a financial statement. They also use a variety of additional data, such as prevailing interest rates and staffing levels, to provide meaningful information required by management.

### Describing Costs

**Cost accounting** is the discipline of identifying and measuring costs and is a unique subset of the accounting profession. However, a general understanding of the terminology helps nonfinancial managers participate in and support the process. There are numerous ways to describe costs, but the most important ones for this discussion are included here.

#### Direct Costs

**Direct costs** are traceable to a specific good or service provided. To a hospital, the cost of a specific medication can be matched to the specific patient to whom it was administered. Room charges are another example. Similarly, to a consulting firm, the hours a consultant coder spends coding are directly linked to the services provided to a specific facility.

#### Indirect Costs

**Indirect costs**, or overhead costs, are incurred by the organization in the process of providing goods or services; however, they are not specifically attributable to an individual product or service. The costs of providing security services at a hospital or customer support at the call center are indirect costs with respect to patient care. To the consulting firm, the cost of CE for its coding staff is an indirect cost of providing services to a particular client.

The classification of costs as direct or indirect depends on the relationship of the cost to the client, department, product, service, or activity in question.

Payroll in the security department is an indirect cost to patient care, but payroll is a direct cost on a nursing floor. Therefore, the distinction between direct and indirect costs is important in understanding the broader financial impact of activities within the facility. In developing capital projects (discussed later in this chapter) such as the development and implementation of an electronic health record, an understanding of the associated costs (and, conversely, the cost savings) is crucial in making realistic financial estimates and projections.

### Fixed Costs

For planning and analysis, it is useful to classify costs as fixed or variable. **Fixed costs** remain the same, despite changes in volume. For example, a manager's base salary does not change, regardless of patient volume or other changes in activity. In figure 25.7, the copy machine depreciation expense does not vary, despite the number of release of information requests.

### Variable Costs

**Variable costs** are sensitive to volume. Medication is a good example. The more patients treated, the more medication used. Release of information requests are another example. The larger the volume of requests for paper records, the more paper is used when printing medical records. In figure 25.8, the cost of paper used to complete release of information requests rises proportionately with the number of requests.

### Semifixed Costs

Costs may behave in a combination of fixed and variable ways, and volume is not the only change agent. For example, consider the coding function. Base coding salaries are fixed. Increases in discharges may require a temporary coding consultant. If the consultant charges on a per-case basis, the cost of coding services rises variably with that volume. Similarly, the combination of personnel and paper costs for release of information has a combined mixed variability, as illustrated in figure 25.9.

On the other hand, nursing base salaries are also a fixed cost. However, hospitals do not staff nursing for full capacity. Therefore, increases in census require the use of part-time or per diem nurses, who are added based on established patient-to-nurse ratios. The full cost of nursing services, then, goes up in steps. Figure 25.10 illustrates this type of personnel cost variability.

### Cost Reports

Prior to implementation of prospective payment systems (PPSs), Medicare reimbursement to hospitals was related directly to the costs incurred by the

**Figure 25.8.** Variable cost

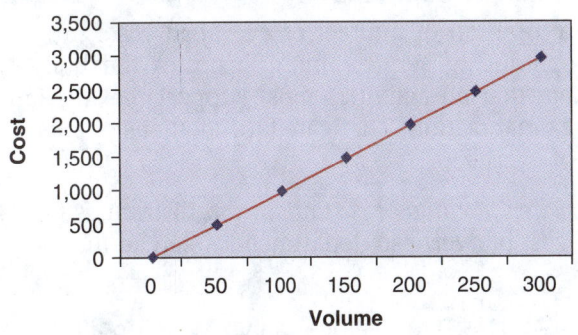

**Figure 25.9.** Mixed cost

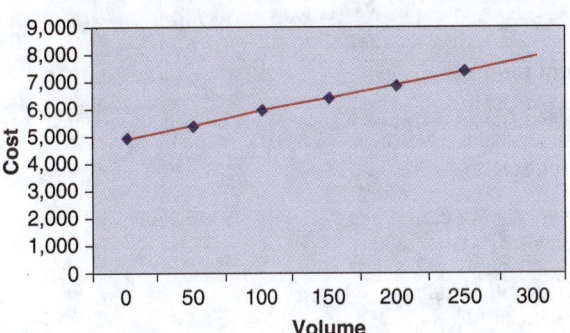

**Figure 25.7.** Fixed cost

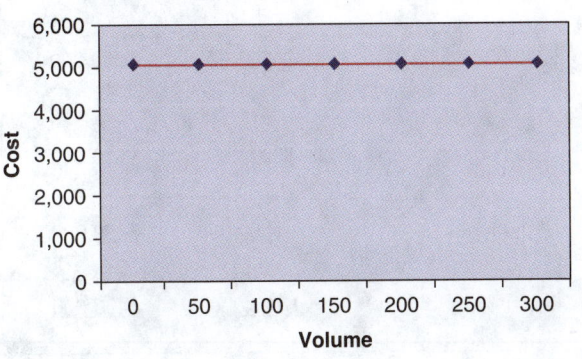

**Figure 25.10.** Step mixed cost

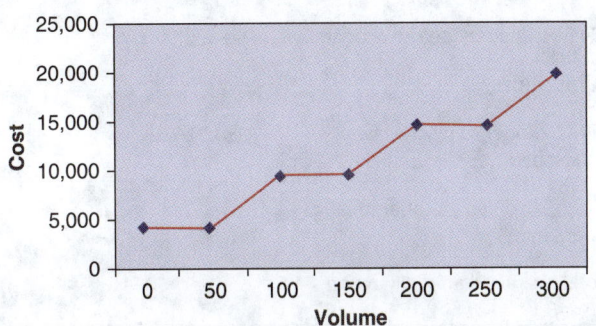

facilities. Individual facility cost reports were submitted to Medicare, identifying the direct and indirect costs of providing care to Medicare patients. Direct costs include nursing and radiology; indirect costs include HIM and information systems.

The expense of non-revenue-producing cost centers is allocated to revenue-producing cost centers to fully understand the cost of providing services. Although cost reporting is no longer used to directly determine Medicare reimbursement for prospective payment facilities, critical access hospitals are reimbursed a specified rate of eligible Medicare costs. In addition, CMS uses cost reports to help determine facility-specific and regional cost adjustment factors for healthcare PPSs.

## Allocation of Overhead

The attribution of indirect or overhead costs to revenue-producing service units illustrates the budget concept that all activities must support the mission of the organization. There are four methods of allocation of overhead:

- *Direct method of cost allocation* distributes the cost of overhead departments solely to the revenue-producing areas. Allocation is based on each revenue-producing area's relative square footage, number of employees, or actual usage of supplies and services.
- *Step-down allocation* distributes overhead costs once, beginning with the area that provides the least amount of non-revenue-producing services. (See figure 25.11.)
- *Double distribution* allocates overhead costs twice, which takes into consideration the fact that some overhead departments provide services to each other.
- *Simultaneous equations method* distributes overhead costs through multiple iterations allowing maximum distribution of interdepartmental costs among overhead departments.

The last three methods of cost allocation listed assume that overhead cost centers (such as housekeeping) perform services for each other and revenue-producing areas. Therefore, overhead costs are distributed among overhead cost centers and revenue-producing areas. Although each of these methods may produce slightly different results, the goal is to

**Figure 25.11.** Direct allocation versus step allocation

|  | Non-revenue-producing department | Revenue-producing department |  |  |
|---|---|---|---|---|
|  | HIM department | Pharmacy | Medicine | Laboratory |
| **Direct method:** |  |  |  |  |
| Overhead costs before allocation | $360,000 | $240,000 | $400,000 | $250,000 |
| **Allocation** |  |  |  |  |
| HIM (number of discharges processed) | ($360,000) |  | $340,000 | $20,000 |
| Business office (number of labor hours used) |  | ($240,000) | $80,000 | $160,000 |
| Total overhead after allocation | $0 | $0 | $820,000 | $430,000 |
| **Step method:** |  |  |  |  |
| Overhead costs before allocation | $360,000 | $240,000 | $400,000 | $250,000 |
| **Allocation** |  |  |  |  |
| HIM (number of discharges processed) | ($360,000) | $50,000 | $300,000 | $10,000 |
| Business office (number of labor hours used) |  | ($290,000) | $90,000 | $200,000 |
| Total overhead after allocation | $0 | $0 | $790,000 | $460,000 |

allocate overhead costs appropriately, enabling the facility to express the full cost of providing services.

## Impact of Accounts Receivable on Financial Statements

Accounts receivable represents a current asset. Delays in processing claims cause receivables to age. Aged receivables can negatively affect a facility's ability to borrow money. Failure to claim and collect receivables affects cash, which in turn negatively affects the facility's ability to discharge its current liabilities, the largest of which is payroll. Therefore, in a facility for which reimbursement is the largest revenue item and payroll is the largest expense, there is a direct relationship between getting paid and paying employees. Thus, the role of HIM becomes a critical component of maintaining the facility's fiscal integrity.

# Internal Controls

In any industry, internal controls must be in place to safeguard assets and to ensure compliance with policies and procedures. Internal controls may be designed to prevent the theft of cash or to ensure a patient receives the correct medication. The three major categories of internal controls are preventive, detective, and corrective controls.

## Preventive

A preventive control is a front-end process that guides work in such a way that input and process variations are minimized. They are implemented prior to the activity taking place because they are designed to stop an error from happening. In financial management, pre-transaction supervisory review and authorization is a preventive control. Data entry validation is another preventive control. Data entry validation prevents the user from entering "64," for example, as a day of the month. Preventive controls are sometimes more costly than their effect warrants. In those cases, other types of controls must be put in place to find and correct errors.

## Detective

Detective controls are processes designed to find errors that have already been made. Detective controls tend to be less expensive than preventive controls and can be implemented at many levels. Quantitative record reviews and computer exception reports are examples of detective controls. In accounting, the summing of debits and credits is a detective control, because the two sums must always be equal. Footing and cross-footing financial reports are another detective control (See figure 25.12.)

The foot is the sum of the columns; the cross-foot is the sum of the rows. Notice that in this example the sums do not match. Footing and cross-footing reports that are supposed to represent arithmetic totals is a very useful detective control, particularly with manually prepared or PC-prepared reports. A simple error in creating a formula in a spreadsheet program can cause an entire report to be incorrect.

## Corrective

When an error or other problem has been detected, action must be taken to correct the error, solve the problem, or design controls to prevent future errors or problems. The error or problem must be analyzed to determine the cause. When a correction can be made, it is documented and implemented. However, if an error cannot be corrected, analysis of the root cause is important so that the error can be prevented in the future. In financial management, very few errors cannot be corrected. Typical errors include posting transactions to an incorrect account, posting transactions that have not been completed, and posting incorrect amounts. Even financial statement errors can be corrected, and the reports redistributed. Problems that cannot always be corrected include theft of assets and failure to invest funds on a timely basis. These problems require analysis and development and implementation of controls for the future.

Corrective controls are designed to fix any problems discovered, frequently as a result of detective controls. Many errors and problems occur routinely, such as failing to complete forms, making computation errors, and wrongly posting transactions. Therefore, procedures must be in place to ensure the timely and accurate correction of the error or solution to the problem. In the HIM department, the incomplete record system is a corrective control. Incomplete records have been detected, the source of the error identified, and the responsible individual contacted for completion of the documentation. In financial management, supervisory review of transactions is typically used to detect errors and problems. The ability to correct errors in journal entries is essential.

Internal controls may be present at every level of the organization. In a service organization, such as a hospital, controls over expenditures are some of the most important responsibilities of individual managers. Two key methods of exerting such controls are through purchasing and analysis of budget variances.

**Figure 25.12.** Footing and cross-footing financial reports

**Summing of debits and credits**

| | | |
|---|---|---|
| Supplies (photocopy paper) | $974 | |
| Supplies (Toner) | $362 | |
| Cash | | $1,345 |

In this journal entry, the debit ($1,345) does not match the credits ($1,336). This means that an error has been made. Reference to the original documentation will reveal the sales tax on the items was not accounted for.

**Footing and cross-footing**

| | January | February | March | Year-to-date (Cross-foot) |
|---|---|---|---|---|
| Payroll | 20,000 | 20,000 | 20,000 | 60,000 |
| Benefits | 6,000 | 6,000 | 6,000 | 24,000 |
| Office supplies | 1,000 | 1,000 | 1,000 | 3,000 |
| Equipment service | 400 | 500 | 600 | 500 |
| | | | | 87,500? |
| Monthly totals | 27,400 (Foot) | 27,400 | 27,400 | 82,200? |

The foot is the sum of the columns; the cross-foot is the sum of the rows. Notice that in this example the sums do not match. Footing and cross-footing reports that are supposed to represent arithmetic totals is a very useful detective control, particularly with manually prepared or PC-prepared reports. A simple error in creating a formula in a spreadsheet program can cause an entire report to be incorrect.

### Check Your Understanding 25.3

Answer the following questions in a separate document.

1. Give four examples each of direct and indirect costs in a hospital.

2. How can the management of accounts receivable affect the financial statements and an organization's financial health? Include the role of HIM in an organization's financial health.

3. Hackers routinely try to gain unauthorized access to healthcare system information technology networks. Strong passwords are an important internal control to avoid unauthorized access. Compare the three types of internal controls, and state which type of internal control strong passwords would be categorized as.

4. When allocating overhead, organizations rely on statistics or metrics that best reflect utilization of overhead; for example, the maintenance department could be allocated based on square footage per department. Formulate a method to allocate overhead for the following departments: human resources, the laundry department, and the finance department.

5. Categorize the following costs as fixed, variable, or mixed, and provide your rationale: wages for RNs in the operating room (OR), monthly lease costs on a surgery center, and disposable supplies for a surgical robot that are required for each case.

## Budgets

Managers must have some understanding of managerial accounting to control the financial aspects of their departments' operations. As stated earlier, managers must work within budgets developed based on their organization's goals and objectives. Therefore, it is not sufficient for a manager merely to review for accuracy the financial transactions generated by the department during the period. Rather, the transactions must be compared to the expected or budgeted transactions to ensure that the goals and objectives of both the department and the organization are being met. **Managerial accounting** is the development, implementation, and analysis of systems that track financial transactions for managerial control purposes; it includes both budget and cost analysis systems.

## Types of Budgets

In addition to the most familiar budgets, operating and capital budgets, organizations develop and monitor other budgets, including financial budgets, cash flow budgets, and incremental budgets. These budgets are the responsibility of the finance department.

The development and monitoring of budgets is guided by the facility's policy and procedures manual and the management styles of the administrative and departmental management team. Therefore, it is important for department managers to understand the facility's budgeting methods, including how administration uses budgets.

A budget is a manager's best guess at the outcomes of future financial transactions. Unexpected events that influence those transactions, such as declining census, increase in interest rates, and staffing changes, create budget variances. Some budgets are specifically designed to take these fluctuations into consideration. A budget can represent virtually any projected set of circumstances. Therefore, there are many different types of budget methodologies. Common methodologies include fixed, flexible, activity-based, and zero-based budgets.

The most common type of budget is a **fixed budget**, in which amounts are based on expected capacity. Fixed budgets do not change when expected capacity changes. For example, the HIM department would budget outsourced coding service expense based on the estimated number of discharges and historical need. When the number of discharges materially increases or declines, the outsourced coding service expense will increase or decrease, thus creating a budget variance.

**Flexible budgets** are based on projected productivity. In this case, the HIM department would budget outsourced coding service expense at several levels of discharges. As the actual discharges become known, the budget reflects the estimate at that level of activity. Used primarily in manufacturing, this method of budgeting also is useful for projecting personnel budgets in service areas, such as nursing units, where increased activity has a direct impact on staffing and supplies.

**Activity-based budgets** are based on activities or projects rather than on departments. Typically used for construction projects, an activity-based budget can be useful for any project that spans multiple budget lines or departments and for projects that span more than one fiscal year. Computer system installation and implementation should be controlled using an activity-based budget.

Different budget methodologies are developed to meet the needs of the organization. Fixed and flexible budgets are characteristic of operating budgets. Activity-based budgets are more often used for capital projects. All three types of budgets can be used by virtually any organization. **Zero-based budgets**, on the other hand, apply to organizations for which each budget cycle poses the opportunity to continue or discontinue services based on the availability of resources. Every department or activity must be justified and prioritized annually to effectively allocate the organization's resources. Professional associations and charitable foundations, for example, routinely use zero-based budgeting.

## Operational Budgets

The purpose of an **operational budget** is to allocate and control resources in a manner consistent with the organization's goals and objectives. These goals and objectives are tied to the organization's mission. Each department should have its own mission, goals, and objectives that identify how it contributes to the organization's overall mission. Every item in the operational budget should have a direct relationship to a departmental goal that supports an organizational goal.

The budget process begins with the board of directors or trustees, which approves the fiscal assumptions for the upcoming year. Those assumptions are quantified and communicated to the department managers, who develop budgets based on those assumptions. Typical assumptions include the desired growth in revenue and targeted cost reductions.

### Budget Cycle

The operational budget cycle generally coincides with one fiscal year. The purpose of the operational budget is the quantification of the projected results of operations for the coming fiscal year. This process begins three to four months before the end of the current fiscal year. Projected budgets should be collected, compiled, reviewed, and approved prior to the start of the new fiscal year.

***Fiscal Period*** An organization's budget year coincides with its fiscal year on file with the IRS. Although the actual operational budget generally only applies to one fiscal year, financial managers often project multiple years of budgets with a variety of scenarios to test the financial impact of current decision-making.

***Interim Periods*** Monthly budget reporting is the most common budget cycle. Any period that represents less than an entire fiscal year is an interim period. Figure 25.13 provides a sample budget report for

**Figure 25.13.** HIM department budget report for May

| Description | May budget | May actual | May variance | YTD budget | YTD actual | YTD variance |
|---|---|---|---|---|---|---|
| Payroll | $25,000 | $22,345 | $2,655 | $125,000 | $110,321 | $14,679 |
| Benefits | $8,000 | $7,360 | $640 | $40,000 | $37,870 | $2,130 |
| Contract services | $5,000 | $8,000 | ($3,000) | $25,000 | $40,000 | ($15,000) |
| Office supplies | $150 | $145 | $5 | $750 | $975 | ($225) |
| Printer paper | $100 | $250 | ($150) | $500 | $500 | – |
| Postage | $95 | $97 | ($2) | $475 | $456 | $19 |
| Travel | $0 | $0 | – | $0 | $0 | – |
| Continuing education | $0 | $0 | – | $0 | $45 | ($45) |

an HIM department for May. The budgeted amounts for each item are listed next to the actual amounts for the month. As is common, the year-to-date (in this case, January through May) budget and actual amounts also are included. It is useful for budget reports to show the *variances*, which are the differences between budgeted and actual amounts. Many budget reports also show the percentage variance for each item, based on the budget. Managers may be required to explain variances that exceed a particular dollar value or a specified percentage.

In the budget report shown in figure 25.13, there is a large variance in May's budgeted expense for printer paper. By following that line item across to the year-to-date amount, it is evident there is no year-to-date variance in the budget. This illustrates a timing difference between the expected expense and the actual expense. The budget may have placed that expense in April even though the actual expense occurred in May. These types of temporary variances are the result of normal business activities; and although they may require explanation, they are usually not of concern.

### Budget Components

The components of an operational budget generally follow the format of the income statement and list revenue items and expense items. Every department is different, depending on its unique activities. However, budget reports tend to be uniform throughout the organization. Therefore, line items that do not apply to a particular department are likely to be listed with zero values rather than be omitted.

**Revenues** There is little, if any, revenue in the HIM department. Occasionally, a facility with excess capacity will contract or outsource transcription or coding services. Copy fees are another potential source of revenue. However, because such fees should be cost-based, they are probably more appropriately considered a reimbursement (reduction of expenses).

**Expenses** The HIM department budget consists primarily of expenses. Expenses may be incurred because of financial transactions outside or within the organization. Some departments, such as housekeeping and facilities maintenance, perform services for other facility departments. Therefore, charges from these departments may appear on the budget. Such charges are generally carried forward through the cost allocation process and usually are not estimated by individual managers.

Ordinarily, the single largest expense in a healthcare facility is payroll. This is typical for service organizations. Payroll can be a difficult expense to project because employees have different anniversary dates and different salary increases. For direct patient care departments, the payroll budget is driven by patient volumes. For example, on a nursing floor, a manager will multiply the number of budgeted patient days times the budgeted hours per patient. As patient days increase or decrease, the number of budgeted nursing hours will change along with the payroll budget. For many indirect departments such as HIM or accounting, the payroll budget is often based on the prior year's actual expenses and adjusted for any staffing changes and pay increases. Because payroll is the largest expense category, there is often pressure from management to reduce payroll expenses.

The cost of employee benefits is part of payroll but is often listed separately. Facilities rarely expect department managers to calculate benefits budgets because this is a human resource-controlled line item. The cost of benefits tracks with payroll, for example as payroll expense increases so does benefits expense.

Supplies are often the next largest expense account. Clinical supplies are a substantial item on the cardiology or radiology department budget, whereas office supplies might be a large item for HIM. Examples of cardiology supplies include stents and $40,000 pacemakers while examples of office supplies includes printer ink, USB devices, pens, and paper.

Cost of goods sold is a manufacturing concept that refers to the underlying cost of making the finished goods. This concept applies to healthcare providers in the sense that there is a cost basis for providing services. For every inpatient treated, there are payroll, utility, office supplies, pharmaceutical, and equipment costs the facility incurs. Unlike manufacturing, in which the cost of producing items is tracked very closely, healthcare facilities historically have not been good at tracking each of the underlying costs of providing services to individual patients. The costs of providing care are often analyzed at a facility-wide level that includes total costs for all patients.

## Management of the Operating Budget

Once the operating budget is developed and approved, it is the responsibility of department management to ensure budget goals are met. As a rule, in meeting goals, revenue should meet or exceed budget, and expenses should meet or be less than budget. However, because expenses support revenues, an increase in revenues (perhaps due to unexpected volume) may signal an expected increase in expenses, such as variable expenses. This is particularly true when the patient census exceeds expectations. Despite the logical and expected nature of these results, managers are required to investigate and explain differences between budgeted and actual amounts on a regular basis.

### Identification of Variances

A variance is the arithmetic difference between the budgeted amount and the actual amount of a line item. Variance analysis places accountability for financial transactions on the manager of the department that initiated the transaction.

Variances are often calculated on the monthly budget report. An organization's policies and procedures manual defines unacceptable variances or variances that must be explained. In identifying variances, it is important to recognize whether the variance is favorable or unfavorable and whether it is temporary or permanent.

*Timing* The problems identified by variance analysis and the action that must be taken depend largely on whether the variance is temporary or permanent. Temporary variances are generally self-limiting. Temporary budget variances are not expected to continue in subsequent months. For example, a department may budget for a large purchase of printer paper in May. When that purchase does not actually take place until July, there will be a temporary variance in the May and July monthly report and a temporary variance in the May and June year-to-date numbers. Figure 25.14 illustrates this point. In this example, the HIM department budgeted $260 per month for department supplies, plus an additional $900 in May for printer paper. This created a temporary, favorable variance in expenditures in May and June.

In contrast, permanent budget variances do not resolve during the current fiscal year. In the preceding example, a variance still would have existed at the end of December (the close of the fiscal year) if the printer paper had been budgeted in November. The department supplies variance then would be a permanent variance during the current and subsequent fiscal year, unless the subsequent year's budget can include the purchase.

*Impact* In addition to identifying whether timing is an issue, the variance analysis is expected to identify whether the variance is favorable or unfavorable. This is often determined from the budget report but should be stated clearly when discussing the variance so that the information is not misinterpreted.

Favorable variances occur when the actual results are better than budget projections. Actual revenue greater than budget is a favorable variance. Unfavorable variances occur when the actual results are worse than what was budgeted. Actual expenditure in excess of the budget is an unfavorable variance. Note that the terms *favorable* and *unfavorable* refer to the impact on the organization rather than to the magnitude or direction of the variance. Sometimes the terms *negative* and *positive* are used instead. This can be confusing because a negative expense variance is favorable. Therefore, it is extremely important to ensure the manager understands and correctly uses the language of the organization.

### Explanation of Variances

The analysis of budget variances is a financial management control. Administration may review the monthly budget report first and then ask questions of the appropriate manager. In other instances, the department managers are automatically required to respond to certain variances.

In general, the reason for a temporary budget variance is the timing of the transaction. Referring to the department supplies and printer paper example in figure 25.14, there is a simple explanation for the temporary

**Figure 25.14.** Examples of budget variances

| | Budget | Actual | Variance | YTD budget | YTD actual | YTD variance |
|---|---|---|---|---|---|---|
| **May budget report** | | | | | | |
| Department supplies | 1,150 | 250 | 900 | 2,150 | 1,250 | 900 |
| **June budget report** | | | | | | |
| Department supplies | 250 | 250 | 0 | 2,400 | 1,500 | 900 |
| **July budget report** | | | | | | |
| Department supplies | 250 | 1,150 | –900 | 2,650 | 2,650 | 0 |

variance. In wording the explanation to administration, the department manager should state the following:

- Nature of the variance (favorable or unfavorable, temporary or permanent)
- Exact amount of the variance
- Cause of the variance
- Any mitigating circumstances or offsetting amounts

Understanding and explaining budget variances is an important aspect for managers to control expenses.

***Amount*** In the analysis of variance, materiality is an issue. Rarely will a manager be required to explain a five-dollar variance. Clearly, the cost of a manager's time to explain such an insignificant amount far exceeds the benefit of knowing why the variance has occurred. In fact, because budgets are largely estimates, it would be quite odd if the actual amounts always matched the budgeted amounts. Therefore, dollar and percentage limits are set in the organization's policies and procedures manual. Variances that exceed these limits must be explained in detail.

***Cause*** For the preceding printer paper variance example, the explanation might be something like the following: In department supplies, the favorable, temporary variance of $900 will resolve in July when the budgeted expenditure for printer paper is processed. For such a temporary variance, no additional explanation is usually necessary.

Temporary variances are not typically of serious concern to administrations. However, permanent variances can be a problem because management of departmental budgets is an important indicator of the competence of department managers.

Whether a variance is temporary or permanent depends on the answers to two questions:

- Are the subsequent transactions that will compensate for the variance likely to occur within the same fiscal year?
- Is it reasonably certain the transactions will occur as predicted?

If the compensating transactions are unlikely to take place during the current fiscal year, the result is a permanent variance in the current budget report. Sometimes the manager may not know when—or if—the transactions will take place. For example, the manager may have budgeted $2,000 for attendance at an unspecified CE conference in June. A conflict with the Joint Commission survey prevented the manager from attending the conference, creating a favorable expense variance. If the manager believes the amount will be spent appropriately at some time during the fiscal year, the variance is temporary. For example, the manager may be able to attend a conference later in the year. However, if the manager knows that there is no chance of attending a conference and appropriately spending the budgeted amount, the variance should be explained as permanent.

Additional explanation may be necessary for a permanent variance. An expenditure that must be deferred until the next fiscal year is particularly important. In that case, the explanation might be as follows: In department supplies, there is a favorable, permanent variance of $900 because a large order of printer paper was planned for this fiscal year but did not occur; this amount is included in next year's budget.

***Circumstances*** Managers may have the opportunity to utilize favorable variances in one line item to offset unfavorable variances in another line item. For example, unused travel budget may be used for CE. The explanation of these circumstances will generally be carried forward through all remaining variance analyses for the remainder of the fiscal year.

The ability to work with the departmental budget as a whole as opposed to justifying line items is entirely dependent on the administration of the budget process. One typical example of offsetting variances occurs when an employee leaves and cannot be replaced immediately. Several things may happen. The vacancy may cause a favorable variance in payroll expense until the position is filled or an unfavorable variance in payroll expense if other employees are paid overtime to help fill the vacancy. Both variances are permanent. Alternatively, the vacancy may cause a permanent, favorable variance in payroll expenses and a permanent, unfavorable variance in consulting expenses when the vacant position is outsourced. In the latter case, the two variances at least partially offset each other, which must be explained in the monthly variance report.

## Capital Budget

Unlike the operational budget, which looks primarily at projected income statement activity for the next fiscal year, the capital budget looks at long-term investments. Such investments are usually related to improvements in the facility infrastructure, expansion of services, or replacement of existing assets. Capital investments focus on either the appropriateness of an investment (given the facility's investment guidelines) or choosing among different opportunities to invest. The capital budget is the facility's plan for allocating resources over and above the operating budget.

Funding for the capital budget may come from diverse sources. For example, donations or grants may fund a building project or retained earnings, or unallocated reserves may fund equipment purchases. Federal and state government funds may be available to offset the cost of capital investments. Regardless of the source of the funds, capital investments are defined by facility policy and selected using financial analysis techniques.

### Large-Dollar Purchases

From a departmental perspective, capital budget items are large-dollar purchases, as defined by facility budget policies and procedures. Capital budget items usually have a useful life more than one fiscal year, making them long-term assets, and a dollar value greater than a predetermined amount—often $500 or $1,000. Common HIM department capital budget items include office furniture, photocopying and scanning equipment, and computer equipment. Some organizations maintain a separate capital budget and process for computer-related equipment and software. In addition, control over the acquisition of the related long-term assets in such cases may rest with the information technology or IS department.

### Acquisitions

The acquisition of long-term assets may be controlled by the purchasing department. The purchasing department may already have a contract with a specific vendor to provide certain types of equipment or furniture. In the absence of an existing contract, it may still be the purchasing department's responsibility to ensure the appropriate acquisition of assets through the request for proposal (RFP) process. The RFP process is a preventive control designed to eliminate bias and to ensure competitive pricing in the acquisition of goods and services.

### Cost–Benefit Analysis

Cost benefit is the concept that the benefit of an action should exceed its cost. For example, an old photocopying machine breaks down at least once a week. Repair of the machine takes up to two days and is increasingly expensive. During the downtime, release of information clerks must use a machine located two floors below the HIM department and shared by three other departments. It seems obvious to HIM department personnel that a new machine is needed and including a new machine in the HIM department's capital budget request is certainly warranted. However, funding for a new machine is based on specific, detailed cost justifications and is weighed in comparison to all departments' requests. Facility administration may be forced to choose between a new copier for the HIM department and several new computers for the patient accounts department. All other factors being equal, increased efficiency and productivity in claims processing is likely to be chosen over increased efficiency in release of information. For this reason, HIM managers should include cost savings calculations in such requests.

### Depreciation

As discussed previously, certain long-term assets, such as equipment and furniture, wear out over time and must be replaced. Such assets contribute to revenue over multiple fiscal periods. Therefore, the cost of these assets is not recorded as an expense at the time of purchase. Rather, the current asset—cash is exchanged for a long-term asset—equipment. A portion of the historical cost of equipment then is moved from asset into expense each fiscal year and cumulated into the contra-account—accumulated depreciation.

Eventually, the cost of equipment has been expensed and equipment account value is zero. The purpose of depreciation is to spread the cost of an asset over its useful life. (See table 25.7 for sample depreciation methods.)

Note that the depreciation of long-term assets does not necessarily have a direct relationship to the activity of using the asset. It is common to depreciate an asset over five years and then continue to use it for another five. For example, a facility whose equipment is fully depreciated and whose current assets are heavily financed with debt obligations may be unable to reinvest in new equipment. This is another example of how ratio analysis affects lending decisions.

## Capital Projects

A facility's ability to invest in capital projects is important to the continued success of its operations. Because buildings deteriorate, equipment wears out, and new technology is important to healthcare delivery, capital improvements must be implemented. Individual departments request equipment purchases and facility improvements as the needs arise. Facility administration must choose among the suggested projects to optimize use of its resources.

In addition to capital improvements, facilities may make capital investments that improve operational efficiency. Some of these capital investments require broader analysis than the cost of the equipment.

**Table 25.7.** Sample depreciation methods

| Method | Description | Formula |
|---|---|---|
| Straight line | The cost of the asset is expensed equally over the expected life of the asset. The estimated sale value of the asset at the end of its useful life is called the residual value and is subtracted from the cost prior to depreciation.<br>**Example:**<br>Copy machine purchased at a cost of $5,000<br>Useful life = 4 years<br>Residual value = $200<br>$$\text{Annual depreciation} = \frac{\$5,000 - \$200}{4} = \$1,200 \text{ per year}$$ | $$\frac{\text{Cost} - \text{residual value}}{\text{Number of years (useful life)}}$$ |
| Units of production | The cost of the asset is expensed over the expected life of the asset, measured in usage. In this case, usage would be the number of copies.<br>**Example:**<br>Copy machine purchased at a cost of $5,000<br>Useful life = 100,000 copies<br>Residual value = $200<br>Annual depreciation = $0.048 times the number of copies made<br>$$\text{Depreciation rate} = \frac{\$5,000 - \$200}{100,000} = \$0.048 \,(4.8 \text{ cents}) \text{ per copy}$$ | $$\frac{\text{Cost} - \text{residual value}}{\text{Number of copies (useful life)}}$$ |
| Accelerated | There are several accelerated depreciation methods, all of which are designed to expense more of the asset's value early in its useful life. One such method is called double declining balance (DDB). DDB expenses the asset at double the straight-line method, based on the book value rather than on the historical cost.<br>**Example:**<br>Copy machine purchased at a cost of $5,000<br>Useful life = 100,000 copies<br>Residual value = $200<br>Straight-line rate $1,200/$4,800 = 25%<br>Annual depreciation = Book value times 50% | Book value times twice the straight-line rate<br>$$\text{Straight-line rate} = \frac{\text{annual depreciation}}{\text{cost} - \text{residual value}}$$ |

*Note:* These examples of depreciation methods are just a few of the acceptable methods in use today for various purposes. The reader should be aware there are other methods and that not all methods are acceptable for income tax purposes or for GAAP. Accounting for income taxes is beyond the scope of this discussion.

Replacing a manual incomplete record tracking system with a computer-based system, for example, involves an analysis of employee time and departmental space allocations as well as the associated equipment and software costs. Medical staff relationship improvement is another factor that is difficult to quantify but should be considered.

Facility administration looks at capital projects differently from how it reviews operational activities. Theoretically, operational activities contribute to the generation of revenue for the facility. For example, all hospital activities either provide healthcare services or in some way support departments that provide healthcare services. A hospital may elect to perform its own printing rather than outsource the printing function. However, it is unlikely to provide printing services to the public. Printing forms supports clinical and administrative services internally, but running a printing business does not. Therefore, the justification for operational budget amounts generally rests on the extent to which the underlying activities support the mission of the facility at the projected productivity levels. Capital projects, on the other hand, although still mission supportive, often leverage the facility to higher levels of productivity, increased efficiency, or expansion of services and capacity.

Departments acquiring capital equipment often work with the finance department to prepare financial analysis reports that review projected revenues, costs, and cost savings and use a variety of financial analysis techniques discussed later in the chapter to determine whether the project meets predetermined levels of return. For example, if the obstetrics department wants to acquire an additional ultrasound machine, the department manager would work with the finance department to project expected patient volumes, reimbursements, and costs that a new ultrasound machine would be expected to generate and compare those returns to predetermined levels set by management.

Finally, budgeted capital funds generally must be expended in the period for which they were approved. Even when allocated, capital budget items may be prioritized and timed so that purchases are made only with administrative approval. Actual funding may not meet anticipated levels, or unforeseen circumstances may change administrative priorities. For capital budgets, supporting the mission of the facility is not sufficient justification. Capital projects also must satisfy predetermined levels of return on the projected investment.

## Cost Justification

All departments in a facility compete for its finite resources. Therefore, department managers must be familiar with cost justification techniques and with their facility's method of analyzing capital projects. Typical cost justifications are based on increased revenue, increased efficiency, improved customer service, reduced liability, and reduced costs. The analysis of a capital project is based on the estimated ROI, including the weight of the costs versus the benefits to be derived from the project. The specific cost–benefit analysis method used by facility administration depends on the characteristics of the project and the preferences of the analyst. When no specific cash inflows are expected, return may be based on depreciation or other cost savings. Sometimes the capital budget includes the allocation of resources for assets whose acquisition will attract or retain valuable personnel or physician relationships. Even in such cases, the acquisition should be analyzed financially, not just politically.

## Payback Period

The **payback period** is the time required to recoup the cost of an investment. Mortgage refinancing analysis frequently uses the concept of payback period. Mortgage refinancing is considered when interest rates have dropped. Refinancing may require up-front interest payments, called points, as well as a variety of administrative costs. In this example, the payback period is the time it takes for the savings in interest to equal the cost of the refinancing:

| Payback period | |
|---|---|
| Investment: | $100,000 |
| Cash in: | $50,000 per year |
| Payback period: | 2 years (100,000/50,000) |

The advantage of using a payback period to analyze investments is that it is relatively easy to calculate and understand. For example, a payback period can be used to describe the time it takes for the savings in payroll costs to equal the cost of productivity-enhancing equipment.

The disadvantage of a payback period is that it ignores the time value of money. Because the funds used for one capital investment could have been invested elsewhere, there is always an inherent opportunity cost of choosing one investment over another. Hence, there is an assumed rate of return determined by administration against which investments are compared and a benchmark rate of return under which a facility will not consider an investment.

## Accounting Rate of Return

Another simple method of capital project analysis is the **accounting rate of return (ARR)**. This method compares the projected annual cash inflows, minus any applicable annual depreciation, divided by the initial investment. Consider the purchase of an ultrasound machine. Reimbursement from use of the machine is the cash inflow. Depreciation is calculated based on the initial investment. The following example shows the ARR for the purchase of a $100,000 ultrasound machine:

| Accounting Rate of Return | |
|---|---|
| Investment: | $100,000 ultrasound machine |
| Straight-line depreciation over five years: | $20,000 per year |
| Cash in: | $50,000 per year |
| ARR: | 30 percent [(50,000 − 20,000)/100,000] |

ARR is another example of a simple method of capital project analysis. However, it also ignores the time value of money. In addition, ARR is based on an estimate. If the analyst incorrectly projects annual cash inflows, the projected rate of return will be incorrect.

### Return on Investment

ROI is most frequently used to analyze marketable securities, or investments in stock, retrospectively. The increase in market value of the securities divided by the initial investment is the ROI. When an income stream is associated with the investment, the income stream is added to the market value of the securities in calculating return. In comparing the ROI among different securities, the tax implications must be considered. Long-term gains are taxed differently than short-term gains. Tax-exempt investments result in different returns than taxable investments.

With respect to capital investments, the equation is similar. Divide the controllable operating profits by the controllable net investment. Operating profits are the cash inflow minus the direct costs of operation. For instance, the ROI for the purchase of $100,000 worth of equipment would be calculated as follows:

| Return on Investment | |
|---|---|
| Investment: | $100,000 in equipment |
| Straight-line depreciation over 5 years: | $20,000 per year |
| Operating costs: | $5,000 per year |
| Cash in: | $50,000 per year |
| ROI: | 25 percent [(50,000 − 25,000)/100,000] |

As with ARR and payback period, ROI is easy to calculate and understand. Similarly, it does not consider the time value of money. Organizations will establish a benchmark ROI required for new investments. In this example, if the benchmark ROI is 15 percent, this investment would be approved because it is projected to generate an ROI of 25 percent.

### Net Present Value

To take into consideration the time value of money, the analyst must establish an interest rate at which money could have otherwise been invested. From that implied interest rate and the projected future cash inflows of the investment, the present value of the cash inflows is calculated. Present value is the current dollar amount that must be invested today to yield the projected future cash inflows at the implied interest rate. Net present value (NPV) is the calculated present value of the future cash inflows compared to the initial investment.

The advantage of using NPV to analyze investments is that it considers the time value of money. When choosing among like investments, NPVs can be reliably compared to determine the financial advantages of the investment. For example, the NPV of $100,000 worth of equipment would be calculated as follows:

| Net Present Value | |
|---|---|
| Investment: | $100,000 |
| Cash in: | $25,000 per year (revenue minus depreciation and operating costs) |
| Interest rate: | 7 percent |
| NPV: | $2,505 (based on 5 years of service) |

As with other analysis tools, analysts may have to estimate the projected cash flows. However, the main disadvantage of NPV is that the interest rate is subjective. Therefore, it is best used to compare multiple investment opportunities rather than to analyze one investment alone. Another disadvantage of using NPV is that it requires some knowledge of mathematics to calculate and to accept its validity and understand its relevance. Fortunately, financial calculators and spreadsheet programs have made the calculation of NPV relatively simple.

### Internal Rate of Return

Internal rate of return (IRR) is the interest rate that makes the NPV calculation equal zero. In other words, it is the interest rate at which the present value of the projected cash inflows equals the initial investment. IRR considers the time value of money. Both individual and multiple investments can be evaluated. As with NPV, knowledge of mathematics is helpful. The main disadvantage is that a project may have multiple IRRs. For example, the IRR of $100,000 worth of equipment would be calculated as follows:

| Internal Rate of Return | |
|---|---|
| Investment: | $100,000 |
| Cash in: | $25,000 per year (revenue minus depreciation and operating costs) |
| NPV: | $0 (based on 5 years of service) |
| Interest rate: | 8 percent |

Management roles in any healthcare facility require some knowledge of accounting and financial management. The ability to read, understand, and interpret pertinent financial reports is a desirable business skill. Because of the close ties between reimbursement and HIM, this basic skill is even more important. Although the financial accounting methodologies of compiling and analyzing financial statements may not be needed routinely, the managerial accounting skills involving budget preparation and analysis are critical. Also important is an awareness of the preventive, detective, and corrective controls managers must implement to ensure financial data accuracy.

## Check Your Understanding 25.4

**Answer the following questions in a separate document.**

1. Compare and contrast financial accounting and managerial accounting. Which type of accounting will you do as an HIM manager? Explain your answer.

2. Compare and contrast operational budgets and capital budgets. What type of items would an HIM manager include in each?

3. Calculating and explaining budget variances is an important management control. Following up and acting on budget variances is also critical. How would you categorize these activities based on the three types of internal controls: preventive, corrective and detective?

4. St. Ava Hospital is evaluating whether to purchase a surgical robot for the urology department for $4,000,000. Cash flow from the robot is expected to average $200,000 per month. On high-tech equipment the hospital expects a payback period of two years or less. Calculate the payback period of the surgical robot. Should St. Ava purchase this equipment based on the payback period?

5. The pharmacy department has a YTD patient revenue budget of $5,000,000 and the actual YTD amount is $4,600,000. Is this a favorable or unfavorable variance? Explain why.

# References

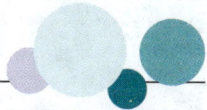

Davis, N., and R. Revoir. 2013. "Financial Management." Chapter 25 in *Health Information Management: Concepts, Principles and Practice*, 4th ed. Edited by K. M. LaTour, S. Eichenwald Maki, and P. Oachs. Chicago: AHIMA.

IRS (Internal Revenue Service). 2023. "Tax Exempt Status for Your Organization. Pub. 557." http://www.irs.gov/pub/irs-pdf/p557.pdf.

# chapter 26

# Project Management

*Brandon D. Olson, PhD, PMP*

## Learning Objectives

- Determine a project's purpose
- Associate organizational and team structures with the project environment
- Determine the deliverables of each of the project management process groups
- Associate the project roles with the activities in the project management process
- Evaluate and apply the skills and abilities needed for project management
- Differentiate among project management, program management, and portfolio management

## Key Terms

Agile approach
Balanced matrix organization
Compliance projects
Consultant
Contractor
Expense projects
Functional manager
Functional organization
Gantt chart
Iterative approach
Matrix organization
Operations
Outsourcing agency
Program
Program management
Project
Project budget
Project champion
Project coordinator
Project expediter
Project failure
Project management
Project management constraints
Project management life cycle
Project manager
Project portfolio management (PPM)
Project portfolio manager
Project schedule
Project scope
Project sponsor
Project stakeholder
Project team
Projectized organization
Requirements document
Revenue projects
Scope creep
Strong matrix organization
Talent triangle
Triple constraint
Users
Variance
Waterfall method
Weak matrix organization
Work breakdown structure (WBS)

The healthcare industry changes rapidly, requiring systems and processes to be revised or replaced and cross-departmental effort to support these changes. The health information management (HIM) professional interacts with many functions across the healthcare organization and is called upon to participate in or lead new initiatives that enable the organization to change. These efforts occur while the day-to-day operations continue. As a result, a separate set of activities occurs outside of the daily work supporting patient care. These additional activities are the projects carried out in response to the changing healthcare industry.

Projects and managing projects are an important part of any industry. Given the evolving environment in healthcare, effective project management is critical to keep up with the amount of change taking place. In this chapter, projects, project management, and the role and attributes of a project manager are introduced, and the methods used to lead projects are discussed. The chapter also introduces concepts that are applied to projects and project management to connect the project with an organization's long-term goals.

# The Project

Projects exist because of the organization's need for or reaction to change. Change may be needed to offer new products or services, respond to new industry trends or regulations, or improve or automate processes. Whatever the reason for change, projects are created to direct and coordinate the organization's efforts and resources to ensure an effective transition from the current state of operating to a new state. In other words, projects are used to make changes in the organization.

Change is common in the workplace and creating change is often a strategic priority for organizations. Projects and the management of these projects are key to achieving long-term goals and critical to an organization's success. A study found that in organizations that were most successful in achieving desired results from projects, 97 percent of the executives consider project management critical to the organization's performance, and 94 percent believe projects enable the organization to grow (PMI 2013). Organizations recognize the importance of project management and realize projects facilitate the change needed to achieve its goals.

## Definition of a Project

Projects are important to organizations, but it may not be clear what a project is and how it differs from the ongoing work taking place in an organization. There are many ways to define projects, and each definition offers additional characteristics to the term. The most widely accepted definition of a project is "A temporary endeavor undertaken to create a unique product, service, or result" (PMI 2023, 5).

Additionally, projects can be better understood through identifying the characteristics that make up a project:

- An established and specific objective with a focus on creating value
- A predetermined lifespan with a defined start and end date
- Multifunctional involvement of several departments and professionals
- Specific time, cost, and performance requirements and constraints
- Reliance on new techniques or processes that are uncommon to the standard operations (Kerzner 2022; Larson and Gray 2021).

Using the accepted definition and the common characteristics of a project, a more comprehensive definition can be derived. A **project** is a temporary and unique instance of work involving specialized individuals working together to achieve a specific goal within resource and time limitations.

It is important to differentiate projects from ongoing, daily operations. While a project is temporary and occurs only once, **operations** do not have a planned end date, and the work is repeated routinely. Additionally, while operations are designed for consistency, each project is designed to address a specific and unique set of goals. Table 26.1 provides examples to illustrate the differences between projects and operations.

The routine work of operations is important to the organization's ability to deliver quality products and services in a consistent manner. Operations are the ongoing and routine work that changes only when the organization's objectives can no longer be met. When these operational objectives can no longer be met, change must occur. These changes are carried out through projects. Projects are the temporary efforts carried out to meet specific objectives and enable change.

The need for change may be requested or required from within or outside of the organization. As a result, a project is created to achieve the outcomes needed and allow the organization to change. These unique and temporary projects are planned and executed to accomplish specific objectives that enable the change. Understanding the objectives is important to determining why the project exists. These project

**Table 26.1.** Differences between operations and projects

| Operations | Project |
|---|---|
| Taking notes in class | Writing a research paper |
| Using an existing electronic health record system | Implementing an electronic health record system |
| Attending team meetings | Planning a professional conference |
| Practicing the piano | Organizing a community concert |
| Capturing provider documentation | Creating a new method to integrate provider documentation into the electronic health record |
| Following a patient registration process | Designing a new registration workflow |

**Table 26.2.** Examples of categorized projects

| Project type | Examples |
|---|---|
| Revenue | • Open a new clinic<br>• Add a sports medicine practice<br>• Extend clinic hours |
| Expense | • Digitize charts in warehouse<br>• Share electronic health records across departments<br>• Create new productivity report |
| Compliance | • Convert to ICD-11 coding standards<br>• Upgrade all computers to a new operating system<br>• Develop and conduct HIPAA training |

objectives or sources are associated with the purpose for the need or desire to change, and understanding the true purpose enables the organization to focus on the important outcomes from the project.

## Determining a Project's Purpose

The objective or purpose of any project can be associated with one of three separate categories. Each project category determines the overall business goal of the project and describes the reason the project exists. The three categories of projects and project examples for each are listed in table 26.2. The three separate categories are as follows:

- Revenue: Projects with the purpose of increasing the organization's income
- Expense: Projects with the purpose of reducing the costs of providing goods or services
- Compliance: Projects with the purpose of meeting the expectations or directives set by an internal or external governing body

There are a few things to note regarding the categorization of projects. **Revenue projects** may include projects that result in new or expanded products or services. In nonprofit and government organizations, these revenue projects may not increase revenue but rather increase the quantity or capacity of its services. **Expense projects** include projects where new and improved information is created. Such projects fall into the expense reduction category since increased access to information and knowledge results in better decision-making and reduced costs from inferior decisions. Finally, it should be noted that **compliance projects** include self-imposed initiatives organizations place on themselves, industry-imposed compliance where organizations must meet a minimum level of stakeholder expectations, and government or regulatory compliance that organizations must meet to remain in business.

Understanding the categorization of a project is important as it determines the ultimate purpose for the change the organization seeks to make. Some projects will have a goal to help the organization increase its revenue or services, other projects will have a goal to reduce inefficiencies and expenses, and some projects will have a goal to comply with an internal or external requirement. In all these situations, the goal becomes a target for the project and projects must be planned and executed to address this goal.

## Check Your Understanding 26.1

**Answer the following questions in a separate document.**

1. Describe an example of a project and an example of typical operations from your own personal or professional life. Include the rationale behind your examples.
2. Using an example, explain why the term "unique" is an important attribute in the definition of a *project*.
3. University Hospital is seeking certification by the American College of Surgeons as a Level 1 Trauma Center. What project category is this? Explain why.
4. There is a project proposal to create a decision support department with a budget to hire three business analysts and three clinical analysts and to purchase and implement new decision support software. What outcomes are expected for this project and what is the cost justification for this project?
5. Is cost savings or revenue generation a measure for a compliance project? Why or why not?

# Project Management

Projects, and various forms of managing them, have existed for thousands of years; but the modern systematic methodology and specific discipline of project management emerged in the mid-20th century. The US Navy's Polaris project of 1956 to 1961 was credited as the first project to refine and apply the project management concepts used today (Kwak 2003). Between the early 20th century and today, project management guided projects in the fields of transportation and telecommunications and matured to lead modern computer automation of business processes and internet-based commerce and systems. Along with this evolution, project tools like the Gantt chart, work breakdown structures (WBSs), and project management software emerged to support the increasing size and complexity of projects.

The project management method has continued to be improved and is used by almost every industry. During this time, project management became a specific discipline with professional organizations like the Project Management Institute (PMI) establishing best practices and promoting the project management field. Today there are more than 700,000 PMI members and more than 1,400,000 professionals holding a Project Management Professional (PMP) certification or other PMI professional certification (PMI 2024). The PMI established the standard for best practices in project management in the Project Management Body of Knowledge (PMBOK). In addition to the PMP certifications, PMI issues several additional certifications to validate expertise in other project-related areas. These additional certifications include the following: Certified Associate Project Management (CAPM), Portfolio Management Professional (PfMP), Program Management Professional (PgMP), Risk Management Professional (PMI-RMP), Scheduling Professional (PMI-SP), Agile Certified Practitioner (PMP-ACP), and Professional in Business Analysis (PMI-PBA).

Project management is defined as "the application of knowledge, skills, tools, and techniques to project activities to meet the project requirements" (PMI 2023, 2). This means that project management is both a set of processes and the application of previous experience and is used to guide the project activities toward achieving the project goals. Perhaps more specifically, project management is an intentional effort to plan, organize, direct, and control the organization's resources toward achieving a specific short-term objective. This short-term effort is the project. The planning, organizing, directing, and controlling take place in the act of managing the project. Using either definition, project management requires expertise to be applied to a set of processes.

## Project Management Process

Project management is achieved through the execution and integration of processes. Based on an evolution of best practices, PMI logically categorized a set of 49 core project management processes into groups (PMI 2023, 21). The processes in this formal categorization are referred to as process groups, and these groups and their relationship to one another is commonly viewed as the project management process. The five process groups are: initiating, planning, executing, monitoring and controlling, and closing. Each of these process groups is required to complete a project, and omitting any of these process groups from the project greatly increases the risk of failure for the project. The process groups are also connected and sequenced for a project. Figure 26.1 illustrates an example of how the process groups may be sequenced in a project.

The process groups are carried out over time. Successful completion of all process groups results in a completed project. Although the sequencing may change for each project, the order of these process groups is important. The output of one process group is often needed for successful completion of the next process group. For instance, the executing process group cannot be completed without some or all results from the planning process group. The exception to the sequencing is that the executing and monitoring and controlling phases may occur simultaneously. Each of the process groups include many individual processes to create the output needed for subsequent process groups. Figure 26.1 represents the sequencing of the process groups but does not indicate the activities taking place within each group. A more detailed explanation of the activities taking place within each process group is provided later in the chapter.

## Alternative Project Methodologies

Each of the process groups may also be considered a phase of a project. The collection of project phases forms the project management life cycle. The traditional method of completing the life cycle is in a sequential order. This sequential method of completing the project phases is commonly referred to as the waterfall method. In this method, the phases are structured so that one phase begins at the end or near the end of the previous phase. This method has been successfully applied for decades and ensures the output from one phase is complete and ready to serve as inputs for the next phase.

The traditional waterfall method ensures the entire project is cohesively planned and executed. The waterfall method is a good fit for complex projects requiring thorough planning or projects having a clear and complete understanding of the specifications for the final output. However, the downside to the waterfall method is that the sequential nature delays delivery of the final project output until the end of the project and does not offer the flexibility needed if the output or design specifications for the project are not clear. The waterfall method requires the planning to be complete prior to executing, and output from the project is not available until the very end of the project. To make project output available sooner, some projects are executed in releases following an **iterative approach** to the project management life cycle (figure 26.2) or through an **agile approach** (figure 26.3) where the life cycle is repeated in many iterations.

The iterative approach to projects is an adaptation of the waterfall method. Rather than a single project life cycle sequence, iterative methods use multiple sequences of planning, executing, monitoring, and controlling in a project. In this iterative approach, the overall project is initiated, and then the project is completed using multiple phases before the entire project is wrapped up with a single closing phase. Using the iterative approach, the project can produce portions of the deliverables earlier than in the waterfall approach, where the deliverables are held until the very end of the project. The iterative model also provides greater flexibility since each phase is planned individually, thus allowing the requirements to evolve as the project is better understood. The flexibility offered through the iterative approach does restrict the ability to have an overall design of the project deliverables, so it may not be a good fit in significantly complex projects or projects where the deliverables cannot be separated out and must be delivered as a single unit.

**Figure 26.1.** Sample process group sequence

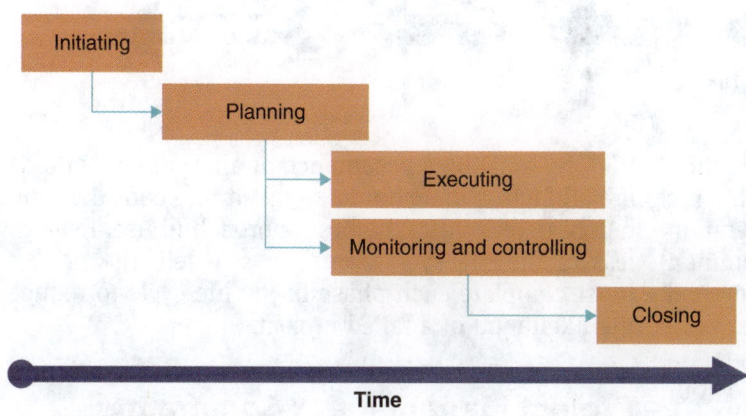

**Figure 26.2.** Sample iterative sequence

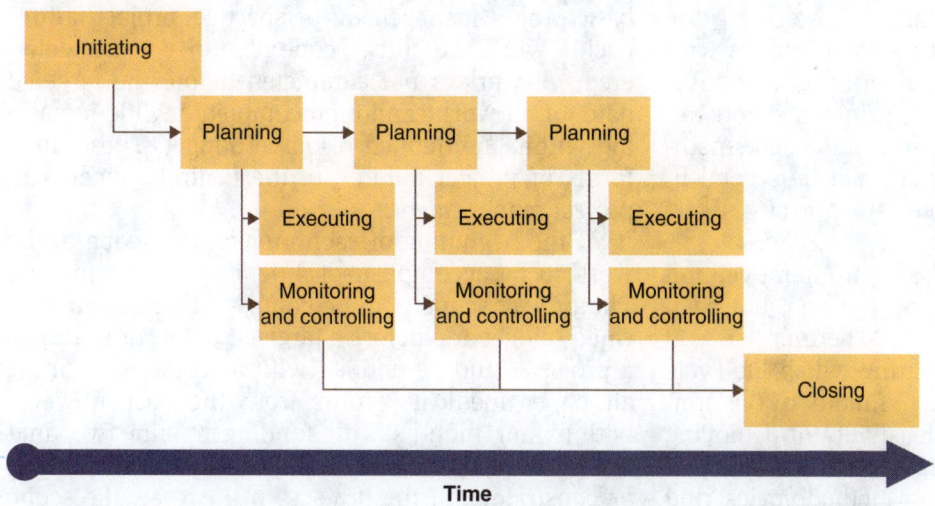

**Figure 26.3.** Sample agile sequence

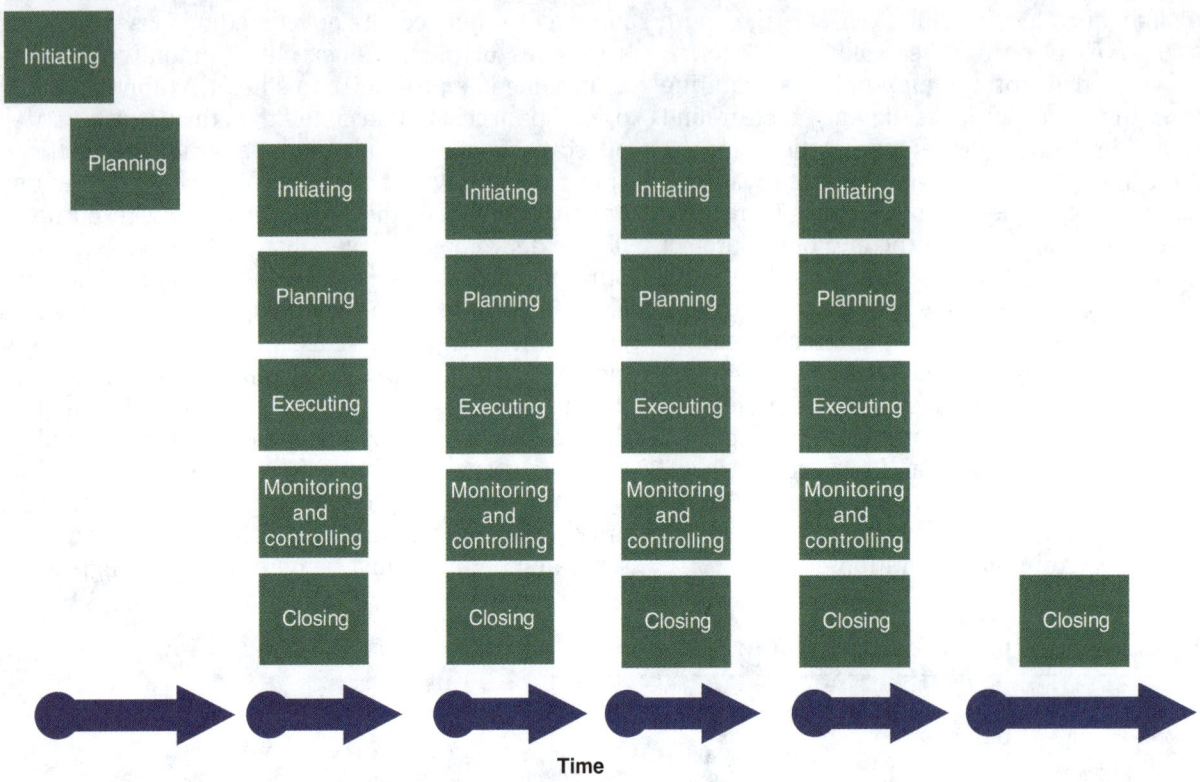

The agile approach is a type of iterative method for projects. In the agile approach, rather than having single initiation and closing processes, each iteration includes initiation and closing processes. A common form of an agile project method is the Scrum method to projects. Scrum projects are dissected into several units called sprints, where each sprint represents a standard period of work ranging from one to four weeks. Using Scrum, the overall project is initiated and includes a high-level plan for the work that will take place in each of the sprints. Each sprint includes initiation and planning work prior to executing the plan for the sprint. Each sprint also concludes with a closing process referred to as a sprint retrospective. The benefits of the iterative project method are increased using the frequent sprints of the agile method, but the agile method may still not be a good fit for complex projects or for projects requiring a single delivery.

Each life cycle approach—waterfall, iterative, and agile—has been applied to many projects, but each approach may not fit all projects. There are several factors to consider when evaluating which life cycle approach to use in a project. The fluidity of the project output specifications, the feasibility of deploying subsets of the project deliverables, the familiarity of the team with alternative project methodologies, and the organization's acceptance of alternative methods are all factors that should be taken into consideration before determining the best approach to use. Regardless of the life cycle approach selected, the project must complete each phase in the life cycle to reduce the likelihood of a failed project.

## Project Management Constraints

Projects sometimes fail. Project failure can have different meanings from different perspectives, but from a basic project management perspective, **project failure** occurs when the entire scope identified is not delivered, all work is not completed before the targeted date, or all work cannot be completed while remaining within the defined resource budget. These three forms of project failure are the central concerns in project management.

At the beginning of each project, the scope of the work to be accomplished is defined for the project. The project scope is to be completed within an allocated budget and before a targeted date. For example, a project could be defined with a scope of scanning all paper medical records from the past 10 years within four months with funding to hire two analysts. These three expectations comprise the limits, or constraints, of the project. In this case, the scope constraint is scanning all paper records from the past 10 years, the time constraint is a four-month period, and the budget constraint is limiting the resources (in this case, human resources) to two full-time analysts. These three constraints are commonly referred to as the **triple constraint** and expressed as a triangle similar to figure 26.4.

The **project management constraints** are typically depicted as a triangle due to the three sides representing the three constraints. The triangle also represents the connectedness of the three constraints where each constraint is dependent upon the other two constraints. The **project scope** determines the work to be completed; the **project schedule** defines target dates for when the scope must be completed and limits the amount of scope that can be completed within the time and given budget; and the **project budget** identifies the resources made available to the project and limits the amount of scope that can be delivered and the amount of time available to complete the project. A project must be managed to maximize the scope while minimizing the schedule and budget. Increased scope may cost more and take more time. Conversely, decreased resource budget or time may limit the amount of scope the project may deliver. The goal of effective project management is to carefully balance the scope, schedule, and budget, which leads to successful projects.

Due to the importance of the project management constraints, most project status reporting centers on progress toward these three constraints. The project begins with an initial set of scope, schedule, and budget expectations. These initial expectations are the baseline for the project. In project management, any deviation from the project's initial baseline expectations is referred to as a **variance**. As the project is underway, the project manager typically reports the current progress and forecasted estimates of the three constraints and identifies any deviation from the project baseline. In addition to reporting the status for the project in respect to these three constraints, the project manager often adjusts the three constraints to correct any variances with scope, schedule, and budget to ensure the project falls within the expected baseline targets.

## Project Members

There are many individuals associated with a project. Anyone with an interest in the deliverables created as part of the project is considered a **project stakeholder**. The project stakeholders frequently rely on results from the project to fulfill some of their operational needs or long-term goals. In addition to the project stakeholders, there are individuals directly involved in specifying, supporting, or creating the project deliverables.

Projects are carried out by several individuals who contribute a specialized skill set or knowledge to complete the project deliverables. The specialized skills and knowledge needed are driven by the type of work required to complete the project. While roles and specialties vary across all projects, there are many roles associated with the project that are clearly defined and required for any successful project. These roles include the project sponsor, users or recipients, project manager, project champion, and the project team members. Each of these roles is directly related to specifying, supporting, and completing the project; and is not a part of the organization's standard operations roles.

### Project Sponsor

Every project begins with a need or desire for change. This need may originate from a functional leader, or it may originate at the top level of the organization. In either case, the organization must determine the functional area(s) within the organization where the project should reside. Either the functional leader expressing the need for change or a leader over the functional area most likely to be affected or benefited by the project often becomes the **project sponsor** or project owner. For example, the manager supervising release of information could serve as the project sponsor for a project where the release of information module is integrated within the electronic health record

**Figure 26.4.** Project management constraints

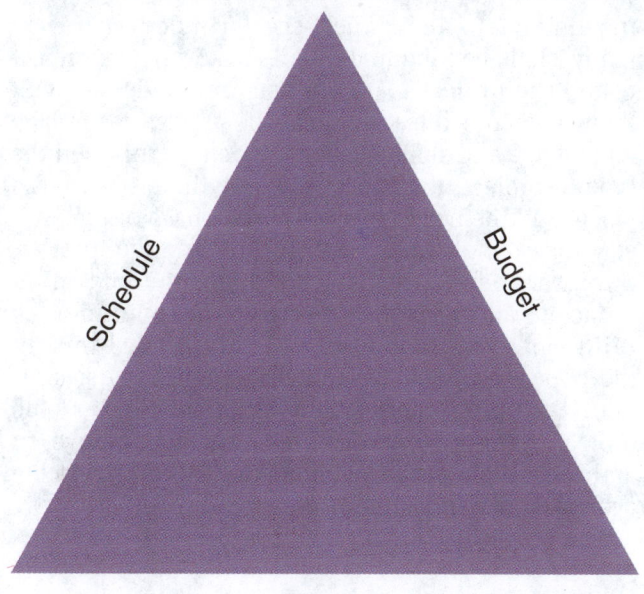

(EHR) system. This individual may be responsible for securing the budget for the project and would provide overall direction for the project and how it fits within the EHR system. The project sponsor secures resource commitments for the project and makes many of the decisions regarding project objectives and scope. The sponsor is a key decision maker for the project and responsible for ensuring the project deliverables effectively satisfy the needs of the organization.

### User or Recipient

Although the project is owned by the project sponsor, it is often executed for the benefit of a group of users or recipients. The **users** are all internal and external stakeholders directly affected by the project deliverables. In the case of a release of information module implementation project, the staff working on release of information who are familiar with the current workflows would serve as users in the project. These individuals offer insight as to how the results from the project affect them or their work and identify the specifications of the project deliverables so the results fulfill their expectations. The project users must be engaged in the project to ensure they are satisfied with the project deliverables and that these products meet their needs. The project sponsor provides the overall direction for the project, but the project users provide the detailed specifications and are best able to determine the acceptability of the project deliverables.

### Project Manager

Every project must have an individual responsible for planning, organizing, directing, monitoring, and controlling the work. The **project manager** is responsible for these activities from the beginning to the end of the project, keeping all stakeholders informed and engaged and ensuring the project is completed within the constraints of scope, schedule, and budget. The project manager may come from within the department or may be a project management specialist from another department. To be successful as a project manager, this individual will possess a wide range of technical and interpersonal skills that are described later in this chapter. However, it should be acknowledged that a project manager is always developing these skills and may be more proficient in some areas than others.

While planning and managing the work is an important responsibility of the project manager, stakeholder communication is the most critical to project success. Project managers must ensure communications exist within the project team and between the project team and the other stakeholders. Through project planning documents, standardized and structured status reports, email messages, tracking logs, and project meetings, the project manager must insist that communications take place so that all project stakeholders are engaged, and the project team is able to receive the information and resources needed to successfully execute the project.

### Project Champion

Projects require support from the organization to meet the organization's needs. This support includes both the continued approval from the organization and sufficient resources to properly complete the project. The **project champion** is an executive in the organization who believes in the benefits of the project and advocates for it. Depending on the overall impact the project has on the healthcare organization, this individual may be the manager of a department, the director over the business unit where the department resides, or the chief operations officer (COO) or another member of the executive team. The project champion is responsible for making sure the project objectives align with the organization's goals and for ensuring the project receives the resources needed to meet these objectives. Without the project champion, organizational support for the project would wane and the project could lose access to the budgeted resources.

### Project Team

In addition to the project-specific roles, there are many skilled individuals who make up the project team. The **project team** consists of individuals with knowledge or skills specific to the project needs. The knowledge and skills needed are dependent upon the type of project, the industry where the project takes place, and the needs specific to the phase of the project. For example, in a paper record scanning project, a software developer may be required to build an interface to allow scanned records to be input into the EHR. However, the developer is not needed to scan the paper records. The knowledge and skill sets required for the project vary at different times of the project. As a result, project team members move on and off the project throughout the entire project life cycle and return to their operational roles once they are no longer needed on the project.

## Check Your Understanding 26.2

**Use the following scenario to answer questions 1 through 4.**

The HIM annual educational conference is being held in the spring. Ryan is the president of the HIM association and Susan is the chair of the conference planning committee, which includes five people on the speaker subcommittee, three people on the food and beverage subcommittee, and two people on the marketing subcommittee.

1. Who are the stakeholders in this project? Explain why.
2. Who is the project sponsor? Explain why.
3. Who is the project manager? Explain why.
4. Susan, the chair of the HIM conference planning committee, was asked to move the date of the conference two weeks earlier than originally planned. What should Susan consider before responding to this request?
5. If a silent auction were added to the annual meeting, would Susan need to acquire additional people to the project team? Why or why not?

## Organizational Structures

Project team members are borrowed from functional departments across the organization to contribute specialized skills or knowledge to the project. Once the project no longer requires their contributions, they return to their role within the functional department. As a result of the temporary nature of projects, no permanent organizational structure exists for the project team. The project exists as a dynamic structure within the existing permanent or semipermanent organizational structure. Some organizational structures support the project environment better than others. The following sections outline several common organizational structures and the corresponding fit for a project environment.

### Functional Organization

The traditional hierarchy in an organization is the **functional organization** where each employee has a single supervisor, and employees are grouped in departments by specialty or subspecialty (see figure 26.5). Each department within the functional organization operates independently of the other departments.

**Figure 26.5.** Functional organization

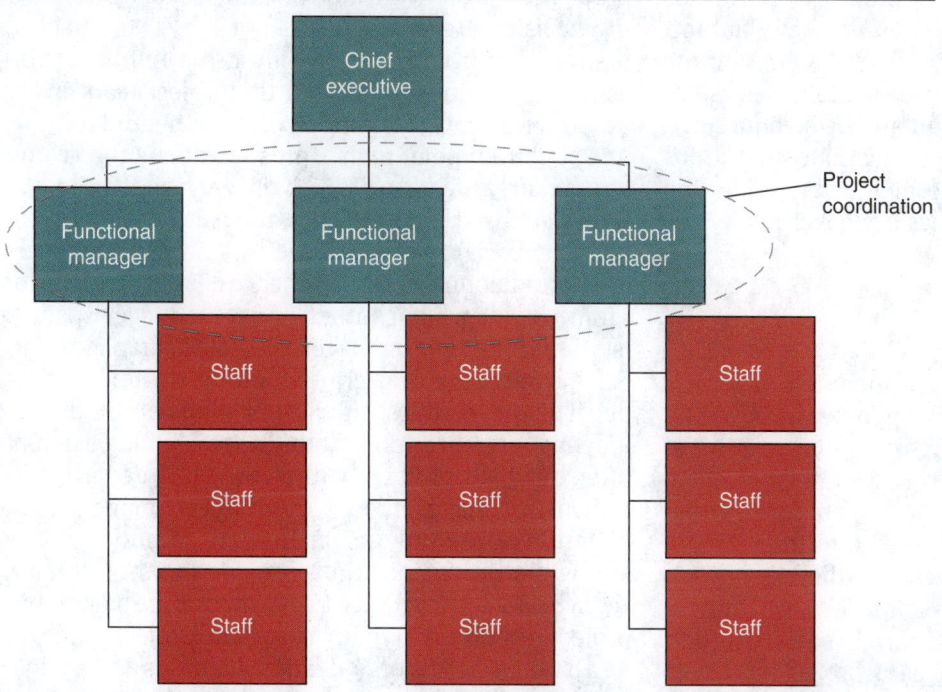

The specialization of the functional organization creates challenges for projects. If a project exists within a single department and only members of the department are affected by the project, a functional organization can support projects. However, many projects span multiple areas of specialty, making it a challenge for the functional organization to manage coordination between departments. This cross-departmental collaboration must take place, but it is counter to the contained department-specific work typically carried out in the functional organization.

Due to the independent nature of the functional organization, the true role of a project manager does not typically exist. A project manager in this structure would have little or no authority, have limited abilities to obtain resources or budget, and would perform project manager duties in addition to department responsibilities. Rather than a true project management role, the functional organization uses what is referred to as a **project coordinator** to facilitate resources and collaboration across the departments participating in the project. The project coordinator, typically a professional with experience working with different departments, works with the functional manager of each department to get work completed. The functional manager is a leader over an organizational unit or department, such as release of information. The functional manager maintains full authority over the staff and the work performed by the unit, and the project is dependent upon the project coordinator's effective collaboration with the participating functional managers and each functional manager's direct authority over the staff completing the project work. In this case, the project coordinator does not have authority over the staff but rather work is directed by the staff's functional manager. For example, a release of information analyst may coordinate the activities of a release of information-related project but cannot prioritize the work of any of the members working on the project since these priorities are governed by the individual's respective managers.

## Matrix Organization

Functional organizations can be modified to form a matrix organization by integrating a secondary project structure. In the **matrix organization**, employees report to a functional manager from their original functional area to carry out their operational work. This **functional manager**, also referred to as an administrative supervisor, carries out the employee's performance reviews and has authority over promotions and terminations. The employee may also report to a different manager, such as a project manager, who oversees their temporary work outside of their operational duties. This secondary manager only oversees work on the special duties and does not have authority over the employee outside of these duties. The matrix organization generally offers a better support structure for projects, but the type of matrix organization also affects the structure's efficacy.

A matrix organization is further classified using subcategories of weak matrix, balanced matrix, or strong matrix. In the **weak matrix organization** (see figure 26.6), the project manager role does not exist, but a **project expediter** role is used to work directly with the functional staff rather than through the functional managers. This modification from the functional organization provides a little more authority and resources for the project expediter, but the budget and resources are still managed by the functional managers. As a result, the project expediter role is part time in addition to operational responsibilities.

The role of project manager does not exist within the purely functional or weak matrix organizations due to inseparability of the project work from the operational work. Balanced matrix organizational structures provide the separation of operations and project work. In the **balanced matrix** organizational structure, a project organization exists within the existing functional hierarchy and a project manager is recruited from one of the functional departments to serve as the leader of the project. In the balanced matrix organization, the project manager has moderate authority and access to resources but must still collaborate with the functional managers to obtain these resources. The work on the project is directed completely by the project manager with the functional managers making decisions regarding project scope. The balanced matrix organizations commonly use a full-time project management role to lead the project team made up of part-time project members (see figure 26.7).

The third type of matrix organization is the **strong matrix organization**, which is very similar to the balanced matrix but includes a department of project managers. In these organizations, project managers are not functional staff members assuming the role of project manager but rather project manager specialists reporting to a manager of project management. For instance, the transcription group within the HIM department includes individuals who reports to the manager of transcription, but these individuals do not often manage projects within the HIM department; projects managers from the project management department are brought in to manage projects. The strong matrix organizations provide the project manager a moderate to high level of authority over the project and project resources. In many cases, the project manager in a strong matrix organization manages the budget and is a full-time project manager (see figure 26.8).

**Figure 26.6.** Weak matrix organization

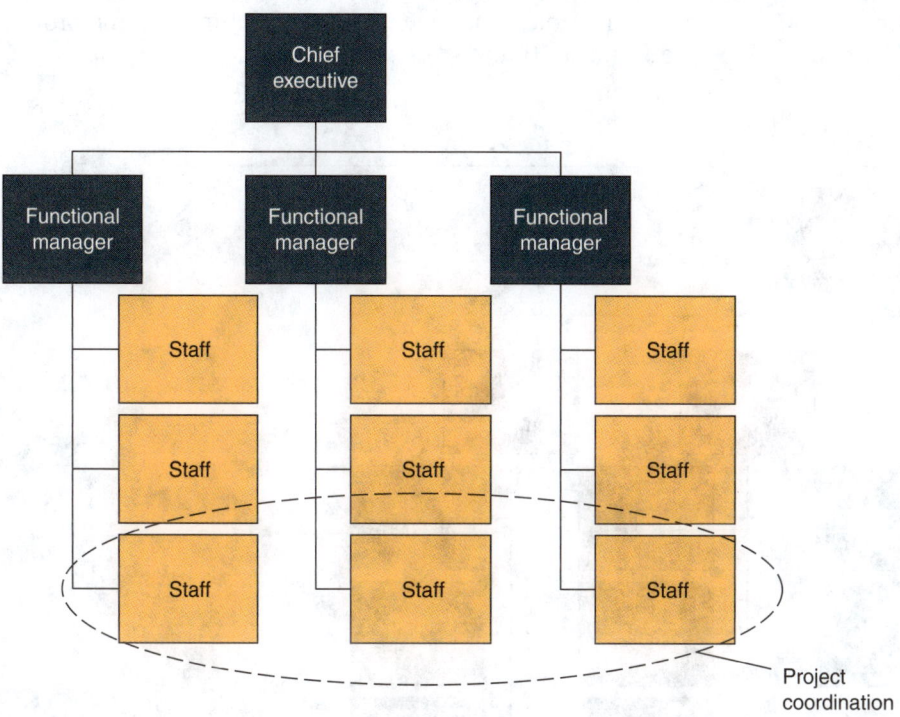

**Figure 26.7.** Balanced matrix organization

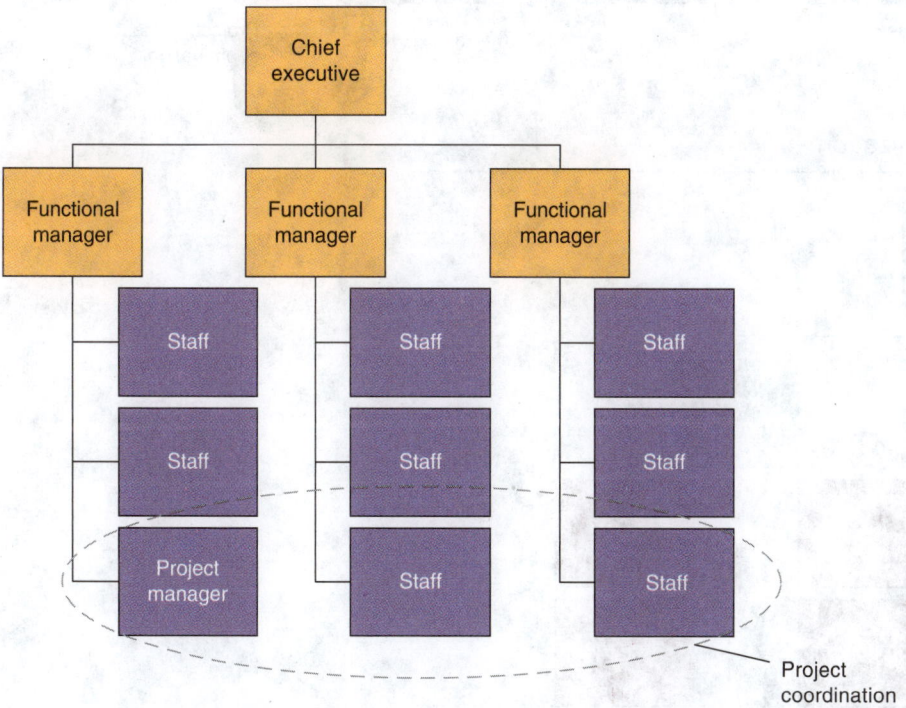

## Projected Organization

The functional and matrix organizations are designed around operational work. For this reason, they are separated by functional areas and any project structure must fit within the operational structure. Some organizations are designed around work in projects rather than operations and for these organizations a projectized structure is applied. In this **projectized organization**, the operational department structures focused on a specialty or subspecialty are replaced by multidisciplinary project teams led by a project manager. (See figure 26.9.) In these projectized organizations, the project manager has almost total authority over the team and access to resources as well as the project budgets. Much like the strong matrix organizational structure, projectized structures also make the project management role full time and the project staff full time.

**Figure 26.8.** Strong matrix organization

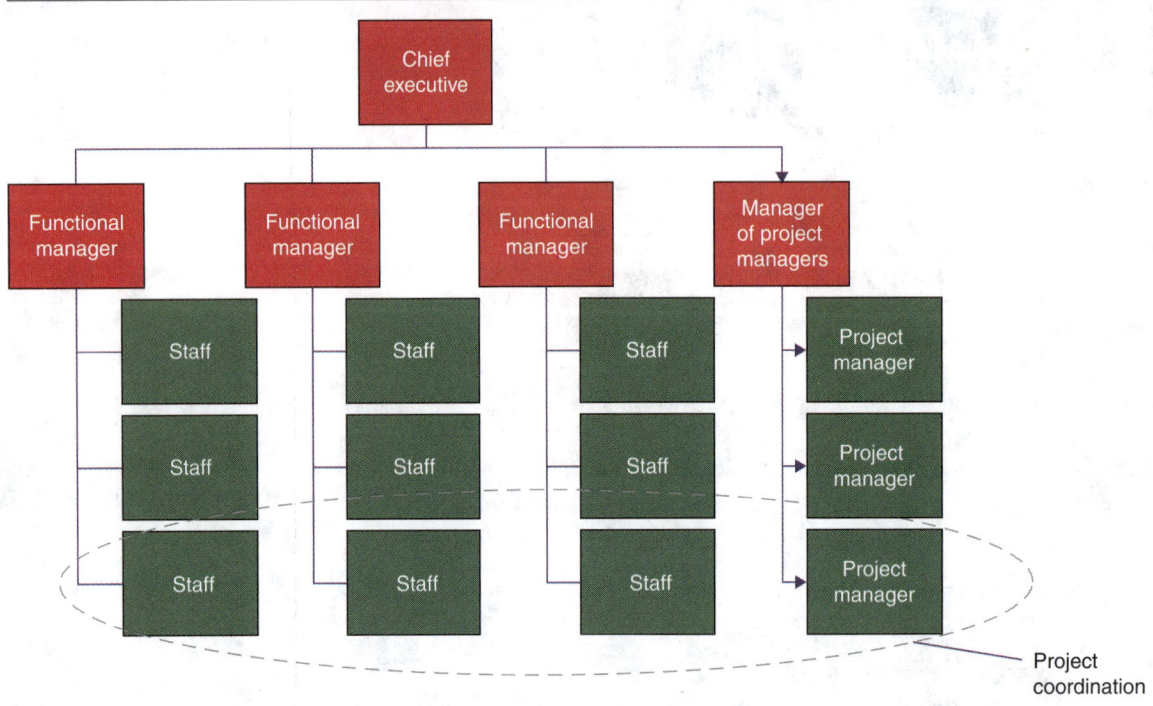

**Figure 26.9.** Projectized organization

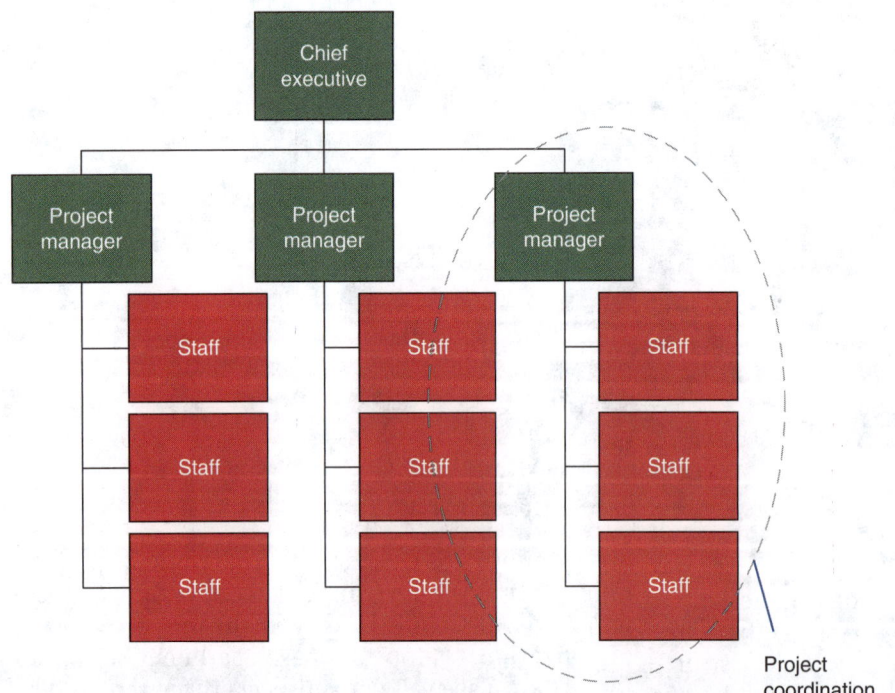

## Summary of Organizational Structures

Each of these organizational structures serves a different purpose, and one or more may exist within the same organization. Also, these structures may evolve over time so any one structure may be a temporary organizational structure based on the organization's needs at the time. In the context of project management, the projectized and strong matrix structures offer the most control and authority to project managers while the balanced and weak matrix organizations reduce the authority and decision-making permissions. Finally, in a true functional organizational structure, project managers exist in the form of a project coordinator or a project expediter who merely coordinates the activities across departments under the direction of the individual department managers.

Organizations that undergo frequent change and wish to promote project management practices adopt a balanced matrix or strong matrix structure to provide the ability to centralize authority of the project and encourage collaboration across departments. Organizations with infrequent change and fewer project needs may continue to adopt a functional or weak organizational structure so they remain focused on operations and the specialization of each department. The projectized structure is adopted by organizations whose work is predominantly centered around projects spanning multiple disciplines or for organizations going through significant change where projects become a focus over operations. See table 26.3 for a comparison of the various project management organizational structures.

## Team Structures

In addition to the structure of the organization, the structure of the team also contributes to the project team dynamics and the role of the project manager. The project team structure characteristics include the physical location of the team members, the time allotted to the team members for the project, and the employment status of the team members. The physical location of the team influences the team communications and management of work. Additionally, the availability of the team members determines project workload and scheduling, and the employment status may impact commitment and expertise. Each of these characteristics influences how the project team interacts and how the project manager leads the team.

### Part-Time Team Members

Often, project team members are assigned to a project in a part-time capacity. This is especially true in functional, weak matrix, and balanced matrix organizations. Even in strong matrix and projectized organizations, project team members may not be permanently assigned to the project since the project's needs vary over its duration. Whether the part-time status is due to the availability of the project team member or to the needs of the project, many project team members are not fully allocated to the project.

As a result of the dynamic makeup of the project team and its members' availability to work on the project, project managers must be able to shift work from one team member to another team member and try to capture and disseminate project knowledge between team members. As new team members are added to the project, the project manager must be able to quickly prepare the new team member with project and process knowledge and integrate them into the team so they are effective. Project managers also must capture any knowledge or information from team members transitioning off the project so this knowledge is not lost and may be transferred to other project team members.

In addition to managing the knowledge of new and transitioning team members, project managers must properly assign work based on availability. Part-time project team members cannot be assigned the same workload as full-time team members. Additionally, members assigned to the team on a temporary basis cannot be assigned work beyond their anticipated time on the project. This work assigned must match the expected availability. Project managers must assign work based on time of day, day of week, or time of year availability and must assign work for only the period when the member is assigned to the team. Proper work assignment requires careful planning and revisions as plans change.

### Vendor Partners

Not all project members are employees of the organization. The organization may partner with outside vendors to bring in additional or specialized expertise to supplement any shortages of employees with a specific skill set. The vendor partners work alongside the organization's employees and become a part of the project team. These vendor partnerships may fall into three separate categories—consultants, contractors, and outsourcing agencies.

An organization may add a consultant to a project team. The role of the consultant is to provide specialized expertise that current employees may not have. These consultants may offer expertise in high-level knowledge areas such as business, process, technology, regulatory, or other knowledge relevant to the project. For example, a professional with experience implementing EHRs may be hired to offer expert advice and direction to the project team. The organization adds the consultant to the project team so the team may learn from the consultant's knowledge and previous experience to make them more effective when encountering a new domain. Consultants may be added to the team for a short period of time or may be brought in for the duration of the project. The length of time the consultant is allocated to the project is based on the project needs, budget, and the consultant's availability.

Like consultants, **contractors** are added to a project team to fill a temporary void. Unlike consultants, who are added for higher-level knowledge, contractors are added to the team for their specialized skills and detailed knowledge not available within the existing employees; or the contractors may be added to increase the work capacity of the existing project team. These contractors should be integrated with the team while their services are needed by the project team. As is the case with part-time team members, onboarding and knowledge capture and sharing should take place with all outside partners.

Consultants and contractors are brought into the project team to fill voids in skill and knowledge areas. These individuals supplement the project team. Another vendor partnership, **outsourcing agencies**, are used to offload a portion of the work rather than being brought in to work directly with the project team. For instance, an outsourcing agency could be contracted to scan and properly dispose of paper records for a digitization project. In this case, the outsourcing agency specializes in this process and could perform the work in a more efficient manner than if the organization attempted to perform the work itself.

### Co-located Teams

The traditional project team is located within the same space. This co-location allows members to carry on ad-hoc conversations and quickly and easily collaborate and share work. Additionally, this frequent interaction allows the team to develop into an effective group where each knows the working and communication styles of the other and they adjust to work as a cohesive team. Unfortunately, this means that the knowledge and skills needed for any given project must be made available in the same location. This is not always possible; especially in balanced or weak matrix organizations where the team members are not fully assigned to the project. Placing the team in a single location simplifies communication and collaboration but limits the selection of specialists who may participate in the team.

### Distributed Teams

Within a more geographically dispersed workforce and national or global businesses, employees may no longer work in the same building, city, or country. It may not be possible to place all members of a project team in the same location. Additionally, the consultants and contractors brought in to participate on the project may work in a separate location from the rest of the project team. In recent years, remote work has increased so it is increasingly common to work as a distributed team with team members located across many different locations. These teams enjoy the different backgrounds and experiences offered by a distributed team and the access to specialists not available at any single location. However, communications and collaboration are more challenging in the distributed team environment. In these distributed team projects, the project manager must prepare a plan to support and promote communication and collaboration so that the team will not be limited in its interactions.

**Table 26.3.** Change and organizational structure

|  | Functional | Weak matrix | Balanced matrix | Strong matrix | Projectized |
|---|---|---|---|---|---|
| Change frequency | Stable | Low | Moderate | High | Continual |
| Project manager's authority | Little or none | Low | Low to moderate | Moderate to high | High |
| Project manager's role | Part-time | Part-time | Part-time | Full-time | Full-time |

*Source:* Adapted from PMI 2023.

### Check Your Understanding 26.3

Answer the following questions in a separate document.

1. An increase in the number of duplicate medical record numbers (MRNs) has been noted recently at the community hospital. The registration manager would like to work on a project to determine the cause and develop potential solutions. This may include retraining of staff in all areas that may assign MRNs. What type of organizational structure (see table 26.3) would work well for this type of project and setting? Explain why.

2. The largest health system in town has several strategic initiatives planned next year and anticipates many projects over the next several years. What type of organizational structure would work well for this type of situation and setting? Explain why.

3. Describe the three categories of vendor partners and describe a situation in which one would use each.

4. A large, multistate health system is planning to merge with another large system in a neighboring region. As part of this merger, the two organizations need to create shared processes, systems, and data. What type of project team would work best in this scenario, co-located teams or distributed teams? Explain your rationale.

5. Managing a geographically distributed team can be a challenge for a project manager. What are the primary challenges facing a project manager leading a distributed team and what can the project manager do to increase the effectiveness of the distributed team?

## The Project Manager

A project manager is critical to the project's success. This individual is responsible for planning and directing all project activities and keeping all stakeholders informed and engaged. While the project manager has responsibility to lead the project team, this functional leadership is often provided without administrative authority. Except for projectized organizations, the project manager is a leader for the project team members while on the project, but the team members continue to report to their administrative supervisor within the functional departments. Within the structure of a matrix organization, the administrative supervisor has the authority to hire, fire, and promote employees and may also remove employees from the project team. This means the project manager often must lead and motivate a project team without the benefit of authority over the team members. As a result, the project manager must possess strong leadership attributes and interpersonal skills in addition to technical knowledge and abilities. A set of common project management skills is listed in tables 26.4 and 26.5 and emphasizes the importance of both the technical and interpersonal skills required for a project manager.

The project manager must possess a set of technical skills to accomplish the work of managing a project. While these skills are important to the project manager, they represent only part of the skills needed. Project managers are proficient in operating projects within the organization, and also must be leaders. As a result, the project manager must possess or develop many interpersonal skills. These skills are needed to lead the project team and engage the project stakeholders while navigating the project through the challenges it faces. Table 26.5 includes several of the interpersonal skills the project manager must possess or develop to direct the project.

Comparing the two sets of skills, technical and interpersonal, it is clear that project managers must be proficient beyond the technical skills of the position. Interpersonal skills play a critical role in project management and the project manager relies significantly on these skills. Project management is more than simply assigning work and tracking the project.

**Table 26.4.** Project manager technical skills

| Technical skills | Description |
| --- | --- |
| Project management processes | Understanding of all project management processes, the inputs needed for each process, and the outputs resulting from each process as well as the ability to execute each process |
| Project management software | Expertise in using project management software and other software tools used in planning and executing the project |
| Project technology | Awareness of the technologies, tools, and techniques used by the project team in producing the project deliverables |
| Business domain | Basic understanding of the functional areas involved in and affected by the project |
| Budgets | Ability to plan, build, maintain, and evaluate a project budget as well as the tools for managing the budget |
| Cost estimates | Expertise to identify, estimate, schedule, and evaluate project costs throughout the project |
| Time estimates | Knowledge of multiple time estimation techniques and the ability to accurately collect and produce task and activity durations |
| Communication tools | Proficiency with many tools used to communicate and collaborate with the project team and project stakeholders |

*Source:* Adapted from PMI 2013; Brewer and Dittman 2022.

**Table 26.5.** Project manager interpersonal skills

| Interpersonal skills | Description |
|---|---|
| Leadership | Guiding a group of individuals within and outside the project team to work together toward a common goal |
| Team building | Forming the project team into a cohesive unit with the ability to work together to accomplish the project tasks while respecting and supporting each other |
| Motivation | Creating an environment where the project team achieves satisfaction through their work while having a common desire to reach the project goals |
| Communication | Conveying oral and written messages and meaning to the project team and project stakeholders while recognizing the proper styles, norms, relationships, and context of the communicated message |
| Influencing | Using interpersonal skills and shared power to obtain cooperation by the team and stakeholders to work toward the project goals |
| Decision-making | Applying the appropriate decision method based on the decision-making factors (time, trust, quality, and acceptance) |
| Political and cultural awareness | Understanding and appreciating the cultural and political landscape of the organization to identify and adeptly make use of the organization's power structures to accomplish the project while being sensitive to differences in organizational and individual cultures |
| Negotiation | Reaching agreements between parties of opposing interests through compromise and identification of mutual benefits |
| Trust building | Demonstrating information sharing, cooperation, and successful problem resolution to create trust across the project team and with the project stakeholders |
| Conflict management | Recognizing that conflict will occur, identifying when conflict is likely to occur, and helping the project team rationally work through disagreements toward the best results for the team |
| Coaching | Empowering and developing the project team and all team members to realize their potential through mentoring or training to increase skills and improve performance |
| Change management | Preparing the organization for the change resulting from the project as well as providing the flexibility to adjust the project based on changing business needs and shifts in the business environment |
| Active listening | Focusing on the speaker to understand the message and reiterating the message to ensure it was properly understood and applying this form of listening to all project team members and stakeholders to build trust and effective communication |

*Source:* Adapted from PMI 2017a; PMI 2017b.

Project managers must lead teams without having authority over the members and make organizational change without having leverage of a functional leadership position. All these skills are needed to support the project manager as they serve multiple roles throughout the project.

## Roles of a Project Manager

Project managers serve multiple roles in the project and are responsible for leading the project to successful completion. Since project management involves planning, organizing, directing, and controlling the organization's resources to achieve the project's objectives (Kerzner 2022), the project manager takes on many responsibilities. These responsibilities can be summarized in six basic functions related to guiding the project to successful completion. That is, to manage resources, scope, quality, schedule, costs, and communications (Brewer and Dittman 2022).

### Manage Resources

The project's resources must be managed to most effectively contribute to the project objectives. This means the project manager must ensure the project team is performing well and the resources for the project are planned and made available as needed without delays. These resources may include record storage space, scanning or photocopying equipment, staff, and budget assigned for the project. The project manager is the steward over the human resources and the project materials and must ensure these resources are not wasted and are applied effectively.

### Manage Scope

The project manager must first determine the project's scope, ensuring that it does not deviate or fall short of producing deliverables to meet the organization's needs. While the project is executed, the project manager must ensure the team delivers the entire scope to satisfy project objectives. Even after the scope is determined for the project, the project manager must monitor the project scope to ensure the project plans are reevaluated if the scope changes. Changes to live projects are common and typically lead to increased scope. These changes could include unplanned functionality added to the EHR system, increasing the number of records included in a digitization project, or including additional departments in a workflow standardization project. While the project is underway, new or revised needs are uncovered. For this reason, the project manager must be aware of changes in the scope so revisions to the project plans may be made if necessary.

### Manage Quality

In addition to ensuring the project's scope is managed, the project manager must implement controls to inspect the project output and evaluate the quality of the deliverables. The project deliverables must align with the scope defined for the project and must meet the stakeholder's quality expectations. Managing project quality at times creates conflicts with the project manager's other functions in terms of completing the project on time and within budget. For instance, adding field validation to a patient's blood type field in the EHR ensures higher quality data but requires additional development time. Producing quality deliverables or reworking deliverables to meet quality expectations requires additional time and cost and, as a result, negatively affects the schedule and budget targets. Due to this conflict in priorities, project managers should attempt to plan quality into the project deliverables to reduce the risk of rework or inferior deliverables.

### Manage Schedule

The timeline goals are established at the beginning of the project. These timelines drive the organization's plans for adopting the project deliverables. Due to this dependency on the deliverables, it is important that the project team complete the work based on the timelines. The project manager must prepare a schedule for the project and guide the project to produce the deliverables on time or provide early communication when they may be delayed. This project schedule and communication allows the organization to plan the adoption of the project deliverables.

### Manage Costs

Similar to the schedule, the project manager must establish, maintain, and communicate the project budget. The project is given a budget, and the project costs must be controlled to not exceed the project budget. If an overage occurs or will occur, the project manager must communicate the cost variance and attempt to secure additional funding or take other actions to reduce costs.

### Manage Communications

Communication is the most important function a project manager performs (Besteiro et al. 2015). Project communication is critical both within and outside the team with all stakeholders. Project managers must provide frequent communications to ensure the project team, and all project stakeholders remain informed and engaged.

Communication is one of the key reasons why projects are important. Projects frequently work across multiple departments with involvement by multiple layers of management in the organization. Working with so many different groups is challenging, and many organizations struggle to do this with multifunctional communications. Organizations are split in many ways, as illustrated in figure 26.10. There are layers of management where each layer views the business through a different perspective. The organization is also broken down into different units or functions. Between the organizational layers and functional units, people work on an operational island where they focus on the function and processes within their own unit and within their own management perspective.

One of the purposes of projects and project managers is to fill the gaps between operational islands so that diverse groups can work together. Much of this collaboration is supported by good communication. The project manager must take steps to connect all necessary groups with each other and with the project team so agreements can be made, expectations are clear, and project work products are adopted. Filling the gaps between the operational islands is an important factor for successfully executing the project.

## Project Management Competencies

There is no such thing as a perfect project manager. Project managers must continually develop their skills

**Figure 26.10.** Operational islands

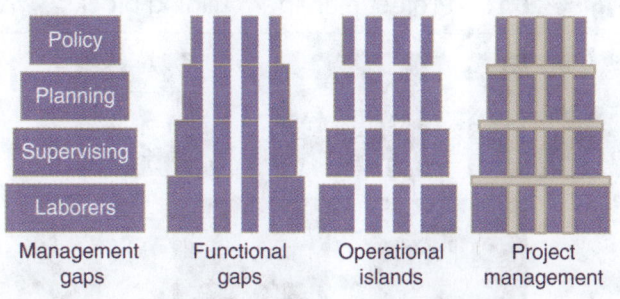

*Source:* Adapted from Kerzner 2022.

and knowledge. Many areas must be mastered, and the field evolves so project managers always have new competencies to develop. Given the need for continued development, PMI proposed a framework to outline the competencies project managers must develop. This framework is referred to as the Project Manager Competency Development (PMCD) framework (PMI 2017b). This framework can also be considered a set of building blocks a project manager develops over time. All of these blocks are connected and build upon each other to form the complete project manager. The individual blocks are professional behaviors, process knowledge, project performance, industry experience, and organizational experience (PMI 2017b).

Figure 26.11 is a model of the project manager building blocks. Each block represents an area of development. Since project management is an applied field, the areas of development specific to project management must be based on a firm foundation of experience within the field. For example, effective project managers in the healthcare field must be familiar with healthcare processes and terminology. They must also have a good understanding of key decision makers and influencers in the organization to effectively apply project management practices. These categories are directly based on the PMCD framework, but direct project management skills and knowledge are separated from supporting skills and knowledge. The industry experience and organizational experience building blocks are needed to emphasize the value of the industry and organizational nuances so the project context is properly understood. Industry and organizational experience provide the foundational building blocks for the project management–specific blocks.

### Industry Experience

Industry experience is a supporting competency for project managers. Competent project managers should have a solid foundational knowledge of the industry. The industry knowledge includes awareness of regulatory and legal requirements, past and future trends within the industry, and experience with projects in the industry. For example, a project manager within the healthcare field should be familiar with HIPAA requirements and history and trends in patient charting. They should also possess the insight gained from previous healthcare projects to understand the sources of project risk in a healthcare project (like communication, regulatory compliance, transportation logistics, and the like).

In addition to industry knowledge, a project manager must also possess the technical skills, or at least an understanding and appreciation for the skills needed, for the work to be carried out in a project within the industry. For example, in an IT project, the project manager should understand the level of difficulty for writing the code for a piece of software and understand the amount of time it takes to design, code, and test the software. The technical experience or technical skill appreciation helps the project manager assign the work to the properly skilled team member and evaluate the schedule needed to complete the work.

Industry experience is not a requirement for successfully managing projects. However, industry knowledge and technical skills are beneficial in understanding projects within the context of the industry. This contextual understanding enables the project manager to better communicate with the project stakeholders, better understand the sources and solutions to project risk within the industry, and improve project decision-making (PMI 2017b).

### Organizational Experience

Similar to industry experience, organizational experience is a foundational competency for project managers. These skills and knowledge are not directly related to project management but provide the background needed for a contextual understanding of the project environment. The previously described *industry experience* building block represented the industry-specific experience that helps project managers understand how projects are successfully executed. The organizational experience, on the other hand, provides the project manager with an understanding of how projects are executed within the context of the organization.

Organizational experience is gained from developing an understanding of the processes an organization follows, recognizing the power structures that exist within and outside of the organization, realizing who has the authority to make things happen, and observing the unwritten rules and expectations an organization has for its employees and supervisors. These organizational factors may be unique in each organization, and it is beneficial for the project

**Figure 26.11.** Project manager building blocks

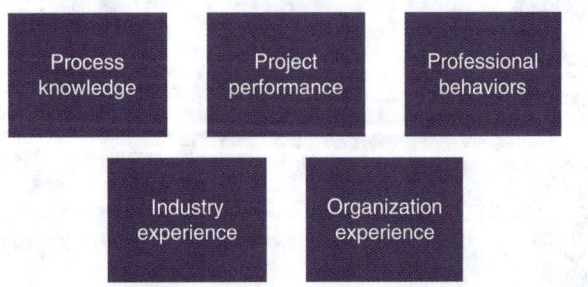

manager to understand these characteristics before initiating a project.

Organizational experience is an important competency to develop for project management consultants who may be experts in the project management field but may be at risk in the role due to insufficient experience with the organization. People unfamiliar with the organization will need to quickly understand the organizational context and apply it to the project (PMI 2017b).

### Process Knowledge

Anyone new to the project management field will begin developing project manager competencies in the *process knowledge* building block. The competencies in the process knowledge building block are developed by identifying and understanding all the processes used across one or more project management methodologies; for instance, becoming familiar with PMI's PMBOK, reading project management textbooks, and discovering project management tools and other resources.

In developing the process knowledge building block, a project manager becomes familiar with common and unique processes and tools and understands how they are applied to the project setting. While the *process knowledge* building block is primarily developed by those new to the project management field, a project manager should continually refine their process knowledge to discover new and changing tools and processes to improve their own project management practice (PMI 2017b).

### Project Performance

The project performance competency building block represents the project manager's ability to apply the project process knowledge and technical skills to the project environment. Project managers must know the project management processes and tools and be able to apply them to real projects. The project performance competency is developed by identifying the performance elements, determining target performance criteria, evaluating the individual's project performance competencies, identifying gaps between performance and target criteria, establishing a development plan, engaging in performance competency development activities, and reevaluating the performance. The evaluation, gap analysis, development plan, and development steps are continually iterated as the project manager develops the project performance competency. This cycle of performance competency development should continue throughout one's career as the project manager constantly learns and gains proficiency in applying project management process knowledge. A project manager needs to determine the elements of project management that are important to evaluate, determine how to measure the performance for each of the elements, define a target goal for each element, and discover ways to improve in the lower performing elements (PMI 2017b).

### Professional Behaviors

The professional behavior building block is based on the personal competencies in the PMCD framework (PMI 2017b). This building block consists of the ability to manage project resources; guide a team through motivation and goal setting; communicate effectively with all project stakeholders; understand the project complexities and the external environments affecting the project; apply good judgment when evaluating the project environment leading to sound decisions; and demonstrate ethical and professional behaviors to achieve the desired project results.

Professional behavior is developed outside project management skills and knowledge. Professional behaviors must be developed through experience, education, and mentoring. A project manager may be technically sound in the knowledge and application of the processes and tools, but without developed professional behaviors they will struggle in leading the team and stakeholders to achieve the desired results.

The *professional behaviors* building block along with all the *project manager* building blocks require continual development. The project environment is always changing, and a project manager can always find ways to learn new techniques or improve existing practices. These building blocks are simply a way to view the different types of skills and knowledge needed to be a successful project manager (PMI 2017b).

## Project Manager Talent Triangle

The building blocks of the PMCD framework were further developed, applied, and presented as the PMI talent triangle (PMI 2023, 58). The talent triangle is derived from the PMCD framework and represents the categorization of three areas of applied expertise project managers possess and must continually develop. The areas of applied expertise are ways of working, power skills, and business acumen. Together these three foundations are used to form the project manager's skillset and guide their development.

### Ways of Working

Each project represents distinctive requirements, constraints, and outcomes. As a result, a project manager must be able to apply a diverse set of methods, techniques, and approaches—the ways of working—to meet each project's unique needs.

A project manager demonstrates the ways of working by understanding the project needs, evaluating the right project practices to address the project needs, and effectively applying these practices. These practices may range from the overall project process to guide the project, to the methods of managing risk, to transforming the organization through the project. Following are a few examples of ways of working practices for project managers:

- Agile or waterfall project methods
- Design thinking
- Earned value management
- Risk management
- Data gathering and modelling
- Governance
- Scope management
- Time, budget, and cost estimates

The ways of working is not limited to strictly core project management practices, borrowing practices from other fields. These practices enable the project manager to effectively guide the project and deliver value to the organization. Developing the ability to apply an increasingly large and diverse set of practices increases the project management toolbox and enables the project manager to adapt to unique project needs and effectively lead a broader range of projects.

### Power Skills

Project management is more than executing project management practices. Projects involve people, and project managers must motivate, guide, and empower the project stakeholders to produce project deliverables and provide additional value to the organization. The power skills are the interpersonal talents needed to lead the project stakeholders and to fulfill the project objectives.

Developing power skills enables project managers to increase their effectiveness on the project and the effectiveness of team members and other project stakeholders. These power skills are applied to engage and lead stakeholders and overcome the challenges that arise throughout the project. Some of the talents associated with the power skills are:

- Active listening
- Communication
- Brainstorming
- Conflict management
- Problem solving
- Teamwork
- Emotional intelligence
- Negotiating

The project manager applies these skills to address the needs of the project and develop an environment where the stakeholders are trusting, engaged, and contributing. These power skills complement the more technical skills of the ways of working and represent the soft skills the project manager demonstrates to support the interactions with project stakeholders.

### Business Acumen

In addition to project and project-related practices, a project manager must possess domain knowledge to understand the environment where the project takes place. The business acumen talents are those that enable an awareness of the context for the project. This includes recognizing the internal and external influences on the project and project goals and the ability to consider the project context and environment factors in making project decisions. Additionally, the project manager must possess a *business acumen* to determine and anticipate the stakeholder needs and concerns and recognize the project's contribution to the organization's strategic objectives.

Unlike the ways of working and power skills talents that focus on activities within the project, the business acumen talents are primarily concerned with factors outside the project operations; the environment where the project operates. These talents guide the interactions of the project with the organization and include:

- Business models and structures
- Benefits management and realization
- Industry domain knowledge
- Competitive analysis
- Market awareness
- Strategic planning, analysis, and alignment

The business acumen talents provide the project manager with a strategic perspective of the project and remove the blinders of a project operations-centric view. These talents enable the project manager to ensure the project achieves the business objectives, delivers enduring value to the organization, and aligns with the organizational strategies.

Together, the ways of working, power skills, and business acumen skills make up the range of talents, skills, and knowledge project managers must develop to increase their effectiveness leading projects and the value these projects deliver to the organization. It is not possible for project managers to master the entire set of talents. Rather, these talents are the areas project managers continually develop to increase their effectiveness as project leaders and enhance the impact their projects have on the organization.

---

### Check Your Understanding 26.4

**Answer the following questions in a separate document.**

1. Why do you think the project manager serves as a functional leader rather than an administrative supervisor?
2. How does the functional leadership structure of a project manager change how they lead a project team when compared to administrative managers leading a team?
3. What are operational islands and what skills can a project manager use to address these islands?
4. A healthcare organization hires a project manager as a contractor, but this individual has project management experience only in the construction industry. Which existing competencies can be leveraged and what must this project manager do to be successful as a project manager in this healthcare organization?
5. A healthcare organization promotes a business analyst with five years of experience in the organization to a project manager. Which existing competencies can be leveraged and what must this new project manager do to be a successful project manager?

---

## The Project Management Process Groups

As noted in the project management competencies, knowledge of project processes is the first area of development for project managers. Understanding the processes of project management provides the foundation for becoming a project manager. Fortunately, over the decades, project management processes have matured, and best practices have emerged. These best practices have been published through PMI as the *Process Groups: A Practice Guide* (PMI 2023). This guide outlines the processes that occur while managing a project. These processes are categorized into five separate and sequential groups—initiating, planning, executing, monitoring and controlling, and closing. As described earlier in this chapter, these processes are executed sequentially in a single iteration or in multiple iterations across the project. Each of the process groups involves several different processes and requires input into the process group and produces some form of project output (see figure 26.12).

To better explain the process groups, a fictitious case study follows. This case is applied across each of the process groups to demonstrate the application of the project management process. While this case is a simplification of project management, it illustrates how the project management process is applied to a project without having to understand the complexities of the project.

### Case Study: Continuing Education Event

*Betsy is a medical records supervisor and a member of a local HIM professional organization. She has always enjoyed learning more about her field and would like to organize a continuing education event for her staff and other HIM professionals in the area. Betsy is also studying to become a project manager so she thought planning and hosting a continuing education event would be a great opportunity to practice her project management skills by treating this event like a project. She decides to begin by initiating the continuing education event and following all process groups through project closing. Betsy cannot wait to connect with her colleagues in the HIM field and hopes the project management process will make this continuing education event successful.*

### Initiating

Projects begin with the initiation process group where the project is first defined. This process group uses a project definition and scope, schedule, and budget estimates as inputs and results in an output of a completed project charter. The purpose of this first phase of the life cycle is to identify the project goals

**Figure 26.12.** Process group framework

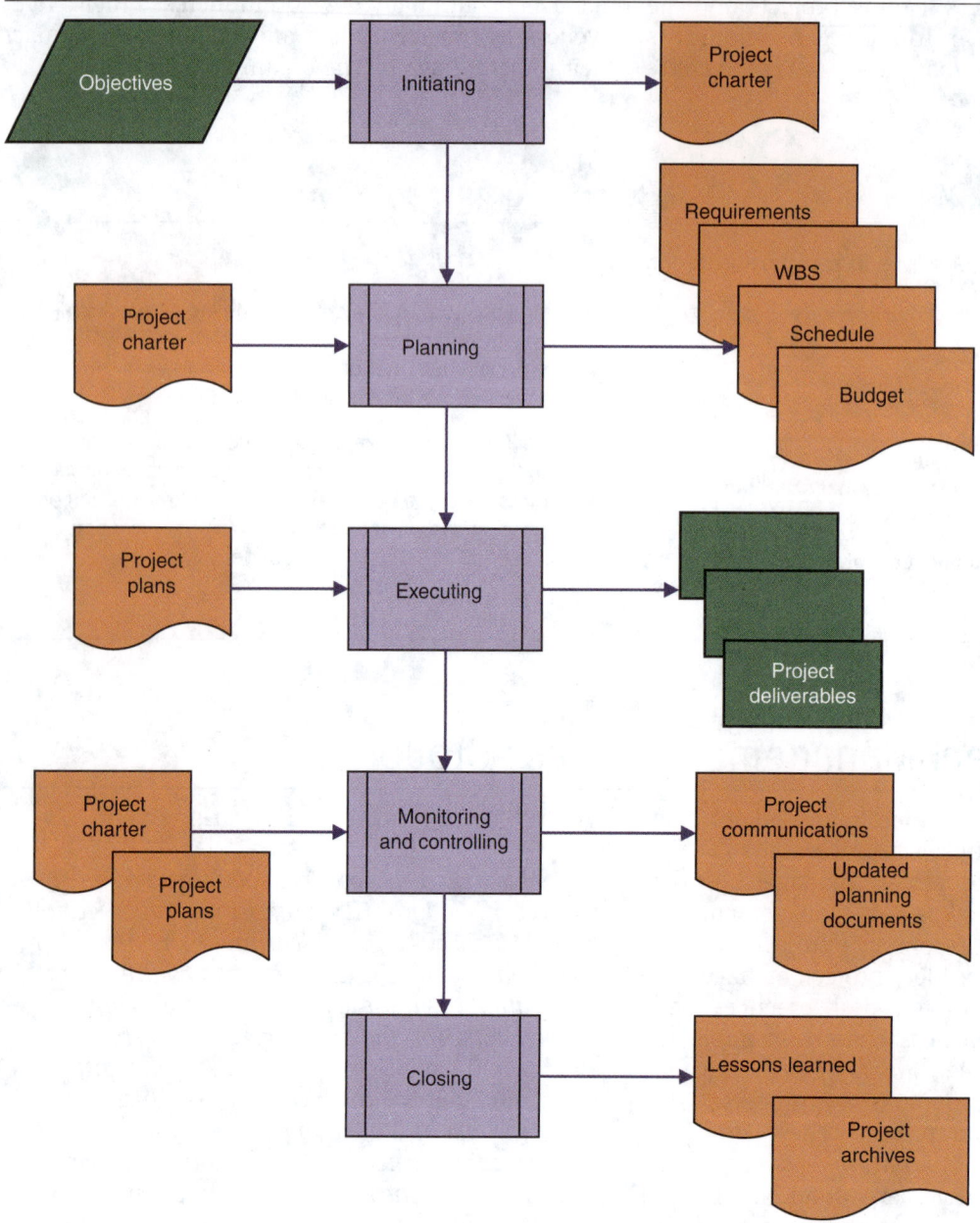

and gain agreement on the project constraints (scope, schedule, and budget). During the initiation phase, the project is formed. Using the definition of a project as being a temporary endeavor executed to reach specific objectives while constrained by time and resources, the initiation phase describes the effort using these attributes of a project. The objectives are determined and limited to fit within a temporary period of time, the timeframe the effort will take is determined, and the type and quantity of resources (human, financial, and other resources) are estimated. All of these factors are required to create a project. Therefore identifying and agreeing upon these factors must be completed at the beginning of any project.

The project objectives are first established to justify the project. The purpose of the project is based on one of the three categories of projects (revenue, expense, compliance) and should be associated with some form of benefit to the organization to help justify the organization's financial investment (Levine 2005). Ideally, the benefits described should include measurable objectives that can be evaluated once the project is completed to evaluate the contributions to the organization.

In addition to the project objectives, the project constraints must be defined. The scope of the project is defined to set the expectations of what will be delivered, and the schedule and budget are defined to express the constraints by which the scope must be delivered.

Once the scope is defined and the time and budget constraints identified, the project schedule can be prepared. A high-level plan is developed to identify the work that must be done to complete the project and deliver the entire project scope. Using this plan, the time required to complete all this work is estimated. These time estimates may be in the form of hours, for a short project, or days or weeks for a longer project. Regardless of the units used for these time estimates, the units should be consistent. For instance, if days are determined to be the best way to estimate some of the work, then the estimation of all the work should be calculated in days. The results of the schedule estimate should be the total amount of time (hours, days, or weeks) required to complete all the work needed to deliver the entire project scope.

The next step is to use the previously defined work to determine the resources needed to complete the project. These resources include the money needed to purchase the raw materials for the project, money needed to pay the additional specialists required to complete the work, and money needed for the tools or project logistics. These cost estimates are calculated for each of the tasks required and then added up to determine the total costs for the project. These costs form the project budget.

Once the project objectives and constraints are determined, a project charter is created. This project charter documents the objectives, benefits, and project constraints so the project manager and project team along with the project owner all have the same baseline expectations. In some organizations this project charter is signed and treated as a binding document while in other organizations it is simply used to document the initial vision for the project.

### Case Study: Project Initiating

*Betsy begins her education event project by first creating a project charter. She does this by simply writing in her notebook the objectives and project constraints. Betsy identifies the project objectives of increasing knowledge of current HIM practices and improved collaboration across local HIM professionals. In her project charter, she identifies the scope as providing a speaker, providing food and beverages for everyone attending the event, and inviting her colleagues and all other members of her local professional association. She estimates she will need approximately 60 days to reserve a conference room, purchase the food and drinks, recruit a speaker, and send out invitations. Betsy does not yet know the menu she will serve or supplies that are needed, but she calculates that $30 per attendee should be enough to cover all expenses and she anticipates 100 people will attend the event. After summarizing the objectives, scope, schedule, and budget for the education event, she decides the effort, time, and costs are worth the benefits she and her colleagues will gain from learning more about the profession and networking with other local professionals. Based on this benefit, Betsy decides to go ahead with the educational event and moves on to complete her detailed planning.*

## Planning

Once the initiation is complete, the planning process group begins. The planning phase uses the completed project charter and several planning tools as input and produces a detailed project plan and updated project constraints as the output for the project planning process. The purpose of this process is to investigate the project further to gain a complete understanding of the project and the work to be completed to establish a detailed plan. The initial project constraints of scope, schedule, and budget from the project charter were educated guesses and must be better defined as the work is planned.

During the planning phase, the project scope specifications can be captured, the work is broken down into individual tasks, a detailed schedule of the tasks is prepared, and all expenses associated with completing the project based on the plan are identified and summarized. Common outputs from the planning phase include a requirements document, WBS, project schedule, and detailed project budget.

The project requirements may be captured in a requirements document or through other means of capturing the attributes of the expected project deliverables. Through interactions with the project owner, project users, and other project stakeholders, the project team establishes a detailed collection of expectations for the project output. To ensure these specifications are communicated correctly, they are expressed in a **requirements document**. There are many forms of requirements documents but one of the most basic forms of capturing these requirements is through a requirements matrix document (table 26.6).

While the requirements are collected, a detailed plan of the work to be completed is prepared. The work is

**Table 26.6.** Sample project requirements matrix

| Requirement ID | Description | Priority |
|---|---|---|
| 1 | Hold event on a weekday evening to maximize the number of attendees | A |
| 2 | Meeting room should hold at least 150 people | B |
| 3 | Meeting location should be within 10 miles from office | B |
| 4 | The meeting location must allow external catering | A |
| 5 | The speaker must have experience related to the educational topic | A |
| 6 | It would be nice if the speaker has never presented at a previous event | C |
| 7 | The food should be healthy | B |
| 8 | The food must be served in individual portions | A |

often broken down into major deliverables or phases, individual components of each deliverable or phase, activities needed to create these deliverables, and individual tasks (referred to as work packages) assigned and carried out during the activity. The **work breakdown structure (WBS)** diagram tool is developed to summarize and illustrate the project work. This form of project artifact (figure 26.13) is commonly used due to the analytical nature where the project is dissected into manageable components. In addition to the ability to dissect the project, the visual nature of this tool provides simplicity for communicating the complex work structure of the project.

Once the WBS is complete and verified, the work can be scheduled. Scheduling the project is commonly planned and managed through a Gantt chart. The **Gantt chart** captures each of the work packages identified in the WBS as tasks for the project team, assigns each task to a project team member, identifies the dates when the work begins and when it will be completed, and identifies any scheduling dependencies with other tasks. The Gantt chart can be used to display the schedule in a hierarchical form like the WBS. The resulting Gantt chart (figure 26.14) is used to communicate the schedule and to monitor the progress of the project during execution.

The project budget must be planned, and the resource expenses captured and calculated to determine the detailed project budget. These resource expenses may include procuring materials for the project, purchasing the tools or project shipping and transportation costs, and employing additional specialists from outside of the organization to complete the work for the project. In many projects where internal employees work on the project, the labor costs for these employees are not included in the budget. However, when projects are conducted on behalf of another organization, the employees' time may need to be captured using a billing rate for each type of team member and the number of hours expected to be used by each role in the project.

Once all material resource estimates and, if appropriate, team resource estimates are collected, a budget is prepared. The expenses are calculated for each work package and are either reported by phase or by the work package for the project. Another method of reporting the budget is to categorize the planned expenses (table 26.7).

In addition to the requirements, WBS, Gantt chart, and project budgets, other outputs may be produced based on the size and complexity of the project. These additional project artifacts include project organizational structure, change management plan, test plans, risk management plan, stakeholder analysis and communications plan, and many other artifacts prepared to address any planning needs anticipated for the project.

### Continuing Education Event Case Study: Project Planning

*After deciding to go ahead with the continuing education event, Betsy begins her detailed project plans. Using a work breakdown structure, Betsy outlines the work to be done to reserve a location, send out invitations, order the food and drinks, and recruit the speaker. She then develops a Gantt chart to schedule the tasks to be completed and delegates the work of reserving a location to her assistant, Emily. Betsy knows that attendance ranged from 75 to 95 people for the past five continuing education events, so she is planning to host a total of 100 people. She decides to serve lasagna, salad, asparagus, water and iced tea, and cupcakes. She also plans to recruit two separate speakers for the event. Betsy now recalculates the budget and finds out that the cost to host 100 attendees will be $2,700 (or $27 per person). Having a better understanding of the effort required, time needed, and costs, Betsy reevaluates her educational event idea and determines the benefits of the event still outweigh the costs and decides to execute her plan.*

**Figure 26.13.** Work breakdown structure (WBS)

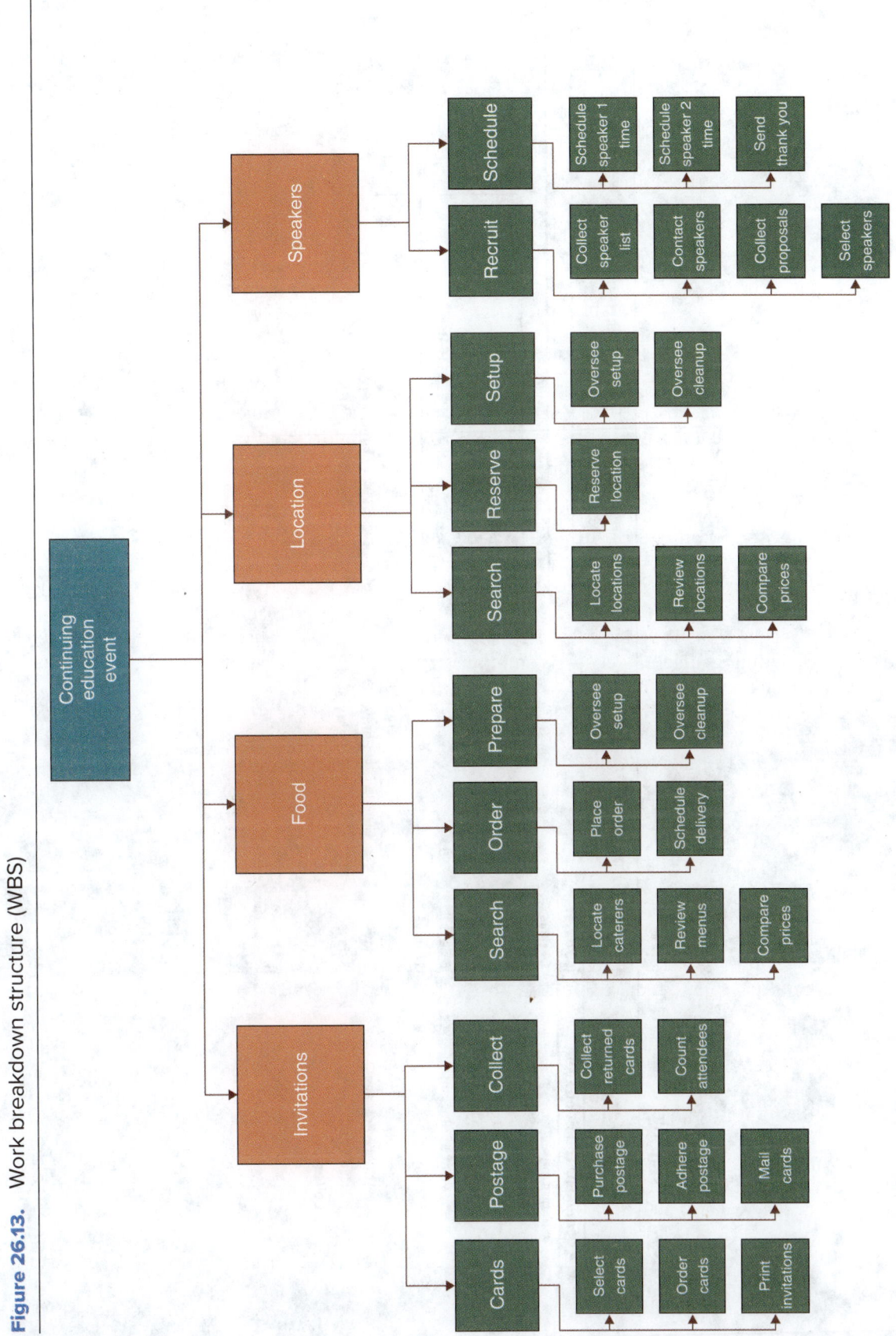

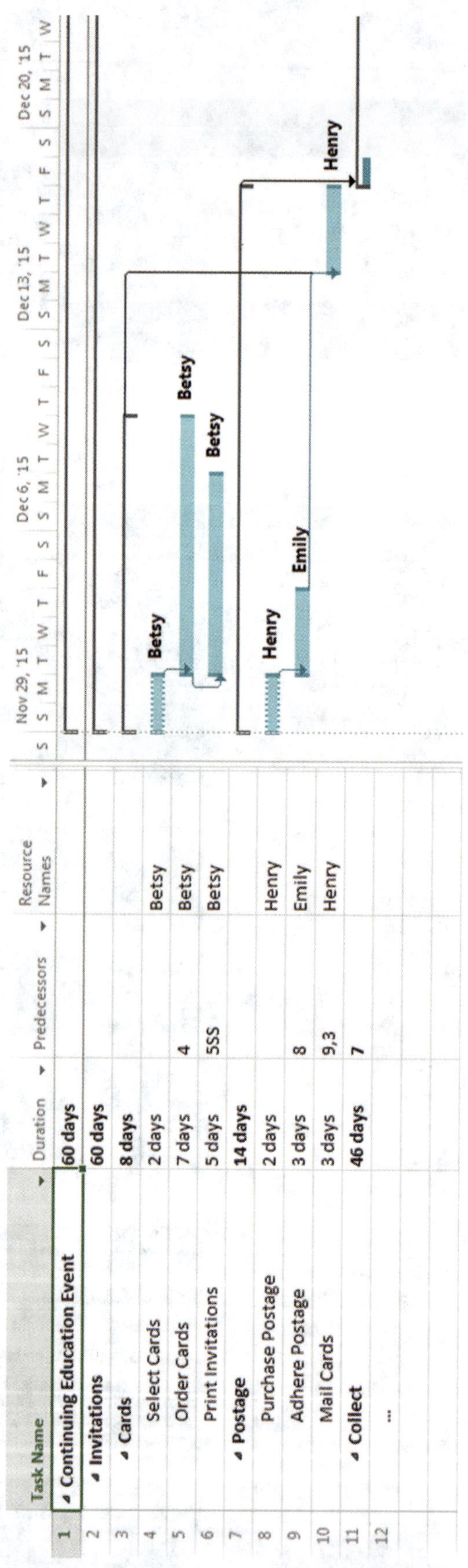

## 746 Chapter 26 Project Management

**Figure 26.14.** Sample Gantt chart

| | Task Name | Duration | Predecessors | Resource Names |
|---|---|---|---|---|
| 1 | ▲ Continuing Education Event | 60 days | | |
| 2 | ▲ Invitations | 60 days | | |
| 3 | ▲ Cards | 8 days | | |
| 4 | Select Cards | 2 days | | Betsy |
| 5 | Order Cards | 7 days | 4 | Betsy |
| 6 | Print Invitations | 5 days | 5SS | Betsy |
| 7 | ▲ Postage | 14 days | | |
| 8 | Purchase Postage | 2 days | | Henry |
| 9 | Adhere Postage | 3 days | 8 | Emily |
| 10 | Mail Cards | 3 days | 9,3 | Henry |
| 11 | ▲ Collect | 46 days | 7 | |
| 12 | ... | | | |

**Table 26.7.** Project resource budget

| Continuing education event | | | |
|---|---|---|---|
| Category | Planned | Actual | Variance |
| Room reservation | $ 400.00 | | |
| Speaker 1 | $ 300.00 | | |
| Speaker 2 | $ 300.00 | | |
| Catering (100 people) | $ 1,500.00 | | |
| Invitations | $ 150.00 | | |
| Postage | $ 50.00 | | |
| **Total:** | $ 2,700.00 | $ – | $ – |

## Executing

Project execution begins during the end of the planning process. The project plans are carried out and the project work products are delivered. This phase includes forming the project team, purchasing supplies and materials for the project, inspecting the project deliverables for quality issues while they are produced, communicating with the project stakeholders, and managing their expectations.

One of the main priorities for the project manager during project execution is to maintain communications with and among the project team members and project stakeholders. This requires publishing project planning documents and updates, frequent project meetings with the project team, maintaining an issues log to track problems and resolutions as they occur, status reporting to communicate current project progress to the project stakeholders, and frequent personal interactions with the project stakeholders to maintain interest and participation in the project.

### Continuing Education Event Case Study: Project Executing

*After reevaluating the continuing education event plans and deciding to go ahead with the event, Betsy begins carrying out her plan. Betsy first sends out social media messages and email messages to all invitees to let them know she is planning the event and informs them that invitations to the event will be sent soon. She then contacts her assistant Emily to ask her to find and reserve a location for the event and gives her some general guidelines, including cost ($200), for selecting a good location. Betsy then prepares her detailed menu and purchases invitations and postage stamps. Next, she recruits her colleague Henry to prepare and send out the invitations for the event. As the event day draws near, Betsy places her order with the caterer and schedules a delivery date and time. When the day of the event finally arrives, she recruits her assistant Emily and colleague Henry to help her welcome the attendees as they arrive. After the event ends, Betsy, Henry, and Emily say goodbye to their attendees and begin cleaning up.*

## Monitoring and Controlling

While the project team executes the project plan, the project is monitored and controlled by the project manager. During this phase of the life cycle, the project is evaluated to ensure it is on track according to the plan; alterations are made to the plans as changes occur, and variances to the baseline are reported. The scope, schedule, and budget are regulated using a change management plan (described later in the chapter), issues are identified and addressed, risks are evaluated, and appropriate contingency plans are made. This project's progress is continually evaluated and any deviations or anticipated deviations from the plan are communicated to the project stakeholders, and appropriate actions are taken to resolve the variances.

The executing and monitoring and controlling phases are very fluid. Although the project begins with detailed plans, changes occur that cause the project to deviate from the plan. The monitoring and controlling phase is when the project manager ensures the plans and project execution are aligned so the project adheres to the project stakeholder's scope, schedule, and budget expectations established in the project baseline.

### Continuing Education Event Case Study: Project Monitoring and Controlling

*While Betsy, Emily, and Henry were preparing for the educational event, Betsy ordered the food and drinks and discovered the food was more expensive than she anticipated. Rather than the $1,500 she budgeted for food and beverages, the total came to $1,650. Discovering that she was $150 over budget, Betsy wrote down this issue in her notebook and decided it was important enough to try to resolve this problem. She then contacted Emily to encourage her to find a location that was less expensive than the original budget of $250. A day later Emily informed Betsy that she was able to reserve a location for $200 rather than the $400 budgeted. Betsy was happy to see that she was now under her budgeted costs, and she made the update to her project budget and captured the result of the issue in her notebook. The rest of the preparation and the event itself went as planned.*

## Closing

The final process group in the project management life cycle is the closing process group. During this phase, the project is reflected upon and evaluated by the project team and all stakeholders, all project expenditures are concluded, and the project documents and other artifacts are archived for future reference or reuse. During this closing phase, it is important for the project manager to identify the lessons learned from the project and document these lessons to help the team, stakeholders, and the organization learn from the project to improve future projects. This final phase also results in the project team disbanding and moving on to a new project or returning to their operational roles.

### Continuing Education Event Case Study: Project Closing

*Once Betsy, Emily, and Henry finished cleaning up after the event, they sat down and enjoyed a beverage and talked about the event and their preparations. Betsy told her colleagues how much she appreciated their help and commended Emily for finding a good location for less than the planned $400. The three of them shared the comments they heard from attendees about the educational event and discussed what they would do differently the next time they planned a similar event and what they thought worked well and will do again. While they talked about their experience with the event and preparations, Betsy took out her notebook and wrote down the comments about the event so she could remember these ideas. Once Betsy returned to work the next day, she placed her notebook in her file drawer to refer to next year when she begins planning the next educational event.*

---

### Check Your Understanding 26.5

Evaluate the Continuing Education Event Case Study on pages 741 to 748 and determine the answers to the following questions in a separate document.

1. What problems would Betsy encounter if she did not complete the project initiating process group?
2. Why did Betsy use a WBS as part of her project planning?
3. What problems would Betsy encounter if she executed the project without referring to the project plan?
4. What problems would Betsy encounter if she failed to follow the monitoring and controlling process group?
5. Why should Betsy carry out the project closing process group?

---

## Managing Project Change

Change is important both prior to and during project management. Earlier in this chapter, change was described as the catalyst for projects. Projects are the response to the organization's need or desire to change. Additionally, change occurs frequently during the project, and the project team must respond appropriately to keep it on track and ensure the project work products remain relevant and valuable to the organization. In this section, change is discussed in terms of the different types of change occurring during the project and how the project manager must respond.

### Types of Change

Project change occurs through several different means. Change may originate from the project team, project owner, project stakeholders, the organization, or the external environment and regulations (see table 26.8). Regardless of the source of the change, the project manager and project team must respond and shift the project plans to accommodate the change.

Also, the project manager must engage the project stakeholders to reset project expectations because of the change.

The project manager must be aware of change and look for it throughout the project, particularly during the monitoring and controlling phase. It must be acknowledged that change will most likely occur, and the project plans will have to be adjusted. However, change must also be appreciated. While change creates more work in project planning and coordinating, change and the project team's response to it provides a great deal of benefit to the organization. The project manager needs to know how to respond to change and reap the benefits of a proper response.

### Benefits of Change

Although not all change is positive, responding properly to change contributes positively toward the project outcomes. For instance, if a project member resigns from the organization, the project manager can

**Table 26.8.** Examples of project change

| Origin of change | Examples |
|---|---|
| Project team | A project team member leaves the organization, and a replacement must be requested from the functional department, resulting in delays in the project products |
| Project owner | A new feature is requested that will benefit the organization |
| Project stakeholders | Disagreements occur between project stakeholders and the project owner over some of the project specifications resulting in more time to collect detailed specifications |
| Organization | Two business units are merged requiring a redesign of the project products |
| External | A new government regulation has been passed adding a new design consideration for the project |

quickly respond to this negative change. They can do so by acquiring another team member from the corresponding functional area and updating the project plans, while informing the stakeholders of any delay resulting from this change in the team. By responding quickly and communicating the change and corresponding effect on the project, the project manager minimizes the delay and maintains the stakeholders' expectations. The stakeholders will be pleased the change was responded to quickly and that they were able to readjust their expectations early rather than later in the project, thus reducing their time to respond.

Recognizing the need for change and responding quickly to this need is essential for meeting stakeholder expectations. Changes in the business environment or changes to functional needs require the project team to revise the project deliverables and will most likely lead to delays and increased costs. However, without a response to this change, the project team would have produced work products that did not adequately meet the needs of the functional department or organization resulting in a decrease in the value of the project. Properly responding to change ensures the project work products continue to provide value to the organization and meet the stakeholder's expectations.

A project manager should accept and be prepared for change. By understanding that change will indeed occur during the project, the project manager responds to ensure project objectives are achieved and the project stakeholder's expectations are met. Lack of a proper response to change detracts from the project value and results in unmet stakeholder expectations. Project managers must be able to negotiate with the project owner and other stakeholders when responding to change to maintain their expectations while meeting the project goals and project constraints.

## Negotiating Change and Managing Expectations

Any change encountered in the project has potential to affect the three project constraints—scope, schedule, and budget. The project manager must monitor the project and the environment to recognize potential changes with the project constraints. As changes occur, the project manager recognizes the relationship between the change and the project constraints and needs to adjust the plans accordingly. Unfortunately, all stakeholders may not understand the relationship between changes to the project and the project constraints. As part of managing the stakeholder expectations, the project manager must educate the stakeholders so they understand this relationship and remain open to changes to the project constraints as they occur.

The project manager should use the project constraint triangle (figure 26.4), to educate the project stakeholders about the relationship between the three constraints (schedule, budget, and scope). The project manager should explain that all three constraints are related and any change to one of the constraints may affect the other two. Using an example of introducing a new addition to the project scope, the project manager should be able to explain how the project team must expend additional work to deliver the new scope, and this work will take time and resources. The change then results in a potential increase to the project schedule and in the project budget. The stakeholders should learn to expect adjustment to the project variables as changes are introduced. Failure to understand this relationship forces the project team to respond to changes without revising the project constraints and results in the inability to meet the expectations of the project stakeholders due to missed scope, delayed delivery, or budget overage.

Project managers establish awareness of the constraint relationships early in the project and use this understanding to renegotiate the project constraints as changes occur during the project. The project stakeholders should learn to anticipate change but expect the project manager to take actions to minimize the effect the change has on the project constraints. Once the constraint relationship awareness is established, the project stakeholders will be open to working with the project team in responding to change during the project.

## Change Management Process

Managing change can be difficult for the project manager and the project team. One of the most significant changes during a project is a change to the project scope. Various stakeholders frequently wish to add new or enhanced project requirements after the initial requirements were gathered, and the schedule and budget were established based on these requirements. Over time, these small changes in scope create significant changes and require more resources and time than originally planned. These incremental changes are commonly referred to as **scope creep**. To best deal with the volume of changes that occur as a result to changes in the project scope, a change management process must be established and enforced.

The change management process illustrated in figure 26.15 outlines the steps to take when a change to the project scope is requested. The process begins by the stakeholder formalizing a request for a new enhancement or new addition to the project scope. The requested change and its benefits to the organization should be clearly explained. Ideally these benefits are assigned a monetary value. The change request is then reviewed by the project manager and project team and a change proposal is prepared. The change proposal reiterates the change and value to the organization and describes the work required to implement the change. This includes the changes to the project scope and the effect the proposed change has on the project schedule and budget. Once the project change proposal is prepared, it is reviewed by the project owner and other stakeholders to determine if the benefits of the proposed change outweigh the changes in project schedule (typically schedule delay) and budget (typically budget increase). If the project owner and stakeholders reject the change proposal, the originator of the change request is notified by the project manager. If the project owner and stakeholder determine the change should be approved, then the project manager adjusts the scope document and updates the schedule and budget to reflect the new project baseline constraints. The updated project plans are then communicated to the stakeholders, so all stakeholders are aware of the revised scope, schedule, and budget.

**Figure 26.15.** Change management process

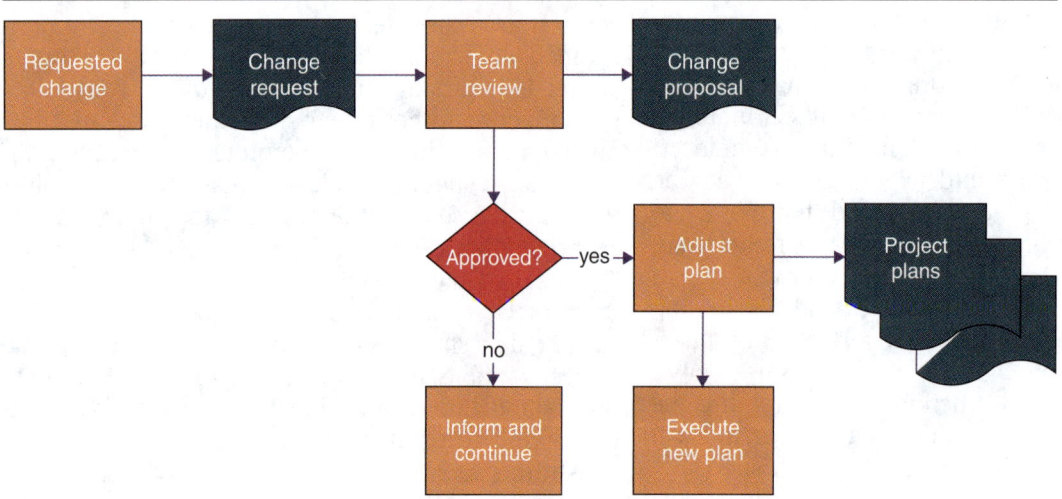

 **Check Your Understanding 26.6**

**Using the Continuing Education Event Case Study on pages 741 to 748, respond to the following questions in a separate document.**

1. What would be the result if Betsy failed to prevent scope creep in her project?

2. If scope creep was observed, how could Betsy respond to manage it?

3. If a change order for attendee gifts was approved for the event with a cost of $25 per attendee, how is the budget affected?

4. After the change order was approved and new plans were made, a second change order was received and approved for a sponsored pre-conference reception event. A local healthcare organization agreed to sponsor a reception the evening before the beginning of the conference and pay the costs for the location, food, and beverages. How does the new change order affect the project plan?

5. Why should Betsy encourage a formalized change order process?

# Beyond Project Management

Every project has a purpose or objective that is associated with some benefit to the organization. The organization will achieve a benefit that in most cases exceeds the cost of the project and places the organization in position to either continue to operate or improve its ability to operate. These projects exist alongside other projects within the organization and in some cases have similar or related objectives. These project objectives are connected to the organization's goals, so the project helps the organization realize its long-term goals. Given the organizational value and connectedness of projects, and the contributions to the organizational goals, it is important to view projects not as isolated work but rather within the context of the entire organization.

Projects and project management are traditionally viewed from an operational perspective. Project goals have been primarily focused on the three variables of scope, schedule, and budget. In the past, a project was successful if the entire scope was delivered on time and within budget. However, this operational perspective of project management is shifting to be combined with a more strategic perspective of project management. Projects are viewed as contributors to the organization's goals and their association with other projects is recognized. As a result, how projects are selected and managed is changing.

## Project Selection

Every organization functions within the limits of its financial resources, employees, and time available to accomplish their goals. These limits restrict the number of projects an organization can complete. The organization must determine in which projects to invest. Given the need to select only a subset of the proposed projects, the organization needs to use a method to select projects to pursue and then delay or turn down other project opportunities. Despite the project selection method used, organizations must recognize not all projects can be pursued and a method of selecting projects is needed. The selection method should reflect the needs, culture, and goals of the organization and be consistently applied to all projects.

## Program Management

Projects become difficult to manage as they become larger and more complex. The scale of the scope and the large resource investments creates a high degree of risk for the organization. These projects become increasingly prone to failure. This means the organization has a greater risk of not achieving the benefits of the project while still investing resources into the project. In order to reduce this risk and increase the likelihood the project will succeed, projects can be broken down into smaller projects where the entire set of projects is referred to as a program. The program is made up of several related projects and each project contributes to the overall objectives of the program.

Program management is used as another layer of management, mostly over projects where a program manager guides and coordinates the set of individual projects to ensure they produce deliverables useful for other projects within the program. The result of a successful program is that the entire set of projects produce complete and integrated deliverables on time and within the overall budget. While the project manager continues to control the individual project and manages the three project constraints, the program manager focuses on connections between the projects and making sure the set of projects are successful in meeting the organization's needs while completing them on time and within the established budget.

## Project Portfolio Management

Project portfolio management (PPM) is a method some organizations use to optimize the benefits gained from limited project resources. PPM is used to identify, select, and prioritize projects and programs in a manner to make best use of the limited resources. The purpose of this method is to leverage the suite of projects and programs to achieve the highest value to the organization. This means the organization distributes resources to the collection of projects that benefit the organization the most.

The PPM method helps the organization better connect the project objectives with the organization's goals. As with the project and program managers, a portfolio also has a manager. The project portfolio manager is responsible for ensuring all projects and programs within the portfolio produce benefits to the organization. Since each project and program begins with clearly stated objectives, the projects and programs are expected to achieve some form of benefit to the organization. The project portfolio manager's role is to monitor, guide, and direct the projects and programs to ensure each project or program within the portfolio produces the benefits promised as part of its objectives. The project portfolio manager is not as concerned with individual budgets and schedules, but rather with the benefits gained from the projects and programs.

As part of managing the suite of projects and programs within the portfolio, the project portfolio manager cancels projects or programs that are no longer able to produce sufficient benefit to the organization. They then shift the resources to another project with potential to deliver a greater benefit. In addition to cancelling projects, new projects and programs are added to the portfolio as existing projects and programs are completed and new resources become available to invest in further projects and programs. As a result, projects and programs are continually added and removed from the portfolio and the portfolio changes to reflect the organization's current goals.

Project management and the related fields of program management and portfolio management are an important function in any organization. Not all organizations have formalized a project management practice, but projects and managing projects occur in almost every organization. Projects and effective management of these projects allow the organization to respond to change and make changes to improve. Change is a certainty in the modern organization and project management exists to help ensure such changes occur.

### Check Your Understanding 26.7

**Answer the following questions in a separate document.**

1. Differentiate between operational and strategic project management by first explaining each, then giving an example to support your perspective.
2. Differentiate a program from a project using an example.
3. How do a program manager's objectives differ from a project manager's?
4. How can a project that is over budget, late, and unable to deliver the entire scope be considered a success by the portfolio manager?
5. Given the following options, which projects should be included in the organization's project portfolio if $800,000 is available to invest in the portfolio?

| Project | Proposed Budget | Financial Benefits |
|---|---|---|
| A | $100,000 | $750,000 |
| B | $950,000 | $2,000,000 |
| C | $600,000 | $1,500,000 |
| D | $200,000 | $100,000 |
| E | $200,000 | $250,000 |
| F | $100,000 | $200,000 |

# References

Besteiro, E., J. Pinto, and O. Novaski. 2015. Success factors in project management. *Business Management Dynamics* 4(9):19–34.

Brewer, J. L., and K. C. Dittman. 2022. *Methods of IT Project Management*, 4th ed. Purdue University Press.

Kerzner, H. 2022. *Project Management: A Systems Approach to Planning, Scheduling, and Controlling*, 13th ed. Wiley.

Kwak, Y. H. 2003. "Brief History of Project Management." In *The Story of Managing Projects*. Edited by E. G. Carayannis, Y. H. Kwak, and F. T. Anbari. West Port, CT: Praeger.

Larson, E. W, C. F. and Gray. 2021. *Project Management: A Managerial Process*, 8th ed. New York: McGraw Hill.

Levine, H. A. 2005. *Project Portfolio Management: A Practical Guide to Selecting Projects, Managing Portfolios, and Maximizing Benefits*. San Francisco: Jossey-Bass.

PMI (Project Management Institute). 2024. "Community You Can Count On." http://www.pmi.org.

PMI (Project Management Institute). 2023. *Process Groups: A Practice Guide*. Newtown Square, PA: PMI.

PMI (Project Management Institute). 2017a. *A Guide to the Project Management Body of Knowledge (PMBOK Guide)*, 6th ed. Newtown Square, PA: PMI.

PMI (Project Management Institute). 2017b. *Project Manager Competency Development Framework*, 3rd ed. Newtown Square, PA: PMI.

PMI (Project Management Institute). 2013. "PMI's Pulse of the Profession: The High Cost of Low Performance." https://www.pmi.org/-/media/pmi/documents/public/pdf/learning/thought-leadership/pulse/pulse-of-the-profession-2013.pdf.

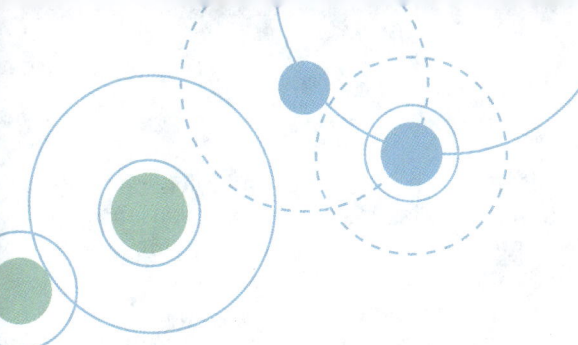

# chapter 27

# Ethical Issues in Health Information Management

*Eric S. Swirsky, JD, MA, MHPE*

## Learning Objectives

- Differentiate fundamental bioethical theories and principles related to healthcare and biomedical sciences
- Evaluate and respond to ethical issues that arise in health information management (HIM) practice
- Evaluate personal values and ethical duties of HIM professionals
- Assess the *AHIMA Code of Ethics* to evaluate essential ethical skills and standards of professional practice
- Utilize an ethical decision-making tool to analyze complex ethical issues and make reasoned decisions
- Determine areas of personal and professional bias that inform HIM practice, including the influence of culture and politics on diversity, equity, and inclusion

## Key Terms

A priori
Altruism
Autonomy
Beneficence
Bias
Bioethics
Blanket authorization
Code of ethics
Cultural humility
Cultural diversity
Deontology
Distributive justice

Double billing
Equity
Ethical lapse
Ethics
Ethics committee
Integrity
Justice
Least harm
Moral agent
Moral courage
Moral dilemma
Moral distress

Morality
Need-to-know principle
Nonmaleficence
Paternalism
Prejudice
Procedural justice
Professionalism
Retrospective documentation
Stereotyping
Utilitarianism
Virtue ethics

Through the millennia, the science and practice of medicine have evolved alongside the moral relationship that exists between caregivers and patients. The movement towards professionalization of medicine, essentially beginning with the work of Hippocrates, served as the vanguard for the subsequent transformation of the healing arts and sciences into a $4.3 trillion healthcare industry in the US—more than

753

18 percent of the Gross Domestic Product (CMS 2021). Of course, the Hippocratic tradition was not part of a professional organization. However, it tried to codify the moral relationship between physicians and their patients in a manner still recognized today. The ancient ethical principles of refraining from harm and protecting patient confidentiality stand among the traditional clinical values that have withstood time. Yet, they have become weathered and worn through the ages.

Technology has expanded and challenged the clinician-patient relationship in many ways. Traditional values have given way to a new set of societal interests in the wake of technological innovation and implementation; in the age of the electronic health record (EHR), for example, the Hippocratic notion of confidentiality has been labeled a "decrepit concept" due to information sharing and the number of clinicians and administrators who access patient records (Siegler 1982, 1518). The widespread implementation of information technologies and novel uses of data have resulted in further challenges to the concept of confidentiality. Information is shared to benefit patient health outcomes. However, information is also shared for the financial benefit of healthcare providers and third-party payers. As such, the clinician-patient relationship is very crowded. From an ethical standpoint, information technologies may have an even more profound impact. Technologies can develop identities that limit the patient experience to the measurable aspects of illness, ignore important human factors and the patient's voice, diminish clinician-patient relationships, and erode clinical skills (Reiser 1978, 229).

Healthcare technology has the potential to improve the quality of human life, but it must be wielded with care. Health information technology (HIT) and attendant professions serve a wide variety of stakeholders in the healthcare system, including patients, clinical and nonclinical healthcare workers, institutions and organizations, third-party payers, state and federal agencies, accrediting organizations, and an array of others. Due to the ubiquity of HIT in clinical environments, HIM and health informatics (HI) stand at the crux of communication in a complex and multidisciplinary health system. As such, these disciplines form the mortar that binds together the bricks of team-based healthcare as information is exchanged to coordinate care of patients. The importance of ethical standards in HIM and HI should not be minimized. Communication issues are among the most common root causes of sentinel events, which are defined by the Joint Commission as unanticipated "patient safety events (not primarily related to the natural course of the patient's illness or underlying condition) that reach a patient and result in death, permanent harm, or severe temporary harm" (Joint Commission 2015, 1). Therefore, professionals working in these fields must abide by their respective ethical codes and standards of professional conduct to avoid medical errors, malpractice, and other risks to patient safety related to the use of HIT and communication of health information and data.

HIM professionals are guided to attend to these issues through the American Health Information Management Association (AHIMA) Code of Ethics so that they may serve as stewards of the profession. Ethical problems arise in scenarios that make us question, "What should I do?" Ethical principles, theories, and codes are tools that help us identify issues, analyze information, and justify options. The study of ethics can help HIM professionals prepare for situations they may not have considered or know how to resolve. It provides tools for making difficult decisions and offers ways to reflect upon competencies related to **professionalism**—the knowledge, skills, and attitudes required to meet the expected standards of deliberate professional practice and excellence through lifelong learning.

## Morality and Ethics in Health Information Management

Like others in healthcare disciplines, HIM professionals must adhere to a **code of ethics**, which is a set of standards regarding business practices and professional behavior. Health information managers may not be directly involved with patient care, but they are indirectly involved in terms of coding, release of information (ROI), data quality, and so forth. Thus, the work of HIM professionals can affect every life in a health system. Moreover, healthcare workers are frequently called to make decisions in situations where there are conflicting standards or values among stakeholders, and understanding one's professional roles and responsibilities will help the decision-making process. To fully comprehend the expectations set out in the *AHIMA Code of Ethics*, it is necessary to understand the theories and principles that provide its moral foundations.

### Morality

**Morality** is the general term used to describe norms, duties, manners, or customs that people use to distinguish between right and wrong; it conveys fundamental communal standards of conduct and character. There are numerous sources of moral standards; for example, they can be derived from an individual's personal attitudes and experiences, societal or cultural beliefs and customs, or from other sources like professional codes or institutional policies.

Professional guidelines can clarify some responsibilities. However, categorizing right and wrong behavior is nuanced in that actions can be morally prohibited, permissible, obligatory, or supererogatory. Immoral actions or omissions are morally prohibited and should be avoided; however, morally right acts are different in that they can be either permissible (not required, but allowable) or obligatory (morally required). Then there are morally supererogatory acts, which go above and beyond what is morally required.

Although they may be related, morals are not the same thing as laws. Laws are formal rules that are defined and uniformly enforced by the government and determine what is *legally* right and wrong based on concepts of justice and equity. Morality is a set of informal personal, group, organizational, or societal norms based in communal ideals of goodness. There are many issues in healthcare that have both legal and moral implications. Consider an act of deception. One may feel morally compelled or justified in lying to a third-party payer so a patient can get treatment they cannot afford. However, falsification of medical records or lying to insurance companies can have legal and professional ramifications. The intersections of ethics, law, and healthcare are nuanced and may change from time to time and place to place. Issues that impact frontline healthcare workers also implicate HIM professionals, such as laws that mandate reporting of infectious diseases, elder abuse, and child abuse that vary by state.

A moral dilemma is a situation in which there is a decision to be made, but the right thing to do may be hard to choose or be unknown because any choice may violate a duty or standard. It can be difficult to identify moral dilemmas when they arise; they are frequently embedded in complex situations, especially in healthcare. Issues may arise among conflicting moral obligations, between moral standards and laws, when there is a barrier that prevents doing the right thing, or when we have a gut feeling that something is wrong, but it is unclear what it is. Moral dilemmas have three common structural features:

- A moral agent—a person with decision-making responsibility for themselves or others
- A course of action—the decision that needs to be made, and the decision-making process used to reach it
- An outcome—the result of taking a particular course of action (Doherty 2021, 55)

A mistake or error in judgment that results in harmful effects relative to ethical standards is referred to as an ethical lapse. For an ethical lapse to occur, one does not have to have a bad intention or deliberately choose to deviate from a standard. All that matters is that one intended the action that resulted in harm.

When an HIM professional is asked to release information to a third party, their decision-making responsibilities are invoked as a moral agent. In this scenario the moral dilemma is related to professionalism and the standards and practices that must be followed. There are decisions that must be made, and professional standards and legal codes dictate the process. The outcomes will be determined by the course of action the professional takes. Dilemmas can arise from any of these structural features individually or in concert. In other words, issues arise for healthcare providers in their position as moral agents (who should decide?), the course of action (what should be done?), and the outcome (were professional responsibilities met?).

## Moral Distress

Situations involving moral dilemmas or lapses can result in moral distress for healthcare professionals. Moral distress refers to the perception of dissonance between one's beliefs and values, standards, and issues they face at work. Situations that evoke moral distress include negative role modeling, witnessing the immoral acts of others, and participating in substandard patient care. Moral distress has been associated with burnout and cynicism when it manifests as humiliation, dehumanization of patients, and witnessing unethical acts, such as blatant falsification of patient health records (Billings et al. 2011, 504). Figure 27.1 illustrates some sources of moral distress. The effects of moral distress build over time, and they begin during training with impacts to relationships, job satisfaction, and professionalism. Few people receive training to deal with their moral distress and therefore lack the agency to participate in controversial cases or report wrongdoing as they progress through training and move into practice. Moral distress impairs a person's moral agency because cognitive-emotional dissonance can prevent the person from responding appropriately when something may be wrong. In the face of these distressing moral dilemmas, health information managers are expected to uphold professional responsibilities, standards, and values. This is referred to as moral courage, defined as the personal trait of individuals who act upon their ethical values to help others despite personal risk, adversity, and professional isolation; despite the consequences, morally courageous people are prepared to do the right thing when others are not (Murray 2010).

# Ethical Theories, Principles, and Concepts

Morality is closely related to the field of ethics, which is the study of morality using the principles, theories, and decision-making frameworks of philosophy. Morality refers to standards of conduct and right and wrong, whereas ethics provides structure to analyze those standards within a particular context. In healthcare, ethics involves formal and informal decision-making frameworks used in the analysis of issues involving diverse and competing perspectives, values, and obligations of stakeholder interests in a common problem. Different ethical theories approach moral questions in different ways, such as focusing on outcomes or character traits. There is no pure ethical theory that controls the others, and there is no hierarchy to settle disputes when theories conflict; each one has its strengths and weaknesses, but understanding them enhances a healthcare professional's decision-making toolbox and abilities. The moral relationship between providers and their patients has been studied by philosophers for thousands of years, resulting in the development of a variety of ethical theories, principles, and concepts. This is sometimes referred to as bioethics, the discipline is concerned with the ethical, legal, and social milieu of healthcare, bioresearch, public health, and environmental ethics. The following is a review of some ethical lenses regularly applied in bioethics.

## Virtue Ethics

Different approaches to bioethics in the West trace their origins to the Hippocratic tradition that emerged from ancient Greek medicine around the fifth century BC—the Age of Virtue Ethics. In determining what is good or right in terms of conduct, the virtue ethics approach considers the character of the moral agent performing the action. How the virtues work is described thoroughly by Aristotle in his work entitled *Nicomachean Ethics*, which provides an account of the gradual progression of human excellence (figure 27.2). Moral excellence begins with having the predisposition and capacity to progress in that way, and the person must work deliberately to attain virtue of character. Aristotle explains that this sort of virtue is not something people are born with. Rather, virtue results from the cultivation of habits over a lifetime of training in the practical application of theoretical knowledge, which leads to character development and expertise, and ultimately mastery in adult life

**Figure 27.1.** Sources and examples of moral distress

- There are multiple options known, but the right action is not clear.
  - E.g., conflicting policies create a situation in which the professional does not know the applicable policies, protocols, and procedures.
- There are multiple options known, but none of the actions feel *right* or they lead to undesirable outcomes.
  - E.g., the professional is hesitant to be a whistleblower due to fears of reprisal.
- Something does not feel right, but we do not know what it is.
  - E.g., a colleague appears to nervously close a patient record and blush when you appear unexpectedly.
- Something does not feel right, but options are unknown.
  - E.g., the professional witnesses unethical behavior but does not know what is morally prohibited, permissible, or required.
- We cannot do what we know to be *right*.
  - E.g., professional policy dictates action or inaction that conflicts with personal values.

**Figure 27.2.** The progression of excellence

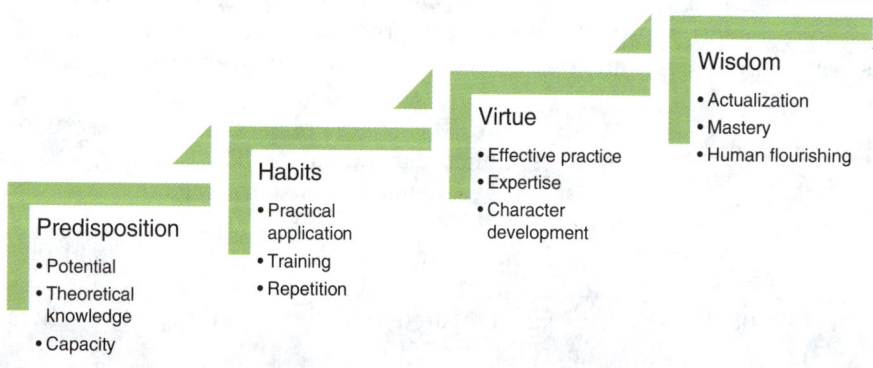

(Aristotle and Irwin 1999, 18). These virtues include things such as courage, honesty, generosity, and temperance. To determine if a particular act is right or wrong, virtue ethics asks, "What would a moral agent with a virtuous character do?" The virtuous moral agent does not act because of a rule or obligation or to achieve a good result. Rather, the virtuous person acts because they are the type of person who behaves in a way that reflects the excellence of character to make proper moral decisions. In other words, good acts are the expression of a good life, or a life well lived. Although this line of philosophical reasoning is thousands of years old, there are modern philosophers who assert the Aristotelian framework is essential to medical practice and the philosophy of technology. As we will see in the pages to follow, these types of professional virtues may be derived from the guidelines established by the *AHIMA Code of Ethics*.

## Deontology

**Deontology**, or Kantianism, is a theory developed by German philosopher Immanuel Kant in the late 18th century that studies the nature of moral obligations. Deontology holds that what is right and good in terms of morality is determined by a moral agent's actions and intentions relative to their duties and obligations. An action is judged good or bad by the nature of the act itself and the moral agent's intentional will to do the act. According to Kant, true happiness is found by leading this sort of principled life, and to choose any other way of life is irrational. There is no good act without good will, and a virtuous act must be done because it is the right thing to do, not out of a sense of duty or ego. This is rational behavior in Kant's philosophy—to act immorally is to behave irrationally because it is irrational to pursue something of lesser value at the risk of the greater (that is, bodily pleasure versus human dignity). So, if a person has the means to make a moral choice and does not, then the person is not only being immoral but also irrational (Kant and Gregor 1998, 37). Moral laws are not supposed to be moral constraints; rather, they are natural behavior of rational beings. There may be duties and obligations, but when the rational moral agent acts, they do so because they believe what they are doing is the right thing to do and not because they must comply with the rules—following rules is not the same as acting morally because moral action flows from free will.

Kant believed in a right way of living and acting, and that was determined *a priori*. That means human knowledge of right and wrong comes through deduction beforehand rather than observation after the fact; a thing is morally right or wrong based upon reason and not consequences. But that is not all: Kant believed a person should always act in a way they hope all people would act in the same situation—what Kant called the categorical imperative. In essence, the categorical imperative states that moral actions are universalizable laws of nature, meaning that an act is always either moral or immoral as determined by rational analysis of the act and the intention of the person doing the action. One such universalizable law dictates that people may not be used as a means towards an end; rather, all people are ends in themselves and deserve to be treated with dignity. In other words, an action that treats people badly to achieve a positive result is immoral—one person cannot be used to benefit another (Kant and Gregor 1998, 31–42).

To demonstrate this, consider the act of lying, which is immoral under the construct of deontology (see figure 27.3). Remember that for an act to be moral it always must be the right thing to do. If lying is

**Figure 27.3.** Kant decision matrix—honesty

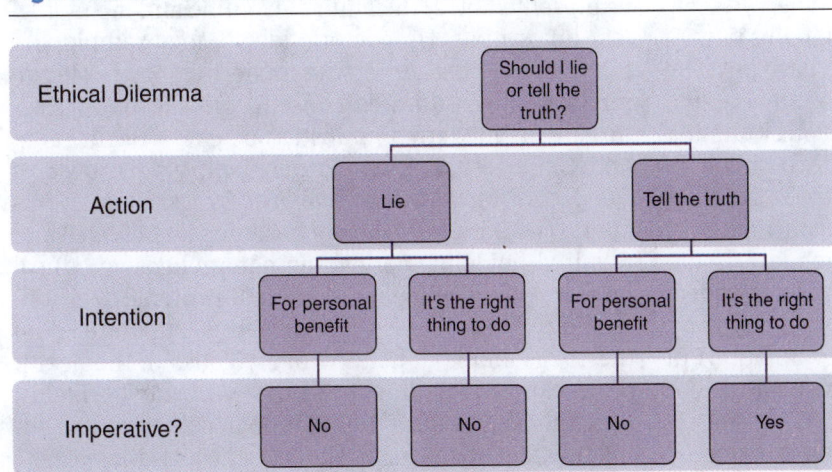

moral, then it must always be morally correct to lie, which leads to an absurd result that strains rationality: if lying were to be the moral standard, then there never would be a reason to believe anything that anyone said. This would defeat a fundamental purpose of communication, which is to convey information. To the contrary, if truth telling is the standard, then we can expect the truth to be told, and we can rely on the information we receive. But veracity is not enough; it must be done with the intention of doing the right thing. Making truth telling a categorical imperative does not belie the fact that people regularly deceive one another; it merely sets a universal morality standard for truth telling. Kant believed in a right way of living and acting, and that way was determined *a priori*, "where we have to do not with assuming grounds for what happens but rather laws for what ought to happen even if it never does" (Kant and Gregor 1998, 36). One can see how deontology applies to HIM in that health information managers have many duties they are expected to follow, including duties to patients, the organizations they work for, and the community at large.

## Utilitarianism

Utilitarianism is one of the most influential approaches to modern medical ethics and in healthcare in general. It provides a basic model for preserving healthcare resources, triage, and disaster response. The general view of classical utilitarianism is the greatest happiness principle, which proposes that to determine the greatest good we look to the consequences of action; that is, "actions are right in proportion as they tend to promote happiness, wrong as they tend to produce the reverse of happiness. By happiness is intended pleasure, and the absence of pain" (Mill 2007, 6). So, according to utilitarian theory, an act is moral to the extent that it produces happiness, and the morally correct action is that which creates the greatest and most good for the largest number of people.

Although there is a sense of hedonism in this pursuit of happiness, it should not descend into base physical pleasures because of the focus on consequences and obtaining the greatest benefit for the greatest number of people. Some kinds of pleasures are more desirable in that they produce more valuable outcomes. In other words, determining the greatest good is a matter of quality as well as quantity, and the standard is not individual happiness but what is best for the collective (Mill 2007, 7–10). Of course, there are many ways to calculate the greatest good, and determinations of utility can lead to all sorts of results. Cost-benefit analyses, for example, can be troubling. For instance, in the 1970s, Ford Motor Company put a value of around $200,000 per life based on deferred future earnings (DFE). It was widely reported that they did not recall their Ford Pinto, which had gas tanks that caught on fire after traffic accidents, because the cost of the recall was more than the DFE. This led to public outrage.

Utilitarianism requires moral agents to consider outcomes in making the determination whether an act is moral or not. In doing so, HIM professionals must consider several different courses of action, their possible outcomes, and which of those results brings about the greatest balance of benefit over harm. This is an essential task in a utilitarian approach, and predicting the future is not easily done. Frequently, utilitarianism requires balancing hypothetical benefits and burdens, and when we look to the greatest benefit for the greatest number of people, the minority can lose out. Still, utility plays an important role in the formulation and assessment of institutional and public policies such as data sharing and interoperability. Yet, in maximizing good outcomes one must be careful to avoid unjust distributions of benefits or burdens (Beauchamp and Childress 2013, 360). For example, utility may support confidentiality as it fosters trust in the provider-patient relationship; if patients do not trust their clinicians, then they may not seek care or suffer poor outcomes and health. In this scenario, the health of the community may suffer, and so it can be said that greater good is upheld when health records are kept confidential. However, there are situations in which the public welfare would not be upheld by maintaining confidentiality, such as preventing an outbreak of a particularly virulent contagion like Ebola or tuberculosis, where it might be important to know who encountered documented carriers of the disease.

## Principlism

Despite centuries of philosophical thought, bioethics has been somewhat ill-equipped to face the challenges presented by 20th century scientific and technological innovation. Hippocratic ideals, for example, are not adequate for addressing modern issues related to public health, informed consent, privacy, and access to care in modern pluralistic societies (Beauchamp and Childress 2013, 1). Principlism, also known as *The Four Principles of Biomedical Ethics*, arose in this context as American society became more diverse and required guidelines providing comprehensive ethical direction while allowing for patient-centered decision-making. This set of guidelines was popularized in the 1970s and is upheld by many codes in the health professions, including the *AHIMA Code of Ethics*. Principlism has four foundational components: autonomy, beneficence, nonmaleficence, and justice.

Often referred to as the right to self-determination, **autonomy** refers to a person's right to decide what does or does not happen to them in terms of healthcare. Autonomy is a core ethical principle of Western medicine, meaning patients have rights to choose their course of medical treatment within accepted standards of care. Two conditions are essential for a person to exercise their autonomy: liberty and agency. That means a person must be free from controlling influences, such as coercion, and have the capacity to make an intentional choice. These are the same conditions necessary for patients to provide informed consent, defined as a person's "autonomous authorization of a medical intervention or of participation in research" (Beauchamp and Childress 2013, 122). The principle of autonomy promotes truth telling because patients cannot meaningfully participate in decision-making unless they have accurate information. At the same time, patients who lack decision-making capacity, such as children under the age of 18 years of age or people living with dementia, may not have the required agency to decide for themselves and must have someone else make decisions for them. This sort of interference with the actions and decision-making of others, when it is done for their benefit, is referred to as **paternalism** and can be ethically controversial.

**Beneficence** refers to the moral obligation of promoting good for or providing services that benefit others, such as releasing health information that will help a patient receive care or ensure payment of services received. Beneficence creates a variety of duties for healthcare providers, including duties to prevent harm, promote rights of patients, and remove conditions that cause harm to others. **Altruism**, the belief that one must make personal sacrifice and benefit other people before oneself, is a related ethical concept. The principle of beneficence holds that good outcomes are determined by balancing benefits with risk for harm or cost so benefits can be maximized to yield a greater good. Beneficence has two distinct aspects: first, positive beneficence requires that people promote the good for others; and second, utility requires people to seek the best possible result. However, utilitarianism and beneficence are different and should not be conflated. For utilitarians, the balance of harms and goods to maximize beneficial outcomes is the primary determinant of ethics. In principlism, the balancing of harm and good is just one of the factors to be weighed in the balance (Beauchamp and Childress 2013, 203).

Whereas beneficence requires providers to promote good, prevent harm, and remove harm, **nonmaleficence** requires them to refrain from actions that cause harm (Beauchamp and Childress 2013, 152). The phrase "first do no harm" is well known in healthcare as a long-standing code of conduct for medical professionals. For thousands of years, this goal has ushered providers to refrain from intentionally harming patients. This is not easily done in clinical environments where providers regularly harm people to heal them through invasive medical interventions such as surgery or chemotherapy. Still, the principle of nonmaleficence requires that we justify harmful actions. These actions are not only related to physical harms, but also harms to individual autonomy, such as the disclosure of protected health information (PHI) and other breaches of professional obligations. This is related to the ethical concept of **least harm**, which applies to situations where two choices may both present necessary, justifiable harms. One should choose the situation that does the least amount of harm to the fewest number of people. For example, in disclosing health information, a health information manager is required by the Health Insurance Portability and Accountability Act of 1996 (HIPAA) to abide by the minimum necessary standard and disclose only that information needed to accomplish the task to those who need to know.

The principle of **justice** refers to the fair and equitable treatment of persons considering what is owed to them; the term **distributive justice** refers to the fair and equitable allocation of goods and harms according to social norms, while **procedural justice** addresses the fairness of policies, processes, and strategies for setting priorities and resolving disputes. There are many theories of justice, and common to all of them is the notion that "equals must be treated equally, and unequals must be treated unequally" (Beauchamp and Childress 2013, 250). This aspect of the principle of justice does not parse out what is equal or unequal, but various theories exist that include distribution according to need, equal shares, effort, or contribution, or to address past or current injustice. Naturally, this leads to problems in policy creation due to disagreements that arise in the conception of justice and fairness in distribution. However, as discussed earlier in this chapter, theories and principles are not hierarchical. In a principlism analysis we look at all the factors that arise to determine which options best fit the situation. Distributive and procedural justice apply to HIM professionals' work in relation to the way information is shared with patients and healthcare providers for certain purposes, and the policies and protocols to follow in making such disclosures. Frameworks for procedural and distributive justice are also necessary for attending to issues of diversity, equity, and inclusion (DEI) in healthcare practice, research, and work environments as described later in this chapter.

The four principles of autonomy, beneficence, nonmaleficence, and justice work simultaneously, and no formal hierarchy or priority exists. But they can be useful in situations where conflicting duties or responsibilities arise. When faced with a moral dilemma, the principles are meant to be considered and balanced to determine the best course of action in the situation. The principles frequently conflict as they compete in the balance; for example, there are times when healthcare providers override autonomy to provide for the welfare of the patient or serve another interest, such as a court order for the release of information. As discussed later in this chapter, ethical decision-making tools are useful in managing the various theories, principles, values, and interests that attend morally charged healthcare decisions. See figure 27.4 for a summary of ethical thinking.

**Figure 27.4.** Thinking ethically in HIM

| | |
|---|---|
| Virtue ethics | What would an experienced HIM professional do in this situation? |
| Deontology | Are the action and intention in accord with AHIMA standards and ethical codes? |
| Utilitarianism | Does the outcome lead to the greatest good for the greatest number of people? |
| Autonomy | Are individuals allowed voluntary self-determination? |
| Justice | Are people being treated fairly? |

### Check Your Understanding 27.1

Answer the following questions in a separate document.

1. Evaluate the characteristics of a virtuous HIM professional.
2. How does the sharing and withholding of health information affect a patient's autonomy? When, if ever, is it ethically acceptable to override a patient's autonomy, and how is that justified?
3. Prepare a 10-minute presentation for peers that identifies and explains three ethical duties that apply to HIM professionals.
4. Drawing from your experience, how does the disclosure of patient health information create conflicts among the four principles of autonomy, beneficence, nonmaleficence, and justice? How can these conflicts be resolved?
5. Within the context of the workplace, do you agree with the statement, "Technologies can have identities of their own"? Justify your perspective.

## Ethical Foundations of Health Information Management

Ethical principles and values have been at the core of the HIM profession since its beginning in 1928. The first ethical pledge was presented in 1934 by Grace Whiting Myers, a visionary leader who recognized the importance of protecting information in medical records. The HIM profession was launched with recognition of the importance of safeguarding health information and the requirement of authorization for its release: "I pledge myself to give out no information from any clinical record placed in my charge, or from any other source to any person whatsoever, except upon order from the chief executive officer of the institution which I may be serving" (Huffman 1972, 135).

Today, patients, rather than administrators, authorize the release of their medical information. On the other hand, the most important values embedded in this pledge are to protect patient privacy and confidential information and to recognize the importance of HIM professionals as moral agents in protecting patient information. HIM professionals have a clear ethical and professional obligation not to disclose information unless a release has been authorized (Rinehart-Thompson and Harman 2017, 78). Professionals working in the HIM field are guided by ethical foundations to protect privacy, maintain confidentiality, and ensure data security. The guidance is detailed in AHIMA's professional code of ethics that outlines the values, roles, and responsibilities for HIM professionals.

## Protection of Privacy, Maintenance of Confidentiality, and Assurance of Data Security

HIM professionals are responsible for safeguarding patient privacy and confidentiality and maintaining the security and control of health records. This is accomplished by adhering to ethical concepts guiding these responsibilities. However, there are important distinctions to consider:

- "Privacy can be defined in terms of having control over the extent, timing, and circumstances of sharing oneself (physically, behaviorally, or intellectually) with others" (OHRP 1993). In the HIM context, privacy refers to the freedom from unauthorized intrusion and includes the right of a patient to control the disclosure of PHI.
- "Confidentiality pertains to the treatment of information that an individual has disclosed in a relationship of trust and with the expectation that it will not be divulged to others, in ways that are inconsistent with the understanding of the original disclosure without permission" (OHRP 1993). Confidentiality is a legal and ethical concept that requires healthcare providers to protect health records and other personal and private information from unauthorized use or disclosure.
- Security is the means to control access and protect information from accidental or intentional disclosure to unauthorized persons and from unauthorized alteration, destruction, or loss.

HIM professionals' responsibilities include ensuring that patient privacy and confidentiality are protected, and that adequate data security measures are used to prevent unauthorized access to information. These responsibilities include ensuring that data release policies and procedures are accurate and up to date and violations are reported to the proper authorities.

## Professional Code of Ethics

A code of ethics is a set of standards and rules an organization adopts to establish minimum expectations for professional responsibility and guide its members in determining right and wrong conduct when they perform their job duties. The *AHIMA Code of Ethics* applies to all AHIMA members and is based on the Association's core values. The preamble to the *AHIMA Code of Ethics* states the following:

> The ethical obligations of the HIM professional include the safeguarding of privacy and security of health information; disclosure of health information; development, use, and maintenance of health information systems and health information; and ensuring the accessibility and integrity of health information. (AHIMA 2019a)

The code acknowledges patients' concerns about security, risks to personal privacy, and challenges to controlling how their health information is used and disclosed in a fragmented health system. This includes considerations of information collection, handling, control, access, disclosure, retention, and disposal (AHIMA 2019a). HIM professionals have ethical and legal responsibilities to perform their job duties in compliance with state and federal regulations and employer policies and procedures; these professional obligations are central to the health information manager's role across employment sites and methods of professional practice. In addition, some information, such as genetic, drug, alcohol, and mental health information, requires additional safeguards to protect vulnerable patients. Other information must be disclosed for the public welfare. Safeguarding health information and data is a core function of the business of healthcare and is essential for interactions with patient populations. HIM professionals have access to sensitive information contained within the health record. Patients must be able to trust that the information they share with their healthcare providers will be protected.

HIM professionals are obligated to demonstrate knowledge, skills, and attitudes that reflect the values and ethical code maintained by the discipline. The six purposes listed in the *AHIMA Code of Ethics* are descriptions of the values and principles used to guide HIM professionals' conduct. (See figure 27.5.)

The code includes core principles and guidelines that are aspirational and enforceable. Alleged violations of ethical principles are taken seriously by AHIMA and reviewed by a team dedicated to that purpose. It is the duty of HIM professionals to maintain professional integrity, not only in performing their own job-related tasks but also in reporting suspected violations of professional standards. For example, AHIMA provides the *Standards of Ethical Coding* to assist coding professionals and managers more specifically in decision-making when it comes to coding situations. It outlines expectations for making ethical decisions in the workplace and demonstrates coding professionals' commitment to integrity during the

**Figure 27.5.** Overview of the *AHIMA Code of Ethics*

**The *AHIMA Code of Ethics* serves six purposes:**
- Promotes high standards of HIM practice
- Summarizes broad ethical principles that reflect the profession's core values
- Establishes a set of ethical principles to be used to guide decision-making and actions
- Establishes a framework for professional behavior and responsibilities when professional obligations conflict or ethical uncertainties arise
- Provides ethical principles by which the public can hold the HIM professional accountable
- Mentors practitioners new to the field to HIM's mission, values, and ethical principles

**Principles**
The following ethical principles are based on the core values of AHIMA, and apply to all of its members, nonmembers with CCHIIM certifications, and HIM students. Example behaviors and situations included for each ethical principle may help to clarify the principle. They are not meant to be a comprehensive list of all possible situations.

| Principle | Example |
|---|---|
| Advocate, uphold, and defend the consumer's right to privacy and the doctrine of confidentiality in the use and disclosure of information. | Safeguard all confidential patient information to include, but not limited to, personal, health, financial, genetic, and outcome information. |
| Put service and the health and welfare of persons before self-interest and conduct oneself in the practice of the profession so as to bring honor to oneself, their peers, and to the health information management profession. | Act with **integrity**, behave in a trustworthy manner, elevate service to others above self-interest, and promote high standards of practice in every setting. |
| Preserve, protect, and secure personal health information in any form or medium and hold in the highest regard health information and other information of a confidential nature obtained in an official capacity, taking into account the applicable statutes and regulations. | Take precautions to ensure and maintain the confidentiality of information transmitted or transferred to other parties through the use of any media or in the event of termination, incapacitation, or death of a healthcare provider. |
| Refuse to participate in or conceal unethical practices or procedures and report such practices. | Act in a professional and ethical manner, and adhere to mandated reporting requirements. |
| Use technology, data, and information resources in the way they are intended to be used. | Use healthcare employer technology resources within the confines of organizational policies. |
| Advocate for appropriate uses of information resources across the healthcare ecosystem. | Educate stakeholders about the need to maintain data integrity and the potential impacts should data integrity not be maintained. |
| Recruit and mentor students, staff, peers, and colleagues to develop and strengthen the professional workforce. | Address DEI to promote a fair and just environment for students, staff, colleagues, and members within professional organizations. |
| Represent the profession to the public in a positive manner. | Be an advocate for the profession in all settings and participate in activities that promote and explain the mission, values, and principles of the profession to the public. |
| Advance health information management knowledge and practice through continuing education, research, publications, and presentations. | Develop and enhance continually professional expertise, knowledge, and skills (including appropriate education, research, training, consultation, and supervision). |
| Perform honorably health information management association responsibilities, either appointed or elected, and preserve the confidentiality of any privileged information made known in any official capacity. | Perform responsibly all duties as assigned by the professional association operating within bylaws and policies and procedures of the association and any pertinent laws. |
| State truthfully and accurately one's credentials, professional education, and experiences. | Claim only those relevant professional credentials actually possessed and correct any inaccuracies occurring regarding credentials. |
| Facilitate interdisciplinary collaboration in situations supporting health information principles. | Foster trust among group members and adjust behavior to establish relationships with teams. |
| Respect the inherent dignity and worth of every person. | Treat each person in a respectful fashion, being mindful of individual differences and cultural and ethnic diversity. |

*Source:* Adapted from AHIMA 2019a.

coding process. The principles and guidelines contained in the code reflect ethical theories and principles discussed earlier:

- Virtue ethics: The Code reflects character traits that should be instilled in the professional, including integrity, advocacy, trustworthiness, altruism, veracity, expertise, life-long learning, reflective practice, loyalty, and being honorable, respectable, competent, and service-minded.
- Deontology: The Code states that "professional responsibilities often require an individual to move beyond personal values. For example, an individual might demonstrate behaviors that are based on the values of honesty, providing service to others, or demonstrating loyalty" (AHIMA 2019a). These expected behaviors result in specific duties, such as safeguarding patient information, taking actions against the unethical conduct of colleagues, and cooperation with lawful authorities as appropriate.
- Utilitarianism: The very existence of the Code is an expression of utilitarianism in that one of its intended purposes is to provide for the common good by providing "ethical principles by which the general public can hold the HIM professional accountable" (AHIMA 2019a).
- Autonomy: HIM professionals are expected to promote self-determination for all patients. That includes duties to educate and assist patients in exercising their rights to health information and protect patient privacy and confidentiality.
- Beneficence: The first two guidelines reflect a professional call to act for the benefit of others through advocacy in the protection of patient rights and altruism by putting service before self-interest.
- Nonmaleficence: Health information managers not only have to work for the benefit of others, but they are also expected to refrain from acts of dishonesty, fraud, and deception.
- Justice: Respecting the inherent dignity of every person requires that HIM professionals "value all kinds and classes of people equitably...[and] ensure all voices are listened to and respected" (AHIMA 2019a).

## Professional Values and Obligations

HIM professionals are ethically responsible for preserving, protecting, and securing health information in all mediums. These ethical obligations include duties to preserve patients' confidentiality and privacy; provide service to patients who seek access to their information; promote quality, advancement, and equity of healthcare with actionable data; and function within the scope of professional roles while working within interprofessional teams. Obligations also include duties owed to employers, such as loyalty; protection of committee deliberations (for example, a committee may make decisions related to who will receive an organ donation from a donation list, and those deliberations are protected much like patient information); compliance with all laws, regulations, and policies that govern the health information system (HIS); recognition of the authority and power of the job responsibilities; and acceptance of compensation only in relationship to work responsibilities. Ethical obligations to the public include advocating change when patterns or system problems are not in the best interest of the patients. Examples follow:

- Reporting violations of practice standards to the proper authorities
- Promoting interdisciplinary cooperation and collaboration
- Ethical obligations to self, peers, and professional associations, including being honest about degrees, credentials, and work experiences
- Bringing honor to oneself by committing to lifelong learning
- Strengthening HIM membership in AHIMA and state associations
- Representing the HIM profession to the public
- Promoting and participating in HIM research. (Harman et al. 2017, 3–31)

HIM professionals are ethically obligated to give back to the HIM community by providing practice opportunities for students, such as being involved in student professional practice experience opportunities. HIM professionals also have a responsibility to maintain their skills through continued learning and to pass on knowledge to new HIM professionals and students.

## Ethical Decision-Making

Health information managers bear numerous roles, responsibilities, and expectations that may change during professional practice. Even if they do not, there could be a conflict between professional duties and patient expectations or between personal and professional values. When a healthcare professional is faced with ethical decisions and dilemmas, many factors are considered in the decision-making process. These include patient preferences; cost; technological feasibility; federal and state laws; medical staff bylaws; accreditation and licensing standards; and employer policies, rules, and regulations. Decision-making in ethically charged situations requires thoughtful reflection and informed professional judgment. This chapter has described theories and principles of ethics that result in even more duties and obligations to act or refrain from action. However, tools are needed to provide a framework for decision-making to keep things in order and ensure nothing is missed. Various tools are available, and it is recommended that HIM professionals use a formal ethical decision-making process to encourage reliable moral judgements in professional practice. An ethical approach to decision-making can help moral agents frame professional relationships, consider professional duties, and further develop their professional identities. Ethical decision-making is an exercise in professionalism, and a holistic process helps HIM workers maintain their integrity.

An example of an ethical dilemma for a healthcare organization benefiting from a decision-making process would be a case involving the handling of advance directives for healthcare, such as living wills and powers of attorney, in the EHR. Advance directives are important documents that state patients' wishes for treatment in the event they lose decision-making capacity and are unable to make their own healthcare decisions. Despite good intentions, it is well established in case law and the experiences of clinicians and patients and families across the country that the inability to locate advance directives within the EHR has led to violations of patient wishes, including resuscitating patients who have expressed the wish not to be resuscitated in the case of cardiac arrest. In such cases, decision-making frameworks help care teams identify the various issues, parties, policies, and interests that need to be considered and addressed.

Health information managers should be guided by the *AHIMA Code of Ethics* in making ethical decisions. An ethical decision-making tool helps provide order to the process. Decisions made to resolve an ethical dilemma should go through a process such as the one identified in figure 27.6.

**Figure 27.6.** Ethical decision-making process

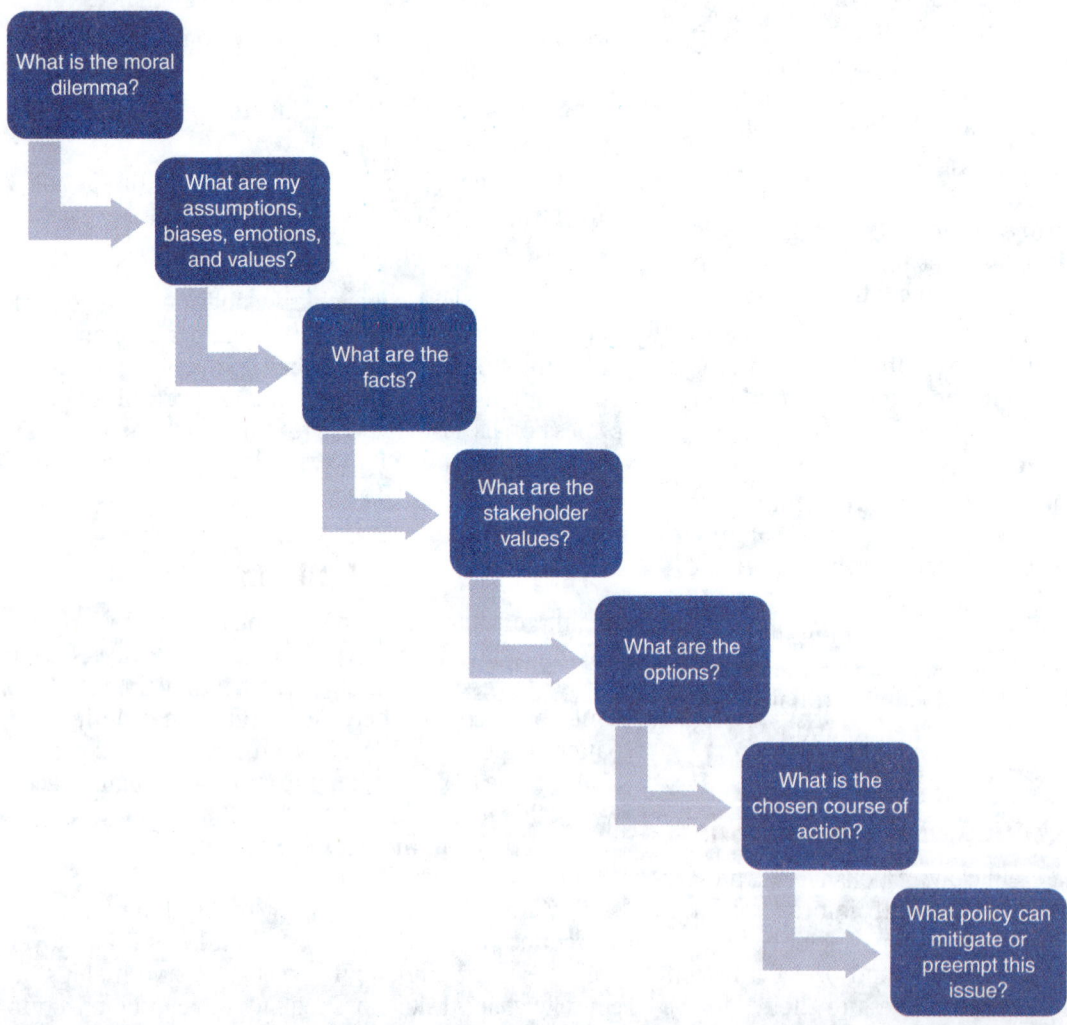

*Source:* Adapted from Doherty 2021; Glover 2017.

Step one prompts us to ask, "What is the ethical problem I am facing?" Frequently, ethically charged scenarios create multiple problems simultaneously, and asking this question at the outset allows a decision-maker to identify and distinguish issues and deal with each individually. Applying the example of advance directives in the EHR discussed above, there are multiple problems that arise, including insults to the agency and autonomy of patients and their families, possible issues in institutional policy and protocol in handling this documentation, and moral distress of patients, families, and healthcare providers and staff that can result from, and lead to, poor outcomes. There are many duties HIM professionals are responsible for, and identifying the questions at hand allows professionals to determine which apply to the situation.

Step two of this process involves the HIM professional's gut reaction to the situation. This is a critical step that allows the decision maker to identify personal assumptions, biases, emotions, and values that may interfere with the decision-making process. Doing this helps us to understand not only our own feelings, but also the distinctions from the other values that should be regarded (Glover 2017, 54). Considering advance directives in the EHR, health information managers may identify with a patient's right to autonomy to make end-of-life decisions in advance. However, they may have personal reservations about an individual's ability to make medical decisions for future health conditions they have not experienced, or they may question whether advance directives accurately reflect a patient's wishes. Explicitly identifying these biases up front helps mitigate their effects during the decision-making process and review of the outcome.

In the third step in the process, we are guided to gather relevant information. In doing so, one must consider facts that are known and work to identify and obtain facts necessary to identify options and make decisions. Some facts will remain unknown, and in those situations, we must proceed with our assumptions duly noted while keeping an eye on how those assumptions impact the analysis (Glover 2017, 54–55). In our ongoing analysis of the issue involving advance directives, there may be few known facts. Suppose that all we know is that the patient has a living will they gave to someone on the care team upon admission. However, it is not in the EHR, and the patient's wishes were not followed as a result. Among the facts to be gathered might be as follows: What does the patient or family want now? Has this happened before? Does the hospital have policies and protocols for handling advance directives, and if so, what are they? If there is a policy, was it followed? If there is no policy, why not? Did the physicians know about the living will and have a legitimate reason for disregarding it? There are many facts to gather in situations like this, and as they are collected, other questions may arise.

Step four asks us to identify the relevant stakeholders—meaning the respective the individuals, institutions, and communities whose values and interests are affected and will be impacted by the decision. Ethical issues frequently impact patients and their families, the clinical care team and other healthcare professionals, HIM professionals and departments, institutions and their administrators, and society at large (Glover 2017, 55). In our advance directives case, consider the following:

- The patient—not just this patient but all patients in the facility have an interest in self-determination (autonomy) and making healthcare decisions at the end of life.

- The care team and other healthcare professionals—the standard of care should be followed using the best available evidence, and the paradigm of patient-centered care requires that patients' wishes be respected when they are known (deontology). Healthcare providers have duties to benefit their patients (beneficence) and avoid harming them (nonmaleficence), thus failing to abide by the terms of a lawfully executed advance directive may violate both. Other providers and staff may be implicated by the outcome as well, including those working on the pastoral service, social workers, house staff, and palliative care and hospice staff. The immediate care team are not the only ones with interests in the well-being of patients at the end of life (beneficence and nonmaleficence).

- The family—end-of-life scenarios are complex events that have wide-ranging impacts with diverse and sometimes incompatible perspectives. In this case, the family may agree with the patient and desire that their wishes be honored. But, as is sometimes the case, families may disagree with patient wishes and may have divergent interests and needs that should be accounted for and addressed. If the advance directive cannot be found, a family member may be called upon to serve as a decision-maker for the patient (autonomy).

- HIM professionals—health information managers share professional duties and values with other members of the care team and have other duties and values unique to the discipline (professional autonomy). Moreover, as described in step two, HIM professionals and everyone else influencing the decision should come to terms with personal interests and biases that may inform the outcome. In this case, the HIM department has an obligation to handle advance directives according to law and professional standards expressed in the *AHIMA Code of Ethics* (deontology), respect a patient's right to choose (autonomy), shield patients from preventable harm, and allocate resources in an equitable manner. Of particular importance are the duties to maintain accuracy, fidelity, and accessibility of information in the EHR (Glover 2017, 55).

- Hospital administrators—these professionals share many of the same values in providing for the welfare of patients as other healthcare providers and staff discussed above, but they also must keep an eye on matters related to risk management and liability of the institution. Policies and protocols are implicated in this case, and the parties responsible for them should be involved in the process to meet the needs of the community the institution serves (utility).
- Society—many jurisdictions provide for advance directives by state law to allow the community at large to make healthcare decisions in the absence of decision-making capacity (utility). As a matter of fairness, the benefits of such laws should be extended to all who are supposed to receive them (justice).

After accounting for the information that must be collected, step five asks us to identify the available options for resolution and how those actions are justified or not justified in terms of professional obligations and legal requirements. The options will flow from the ethical issue being considered but remember—by the nature of the definition of a moral dilemma there should be two or more justifiable options. Suppose the question at hand is the ethical status of the institutional policy on handling advance directives in the EHR. Options might include doing nothing at all until there has been an investigation, providing training for staff on entering this sensitive information in the record, working with the vendor to determine if there is an HIS solution, and revising policy. Each option should be considered on its own merits, regarding how it may be justified (or not) based on the facts of the case and stakeholder interests.

The sixth step asks us to make a choice and complete the chosen course of action based on its ethical justification. In so doing, HIM professionals should pay careful attention to the impacts and outcomes that result from the action, because institutional policies should reflect diverse professional values and stakeholder interests. Professionals are responsible for their own behavior, and the standards they set should not be contrary to the values of the institutions and communities they serve (Glover 2017, 56).

Finally, the seventh step of the ethical decision-making process calls for reflection on the process, outcome, and policy for future occurrences of the problem. Reflecting on what happened helps HIM professionals avoid or lessen the effects of the problem in the future, determine if additional action is necessary to achieve a more desirable outcome, and develop new or amended policies and procedures for the handling of advance directives in the institution so these types of problems do not arise. This is a complex set of issues that requires addressing the needs of patients, families, healthcare providers and staff, the institution, and the community at large. Many different needs and values must be considered and attended to, and in some cases the work of a health information manager may affect them all. See figure 27.7 for an illustration of this process.

## Breach of Healthcare Ethics

As discussed earlier in this chapter, a breach of healthcare ethics is a situation in which requirements established by a code of ethics are violated, intentionally or accidentally. In other words, a breach means an ethical lapse has occurred, and the code states explicitly that its principles and guidelines are both aspirational and enforceable (AHIMA 2019a). Many healthcare facilities have an institutional **ethics committee**, which is a committee within the organization tasked with reviewing ethics questions and policies, suggesting acceptable courses of action in ethically charged situations. Different committees have different rules and requirements for membership. Some require formal applications with references for specific qualifications, while others do not. Most ethics committees involve people from diverse backgrounds and practice areas, such as physicians, nurses, palliative care workers, surgeons, social workers, attorneys, bioethicists, chaplains, risk managers, case managers, and other nonclinical staff. Diversity is valued on ethics committees, many of which work to include representation across racial, gender, ethnic, religious, and community values, but this is not always the case (Prince et al. 2017, 168).

Ethics committees have three major functions: providing clinical ethics consultations to patients, families, care teams, researchers, and administrators; developing policies pertaining to clinical ethics; and facilitating education on topical issues in clinical ethics. The goals of the ethics committee include identifying and ensuring the rights of patients, establishing processes to ensure shared decision-making between patients and clinicians, and ensuring the process does not interfere with the ethical practices of the facility (Pearlman 2013). Although not traditionally recognized as core members of these committees, HIM professionals should seek membership on these committees to ensure their professional duties owed to patients are part of the deliberations and that matters related to the management of health information are adequately addressed for the benefit of all stakeholders.

The *AHIMA Code of Ethics* applies to AHIMA members and other credentialed HIM professionals and requires that they act in a professional manner and as stewards of the profession. The governance structure of this professional association includes the AHIMA Professional Ethics Committee (PEC). The code establishes standards whereby HIM professionals shall "refuse to participate in or conceal unethical practices or procedures and report such practices," and in those situations they are guided to follow the policies of the PEC (AHIMA 2019a). An example of a violation of the *AHIMA Code of Ethics* is the use of an AHIMA credential despite lack of evidence of passing a required credentialing exam. The PEC, which is composed of AHIMA members, leadership, and advisors, reviews complaints of professional ethics breaches, sets the rules for the complaint and response filing procedure, and sets the processes for ethics reviews, hearings, disciplinary actions (see figure 27.8), and appeals (AHIMA 2019b). Health information managers who do not report known or suspected violations of the *AHIMA Code of Ethics* are themselves committing an ethical lapse in breach of their duty to report unethical conduct.

**Figure 27.7.** Ethical decision-making breakdown

---

**Case: Living will in the EHR**

- What is the moral dilemma?
  What should I do about my institution's policies and protocols on handling advance directives in the EHR?
- What are my assumptions, biases, emotions, and values?
  This is personally and professionally disturbing. Patients have an ethical and legal right to make healthcare decisions, and providers have corresponding duties to respect patient requests to withhold life support.
- What are the facts?
  Known: patient has a living will that was given to someone on the care team upon admission, but it is not in the EHR, and the patient was resuscitated.
  Unknown: What does the patient or family want now? Has this happened before? What are the policies and protocols for entering advance directives into the EHR, and were they followed? Are advance directives easily accessible in the EHR? Did the doctors have clinical or other reasons for ignoring the living will?
- What are the stakeholder values?
  Patients: vulnerable at the end of life; want their wishes met when making healthcare decisions in advance directives.
  Care teams: meet the standard of care and abide by patient requests to withhold treatment when appropriate; EHRs that meet the demands for usability in clinical environments.
  Family: want competent care for their loved ones; have healthcare decisions honored.
  HIM professionals: prevent harm; maintain accuracy and accessibility of information in the EHR; maintain the trust of institutional and local community.
  Hospital administrators: welfare of the community; risk management and liability; maintenance of policies; EHRs that meet needs of the system.
- What are the options?
  (1) Do nothing; (2) train staff on timely recording of advance directives; (3) research the problem and make changes to policy to meet the needs of patients, healthcare workers, and institutional workflows.
- What is the chosen course of action?
  Assuming there are appropriate policies in place, it will be important to investigate the issue to see exactly what happened in this case. If this is a matter of training, that can be facilitated in several ways. It may be advisable to perform a needs assessment to see if this is a larger problem than this case.
- What policy can pre-empt or lessen the effects of this issue?
  If this happens to be a recurring issue it may be necessary to make changes to policy. This is a complex set of issues that requires addressing the needs of patients, families, healthcare providers and staff, the institution, and the community at large.

---

**Figure 27.8.** AHIMA professional ethics committee possible disciplinary actions

---

- No action;
- Issue a Letter of Censure (a written reprimand expressing disapproval of conduct);
- Deny or expel Respondent from membership in AHIMA, permanently or for a specified period of time;
- Recommend that AHIMA take legal action against the Respondent;
- Assess a disciplinary fine; or
- Take a combination of any of the above actions or such other action that may be deemed appropriate in the particular circumstances.

---

*Source:* AHIMA 2019b.

### Check Your Understanding 27.2

Answer the following questions in a separate document.

1. Evaluate the effectiveness of the *AHIMA Code of Ethics* in serving its six purposes. Give examples to support your evaluation.
2. Using examples from experience, news reports, or hypothetical scenarios, assess three professional ethical duties that are created by the *AHIMA Code of Ethics*.
3. Assuming the role of a member of the AHIMA Professional Ethics Committee, compose a recommended disciplinary action for an HIM professional who used a coworker's credentials to access a patient record.
4. In a scenario where patient information has been disclosed inappropriately, how do you determine whether confidentiality, privacy, or both have been violated?
5. Evaluate the effectiveness of using the ethical decision-making framework presented in this chapter.

## Important Health Information Ethical Problems

Some areas in HIM have specific ethical problems, such as documentation, privacy, coding, ROI, DEI, public health, and social media. This section introduces a variety of issues that HIM professionals may face.

### Ethical Issues Related to Documentation and Privacy

It is the responsibility of an HIM professional to ensure patient documentation is accurate, timely, and created by authorized parties. This is accomplished by developing policies and procedures, in accordance with laws and regulations, to ensure the integrity of patient information is upheld by the organization. Healthcare providers are required to document their decision-making processes. This means educational sessions are necessary to provide training on documentation that can help protect against unintended unethical behaviors. By providing training on documentation of clinical decisions, healthcare organizations may protect themselves from malpractice claims resulting from related ethical lapses.

An example of documentation an HIM professional can help with is retrospective documentation practice. **Retrospective documentation** refers to the addition of documentation related to clinical intervention after care has been given. Although there are permissible reasons to document retrospectively, providers could do this to increase reimbursement or avoid a medical legal action. There should be policies and procedures in place to deal with these scenarios. Training can also mitigate the consequences of mistakes. HIM professionals can contribute to the professional development across the organization by providing education sessions on documentation.

### Ethical Issues Related to the Release of Information

ROI specialists should embody the value of integrity. The HIM professional must "release information only with valid authorization from a patient or a person legally authorized to consent on behalf of a patient" (AHIMA 2019a). There are two primary ethical issues that arise from ROI—the need-to-know-principle and blanket authorizations. The **need-to-know principle** is based on the minimum necessary standard; for example, if there is a request to verify an admission for lap-band surgery and the ROI specialist gives out the history and physical, labs, discharge summary, and operative report to an insurance company, the documentation could reveal a lot more information than requested, which in turn results in the patient's privacy being violated because more information is being released than just the verification of the admission. An ROI specialist must only give out the need-to-know or the least amount of information necessary, in this case just the admission information.

The other ethical concern for ROI is misuse of the **blanket authorization**, which is when the patient signs an authorization allowing the ROI specialist to release all information from that point forward. This is an issue because under a blanket authorization the patient is giving authorization for future diagnosis and treatment, one of which they may not want authorized. For example, assume the patient signs the blanket authorization today to release their annual examination to their employer. In five years, the patient is diagnosed with cancer. The employer could find out about the cancer because the information was automatically released to them, and the patient may not remember they signed the blanket authorization five years prior. HIM professionals must be aware of this dilemma and help with the education of the patient to what the blanket authorization means.

## Ethical Issues Related to Coding

Codes are associated with reimbursement rates and, therefore, there are inherent incentives to code in such a way allowing healthcare facilities to receive the highest reimbursement dollar amount possible. Coding professionals must be guided by ethical coding practices because, for example, they may be asked by a provider to fraudulently code to receive higher payment for services rendered. A coder must only assign codes where data are clearly stated in the health record. If more information is needed, or the information has to be clarified, a query should be sent to the physician.

The *Standards of Ethical Coding* (see appendix C) are based on AHIMA's *Code of Ethics* with the guidelines outlining eleven standards for ethical coding. Some examples of coding ethical dilemmas are upcoding, downcoding, unbundling, and double billing. Upcoding and downcoding are the practices of assigning diagnostic or procedural codes that represent higher or lower payment rates than the codes that accurately reflect the services provided to patients through the documentation. For example, a physician examines a patient briefly for the flu, but the bill submitted for the visit includes an hour-long, complex exam that did not occur. Unbundling is the practice of using multiple codes to bill for the various individual steps in a single procedure rather than using a single code including all the steps. For instance, a patient goes in for a new cast on a broken leg and instead of billing for one bundled visit (all services related to treating the fracture are billed as one service), the provider lists on the bill codes for each step as individual procedures, resulting in a larger reimbursement. **Double billing** is when two providers bill for one service provided to one patient. An example of this is if a surgeon who was an assistant for a procedure bills Medicare as if she were the primary surgeon, with the primary surgeon also billing Medicare for the same surgery on the same patient.

## Ethical Issues Related to Public Health and Sensitive Health Information

HIM professionals, like others working in healthcare, are in a position where they are required to advocate the interests of the public, the profession, and patients. While health information managers may work primarily with the clinical use of data, public health is another field where the information is used. An example of this is global infections, or bioterrorism, where one must balance protecting the privacy of those injured or affected and delivering information to the government and healthcare professionals so the crisis can be resolved. Government access and use of health-related information is of critical importance to the protection and maintenance of public health. However, there are countervailing interests in confidentiality and privacy as we move across stakeholders.

All health information must be protected; however, some information requires special attention because it is considered sensitive health information, such as genetic, adoption, drug, alcohol, sexual health, and behavioral information. This type of information not only often has stricter rules and regulations but provides a ethical gray area when it comes to releasing and providing records. When developing policies and procedures for ROI that can contain substance abuse, sexually transmitted disease, and mental health information, extra caution is required on the HIM professional's part because there may be competing interests between public safety and patient privacy. Federal and state legislation provides some guidance, but legal counsel may be needed in most cases.

In some jurisdictions the release of sensitive information is required due to public health concerns. For example, some states have sexually transmitted diseases programs that include contact tracing and partner notification; this means public health authorities collect reports from health clinics, physicians, hospitals, prisons, and blood banks to contact, interview, and counsel infected individuals. Authorities will also seek to search for and contact partners for counseling and treatment when necessary. Programs such as these illustrate the difficulty of maintaining patient confidentiality while serving the interest of maximizing the public good (Neuberger and Swirsky 2017, 242).

## Ethical Issues Related to Research

Research is essential for the growth and advancement of the healthcare profession. Institutional Review Boards for the Protection of Human Subjects (IRBs) are committees overseeing the clinical research conducted for healthcare who have responsibility over the ethical application of research (Adams and Callahan 2013). Without research, common medications and medical interventions would not exist. However, with research comes ethical obligations to provide patient safety and other protections. These obligations are cited in the Belmont Report, which provides the foundation for ethical research. The intent of the Belmont Report is to protect the autonomy, safety, privacy, and welfare of human research subjects (Adams and Callahan 2013). The Belmont Report provides three primary ethical principles:

- *Autonomy:* Defined earlier, autonomy includes the informed consent process for human research subjects and starts with a full disclosure of the nature of the study, the risks, and the benefits, and gives the participant the opportunity to back out of the study if he or she wants. The idea behind this is that the potential participant has full knowledge of what he or she is doing, and can confidently say yes or no.
- *Beneficence:* Defined earlier, beneficence is when a researcher determines what the maximum potential is for society, compared to the minimum risk of harm done to the participants in the research study. An example would be a researcher looking at a trial for finding a cure for the common cold. The risk to the research participants would be low and the maximum potential for the trial is high because the common cold affects a large number of people each year.
- *Justice:* Defined earlier, this principle involves impartial selection of participants in a research study. The research study must stay within the law when choosing participants. It is important to avoid unfairly coercing participants, such as prisoners who have historically been coerced into taking part in medical research against their will. (Adams and Callahan 2013)

The HIM department is involved in the IRB process by making the health records of patients enrolled in a research study available to external monitors and auditors. Agreements between the HIM department and researchers ensure patient consent and other policies and procedures are followed. In the case of electronic health information there are agreements outlining the exact information to be released to researchers. The HIM department offers training to researchers and HIM staff for the procedures in place for the consent process and maintenance of the records.

Aside from researcher access to patient records, there is the matter of whether research data should be included in the EHR. Some research protocols collect patient reported outcomes (PROs) as a narrative of patient experience of clinical care. PROs represent the patient's voice and appeal to the values of autonomy, as they incorporate the patient's perspective, but if collected by independent investigators, there is a question of whether the data should be included in the EHR. Moreover, if the patient is at risk, there may be a duty to report the information to their primary care physician. This should be done with the patient's prior approval, which means that the research protocol should be structured in such a way that participants are notified during the informed consent process that they will be asked sensitive questions, that the results will be entered in their records, and that other members of the care team will be notified if necessary. For example, consider a research protocol for studying the efficacy of complementary and integrative therapies for people living with chronic pain from sickle cell disease. This patient population is at risk for depression and suicidal ideation, and so investigators design a protocol that collects PRO information through psychometric evaluations that assess changes in mood, anxiety, and other conditions. If patients express suicidal ideation and thoughts of harming themselves, then there may be a duty to report that information and the research data and patient record must be interoperable (Swirsky et al. 2023). HIT and information governance feature prominently in IRB approval and research operations because evidence-based medicine requires access to accurate healthcare data. Health information managers play a vital role in the protection of research participants.

## Ethical Issues Related to Diversity, Equity, and Inclusion

Human values include social and cultural belief systems of people and the healthcare organizations they work for and are certified by. Culture is learned, shared, social in nature, dynamic, and changing—meaning people generally have similar beliefs and values based on their upbringing, what they were taught by parents, peers, and surroundings. The values of an individual can shift over time based on changing environments, social networks, and attitudes. For example, a student who leaves home for the first time to go away to college will be exposed to new and different experiences, and, as a result, over time the values developed at home may shift and reflect those from the college environment.

People are guided by their own sets of values and ethical principles according to their personal beliefs and cultural upbringing. Therefore, it is important for HIM professionals to understand cultural competency and diversity to help guide their actions and interactions in the workplace and when representing the profession. Understanding a person's background, culture, beliefs, and values makes it possible to comprehend why they act a certain way and can help guide professional interactions. **Cultural humility** is the process of self-reflection and critique on beliefs and values combined with an acceptance of other people and groups and is vital to the overall culture of an organization, whereas **cultural diversity** is the perceived or actual difference among people. In the context of DEI in healthcare, the term **equity** refers to the fair and just distribution of resources, opportunities, and advantages within a given organization or system. It involves recognizing and addressing historical and systemic disparities to ensure all individuals, regardless of their background or characteristics, have equal access to opportunities and receive fair treatment. Equity in this sense goes beyond treating everyone the same; it acknowledges and seeks to rectify past and existing inequalities to create conditions where everyone can reach their full potential. In DEI discussions, equity is often emphasized as a fundamental principle to counteract discrimination and promote a more just and inclusive society or workplace. Inclusion in DEI emphasizes valuing diverse perspectives, creating spaces where everyone feels welcomed and respected, and fostering a just and equitable environment.

Considering the interplay of diversity and equity, some consider the concept of cultural competence as flawed because culture is socially and contextually constructed. Therefore, it is of greater importance to practice cultural humility and be aware of personal attitudes and "cultural baggage" to limit their impact on professional work (Dean 2001). Attitudes that affect one's cultural competence include prejudice, stereotyping, and bias. **Prejudice** is judgment of a person based on cultural elements without reviewing all the information; for example, disliking a person because of their national origin or ancestry. **Stereotyping** is an assumption that everyone within a certain group is the same; for example, believing surgeons are difficult to communicate with. A **bias** prevents a person from having an impartial judgment; for example, an HIM professional who prefers to work with only women. Healthcare professionals should be mindful of the differences in culture, beliefs, and values of other people, particularly coworkers and patients, and avoid prejudice, stereotyping, and bias. One way to become more mindful is by exploring different cultures, values, and beliefs, and remaining sensitive to the ways other people conduct their lives (Simmers et al. 2014). For example, ethics issues can arise amid misunderstanding or insensitivity to the postmodern conceptions of gender that affect demographic data for a vulnerable population because many EHRs are not designed to collect nuanced data on gender identity or transgender status. Transgender patients' gender or personal identity does not correspond with sex assigned at birth. Thus, a person born with typically male anatomy may identify as being female, may be in the final stages of transitioning to female, or may not be considering transitioning at all (Coleman et al. 2012). Moreover, some transgender patients do not accept the male-female binary gender identity, have preferred or legally changed names, or have other needs regarding the demographic information contained in their health records. The failure to record this information and identify transgender patients accurately in clinical environments impacts the quality of care provided (Deutsch et al. 2013). Of course, gender status may be irrelevant to the patient's immediate healthcare needs, such as visiting a dental clinic for a root canal, but the same may be said of other patients and information contained in the EHR. While acknowledging barriers to collection, the sensitivity of this information, and the need for adequate privacy and security protections, the Institute of Medicine has recommended that the Office of the National Coordinator for Health Information Technology include data on gender identity in required demographic data sets (IOM 2011). While there has been increasing recognition of the importance of this data in addressing social determinants of health, significant health data gaps remain and create barriers for improving outcomes (SHADAC 2024).

## Ethical Issues Related to Electronic Health Record Systems

The access to EHR systems is a complex challenge regarding record integrity, information security, linkage of information for continuum of care within different e-health systems, and the development of software for HIM purposes. HIM professionals need to be part of the implementation team to provide their unique understanding of the federal rules and regulations regarding privacy and security and can help facilitate a successful core in the implementations of these issues. HIM professionals are trained in the ethical issues related to EHR systems because staff may have access to more information than what is needed to do their job. Employees accessing the record should not explore information out of curiosity; this would be unethical. When a patient's health information is shared or linked within an EHR without his or her knowledge, the patient's autonomy is breached.

The information and data contained in health records are disembodied aspects of patients, which can become objectified and medicalized. People are more than data points, yet patient information in EHRs is often reduced to data with and without patients' knowledge, and usually in a form or format that is not accessible to the average patient. For example, patient narratives are rarely incorporated into the patient record. Instead, the record includes structured notes that can be quantified because evidence-based medicine prefers quantitative data over qualitative data. The EHR reflects the work that was done, lab values, and what was billed. However, many physicians lament EHR systems that tell them little about what is going on with the patient as a whole person. Additionally, the quality of notes is under scrutiny; a recent study showed that an EHR's progress notes are about 50 percent copy-pasted material and possibly containing inaccurate representations of the patient's condition or the care they received (Wang et al. 2017).

In this field, we sometimes use data (and, therefore, personal information) for some purpose other than the care of the patient to whom the data refer. This may be justifiable in terms of utilitarianism and serving the greater good but problematic in a deontological sense because people should never be used as a means towards some other end—all people are supposed to be ends in themselves. This means that people should always be treated with inherent dignity, rather than as instruments to achieve someone else's goals. This respects autonomy and ensures their rights and interests are not disregarded or exploited. For example, deidentification dehumanizes patient data such that it can be used for many purposes, values, and forces other than the needs of the individual patient contributing the data (Swirsky 2017). We see this means and ends problem exemplified in cases of upcoding, as explained earlier in this chapter. In a deontological analysis, people cannot be used as a means to some end, so the ethical acceptability depends upon what the end is. The end for the patient is still clinical care and personal well-being, but in the US healthcare system there are other considerations, such as population health, profitability, and resource management. These ends get confused and convoluted, and sometimes there are trade-offs.

Clearly, if EHRs are implemented for the purpose of billing and increased profitability for the provider, then there is a problem of a system that does not reflect a patient's humanity and treats them as a means toward some end. The patient-centric focus is lost, and the EHR is increasingly populated by structured data meant to justify billing at certain rates; the EHR becomes the means of commoditizing the patient-clinician encounter. Moreover, if health information systems are not designed with diversity in mind, they may inadvertently perpetuate biases present in the data, leading to inaccurate representations of certain demographic groups. This starts with the very architecture of EHR systems, which is influenced by a wide variety of clinical, financial, business, and information technology concerns. EHRs place cognitive constraints upon clinicians that impact coverage, sequencing, categorization of care; clinical decision-making; and satisfaction with these systems among providers (Scott and Purves 1996, 355). These issues of useability create persistent issues associated with poor patient outcomes, higher rates of readmission, and provider burnout (Kutney-Lee et al. 2021).

Clinicians may observe a dissociation among the architecture of these systems and clinical workflows, note content standards, and usability considerations caused by the need for structured data and financial concerns. The history of the development of HIT supports this claim, as early decision support systems were largely ignored in favor of financial and administrative systems (Singer et al. 2006, 818). This is a chronic problem. There is a fundamental rift between legislators' expectations of EHRs and the experience of providers in terms of an EHR's ability to support coordinated care, in part because system design is disproportionately influenced by billing and documentation needs at the expense of patient and provider needs that aim at improved outcomes (O'Malley et al. 2009, 183).

Financing has been among the most influential factors when it comes to implementation and use of HIT. Implementation rates were low until Congress enacted Meaningful Use, which threatened Medicare reimbursements; the needs of payers and healthcare providers to justify billing at the highest rates is a primary factor. While financing features prominently in implementation decisions, it is not necessarily for the purpose of making care more affordable; implementations took a sharp upturn only after the Meaningful Use incentive program started. As of September 2009, approximately only 8 percent of US hospitals had implemented a basic EHR system, and by 2014 adoption rates rose to over 40 percent for basic systems and 34 percent for comprehensive systems (Jiang et al. 2023). Healthcare providers needed the financial incentive to implement EHRs because they are expensive and do not immediately lead to return on investment. As a result, leadership may prioritize organizational needs and dynamics ahead of clinical functionality and an evidence base for efficacy (Koppel 2013, 1).

Claims have been made purporting the benefits of EHR implementation, but many remain aspirational. Research suggests that many areas of IT application are understudied and that the majority of studies result in mixed or insignificant findings with regard to patient outcomes (Brenner et al. 2016). According to some researchers, the proposition that EHRs will reduce the cost of healthcare is a fallacy (Soumerai and Koppel 2012). It can be argued that EHRs increase costs because they ease a clinician's ability to upcode Medicare patient billings (Schulte 2014).

They can also make it easier to scour the record for charge capture and reduce billing errors, which in the past generally favored patients.

There has been significant public and private investment in EHRs, which has led to bias, particularly by the federal government and major corporate stakeholders seeking return on investment. The triple aim of healthcare—efficiency, cost-effectiveness, and improved outcomes—is firmly grounded in business values than clinical values. In some sense, healthcare is a business term that creates an adversarial relationship between providers and patients (Sawyer 2018). Business values such as efficiency, quality, and cost savings tend to reap business rewards, and business values control many HIT architecture and implementation decisions. For example, cost-effectiveness has led to increased revenues and executive compensation; the cost of care per procedure continues to rise because cost savings relate to profit and not cost to consumer. Healthcare is a business, and the implementation of information technology serves as a vanguard of commoditization of the patient-provider encounter. Like social media companies discussed below, healthcare institutions routinely commoditize patient data through the practice of data-blocking to improve revenue (Adler-Milstein and Pfeifer 2017, 133). Data-blocking, the deliberate and unreasonable interference with the exchange of electronic health information, is ethically unacceptable, is inconsistent with legislation intended to promote the rapid adoption of interoperable HITs and frustrates efforts to improve care and efficiency in the US healthcare system (ONC 2015). Beginning September 1, 2023, information blocking provisions of the 21st Century Cures Act went into effect establishing penalties up to $1 million per violation and carving out exceptions for certain nondisclosures such as preventing harm to patients, protecting an individual's privacy, or safeguarding security of electronic health information (OIG 2023).

## Ethical Issues Related to End-of-Life Care

Patients have the right to accept or refuse lifesaving medical treatment; one of the primary tenets of patient-centered care is incorporating the desires of patients and their families for end-of-life care and resuscitation needs into care plans. Since 1990, this "right to self-determination" has been legally codified in the Federal Patient Self-Determination Act, and healthcare organizations across the United States have been challenged with identifying effective means of supporting this expression of patient autonomy. Many different approaches have been attempted to combat this potential misplacement of important information, from taping documents to one's refrigerator, to tattooing wishes on one's chest, to the creation of mobile apps allowing for access virtually anywhere. Various documents are available that differ by jurisdiction, such as powers of attorney, also known as healthcare proxies; living wills; and the newer POLST form, which presents a different paradigm of end-of-life decision-making.

As mentioned previously, the nonexistence of or inability to locate advance directives has led to lifesaving actions that were taken unknowingly against patients' wishes and contribute to medical waste. It is estimated that 25 percent of Medicare expenses are incurred during the last twelve months of life, and advance directives present an opportunity to lower out-of-pocket expenses and improve care (Zhu and Enguidanos 2022). Momentum has gathered in getting patients to complete these documents; however, research suggests that they are present in EHRs 4 to 13 percent of the time, and when present can be difficult to access or interpret (Pyles et al. 2022). EHRs contribute to these problems due to a lack of standardization, making documentation difficult to locate, leading to invalid documentation, and misidentification of documentation by user error (Caurdy-Bess et al. 2021). Even if hospitals and other organizations work to fill in dangerous gaps in their EHR systems, lack of interoperability means that patients who move from system to system frequently do not have their documents follow them unless they or their loved ones hand carry them. At the same time, this is an important and emerging area of research that provides evidence of how certain "EHR interventions, such as documentation templates, order sets, and prompts, may improve the incidence and quality of advance care planning" (Huber et al. 2018, 538). As a matter of patient safety and quality improvement, HIM professionals should address this matter at their home institutions.

## Ethical Issues Related to Disparities and Literacy

Many factors influence health and healthcare, including health status, disease risk factors, access to healthcare, and culture. The World Health Organization (WHO) defines the social determinants of health as "the conditions in which people are born, grow, work, live, and age, and the wider set of forces and systems shaping the conditions of daily life" (WHO 2019). These same social determinants are largely responsible for health disparities that exist disproportionately across populations. For example, people who live in low-income neighborhoods have less access to quality healthcare than people who live in high-income neighborhoods. Data show that residents of underrepresented communities have lower socioeconomic status, greater barriers to healthcare access, and greater risks for disease compared with the general population (Meyer et al. 2013). As described in a report commissioned by the Institute of Medicine, addressing these disparities requires that providers deal with patient health literacy:

> The U.S. health care system, with its myriad public and private programs, institutions, services, products, and information, poses a significant challenge to those seeking access to affordable, quality healthcare. Understanding the complexities of insurance eligibility, therapeutic guidance, medical technology, prescription medication, disease management, prevention, and lifestyle modification are difficult for any consumer, let alone one with compromised levels of literacy or numeracy. An individual seeking to participate successfully in the health system requires a constellation of skills—reading, writing, basic mathematical calculations, speaking, listening, networking, and rhetoric—the totality of which defines health literacy. (Somers and Mahadevan 2010, 5)

Health literacy presents a complex problem for healthcare. Low literacy is prevalent among those with low education levels, the elderly, underrepresented racial and ethnic groups, and those living with chronic diseases. The literature describes myriad health consequences of limited literacy. It is a risk factor for worsened health status, hospitalization, mortality, increased incidence of chronic illness, and decreased use of preventative services. The shift toward shared decision-making and patient autonomy has served to exacerbate the complexity of a healthcare system not well suited for those with low literacy. Many people who suffer from literacy barriers would not be so limited if the system was simplified, and the addition of technology can exacerbate and create disparities. Ethical concerns related to health literacy are manifold and can be identified through the ethical lens of principlism:

- Autonomy: Low health literacy impairs a patient's abilities for self-determination because lack of knowledge limits a person's ability to make decisions or act on information needed for self-care.
- Beneficence: A clinician's duty to do good and maximize health includes patient education, which can be stymied by gaps in communication. These gaps can leave providers with inadequate knowledge of patient needs and result in patients who lack skills for self-efficacy needed for optimal health outcomes.
- Nonmaleficence: The invocation to do no harm includes harms related to the use, misuse, and nonuse of information. Low health literacy can have a negative influence on health outcomes due to problems such as misunderstanding treatment instructions, poor adherence, loss of access to care, limited use of preventative measures, and unwarranted apprehension of care that leads to higher rates of mortality.
- Justice: Considerations for social justice and the equitable distribution of resources require that providers use reasonable and nonarbitrary bases in the allocation of healthcare resources. Discrimination, stigmatization, and unequal access can result from limited health literacy, which increases the health disparities between the advantaged and disadvantaged. (Sorensen et al. 2013, 75)

The US Department of Health and Human Services Office of Minority Health (OMH) established national standards for culturally and linguistically appropriate services (CLAS) in health and healthcare with the intention to advance health quality, improve the quality of the healthcare provided, and help eliminate healthcare disparities in the US. The principal standard is to provide effective, equitable, understandable, and respectful quality care while being responsive to diverse cultural beliefs and practices, preferred languages, health literacy, and other communication needs (OMH 2015). When providers deliver services in this way, patients feel they are respected and understood, and they can understand the medical care direction their provider is asking them to take. As byproducts of the patient-provider relationship, the complex barriers to health literacy should be addressed through the systems and dynamic relationships that affect health institutions, clinical encounters, and communication in general.

## Ethical Issues Related to Social Media Use

The use of novel communication technologies creates a variety of professional ethical issues for patients and those working in clinical environments. It is estimated that from 2000 to 2023 the percentage of American adult internet users rose from 52 percent to 95 percent (Pew 2024). Healthcare-related information searches are a common activity among users, and healthcare information seeking among older adults has increased significantly over the past decade (CDC 2023). Since social media plays an important role in patient education and public health due to its ability to facilitate expedited information sharing and accessibility of unrestricted information to a wide audience, patient education on locating, evaluating, and using online health information can be beneficial to users (CDC 2023). As such, social media has opened many new channels for patient-provider communication and community engagement; however, despite the actual and potential values of these technologies, ethical issues thrive in the gap between the intentions and actions of patients, providers, and industry and governmental agencies in the use and surveillance of health data, including the following:

- Confidentiality and privacy: There are conflicts in the ownership interests in the data between patients and for-profit social media companies.
- Accuracy: The lack of authentication for some social media data raises issues related to accuracy, veracity, and reliability of information.
- Scientific merit: The validity of information posted to social media sites may not reflect peer-reviewed scientific research.
- Professionalism: There can be a disconnect between personal use and fidelity to professional values, which can have a negative impact upon the community's trust. For example, providers who depict patients or the profession in a negative light on personal social media pages can damage the reputation of the employer or the HIM profession.
- Digital divide: As ubiquitous as internet access is in many communities, large swaths of the global population remain untouched. Like other electronic means of patient engagement, the use of social media as an outlet for information may serve to increase disparities if the information is not presented in a way that is accessible and targeted to meet the needs of the intended audience. (Neuberger and Swirsky 2017, 258)

Similarly, there are clinical, legal, and ethical implications of using mobile technologies in clinical environments, such as text messaging initiatives between providers and patients. These initiatives may serve as a novel way to increase communication, trust, compliance, and fidelity in clinical encounters, particularly with younger patient populations. There are, however, many technical, legal, and ethical issues associated with use of mobile technologies in healthcare. For example, without proper administrative and technology safeguards, this channel of communication can quickly run afoul of security policies, documentation requirements, and basic notions of patient confidentiality and privacy. Furthermore, in today's HIPAA-ruled environment, healthcare providers may face penalties or costly corrective actions for data breaches. There are real and potential benefits to using this technology. However, we cannot ignore the burdens to patients and risks to healthcare providers. Since 2009, the Office of Civil Rights' breach portal research report indicates that approximately 500 million individuals have been affected by information breaches; approximately 11 percent of those breaches were related to use of laptops, email, and other portable devices (OCR 2023). Excessive use of social media by providers while on duty also raises concerns for patient care and health outcomes (Black et al. 2013). Although patients and healthcare providers have been empowered by access, the application of mobile technologies to clinical encounters must be guided by sound policy development and standards of professionalism.

## Ethical Issues Related to Artificial Intelligence

There are many benefits to the use of technologies powered by artificial intelligence (AI); however, deployment of AI in healthcare has resulted in some crosscutting ethical issues with the propensity to worsen some of the dilemmas described above. AI, defined as the high-level information technologies used in developing machines that imitate human qualities such as learning and reasoning, creates challenges related to bias due to a lack of clear standards of fairness in automation. Technology creates new decisions across the continuum of healthcare and serves a variety of values that can be difficult to reconcile, and standards of fairness that extend from the patient to the payor serve competing interests. For example, insurance giant Cigna developed the *PxDx* ("procedure-to-diagnosis") system to automate claims review in large batches. Federal lawsuits allege that Cigna used this system to deny more than 300,000 claims in approximately 1.2 seconds, calling fairness into question (*Kisting-Leung vs. Cigna Group*, Case 2:23-at-00698 (E. Dist. Cal.); *Van Pelt v. The Cigna Group*, Case No. 3:23-cv-01135 (Dist. Conn)).

There are also large gaps in data due to underrepresentation of racial and ethnic populations. Thus, AI models are regularly trained with poor quality datasets representing predominantly non-Hispanic White patients. If health information systems are not designed with DEI in mind, they may inadvertently perpetuate biases present in the data, leading to inaccurate representations, disparities in healthcare delivery, and health outcomes for certain demographic groups (Boyd et al. 2023). To address these and other concerns related to algorithmic discrimination, The White House issued a Blueprint for an AI Bill of rights in 2022 that called for safe and effective systems, algorithmic discrimination protections, enhanced data privacy, accessible notices of system use and explanations of system outcomes, and appropriate opt-outs and human alternatives (The White House 2022).

The complexity of AI systems also creates problems related to understandability and explainability. This is sometimes referred to as "black box technology" because users can produce results but not how the system works. Black box medicine refers to "the use of opaque computational models to make decisions related to health care," which are difficult to understand and explain (Price 2015). Use of black box systems and computational models frustrates transparency, reproducibility, and validation; hinders accountability due to difficulties in attributing error; exacerbates biases present in training data; and challenges the exercise of autonomy through informed consent as providers and patients may not fully understand or trust the application. Moreover, the inherent qualities of black box systems allow them to be deliberately trained to mask training data and allow plausible deniability of intentional bias or unethical business practices (Moreau et al. 2020; Rass et al. 2022).

### Check Your Understanding 27.3

Answer the following questions in a separate document.

1. Describe some ways that diversity, equity, and inclusion can be incorporated into HIM organizational policies and procedures?
2. What judgment would you make about a provider who generally enters procedural codes that represent higher payment rates?
3. Is it justifiable for a healthcare institution to prohibit social media use by employees during work hours? What are the possible consequences?
4. How do HITs impact health literacy?
5. Appraise HIM professional responsibilities and duties related to DEI in the context of patient data, work environments, and the HIM profession.
6. Create a 10-minute presentation that compares and contrasts three fundamental ethical principles or theories that justify the use of AI in healthcare.

# References

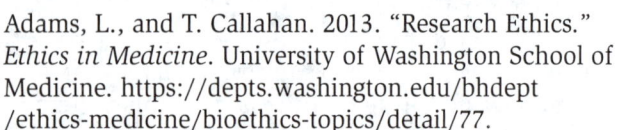

Adams, L., and T. Callahan. 2013. "Research Ethics." *Ethics in Medicine*. University of Washington School of Medicine. https://depts.washington.edu/bhdept/ethics-medicine/bioethics-topics/detail/77.

Adler-Milstein, J., and E. Pfeifer. 2017. Information blocking: Is it occurring and what policy strategies can address it? *The Milbank Quarterly* 95(1):117–135.

AHIMA (American Health Information Management Association). 2019a. *AHIMA Code of Ethics*. https://bok.ahima.org/doc?oid = 105098.

AHIMA (American Health Information Management Association). 2019b. Policy and Procedures for Disciplinary Review and Appeal. https://www.ahima.org/media/4sylhr31/ahima_-disciplinary-review-and-appeals_rev1-9-19.pdf.

Aristotle, A., and T. Irwin. 1999. *Nicomachean Ethics*, 2nd ed. Indianapolis: Hackett Pub. Co.

Beauchamp, T. L. and J. F. Childress. 2013. *Principles of Biomedical Ethics*, 7th ed. New York: Oxford.

Billings M. E., M. E. Lazarus, M. Wenrich, J. R. Curtis, and R. A. Engelberg. 2011. The effect of the hidden curriculum on resident burnout and cynicism. *Journal of Graduate Medical Education* 3(4):503–510.

Black, E., J. Light, N. P. Black, and L. Thompson. 2013. Online social media use by health care providers in a high traffic patient care environment. *Journal of Medical Internet Research* 15(5):e94.

Boyd, A. D., R. Gonzalez-Guarda, K. Lawrence, C. L. Patil, M. O. Ezenwa, E. C. O'Brien, H. Paek, J. M. Braciszewski, O. Adeyemi, A. M. Cuthel, et al. 2023. Equity and bias in electronic health records data. *Contemporary Clinical Trials* 130:107238–107238.

Brenner, S. K., R. Kaushal, Z. Grinspan, C. Joyce, I. Kim, R. J. Allard, D. Delgado, and E. L. Abramson.

2016. Effects of health information technology on patient outcomes: A systematic review. *Journal of the American Medical Informatics Association* 23(5):1016–1036.

Caurdy-Bess, L., S. Damiano, A. Fresch, M. Begle, S. Yedavally-Yellayi, H. A. Eraqi, and A. H. Mahmood. 2021. When we know better, we do better: Maintaining and retrieving advance directive documents in the electronic health record. *Collaborative Case Management* 80:5–11.

CDC (Centers for Disease Control and Prevention). 2023. "Use of Online Health Information." https://www.cdc.gov/healthliteracy/developmaterials/audiences/olderadults/online.html.

CMS (Centers for Medicare and Medicaid Services). 2021. "National Health Expenditure Fact Sheet." https://www.cms.gov/data-research/statistics-trends-and-reports/national-health-expenditure-data/nhe-fact-sheet.

Coleman, E., W. Bockting, M. Botzer, P. Cohen-Kettenis, G. DeCuypere, J. Feldman, L. Fraser, J. Green, G. Knudson, W. J. Meyer, et al. 2012. Standards of care for the health of transsexual, transgender, and gender-nonconforming people. *International Journal of Transgenderism* 13(4):165–232.

Dean, R. G. 2001. The myth of cross cultural competence. *Families and Society: The Journal of Contemporary Social Services* 82(6):623–630.

Deutsch M. B., J. Green, J. Keatley, G. Mayer, J. Hastings, A. M. Hall, R. Allison, O. Blumer, S. Brown, M. K. Cody, et al. 2013. Electronic medical records and the transgender patient: Recommendations from the world professional association for transgender health EMR working group. *Journal of the Medical Informatics Association* 20:700–703.

Doherty, R. F. 2021. *Ethical Dimensions in the Health Professions*, 7th ed. St. Louis, MO: Elsevier.

Glover, J. J. 2017. "Ethical Decision-Making Guidelines and Tools." Chapter 2 in *Ethical Health Informatics: Challenges and Opportunities*, 3rd ed. Edited by L. B. Harmon and F. H. Cornelius. Burlington, MA: Jones and Bartlett.

Harman, L. B., V. L. Mullen, and F. H. Cornelius. 2017. "Professional Values and the Code of Ethics." Chapter 1 in *Ethical Health Informatics: Challenges and Opportunities*, 3rd ed. Edited by L. B. Harman and F. H. Cornelius. Burlington, MA: Jones and Bartlett.

Huber, M. T., J. D. Highland, V. R. Krishnamoorthi, and J. W. Tang. 2018. Utilizing the electronic health record to improve advance care planning: A systematic review. *American Journal of Hospice and Palliative Medicine* 35(3):532–541.

Huffman, E. K. 1972. *Manual for Medical Record Librarians*, 6th ed. Chicago: Physician's Record Company.

IOM (Institute of Medicine). 2011. *The Health of Lesbian, Gay, Bisexual, and Transgender People: Building a Foundation for Better Understanding*. Washington, DC: National Academies Press. https://www.nap.edu/catalog/13128/the-health-of-lesbian-gay-bisexual-and-transgender-people-building.

Jiang J. X., K. Qi, G. Bai, and K. Schulman. 2023. Pre-pandemic assessment: A decade of progress in electronic health record adoption among U.S. hospitals. *Health Affairs Scholar* 1(5):qxad056. https://doi:10.1093/haschl/qxad056.

Joint Commission. 2015. *Root Cause Analysis in Health Care: Tools and Techniques*, 5th ed. Oak Brook, IL: Joint Commission Resources. https://www.jcrinc.com/assets/1/14/EBRCA15Sample.pdf.

Kant, I., and M. J. Gregor. 1998. *Groundwork of the Metaphysics of Morals*. Cambridge, UK: Cambridge University Press.

Koppel, R. 2013. Is healthcare information technology based on evidence? *Yearbook of Medical Informatics* 8:7–12.

*Kisting-Leung vs. Cigna Group*, Case 2:23-at-00698 (E. Dist. Cal.).

Kutney-Lee, A., M. Brooks Carthon, D. M. Sloane, K. H. Bowles, M. D. McHugh, and L. H. Aiken. 2021. Electronic health record usability: Associations with nurse and patient outcomes in hospitals. *Medical Care* 59(7):625–631.

Meyer, P., P. Yoon, and R. Kaufmann. 2013. Introduction: CDC Health Disparities and Inequalities Report. http://www.cdc.gov/mmwr/preview/mmwrhtml/su6203a2.htm?s_cid=su6203a2_w.

Mill, J. S. 2007. *Utilitarianism*. New York: Dover Publications.

Moreau J. T., S. Baillet, and R.W. Dudley. 2020. Biased intelligence: On the subjectivity of digital objectivity. *BMJ Health & Care Informatics* 27(3):e100146.

Murray, J. S. 2010. Moral courage in healthcare: Acting ethically even in the presence of risk. *The Online Journal of Issues in Nursing* 15(3):Manuscript 2. http://ojin.nursingworld.org/MainMenuCategories/EthicsStandards/Resources/Courage-and-Distress/Moral-Courage-and-Risk.html.

Neuberger, B. J., and E. S. Swirsky. 2017. "Public Health and Informatics." Chapter 9 in *Ethical Health Informatics: Challenges and Opportunities*, 3rd ed. Burlington, MA: Jones and Bartlett.

OCR (Office for Civil Rights). 2023. Breach Portal: Notice to the Secretary of HHS Breach of Unsecured Protected Health Information. Research Report. https://ocrportal.hhs.gov/ocr/breach/breach_report.jsf.

OHRP (Office for Human Research Protections). 1993. "IRB Guidebook." https://www.hhs.gov/ohrp/education-and-outreach/archived-materials/index.html.

OMH (Office of Minority Health). 2015. "What Are the National CLAS Standards?" https://thinkculturalhealth.hhs.gov/assets/pdfs/EnhancedNationalCLASStandards.pdf.

OIG (Office of Inspector General). 2023. Grants, Contracts, and Other Agreements: Fraud and Abuse; Information Blocking; Office of Inspector General's Civil Money Penalty Rules. *Federal Register* 88(126):42820–42841.

ONC (Office of the National Coordinator for Health Information Technology). 2015. Report to Congress – Report on Health Information Blocking. https://www.healthit.gov/sites/default/files/reports/info_blocking_040915.pdf.

O'Malley, A. S., J. M. Grossman, G. R. Cohen, N. M. Kemper, and H. H. Pham. 2009. Are electronic medical records helpful for care coordination? Experiences of physician practices. *Journal of General Internal Medicine* 25(3):177–85.

Pearlman, R. 2013. Ethics Committees, Programs and Consultation. Ethics in Medicine, University of Washington School of Medicine. https://depts.washington.edu/bhdept/ethics-medicine/bioethics-topics/detail/64.

Pew Research Center (Pew). 2024 (January 31). "Internet Broadband Fact Sheet." https://www.pewresearch.org/internet/fact-sheet/internet-broadband/.

Price, W. 2015. Black-box medicine. *Harvard Journal of Law & Technology* 28(2):419–468.

Prince, A. E., R. J. Cadigan, W. Whipple, and A. M. Davis. 2017. Membership recruitment and training in health care ethics committees: Results from a national pilot survey. *AJOB Empirical Bioethics* 8(3):161–169.

Pyles, O., C. M. Hritz, P. Gulker, J. D. Straveler, C. R. Grudzen, C. Briggs, and L. T. Southerland. 2022. Locating advance care planning documents in the electronic health record during emergency care. *Journal Of Pain and Symptom Management* 63(5):e489–e494.

Rass, S., S. König, J. Wachter, M. Egger, and M. Hobisch. 2022. Supervised machine learning with plausible deniability. *Computers and Security* 112:102506.

Reiser, S. 1978. *Medicine and the Reign of Technology.* Cambridge: Cambridge University Press.

Rinehart-Thompson, L. A., and L. B. Harman. 2017. "Privacy and Confidentiality." Chapter 3 in *Ethical Health Informatics: Challenges and Opportunities*, 3rd ed. Burlington, MA: Jones and Bartlett.

Sawyer, N. T. 2018. In the U.S. healthcare is now strictly a business term. *The Western Journal of Emergency Medicine* 19(3):494–495.

Schulte, F. 2014. "Electronic Medical Records Probed for Over-Billing." The Center for Public Integrity. https://www.publicintegrity.org/2013/02/14/12208/electronic-medical-records-probed-over-billing.

Scott, D., and I. N. Purves. 1996. Triadic relationship between doctor, computer and patient. *Interacting with Computers* 8(4):347–363.

Siegler, M. 1982. Confidentiality in medicine—A decrepit concept. *The New England Journal of Medicine* 307(24):1518–1521.

Simmers, L., K. Simmers-Nartker, and S. Simmers-Kobelak. 2014. *Simmers DHO Health Science*, 8th ed. Stamford, CT: Cengage Learning.

Singer, S., A. Enthoven, and A. Garber. 2006. "Health Care Financing and Information Technology: A Historical Perspective." Chapter 23 in *Biomedical Informatics: Computer Applications in Health Care and Biomedicine*, 3rd ed. Edited by E. H. Shortliffe and J. J. Cimino. New York: Springer.

Somers, S. A. and R. Mahadevan. 2010. "Health Literacy Implications of the Affordable Care Act." Hamilton, NJ: Center for Health Care Strategies, Inc. https://www.chcs.org/media/Health_Literacy_Implications_of_the_Affordable_Care_Act.pdf.

Sorensen, K., B. Schuh, G. Stapleton, and P. Schroder-Back. 2013. Exploring the ethical scope of health literacy—A critical literature review. *Albanian Medical Journal* 2:71–83.

Soumerai, S., and R. Koppel. 2012. (September 17). A major glitch for digitized health-care records. *The Wall Street Journal*. https://www.wsj.com/articles/SB10000872396390443847404577627041964831020.

SHADAC (State Health Access Data Assistance Center). 2024 (March 11). Sexual orientation and gender identity data: New and updated information on federal guidance and Medicaid data collection practices. https://www.shadac.org/sogi-data-collection-medicaid-SHVS-updated-brief.

Swirsky, E. S. 2017. A billion tiny ends: Social media, nonexceptionalism, and ethics by association. *The American Journal of Bioethics* 17(3):15–17.

Swirsky, E. S., A. D. Boyd, C. Gu, L.A. Burke, A. Z. Doorenbos, M. O. Ezenwa, M. R. Knisely, J. W. Leigh, H. Li, M. W. Mandernach, et al. 2023. Monitoring and responding to signals of suicidal ideation in pragmatic clinical trials: Lessons from the GRACE trial for Chronic Sickle Cell Disease Pain. *Contemporary Clinical Trials Communications* 36:101218.

The White House. 2022. "Blueprint for an AI Bill of Rights: Making Automated Systems Work for the American People." https://www.whitehouse.gov/ostp/ai-bill-of-rights/.

*Van Pelt v. The Cigna Group*, Case No. 3:23-cv-01135 (Dist. Conn).

Wang M. D., R. Khanna, and N. Najafi. 2017. Characterizing the source of text in electronic health record progress notes. *JAMA Internal Medicine* 177(8):1212–1213.

WHO (World Health Organization). 2019. "Social Determinants of Health." https://www.who.int/social_determinants/sdh_definition/en/.

Zhu, Y., and S. Enguidanos. 2022. Advance directives completion and hospital out-of-pocket expenditures. *Journal of Hospital Medicine* 17(6):437–444.

# Odd-Numbered Answer Key

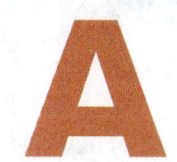

APPENDIX A

 **Check Your Understanding 1.1**

1. Late 1700s—First hospital was developed to care for the sick; 1760—First licenses to practice medicine were issued; 1847—the AMA was established to represent physicians; 1876—the AAMC was established to standardize medical school curriculum and encourage licensing physicians; 1910—review of medical curricula reported poor quality of medical training prompting reforms; 1913—The American College of Surgeons was formed to assist with hospital reform; 1917—Adoption of Minimum Standards for hospital care marking the beginning of the modern accreditation process sponsored by the ACS; mid-1900s—Modern diagnostic and therapeutic technology prompted the growth of allied health professionals; 1952—The Joint Commission on Accreditation of Hospitals was formed and took over for the ACS in performing accreditation surveys. ASAHP formed in 1967, and HPAC in 2014, with both encouraging IPE. Each of the major milestones incrementally increased standardization, education, and oversight for the provision of medical care. Professional licensure and facility accreditation are expected in current practice.

3. To be a pediatrician, one must have a bachelor's degree, complete medical school, pass a licensure exam administered by the state medical board, complete the required residency, complete further residency for any pediatric specialty, and pass the board certification exam.

5. Professionals from two or more disciplines must learn *from*, *with*, and *about* each other. Healthcare is delivered by a team of specialized professionals which must communicate and perform effectively to optimize outcomes for patients.

 **Check Your Understanding 1.2**

1. b
3. a
5. c
7. e

9. There is an obvious trend in legislation to try to control healthcare costs, particularly in Medicare and Medicaid programs. Many efforts are made, yet it seems that costs continue to rise. Another recent trend in healthcare legislation is a focus on increasing quality and access to care. This is a positive trend, yet its level of success is unclear.

11. Research using messenger ribonucleic acid (mRNA) beginning in the 1960s led to significant advances in vaccine technology in the 21st century during the global COVID-19 pandemic, laying the foundation for the quick development of mRNA-based COVID vaccines.

## Check Your Understanding 1.3

1. c. The patient's diagnosis and treatment required hospitalization with 24-hour nursing care, and then quickly resolved.

3. a. VA hospitals are owned by the government and serve retired military personnel and their families.

5. b. The speech-language pathologist's scope of practice uniquely includes assisting patients with speech, language, and swallowing/feeding impairments associated with a variety of etiologies including traumatic brain injury.

7. b. The chief executive officer is responsible for working with the board and senior leaders to develop the strategic plan for an organization.

## Check Your Understanding 1.4

1. Since it is a weekend and many primary physician offices are closed, the most appropriate settings for a nonemergent health concern such as a sore throat and fever are an urgent care center (one that is part of the individual's healthcare system or is freestanding) or a local retail clinic that does not require appointments.

3. The most appropriate care setting would be an ambulatory surgical center where an anesthesiologist is on staff to provide general anesthesia but does not provide 24-hour care and is less expensive than the services of a hospital.

5. Since there is no one available to drive the person to therapy, home healthcare services is a good option. The PT will come to the house and provide therapy services, so transportation is not an issue.

## Check Your Understanding 1.5

1. Hospice care would be the best option as services are offered in the patient's home and include both medical support for the patient and spiritual and social support for the patient and family.

3. An IDS combines financial and clinical aspects of healthcare within a group of healthcare providers to furnish comprehensive care across the entire continuum. This includes primary, secondary, and tertiary care, long-term care, and hospice.

## Check Your Understanding 1.6

1. The difference is that licensure is required, and accreditation is voluntary. Licensure requirements must be met to operate. Normally, licensure is awarded for one year where accreditation may be awarded for multiple years. Accreditation standards are set above the minimum required for operation and define high-quality patient care.

3. The Healthcare Quality Improvement Act created legislation to moderate the incidence of malpractice and improve the accuracy of malpractice information. It also indicated a readiness to weed out medical incompetence and required hospitals to request malpractice information when hiring, reviewing, or offering medical practice privileges to healthcare providers.

5. Organizations may be surveyed by Medicare, or they may be surveyed by an accreditation agency such as the Joint Commission or AOA, with "deemed status" ensuring the organizations meets federal government requirements of CoPs and CfCs.

### Check Your Understanding 1.7

1. Because the HSA is intended to be a savings account for healthcare costs in the future, young and healthy individuals would benefit most since they could build up their savings over time due to low utilization. Those nearing retirement now also benefit, as it is a way to save money for future healthcare costs. Both groups would receive the benefit of paying less in taxes.

3. Artificial intelligence is commonly used to automate decisions previously made by humans whereas augmented intelligence enhances human intelligence and underscores the continued human involvement.

### Check Your Understanding 2.1

1. The students' answer should be in their own words, but it should address the purpose of the term and cover the primary functions. The two definitions should be different from each other.

3. Any five of the ten IG competencies can be selected; the student's rationale should include solid knowledge of each competency listed. The strongest replies will substantiate their selection.

5. The GARP principle used is accountability. It requires that an IG program is overseen by a senior executive.

### Check Your Understanding 2.2

1. c. The data life cycle management domains include the DG function of setting standards for data retention and storage.

3. The student may describe data breaches due to unauthorized access, accidental or intentional modification, destruction, or use. Steps the office can take to minimize risk are to develop and implement policies and procedures addressing the use of data by patients, providers, employees and contractors; require and deliver employee security awareness training; monitor audit trails to identify potential and actual security violations; and develop a risk management program including a business continuity plan.

5. To ensure AI is used effectively and responsibly, it is important to have a strong DG framework. This includes having a clear understanding of the data being used to train AI models, ensuring the data is of high quality and free from bias, and having processes in place to monitor and manage AI workflows.

### Check Your Understanding 2.3

1. a. The business case should identify the purpose and value of the program and the benefits and value for the organization implementation of the DG program can obtain by anticipating a positive change from the current status. None of the other distractors provide a specific result that can be measured vis-à-vis the value in monetary or quality terms to the organization.

3. In developing a governance program, identifying the purpose of the program helps to identify the benefits and value for the organization that implementation of the DG program can obtain. The business case is sometimes called the value proposal because it clearly articulates why the effort should be made showing the benefits and the risks.

5. Once the mission and scope of the program are established, resources need to be identified and organized. This includes funding and human resources. Identifying what roles are needed and ensuring individuals are in those roles and appropriately organized is important too, as is securing funding to move forward.

### Check Your Understanding 2.4

1. b. A DG framework assists an organization in determining what constitutes the DG mission and scope, DG responsibilities, authority, organizational structure, and governance processes.
3. b. A stakeholder analysis assesses stakeholder needs. It identifies and analyzes the attitudes or opinions of stakeholders.
5. Assignment of decision rights consists of appointing authority to specific individuals or categories of individuals to make data-related decisions and designating when and how those decisions are made.

### Check Your Understanding 2.5

1. c. Governance is implemented through a formal organizational structure with both authority and responsibility for managing an organization's data assets. The IG council has executive functions; the other distractors are operational in nature and granting authority to HIM professionals or registration personnel, or physicians and nurses for information would be handled at lower levels of the organization.

3. 
- Level 1 (Substandard): Principle is minimally addressed, not addressed, or sporadically addressed. Organization likely does not meet legal, regulatory, or business requirements.
- Level 2 (In Development): Recognition that the principle has an impact on the organization, but practices are ill-defined, incomplete, marginally effective, or insufficiently developed leaving the organization vulnerable to legal or regulatory risks.
- Level 3 (Essential): There are defined policies and procedures and implementation processes that support the principle, but there are additional opportunities for streamlining business processes and controlling costs.
- Level 4 (Proactive): Supports the principle with a focus on continuous improvement with IG issues routinized and integrated into business decisions.
- Level 5 (Transformational): IG is embedded into the organization's infrastructure and business processes such that compliance with the organization's policies and legal and regulatory responsibilities is routine.

5. Stakeholder consultation is important because it ensures communication regarding the unique impact of IG on each department and employee across the enterprise will occur regularly. Students may add that such communication helps staff feel involved and have bought into the IG process.

### Check Your Understanding 3.1

1. The patient health record was initially a brief documentation of the patient's name and illness because there was likely one care provider who took care of the community and held all the records. As more providers became involved, communities grew, and medicine advanced; more details needed to be documented and stored. The development of quality initiatives, rules, regulations, and standards along with a mobile population prompted the need for electronic records. The benefits of EHRs include the ability to treat patients at multiple locations while having all the patient documentation available, simultaneous viewing of patient documentation for providers and staff, and the ability to document remotely. There are many more benefits related to aggregating data, reimbursement, and research. Challenges include privacy and security, data integrity, system downtime, interoperability, provider acceptance and training, and patient education.

3. Patient health record data can be used to determine if a particular clinical service is profitable or not; it can be used to review what types of conditions are most common in the emergency department; it

can assist with looking for trends in patients who are readmitted to the hospital; and it can be used to educate providers on the effectiveness of treatments.

5. The health record facilitates ongoing care and treatment, supports clinical decision-making, captures the provider's documentation to support reimbursement, tracks patient outcomes to improve patient care, supports medical research and acts as a resource for training healthcare students, and serves as legal documents to defend the care they provided and demonstrate compliance with legal and regulatory requirements.

## Check Your Understanding 3.2

1. d
3. j
5. g
7. i
9. The MDS 3.0 is a standardized assessment tool used to measure the health status of residents in SNFs. It encompasses a wide range of health indicators, including physical, psychological, and psychosocial domains. The CAA complements the MDS by focusing on specific areas where residents may require assistance, such as activities of daily living, cognition, mobility, and continence. Together, these assessments provide a holistic view of a resident's health and needs. The MDS is completed every three months or more frequently if the resident's health status changes. Continuous monitoring through the MDS and CAA helps in maintaining up-to-date and accurate clinical records. The detailed and systematic data collected through the MDS and CAA form the basis for developing individualized care plans tailored to meet the specific needs of each resident. The MDS and CAA play a crucial role in fulfilling CMS documentation requirements. The MDS and CAA assessments are foundational to determining the reimbursement rates from Medicare. Reimbursement rates are based on the level of care required by residents, as determined by the MDS and CAA.
11. Certification by the patient's attending physician and the hospice organization that the patient has a terminal illness.

## Check Your Understanding 3.3

1.a. Quantitative: Whether documentation is signed or not is considered a "yes" or "no" question and is, therefore, quantitative in nature.

1.b. Quantitative: Whether documentation was dictated and placed on the chart or not is considered a "yes" or "no" question and is, therefore, quantitative in nature.

1.c. Qualitative: When documentation must be reviewed and compared against a standard to determine whether all elements are present and adequately described, the analysis is considered qualitative in nature.

1.d. Qualitative: When documentation must be reviewed to ensure descriptors, the analysis is considered qualitative in nature.

1.e. Quantitative: Whether all ordered labs have reports or not is considered a "yes" or "no" question and is, therefore, quantitative in nature.

3. Incomplete records can hold up a facility's billing process and affect the timely reimbursement for patient care. Reimbursement is necessary for the viability of the organization. That is, to meet payroll obligations, pay bills, and maintain liquidity for necessary expenses.

5. Qualitative analysis involves a detailed review of the health record to ensure compliance with facility policies, licensing, accrediting bodies, and government requirements. It includes reviewing the completeness, accuracy, and adherence to documentation standards both concurrently (during the patient's stay) and retrospectively (after discharge).

7. Front-end speech recognition allows providers to dictate reports into a microphone and see the text in real time, editing it immediately. In contrast, back-end speech recognition involves storing the dictation as a digital voice file, which is then processed by the software to create a draft document that a transcriptionist reviews and edits.

### Check Your Understanding 3.4

1. The MPI is the key locator for records in a numerical filing system because it contains the patient numbers by which the records are filed. Accurate information in the MPI ensures the correct identification of both the patient and the record.

3. The consequence of a patient having duplicate health record numbers is that providers will not have the correct information for patient care, resulting in duplicate testing and poor-quality healthcare.

5. AHIMA recommends that retention of health information be based on the needs and requirements of the facility, such as legal requirements, continued patient care, research, education, and other legitimate uses. The Joint Commission asserts that the length of health record retention depends on laws, regulations, and the use of health records for care and for other purposes such as research and education.

   State laws, CMS regulations, and other federal regulations, accreditation standards, and facility policies and procedures must also be reviewed when establishing a retention schedule. The HIM professional must adhere to the strictest time limit if the recommended retention period varies among different laws and regulations. In addition to the length of time for maintaining health records, the HIM professional must consider the required length of retention for other documentation such as immunization records, mammography records, x-rays, and radiographs. It is important to realize that the retention periods are different for the records of minors and incompetent patients.

   CMS requires health records to be maintained for at least five years, according to 42 CFR 482.24(b)(1). This requirement includes committee reports, physician certification and recertification reports, radiologist records (printouts, films, scans, and other images), home health agency records, long-term care records, laboratory records, and any other records that document information about claims. OSHA (29 CFR 1910.1020) requires records of employees with occupational exposure to be maintained for the duration of employment plus 30 years. The statutes of limitation (deadline for filing a lawsuit) in various types of legal actions are important considerations in developing a retention schedule.

7. The four primary steps in an effective record retention program are conducting inventory, determining storage format and location, assigning retention periods, and destroying unnecessary records. First, John must find out how many records are being stored and what condition they are in. Depending on whether the warehouses were climate controlled or not, some records might be in a state of decay. Did the hospital keep an inventory list of information such as patient names, patient type, and dates? If so, John must determine which records can be purged based on patient care needs, facility retention policies, state laws, Joint Commission standards, and CMS rules. Records deemed ready for destruction can then be purged, and an estimation of how many records will be retained can be given to the CFO.

9. Key considerations for health record storage include ensuring sufficient, conveniently accessible space; maintaining environmental conditions to prevent damage from flooding, fire, pests, mold, and dust; ensuring physical security safeguards for paper records; and, for electronic records, following HIPAA privacy and security standards with role-based access controls and conducting access audits.

### Check Your Understanding 4.1

1. A clinical classification is typically identified in a standardized format using names or symbols (codes). The intent of using this format is to provide easily accessible data for transmitting and comparing data. A *terminology*, on the other hand, is set of terms representing a system of concepts.

This is often referred to as a *lexicon*, referring to a listing of words and definitions. A vocabulary differs from a clinical classification in that it is a list of preferred terms and is less specific than terminologies. The incorporation of clinical classifications, vocabularies, and terminologies is important because each has a different intent. For example, a clinical classification is intended for use in billing, quality reporting, and public health. Terminologies function to capture data and information within an EHR at the time of documentation. They represent health information ranging from laboratory data, to nursing documentation, to medical devices, and can be used for functions such as clinical decision support and EHR alerts. One cannot be used for all functions within an EHR. However, they must work together to be impactful. One way is through mapping, or bridging, the similarities of each to enhance the functionality of the EHR (such as data capture and use).

3. LOINC

5. Standardized data is necessary for comparing data for outcomes measurement, quality improvement, resource utilization, medical research, reimbursement, and patient safety. Standardization is key to the success of these initiatives and can begin with standardization of terminology within the EHR.

## Check Your Understanding 4.2

*Instructions: Answer the following questions in a separate document.*

1. T40.0X6D. Be sure to use the number "0" and not the letter "O." Also, it is necessary to select a seventh character, in this case "D" for subsequent encounter, for the code to be valid.

3. The purpose of HCPCS and CPT codes is to capture services and supplies in the outpatient setting (ambulatory). CPT is considered Level I of HCPCS. CPT's intent is similar to the intent of ICD-10-PCS, meaning the capture of services provided, versus just diagnostic, and the outpatient setting. CPT codes must correlate to an ICD-10-CM diagnostic code, indicating medical necessity for the service, to be submitted for reimbursement. Some settings where HCPCS and CPT codes are used include clinics, emergency departments, outpatient surgery centers, and outpatient services within a hospital setting.

5. This directory serves as a universal product identifier for human drugs. It includes the labeler or vendor, product, and trade package size. It is the approved HIPAA billing and financial transaction code set for reporting drugs and biologicals.

   NDC: 0777 – **3105** – 02

   **3105** would be considered the "Product Code or Second Segment"

   The Second Segment, or the Product Code, would include the specific strength (that is, 20mg), dosage form (that is, capsules), and the drug formulation of the specific manufacture (that is, Prozac).

## Check Your Understanding 4.3

1. Interoperability is the ability to exchange information between computer systems. The use of clinical terminologies in EHRs provide standardized data essential to achieving semantic interoperability. Reference terminologies provide a common source while an interface terminology provides a limited set of words and phrases consistent with a provider's thought process. Semantic interoperability provides a means for clinical documentation to be placed and transmitted in an understandable standard structure. Mapping the two allows interface terminologies to be mapped to reference terminologies, which allows for a common reference point for data collection and comparison.

3. (a) LOINC, (b) CCC, (c) SNOMED-CT. *Not* all-inclusive but most common type of examples.

5. Lab LOINC and Clinical LOINC. Lab LOINC provides distinct laboratory observation, characteristics, and attributes of laboratory tests. Clinical LOINC focuses on vital signs, intake and output, EKG, obstetric ultrasound, cardiac echo, urologic imaging, gastroendoscoptic procedures, and more.

### Check Your Understanding 4.4

1. The importance of data standardization is to support the improvement of care coordination, interoperability for health information exchange, and other important healthcare functions. The use of standardization facilitates electronic data collection at the point of care; retrieval of relevant data, information, knowledge; and the reuse of the data for multiple purposes.

3. Patient data is transferred from the EHR to the AI coding assistance system through system integration. The AI system processes the data and suggests appropriate codes, which are then reviewed and validated by the healthcare provider. This integration enhances the accuracy and efficiency of clinical documentation, ensures standardized coding, and supports better decision-making for patient care.

5.

| Healthcare Informatics Standard | Key Components |
|---|---|
| Health Level Seven (HL7) | Provides a set of international standards for the exchange, integration, sharing, and retrieval of electronic health information. It is used widely for clinical messaging, while HL7 FHIR is a modern standard designed to facilitate web-based healthcare data exchange. |
| Clinical Documentation Architecture (CDA) | A HL7 standard that specifies the structure and semantics of clinical documents for exchange. It ensures that clinical content can be shared and understood by different systems. |
| ASTM E2369 Continuity of Care Record (CCR) | CCR is an ASTM standard that specifies the structure of a patient summary record, facilitating the transfer of health information between providers, systems, and settings. |
| LOINC | Universal standard for identifying medical laboratory observations. It enables the seamless exchange and understanding of lab results across different health systems. |
| ISO/IEC 27000 Series | Set of standards that provides guidelines for information security management systems. It ensures healthcare organizations implement appropriate controls and protect patient data against breaches and cyber threats. |
| SNOMED-CT | Comprehensive clinical terminology that provides codes, terms, synonyms, and definitions for clinical documentation. Helps in precise recording of patient data, facilitating interoperability and analysis. |
| ICD | Used globally for coding a wide range of diseases and health conditions. Critical for standardized diagnosis coding, billing, and epidemiological research. |

### Check Your Understanding 5.1

1. An operative report is a primary data source. A primary data source is created by the healthcare professionals providing the care. The medical record is considered a primary data source. A secondary data source is made up of data taken from a primary data source and put in a different format, such as a registry.

3. Secondary data sources are used in research to help determine the effectiveness of treatment, provide alternative methods, and aid in identification of trends.

5. Secondary data sources are created to put the data from the primary record into a format that is easier to query and manipulate. For example, it is difficult and time-consuming for a cancer registrar to determine the number of patients with each type of cancer by looking at individual records. A database, which is a secondary record, can be queried to provide this information in a report from the secondary data that have been entered, thus accelerating the process.

 **Check Your Understanding 5.2**

1. HIM departments use indices to locate data as requested by internal and external users. The operation index, for example, could be used to locate medical records for patients with a specific operation for a quality assessment study. It could also be used to provide information to external users. For example, resident physicians often must provide data on the types of operations they have performed during their residency to the appropriate board for certification in their specialty.

3. He would use a disease index. The disease index allows users to find medical records of patients with a particular diagnosis. At a minimum, it will include the patient's health record number and diagnosis codes and possibly the attending physician and date of discharge.

5. They would use the physician index. The purpose of the physician index is to locate medical records of patients who have been treated by a particular physician. It must, at a minimum, include the physician's name or a code number assigned and the patient's name or health record number.

 **Check Your Understanding 5.3**

1. Is it facility-based, population-based, or both?
3. What methods of follow-up are used?
5. What education is required for registrars?

The student will use the information to integrate into a comparison table.

| Healthcare Informatics Standard | Cancer | Trauma | Diabetes | Transplant | Immunization |
|---|---|---|---|---|---|
| Facility or Population Based (or both) | Both | Facility | Both | Population | Population |
| Follow-up | Reviewing medical records for treatment in the last year; contacting the patient's physician; contacting the patient, newspaper obituaries, or websites | Follow-up is done by some, but not all, registries; emphasis is on patient's quality of life | Done to ensure appropriate continued care | At intervals throughout the first year and then annually. *Living donor:* Complications of the procedure, length of hospital stays. *Recipient:* Status at time of follow-up, functional status, graft status, treatment | Follow-up reminders that immunizations are due, by postcard, telephone call, |
| Education requirements | On-the-job training, seminars, and/or cancer registry program in a college; AHIMA's online Cancer Registry program | Varies; may use RHITs, RHIAs, RNs, LPNs, EMTs, or other health professionals or workshops and on-the-job training | None specified (not specified) | None specified (not specified) | None specified (not specified) |

7. a, b, and d are correct. Training new staff is not directly related to managing the new trauma case; the other three are related.

## Check Your Understanding 5.4

1. Database design contains three phases: conceptual, logical, and physical. The conceptual design phase consists of designing a database without any physical implementations. In this phase, there is no thought of hardware, software, or any physical entities; instead, it focuses on the thought process of the design and serves as a model. The phase is necessary as it supports the logical design phase. The logical design phase is based on the results conceptual model, and a DBMS has been selected. It takes the data from the conceptual model, normalizes the data, and tests the data for accuracy. The physical database design takes the logical design and adds the DBMS assigned for the enterprise. It designs the physical layout of the system including creating tables, relationships, and constraints, to setting security protocols.

   There are several potential benefits of separating the database design tasks into phases that students might identify. One advantage of having a conceptual phase is that a model can be made before any decision about the management system is defined. Database designers may start the process early and make decisions for the logical and physical phases based on the conceptual one. Another advantage is that the conceptual can be easily understood, which can help database designers effectively communicate with their clients regarding specifications. Separating tasks into the logical and physical design phases is also beneficial because it allows the designer to identify the exact data needs before a specific system is selected. Then, they can select the best DBMS to meet their requirements or make changes before the final implementation.

3. A one-to-one relationship indicates that each patient has only one medical record number, and each medical record number is linked to only one patient.

5. Both PCORnet and OMOP are data models designed to standardize and organize healthcare information for research and analysis. Here's a comparison and contrast between the two based on the information provided:

   PCORnet:
   1. **Focus on Patient-Centric Approach:**
      - **Pro:** PCORnet emphasizes a patient-centric approach, capturing patient-reported outcomes and incorporating patient-generated health data.
      - **Con:** While patient-centricity is a strength, it may potentially limit the focus on other clinical and administrative data elements.
   2. **Data Sources:**
      - **Pro:** PCORnet's Common Data Model (CDM) harmonizes data from diverse sources, including electronic health record (EHR) systems, claims databases, and other healthcare sources.
      - **Con:** The inclusion of various data sources may lead to challenges in standardization and consistency.

   OMOP:
   1. **Observational Research Focus:**
      - **Pro:** OMOP is designed specifically to support observational research, enabling the harmonization of disparate data sources for large-scale studies.
      - **Con:** The focus on observational research might limit its suitability for certain studies requiring a more detailed capture of patient-reported outcomes.
   2. **Data Integration:**
      - **Pro:** OMOP enables data integration from diverse healthcare systems, allowing researchers to conduct analyses that reflect real-world variations in healthcare practices.
      - **Con:** The complexity of integrating data from diverse sources may pose challenges in maintaining data quality and consistency.

Commonalities:
1. **Standardization:**
   - PCORnet and OMOP are designed to standardize healthcare data, facilitating interoperability and data exchange.
2. **Diverse Data Sources:**
   - Both models recognize the importance of harmonizing data from various sources, such as EHR systems and claims databases.
3. **Large-Scale Research:**
   - Both models aim to support large-scale research by providing a consistent format for data representation.

While both PCORnet and OMOP share common goals of standardizing healthcare data for research, they differ in their specific focuses, with PCORnet prioritizing a patient-centric approach and OMOP emphasizing observational research and real-world evidence generation. The choice between them may depend on the research's specific goals and nature.

## Check Your Understanding 5.5

1. HIM professionals use databases like MEDLINE and systems like the Unified Medical Language System (UMLS) to support their roles in quality improvement, medical research, and integrating information systems. MEDLINE provides access to a comprehensive array of medical literature, enabling HIM professionals to stay informed about developments and best practices. UMLS integrates biomedical concepts from various sources, supporting the linking of different EHR systems using standardized vocabularies. This ensures accurate and consistent patient records and improves system interoperability. Together, these tools enhance the quality and effectiveness of healthcare information management.

3. HCUP includes data on inpatients from a variety of payment sources including demographic information, diagnoses and procedures, admission and discharge status, payment sources, total charges, LOS, and facility information. A limitation may be that some of the data are from a sample of states and not all. The student may offer a study using any of the data elements listed here, for example, average total charges by payer or ALOS for patients with total hip replacement

5. The NPDB provides information on malpractice and loss of license. It helps ensure that during the hiring process, organizations can identify applicants who are charged with abuse, fraud, or other misconduct. This helps protect patients by helping ensure clinicians who have committed harmful acts cannot continue to practice.

## Check Your Understanding 5.6

1. Data that should be electronically incorporated into a registry if possible are patient demographic data. This is critical to ensuring data integrity between the facility system and the registry and it is faster and more efficient than manual abstraction of data. There is less possibility for human error when using electronic system.

3. Increased use of automated data entry is a current trend in the collection of secondary data. Developing the electronic patient record will ensure less data must be abstracted from the health record into secondary records. Emphasis by stakeholders on issues such as ownership of secondary data has also increased. This may impact the HIM professional should the registry staff be needed less for manual abstraction into separate registries and databases and more for data analysis and reporting. The HIM professional will need to use skills and knowledge related to primary data with secondary data even more.

5. HIM professionals are often integral staff members within privacy initiatives. These workers can champion privacy, first and foremost, by having an in-depth knowledge of the policies and procedures associated with protecting patient privacy. They can also help oversee yearly training

and documentation of all employees who deal with patient data. Finally, they can promote and help manage a yearly initiative for all staff members to review and update privacy training and policy compliance statements.

### Check Your Understanding 5.7

1. The major difference between AHIMA's data quality model and the CMS Documentation Matters Toolkit is their scope and approach. The CMS Toolkit provides specific guidelines and practical advice for enhancing documentation practices in healthcare settings, tailored to different healthcare roles. In contrast, AHIMA's data quality model offers a broad framework for managing data quality across various contexts, without specific instructions. Despite these differences, they are compatible: the CMS Toolkit's detailed guidelines support the broader data quality principles of AHIMA's model, making them complementary tools for ensuring high-quality healthcare documentation and data management.

3. Some potential answers are: a definition of first name (for example, the first name should be the full patient first name, not a nickname or initial), the data type (for example, text or numeric), the size of the field (for example, 25 characters), or whether it is required. By having a standard way of collecting the patient first name, it is more likely the patient will be identified in the database each time an individual tries to access the record, reducing errors such as creating a duplicate medical record number.

5. 
   - Design a plan: Preplan the development, implementation, and maintenance of the data dictionary.
   - Develop an enterprise data dictionary: Integrate common data elements across the entire institution to ensure consistency.
   - Ensure collaborative involvement: Make sure there is support from all key stakeholders.
   - Develop an approvals process: Ensure a documentation trail for all decisions, updates, and maintenance.
   - Identify and retain details of data versions: Version control is important.
   - Design for flexibility and growth.
   - Design room for expansion of field values.
   - Follow established International Organization for Standards (ISO)/International Electrotechnical Commission (IEC) 11179 guidelines for metadata registry: To promote interoperability, follow standards.
   - Adopt nationally recognized standards.
   - Beware of differing standards for the same concepts.
   - Use geographic codes and conform to the National Spatial Data Infrastructure and the Federal Geographic Data Committee. This committee provides standards on acquiring, accessing, storing and distributing geospatial data.
   - Test the IS: Develop a test plan to ensure the system supports the data dictionary.
   - Provide ongoing education and training.
   - Assess the extent to which the data elements maintain consistency and avoid duplication.

### Check Your Understanding 6.1

1. Medicare Part A recipients are provided inpatient hospital care and skilled nursing care when such care is medically necessary; home healthcare and hospice care are also covered under Medicare Part A. Medicare Part B covers services by a variety of providers including podiatrists, chiropractors, and dentists, among others; outpatient visits, diagnostic tests, therapy, DME, certain drugs, and preventive services. The major difference between the two parts is generally the settings that the services are provided in. Most of the services provided under Part A are provided to inpatients while most of the services provided under Part B are outpatient services. The infographic prepared will vary by student.

3. Integrated Delivery System (IDSs) and Integrated Delivery Networks (IDNs) are both terms used in the healthcare industry to describe organizational structures that Provide a coordinated and comprehensive approach to healthcare delivery. While the terms are sometimes used interchangeably, they can have slightly different meanings in different contexts. An IDS typically refers to a healthcare organization or entity that seeks to integrate various components of healthcare services within its own system. An IDN is a broader concept that encompasses multiple healthcare organizations working together to deliver a coordinated and comprehensive approach to healthcare delivery within a specific geographic area or community.

5. Private commercial insurance plans are financed through the payment of **premiums.** When a claim for medical care is submitted to the insurance company, the claim is paid out of the fund's reserves. Before payment is made, the insurance company reviews every claim to determine whether the services described on the claim are covered by the patient's policy. The company also reviews the claim to ensure services provided were medically necessary. Payment is then made to either the provider or the policyholder.

Most insurance policies include the following information:

- What medical services the company will cover
- When the company will pay for medical services
- How much and for how long the company will pay for covered services
- What process is to be followed to ensure covered medical expenses are paid

The cost of employer-based self-insurance funding is lower than the cost of paying premiums to private insurers because the premiums reflect more than the actual cost of the services provided to beneficiaries. Private insurers build additional fees into premiums to compensate them for assuming the risk of providing insurance coverage. In self-insured plans, the employer assumes the risk. By budgeting a certain amount to pay its employees' medical claims, the employer retains control over the funds until the time when group medical claims need to be paid.

Employer-based self-insurance has become a common form of group health insurance coverage. Many employers enter administrative services only (ASO) contracts with private insurers and fund the plans themselves. The private insurers administer self-insurance plans on behalf of the employers. Generally, self-insurance plans will be less expense for the employer.

## Check Your Understanding 6.2

1. FFS reimbursement methodologies issue payments to healthcare providers on the basis of the charges assigned to each of the separate services performed for the patient. The total bill for an episode of care represents the sum of all itemized charges for every element of care provided. Independent clinical professionals such as physicians and psychologists who are not employees of the facility issue separate itemized bills to cover their services after the services are completed or monthly when services are ongoing. Managed fee-for-service reimbursement methodology is when the managed care plan controls costs by managing the use of services by its members. Both prospective and retrospective review is used to ensure services provided were necessary and at the lowest cost. Managed care systems generally are more effective in keeping healthcare costs down due to the utilization controls that are part of the system.

3. Professional component: Injection of contrast material into the uterus by the OB-GYN

   Technical component: X-rays of the uterus and fallopian tubes (hospital-employed technician); interpretation of the x-rays (hospital-employed radiologist)

   Global payment: The facility received a lump-sum payment for the procedure and paid for the services of the OB-GYN from that payment. The hospital-employed technician and radiologist were paid their normal salary from the facility.

5. The capitated managed care plan negotiates a contract with an employer or a government agency representing a specific group of individuals. According to the contract, the managed care organization agrees to provide all the contracted healthcare services the covered individuals need over a specified period (usually one year). In exchange, the individual enrollee or third-party payer agrees to pay a fixed premium for the covered group. Like other insurance plans, a capitated insurance contract stipulates as part of the contract exactly which healthcare services are covered and which ones are not. This type of managed care plan provides a steady flow of income each month of the year.

## Check Your Understanding 6.3

1. A hospital's CMI (types or categories of patients treated by the hospital) is based on the relative weights of the MS-DRG. A hospital may relate its CMI to the costs incurred for inpatient care. As the CMI increases or decreases, the cost of care will shift, possibly affecting reimbursement and the resources needed or available to do business.

3. The high-cost outlier for acute care allows a hospital to seek additional payment for extreme cases where the cost of care is exceptionally higher compared to other cases in the same DRG. The additional payment amount is 80 percent of the difference between the hospital's entire cost for the stay and the threshold amount. There are reasons for add-on payments if the hospital treats a high percentage of low-income patients, if the hospital is an approved teaching hospital, or if the hospital can demonstrate the use of new technology that is a large clinical improvement over other existing technology. The student may then offer their opinion of the appropriateness of this cost outlier threshold that changes annually. They may mention that this cost outlier process allows facilities to treat patients needing a large amount of care without the fear of losing a lot of money.

5. Like the inpatient prospective payment system (IPPS), the long-term care hospitals (LTCH) PPS classifies patients into distinct diagnosis groups based on clinical characteristics and expected resource use and is paid based on this group. IPPS calls their groups MS-DRGs and LTCH-PPS calls their groups MS-LTC-DRGs. Both systems have methods to deal with high-cost outliers. Differences are the ALOS, types of cases, and types of outliers.

## Check Your Understanding 7.1

1. The revenue cycle is the sequence of activities that occur from patient account creation to closing. Revenue cycle management (RCM) refers to the strategy used to direct the associated activities. The key difference is specific actions versus approach to those actions. Individual department or team operations with segmented activities of the revenue cycle are a practice of the past. A patient-centric approach involving a focus on quality care with full communication and collaboration industry-wide is necessary for RCM success.

3. The organization must initially have a policy and procedure in place to establish guidelines for payment or discounting of patient accounts. Financial counselors must be able to evaluate the patient's financial status against eligibility criteria as written in the organization's policy. Depending on the eligibility criteria, counselors may then offer charity care, a scaled discount to the total billed charges on the account, or a structured payment plan for paying the bill balance.

5. The process of preauthorization for this service is necessary for determining if the patient is eligible for bariatric service benefits based on the documented condition available under the patient's insurance plan. In addition, the staff must determine what those benefits will cover. Patient access staff should review the patient's insurance to determine the payer's specific preauthorization

requirements for this procedure. Without following the payer's requirements for preauthorization, the service may be denied for payment. If it was determined the bariatric procedure was not covered under the patient's insurance, the first decision is whether to proceed with the procedure. If the patient elects to undergo the procedure, the patient needs financial counseling. The insurer may have options available for elective procedures, or the healthcare organization may have specific payment options for elective procedures.

### Check Your Understanding 7.2

1. Complete and accurate charges must be posted to the claim because reimbursement rates are often related to the individual charges, the charges posted to the claim can drive specific prices and reimbursement rates, and payers also use historical claim information to set current and future reimbursement rates. The charges reflect the resources used to provide the services and they help organizations measure labor costs and staff productivity. Poor charge capture processes could result in underpayments and unrepresentative future payment rates. Poor charge capture processes can also reflect inaccurate labor costs and staff productivity, resulting in understaffing which directly affects patient care. In addition, significant rework and delays in billing often result from inadequate charge capture practices, causing an increase in resource utilization costs to the organization and potential compliance risks by not following regulatory requirements.

3. Soft-coding refers to human interaction with code assignment by reviewing clinical documentation to select the most appropriate code. In order for the soft-code to be assigned to the claim, a charge for the service or item must be charged through the chargemaster. The item will not have an associated CPT or HCPCS code. Rather, that field is blank and then populated when the soft-code is transferred from the HIM department. Example 1 involves operating room time charges in which no hard-code has been assigned. The charge for the OR time would pass from the CDM and then HIM would review the clinical documentation and provide the most appropriate CPT or HCPCS code to represent what was provided during that OR time. The OR charge item would be charged to the account and HIM would assign the CPT/HCPCS code field, such as 42700, drainage of tonsil abscess.

   Hard-coding refers to a chargemaster line item where the CPT or HCPCS code is directly placed in the chargemaster file. This is commonly done in service areas where services or items can be described and coded without requiring review of documentation. HIM can be of assistance for hard-coding by collaborating to determine if a code assigned in the chargemaster is accurate and current based on the chargemaster description associated. In example 2, HIM may review the code assignment and inform the chargemaster department that 97001 was discontinued at the end of 2016 and the code *and* the item description should be changed. 97001 has now been expanded into three physical therapy evaluation codes based on complexity and time (97161, 97162, 97163).

5. CDI programs aim to educate physicians and other clinical staff on opportunities to enhance patient encounter documentation. Artificial intelligence, using EHRs with cross-platform communication, could eliminate the need for queries and manual audits. Documentation suggestions with automatic links to codes and/or computer-assisted coding create more efficient workflows. With these enhancements, CDI specialists and coders should expand and assume research and data analysis roles and programs.

### Check Your Understanding 7.3

1. The greater the number of bill hold days and the lower the percentage of clean claims, the higher the A/R days. Conversely, the shorter the bill hold days and the higher the clean claims submission, the lower the A/R days. The lower the A/R days, the higher the cash flow.

3. Under the No Surprises Act, if the patient had no choice but to receive services from an out-of-network provider, that provider cannot bill the patient a surprise balance bill for emergency

treatment or out-of-network care given at an in-network hospital. The patient may only be charged regular in-network, cost-sharing prices.

5. Contract terms are examined and used to select claims that should be audited to determine whether proper reimbursement was received. It is important to balance resources available and return on investment (ROI) of those resource hours. Prioritizing audits based on claims with high dollar amounts, high rates of denial, or with codes that have high volumes produce the best direct ROI.

## Check Your Understanding 7.4

1. Providers should focus on three areas when building patient relationships: patient engagement, transparency, and demonstrating consumer-centric practices. The patient experience is important for healthcare organizations as the healthcare industry moves toward value-based care. Patient satisfaction even after healthcare services are provided is a primary goal, and the experience with getting their bill paid is the last thing they will remember about their visit. Treating patients with respect and dignity despite their account status builds patient loyalty, which brings the patient back for their continued care needs.

3. The component lacking in this contract is the contract language specifying the administration of the contract. A potential discrepancy triggering the payment variance may be from unclear language. T. J. should work collaboratively with the payer and identify areas of variance where actual payment is not consistent with T. J.'s interpretation for basis of payment agreed upon and written in the contract. Payment variance could be a result of payer or provider interpretation of the contract language for basis of payment if the language is not clear and understood by both parties. T. J. should establish routine meetings with the payer, clarify the language or remove unclear language, monitor future payments, and, if required, renegotiate future language to be proactive.

5. The value for C. Lewis Medical Center's point-of-service (POS) cash collection is favorable because the value is increasing and is currently higher than the median benchmark of high performance in the revenue cycle. The formula for POS cash collection KPI is patient POS payments divided by total self-pay cash collected. This KPI reflects greater cash flow, and a higher ratio suggests a reduction of bad debt by collecting payments upfront. However, the organization still has an opportunity for improvement in the collection of patient cash prior to or at the time of a new service.

## Check Your Understanding 8.1

1. CDI is a process to facilitate the accurate representation of a patient's clinical status in the patient health record, which is then transformed into coded data. This is important for quality patient care, reimbursement, and reporting. The data are used not only for payment but in quality metrics which reflect upon the provider's practices. Accurate documentation also supports better communication between care providers for current and future treatment. CDI is not about maximum payment but having the complete documentation available for both facilities and providers to receive the most accurate reimbursement for services provided.

3. Clinical documentation is the foundation for communication between providers and multiple reimbursement, quality, and public health measures. Each stakeholder has a different part in the process. Information is used by many people for many functions and having each perspective represented promotes a better understanding and more inclusive approach. It also helps garner support for the CDI process from multiple areas of the organization.

5. Composition of the CDI staff, alignment of the CDI program, identification of the types of records to review, frequency of reviews, budget, training needs, reporting, and performance monitoring are factors to be considered when planning to implement a CDI process. Students can elaborate on each factor's importance rather than provide a list; each student may have varying justification for the importance of each component and what they see as potential issues accompanying each factor.

7. Answers will vary by student.

9. "The relationship isn't perfectly linear. Sometimes sending queries will have a negative impact on CMI, for instance, and eventually CMI will have to stop increasing and should level off. Looking at CMI metrics over time provides a much better picture of CDI impact, but even then, there can be outliers. To see CDI impact more accurately, they recommended that higher-weighted DRGs be removed when measuring, as they can greatly skew metrics. The DRG relative impact can also be measured by looking at pre- and post-CDI DRGs to more accurately calculate DRG weight."

https://acdis.org/articles/acdis-update-quarterly-call-covers-how-cdi-efforts-affect-cmi

## Check Your Understanding 8.2

1. Compliance means adhering to rules, laws, standards, or regulations. A compliance plan is needed to identify applicable rules, implement strategies to adhere, monitor, and improve adherence. Participating in Medicare requires providers to formulate a compliance plan, and a coding compliance plan as part of the overall compliance strategy ensures the information submitted as claims is accurate. The coding compliance plan will help prevent deliberate fraud and includes education components to support employees in avoiding practices which may be abuse.

3. Optimization seeks the most accurate documentation, coded data, and resulting payment in the amount the provider is rightly and legally entitled to receive. This is as opposed to maximization, which focuses on collecting the highest rate of payment. In some cases, the optimization of reimbursement payment—what the organization is rightly and legally entitled to—is the maximum amount available if supported by documentation of the actual treatment provided. In other cases, a conflict exists if obtaining maximum reimbursement payment is only possible by using codes that do not accurately describe the documentation or actual services provided using the coding conventions of each system (ICD-10-CM/PCS, CPT, or HCPCS).

5. Exclusion is significant because the government is the largest purchaser and provider of services in the US. Patients may choose care elsewhere if the healthcare provider is excluded, and no reimbursement would be received from federal programs for care that is provided.

7. Students should submit a memo format that includes the following:
   1. Include reasonable policies and procedures to identify the red flags of identity theft
   2. Design the program to detect red flags identified in step 1
   3. Detail appropriate actions when red flags are detected
   4. Detail how to keep the plan current and to reflect new and emerging threats. The best way to prevent medical identity theft is by incorporating these items into the day-to-day activities by alerting staff to watch for red flags.

9. External drivers include whistleblower incentives, data mining and data validation, working with RAC, and other audits. Internal drivers include proactive review of coding, contracts, repayment, post-payment, and the monitoring of third-party transaction.

## Check Your Understanding 9.1

1. Common law (also known as judicial law, judge-made law, or case law), is created by courts that resolve disputes. Statutory (legislative) law is written law established by federal and state legislatures. It may be amended, repealed, or expanded by the legislature. Administrative law controls the government's agency, or administrative, operations and provides rules established by statute. It consists of regulations, which are rules derived from or brought forward by administrative agencies after the passage of statutes. The regulations establish how statutes are to be carried out. Constitutional law includes constitutions at different levels of government (for example, federal, state and local). The Constitution of the United States is the highest law in the land. It takes precedence over constitutions and laws in the individual states and local jurisdictions.

3. Civil law involves relations between individuals, corporations, government entities, and other organizations. The typical remedy for a civil wrong is monetary. Criminal law involves matters between individuals or groups of people and the government. Criminal law addresses crimes, which are wrongful acts against public health, safety, and welfare. It also addresses punishment for offenders.

5. Preponderance of the evidence is the "more likely than not" standard that means there is enough evidence to tip the scales, even slightly, in favor of the plaintiff's case. This is a substantially lower standard than a criminal case, in which the government must prevail beyond a reasonable doubt. The standard of proof is higher in criminal cases because the stakes and the potential penalty (confinement) are higher.

7. Subject matter jurisdiction limits what cases can be brought in federal courts. The first type of subject matter jurisdiction is federal question jurisdiction, which is a claim related to federal law, including federal crimes; constitutional issues; and other federal laws. The second type of subject matter jurisdiction is diversity jurisdiction, where no plaintiff is from the same state as any defendant in a case. Other civil and criminal cases are brought in the state court systems.

## Check Your Understanding 9.2

1. Malfeasance: performance of a wrongful act, and the act may be unlawful

   *Example:* using a joint replacement device the physician knows may be problematic.

   Misfeasance: improper performance of a lawful act that causes injury to another.

   *Example:* accidentally cutting an adjacent organ when performing surgery.

   Nonfeasance: failure to perform an act a person has a duty to perform and which a person of ordinary prudence would have done in similar circumstances.

   *Example:* not ordering an x-ray when one's symptoms are indicative of a fracture.

   Examples given will vary.

3. Assault is conduct, along with apparent ability, causing apprehension that physically harmful or offensive contact will occur. Battery is the intentional and nonconsensual touching of another person's body. False imprisonment is intentional confinement of someone against their will. This cause of action includes the defendant's lack of legal authority or justification to confine a person. Defamation of character is a false communication about someone to a person other than the subject that may injure the subject's reputation. Fraud is "an intentional deception or misrepresentation made by a person with the knowledge that the deception could result in some unauthorized benefit to himself or some other person. Invasion of privacy is the intrusion upon one's solitude, including the unlawful disclosure of a patient's health information. The intentional or reckless infliction of emotional distress for which a person can be held liable includes mental suffering resulting from such things as despair, shame, grief, and public humiliation.

5. Often, when a patient experiences a bad outcome, a healthcare provider will express remorse, sorrow, sympathy, empathy, or some other type of compassionate response that can take the form of an apology. However, a common fear of healthcare providers is that apologies or expressions of sympathy made to a patient or patient's family members will be considered an admission of liability and used against providers named as defendants in lawsuits. Many states have created apology statutes ("I'm Sorry" laws) that protect a healthcare provider's apology from being admitted into evidence as an admission of liability during a court proceeding (Rinehart-Thompson 2023b, 81). Apology statutes are not a type of defense but, instead, protect apologies from being admitted as evidence.

7. Contributory negligence: The plaintiff's conduct contributed in part to the injury the plaintiff suffered and, if found to be sufficient, can preclude the plaintiff's recovery for the injury.

Comparative negligence: The plaintiff's conduct contributed in part to the injury the plaintiff suffered, but the plaintiff's recovery is reduced by some amount based on his or her percentage of negligence.

Contributory negligence can much more readily bar complete recovery for the plaintiff. As such, it is more punitive in nature to a plaintiff who has also committed negligence in addition to the defendant.

## Check Your Understanding 9.3

1. Licensure is offered through governmental bodies. It is vital because an organization must be licensed to operate. Accreditation is offered through nongovernmental organizations. Accreditation is considered voluntary and is not legally mandated, but it is very important to healthcare organizations because it provides an organization with a designation as a high-quality healthcare provider.

3. Risks:
   - Inaccurate or outdated information that may adversely impact patient care by compromising interaction among healthcare team members
   - Redundant information, which causes the inability to determine current information
   - Inability to identify the author or intent of documentation
   - Inability to identify when the documentation was first created
   - Inability to accurately support or defend E/M codes for professional or technical billing notes
   - Propagation of false information or documentation services not rendered
   - Internally inconsistent progress notes
   - Unnecessarily lengthy progress notes
   - Potential for fraud and abuse allegations
   - Compromised integrity of legal EHR

   Student responses will vary on which one of these they believe presents the greatest risk and why.

5. An individual has the right to access his or her own health record, but the organization that created and maintains the physical record is responsible for its integrity and security as the legal custodian. In other words, the organization owns the record and controls the physical health record, and the patient has rights to the information contained in it. Because of electronic access, the ownership issue may appear murky. Nonetheless, the organization is still responsible for its integrity and security, regardless of what format it exists in.

7. Preemption is a legal concept whereby federal law is given precedence over conflicting state law. With respect to access to one's own health information, state laws must provide individuals with at least the same degree of access that HIPAA allows; otherwise, it will be superseded by HIPAA.

## Check Your Understanding 9.4

1. A durable power of attorney for healthcare decisions is a document in which an adult—while competent—designates another person (proxy) to make healthcare decisions consistent with the individual's wishes on the individual's behalf if he or she is unable. The term *durable* indicates that the document is in effect when the individual is no longer competent.

    A living will is executed by a competent adult, expressing the individual's wishes to limit treatment should the individual become afflicted with certain conditions (for example, a persistent vegetative state or a terminal condition) and no longer able to communicate on his or her own behalf. Living wills often address extraordinary lifesaving measures such as ventilator support and either the continuation or removal of nutrition and hydration.

    A do-not-resuscitate (DNR) order directs healthcare providers to refrain from performing the otherwise standing order of CPR should the individual experience cardiac or respiratory arrest.

The first is unique because it defers decision-making to another (a proxy), although decisions should be made according to the will of the individual. The other two are more specific. The third is generally initiated by a physician, whereas the first and second are created by the individual.

Comparison of advance directives

| Durable power of attorney for healthcare decisions | Executed by a competent adult on his or her own behalf |
| --- | --- |
| | Designates another person (proxy) to make healthcare decisions consistent with the individual's wishes on the individual's behalf |
| Living will | Executed by a competent adult on his or her own behalf |
| | Expresses one's wishes to limit treatment if a medical condition renders the individual unable to communicate on his or her own behalf |
| | May be limited to certain medical conditions (for example, vegetative state), depending on state law |
| Do-not-resuscitate order (DNR) | Most often used by the elderly or chronically ill |
| | Directs healthcare providers to refrain from CPR if the individual experiences cardiac or respiratory arrest |

3. Information that is subject to an e-discovery request can reside in many different locations; exist on different media types; and enter a system by various points of entry. All these must be accounted for in the e-discovery preservation process. Individual student responses will vary, but examples include information created and stored on laptop and desktop computers; information on mobile devices such as tablets and smart phones; storage on servers that may be local, remote, cloud-based, or removable (for example, flash drives).

One must also consider the location of information, such as in various systems. In addition to the EHR, information may be in ancillary service systems, personal equipment, instant messages, and email. One should know whether ancillary service information is integrated into the EHR or maintained separately. Data residing on devices such as imaging equipment, IV medication pumps, and dictation systems must also be accounted for, for inclusion in an inventory of ESI that can serve as evidence.

5. Waiver is a critically important concept for a provider seeking to defend him- or herself in a legal action. A patient who places his or her treatment at issue through the filing of a lawsuit waives the privilege that protects the information. This is necessary so the defendant-provider can testify regarding the information previously considered confidential.

7. Spoliation is "intentional destruction, mutilation, alteration, or concealment of evidence." It is intentional and illegal. Other types of health record destruction may be intentional (but legal), such as record destruction per a formalized destruction process, or unintentional (either legal, meaning it was not intended but did not violate any laws, or illegal, meaning it was not intended but it nonetheless violated one or more laws). The legality of health record destruction depends on applicable record retention laws.

## Check Your Understanding 9.5

1. Categories include behavioral health, substance use disorder (SUD), HIV and AIDS, genetic testing, and adoption records. The first three are stigmatic in nature and can lead to discrimination. The same is true of genetic testing *if* the testing reveals a propensity for a disease or condition. Adoption records are generally not viewed as stigmatizing, but they may contain information about birth parents who wish for their identity to remain concealed from the child who was given up for adoption or the child's adoptive parents.

3. External medical identity theft is committed by individuals from outside an organization. Perpetrators can include uninsured individuals who use another's insurance to obtain services or technically savvy individuals who introduce malware or ransomware into a system. Internal medical identity theft is committed by individuals inside an organization who have access to vast amounts of patient information. These individuals may act alone or as part of a larger crime ring that has intentionally infiltrated the organization to gain access to information.

5. Concurrent quality review activities are carried out as treatment is being provided. Retrospective quality review activities are carried out after an encounter has ended.

7. The federal Genetic Information Non-Discrimination Act of 2008 (GINA) protects individuals from being discriminated against by health insurers and employers based on genetic information. Note that not all insurers are regulated by GINA, such as life and disability insurers. In the insurance realm, the scope of the law is limited to health insurance.

## Check Your Understanding 10.1

1. Physical safeguards—intended to manage administrative actions, policies, and procedures to prevent, detect, contain, and correct security violations. Examples include policies, procedures, door locks, and backup hard drives.

   Technical safeguards—protects access and control of ePHI. Examples include automatic log-off, unique user identification, encryption, and audit controls.

   Organizational safeguards—protect ePHI between organizations. Examples include business association agreements, identification of a security official, minimum necessary access controls, and contingency plan.

3. Privacy is the right of an individual to be let alone; it also refers to who should have access, what constitutes the patient's rights to confidentiality, and what constitutes inappropriate access to health records.

   Confidentiality is when data or information is not made available or disclosed to unauthorized persons or processes. It also establishes how the records (or the systems that hold those records) should be protected from inappropriate access.

   Security is how the privacy and confidentiality of information is maintained.

   Privacy is critical when determining who should have access to PHI and a patient's rights related to accessing their PHI, while confidentiality ensures PHI is protected from unauthorized use or disclosure. Security provides the controls necessary to ensure appropriate access, use, and disclosure.

5. d. The Breach Notification Rule was developed in response to the HITECH Act which required mandatory reporting of breaches. The minimum necessary standard is included as part of the Privacy Rule.

## Check Your Understanding 10.2

1. Because Vermont law is more stringent than HIPAA with respect to the rights of the patient to access to their medical record, state law takes precedence over HIPAA.

3. As a patient, you have the right to agree or object to the disclosure of your PHI within the facility directory. If you agree, your PHI will be included in the directory and will only be disclosed to individuals such as family members and clergy. The only PHI disclosed in the directory is your name, your location in the facility, your condition described in general terms that do not communicate specific medical information about the you, and your religious affiliation. The disclosure of this information will only be for the purpose of releasing the information to clergy or to an individual who asks for you by name, and we will only disclose the information as long as it is consistent with your expressed preferences, or it is in the best interest of the patient based on professional judgement.

5. Answer should include the following:
   - Documentation to release records:
     - Authorization for Disclosure of PHI signed by the patient (or representative)
   - Verification:
     - Identification of attorney
     - Link to the law firm by attorney (request on letterhead, business card, and such)

### Check Your Understanding 10.3

1. Mitigate the risk: the process of reducing or eliminating the risk by implementing a control, used when the risk is high, and action is required. An example is implementing role-based access.

   Transfer the risk: outsourcing or insuring the risk against any potential loss to the organization, used when the risk is medium to high, and the most efficient course of action is to shift the repercussion of the risk to another party. An example is moving data from local servers to the cloud.

   Accept the risk: accept that risk remains even with safeguards in place, used when the risk is low. An example is when new technology is cost prohibitive and does not substantially reduce the risk to the organization.

3. HIPAA defines data encryption in two separate, addressable requirements. Data at rest are in storage within a database or on a server no longer in use or accessed. Data in motion are data in the process of being transmitted from one location to another location such as an email. Because these are addressable requirements, the covered entity and business associate may evaluate and determine if they are going to implement the technical safeguard. If the covered entity chooses not to implement the encryption safeguards, other safeguards to protect the information must be documented, including the reason for not implementing the encryption.

5. Answer should include:

   The criticality analysis determines how different systems of the organization are crucial to day-to-day healthcare operations and patient care. The goal of the criticality analysis is to

   (1) create a listing that prioritizes all systems to allow for the successful restoration of critical systems more efficiently after an unexpected or expected downtime.

   (2) understand where the critical information system and data exists to create and implement proper safeguards for protection of the data

### Check Your Understanding 10.4

1. Healthcare organizations should evaluate and implement proper security measures to safeguard information being accessed on mobile technology. Considerations include identification of device ownership, personal device use within the organization, required authorization for mobile technology use, conditions under which ePHI is allowed on mobile devices, acceptable behaviors and use of ePHI on mobile technology, safeguards to protect ePHI, procedures for reporting lost or stolen devices, and evaluation and scanning of mobile technology on a regular basis.

3. Benefits: timely and efficient communication among healthcare providers (potential impacts: increased patient satisfaction and provider satisfaction), improve quality of care (potential impacts: better patient outcomes, less unnecessary hospital visits), reduce healthcare costs (potential impacts: reduced health insurance premiums, increase in payments).

   Risks: ensuring correct patient identity (potential impacts: care provided to the incorrect patient, incorrect data used to treat a patient), increased cost (potential impacts: higher healthcare premiums, increased amount of accounts written off to bad debt or unpaid), requires all healthcare organizations to participate (potential impacts: patients having to sign multiple authorization forms, sharing of information for nontreatment purposes, unauthorized access to information).

5. Answer:
   - Process for consent and authorization
   - Process for education to patients and families
   - Process for adequate patient searching and patient matching

- Process for assurance of selection of the correct patient
- Process for patient information to be utilized to support care
- Process for processing patient information if used to support care
- Process for reporting any issues or concerns with the HIE and data being used
- Information regarding the organization's evaluation of audit trails and supporting of patient care for accessing PHI in the HIE

### Check Your Understanding 10.5

1. Employees, volunteers, trainees, students, interns, medical students, and any other individual the covered entity or business associate has direct control over through daily tasks and responsibilities, whether they get paid or not by the covered entity or business associate.

3. Answers will vary, but should include the following:

   Privacy Rule—train all workforce members in the organizational policies and procedures and the uses and disclosures of PHI and patient's rights under HIPAA.

   Security Rule—implement a security training program on the organizational policies and procedures and established technological safeguards of ePHI, including protection from malicious software, login monitoring, and password management. In addition, provide periodic security updates throughout the year.

   Breach Notification Rule—train all workforce members on the organizational policies and procedures for unauthorized uses and disclosures of PHI, including the need to report to the organization upon discovering a potential data breach.

5. Periodic security updates, procedures for guarding against, detecting, and reporting malware, procedures for monitoring login attempts and reporting discrepancies, and procedures for creating, changing, and safeguarding passwords.

### Check Your Understanding 11.1

1. d. The scenario reflects an instance where a process did not work as it ordinarily does and needs to improve so the desired outcome of timely medication administration occurs. In performance improvement, study and adaptation occurs to increase the likelihood of achieving a desired outcome. To improve performance, a meeting with key stakeholders is common to evaluate what happened and why, and what steps are necessary for improvement to occur.

3. d. Adverse events refer to instances in which medical care causes injury. A variety of examples exist which illustrate the concept of adverse events.

5. Because the provider is receiving reduced reimbursement due to low scores for a preestablished measurement, meaning the health status of the patient on the measure was not ideal. In this instance, a higher score among the patients would have suggested better outcomes and not resulted in payment reduction.

### Check Your Understanding 11.2

1. No, it is not external benchmarking because the comparison among needle stick rates is made between units within the hospital. Instead, this is an example of internal benchmarking.

3. It is important for the organization to know if there have been licensure issues with the physician. Depending on the issues, the physician may not be eligible for hire or may be considered too high risk to join the medical staff if negative actions are on his or her record.

5. The correct answer is a. sentinel event. Sentinel events are serious events which occur in care processes and require immediate investigation; the investigation goal is twofold: (1) identify what happened and how it happened and (2) prevent future occurrence.

### Check Your Understanding 11.3

1. A hip fracture is a relatively common injury and should not frequently lead to death. Therefore, a quality analyst would review medical records from hip fracture patients who expired to identify the presence of comorbidities contributing to death or issues in the medical care provided that contributed to unfavorable outcomes.

3. Answers to this question will vary. An example of a correct answer is charges among similar hospitals in different geographic locations for total hip arthroplasty procedures. The HCUP database would be a good resource to examine this topic because it contains vast amounts of claims data to illustrate charges for procedures.

5. d. Answer choices a and c are both correct answers

### Check Your Understanding 11.4

1. Interprofessional education inspires diverse health professionals to improve communication and cooperation among the varying health professions. Increased communication among a diverse care team may decrease the likelihood of errors. One example is ensuring all medication allergies are documented immediately upon patient admission so all caregivers know what medications are not to be administered. By ensuring interprofessional education, all caregivers will understand the importance of clear and prompt communication.

3. Clinical pathways help standardize types of care for common conditions. If providers reduce variance in their approach to treating common conditions, it may reduce errors or inconsistencies.

5. The Certified Professional in Healthcare Risk Management (CPHRM) would be an ideal choice if they plan to continue working in risk management.

### Check Your Understanding 12.1

1. Informatics applies information management in the context of computer-based systems designed to support specific types of users in performing their work (for example, decision-making support). Information management, however, is a more generalized discipline with similar aims that are applied in both paper-based and computer-based environments.

3. Healthcare professionals use data and information constantly throughout their day to perform work for patients. They need to review previous and current clinical, financial, and demographic patient data and information and document new findings. Patient information is crucial for sharing and planning patient care with the healthcare team of professionals, for proper consultation and appropriate referrals, and for appropriate patient interaction from patient visits to patient billing.

5. The government influences the level of health IT utilization by offering monetary incentives for adopting and using it well; they can offer guidance regarding best practices for implementation and use of health IT; and they can oversee progress toward adoption to ensure an organization stays on track.

### Check Your Understanding 12.2

1. When data is unstructured, it is difficult for a search engine to find, retrieve, and manipulate the data element. Unstructured data does not have limits and defined fields, making healthcare data collection, reporting and analysis difficult. NLP can capture unstructured data elements from the EHR, analyze and obtain meaning from their grammatical structure, and summarize information for

use in further analysis. This is particularly helpful with a large amount of unstructured healthcare data that needs to be transformed into usable information.

3. Speech recognition technology employs basic NLP capabilities as it translates spoken words (natural language voice bytes) into text. However, speech recognition technology does not yet employ the advanced capabilities of NLP; for instance, speech recognition technology is not yet capable of taking two sound-alike terms (such as ileum and ilium) with different meanings and then selecting the correct term based on an analysis of the context.

NLP technology and Boolean searching differ from each other in that the former considers sentence structure (synTaxonomy), meaning (semantics), and context to accurately extract data from free text. For example, "no shortness of breath, chest pain aggravated by exercise" and "no chest pain, shortness of breath aggravated by exercise" look the same to a Boolean word search engine when it identifies occurrences of *chest* and *pain* in the same sentence. NLP technology, however, would discern the syntactical and semantic differences between these two phrases. Students should discuss benefits and disadvantages of these technologies, and how the technologies could help or hinder the use of the tool. Students should explain their answers using what they have learned from this textbook.

5. Students may provide different practical examples. Following are some possible answers.

- Document imaging technology electronically captures, stores, identifies, retrieves, and distributes documents that are not generated digitally or are generated digitally but stored on paper.

Example: Document imaging can be used to scan paper consent forms into the patient record.

- Workflow/BPM technology allows computers to add and extract value from document content as the documents move throughout an organization. The documents can be automatically assigned, routed, activated, and managed through system-controlled rules that mirror business operations.

Example: Workflow technology can be used to route the electronic patient record from the record analysis and completion area to the coding area.

- Automated forms processing technology allows users to electronically enter data into online forms and electronically extract the data from the online forms for data manipulation. The form document is stored in a form format, as the user sees it on the screen, for ease of interpretation.

Example: Automated forms processing technology can be used when a patient wishes to electronically complete a patient satisfaction or clinical assessment form.

- Digital signature management technology offers both signer and document authentication for analog or digital documents. Signer authentication is the ability to identify the person who digitally signed the document. Document authentication ensures the document and the signature cannot be altered.

Example: Digital signature management technology can be used when a provider needs to sign a medication order in the EHR from a remote location.

 **Check Your Understanding 12.3**

1. Answers will vary. They should include functionality such as the ability to see and pay their bills online and to securely view all or portions of their provider-based EHR, such as current medical conditions, immunization records, medications, allergies, and test results. They may also include functionality, such as the ability to see and schedule appointments, refill prescriptions, or send a message to their provider.

3. The clinician portal provides the clinician with a single point of access with a common user interface (and a single login password) to launch and view information from disparate applications. In this case, the on-call physician can access the clinic system to pull up the patient's record to verify the patient's problem list; determine what prior instruction and care was recently provided, if any; and see what medications have been prescribed to the patient. The physician may need to access the hospital system to determine if any emergency room visits have occurred, as they may impact his

suggested treatment. The physician may also need to access an external decision support system to check on potential treatments, side effects, and contraindications to planned treatment. The physician may also need to access a directory of 24-hour behavioral health centers for assistance to the patient. Once advice is given to the patient, the physician may then need to access his email to let the attending physician know about his patient's problem and how it was handled.

5. Benefits of open-source technology: it is freely available, can be customized, and the collaborative nature of this technology allows users and developers to interact and improve upon the product. Drawbacks include the need for skilled developers within the organization to make it work as required for the organization's needs and the lack of technical support for the product. Even though the cost is free to obtain open-source software, the student should not recommend it to ABC Clinic because they do not have the necessary IT staff to ensure its functionality.

### Check Your Understanding 12.4

1. Distinct examples of diagnostic tests involving physiological signal processing include electrocardiograms (EKGs), electroencephalograms (EEGs), electromyograms (EMGs), fetal tracings, digital blood pressure (BP) monitors, and digital thermometers. These diagnostic tests provide markers that may indicate other things happening that could provide evidence of underlying issues that should be considered within the overall patient's observation.

3. Some of the barriers to consider include the lack of systems interoperability, broad bandwidth limitations, physician resistance, lack of proven cost-effectiveness; lack of proven medical effectiveness; concerns for safety; and challenges related to reimbursement for services provided.

5. Based upon the definitions provided by NAHIT, the major difference between an EHR and EMR is whether the system conforms to nationally recognized interoperability standards. The impact is that an EMR cannot be shared outside of the organization, creating continuity of care and efficiency issues when the patient information is needed elsewhere.

### Check Your Understanding 12.5

1. f
3. a
5. e
7. e

### Check Your Understanding 12.6

1. HIE is intended to facilitate access to and retrieval of clinical data to provide safe, timely, efficient, effective, equitable, patient-centered care. Care quality is intended to be improved by making critical patient information available at the point of care delivery and through the aggregation and mining of data to determine best practices in diagnosis and treatment. Student answers will vary. Examples of when HIE is beneficial are when a patient presents to an ED while on vacation and all the patient's records are from another facility. With HIE, those records can be accessed. If a patient is in an accident and is brought to a facility that has no medical records for her there, they can access them through HIE.

3. Interoperability is the ability of different IT systems and software applications to communicate, exchange data, and use the exchanged information. Before IT gets involved, it is critical to have trust and a cultural commitment between the organizations to determine how standards will be used and implemented.

5. The ability for medical devices and systems to exchange information, although complex, can offer advantages. Devices such as vital signs monitors, infusion pumps, and the like can send the information collected from patients directly to EMR systems, which helps with documentation automation. This auto-documentation eases the burden of nurses to ensure information is collected in a timely and accurate way. It also gives the care provider more time to care for their patients rather than documenting. Auto-documentation also allows for things like start and stop times that must not be missed, to meet billing protocols and ensure hospitals receive proper healthcare reimbursements.

## Check Your Understanding 12.7

1. The student may note the timeline from approximately 2004 to present, and they may see that as either satisfactory or slow progress depending on their perspective. They may note the federal funding has been consistent and participation is good. They may note the development of standards and guidelines as a success. Interoperability and sustainability issues are a challenge.

3. If Sandy does not want to participate in an HIE, she must opt out with her healthcare provider. Opting out keeps her information from being shared in the HIE. Ensure Sandy understands the benefit of participating in an HIE before she makes her decision. Indicate that if she opts in to an HIE, her health information would be shared with another participant immediately if she needed emergency treatment or care at another facility.

5. Both the Sequoia Project and TECFA are initiatives promoting interoperability and health information exchange nationwide. A difference is that The Sequoia Project is an independent, private company and TECFA is a government initiative under the ONC.

## Check Your Understanding 12.8

1. Student answers may vary. They should choose a benefit such as timely and secure sharing of important patient information at the point of care, a more complete patient health record, an increased ability for better decision making, a lower readmission rate, fewer medication errors, accurate diagnoses, reduced duplicate testing, fewer medical errors, and possibly stronger patient engagement. Students should include an example, either hypothetical or from their personal experience or research. For instance, by having a patient's medication list available at the point of care in the ER, an adverse reaction can be avoided. Or by having the patient's problem list available in the ER, better decisions can be made regarding next steps in the patient's treatment.

3. The MPI is a patient-identifying directory referencing all patients related to an organization, which also serves as a link to the patient record or information, facilitates patient identification, and assists in maintaining a longitudinal patient record from birth to death. In the context of an HIE, the MPI will rely on algorithms that match elements of patient demographic information to determine relationships in patient identity. During the testing stages of the implementation, these algorithms and criteria will be adjusted until a designated performance metric for accuracy is met.

5. Once organizations have agreed to exchange patient data, the establishment of policies, procedures and the metrics against which to monitor their progress toward their stated goals must be established.

## Check Your Understanding 13.1

1.a. To meet the need to achieve quality and cost improvements in healthcare, physicians must be aware of the quality and pricing of the physicians to whom they make referrals. (1) Recognizing the challenge that selective referrals can be an issue relating to Stark Laws that aim to prevent kickbacks. (2) Clinically integrated networks are being legally created to collectively monitor and control utilization of health services, hence overcoming antitrust issues (American College of Surgeons,

2019). (3) Integrating the clinical and financial data, and to make such data accessible at the point of care, including across providers to whom physicians may refer patients, is yet another element that requires strategic planning.

1.b. Mergers and acquisitions among healthcare providers (and nonhealthcare providers) are a growing trend to achieve economies of scale. Considerable planning must be undertaken. This includes (1) the need to identify the appropriate stakeholders from all parties to the merger to provide governance, (2) determining where there is a need to combine departments or keep them separate, (3) renegotiation of contracts with vendors for services where the larger contracts should reduce cost, and (4) planning for integration of HISs. Even where the parties to a merger may have the same vended IS product, there are different configurations and data issues to address.

1.c. While a construction project may not seem to require strategic planning, today's healthcare facilities face much more complex tasks than simply building with bricks and mortar. (1) Creating a strategic plan that assures appropriate governance by not only architects and building contractors, but also information technologists (to ensure appropriate cabling, making decisions on data storage, and many other technical issues), legal analysts, and others. (2) There are many challenges in renovating a healthcare facility, such as recognizing areas prone to natural disaster. (3) Designing a building not only to make it weather external conditions, but to think about and incorporate how medicine may be practiced in the future, such as in a "hospital in the home" environment and with much less invasive surgery, which may require very specialized equipment, is very important.

3.a. Does not belong on migration path because it is part of an implementation plan.

3.b. Does belong on the migration path under applications—customer relationship management systems are aids for care coordination, as they help track patients' needs when they are at home and maintain community service contacts.

3.c. Does belong on a migration path under operations. If a provider organization simultaneously undertakes many major projects, a project management office is a way to aid in coordinating projects to optimize resource utilization and reduce the risk of two or more projects attempting to achieve the same purpose.

3.d. Does belong on a migration path under technology—whether the provider organization is actually developing the apps or analyzing them for provider use with patients.

3.e. Does belong on the migration path under applications. The health insurance provider network will determine eligible providers in-network and out-of-network for that health insurance

5. Applications: Master person index, coding, clinical documentation integrity, consent management, release of information, electronic document management system, record analysis, and quality reporting.

Technology: Human-computer interfaces, scanners, databases, registries, HIM applications in EHR, patient portal access to view health information

Operations: Project management, data and information governance, data administration, data analysis, compliance, and strategic planning for applications specified above.

7. a. This option can be achieved through an environmental scan because it involves looking at internal and external factors. This specific barrier could be achieved through a survey.

## Check Your Understanding 13.2

1. g
3. h
5. a
7. f
9. i

 **Check Your Understanding 13.3**

1. Quality measurement staff may need to work with both IT staff (for example, a clinical data analyst) and the chief medical informatics officer (CMIO) to investigate the issue more closely. It may be necessary to create a report on the number of times the comment field is used, for what specific purposes it is used, which physicians use it the most, and how frequently use of the comment field impacts quality measurement. It may also be necessary to survey nurses to determine how frequently there are calls from the pharmacy to clarify orders.

3. Public health data is collected and analyzed to prevent the spread of disease. For example, if people are getting sick from eating lettuce, there will likely be investigations to find the source of the bad lettuce and corrective action. Population health data is a collection of healthcare quality, cost, and risk data on a specific set of individuals used to study trends on that population to determine best practices that providers in a community can use to improve; for example, if a community has a lot of patients with diabetes and heart disease and correspondingly high healthcare costs, population health data could identify the need and help lobby for a grocery store that stocks fresh produce and other healthy food choices.

5. Administrative metadata should be reviewed to investigate a potential breach. This type of metadata provides information about how and when data was used. An example of administrative metadata is audit logs, which record the actions taken on data within a system including who accessed what and when. This would be very helpful in investigating the details of a potential breach.

 **Check Your Understanding 14.1**

1. Organizations promote patient-focused websites, offer tools for health information tracking and sharing for both patient and organization-generated data, and encourage patients to respond to patient satisfaction surveys. The student can add other ideas of their own beyond chapter content, such as the use and sharing of Fitbit-type technology, email communications with providers, and the like.

3. Medical paternalism refers to the patient care approach in which providers are the center of the clinical experience, they make the decisions using their knowledge and training and determine the best care for the patient from their perspective. The patient-centered care approach places the patient at the center. It includes them and their family in the decision-making process, and considers the patient and family's wishes along with interprofessional collaboration when determining the best plan of care. The main motivation for the shift to patient-centered care is to improve the outcome for the patient. Including the patient, the family, and appropriate healthcare professionals assists the provider in determining the best care plan for the specific patient and their specific needs.

5. Patient experience accounts for a significant percent of the Hospital VBP Program because the satisfaction and engagement of patients has been shown to positively impact patient outcomes potentially due to improved compliance and coordination of care. An efficient and effective patient experience improves outcomes and decreases extra costs.

 **Check Your Understanding 14.2**

1. The student should include in the answer any mention of obtaining, understanding, and processing health information and services. They may also include concepts related to the ability to use and understand the purpose of technology; the ability to hear and act on information given; and the ability to make decisions based on their own health and related information. Examples may be the difficulty in reading instructions on where to go for an appointment or when to call with questions; inability to make decisions related to taking medication—that is, time, dose, interactions with other meds; and inability to know which care setting is appropriate.

3. The student may discuss their current education and experience related to healthcare, technology they use or know about, a personal or experience they have learned from, their results on a literacy measurement tool, and so forth.

5. The student may try to determine the existing level of health literacy by administering an assessment tool such as the SAHL–S&E or conducting focus groups or interviews. The results can inform the educator about community needs and when educational sessions at various locations, dates, and times can be conducted.

### Check Your Understanding 14.3

1. It is estimated that nearly five percent of all web searches are health related and that more than 70 percent of all US adults conduct health-related web searches each year. There are several reasons health-related web searches are so frequent by American adults. One of the primary reasons is we are all humans who become ill or patients who typically have little or no clinical training. The internet provides a useful tool for investigating symptoms or researching clinical diagnoses.

3. The PAM has four levels. The fourth level refers to an individual maintaining behaviors and pushing further. They are active health advocates. Individuals who fall into this category have greater likelihood of engaging in healthier behaviors and adhering to recommended clinical practices. If individuals are more active in their care and better adhere to clinical practices recommended by their providers, their health will more likely improve.

5. Providers may not want to promote the use of online health information resources because an individual may not have a strong level of clinical knowledge and may misinterpret the information causing them to take action that is unnecessary or not helpful, they may become overly anxious, or they may try to treat themselves rather than ask a clinician.

### Check Your Understanding 14.4

1. Sally would likely access her provider's patient portal where her recent labs are stored. If she collects and stores her visit data in some way herself, she may refer to her PHR.

3. Joe could create a PHR for each resident to document daily information to share with the provider as needed. The PHR could be paper documents, a spreadsheet, or specific PHR software.

5. Telehealth offers an alternative to receiving care and advice that may be more convenient or accessible to some individuals. For example, an individual may not have transportation or time to go to their provider or possibly they do not feel well enough to go out. Telehealth offers an option to traveling to an appointment for care. Some may seek care through telehealth where they may not have otherwise. Another example is that an individual may want privacy regarding a condition and does not want to be seen at a particular provider or clinic. Telehealth offers more individual privacy if care can be offered in one's own home.

### Check Your Understanding 14.5

1. PGHD is collected by a patient or the family of a patient to address a health concern. This data can be organized and stored in a PHR, which the patient owns and controls access to.

3. By focusing on very specific personal health attributes, a person could tailor their lifestyle accordingly. For example, if an individual discovered they were susceptible to heart disease they may focus their diet away from red meat and may make exercise a priority. Or if a woman learns she is susceptible to breast cancer, she may choose an elective, preventive mastectomy. The students may offer other examples related to other health conditions. The students should also give an example specific to themselves.

5. Student answers will vary. If age is described as an issue, ideas may include having a one-on-one education session with the patient or a family member, so they can use the patient portal together. If resources, such as access to a computer or internet are a barrier, investigate public areas where computers and internet could be placed, such as a library, church, or community center. If health literacy or education level is a barrier, develop appropriate educational sessions.

## Check Your Understanding 15.1

1. The ratio is 30:10, but since both numbers can be divided by 10 this can be reduced to the smallest numbers possible. 30/10 is 3 and 10/10 is 1, therefore the simplified ratio is 3:1. This information may be used by the clinic administrator to determine scheduling needs in terms of physicians who specialize in adults versus children (additional data may also be required). It can inform strategic planning and the need to determine if another pediatric physician may be needed in the future; this ratio may be used to determine where to increase or decrease staff; or it may be used when planning the supply budget or staff coverage during physician days away. It could also be used to determine skill sets needed when hiring support staff.

3. The average (mean) age is 31.86. 26 + 32 + 29 + 36 + 28 + 40 + 32 = 223. 223 divided by 7 = 31.86. The average age may indicate when females most often see an OB/GYN specialist, which may allow some target marketing within that age group, or the information may possibly indicate a need for an awareness campaign for the younger women or those in their later years. The average age may also be used with other statistical information, such as OB/GYN patients with diabetes, those who are pregnant, or those with related cancer, to determine clinical needs or the need for awareness initiatives.

5. The mode is 32. List the patient ages in order: 26, 28, 29, 32, 32, 36, 40. The mode is the number appearing most often, which is 32. This indicates that the most common age for the OB/GYN group noted is 32. This is in line with the mean and the median. If the mode were different, decisions related to the mean age of this group should be reviewed and may be revised to ensure that most of the patients in the group were considered in any actions taken.

## Check Your Understanding 15.2

1. This patient should be included in the daily census since the daily census includes all inpatients at a certain time of day (such as midnight) plus patients admitted and discharged (including deaths) in the same day. It is common for a patient to be admitted and discharged on the same day. In this case, regardless of how many hours they were an inpatient, the LOS is one day.

3. The daily inpatient census for July 16 is 247. At midnight on July 15 there were 239 inpatients; and 91 admissions are added (you count the 24 A&Ds in the admissions) and 83 discharges (you count the 24 A&Ds in the discharges) are subtracted.

5. 

| Date | Number of patients discharged | Discharge days | Average length of stay |
|---|---|---|---|
| June 2 | 16 | 86 | 5.38 |
| June 3 | 22 | 119 | 5.41 |
| June 4 | 12 | 54 | 4.50 |
| June 5 | 19 | 109 | 5.74 |
| June 6 | 15 | 45 | 3.00 |
| June 7 | 24 | 128 | 5.33 |
| June 8 | 18 | 68 | 3.78 |

### Check Your Understanding 15.3

1.

| Cases | Gross death rate | Net death rate |
|---|---|---|
| City Hospital reported 49 deaths in June. There were 489 discharges. Eight of those deaths occurred within 48 hours of admission. | 10.02% | 8.52% |
| County Hospital reported 62 deaths in May. There were 524 discharges. Seventeen of those deaths occurred within 48 hours of admission. | 11.83% | 8.88% |

The net death rate represents the quality of care more adequately because the deaths that occurred within 48 hours of admission are excluded from the calculation (both the numerator and the denominator). It is believed that if the patient was so ill they died within 48 hours of being admitted, the hospital did not have enough time to mitigate the illness.

3. The postoperative infection rate for this group of admissions is 1.23 percent. By tracking this rate for orthopedic procedures over time, a variance may be identified specifically in the orthopedic area, which may indicate a potential issue that should be investigated. The rate may also be compared against a designated target or benchmark within the orthopedic area or among all surgical patients, again allowing a way to identify any variances that may indicate a care quality issue. This measure may also be used to assess healthcare provider practice regarding medical staff credentialing.

### Check Your Understanding 15.4

1. A DRG indicates the level of resources given to a patient for an acute-care inpatient hospital episode of care. Case mix looks at the complexity of cases for the overall hospital, not just one episode of care. Both the DRG and case mix can be used for organizational planning and benchmarking. A CEO can look at the common DRGs assigned for an organization's service line to estimate future reimbursement, determine where there is opportunity for growth, and see where the organization is not as profitable or needs more marketing or competitor analysis. Case mix can assist the CEO in the same way with a focus on the organization as a whole and the level of resources required for the type of care provided in the community. Case mix may assist the CEO with payer contracting, resource planning, and profitability measures.

3. The public health officials in cities with a high mortality rate due to lung cancer may choose to do additional research to gather more data specific to their city, such as environmental and industry factors that may affect air quality, the age of homes and buildings which may have asbestos or radon, or if certain neighborhoods have a higher mortality rate from lung cancer than others. They may budget dollars to enhance community education on the dangers of smoking and the value of checking homes for asbestos and radon as well as promote programs for removal of hazardous substances. They may check on air quality and promote education in area industry as well.

5. Vital statistics data can help public health officials determine where they can make the largest impact on improving public health, where more research is needed, and where more resources (financial and human) are needed immediately and moving forward.

### Check Your Understanding 16.1

1. a. Type II error is when the null hypothesis is not rejected when it is false. Type I error is the probability of incorrectly rejecting the null hypothesis, or rejecting the null hypothesis when it is true. Type IV error does not exist.

3. c. Patient gender is nominal data—it is a category that represents names of items but does not have a natural order. Ordinal data are also expressed as categories but do have a natural order. Ratio and interval data take on a continuum of values instead of discrete categories. Their values can be added and subtracted for comparison.

## Check Your Understanding 16.2

1. b. The mean is the arithmetic average of a set of values. It is an estimate of the center of a distribution of a continuous variable. The variance, standard deviation, and range are measures of spread of a continuous variable.

3. b. The one sample t-test is used to compare a population to a standard value. Answer b is the only option comparing the actual length of stay with a standard, in this case the standard negotiated in a contract.

5. a. A larger sample size results in a narrower or more precise interval. Sample size selection is directly related to the precision of the desired confidence level.

## Check Your Understanding 16.3

1. c. The standard error of a proportion is the standard deviation divided by the square root of the sample size. The standard deviation is p*(1-p) where p is the proportion estimated from the sample.

3. b. The alternative hypothesis is the research hypothesis—the state that is to be tested. The **null hypothesis** is typically the status quo (White 2021, 76). The **alternative hypothesis** is sometimes called the research hypothesis and is a conclusion that typically requires some action to be taken (White 2021, 76).

5. c. This may be derived from the standard normal table found in most statistics textbooks or from using the following formula in Excel: = NORMSINV(0.005). NORMSINV(0.005) will return a z score that represents the point for which 0.5 percent of the curve is outside $+/-$ that point. The argument 0.005 is used because the type I error level was set to 0.01 and this is a two-sided test (0.01/2 = 0.005). The value will be 2.57. Since 3.45 > 2.57, reject the null hypothesis.

## Check Your Understanding 16.4

1. b. A positive correlation value means the two variables increase and decrease together. In other words, as BMI increases so does long volume.

3. c. The coefficient of determination is used to measure the explanatory power of the linear regression line. As previously calculated, the $r^2$ = 0.68. The years of experience of a coder explains 68 percent of the variance in coding time.

5. b. The interpretation of this relationship is that the predicted cost for a patient with a 0 LOS is $2,500. This value, $2,500, is referred to as the y-intercept of the line. The y-intercept of the regression line is the value of the dependent variable (cost) when the independent variable (length of stay [LOS]) is zero.

## Check Your Understanding 16.5

1. c. Data mining is a technique of data analytics where the analyst determines any trends and identifies patterns in the data.

3. d. Predictive modeling is a type of technique of data analytics in which statistical methods are applied to historical data to learn the patterns of the data which are used to create models of what is most likely to occur.

5. The student may choose from a variety of reasons including knowledge of the health record, code sets, reimbursement rules and regulations, communications skills, process improvement techniques, database structures, quality measures, compliance, and statistics.

### Check Your Understanding 17.1

1. A scatterplot is a chart that uses length, direction, and angle in the display. The display is developed by plotting the relationship between two quantitative variables. For example, the student can construct a scatterplot showing the relationship between the cost of care and the length of stay for a hospital's inpatient visits.

3. A line chart should be used to display this data since it is presenting data over time.

### Check Your Understanding 17.2

1. The student should create a line plot rather than use a table, because the task requires the user to view a trend over time. A table supports a task of identifying the discrete value, while a chart such as a line plot will support the task of viewing a trend over time.

3. An example of when a symbolic representation is preferred is when a patient wants to obtain their BMI level from their annual physical on January 15, from the prior year A symbolic representation of data is used when the intent is to emphasize a discrete data value. Therefore, a table is an example of a symbolic representation. If a task requires an accurate interpretation of a specific value, tables are better suited than charts.

5. The student will create both a table and a chart for this dashboard. A chart will be used to show the trend of patients who do not show up for appointments per day, and a table may be used to display the exact patient and time of the appointment for further research.

### Check Your Understanding 17.3

1. A line chart is intended to show changes in a value over time. Since the problem is asking to show the changes in revenue over a period, the line chart is the optimal graph to utilize.

3. If the data are skewed, the average will also be skewed and may not be an appropriate metric of the center of the data. In these circumstances, the median is a more appropriate measure of the center of the data, since the median is less sensitive to outliers. Therefore, one should disagree with Connie, the median is entirely appropriate.

5. The student should use a line plot to show the charges and payments by year and month. There will be two lines on the plot, one for the charges and another for payments. The total number of claims by insurance carrier is best displayed on a bar plot where the count of claims are displayed for each insurance company. The average number of days in accounts receivable and the average days to bill can be displayed as an indicator against the benchmark such as an arrow indicating if the measures are above, meeting, or below the benchmark. The total dollars in accounts receivable by age group is best displayed as a bar plot.

### Check Your Understanding 18.1

1. A qualitative research approach is suitable for assessing EHR users' satisfaction as it aims to gather in-depth insights into users' opinions, experiences, and satisfaction levels, providing an understanding of the underlying reasons and motivations related to EHR system usage.

3. This study would be categorized as applied research because it aims to solve a practical problem by determining effective strategies to increase physician engagement with EHR systems. Applied

research focuses on implementing theories into daily practice to address specific challenges, in this case, improving how physicians interact with EHR systems to enhance documentation accuracy and healthcare delivery.

5. This study intends to collect data about mobile app users' perceptions and satisfaction level by observing mobile users to interpret their app usage performance and actions related to diet and weight loss. Data collection methods can use direct observations and interviews. This is a qualitative study design with a direct observation and interview. This approach collects data by observing mobile phone app users in natural situations or predesigned settings and asks questions of users' perceptions and opinions related to app use.

## Check Your Understanding 18.2

1. The researcher should start by precisely delineating the issue of patient portal underutilization, employing the "five Ws" framework to detail who is affected, what the issue is, where it occurs, when it takes place, and why it is a concern. An illustrative problem statement could be: "In Community Health System X, the patient portal's low usage has led to an increased volume of patient inquiries by phone, undermining patient satisfaction with lab result communications and impairing staff efficiency."

3. The researcher needs to begin with creating a problem statement and research questions (EHR acceptance by physicians and the level of EHR use is unknown). Using the criteria for a well-developed research question, a possible research question may be "What is the level of EHR acceptance by physicians as determined by their level of use for each patient they see?" The researcher needs to define the purpose of the study (determine the level of EHR acceptance by physicians) and identify the gaps between the current state and desired goal (where is the acceptance level compared to the goal of full EHR use?).

5. This study is qualitative purpose research by using semi-structured interview to assess EHR users' perceptions and recommendations. The research questions should be related to the qualitative approach. An example of a question is "What do you think the benefits are of using EHRs in your practice?"

## Check Your Understanding 18.3

1. The researcher will gain knowledge (1) to orient readers to the issue and to persuade them of the necessity for the research study, (2) to assure the reader that the researcher has conducted a thorough review of all aspects of the topic, and (3) to build the researcher's knowledge of the topic. Answers may vary since there are many options, but the rationale for the choices should include the resources focused on healthcare systems, healthcare management, or other health or technology-related topics. Examples may be PubMed, since it focuses on topics in biomedicine and health; MEDLINE, since it includes topics on healthcare systems; the AHIMA Body of Knowledge, since it focuses on HIM and systems; AHRQ, since it includes content on health and healthcare interventions; and CINAHL, since it includes content on consumer health.

3. The literature review can be written in different ways and can vary in length. However, basic rules should be followed. First, a literature review should be based on the purpose of the study, so it is important to identify the purposes of the study, which in this case is to compare EHR documentation errors with patient safety issues. Second, decide what type of data (primary or secondary) is used for literature review—primary sources, such as journal articles, are recommended as much as possible. Third, search databases and identify the sources that are most appropriate and available to use. Databases such as PubMed, Google Scholar, and MEDLINE are examples of places to find primary sources on documentation errors and patient safety.

5. Focusing on primary sources is crucial for the researcher because these sources provide original, firsthand accounts of research, offering the most direct evidence about the topic being studied. For a

literature review on AI technology in diagnostics, primary sources such as clinical trials and original research articles are essential. They provide detailed data on the effectiveness and outcomes of AI implementations. The researcher should look for statistical results and insights into operational changes following AI integration to understand the practical implications of AI technologies in healthcare.

## Check Your Understanding 18.4

1. The researcher should use an "evaluation research" design for this study. This design is ideal because it allows for a systematic examination of how the introduction of mobile devices affects specific outcomes, such as the accuracy of patient data entry and the speed at which it is done. By using evaluation research, the researcher can gather both quantitative data (for example, error rates in data entry, time taken for data recording) and qualitative feedback (for example, user satisfaction, perceived ease of use) from healthcare providers. This comprehensive approach provides a holistic view of the mobile devices' effectiveness and efficiency in a high-pressure environment like an emergency department.

3. Answers may vary, but there should be two variables—one described as independent (the one that is adjusted or manipulated in the study), and one described as dependent (the one being measured to see if and how it changes as the independent variable is manipulated). For example, if the independent variable is the hours spent studying and the dependent variable is the grade on an exam, the number of hours spent studying can be adjusted (independent variable) and the exam grade can be measured accordingly (dependent variable).

5. Evaluation research design is a type of applied research best used in a real-world experience. The answers from this question vary based upon each student's experience or research and variation of the setting and type of EHR systems. They may identify user training, availability of support and assistance, level of staffing, time for users to complete a task, functionality of the system, and the like.

## Check Your Understanding 18.5

1. To evaluate the effectiveness of newly implemented telehealth services in a specialty clinic, the researcher should use surveys for quantitative insights on user satisfaction and operational metrics, and interviews for qualitative feedback on user experiences and challenges. This mixed-methods approach ensures a comprehensive understanding of the telehealth system's impact, capturing both broad trends and in-depth user perspectives.

3. The researcher could opt for a four-point scale to quantify confidence levels. However, a Likert five-point scale would be more effective as it allows respondents to express varying degrees of agreement or disagreement, providing a nuanced understanding of their confidence in EHR use. For even more detailed responses, an expanded Likert scale might be appropriate.

5. Interviews are best used when the need is for in-depth information from individuals. Observations provide direct viewing and experience in using the electronic display boards. Both methods are appropriate to use for this study, as interviews of clinicians for assessing their perceptions and experiences from using the device, and observation studies to get real measured facts.

## Check Your Understanding 18.6

1. Content analysis is essential in HIM because it provides a systematic way to review and interpret data within EHRs. This process helps identify significant trends and patterns in health data, which are critical for informed clinical decision-making. By understanding these patterns, healthcare providers can make better decisions that enhance patient care, ensuring the data used is both relevant and of high quality. This supports effective and efficient healthcare delivery, optimizing patient outcomes and resource utilization.

3. Grounded theory methods are particularly valuable when the topic of interest has not previously been studied; for example, to study a new technology or device applied to a weight-loss program. Grounded theory can be applied to bring structure and rigor to the analysis of qualitative data. In the case of hard-to-reach populations, the ability for direct observation and data gathering is particularly challenging, making use of grounded theory more difficult since this technique relies on analysis of the data as it is collected, that is, grounded in data.

5. NVivo is a qualitative data analysis software that aids in organizing, categorizing, and visualizing data, which can streamline the analysis process. However, it is important to clarify to the quality director that while NVivo can enhance the efficiency of data handling, the critical tasks of analysis and interpretation still rely on the researcher's expertise and judgment. NVivo supports the process but does not replace the researcher's analytical role.

### Check Your Understanding 18.7

**Instructions: Answer the following questions in a separate document.**

1. To understand the interpretation of Dr. Smith's study results, the HIM student should refer to the "Discussion" section of the research paper. This section goes beyond stating the findings and includes the researcher's insights, implications of the results, and how they tie into the broader context of the field, providing a comprehensive interpretation.

3. The director of HIM should include on the poster the purpose (evaluating the use of the organizations' patient portal), methods used (she may have held focus groups or distributed surveys, and possibly she looked at utilization data showing overall numbers and characteristics of users), and results of her study (results may include the percent of the patient population using the portal, the geographic region or age of those using the portal versus those not using the portal, the reasons patients do not use the portal, the value that patients see in the portal, and the like). She should also include a discussion of the results and conclusion (limitations in the results and ideas for further study). The poster should be attractive, colorful, and easily readable (large font, white space, and some color). She may also want to have a copy of the research report or a summary available to distribute to those interested.

5. Incorporating multimedia elements such as charts, graphs, and videos can significantly enhance the dissemination of research results on social media by providing clear visual summaries of key points. These elements make complex information more accessible and engaging for a wider audience, thereby increasing the impact and reach of the content. This visual approach can also prompt more shares and discussions, extending the visibility of the research findings within and beyond the health information management community.

### Check Your Understanding 19.1

1. The evolution of ethical guidelines from the Nuremberg Code to the Declaration of Helsinki significantly enhanced the integrity and public trust in medical research by prioritizing the protection of human subjects. These guidelines established rigorous standards for informed consent and independent ethical review, ensuring transparency and participant safety. Consequently, this fostered a more ethical research environment, leading to more credible and trustworthy research outcomes.

3. The major changes are (1) informed consent documents that are shorter and clearer and (2) increased focus on studies that pose more risk. A possible benefit is that potential research subjects can more readily understand the research study and what the study entails. This has ethical implications—subjects obviously will be better informed, and this may impact the number of subjects participating in research studies.

5. The Office for Human Research Protections (OHRP) of the HHS provides leadership and educational programs in this area. The OHRP website has developed online programs such as miniature tutorials and videos that can be adapted for organizational use related to human research protection.

## Check Your Understanding 19.2

1. This research may qualify for exempt status under the HHS Federal Policy regulations, specifically due to its educational context and nature.

3. IRB approval influences the design and implementation of COVID-19 vaccine trials by ensuring ethical considerations are integrated into every aspect of the study. This includes safeguarding participant consent, assessing risk-benefit ratios, and ensuring confidentiality of data. Specific examples of ethical considerations addressed by the IRB include ensuring informed consent is comprehensible, monitoring for adverse effects, and making provisions for vulnerable populations to prevent exploitation and ensure equitable participation.

5. The prisoner can legally participate in the research study even though he or she is considered a vulnerable subject; however, there may need to be additional safeguards included in the study to protect the participant.

## Check Your Understanding 19.3

1. The individuals who were exposed (the case) are 3.7 times more likely to have the disease than those not exposed to the environment factors (the control).

3. 
|  | With Hypertension (cases) | Without Hypertension (controls) | Total |
| --- | --- | --- | --- |
| Fast Food >2 times/wk | 50 | 50 | 100 |
| Fast Food <=2 times/wk | 100 | 100 | 200 |
| Total | 150 | 150 | 300 |

Odds of exposure for cases = 50/100 = 0.5
Odds of exposure for controls = 50/100 = 0.5
Odds ratio = 0.5/0.5 = 1.0

5. Authorization for release of data for research purposes. A signed authorization from subjects is required. This authorization must be specific to a specific project with a specific purpose. The research is violating the Privacy Rule because the data that has been authorized for one project is now being used for a different project that the subject has not explicitly authorized in writing.

## Check Your Understanding 19.4

1. Blue Cross would likely prioritize NCQA measures in their contract discussions. NCQA's performance measures are specifically designed to inform healthcare purchasers, including insurers like Blue Cross, about the quality and cost-effectiveness of healthcare organizations. These measures help them determine the value of contracting with specific providers. While the Joint Commission's measures focus on organizational performance improvement and comprehensive care quality, NCQA measures align more closely with the interests of healthcare payers in terms of cost and quality assurance.

3. A priority of the National Quality Strategy in Person and Family-Centered Care is to increase the use of EHRs by integrating patient-generated data in EHRs and routinely measuring patient engagement, self-management, shared decision-making, and patient-reported outcomes. One of its indicators for doing this is to collect the percentage of patients asked for feedback. This is an example of how the EHR will be used to demonstrate at what rate the patient is involved in his or her care, and patient-centered outcomes research will be a major component in this data analysis.

5. Patient-centered outcomes research will include research important to the patient and include data elements related to survival, functional status, health-related quality of life, and such, instead of just

clinical data elements collected by investigators. It will also ask questions most important to patients such as, what are the benefits and harms related to different treatment options provided?

## Check Your Understanding 20.1

1. Theory X may be appropriate in a repetitive assembly line type of job where production is valued over creativity. In this situation, employees may be more effective with clear guidelines and goals.

3. Organizations who utilize the SEAM model focus on the worth of the individual employee. Feeling respected and valued may increase employees' productivity since they feel their contribution matters. They will feel more invested in their work and in the success of the organization if they are asked for their input and listened to.

5. Use a grid to break the project down into discrete steps and list them vertically on the left side. On the upper line of the chart, designate the days over time horizontally to complete the project. Then draw a bar from the beginning date to the end date of each task as the tasks progress across the time grid.

## Check Your Understanding 20.2

1. The student should list each task and identify it as conceptual, interpersonal, or technical. Given the level of the job (front-line, supervisor, middle management, and so forth), an estimate of the appropriate percentage of each type of skills should be noted.

3. As work has become more complex and requires people at all levels to be accountable and responsive, and as they have become better trained, some leadership functions have been distributed more widely throughout the organization according to the competency level of the person.

5. Students' answers will vary, but they should choose three of the paradigms from the table, identify if their organization falls more in the traditional or modern management paradigm, and offer reasons why they made that determination.

## Check Your Understanding 20.3

1. The students will identify two different situations such as a work team at their job and a sports team, or a work team and a project team in a course, or others. For each situation, personal traits and skills will be listed with an indicator such as a plus or minus next to each, depending on whether it is an advantage or disadvantage in that situation. A brief explanation of the skills needed for each situation is included in the response with rationale for why some traits are more or less advantageous in these different situations.

3. The student should describe a situation where they recognize effective leadership and a situation where they recognize ineffective leadership. The student could make two columns—one for effective and one for ineffective leaders—and identify the traits of each in the appropriate column. Each student and situation will be different, but they may list effective traits such as caring, empowering, and being a good listener; and ineffective traits such as being self-serving, disengaged, disrespectful, and such.

5. Some of the unintended consequences may be that even though the manager's intent was to show that the staff are valued, they now need to find time to do extra work in the day in addition to their daily duties so that may cause resentment, frustration with the manager or co-workers, fatigue, less quality in their daily work, and/or a less than quality solution to their task. In addition, other departments may be affected by either process or staffing changes. Staff may not actually want to change their hours; they were tasked with completing a task they have not bought into.

### Check Your Understanding 20.4

1. Each of the roles involves a special skill at a key time period in innovation. The inventor role occurs when the idea is created, but the inventor may not have the skill or authority to move further with it. The champion role is important and next in sequence since it involves recognition of the value of the idea and provides resources for development. The sponsor provides authority and legitimacy, while the final role of critic ensures it is thought through clearly.

3. Each adopter group is motivated by different values and outcomes. By identifying each one and their unique needs, the innovation can be presented in ways that are meaningful to them and engender less resistance to the innovation.

5. The manager can create a list of the benefits of the new software, identify the existing skill sets of the staff compatible with the new system, describe the new system and the process to implement as simply as possible so staff are not overwhelmed, provide an opportunity to demonstrate and possibly even use the system prior to implementation (or even prior to selection), ask for input and feedback often, and move slowly through the process. These are ideas identified as factors that may enhance responsiveness to change.

### Check Your Understanding 20.5

1. People may resist change due to not knowing what will happen to their jobs, not knowing whether they will lose prestige or turf, feeling they have lost control, feeling they do not have time to get used to the change, the change being suddenly presented without warning, concerns about competence, feeling overwhelmed with the prospect of more work, and such. For all these reasons, managers and leaders need to prepare them early for change, let them know what will be the same and what will be different, reassure them that they will get through the change, provide training for new skills, and the like.

3. People may react with anxiety regarding whether they are qualified for the new position; they may wonder whether they are targeted to be forced out; or they may take it as a message to look elsewhere for a job. Management can reduce the stress by explaining why the position is being restructured, identifying the skills required, and holding information sessions on the pending change. Possibly management would offer information about open positions that a displaced employee could apply for.

5. The student should include a list of the culture characteristics of each organization and identify the similarities and differences. For example, if one culture runs loosely relying on experienced employees to make independent decisions, and the other tends to be more closely supervised and directive, this would be a source of potential conflict. By identifying shared culture characteristics, they have a common core from which to negotiate the more diverse characteristics.

### Check Your Understanding 21.1

1. In strategy development it is just as important to determine what not to do as it is to determine what your key priority strategies are going forward. For example, a college might decide to focus on traditional, on-campus students rather than adding online programs. This decision may be made if the needs of the community served cannot be maintained due to high demand. Another example—an organization might strategically decide to not purchase a company for sale because it determines the company does not fit their strategic profile.

3. Students will evaluate and explain the importance of the role of some of the following individuals: customer, patients, managers, employees, board of trustees, clinicians, and community stakeholders. Their examples will vary but the student may identify key stakeholders for an EHR upgrade as the

patient who is concerned with the quality of their experience, the clinicians who are concerned with the speed and access to their documentation, and the board of directors who may be concerned with the reputation of the facility and the related financial status.

5. Phase I: Environmental Assessment (which includes the elements of organizational overview, strategic profile, internal and external assessments, competition, areas of excellence, and key planning assumptions) is a research phase of gathering information both externally and internally; Phase II: Identify Organizational Direction (which includes the elements of future vision, mission and values, future organizational direction, and areas of excellence) is taking the information from the research found in phase I and focuses on making a vision and direction for the future; Phase III: Strategy Formulation (which includes the elements of scenario building, future critical success factors, future strategic profile, competitive analysis, and new strategies, strategic goals, strategic objectives, and innovations) is different from phase II because it begins translating the new vision into strategy and testing that strategy using new tools; Phase IV: Implementation Plan (which includes the elements of implementation framework, implementation plan, and next steps) takes the new strategy and creates a detailed implementation plan.

### Check Your Understanding 21.2

1. Review healthcare industry forces and primary market research; assess market forecasts; analyze competitors; identify potential collaborators and demographics; and assess market trends. One example is identifying external changes that may impact HIM department planning, which would include the need to determine how technology, governmental regulations, and mergers may impact the HIM department (forces in the healthcare industry and primary market research). Identifying potential collaborators such as the IT division and regional or state health information exchange (identify potential collaborators). Researching the demographics in the student's region will be important (demographics).

3. Clear trends (Apply: how electronic medical records are showing increased consumer interest in accessing their PHR electronically, too); Unknown knowable (Apply: how many patients are retiring and moving out of the area each year?); Residual uncertainty (Apply: will legislation regarding price transparency be passed in the next legislative session?).

5. The strengths and weaknesses of an organization, department, or college are helpful internal environmental assessment tools in the SWOT analysis, while the opportunities and threats describe external environmental aspects of an organization or college. Review the individual responses to their SWOT analysis of their organization, department, or college.

### Check Your Understanding 21.3

1. An effective vision statement includes three of these:
   - Conveys a memorable and simple picture of the future
   - Evokes strong emotion and creates a strong sense of urgency
   - Is clear enough to provide guidance in decision-making
   - Is flexible so alternative strategies are possible as conditions change
   - Is easy to describe and communicate

   Example HIM Vision: *All members of the care team and management will have immediate access to complete and accurate information for each resident to improve patient care, quality, and timeliness.*

3. An area of excellence refers to a describable skill, competency, or capability an organization cultivates to be of the highest quality. Examples might include recruiting excellent HIM professionals, providing accurate coding services, or collaborating with the IT division. Explain why they are

important. For example, turnover will be reduced with the ability to recruit strong HIM professionals; coding denials and revenue collections will be improved with accurate coding services; and implementation will be more effective by collaborating with the IT division.

5. A strategy is an action or set of actions that moves the organization toward its vision—a picture of the desired future state of the organization. Strategic management identifies the set of activities to help realize the vision. Strategic management helps define strategies and related activities therein.

### Check Your Understanding 21.4

1. Describe scenario building and storytelling. (1) Storytelling about possible future states suggested by the external and internal assessment of trends of the department, organization, or college can help build an understandable and emotional story that creates long-lasting value for a business. One story example might be about "What if the HIM department at College XYZ developed a doctoral degree in which current educators and professionals could advance their education and research?" This story can be elaborated on with insights from HIM alumni and other stakeholders. (2) Scenario building can be used to develop different future states and test them against the critical success factors, such as, "What if this doctoral degree was in HIM governance, health data security, or data analytics?" Reflect on the different alternatives and their risks and opportunities in each scenario.

3. A college might offer graduate programs (current products offered) and determine in the future they want to offer undergraduate programs (future products offered). They may serve traditional students (current customers) and decide to begin to also serve nontraditional students (future customers). They may currently serve the X region (current geographic location) and now they want to add in a new region for their college (future geographic location). The industry is higher education, and the market is graduate program (current), and the future industry is still higher education and the future market is now graduate and undergraduate programs.

5. Deciding what to do (and therefore not to do) sets the direction for an organization. By deciding a set of strategies, it demonstrates importance to an organization and prioritizes what to resource. This is critical and has implications for existing programs and services.

### Check Your Understanding 21.5

1. For effective implementation within a busy organization, understanding who will be accountable, timelines, allocation of resources, and measurements are important to ensure success. For example, each step in the plan should have a timeframe and deadline for completion, each task should be assigned to an individual who is accountable to complete it, there should be enough resources including staff to achieve the plan, and there should be specific measures which will indicate whether tasks are being met as expected.

3. A well-defined strategy leads to detailed strategic goals and objectives that include timelines, who's responsible, and resources needed. Ideally, each student will have a unique response. Examples of a response might include:

   a. AHIMA will utilize evidence-based research to determine the quality and variation of the data elements being entered into EHRs throughout the patient's care process from registration to discharge.

   b. Develop a patient process and data map that describes the key data elements collected from admission to discharge. Then, conduct a meta-analysis of all evidence-based literature on the accuracy of the key data elements.

   c. With a process mapping consultant, gather a multidisciplinary team of caregivers and patients to determine the key data elements throughout the patient's care process from admission to discharge. Person(s) responsible: quality director and HIM director, first quarter 2020 (January 1 to March 31, 2020); resource needs: process mapping facilitator ($2,500), mapping software ($200), committee full-day retreat (room rental, food, and staff time are $200, $450, and 64 hours at $35 per hour on average for all staff time).

### Check Your Understanding 21.6

1. Change management refers to the tools and approaches that help the team work together successfully to implement the changes identified during the strategic planning process. Collaboration is one change management technique for managing the political dimensions of change. The use of collaborations can be a force for positive change, and leaders can use collaboration to build support for change because they engage other important stakeholders in the process. If an organization recognizes the need for change, it can use tools and techniques such as collaboration to ensure successful implementation of strategic planning outcomes.

3. The four perspectives are customer, financial, internal process, and learning and growth. Examples of *customer* would be implementing a PHR consumer advisory board; *financial* perspective could be defined as showing a reduction in the total cost of care because of consumers getting engaged in their care using the PHR; *internal process* would be finding ways for clinicians to engage and utilize the PHR more extensively to support their patients; and *learning and growth* might include a focus on physicians' and clinicians' use of the PHR more effectively.

5. c. The more all key stakeholders can be involved in the strategic planning process from the early stages, the more likely the plan will be supported and implemented. Communicating with the stakeholders throughout the planning process is critical. Stakeholders will support what they help create.

### Check Your Understanding 22.1

1. Answers will vary. An aging workforce can impact staffing as employees reach retirement; compounding the impact of an aging workforce is a continually changing workplace in healthcare. For example, many coders retired earlier than they may have otherwise when ICD-10 was implemented. The same could hold true as computer-assisted coding and ICD-11 are implemented. The existing staff in HIM are finding that with the electronic health record (EHR) there is a greater need for skills related to technology and data analytics. Constant changes in regulations require continuous training for CDI staff, and training on processes and reimbursement; for example, in Accountable Care Organizations (ACOs) and healthcare homes. HR is challenged with staff turnover through retirements, retaining staff through the technology and regulatory changes, recruiting staff with the adequate skills and knowledge, training managers on managing change and transition, and assisting managers with skills to manage a variety of age groups and cultures to ensure high motivation and morale.

3. The Occupational Safety and Health Act (OSHA) is designed to assess and address health-related hazards associated with the use of technology and workstation ergonomics. Ashley should work with the HR department to determine how to proceed to have Eva's workstation assessed for comfort.

5. Larry should tell her about the Family Medical Leave Act (FMLA) of 1993 This allows unpaid leave for certain health reasons related to one's family or self without fear of losing one's job.

### Check Your Understanding 22.2

1. The student should use the template in figure 22.2 to create this job description.

3. As the hiring manager, you will decide if you'd like to post the position internally first or not. You may want to discuss this with your management team or HR. Once you have decided, you will post the position using information from the job description. While you wait for applications to become available, you will develop selection criteria to use with each candidate. Possibly you will use the interviewing and selection worksheet or the decision matrix. When a sufficient pool of applications has been received, you will review the cover letters, resumes, or applications and determine three to four candidates to interview. You will interview each, being careful not to ask any unlawful

questions, and document each candidate's qualifications. You will perform background and reference checks on the qualified candidates and once you have all the information from the interviews and background or reference checks, you will decide.

5. Any question violating discrimination law. Examples are as follows: What year did you graduate from high school? (Age discrimination.) Do you plan on having more children? (Pregnancy discrimination.) Do you belong to any groups in town? (Could be getting at religion, national origin, race, sex, or age discrimination.)

### Check Your Understanding 22.3

1. Constructive confrontation brings the conflicting parties together with an objective third-party to moderate a conversation about their perceptions and feelings with the intent of arriving at an understanding of each employees' perspectives and fostering understanding.

3. Tom has reached the end of the probationary period and is very close but has not achieved the required quality level. If this is the first time the supervisor has officially met with Tom related to his performance, she may want to discuss the quality level concerns with Tom and ask him what resources he needs to meet the quality level. She can begin the progressive discipline process with a verbal warning if she has not already discussed concerns with him. Then she will set up a plan with his input to follow throughout the month to increase his quality to the required 95 percent level. If she has discussed his performance before this time, she may be further in the progressive discipline process—possibly issuing a written warning. If Tom is unable to meet the quality standards moving forward, per the progressive discipline policy, it will result in suspension or termination.

5. Because Bernice is meeting performance expectations at work and has not shown any indication of alcohol use during work hours, the supervisor should do nothing. Employers need to stay out of the personal lives of employees unless there are job-related issues to address. The supervisor may want to also work on enhancing a positive culture in the department in which employees support each other.

### Check Your Understanding 23.1

1. A potential plan for John's development may be as follows:

   | | |
   |---|---|
   | Week 1 | Organization and departmental orientation |
   | Week 1–4 | Training on the new job |
   | Ongoing | In-service education on developing new skills |
   | Month 6 | Participate in CE in inpatient coding |
   | Year 1 | Move to an inpatient coding position (career development) |
   | Year 2 | Advance to a lead coding position (career development) |

3. Answers should address such items as the curriculum, budget, who will teach the program, materials to be developed, location, and method of delivery. These should be based on the results of the needs assessment.

5. Answers will vary.

   Reaction:
   - Are members of the audience asking questions regarding the content which indicates interest?

   Learning:
   - Can the audience members answer appropriately when given scenarios based on ROI cases?
   - Can they give examples of inappropriate behavior regarding patient privacy? (for example, talking about patients in common areas).

Behavior:
- Have incidents of improper disclosure been reduced?

Results:
- Did all employees of the organization receive the training?

## Check Your Understanding 23.2

1. An employee orientation program introduces employees to the following:
   - Organization's mission, policies, rules, and culture
   - Department or work unit
   - Specific job he or she will be performing

   The orientation program also provides a period of socialization in which the employee learns the values, behavior patterns, and expectations of the organization. This is important to retaining staff since key pieces of employee satisfaction are feeling knowledgeable, competent, and welcome.

3. The components of orientation and in-service education programs that are similar include:

   Relevance to the job: In both new employee orientation and in-service training for experienced employees, education is most beneficial when the content specifically applies to the employee's work.

   Quality: When evaluating any educational program, it is important to obtain audience feedback on the quality of the content and presentation.

   Content: Audience evaluation of most and least useful sections of orientation and continuing in-service education sessions is used to improve future programs.

   Length: Depending on the content and the delivery method used, program length may contribute to lost interest and boredom if the session is too long, or frustration if it is too short. Either way, the learning conditions are not optimal.

   Instructor Rating: Instructors are evaluated on presentation skills, such as clarity of voice, speed of the presentation, knowledge of the subject matter, and willingness to answer questions.

   Training Materials: Were handouts relevant to the topic(s)? Handouts should be clearly organized and written at an understandable reading level. They should also pertain to the topics covered.

   Components that are different:

   Delivery method: Hands-on training would likely not be included in an in-service. In-service programs build on the basic skills learned through new employee orientation. Hands-on training would be used during orientation to the job.

   Registration: Orientation is coordinated by the employer and registration is typically not necessary. In-service education may require registration, especially if conducted outside the organization.

   Logistics (location, parking, accessibility): Most components of an orientation take place on-site at the employee's place of work. In-service opportunities may be internal or external to the organization.

## Check Your Understanding 23.3

1. The student should provide their own example and should include some of the following information: Diversity training programs might include topics such as review of other cultures from a social studies perspective, cultural norms such as communication styles, behaviors that may be considered offensive in one culture and not another, and perspectives on other cultures on privacy issues. Some employees may need training in English reading and writing skills, interpersonal communication skills, and customer service. Anti-harassment training should also be included.

3. Answers may vary but should reference the need to consider individual employee needs regarding personal responsibilities, job requirements, and career goals. Employees may not be able to attend that early or on Saturday if they have childcare to consider, for example. By calling attention to the relevance of training to specific needs and connecting the knowledge learned with a work goal, training can be facilitated for each employee. Incentives such as overtime pay or time off in the future would show that administration values an employee's contribution to the work of the medical center.

5. The best combination of learning methods is a combination of verbal instruction, demonstration, and hands-on experience. Sarah should explain the policies on confidentiality, demonstrate through example how to keep data secure and how data may be at risk, then provide scenarios for the coders to role play correct behavior.

## Check Your Understanding 23.4

1. Since the employees are geographically dispersed, an e-learning method, such as an interactive webinar, would provide trainees with the opportunity to interact, and would apply to learners of various skill levels, and reduce costs. Use of simulations, such as a MUVE, would also be appropriate, and provide employees with the opportunity to act out decisions through avatars. A disadvantage might be the possibility of a technical problem and finding a time convenient for all.

3. Mobile learning (m-learning) would be suitable for delivering short content, key points, and updates to many learners who need anytime and anyplace learning quickly. Participants can respond using social media or discussion. It is not effective for long courses with a large amount of material. Live or recorded webinars would also be appropriate for asynchronous delivery in a convenient form.

5. Janice might use a case study followed by role playing. Case studies present opportunities for problem solving, critical thinking, and decision-making using a simulated scenario. Role playing permits learners to practice interviewing by acting out a response to a hypothetical situation.

7. Mentoring is a proactive approach where an employee chooses someone from within the organization for guidance. Coaching is generally initiated by the manager or supervisor to adjust certain behaviors. Other differences include:

   - Coaching is for a short term, while mentoring lasts for a longer duration.
   - Coaching is well planned and structured, while mentoring is informal.
   - In coaching, coaches give clear and intentional feedback and regularly supervise your performance on tasks. In a mentorship, supervision is less formal.

## Check Your Understanding 23.5

1. The supervisor could provide time and support for David to work on the changes, delegate decision-making for the design of the form, and suggest resources or classes on screen design.

3. John should offer suggestions for where Julie might find the knowledge she needs. A better response would be, "Review this material and then try deciding on your own. I'll ask Lisa [another more advanced coding professional] to work with you on these records. She has a great deal of background in coding cardiology charts and can provide feedback to help you do better."

5. Answers may vary but could include the following: (1) location—should be accessible to those with mobility issues—ADA 1990; (2) access to CBT for those that have sight challenges—ADA, Rehab Act of 1973; (3) fire evacuation procedures—OSHA of 1970.

### Check Your Understanding 24.1

1. John should ask the staff (both those able to work remotely and those staying on-site) what their needs and ideas are. John should also check in with facility planners to determine if there are any structural or design constraints. The student answers may vary on how the space should be redesigned, but ideas include adding meeting space for staff and removing stationary desks and replacing them with more temporary, flexible workstations, along with plenty of outlets to accommodate remote workers when they need to be on-site occasionally. Workstations for on-site workers may need to move to accommodate workflow and process changes due to fewer people as well any changes due to the new EHR functionality. Since the work environment would change, this is an opportunity to ensure proper wall color, lighting, and ergonomics are assessed.

3. The student should develop two diagrams—one using the existing workflow and one with an improved workflow. They should move furniture or equipment as necessary in the improved workflow and adjust the movement lines, accordingly, using figure 24.1 as a guide to illustrate the improvement.

5. Lighting should be sufficiently bright; exposure to natural light is easiest on the eyes, and desk or task lighting is more physically supportive than overhead fluorescent lighting. Glare from light or PC screens should be avoided. Color influences how people feel. For instance, neutral colors have a calming effect. Certain kinds of music can reduce tension, and soundproofing can make an office less noisy. Carpeting, drapes, and partitioning all affect the noise level because they absorb sound. Air that is too warm or cold can be distracting, so temperature is also important for an effective workspace. The student should then state whether remote work should be a consideration for staff considering these factors and the ability to meet aesthetic best practices.

### Check Your Understanding 24.2

1. Since there do not appear to be acceptable applicants even after a month's time and there is a three-person shortage, the option to continue to handle the work internally with extra hours does not seem like a viable option. Even though there is an increased level of productivity and quality control with internal staff, the ability to obtain and retain experienced staff and meet productivity needs is an issue. Temporarily outsourcing may be a good option if there is an expectation for getting strong applicants soon. Permanently outsourcing may be a good option if staffing in this area is a consistent problem. When outsourcing, it is critical to evaluate the cost compared to internal (should the staffing be acceptable) and to ensure quality, confidentiality, and control over the work product.

3. Angela should conduct a work distribution analysis that documents what employees are spending their time on to reveal potential problem areas such as the following:

   - There is too much or too little job function specialization.
   - There is duplication of efforts of functions.
   - Some employees are overloaded while others do not have enough work to keep them busy.
   - Large amounts of time are spent on functions of minor importance.
   - Small amounts of time are spent on functions of key importance.

   Depending on what Angela discovers in the work distribution analysis, she may need to look at revisions to job training, workflow, process and procedures, and employee performance.

5. Cyclical staffing should be explored to rotate less desirable evening and weekend shifts across the staff. There may be an opportunity to explore shift differential so staff could make more money for the new shifts. Other alternative staffing methods could also be explored, such as a compressed work week. It will be important to be in constant communication with staff, allowing them to ask questions and voice concerns to help ease their concerns and gain buy-in as well.

### Check Your Understanding 24.3

1. When benchmarking, it is important to evaluate others in relevant situations. Different hospitals may have different service lines and complexity of cases. A regional medical center with a newborn intensive care unit (NICU) will have more complex cases that take longer to code than a community hospital that focuses on normal deliveries and newborns. Possibly, one hospital has implemented computer-assisted coding and another has not, affecting expected coding standards. Varying processes and staff experience levels may make a difference.

3. The student should offer a quantitative standard which addresses productivity (work done over time or the amount of time to do work) and a qualitative standard which addresses level of service (such as turnaround time or accuracy rates). An example for a student may be: Quantitative—Read three pages per minute; Qualitative—Receive 95 percent of the points on each assignment.

5. The staff may welcome a work measurement study to assist with setting realistic production standards and possibly an incentive pay system. It may also help with ensuring proper staffing levels. The student answers may vary but some may feel intimidated if work measurement is being done in their work unit, possibly fearful performance is not as expected, unwelcome changes may be made, or they will be admonished in some way. Others will be neutral or excited that the results may help with improving the work environment through better process, equipment, staffing, or pay.

### Check Your Understanding 24.4

1. Preventive controls are put in place at the front end of a process to ensure an error is not made, such as edits in a computer system or employee training. Feedback controls occur after a task is done, offering information regarding the performance, such as an employee review or a customer satisfaction survey. Answers may vary. One example of a preventive control may be to schedule time each day on the calendar for studying so that you save the time and receive a reminder from your calendar. One example of a feedback control is to review each assignment grade and instructor comments.

3. Performance measurement is a fundamental management activity that supports two basic functions of management—planning and controlling. The manager defines objectives, goals, and expectations of performance as a part of the planning function. Performance measurement is the process of comparing the outcomes of an organization, work unit, or employee to those preestablished performance standards as a part of the controlling function.

5. The manager may want to start with communication with the employees, asking for their input on why the variance may be occurring. Depending on that discussion, examples of changes to address performance issues could be additional staff training, modifications in procedures, adjustments in workflow, revision of policies, or purchase of updated equipment.

### Check Your Understanding 24.5

1. Sam has a good process, but she did not take the time to determine who are the customers of each key process so the customers' expectations could be met. Once she begins to measure what is important to the customer, complaints are likely to decrease.

3. The ROI function can be illustrated using the system diagram. *Inputs:* The request for records goes to the ROI staff and is logged (standards and controls). *Process:* Staff ensure request is complete and valid (using ROI regulations which are controls and standards) and obtain and process the records for release. *Outputs:* The records are sent to the requestor and the request is documented as complete (standards and controls). *Feedback:* Productivity and status tracking of requests. External environment: State and federal laws impacting what and how records can be released.

5. The board of directors is an internal customer because they may request information that assists them with strategic decision making for the facility. Registration staff may be an internal customer if they are seeking assistance or information to help identify an incoming patient. An attorney or law enforcement official is an external customer seeking authorized release of patient information. A bond agency may be an external customer who seeks organization performance information to assign a bond rating for seeking loans or financing.

## Check Your Understanding 24.6

1. Since the group is vocal, they want their ideas heard; and because they are a varied team, they may have differing perspectives so they may need to come together on all their ideas. Recommended tools would be brainstorming so all are heard, possibly affinity grouping so they could work toward common themes, and NGT to help bring to them to agreement on lab system-related processes and priorities.

3. The swimlane diagram is a basic visual tool to show each step of a process, the sequence of the steps, and who is doing each.

5. The coding manager should use a run chart to show how productivity and quality are (hopefully) increasing from week to week. If the results are not showing the increase expected or desired (or even if they are), the coding manager may wish to ask the staff what issues are occurring, possibly using a brainstorming technique to get communication flowing, or a fishbone diagram to look at possible cause and effect.

## Check Your Understanding 25.1

1. The HIM department is often the area responsible for the coding of the records. While this is important in the billing process, the actual claims are filed by the patient accounts department. Therefore, the insurance company should be referred to the patient accounts department for resolution. If there is an individual who is specifically responsible for handling billing audits, that individual is an appropriate referral. Part of the claims audit may involve a review of the medical records. In that case, the HIM department will provide access to the records in the department, if necessary. Depending on the organization's structure, the compliance department may also be involved.

3. This is not a good strategy as it violates the matching principle (figure 25.2). While the hospital should certainly make every effort to capture all the associated expenses for this fiscal year, next year's expenses must be booked next year. If some of next year's expenses are actually paid this year, they would not be recorded as expenses but rather as assets under the heading *prepaid expenses*.

5. Clinic B would consider this to be a material error because it represents a 12.5 percent (10,000/80,000) error and could affect decision-making, while for Clinic A, this is an immaterial amount and will not affect decision-making.

## Check Your Understanding 25.2

1. 12/31/23: 50/600 = 0.083 or 8.3 percent, 12/31/24: 100/785 = 0.127 or 12.7 percent. The total margin ratio indicates that for every dollar of revenue, the organization earned a profit of 0.12 cents in 2024. The 12/31/24 total margin ratio is higher than 12/31/23 and therefore more favorable.

3. The three key reports are the income statement, statement of retained earnings or net assets, and balance sheet.

The income statement includes revenues and expenses. The statement of retained earnings or net assets expresses the change in retained earnings from the beginning of the balance sheet period to the end. Net income and loss are carried forward from the income statement. The balance sheet lists the major account categories grouped under their equation headings—assets, liabilities, and retained earnings or net assets—and employs the equation: assets = liabilities + retained earnings or net assets. The ending balance in retained earnings or net assets is then reported on the balance sheet.

5. The best ratio to use for this analysis is the current ratio—an organization's ability to pay current liabilities with current assets is important to lenders. Current assets implicitly will be (or could be) converted to cash at some point within a year, either through collections, sales, or other business activity. The current ratio compares total current assets with total current liabilities.

### Check Your Understanding 25.3

1. Examples of direct costs include nursing salaries, bedding supplies, pharmacy, physician salaries. Indirect costs include security, maintenance, human resources, accounting, billing.

3. The three major categories of controls are preventive, detective, and corrective. Strong passwords are an example of a preventive control because it prevents unauthorized users from accessing a network.

5. Monthly lease costs on a surgery center would be fixed because the amount remains constant regardless of the volume. Disposable supplies for a surgical robot are variable based on the number of surgeries performed. Wages for RNs in the OR would be mixed because a certain number of RNs will be required to operate the OR regardless of volume; however, when volume increases, the number of RNs will increase as well.

### Check Your Understanding 25.4

1. Both branches of accounting deal with the recording, reporting, and analysis of transactions. However, financial accounting focuses on the financial statements and the needs of the users of those statements. Managerial accounting focuses on internal measurements of financial performance, such as budgets. An HIM manager is most likely to participate in managerial accounting, such as personnel and operational budgeting and capital budgeting as well.

3. Calculating and explaining variances would be both preventive and detective controls. Following up on budget variances can be both preventive and corrective so that a department does not exceed budget in future months.

5. This is an unfavorable variance because revenue is $400,000 less than budgeted.

### Check Your Understanding 26.1

1. The student may answer with a variety of examples (outside of the list in the chapter) but their rationale needs to include that the example projects are temporary, with limited budgets, using resources from multiple disciplines, with a start and end date to achieve specific goals. Operations are ongoing and routine, there is no end date, and they only change when operational objectives can no longer be met.

3. This is considered a revenue project since the long-term goal is to expand the volume of trauma patients and services provided and result in increased revenue. Alternatively, this could also be considered a compliance project since the immediate purpose is to comply with the standards for certification.

5. No. While some compliance projects may yield a cost savings or increase revenue, the primary purpose of a compliance project is to deliver the change needed to satisfy the internal or external expectations.

### Check Your Understanding 26.2

1. The stakeholders are the attendees of the conference because they are the recipients of the results of this project, which they need to further their education. Stakeholders also include the project team, project champion, project sponsor, and anyone else affected by the project outcomes.

3. The project manager is Susan since she is working with the project team to ensure the project is completed within the constraints of scope, schedule, and budget. Susan is also responsible for coordinating communication and collaboration with the speaker subcommittee, the food and beverage subcommittee, and the project sponsor.

5. Yes or no. While additional people may be required to support the silent auction, the more important point is that additional expertise may be needed to support this new function. Team members are needed who are skilled at soliciting donations for the auction, and other roles are added for specialists who can set up the auction items and collect money from the winning bidders. The addition of the silent auction requires new specialties and may require additional team members, or the new responsibilities may be distributed among existing team members who possess these specialties.

## Check Your Understanding 26.3

1. This project may be handled best under the functional organization, since it is primarily within a single department (registration) and any cross-departmental collaboration could be done among affected functional managers.

3. The three categories of vendor partners are consultant, contractor, and outsourcing agencies.

   A consultant is used when a temporary and specialized expertise is needed at a high level and current employees do not have that expertise. For example, a consultant may be hired in the coding department to plan for implementation of ICD-11.

   A contractor is hired on a temporary basis for their expertise in specialized skills and detailed knowledge that may not be available in existing staff; or they may be hired to work with the project team. For example, a contractor may be hired to work with the project team to develop a plan to get caught up on the coding backlog before implementing computer-assisted coding.

   An outsourcing agency is used to get a segment of the work done outside the project team. For example, the coding backlog may be outsourced to a group of coding specialists to complete the coding process of the entire backlog before implementation.

5. The primary challenges described in the chapter are communication and collaboration. The team must be able to communicate well and work together. Project managers must ensure all team members have the tools to communicate as needed and the team is able to work together on the project deliverables. Tools such as web conferencing, collaborative productivity software, and shared workspaces can support the team's communication and collaboration needs. Also, the project manager must conduct project team meetings in a manner that engages both the co-located and distributed team members.

## Check Your Understanding 26.4

1. One of the main characteristics of a project is that it is temporary. This means the project team and project structure exist only for the duration of the project. Once the project is completed, the team is disbanded, and the project structure no longer exists. This temporary nature of the project team requires a temporary leader for the team serving the temporary functional team. The long-term supervisor role required for hiring, promoting, and firing is not relevant to this temporary team leadership role.

3. Organizations are separated by layers of management and functional silos. These boundaries form islands of groups with a specific operational focus. These islands allow the groups to specialize a specific function but make it challenging to communicate and coordinate work with other areas. Project management is used to cross these boundaries and coordinate work and communications across the layers of management and functional silos. The project manager may use technical skills

such as project management software and communication tools to communicate and collaborate with groups. The project manager will also need to use interpersonal skills such as leadership, team building, motivation, communication, influencing, and political and cultural awareness to bring people and groups together to work collectively to achieve the objectives of the project.

5. The new project manager can leverage existing competencies in organizational experience, industry knowledge, and professional behaviors that were developed through years of business analyst experience in the organization. However, being new to the role as project manager, the individual must develop a deeper understanding of projects to develop project process knowledge expertise and gain experience leading projects to improve project performance capabilities. Also, while professional behavior competencies were developed in the role of a business analyst, additional professional behavior competencies, such as motivation and stakeholder communications, must be further developed for the new role of project manager.

## Check Your Understanding 26.5

1. Without the project initiation, Betsy may not understand why the event is needed and may design the event in a manner that does not meet the needs of the stakeholders. Additionally, without understanding the constraints, she may exceed the available funds to offer the event, omit important features of the event, or may not have everything ready in time for the event.

3. The project plan was established in the planning process group to identify what all needs to be done, the order in which it must be done, and when it must be done. If the plan is not followed during execution, tasks may not be completed, rework may be required due to missed steps, or the tasks may not be completed on time.

5. Without the project closing group, Betsy would miss the opportunity to learn from her experience in planning the event and would repeat the same mistakes in future projects or would have to recreate the entire plan for future events.

## Check Your Understanding 26.6

1. Scope creep would happen if new features were added to the event, such as gifts for all participants. If this level of scope creep occurred, the costs of the event would exceed the funds available and may have also introduced delays in completing the entire project before the date of the event.

3. Betsy planned the budget based on charging $30 per attendee and assumed 100 people attending the event. The $25 gift for each attendee requires a revised cost of $55 for each attendee to cover the increased cost for the gift. This changes the event budget from $2,700 to $5,200.

5. Betsy should encourage, or require, a formalized change process so that any changes to the project constraints (scope, schedule, or budget) can be evaluated or recalculated, and plans can be revised. Additionally, the formalized process allows for key project stakeholders to have a voice in any changes that affect these project constraints.

## Check Your Understanding 26.7

1. Operational project management focuses on managing the project constraints by ensuring the entire scope is delivered on time and within budget. On the other hand, strategic project management also considers the purpose and goals of the project to ensure the project properly addresses the purpose and maximizes the goals or benefits. Operational project management closely tracks the project budget and will revise the project to ensure the project remains within the allocated budget. Whereas strategic project management focused on an expense reduction project will closely monitor how the project deliverables contribute to reducing the expenses of the organization and alters the project to optimize the deliverables' contribution to reducing expenses. Another example is when an additional task is requested, the project plan will be adjusted to meet the existing budget and schedule or to

extend these resources to include the additional task in operational project management. In strategic project management, there will be a determination on if the additional task helps meet the project purpose and goals before the task is assigned and the schedule and budget are adjusted. Students may add their own examples such as determining whether to add another course to achieve an academic minor in addition to their major. Operational project management would fit it in where credits allow or add another semester to the schedule; strategic project management would decide if it would be advantageous to the goal of graduating or getting a job before adding the course.

3. A project manager is typically concerned with the scope, schedule, and budget for the individual project and executing the project within these constraints. The program manager encourages individual projects to manage these constraints but is more concerned with the output of each project and ensuring the output meets the needs of the overall program. For instance, the program manager of the training program is primarily concerned that individual training sessions are offered as scheduled, and the attendees of these training sessions achieve the skills and knowledge promised by the training program.

5. Projects A, C, and F are funded to make use of the entire budget of $800,000 and to maximize the financial gain of $2,450,000.

### Check Your Understanding 27.1

1. Virtue theory should be applied and evaluated regarding how it informs or should inform professional practice in HIM. The relevant codes, laws, and policies; customs of right and wrong conduct; and any applicable duties, principles, or standards that dictate good or right conduct or character for HIM professionals could be considered. Views outside these norms should be described and opinions offered on what the virtuous character traits should be if they differ from known standards.

3. Ethical duties should be identified, explained, and examined to determine how they apply to the HIM professionals. The analysis should assess the justification for these duties, identify known or potential conflicts, and describe when and how these duties apply to HIM practice. It may be helpful to provide examples of how these duties might play out in professional practice and evaluate possible outcomes that may result. A conclusion may include that there are duties not established by any code or professional practice guidelines; if that is the case, the AHIMA Code of Ethics should be assessed to determine what, if anything, is missing or should be amended.

5. Learners must defend their own position, or at least the one they are considering. While it is preferable for learners to take a position, newer learners may not have developed the agency to take a firm stance one way or another. What is important is that learners base their evaluation on ethical criteria and standards. There are no right or wrong answers per se—arguments may vary in construction or ethical justification. This is not an exercise in entertaining learner opinions; rather, it is a reflection on the material and the learner's progress in metacognitive integration.

### Check Your Understanding 27.2

1. The answer should include an evaluation of the standards of the AHIMA Code of Ethics that create specific duties and responsibilities for HIM professionals. It should explicitly state the code's effectiveness in guiding professional practice using examples to rationalize the answer, present and defend opinions by making judgments about information, validity of ideas, or quality of work based on a set of criteria.

3. This question is purposefully vague. A lot of information is required to make a full determination, and responses should be structured by application of the ethical decision-making framework provided in the chapter. What is the ethical question? What information is needed to respond to it? For example, it might be helpful to know what was done with the information, whether the coworker had a legitimate need to be in the patient's record, and how the credentials were obtained. Based

on relevant facts, which can be elaborated in formulating their answers, students should select and justify their choice of disciplinary action. Learners are challenged to solve problems to new situations by applying acquired knowledge, facts, techniques and rules in a different way.

5. While it is advisable to use such a framework, the fact is that many professionals prefer other models or use no model at all. In evaluating the framework in this chapter, responses to this question should explain and justify the position taken. Some may reckon the framework is too narrow or constricting, while others may find benefit in the order it can provide for unwieldy ethical dilemmas. There are no right or wrong answers, but responses should provide a thorough evaluation of the decision-making framework. Learners must present and defend opinions by making judgments about information, validity of ideas, or quality of work based on a set of criteria.

## Check Your Understanding 27.3

1. Personal and professional knowledge should be synthesized to devise a plan for future practice. Cultural competence can be defined in different ways, and there are differing needs across communities; for example, rural border towns may face different issues than those in large cities, or they may face similar problems that require different solutions to suit the needs of their respective communities.

3. Learners must examine and break information into parts by identifying motives or causes. Due to the ubiquity of social network accessibility, many healthcare institutions have social media policies for their employees. Likewise, professional associations offer guidance to their members to help them avoid the risks while leveraging the many benefits of social media technologies. This question asks students to defend a position for or against banning social media use. Many issues could arise from such a policy, such as enforceability, diminished patient-provider communication, and a loss of communication to the community at large. The answer to this question can change based on the needs of the institution, the community served, the size of the organization, and other factors raised by the learner.

5. Learners must present and defend opinions by making judgments about information, validity of ideas, or quality of work based on a set of criteria. Many issues can be addressed here. The triple aim of healthcare technology (efficiency, cost savings, improved health) does not always work to the benefit of patients. For example, keeping costs down may require changes in the way care is provided, what services are offered and to whom, and other aspects of patient care and community engagement. Likewise, usability for provider can be affected. Learners should elaborate and justify the response using the conceptual frameworks offered in the chapter.

# Glossary

*a priori*  Term that means human knowledge of right and wrong comes through deduction beforehand rather than observation after the fact.

**A&C**  Abbreviation for adults and children.

**A&D**  Symbolizes patients admitted and discharged on the same day.

**Abbreviated Injury Scale (AIS)**  A scale that reflects the nature of an injury and the severity (threat to life) by body system. It may be assigned manually by the registrar or generated as part of the database from data entered by the registrar.

**Abuse**  Practices or incidents inconsistent with sound fiscal, business, or medical practices which result in improper payments from Medicare.

**Accept the risk**  Understanding that residual risk will exist as no additional controls would be implemented.

**Acceptance**  Requires a meeting of the minds between the parties about terms that are sufficiently definite and complete.

**Accession number**  A number used to identify the patient when a case is first entered in the registry.

**Accession registry**  A list of patients in accession number order provides a way to monitor that all cases have been entered into the registry.

**Accountability**  Duty of an individual, group, or organization to be answerable for specific activities.

**Accountable care organization (ACO)**  A group of service providers that work together to manage and coordinate care of Medicare fee-for-service beneficiaries.

**Accountable Care Organizations (ACOs)**  ACOs are designed to encourage coordination and cooperation among various healthcare providers to improve the quality of care for patients, while reducing unnecessary costs.

**Accounting**  An activity that involves the collection, recording, and reporting of financial data.

**Accounting of disclosures**  Information that describes a covered entity's revealing of PHI other than for TPO; disclosures made with authorization; and certain other limited disclosures.

**Accounting rate of return (ARR)**  A method of capital analysis that compares the projected annual cash inflows, minus any applicable annual depreciation, divided by the initial investment.

**Accounts payable**  A liability created when the organization has received goods or services but has not yet remitted the compensation (that is, paid for the goods or services).

**Accounts receivable**  A list of the amounts due from various customers (in healthcare's case, patients).

**Accounts receivable (A/R) days**  The average number of days between the discharge date and the receipt of payment for services rendered as a measure of revenue cycle success.

**Accreditation**  Refers to a voluntary process of organizational review in which an independent body created for this purpose periodically evaluates the quality of the entity's work against preestablished written criteria.

**Accreditation**  A voluntary process of organizational review in which an independent body created for this purpose periodically evaluates the quality of the entity's work against preestablished written criteria.

**Accrue**  A common business practice to record liabilities as they are incurred.

**Acquittal**  When a defendant is found not guilty.

**Activity-based budgets**  Budget based on activities or projects rather than on departments.

**Actors**  Those regulated by the information blocking rule, including healthcare providers, health information network (HIN) or health information exchange (HIE), and Health IT Developer of Certified Health IT.

**Actual causation**  That the defendant's conduct caused the harm.

**Acute care**  Short-term care provided to diagnose and treat an illness or injury.

**Acute-care prospective payment system**  The reimbursement system for inpatient hospital services provided to Medicare and Medicaid beneficiaries based on the use of diagnosis-related groups (DRGs) as a classification tool.

**ADDIE model** Analyze, Design, Develop, Implement, Evaluate—This method emphasizes the how, what, why, where, who, and when of training.

**Addressable standards** Allow the organization to implement the standard based on the size and complexity of the covered entity or business associate; the organization's technical infrastructure, hardware, and software security capabilities; the costs of security measures; the probability and criticality of potential risks to ePHI.

**Adhesion contract** A contract provision that places a healthcare provider in a significant position of power over a patient who relies on the provider's services may be deemed this and found to be against public policy.

**Adjudicated** Formally decided through the trial court (and, if applicable, appellate courts).

**Administrative applications** Technologies and software used to gather and organize administrative data.

**Administrative branch** Government branch that controls governmental administrative operations and operates through administrative agencies that enact regulations.

**Administrative data** Facts associated with identifying patients, location of care, healthcare professionals, and more. These data are vital for organizational operations and ensuring accurate patient documentation.

**Administrative law** The branch of law that controls a government's agency, or administrative, operations.

**Administrative management theory** Proposes a rational approach to designing organizations, with formal structure, clear division of labor, and use of delegation.

**Administrative metadata** Metadata programmed to be generated by IT that provides information about how and when data were created and used.

**Administrative safeguards** Policies and procedures to manage administrative actions, policies, and procedures to prevent, detect, contain, and correct security violations.

**Administrative services only (ASO) contracts** A form of group health insurance coverage where employers enter with private insurers and fund the plans themselves.

**Admit-discharge-transfer (ADT) message** Messages used to communicate patient demographics and visit information and to track patient status at a healthcare facility.

**Adoption** The stage where every intended user is fully using the basic functionality of the system.

**Advance beneficiary notice of noncoverage (ABN)** A written notice to inform patients when an outpatient item or service is not considered reasonable and necessary or may not be covered.

**Advance directive** A special type of written consent that communicates an individual's wishes to be treated or not to be treated should the individual become incapacitated and unable to communicate on his or her own behalf.

**Adverse determination** When a healthcare insurer denies payment for proposed or already rendered healthcare service.

**Adverse event** Incident when a medical event causes injury.

**Affinity diagram** A diagram that allows the team to organize and group similar ideas together.

**Age Discrimination in Employment Act (ADEA) of 1967** The federal act that states it is unlawful for an employer to discriminate against an individual in any aspect of employment because that individual is 40 years old or older, unless one of the statutory exceptions applies, such as the capacity to safely perform the job at a particular age.

**Agency for Healthcare Research and Quality (AHRQ)** An agency that looks at issues related to the efficiency and effectiveness of the healthcare delivery system, disease protocols, and guidelines for improved disease outcomes.

**Aggregate data** Data on groups of people or patients without identifying any patient individually.

**Agile approach** An approach where the project management life cycle is repeated in many iterations.

**Allied health professions** The expanding team of health professionals who work with physicians, nurses, dentists, and pharmacists

**Alternative hypothesis** Sometimes called the research hypothesis; a conclusion that typically requires some action to be taken

**Altruism** The belief that one must make personal sacrifice and benefit other people before oneself.

**Ambulatory care** The provision of preventative or corrective healthcare services on a nonresident basis in a provider's office, clinic setting, or hospital outpatient setting.

**Ambulatory surgery center (ASC)** For Medicare purposes, an ASC is a distinct entity that operates exclusively for the purpose of furnishing outpatient surgical services to patients.

**Americans with Disabilities Act (ADA) of 1990** Federal legislation that ensures equal opportunity for and elimination of discrimination against persons with disabilities.

**Ancillary systems**  Clinical department applications that collect and organize tests and procedures ordered by a practitioner to provide information for use in patient diagnosis or treatment; they include laboratory information systems (LISs), radiology information systems (RISs), pharmacy information systems, and others.

**Answer**  Also known as a response, prepared by the defendant or an attorney on the defendant's behalf that addresses the allegations made against the defendant.

**Anti-Kickback Statute (AKS)**  Legislation that makes knowingly offering, paying, soliciting, or receiving any remuneration that rewards referrals for services reimbursable by a federal program a criminal offense.

**Apology statutes**  Also known as "I'm Sorry" laws. Laws that protect a healthcare provider's apology from being admitted into evidence as an admission of liability during a court proceeding.

**Appellate court**  Also known as a court of appeals. An intermediate court. State appellate courts have general jurisdiction. The federal appellate level is composed of 13 federal courts of appeals.

**Application Programming Interface (API)**  Set of defined rules and protocols explaining how applications talk to one another.

**Application service provider (ASP)**  Vendors that provide the servers, load the organization's software and data on these servers, and provide the organization's users with the data and functionality through a secure connection.

**Application software**  The set of instructions that cause the computer hardware to perform tasks.

**Applied research**  Answers the questions "What?" and "How?" and focuses on the implementation of theories into practice.

**Arbitration**  When an objective third party is brought in to make a binding decision in a case where the parties cannot come to agreement.

**Areas of excellence**  Refers to describable skills, competencies, or capabilities that a department or company cultivates to a level of proficiency greater than anything else it does

**Arraignment**  When the defendant appears before the court, and the prosecutor informs the defendant of the charges.

**Artifacts**  Data models, use cases, data flow diagrams, and data dictionaries developed through data architecture management.

**Artificial intelligence (AI)**  High-level information technologies used in developing machines that imitate human qualities such as learning and reasoning

**Assault**  Conduct, along with apparent ability, that causes apprehension that physically harmful or offensive contact will occur.

**Assessment**  A complete and accurate review of the potential risks and vulnerabilities to the confidentiality, integrity, and availability of ePHI at an organization.

**Asset**  Something that is owned or due to be received.

**Assumption of risk**  If the plaintiff, with knowledge and understanding of a danger, voluntarily undertook the risks of that danger, the plaintiff may not recover damages for the resulting injury.

**Asynchronous**  Training delivery method where learners and instructors interact through email or discussion forums.

**Attributable risk (AR)**  A measure of the public health impact of a causative factor on a population.

**Attributes**  Describe characteristics represented as circles.

**Audit**  A function that allows retrospective reconstruction of events, including who executed the events in question, why, and what changes were made as a result.

**Audit log**  A chronological record of electronic system activities of individual user activity over a period, and a record of different actions a user takes within the system.

**Authentication**  Validates content and proves authorship. In paper records, authentication can be accomplished by a handwritten signature or initials, both in ink. Electronic or digital signatures and computer keys are types of authentication methods in EHRs.

**Authenticity**  Means a record is genuine and "is what it purports to be."

**Authority**  The right to act in ways necessary to carry out assigned tasks.

**Authorization**  A document that gives covered entities permission to use PHI for specified purposes or to disclose PHI to a third party specified by the individual.

**Autocratic leadership**  Where a manager makes decisions without others' input and gives very specific direction.

**Automated drug dispensing machines**  Secure devices that make drugs specific to patient orders readily available to nursing staff. These machines are typically filled by pharmacy department staff based on the physician orders.

**Autonomy**   Often referred to as the right to self-determination, autonomy also refers to a person's right to decide what does or does not happen to them in terms of healthcare.

**Autopsy**   A postmortem examination and study of a dead body to determine the cause of death.

**Avatars**   User-generated electronic representations of themselves in a multi-user virtual environment.

**Average daily census**   The mean number of hospital inpatients present in the hospital each day for a given period.

**Balance sheet**   A snapshot of the accounting equation at a point in time.

**Balanced Budget Refinement Act (BBRA) of 1999**   Act amended by the Benefits Improvement Act of 2000, that mandated the establishment of a per-discharge, DRG-based PPS for longer-term care hospitals beginning October 1, 2002.

**Balanced matrix**   Organizational structure in which a project organization exists within the existing functional hierarchy and a project manager is recruited from one of the functional departments to serve as the leader of the project.

**Balanced scorecard**   A framework for measuring organizational performance across customer, financial, internal process, and learning and growth perspectives.

**Bar plot**   Used for presenting data as a position along a common scale.

**Bar-coding technology**   A method of encoding data that consists of parallel arrangements of dark elements, referred to as *bars*, *light elements*, and *spaces*, and interpreting the data for automatic identification and data collection purposes.

**Basic interoperability**   The ability to successfully transmit and receive data from one computer to another.

**Basic research**   Research that answers the question "Why?" with the intent of increasing the scientific knowledge base, focusing on the development of fundamental theories and their refinement.

**Batch processing**   Describes a high-volume of repetitive data jobs that run without manual intervention.

**Battery**   The intentional and nonconsensual touching of another person.

**Bed count**   The number of inpatient beds set up and staffed for use on a given day.

**Bed turnover rate**   A measure of volume of service and utilization at a hospital that indicates how many times a bed was occupied in a given period.

**Behavioral description interviews**   Requires applicants to give specific examples of how they have performed a specific procedure or handled a specific problem in the past.

**Bench trial**   A case made before a judge rather than a jury.

**Benchmarking**   The systematic comparison of the products, services, and outcomes of one organization with those of a similar organization, or the systematic comparison of one organization's outcomes with regional or national standards such as professional associations and standard-setting organizations.

**Benchmarks**   Measures and performance statistics that allow comparison of one's own results with the results of other individuals, departments, or organizations.

**Beneficence**   A term that refers to the moral obligation of promoting good for or providing services that benefit others.

**Benefits realization**   A formal process of studying whether the value (for example, cost savings, productivity improvements, revenue enhancements, improved quality of care and patient safety, and patient and provider experience of care satisfaction) was worth the investment of time, energy, and money.

**Best of breed**   An approach to acquisition that selects a vendor for each type of technology throughout the migration path, potentially resulting in several different vendors.

**Best of fit**   An approach to acquisition in which the goal is to minimize the number of vendors.

**Beyond a reasonable doubt**   A standard of proof the government must meet to establish the defendant's guilt.

**Bias**   A personal belief that prevents a person from having an impartial judgment.

**Bibliographic databases**   Databases of published literature such as journals, magazines, newspaper articles, books, book chapters, and other information sources.

**Big data**   Data sets so large or complex they are difficult to process using traditional methods.

**Bill hold period**   The number of days in which accounts will be held from billing so charges can be entered after the patient is discharged.

**Binding authority**   After a court establishes a new common-law principle, that principle sets a precedent for future cases that address the same issues in that court system.

**Bioethics**   The discipline concerned with the ethical, legal, and social milieu of healthcare, bioresearch, public health, and environmental ethics.

**Biomedical research**   The process of systematically investigating subjects related to the functioning of the human body.

**Biometric authentication**   Allows a user to be uniquely identified and access the system based on one or more biometric traits such as fingerprints, hand geometry, retinal pattern, or voice waves.

**Biotechnology**   "The manipulation (as through genetic engineering) of living organisms or their components to produce useful usually commercial products (such as pest resistant crops, new bacterial strains, or novel pharmaceuticals)" (Merriam-Webster n.d.)

**Blanket authorization**   When the patient signs an authorization allowing the ROI specialist to release all information from that point forward.

**Blended learning**   Uses several delivery methods, thereby gaining the advantages and reducing the disadvantages of each method by itself.

**Blogs**   A web page where users can post text, images, and links to other websites.

**Boxplot**   Displays the descriptive statistics of a continuous variable including the minimum, first quartile, medium, third quartile, maximum, and potential outlier values.

**Brainstorming**   A technique used to generate many creative ideas free of criticism and judgment.

**Breach**   "An acquisition, access, use, or disclosure of protected health information in a manner not permitted under subpart E is presumed to be a breach unless the covered entity or business associate, as applicable, demonstrates that there is a low probability that the protected health information has been compromised based on a risk assessment" (HHS 2013, 71).

**Breach notification**   One of the largest regulation provisions to privacy and security under the HITECH Act required notification of patients if their personal health information was breached.

**Breach Notification Rule**   Requires covered entities and business associates to establish policies and procedures to investigate an unauthorized use or disclosure of unsecured PHI to determine if a breach occurred, conclude the investigation, and to notify affected individuals within 60 days of date of discovery of the breach.

**Breach of confidentiality**   Causes of action for wrongful disclosure may be based on where a breach exists because of a relationship of trust and obligation between the provider and the patient.

**Breach of warranty**   A broken promise.

**Bring your own device (BYOD)**   Refers to personal devices that are allowed to be used within a healthcare organization and interact with ePHI.

**Bundled payments**   Payments covering multiple services that may involve multiple providers of care.

**Burden of proof**   The obligation to prove a case that lies with the plaintiff to meet the four elements of negligence, except in cases where the facts or circumstances allow for an inference of the defendant's negligence.

**Bureaucracy**   Clear hierarchies of roles, relationships, rules, and regulations to standardize behavior, and the use of trained specialists for jobs typified this form of organization.

**Business associate (BA)**   A "person or organization, other than a member of a covered entity's workforce, that performs certain functions or activities on behalf of, or provides certain services to, a covered entity that involve the use or disclosure of individually identifiable health information" (HHS 2022a).

**Business associate agreements (BAA)**   Contracts between a covered entity and a business associate that establish the permitted and required uses and disclosures of PHI by the business associate.

**Business case**   Lays out the benefits and value for the organization that implementation of the data governance program can obtain by anticipating a positive change from the status.

**Business Continuity Plan (BCP)**   Incorporates policies and procedures for continuing business operations during computer system down time.

**Business intelligence (BI)**   The end product or goal of knowledge management.

**Business process**   A collection of interrelated work tasks initiated in response to an event that achieves a specific result for a customer of the process.

**Business process redesign (BPR)**   A focus strategy for rethinking and drastically improving and sustaining overall performance, not a strategy for cutting costs.

**Business process reengineering (BPR)**   Also known as business transformation and process change management; proposes the radical redesign of the organization and its business processes to reduce costs, streamline operations, and improve quality of service.

**Business record** Documentation created and kept in the usual course of business.

**Business records exception** The prohibition against admitting hearsay evidence will often permit a health record to be admitted.

**Bylaws** Outline the content of patient health records, identify the exact personnel who can enter information in health records, and may restate applicable Joint Commission and CMS requirements.

**Cancer staging** The process of determining the size and extent of spread of the tumor throughout the body.

**Capital budget** A budget that looks at long-term investments.

**Capitation** Reimbursement method based on per-person premiums or membership fees rather than on itemized per-procedure or per-service charges.

**Cardinality** The main rule used to determine table structure based on the maximum number of occurrences of each entity that occurrences of other entities can link to.

**Care Area Assessment (CAA)** A comprehensive assessment of a resident's needs in specific areas or care domains, such as medical, functional, cognitive, psychosocial, and behavioral. These assessments help care providers identify the resident's strengths, weaknesses, preferences, and potential areas for improvement.

**Care coordination** The act of "organizing patient care activities and sharing information among all of the participants concerned with a patient's care to achieve safer and more effective care" (AHRQ 2018).

**Career plan** A strategic plan for an individual, providing direction, goals, and an action plan to reach those goals.

**Case definition** A process in which a registry must determine the cases that are to be included.

**Case finding** The methods used to identify the patients who have been seen and treated in the facility for the disease or condition of interest to the registry.

**Case management** A means for achieving client wellness and autonomy through advocacy, communication, education, identification of service resources and service facilitation. The ongoing, concurrent review performed by clinical professionals to ensure the necessity and effectiveness of the clinical services being provided to a patient.

**Case mix** A description of a patient population based on characteristics including age, gender, type of insurance, diagnosis, risk factors, treatment received, and resources used.

**Case study** When researchers conduct an in-depth investigation of one or more examples of a phenomenon, such as a trend, occurrence, or incident.

**Case-control (retrospective) studies** A major component of epidemiological research. Persons with a certain condition (cases) and persons without the condition (controls) are studied by looking back in time.

**Case-mix group (CMG) relative weight** An appropriate weight assigned to each CMG measuring the relative difference in facility resource intensity among the various groups.

**Case-mix groups (CMGs)** The IRF PPS uses information from the IRF-PAI to classify patients into distinct groups based on clinical characteristics and expected resource needs. Data used to construct these groups include rehabilitation impairment categories (RICs), functional status (both motor and cognitive), age, comorbidities, and other factors deemed appropriate to improve the explanatory power of the groups.

**Case-mix index (CMI)** Types or categories of patients treated by the hospital, based on the relative weights of the MS-DRG.

**Causal relationships** Relationships that show cause and effect.

**Causal-comparative research** A type of quasi-experimental design that resembles experimental research by having many, but not all, of its characteristics, lacking manipulation of treatment and random assignment to a group; also called ex post facto, meaning retrospective, because some past variable or phenomenon has already occurred.

**Centers for Medicare and Medicaid Services (CMS)** The federal agency overseeing Medicare, Medicaid, Children's Health Insurance Program, and the Health Insurance Marketplace and setting standards for healthcare quality.

**Centralized model** Health information exchange model in which all data are stored in a shared data repository.

**Certification** The process by which government and nongovernment organizations evaluate educational programs, healthcare facilities, and individuals as having met predetermined standards.

**Champion** Someone in an organization who believes in an idea, acknowledges the practical problems of financing and political support, and assists in overcoming barriers.

**Change agent** A specialist in organization development who facilitates the change brought about by an innovation.

**Change control** A formal process of documenting what change in an information system is needed, the rationale for the change, necessary approvals (for example, the stakeholder workgroup's approval to turn off a specific CDS system alert), when the change was made, who made the change, that related documentation (for example, data model, data dictionary, policy, and procedure) has been updated to reflect the change, and that monitoring for a period of time was performed.

**Change drivers** Large-scale forces such as demographic, social, political, economic, technical, and more recently, global and informational factors that require organizations of all sizes to revise how they operate.

**Change management** The formal process of introducing change, getting it adopted, and diffusing it throughout the organization.

**Charge capture** A method of recording services and supplies or items delivered to the patient and directing them to be billed on a claim form.

**Charge description master (CDM)** Commonly referred to as a chargemaster; an electronic file that represents a master list of all services, supplies, devices, and medications charged for inpatient or outpatient services.

**Charitable immunity** Doctrine that served as a defense that protected charitable institutions (such as hospitals) from tort liability. Precipitated by the landmark case *Darling v. Charleston Community Memorial Hospital* (1965), however, this doctrine has effectively been extinguished because of the increasing business nature of most healthcare organizations.

**Charity care** Healthcare services that have been or will be provided but are never expected to result in cash inflows.

**Chart** A visual display of data that uses symbols on a graph.

**Chart conversion** Refers to moving from paper to an electronic system

**Check sheet** A data collection tool that permits observations or occurrences to be recorded and compiled.

**Chief executive officer (CEO)** Officer responsible for implementing the policies and strategic direction set by the hospital's board of directors

**Chief financial officer (CFO)** The senior manager responsible for the fiscal management of an entity.

**Chief information officer (CIO)** An executive-level role responsible for the management, implementation, and usability of information and computer technologies for an entity.

**Chief medical informatics officers (CMIOs)** Physicians with a special interest in technology implementations and advanced analytics.

**Chief operating officer (COO)** An executive-level role responsible at a high level for day-to-day operations of an entity.

**Chief technology officer (CTO)** An executive-level role responsible for overseeing current technology and creating relevant policies for its use.

**Children's Health Insurance Program (CHIP)** Title XXI of the Social Security Act. A program initiated by the Balanced Budget Act (BBA). CHIP became available in 1997 and is jointly funded by the federal government and the states. Following broad federal guidelines, states establish eligibility and coverage guidelines and have flexibility in the way they provide services. CHIP allows states to expand existing insurance programs to cover children up to age 19.

**Cipher text** Unreadable or indecipherable text due to encryption.

**Circuit** Courts covering a geographic area. The US Courts of Appeals are also called circuit courts.

**Circuit courts** Courts that have the power to hear appeals of district courts' final judgments.

**Civil law** Addresses noncriminal legal matters and involves relationships among individuals and other entities, including a government.

**Civil Monetary Penalties Law** Legislation that provides punitive fines imposed by a civil court to organizations that profit from illegal or unethical activities.

**Civil Rights Act of 1964, Title VII** Federal legislation that prohibits discrimination in employment on the basis of race, religion, color, sex, or national origin.

**Civil Rights Act of 1991** Federal legislation that focuses on establishing an employer's responsibility for justifying hiring practices that seem to adversely affect people because of race, color, religion, sex, or national origin.

**Civilian Health and Medical Program–Veterans Administration (CHAMPVA)** A healthcare program for dependents and survivors of permanently and totally disabled veterans, survivors of veterans who died from service-related conditions, and survivors of military personnel who died in the line of duty.

**Claim** A statement of services submitted by a healthcare provider to a third-party payer (for example, an insurance company or Medicare).

**Claims adjudication** A process by which payment is received from third-party payers and the discounts and adjustments are applied to the balance on the account, but there may still be a portion the patient owes (related to deductibles, coinsurance, and copayments).

**Claims scrubber software** Software that contains a series of edits to determine if the claim is ready to be submitted.

**Clean claims** Refers to when most billing systems are programmed to automatically submit claims to payers after the bill hold time frame if the account is not being held for any type of edit resolution.

**Clinical** Term that refers to work done with real patients, about or relating to the medical treatment given to patients in facilities such as hospitals and clinics.

**Clinical Care Classification (CCC) systems** A free empirically developed system consisting of (a) standardized coded nursing terminology and (b) information model designed for documenting the essence of care in EHR systems.

**Clinical classification** A clinical vocabulary, terminology, or nomenclature that lists words or phrases with their meanings; provides for the proper use of clinical words as names or symbols; and facilitates mapping of standardized terms to broader classifications for administrative, regulatory, oversight, and fiscal requirements.

**Clinical data** Facts produced by healthcare providers when diagnosing and treating patients.

**Clinical data analysts** Professionals who ensure protocol is followed when research data is collected and analyzed. They also provide reporting and share results of the analysis while ensuring the data management processes are followed.

**Clinical decision support (CDS) systems** Interactive programs designed to assist clinicians in making patient care decisions.

**Clinical Document Architecture (CDA)** Used as the standard for document exchange. HL7 defines the CDA as "a document markup standard that specifies the structure and semantics of 'clinical documents' for the purpose of exchange between healthcare providers and patients" (HL7 n.d.b). Provides an exchange model for clinical documents (such as discharge summaries and progress notes).

**Clinical documentation integrity (CDI)** Previously referred to as clinical documentation improvement. A "process an organization undertakes that will improve clinical specificity and documentation that will allow coding professionals to assign more concise disease classification codes" (AHIMA 2017, 45).

**Clinical Laboratory Improvement Amendments (CLIA)** Enacted to "ensure quality laboratory testing" (CMS 2024b).

**Clinical pathways** Also known as critical pathways; guide evidence-based care and help "translate clinical practice guideline recommendations into clinical processes of care within the unique culture of a healthcare institution" (Rotter et al. 2019).

**Clinical privileges** Permission granted by a healthcare organization's governing board to a member of the medical staff, enabling the physician to provide patient services in the organization within specific practice limits.

**Clinical research** Involves direct interaction with human subjects or human-origin materials to explore health and illness, covering areas such as disease mechanisms, therapeutic interventions, and clinical trials, while excluding in vitro studies not linked to living individuals

**Clinical terminology** A set of standardized terms and their synonyms that record patient findings, circumstances, events, and interventions with sufficient detail to support clinical care, decision support, outcomes research, and quality improvement.

**Clinical transformation** Process that requires "assessing and continually improving the way patient care is delivered at all levels in an organization" (Sensmeier 2011).

**Clinical trials** A structured methodology for testing and validating new clinical or biomedical interventions.

**Clinical vocabulary** A formally recognized list of preferred medical terms.

**Clinician web portals** Sometimes referred to as physician web portals, a way for clinicians to easily access (through a web browser) the healthcare organizations' multiple applications and internal and external data sources.

**Closed records** Records of discharged patients.

**Closed system** A system that operates in a self-contained environment, unaffected by outside factors.

**Closed-record review** Qualitative review done retrospectively following discharge or termination of treatment.

**Cloud computing** On-demand access, through the internet, to computing resources—applications, servers (physical servers and virtual servers), data storage, development tools, networking capabilities, and more—hosted at a remote data center managed by a cloud services provider.

**Cluster sampling** When the population is divided into subsets, called clusters, which are then randomly selected, and all units within the randomly selected clusters are included in the sample.

**Coaching** When an experienced worker observes or reviews the work of the employee in a nonthreatening manner, offering advice and suggestions for revising techniques to improve productivity and efficient work performance.

**Code of ethics** A set of standards regarding business practices and professional behavior.

**Code of Federal Regulations (CFR)** A compilation of federal administrative regulations.

**Coding optimization** Seeks the most accurate documentation, coded data, and resulting payment in the amount the provider is rightly and legally entitled to receive.

**Coefficient of determination** When Pearson's $r$ may be converted to $r^2$. The $r^2$ measures how much of the variation in one variable is explained by the second variable.

**Cognitive complexity** The ability to see the many parts of a problem, process conflicting information, and integrate that diversity into a coherent picture.

**Cohort study** A prospective study in which the investigator selects a group of exposed individuals and unexposed individuals who are followed for a period to compare the incidence of disease in the two groups.

**Common cause variation** A variation caused inherently by the system.

**Common law** Also known as judicial law, judge-make law, or case law—it is created by courts in the resolution of disputes.

**Comorbidity** A condition that existed at admission thought to increase the length of stay (LOS) at least one day for approximately 75 percent of patients.

**Comparative effectiveness research (CER)** Research that generates and synthesizes "evidence that compares the benefits and harms of alternative methods to prevent, diagnose, treat, and monitor a clinical condition, or to improve the delivery of care" (IOM 2009, 13).

**Comparative negligence** If the plaintiff's conduct contributed in part to the injury the plaintiff suffered, the plaintiff's recovery is reduced based on his or her percentage of negligence.

**Compensable factor** "A characteristic used to compare the worth of jobs" (Myers 2011, 691).

**Complaint** A legal document that sets forth the facts and claims, in the appropriate court.

**Complex adaptive systems** Refers to the complexity of structures and processes involved in healthcare, and the ongoing changes and rearrangements of these structures and processes.

**Compliance** Abiding by rules, laws, standards, or regulations.

**Compliance projects** Self-imposed initiatives organizations place on themselves, industry-imposed compliance where organizations must meet a minimum level of stakeholder expectations, and government or regulatory compliance that organizations must meet to remain in business.

**Complication** A secondary condition that arises during hospitalization, thought to increase the length of stay (LOS) by at least one day for approximately 75 percent of patients.

**Compound authorizations** Combine the use and disclosure of PHI with other legal permissions, such as consent for treatment, which is prohibited by the current HIPAA Privacy Rule.

**Compressed workweek** A week in which more hours are combined within fewer days.

**Compromise** A conflict management method in which both parties must be willing to lose, or give up, a piece of their position.

**Computer-assisted coding (CAC)** A tool intended for improved efficiency of the coding and claims submission process. Also, an emerging technology used in the coding process.

**Computer-based training (CBT)** A method designed to provide individual learners with electronic training at their own pace.

**Computerized provider order entry (CPOE)** Systems that enable ordering of everything from patient admission, laboratory tests, x-rays and other diagnostic studies, dietary and food and nutrition, therapies, nursing services, and consults to discharge of patient, referrals, and even building personal task lists, as well as entering orders for medications.

**Concept** The most granular unit within a terminology. In SNOMED CT, it represents a "unique clinical meaning, which is referenced using a unique, numeric and machine-readable SNOMED CT identifier" (SNOMED 2023).

**Conceptual skills** Include such competencies as visioning, planning, decision-making, problem solving, creativity, and conceptualizing the connections among parts of a complex organizational system, or systems thinking.

**Concurrent analysis** Quantitative analysis done while the patient is in the facility.

**Concurrent review** Review of the record that occurs while the patient care is ongoing.

**Conditions for Coverage (CfCs) and Conditions of Participation (CoPs)** Conditions that "healthcare organizations must meet in order to begin and continue participating in the Medicare and Medicaid programs" (CMS 2023a).

**Confidence interval** A range of values, such that the probability of that range covering the true value of a parameter is a set probability or confidence.

**Confidentiality** Establishes the healthcare provider's responsibility for protecting health records and other personal and private information from unauthorized use or disclosure.

**Confidentiality of Substance Use Disorder Patient Records** Provides special protections for SUD records. Health records that contain one's identity, diagnosis, prognosis, or treatment information where alcohol or drug abuse is either the primary or secondary diagnosis are included in restrictions on disclosure and redisclosure.

**Conflict management** Focuses on working with the individuals involved in a disagreement to find a mutually acceptable solution.

**Confounding variables** Extraneous factors that can affect the study's outcome.

**Consent** Where the defendant claims that the plaintiff gave permission or agreed to the now-alleged wrongful action.

**Conservatism** Financial data must comply with and fairly represent the financial results of the period and not overstate or understate information in a significant (material) way.

**Consideration** What the parties will receive from each other in exchange for performing the obligations of the contract.

**Consistency** In accounting, principle that requires that the method not change over the life of the asset.

**Constitutional law** Many of the rights and obligations of government, which subsequently affect the rights and obligations of individuals and entities, are set out in federal and state constitutions.

**Constructive confrontation** A conflict management method in which both parties meet with an objective third party to explore their perceptions and feelings. The desired outcome is to produce a mutual understanding of the issues and to create a win-win situation.

**Consultant** Provides high level, specialized expertise to a project that may not exist within the current employees.

**Consultation** The opinion of a physician with specialty training beyond general board certification such as an oncologist, cardiologist, or dermatologist.

**Consumer health informatics** A field devoted to informatics from multiple consumer or patient views; Focused on developing tools and processes to empower patients. By creating, using, and sharing health information, consumers are more engaged in their health and healthcare, which can lead to overall improvements in individual and population health outcomes.

**Consumer-mediated exchange** Provides patients with access to their health information, allowing them to manage their healthcare online in a similar fashion to how they might manage their finances through online banking.

**Content analysis** The systematic and objective analysis of communication to describe and to make inferences about behaviors.

**Content management** Encompasses managing both structured data (for example, data stored in databases) and unstructured data (such as data contained in text documents).

**Contingency plan** Also known as a disaster plan; a plan that prepares organizations for a potential event that could impact the ability to access patient information, the integrity of the information, or the confidentiality of information.

**Contingency planning** A component of a broader emergency preparedness process that includes an understanding of business practices, operational continuity requirements, and disaster recovery planning.

**Continuing education (CE)** A requirement for most credentialled professionals, including those in HIM. It usually requires a person to complete a certain number of hours of education within a given period to maintain a credential or license status.

**Continuity of Care Document (CCD)** An implementation guide for sharing CCR patient summary data using the CDA. The CCD was recognized as part of the first set of interoperability standards.

**Continuity of care record (CCR)** A core data set of the most relevant administrative, demographic, and clinical information about a patient's healthcare, covering one or more healthcare encounters.

**Continuous data** Data that can take on a continuum of values, such as fractions and decimals, as opposed to discrete categories.

**Continuous quality improvement (CQI)** A management philosophy that emphasizes the importance of knowing and meeting customer expectations, reducing variation within processes, and relying on data to build knowledge for process improvement.

**Continuous speech input** Process that does not require the user to pause between words to let the computer distinguish between the beginning and ending of words.

**Continuous variables** Interval and ratio scales. Examples in healthcare include length of stay, charges, reimbursement, wait time, patient body mass index (BMI), and minutes to code a health record.

**Continuum of care** Patients are provided care by different caregivers at several different levels of the healthcare system.

**Contract** An agreement that in most cases is enforceable through the legal system.

**Contract law** Law addressing the creation of contracts and the resolution of contract disputes.

**Contract negotiation** The process of identifying and discussing issues with the vendor until all are resolved to the satisfaction of both parties.

**Contractors** Individuals added to a project team to fill a temporary void. Unlike consultants, who are added for higher-level knowledge, contractors are added to the team for their specialized skills and detailed knowledge not available within the existing employees; or they may be added to increase the work capacity of the existing project team.

**Contrary** When two laws are unable to be properly complied with, the state law is either considered to be contrary or more stringent. State law is considered when (1) a covered entity determines it is impossible to comply with both the federal and state privacy regulations; or (2) compliance with the state law would create a barrier to compliance with the federal regulations under HIPAA.

**Contributory negligence** If the plaintiff's conduct contributed in any part to the injury the plaintiff suffered, the plaintiff is barred from recovering any damages from the defendant.

**Control** A conflict management method in which interaction may be prohibited until the employees' emotions are under control.

**Control chart** Displays data points over time like a run chart except it has a line displayed at the top, called an upper control limit (UCL), and a line displayed at the bottom, called a lower control limit (LCL). These lines represent two standard deviations above and below the mean, indicating whether the process is stable or out of control.

**Control group** Comprises the control subjects who do not receive the intervention.

**Controls** Measures and functionality established for the purpose of preventing and mitigating risks.

**Controlling** Refers to managerial function of monitoring performance and using feedback to ensure efforts toward achieving prescribed goals are on target, and making course corrections as needed.

**Conviction** A declaration of guilt.

**Corporate governance** Terminology most often used to describe the roles and responsibilities of boards of directors who protect shareholders' interests in publicly held companies.

**Corporate integrity agreements (CIAs)** "As part of the settlement of federal healthcare program investigations, providers or entities agree to the obligations in exchange for the OIG to not seek their exclusion from participation in federal healthcare programs" (OIG n.d.a).

**Corporate negligence** An organization may be liable for the consequences of any unauthorized disclosure under this doctrine, whether by employees, agents, or medical staff members, because the organization breached its duty to maintain information in a confidential manner.

**Corporation** A legal entity that exists separately from its owner(s). Corporations pay their own taxes and have their own legal rights and responsibilities.

**Correlation** The statistic used to describe the association or relationship between two variables.

**Correlational research** Detects the existence, the direction, and the degree of relationships among factors.

**Cost accounting** The discipline of identifying and measuring costs and a unique subset of the accounting profession.

**Cost-outlier** To qualify for a cost outlier, a hospital's charges for a case (adjusted to cost) must exceed the payment rate for the MS-DRG by a fixed dollar amount, which changes each year.

**Counterclaim** When a defendant brings a claim against the plaintiff.

**Courts of appeals** Appellate courts, of which there are 13 at the federal level, each covering a circuit.

**Covered entity (CE)** A "health plan, healthcare clearinghouse, or healthcare provider that transmits information in electronic form in connection with a transaction" (HHS 2022a).

**Credentialing** A screening process to evaluate and validate a healthcare provider's qualifications for medical staff membership, allowing them to provide care to patients within the facility. This process is also used by third-party payers before allowing healthcare providers to deliver services to patients covered by their plans.

**Crimes** Prosecutable wrongful acts against public health, safety, and welfare.

**Criminal law** Addresses the punishment of persons or entities who commit crimes.

**Criminal negligence** If defined by criminal statute, gross negligence that represents reckless disregard or deliberate indifference to another's safety may constitute this.

**Critic** A role that challenges the innovation for shortcomings, presenting strong criteria, and, in essence, providing a reality test for the new idea.

**Criticality analysis** An analysis that consists of evaluating each of the different systems of the organization to determine how crucial the information in the system is to day-to-day healthcare operations and patient care.

**Cross-functional** Composed of individuals who represent different business units.

**Cross-sectional study** Study in which both the exposure and the disease outcome are determined at the same time in each subject.

**Cross-training** Process by which the employee learns to perform the jobs of many team members.

**Crossclaim** When one party brings a claim against another party on the same side of the litigation.

**Cryptographic key** A tool applied to the data to turn the information into cipher text or convert the data from cipher text back to plaintext.

**Cultural diversity** The perceived or actual difference among people.

**Cultural humility** The process of self-reflection and critique on beliefs and values combined with an acceptance of other people and groups vital to the overall culture of an organization.

**Current Dental Terminology (CDT)** A reference manual maintained and updated annually by the American Dental Association (ADA).

**Current Procedural Terminology (CPT)** "A uniform language for coding medical services and procedures to streamline reporting, increase accuracy and efficiency" (AMA n.d.).

**Current ratio** Compares total current assets with total current liabilities.

**Curriculum** The subject content of the program to be taught, including the sequence, activities, and materials.

**Customer data platform** Data is consolidated in one external view seen by customers

**Cybernetic systems** Systems that have standards, controls, and feedback mechanisms built into them.

**Cyclical staffing** The rotation of work schedule for a group of employees to allow for a fair distribution of day, evening, and weekend shifts for each person within the group.

**Damages** A remedy (often an dollar amount) awarded to a plaintiff due to the found liability in a civil case.

**Dashboard** A method developed for presenting a variety of data on a single display in an easy-to-read format.

**Data** "Qualitative or quantitative statements or numbers assumed to be factual, and not the product of analysis or interpretation" (Caldicott 2013, 24).

**Data administrators** Individuals who apply domain expertise to the logical design of a database, establish policies and standards governing creation and use of data, maintain data dictionaries, and manage data quality. Data administrators may have backgrounds in HIM or health informatics.

**Data analytics** Describes a variety of approaches to using data to make business decisions.

**Data architecture** Specifications used to describe existing state, define data requirements, guide data integration, and control data assets as put forth in a data strategy.

**Data at rest** Data in storage within a database or on a server that are no longer being used or accessed.

**Data augmentation** When training data is artificially derived from existing data without collecting new data.

**Data backup plan** Document that defines how the system is being backed up, the method of backing up the data, location of the backup, frequency of the backup, and testing of the backup.

**Data capture** Collecting data.

**Data center** Where the hardware and software for the electronic information systems are held.

**Data cleanroom** A virtual environment to ensure personal identifiable information is anonymized

**Data conversion** Implementation process of taking data already in one automated system and putting it into a new system.

**Data dashboard** Interface that provides a visual expression of the output (charts, graphs, and so on).

**Data democratization** When data are made available without barriers.

**Data dictionary** A descriptive list of the names, definitions, and attributes of data elements to be collected within an information system or database whose purpose is to standardize definitions and ensure consistent use.

**Data governance (DG)** Overall administration, through clearly defined procedures and plans, that assures the availability, integrity, security, and usability of the structured and unstructured data available to an organization.

**Data governance office (DGO)** Individual responsible for providing centralized communication and archive for DG initiatives, working with stakeholders, coordinating DG initiatives, facilitating and coordinating data steward committees, task forces, and meetings, supporting the data governance council, and collecting and analyzing DG metrics.

**Data governance steering committee** Composed of representatives from various business or functional organizational units and serves as the coordinating body for the DG program.

**Data, information, knowledge, and wisdom (DIKW) hierarchy** An essential principle of computer information and library sciences.

**Data in motion** Data in the process of being transmitted from one location to another location, such as an email.

**Data interoperability** The ability of different information technology systems to exchange data accurately, effectively, and consistently so information can be used

**Data lake** Holds data in its raw format.

**Data life cycle** Stages of data planning, data inventory and evaluation, data capture, data transformation and processing, data access and distribution, data maintenance, data archival, and data destruction

**Data mining** When the analyst performs exploratory data analysis to determine trends and identify patterns in the data set. Data mining is sometimes referred to as knowledge discovery.

**Data model** Used to describe how data elements are used in processing data, including the various attributes and relationships between data.

**Data modeling** A fundamental aspect of database design, involving formalizing data requirements and structuring data to meet specific needs.

**Data provenance** The historical record of data and its origins.

**Data quality management** "A continuous process for setting standards, building quality into the processes that create, transform, and store data, and measuring data against standards" (DAMA 2017, 454).

**Data quality measurement** "A mechanism to assign a quantity to quality of care by comparison to a criterion (Davoudi et al. 2015)."

**Data repository** A special open-structure database which is not dedicated to the software of any specific vendor or data supplier and stores data from diverse sources to achieve an integrated, multidisciplinary view of the data

**Data security** The process in which organizations implement protection measures and tools for safeguarding data and information from unauthorized, accidental, or intentional modification, destruction, or use.

**Data security management** Policies and procedures that address confidentiality and security concerns of organizational stakeholders (for example, patients, providers, and employees), protecting organizational proprietary interests, and compliance with government and regulatory requirements, while accommodating legitimate access needs.

**Data stack** A complete suite of tools focused on loading, transforming, warehousing, and analyzing data.

**Data stakeholders** Those who have an interest or stake in organizational data.

**Data steward** An individual appointed with responsibility and accountability for data, usually in a specific domain.

**Data Use and Reciprocal Support Agreement (DURSA)** A legally binding contract that draws from federal and local laws and defines the requirements for participation in the eHealth Exchange national network.

**Data visualization** A process of formatting data into patterns to support the interpretation of information.

**Data warehouses** Databases that make it possible to access data from multiple databases and combine the results into a single query and reporting interface.

**Database administrators** Technical staff members within IT departments who design and manage the technical implementation and maintenance of databases.

**Database management systems (DBMSs)** Software tools used to store, analyze, modify, and access data.

**Days in accounts receivable** Ratio that reflects how long it takes for an organization to collect its accounts receivable.

**Debt ratio** Total liabilities divided by total assets.

**Debt service** The extent to which financial obligations are loans.

**Decision rights** Appointing authority to specific individuals or categories of individuals to make data-related decisions and designating when and how those decisions are made.

**Decision support** Rules programmed into software to recognize various combinations of data being captured in IT and to generate various types of actions by the technology according to the rule requirements.

**Decryption** The process of transforming the information from cipher text to plaintext.

**Deductive reasoning** Also known as deduction; involves drawing conclusions based on generalizations, rules, or principles.

**Deemed status** "In order to participate in and receive federal payment from Medicare or Medicaid programs, a healthcare organization must meet the government requirements for program participation, including a certification of compliance with the health and safety requirements called Conditions of Participation (CoPs) or Conditions for Coverage (CfCs), which are set forth in federal regulations" (Joint Commission n.d.).

**Defamation of character** A false communication about someone to a person other than the subject that may injure the subject's reputation.

**Default judgment** If the defendant fails to file a timely answer, the court will find in favor of the plaintiff and enter a default judgment against the defendant.

**Defendant** The party who is accused of committing the wrong.

**Deidentification** Refers to health information that has had identifiers removed, also removing the capability to reasonably identify the individual to which the information belongs.

**Delegation** The process by which managers distribute work to others along with the authority to make decisions and take action.

**Delinquent health record** A record that is not completed within the specified time frame (for example, within 14 days of discharge).

**Democratic leadership** Involves members making decisions, leading them to perform well whether the leader was present or absent, and increased member satisfaction.

**Denials** A payer's refusal to provide partial or full payment.

**Deontology** A theory developed by German philosopher Immanuel Kant in the late eighteenth century that studies the nature of moral obligations, and holds that what is right and good in terms of morality is determined by a moral agent's actions and intentions relative to their duties and obligations.

**Dependency** Exists when one component cannot operate without another component.

**Dependent variable** Measured variable that depends on the independent variable and is the outcome or variable to be predicted.

**Depositions** Sworn statements from witnesses.

**Depreciation** An estimate of the decrease in value of an asset over time.

**Descriptive metadata** Data that describes each data element to be captured and processed by IT.

**Descriptive research** Determines and reports the current status of topics and subjects.

**Descriptive statistics** Meant to describe a large amount of data by illustrating the data with charts, graphs, and tables in a way that the data are summarized and organized. Descriptive statistics are not used to draw conclusions about the population the data are describing.

**Designated record set** A group of records maintained by or for a covered entity that may include patient medical and billing records; the enrollment, payment, claims, adjudication, and cases or medical management record systems maintained by or for a health plan; or information used in whole or in part to make care-related decisions.

**Detective controls** Processes designed to find errors already made.

**Development** In traditional management theory, a process for maintaining or upgrading competencies for management staff who needed to improve skills such as decision-making and interpersonal communication.

**Diagnosis-related groups (DRGs)** A DRG is a unit of case-mix classification adopted by the federal government and some other payers as a prospective payment mechanism for hospital inpatients in which diseases are placed into groups because related diseases and treatments tend to consume similar amounts of healthcare resources and incur similar costs.

***Diagnostic and Statistical Manual of Mental Disorders,* Fifth Edition (DSM-5-TR)** The handbook used by healthcare professionals as a guide to diagnose mental disorders, first published by the American Psychiatric Association (APA) in 1952.

**Direct costs** Costs traceable to a specific good or service provided.

**Direct maternal death** The death of a woman resulting from obstetrical (OB) complications of the pregnancy state, labor, or puerperium (the period within 42 days following delivery).

**Directed exchange** Used by providers to easily and securely send patient information directly to another healthcare provider over the internet; it is compared to sending a secured e-mail.

**Disaster recovery plan** A document that defines the processes for recovery of data in the event of a disaster.

**Discharged, not final billed (DNFB)** A bill cannot be generated until the coding is complete, so organizations routinely monitor the days.

**Discharge summary** Provides details about the patient's stay while in the facility and is the foundation for future treatment. It is prepared when the patient is discharged or transferred to another facility or when the patient dies.

**Discipline** A field of study characterized by a knowledge base and perspective distinctive from other fields of study.

**Disclosure** The release, transfer, provision of access to, or divulging in any manner of information outside the entity holding the information.

**Discounting** Applies to multiple surgical procedures furnished during the same operative session. For discounted procedures, the full APC rate is paid for the surgical procedure with the highest rate, and other surgical procedures performed at the same time are reimbursed at 50 percent of the APC rate.

**Discovery** Consists of both the pretrial period and the activities by which both the plaintiff(s) and defendant(s) will obtain information held by other parties to assess the strengths and weaknesses of each party's case.

**Discrete data** Ordinal and nominal data that take on categorical values and cannot be added together or divided.

**Discrimination** Practices that result in people being treated differently based solely on their personal distinctions.

**Disease index** A list of diagnosis codes in numerical order for patients discharged from the facility during a particular period.

**Disposition** The process of destroying the records once the end of the retention period is reached.

**Distributive justice** Refers to the fair and equitable allocation of goods and harms according to social norms.

**District courts** Following a three-level hierarchy, the 94 trial courts in the federal court system. District courts hear cases involving federal question jurisdiction or diversity jurisdiction.

**Diversity jurisdiction** Where no plaintiff is from the same state as any defendant in a case.

**Diversity training** Facilitates an environment that fosters inclusion and appreciation of individual differences within the organization's workforce.

**DMAIC** A scientific methodology for quality improvement that involves the following steps: define, measure, analyze, improve, and control.

**Do-not-resuscitate (DNR) order** A document which specifies an individual's wish not to receive treatment (specifically, cardiopulmonary resuscitation or CPR).

**Dot plot** A system that presents the frequency or means to compare many groups using dots.

**Double billing** When two providers bill for one service provided to one patient.

**Double-blind studies** Randomized clinical trials (RCTs) in which neither the investigator nor the subjects know who is in the treatment or control group until the end of the study.

**Due diligence** Steps taken to confirm various facts about the product.

**Duplicate** When two or more medical record numbers are created for the same person, causing them to have two or more records.

**Durable power of attorney** An advanced directive in which the patient names another person to make medical decisions on his or her behalf in the event he or she is incapacitated.

**Durable power of attorney for healthcare decisions** A document in which an adult—while competent—designates another person (proxy) to make healthcare decisions consistent with the individual's wishes and on the individual's behalf if the individual is unable.

**E-discovery** A pretrial process through which parties obtain and review ESI.

**E-learning** Training courses delivered in a variety of electronic formats.

**E-Rx (e-prescribing)** A special type of CPOE application used to write prescriptions and transmit them to retail pharmacies through the National Council for Prescription Drug Programs (NCPDP) SCRIPT standard sent through a pharmacy information exchange.

**Early adopters** Individuals with a high degree of opinion leadership. They are more localized than worldly, and often look to the innovators for advice and information. These are the leaders and respected role models in the organization, and their adoption of an idea or practice does much to initiate change.

**Early majority**   Usually not leaders, but the individuals in this group represent the backbone of the organization, are deliberate in thinking about and accepting an idea, and serve as a natural bridge between early and late adopters.

**Economic compensatory (special) damages**   Damages that are objectively verified and calculable. They include losses such as medical expenses or lost wages.

**85/15 rule**   Rule of TQM that proposes 85 percent of problems encountered are the result of faulty systems and only 15 percent are due to unconscientious or unproductive employees.

**eHealth Exchange**   A group of federal agencies and nonfederal organizations that came together under a common mission and purpose to improve patient care, streamline disability claim benefits, and improve public health reporting through secure, trusted, and interoperable HIE.

**Electronic document/content management (ED/CM) system**   Any electronic system that manages an organization's analog and digital documents and content (that is, not just the data) to realize significant improvements in business work processes.

**Electronic health information (EHI)**   All electronic protected health information (ePHI) in the designated record set (DRS).

**Electronic health record (EHR)**   "An electronic record of health-related information on an individual that conforms to nationally recognized interoperability standards and that can be created, managed, and consulted by authorized clinicians and staff across more than one healthcare organization" (NAHIT 2008).

**Electronic medical record (EMR)**   "An electronic record of health-related information on an individual that can be created, gathered, managed, and consulted by authorized clinicians and staff within one healthcare organization" (NAHIT 2008).

**Electronic remittance advice (ERA)**   Digital distribution of final individual claim adjudication and payment information used by government and many commercial payers.

**Electronic signature**   Also known as an e-signature; a computer data compilation of any symbol or series of symbols executed, adopted, or authorized by an individual to be the legally binding equivalent of the individual's handwritten signature.

**Emergency Medical Treatment and Labor Act (EMTALA)**   A statute protecting any patient seeking emergency care in a Medicare-participating hospital, requiring they be appropriately evaluated for an emergency medical condition regardless of the ability to pay.

**Emergency mode operation plan**   A plan that creates processes and procedures to support the continuation of critical business and patient care operations while protecting the security of ePHI in the event of a disaster.

**Emotional intelligence (EI)**   The sensitivity and ability to monitor and revise one's behavior based on the needs and responses of others.

**Employee handbook**   A reference document that presents policies and requirements all employees must know.

**Employee self-logging**   A form of self-reporting in which the employees track their tasks, volume of work units, and hours worked.

**Employer-based self-insurance**   A common form of group health insurance coverage. Many employers enter administrative services only (ASO) contracts with private insurers and fund the plans themselves.

**Employer-based self-insurance**   When companies provide and pay for employee health plans rather than employees purchasing coverage from private insurers.

**Employment-at-will**   Concept that either an employer or an employee can terminate an employment relationship without providing either notice or reason.

**Empowerment**   The concept of providing employees with the tools and resources to solve problems themselves.

**Encryption**   A mathematical method for the transformation of data from plaintext into cipher text, allowing no individual or machine to get access and decipher the original information.

**End users**   Those using the system for everyday tasks.

**Enterprise governance**   Visible in every aspect of an organization through establishment, application, and monitoring of strategies, policies and procedures to all organizational entities and levels.

**Enterprise master patient index (EMPI)**   Provides access to multiple repositories of information from overlapping patient populations maintained in separate systems and databases.

**Entity**   A class of objects that exist in the real world and have related properties.

**Entity relationship diagram (ERD)** A type of conceptual modeling that has three basic graphical symbols: entities, attributes, and relationships.

**Environmental scan** Part of the strategic planning process where an organization identifies external opportunities and threats that could impact the business in the future.

**Epidemiological study** A study intended to compare one group or population with the risk factor of interest to one group or population without it.

**Epidemiology** The study of the distribution and determinants of health-related states or events in specified populations and the application of this study to control health problems.

**Episode-of-care (EOC) reimbursement** Method used to issue lump-sum payments to providers to compensate them for all the healthcare services delivered to a patient for a specific illness or over a specific period. Also called bundled payments.

**Equal Employment Opportunity Act of 1972** The amendment to the Civil Rights Act of 1964, prohibiting discrimination in the workplace based on age, gender, race, color, religion, sex, or national origin.

**Equal Employment Opportunity Commission (EEOC)** Agency created by Title VII of the Civil Rights Act of 1964 to investigate discrimination claims.

**Equal Pay Act (EPA) of 1963** Requires equal pay for men and women performing substantially the same work.

**Equity** The fair and just distribution of resources, opportunities, and advantages within a given organization or system; In finance, the arithmetic difference between assets and liabilities.

**Ergonomics** A discipline of functional design associated with the employee in relationship to his or her work environment, including equipment, workstation, and office furniture adaptation to accommodate the employee's unique physical requirements with a goal to facilitate effectiveness of work functions.

**Esprit de corps** A work climate in which harmony, cohesion, and high morale promote good work.

**Ethical lapse** A mistake or error in judgment that results in harmful effects relative to ethical standards.

**Ethics** The study of morality using the principles, theories, and decision-making frameworks of philosophy.

**Ethics committee** A committee within the organization tasked with reviewing ethics questions and policies, suggesting acceptable courses of action in ethically charged situations.

**Ethnography** The investigation of a culture by collecting data and making observations while being in the field (naturalistic setting).

**Evaluation research** Research that examines the effectiveness of policies, programs, or organizations.

**Evidence** Supporting information the plaintiff presents before a judge or a jury.

**Evidence-based clinical practice guideline** An explicit statement that guides clinical decision-making systematically developed from scientific evidence and clinical expertise to answer clinical questions.

**Evidence-based management** Also known as information-based management, in which more informed decisions are made based on the best clinical and research evidence that proposed practices are valid.

**Evidence-based practice** The "integration of clinical expertise, patient values, and the best research evidence into the decision-making process for patient care" (Sackett et al. 1996).

**Exchange relationship** A leader offers greater opportunities and privileges to an employee in exchange for loyalty, commitment, and assistance.

**Exclusion provisions** A component of the Social Security Act that indicates the OIG has the authority to "exclude individuals from participating in federal healthcare programs and will not pay for items or services furnished by an excluded individual or entity" (Social Security Act 1996).

**Exclusive provider organizations (EPOs)** Similar to PPOs except that EPOs provide benefits to enrollees only when the enrollees receive healthcare services from network providers, healthcare professionals who are members of a managed care network.

**Executive dashboard** An information management system providing decision makers with regularly updated information on an organization's key strategic measures.

**Executive data governance council** A group of executives and senior-level managers responsible for making the business case for the DG program, providing the authorization for the DG program, establishing the program's mission and scope, setting the program's strategic direction, securing funding and resources for the program, and evaluating and measuring the overall program success.

**Exempt employees** Those who are exempt from some or all of the FLSA provisions and who are paid a salary per pay period.

**Exit interviews** An interview conducted by an HR representative and the direct supervisor with employees who leave the organization to obtain information on how employees feel about their jobs and what issues cause them to leave.

**Expectancy theory of motivation** Proposes that one's degree of effort is influenced by the expectation that the effort will result in the attainment of desired goals and meaningful rewards.

**Expense projects** Projects where new and improved information is created.

**Expenses** Represent the utilization of resources by the organization to generate revenue.

**Experimental (study) group** Comprises the research subjects who receive the study's intervention.

**Experimental research** A design in which the researcher directly manipulates factors in carefully controlled interventions according to strict protocols (detailed sets of rules and procedures).

**Experimental study** A study wherein the exposure status for everyone in the study is determined and the individuals are then followed to determine the effects of the exposure.

**Expert determination method** A method of deidentification in which data elements that could identify an individual are removed from the data and then an expert the organization hires, such as a statistician, applies scientific methodology to determine the likelihood of identification of the individual and provides documentation of the probability that the information would be identified. If there is low probability that the information can be identified, the information is considered deidentified.

**Explanation of benefits (EOB)** Document also known as an explanation of payment (EOP) provided by the payer to describe the payment made on the claim.

**Explicit knowledge** Includes documents, databases, and other types of recorded and documented information.

**Express warranty** Specific promises a seller makes to the buyer.

**External benchmarking** Occurs when an organization compares similar processes, services, or outcomes with other organizations.

**External customers** Customers that reside outside the organization.

**External validity** The generalizability of the study's findings to other people or groups, such as patients, hospitals, and countries.

**Extract > transform > load (ETL)** Process that collects and processes data from various sources into a single data store.

**Extranets** Internet technologies designed to enhance communication among an organization's external business partners.

**Extrapolation method** Wherein auditing claims look at a small sample of records and apply the correction in reimbursement across many claims in a period or service area.

**Facility-based registry** A registry located within a facility such as a hospital or a clinic.

**Factor comparison method** A complex quantitative method that combines elements of both the ranking and point methods. Factor comparison results indicate the degree to which different compensable factors vary by job, making it possible to translate each factor value more easily into a monetary wage.

**Fair Labor Standards Act (FLSA) of 1938** Federally enacted minimum wage and overtime payment regulations.

**False imprisonment** The intentional confinement of someone against that person's will.

**Family and Medical Leave Act (FMLA) of 1993** Federal legislation that allows full-time employees time off from work (up to 12 weeks) to care for themselves or their family members with the assurance of an equivalent position upon return to work.

**Fault** Error

**Favorable variances** Variances that occur when the actual results are better than budget projections.

**Federal False Claims Act of 1863** A federal law that seeks to protect governmental programs from fraud by individuals and companies.

**Federal question jurisdiction** A claim related to federal law, including federal crimes (for example, racketeering); constitutional issues (for example, interpretations of the US Constitution); and other federal laws (for example, bankruptcy law).

*Federal Register* A daily publication issued by the Office of the Federal Register, that makes the rules, opinions, orders, records, and proceedings from administrative agencies available to the public.

**Federated model**  Health information exchange model without a centralized database of patient information.

**Fee-for-service (FFS) reimbursement**  Methodology that issues payments to healthcare providers based on the charges assigned to each separate service performed for the patient.

**Feedback controls**  Back-end processes that monitor and measure output and then compare it to expectations and identify variations.

**Felony**  The more serious of the two categories of crimes (the other being misdemeanor), subject to imprisonment for more than one year.

**Fetal death**  "Death before the complete expulsion or extraction from the mother of a product of human conception, irrespective of the duration of pregnancy that is not an induced termination of pregnancy" (Barfield et al. 2016).

**Fetal death rate**  The total number of early and late fetal deaths for the period divided by the total number of live births and early and late fetal deaths for the same period.

**Fiduciary duty**  Exists because of a relationship of trust and obligation between the provider and the patient.

**Financial Accounting Standards Board (FASB)**  An independent organization that sets accounting standards for businesses in the private sector.

**Financial counselors**  Staff dedicated to helping patients and physicians determine sources of reimbursement for healthcare services.

**Financial data**  Facts associated with healthcare produced by and often exchanged between healthcare providers and health plans, including eligibility and benefits information, healthcare claims, and the like.

**Fiscal year**  Also called the financial year; defined by the tax year.

**Fishbone diagram**  Also known as a cause and effect diagram, it helps determine the root causes of a problem.

**Fixed budget**  Budget in which amounts are based on expected capacity.

**Fixed costs**  Costs that remain the same, despite changes in volume.

**Flexible budgets**  Budget based on projected productivity.

**Flexible spending account (FSA)**  A personal savings account where pretax dollars are deposited for health expenses in a given year. Unused money from one year cannot be rolled over to the next year.

**Flextime**  Work schedule wherein employees choose their arrival and departure times around a fixed core work time.

**Float employees**  Staff who are cross trained in several departmental functions.

**Flowchart**  A visual illustration of a procedure using standard flowcharting symbols to chart the steps.

**Focus group**  A data collection method in which researchers and a small number of participants have a group interview on the researchers' topic to uncover information through the participants' discussion of their thoughts and experiences.

**For-profit healthcare organizations**  Privately owned entities wherein excess funds are paid back to the managers, owners, and investors in the form of bonuses and dividends.

**For-profit organizations**  Sole proprietorships, partnerships, or corporations that may be privately or publicly owned that increase the wealth of the owners through profits.

**Force-field analysis**  Using a T formation, this process visually displays data generated through brainstorming, enabling team members to identify factors that support or work against a proposed solution.

**Foreign keys**  Keys that further determine how tables will be linked as unique identifiers.

**Framework**  A conceptual structure for classifying, organizing, and showing interrelations among activities used as a guide for taking and coordinating action to achieve a goal.

**Fraud**  Willful and intentional deception that could result in harm to a person or to property.

**Freedom of Information Act of 1967 (FOIA)**  A federal law through which individuals can seek access to information without the authorization of the person to whom the information applies.

**Functional interoperability**  Sending messages between computers with a shared understanding of the structure and format of the message.

**Functional manager**  Also referred to as an administrative supervisor, individual who carries out the employee's performance reviews and has authority over promotions and terminations.

**Functional organization**  The traditional hierarchy in an organization where each employee has a single supervisor, and employees are grouped in departments by specialty or subspecialty.

**Gantt chart**  Captures each of the work packages identified in the work breakdown structure (WBS) as tasks for the project team, assigns each task to a project team member, identifies the dates when the work begins and when it will be completed, and identifies any scheduling dependencies with other tasks.

**General consent** Also known as battery consent; consent from patients at the beginning of an encounter to permit providers to perform routine treatment.

**General jurisdiction** When a trial court may hear various types of cases.

**General ledger** A list of all the individual accounts.

**Generalizability** When objective knowledge can be applied to other, similar situations and populations.

**Generally accepted accounting principles (GAAP)** Financial Accounting Standards Board (FASB) rules by which financial data are compiled, reported, reviewed, and audited.

**Genetic Information Nondiscrimination Act (GINA) of 2008** Legislation which prohibits genetic information discrimination against employees or applicants.

**Geographic practice cost index (GPCI)** A number used to multiply each relative value unit (RVU) so it better reflects a geographical area's relative costs.

**Gesture recognition technologies** Collective term for intelligent character recognition (ICR) and mark sense technology.

**Global payments** Lump-sum payments distributed among the physicians who performed the procedure or interpreted its results and the healthcare facility that provided the equipment, supplies, and technical support required.

**Global surgery payment** Payment that covers all the healthcare services entailed in planning and completing a specific surgical procedure.

**Goal** A generalized statement of a unit, department, or organization standard; Statements of intended outcomes that provide a source of direction and motivation as well as a guideline for performance, decision-making, and evaluation.

**Going concern** When analysis of an entity's financial data shows the organization can continue to operate for the foreseeable future.

**Go-live** The final step in turning over the information system to the end users.

**Good Samaritan statutes** A form of immunity that protects against liability for ordinary negligence committed by those assisting with emergency care in settings outside of healthcare facilities (such as motor vehicle accident sites, at sporting events, and so forth) where medical equipment is not generally available, and services are not charged.

**Governance** The establishment of policies and the continual monitoring of their proper implementation for managing organization assets.

**Governmental (sovereign) immunity** Governments of various levels (federal, state, local and tribal) enjoy a degree of protection from tort lawsuits.

**Grand jury** A group of citizens that must return an indictment, or formal charge, for a felony crime to be prosecuted. The grand jury has the authority to issue subpoenas for its investigative process, and all evidence considered by the grand jury remains confidential unless an indictment is returned.

**Graphical perception** The visual interpretation process; originally described as the ability to unconsciously extract information from graphics.

**Great person theory** Theory based on the belief that outstanding historical individuals proved leadership as an inborn ability, sometimes passed down through family, position, or social tradition, as in the cases of royal families in many parts of the world.

**Grey literature** Materials available in print or digital formats but not published through traditional commercial publishing channels, including journals.

**Grievance** When a complaint is documented in writing and brought to the attention of management or union representatives.

**Grievance procedures** Procedures that define the steps an employee can follow to seek resolution of a disagreement they have with management on a job-related issue.

**Gross autopsy rate** Includes all of the deaths that occurred with inpatients, and indicates the proportion of those on which an autopsy was performed.

**Gross death rate** The number of all hospital discharges compared to the number of deaths from that same group of patients.

**Gross negligence** An extreme departure from the ordinary standard of care that shows a reckless disregard toward others.

**Grounded theory** Comprises both the theories generated using the analytical technique and the technique itself.

**Group discussion** When learners form smaller groups to generate ideas through interactive sharing of ideas.

**Group model HMO** When an HMO contracts with an independent multispecialty physician group to provide medical services to plan members.

**Harassment** Practices that create a hostile work environment that can include physical, verbal, or emotional harassment.

**Hawthorne effect** Also called the observer effect; based on the principle that what gets attention and measured is what gets improved.

**Hay method of job evaluation** A modification of the point method that numerically measures the levels of three major compensable factors: the know-how, problem-solving, and accountability requirements of each job.

**Health Care Quality Improvement Act of 1986 (HCQIA)** A federal law that established standards and requirements related to peer review among physicians.

**Health data** The raw facts or figures processed into useful health information.

**Health data stewardship** Responsibilities that best ensure appropriate use of health data.

**Health informatics** A scientific discipline concerned with the cognitive, information-processing, and communication tasks of healthcare practice, education, and research, including the information science and technology to support these tasks.

**Health information** Data that supplies value to the management of illness or injury or the maintenance of health and wellness. Health information is also used to design and support payment strategies for healthcare.

**Health information exchange (HIE)** The exchange of health information, electronically, between providers and others with the same level of interoperability.

**Health information system (HIS)** A set of many individual information systems focused on various aspects of health services that must work together to support delivery of quality healthcare, at a reasonable cost, and with a positive experience for both users and patients.

**Health information technology (HIT)** Describes computer systems and associated components such as networks, software, and end-user devices used to process health data into health information.

**Health Information Technology for Economic and Clinical Health (HITECH) Act** Legislation created to promote the adoption and meaningful use of health information technology (HIT) in the US.

**Health Insurance Portability and Accountability Act of 1996 (HIPAA)** Originally established to ensure health insurance continuity (also known as portability), set standards for electronic claims and national identifiers, and protect against fraud and abuse. It was subsequently expanded to establish national standards for the protection of privacy and the assurance of the security of health information.

**Health Level 7 Fast Healthcare Interoperability Resources (HL7 FHIR)** A standard that defines how healthcare information can be exchanged between computer systems regardless of how it is stored in those systems.

**Health Level Seven International (HL7)** A not-for-profit, ANSI-accredited standards-developing organization founded in 1987, dedicated to providing a comprehensive framework and related standards for the exchange, integration, sharing, and retrieval of electronic health information that supports clinical practice and the management, delivery, and evaluation of health services.

**Health maintenance organization (HMO)** A prepaid voluntary health plan that provides healthcare services in return for the payment of a monthly membership premium and usually only pays for care within its own network and the primary care doctor coordinates care.

**Health record banking model** An organization with information-sharing agreements between a group of healthcare providers that enables the aggregation and delivery of patient information to the patient under the control of the patient.

**Health reimbursement account (HRA)** A health reimbursement arrangement or employer-funded health plan that helps employees pay for their qualified medical expenses.

**Health Research Extension Act of 1985** Requires the secretary of HHS to issue a regulation requiring applicant or awardee institutions to establish an administrative process to review reports of scientific fraud and report to the Secretary any investigation of scientific fraud which appears substantial.

**Health savings account (HSA)** A personal savings account, but the money deposited into it can be used only for healthcare expenses.

**Health services research** Examines the quality, accessibility, cost, and efficiency of healthcare services to improve the overall patient care standards.

**Health statistics** Providing information for understanding, monitoring, improving, and planning the use of resources to improve the lives of people, provide services, and promote their well-being.

**Health technology assessment (HTA)** The evaluation of the usefulness (utility) of a health technology in relation to cost, efficacy, utilization, and other factors in terms of its impact on social, ethical, and legal systems.

**Healthcare Common Procedure Coding System (HCPCS)** Used to report services and supplies primarily for reimbursement purposes in the outpatient or ambulatory setting.

**Healthcare Cost and Utilization Project (HCUP)** A major initiative for the Agency for Healthcare Research and Quality (AHRQ). HCUP uses data collected from nationwide databases and state-specific databases at the state level from either claims data from the UB-04 or discharge-abstracted data, including UHDDS items reported by individual hospitals and, in some cases, by freestanding ambulatory care centers.

**Healthcare data analytics** The practice of using data to make business decisions in healthcare. More specifically, healthcare data analytics is the application of statistical techniques to allow informed decisions to be made based on the data.

**Healthcare Effectiveness Data and Information Set (HEDIS)** Developed by the NCQA, a set of standardized measures used to compare managed care plans in terms of the quality of services they provide.

**Hearsay** A statement made outside of court that can be used in court to prove the truth of a claim, the business records exception to the prohibition against admitting hearsay evidence will often permit a health record to be admitted

**Hierarchical Condition Categories (HCCs)** HCCs categorize diseases and health conditions for the purpose of risk adjustment in healthcare. HCCs are hierarchical in nature, meaning they are organized to reflect the complexity of diseases and the costs associated with those diseases.

**Histogram** A data analysis tool used to display frequencies of response or density distribution of a single numeric variable.

**History** A summary of the illness or injury from the patient's point of view. Its purpose is to allow the patient or the patient's authorized representative to give the practitioner as much background information about the patient's illness as possible.

**Historical research** Investigates past events to draw associations and develop predictions for present and future events.

**HITECH-HIPAA Omnibus Privacy Act** Also known as the Omnibus Rule, strengthened the privacy and security of patient information, modified the Breach Notification Rule, strengthened privacy protections for genetic information by prohibiting health plans from using or disclosing such information for underwriting, made BAs of HIPAA covered entities liable for compliance, strengthened limitations on the use and disclosure of PHI for marketing, research, and fundraising, and allowed patients increased restriction rights.

**Holding** A court's decision.

**Home health agency (HHA)** A program or organization that provides a blend of home-based medical and social services to homebound patients and their families. It may be provided part-time in a homebound beneficiary's home when intermittent or part-time skilled nursing or certain other therapy or rehabilitation care is needed.

**Home Health Resource Groups (HHRGs)** Represents the classification system established for the prospective reimbursement of covered home care services to Medicare beneficiaries during a 60-day episode of care.

**Home healthcare** A wide range of healthcare services that can be delivered in the home.

**Hospice** An interdisciplinary program of palliative care and supportive services that addresses the physical, spiritual, social, and economic needs of the terminally ill and their families.

**Hospital** Applied to any healthcare facility that has an organized medical staff, permanent inpatient beds, around-the-clock nursing services, and diagnostic and therapeutic services.

**Hospital autopsy rate** A type of autopsy rate that includes anyone who had an autopsy at the hospital and any former patients who died when they were not a hospital inpatient.

**Hospital death rate** A measure of quality of care and patient demographic for each hospital calculated using the number of patients discharged from the hospital (both alive and dead) during a specific time.

**Hospital inpatient** "A patient who is provided with room, board, and continuous general nursing service in an area of an acute-care facility where patients generally stay at least overnight" (IHS n.d.).

**Hospital newborn inpatient** A patient born in the hospital at the beginning of the current patient hospitalization.

**Hospital outpatient** A patient who receives hospital services without being admitted for inpatient care.

**Hospital Value-Based Purchasing Program** This program allows Medicare to adjust payments to hospitals through the Inpatient-Prospective Payment System, a Medicare program reimbursement methodology. It also emphasizes improved quality of care and hospitalization experiences for patients with Medicare.

**Hospital-acquired conditions (HACs)** CMS identified conditions not present on admission and identified as reasonably preventable; hospitals will not receive additional payment for cases in which one of the eight selected conditions was not POA.

**Hospital-issued notice of noncoverage (HINN)** A notice provided to patients when an inpatient service has been deemed noncovered due to medical necessity.

**Human subjects** Defined by the Common Rule as "living individual[s] about whom an investigator (whether professional or student) conducting research obtains (1) data through intervention or interaction with the individual, or (2) identifiable private information" (45 CFR 46.102).

**Human–computer interface (HCI)** Term used to describe technologies that are the construct that enables exchange of data between the human and the computer.

**Hung jury** Occurs if all individuals on a jury cannot agree.

**Hybrid model** A cross between the centralized and the decentralized health information exchange model.

**Hypothesis** A statement that describes a research question in measurable terms.

**Hypothesis test** Test that allows the analyst to determine the likelihood a hypothesis is true given the data present in the sample with a predetermined acceptable level of making an error.

**Identity theft** "A fraud attempted or committed using identifying information of another person without authority" (FTC 2021).

**Implementation** The process in which hardware is installed; software is loaded to the organization's servers, to the ASP environment, the SaaS environment, or a combination of these; special tools supplied by the vendor are used to customize the system in order to meet a specific organization's needs; data from a preexisting system are converted and loaded to the new system; paper chart conversion is performed through scanning or direct data entry; and policies and procedures are updated with new process and workflow requirements.

**Implementation plans** Used to manage the thousands of tasks involved in selecting, acquiring, implementing, adopting, and optimizing the use of the various hardware, software, and operational components of the HIS.

**Implied warranty** When the facts lead to an inference that an express warranty exists "as a matter of public policy" to protect the public from harm.

**In-group** Those employees who form a group around the leader.

**In-service education** Continuous employee development process that builds on the basic skills learned through new employee orientation and on-the-job training.

**Incentive pay** A form of positive reinforcement. The higher the quality and quantity of work, the better the pay increase given.

**Incidence** The number of new cases of a disease.

**Incidence rate** A statistic that measures frequency.

**Incident** An occurrence that is inconsistent with the standard of care.

**Incident report** A tool staff can use to report unusual incidents to administration, initiate investigations, and provide appropriate feedback to staff involved in an incident.

**Income statement** A summary of the organization's revenue and expense transactions during the fiscal year.

**Independent practice association (IPA)** A model in which the HMO contracts with an organized group of physicians who join for purposes of fulfilling the HMO contract but retain their individual practices.

**Independent variables** Antecedent or prior factors researchers manipulate directly that are the variables used to predict; they are also called treatments or interventions.

**Index** A report from a database that enables health records to be located by diagnosis, procedure, or physician, indices are computerized reports available from data included in databases routinely maintained in the healthcare facility.

**Indian Health Service (IHS)** An agency within the HHS responsible for providing healthcare services to American Indians and Indigenous People of Alaska.

**Indictment** A formal charge for a felony crime

**Indirect costs** Also known as overhead costs, they are incurred by the organization in the process of providing goods or services and are not specifically attributable to an individual product or service.

**Indirect maternal death** The death of a woman from a previously existing disease or a disease that developed during pregnancy, labor, or the puerperium not due to obstetric causes, although the physiologic effects of pregnancy were partially responsible.

**Indirect standardization**   A more straightforward method for calculating a RSMR to derive the expected rate for an outcome variable. Indirect standardization is appropriate to use for risk adjustment when the risk variables are categorical and the rate or proportion for the variable of interest is available for the standard or reference group at the level of the risk categories.

**Individually identifiable health information**   Information that identifies the individual, or there is reasonable belief it can be used to identify the individual, and relates to the individual's past, present, or future physical or mental health or condition; the provision of healthcare to the individual; or the past, present, or future payment for the provision of healthcare to the individual.

**Inductive reasoning**   Also known as induction; involves drawing conclusions based on a limited number of observations.

**Infection rates**   Calculation of infection in healthcare facilities.

**Inferential statistics**   Used to test a hypothesis and draw conclusions about the population.

**Infliction of emotional distress**   Intentional or reckless behavior for which a person can be held liable that includes mental suffering resulting from despair, shame, grief, and public humiliation.

**Informatics**   A field of study focusing on the use of technology to improve access to, and utilization of, information. It uses computers to manage data and information and support decision-making activities.

**Information**   "The output of some process that summarizes, interprets, or otherwise represents data to convey meaning" (Caldicott 2013, 24).

**Information governance (IG)**   Employs policies, procedures, and multi-disciplinary arrangements to manage and optimize an organization's information for its immediate and future needs including regulatory, legal, risk, environmental, and operational requirements

**Information management**   The generation, collection, organization, validation, analysis, storage, and integration of data, and the dissemination, communication, presentation, utilization, transmission, and safeguarding of information.

**Information overload**   Difficulty in making decisions due to the presence of excessive amounts of information.

**Information system**   "An automated system that uses computer hardware and software to record, manipulate, store, recover, and disseminate data (that is, a system that receives and processes input and provides output)" (Sayles and Kavanaugh-Burke 2021, 1).

**Informed consent**   This ensures a patient has a basic understanding of his or her diagnosis; the nature of the treatment or procedure along with the risks, benefits, and alternatives (to include opting out of treatment); and names of individuals who will perform the treatment or procedure.

**Injunction**   An order to generally stop some action.

**Injury Severity Score (ISS)**   An overall severity measurement calculated from the AIS scores for the patient's three most severe injuries.

**Innovators**   A venturesome group comprised of individuals eager to try new ideas. These individuals tend to be worldly and sophisticated, seek out new information in broad networks, and are more willing to take risks.

**Inpatient**   A person who is provided with room, board, and continuous general nursing services in an area of an acute care facility where patients generally stay at least overnight.

**Inpatient admission**   An acute-care facility's formal acceptance of a patient who is to be provided with room, board, and continuous nursing service in an area of the facility where patients generally stay overnight.

**Inpatient bed occupancy rate**   The percentage of official beds occupied by hospital inpatients for a given period.

**Inpatient census**   Indicates the number of inpatients present in the hospital at a particular point in time.

**Inpatient discharge**   The termination of hospitalization through the formal release of an inpatient by the hospital.

**Inpatient service day (IPSD)**   The unit of measure denoting the services received by one inpatient in one 24-hour period.

**Installation**   The process used to set up hardware and load software onto the acquired hardware.

**Institute for Healthcare Improvement (IHI)**   A healthcare improvement organization that focuses on the "values of courage, love, equity, and trust to improve health and healthcare worldwide so that everyone has the best care and health possible" (IHI n.d.a).

**Institute of Medicine (IOM)**   Established in 1970, the present-day National Academy of Medicine, a branch of the National Academy of Sciences, that exists "to advance science, inform policy, and catalyze action to achieve human health, equity, and well-being" (National Academy of Medicine n.d.).

**Institutional Review Board (IRB)** An HHS-mandated committee established (within a hospital or university, for example) to protect the rights and welfare of human research subjects involved in research activities.

**Instrument** A standardized, uniform way to collect data.

**Insurance verification** Part of the prearrival process for scheduled patients that entails validating that the patient is a member of the insurance plan given and is covered for the scheduled service date, whether the patient's insurance plan is in-network versus out-of-network, whether the scheduled service expenses will be covered, whether a referral or an authorization is required prior to the service being rendered, and whether the patient will incur an out-of-pocket expense.

**Integrated delivery system (IDS)** A system combining the financial and clinical aspects of healthcare using a group of healthcare providers across facilities within the same system, selected according to quality and cost management criteria, to furnish comprehensive health services throughout the continuum of care.

**Integrated Outpatient Code Editor (IOCE)** Editor that validates complete and accurate outpatient claims.

**Integrity** To behave in a trustworthy manner, elevate service to others above self-interest, and promote high standards of practice in every setting.

**Intelligent document recognition (IDR) technology** Technology that trains itself to identify document or form types and sorts the information accordingly for subsequent data entry, eliminating the need for barcodes or other identifying characters and symbols.

**Intent** Means the person committed an act deliberately, intending to cause harm, or knowing that harm would likely occur.

**Interface** Software that works between two or more systems to enable the two systems to share data.

**Interface terminology** Terminology concerned with facilitating clinician documentation within the standardized structure (for example, menus, drop-down boxes) needed for an EHR.

**Internal benchmarking** Compares similar processes, services, or outcomes across internal departments of an organization; it may also track changes within the organization over time.

**Internal customers** Customers located within an organization.

**Internal rate of return (IRR)** The interest rate that makes the NPV calculation equal zero. In other words, it is the interest rate at which the present value of the projected cash inflows equals the initial investment.

**Internal Revenue Service (IRS)** The federal agency that regulates and collects federal taxes.

**Internal validity** An attribute of a study's design that contributes to the accuracy of its findings.

**International Classification of Diseases (ICD)** A classification system that facilitates the storage and retrieval of diagnostic information and serves as the basis for compiling mortality and morbidity statistics reported by WHO members.

**International Classification of Diseases for Oncology (ICD-O-3)** Currently in its third edition via the WHO, this classification system is used for coding diagnoses of neoplasms in tumor and cancer registries and pathology laboratories.

**International Classification of Diseases, Tenth Revision, Clinical Modification (ICD-10-CM)** System for the reporting of morbidity data and reimbursement in the US. It is based on the WHO's ICD-10 system and was modified by CMS and NCHS.

**International Classification of Diseases, Tenth Revision, Procedure Coding System (ICD-10-PCS)** Seven-character alphanumerical system used for inpatient procedure coding in the US. It includes the use of standardized definitions, ease of expandability, ease of use, and comprehensiveness.

**International Classification of Diseases, Eleventh Revision (ICD-11)** A classification system designed to include linkages to standardized healthcare terminologies to facilitate processing and use of the data for a variety of purposes, such as research.

**International Classification of Primary Care (ICPC-3)** A coding terminology for the classification of primary care developed by the Academic Associations of General Practitioners /Family Physicians (WONCA) International Classification Committee (WICC).

**International Classification on Functioning, Disability, and Health (ICF)** A classification, developed by the WHO, of health and health-related domains that describe body functions and structures, activities, and participation that is used within the US.

**International Health Terminology Standards Development Organization (IHTSDO)** An international nonprofit organization based in Denmark that owns, maintains, and distributes SNOMED CT.

**Internet forum** A "web application for holding discussions and posting user-generated content, also commonly referred to as web forums, newsgroups, message boards, discussion boards, bulletin boards, or simply a forum" (Ho 2009, 187).

**Internet of Medical Things (IoMT)** A network that describes a network of physical objects or "things" integrated to exchange healthcare data between devices and systems over the internet.

**Interoperability** Ability to exchange information between computer systems and the capability of different information systems (ISs) and software applications to communicate and exchange data; The ability of different information technology systems and software applications to communicate; to exchange data accurately, effectively, and consistently; and to use the information that has been exchanged.

**Interpersonal skills** The ability to work with and through others to accomplish goals.

**Interprofessional education (IPE)** When individuals from "two or more professions learn about, from, and with each other to enable effective collaboration and improve health outcomes" (WHO 2010, 13).

**Interrater reliability** Different persons completing the test will have reasonably similar findings.

**Interrogatories** Discovery devices consisting of a set of written formal questions given to a party, witness, or other person who has information needed in a legal case.

**Interval data** Naturally numeric data where the distance between two values has meaning, but multiplying values and zero value has no interpretation.

**Interviews** When a researcher wants to understand a patient's impressions and experiences, interviews can be applied to gain more insight through telephone calls or face-to-face interactions.

**Intranets** Use internet technologies but are protected with security features and designed to enhance communication among an organization's internal employees and facilities only.

**Intrarater reliability** The same person repeating a test will have reasonably similar findings.

**Invasion of privacy** Intrusion on one's solitude.

**Inventor** Also called an innovator. The individual who develops a new idea or practice in the organization.

**Investor-owned hospital chains** Publicly traded for-profit groups of hospitals.

**Iterative approach** An approach to make project output available sooner by executing projects in releases following the project management life cycle.

**Job classification method** Involves matching a job's written position description with a description of a classification grade.

**Job evaluation** The process of applying predefined compensable factors to jobs to determine their relative worth.

**Job procedure** A structured, action-oriented list of sequential steps involved in carrying out a specific job or solving a problem.

**Job ranking** The simplest and the most subjective method of job evaluation. It involves placing jobs in order from highest to lowest in value to the organization.

**Job rotation** Technique in which an employee moves from job to job at planned intervals, usually three to six months.

**Job sharing** Work schedule that divides one job between two part-time employees, each with partial benefits (as they apply).

**Job specification** A document (or a section of the job description document) focused on the knowledge, skills, abilities, and characteristics required of an individual to perform the job.

**Joinder** If a defendant brings a claim against an outsider as a codefendant.

**Joint Commission** The successor organization to the American College of Surgeons (ACS) in the area of standardization; was initially responsible for the accreditation of hospitals and has since expanded its accreditation process to home health, long-term care, and other types of healthcare facilities.

**Judicial branch** The court system, which provides an avenue to enforce rights and obligations through the resolution of disputes.

**Jurisdiction** The power to hear and decide the controversy in a given case.

**Just-in-time training** Content is taught in small, relevant portions where and when the learner can use it most readily.

**Justice** Refers to the fair and equitable treatment of persons considering what is owed to them.

**Key indicators** Current measurement thresholds that alert a department or work unit to its existing level of service.

**Key performance indicators (KPIs)** Goals that allow healthcare facilities to measure and benchmark their data against best practice.

**Labor relations** HR management activities associated with unions and collective bargaining.

**Labor-Management Relations Act (Taft-Hartley Act) of 1947** Federal legislation passed in 1947 that imposed certain restrictions on unions while upholding their right to organize and bargain collectively.

**Labor-Management Reporting and Disclosure Act (Landrum-Griffin Act) of 1959** Federal legislation passed in 1959 to ensure union members' interests were properly represented by union leadership; it also created, among other things, a bill of rights for union members

**Laggards** The traditional members of this group are usually the last ones to respond to innovations.

**Late majority** This skeptical group usually adopt innovations only after social or financial pressure to do so.

**Latency** Describes the amount of time it takes to answer a question.

**Layoffs** Unpaid leaves of absence initiated by the employer as a strategy for downsizing staff in response to a change in the organization's status.

**Leader–member exchange (LMX)** A theory that focuses on dyadic relationships and describes mentoring relationships between leaders and groups.

**Leadership** The "activity of guiding a group of people to a definite result" (Kelly and Greenstone 2019, 913).

**Lean** A management strategy in which the core idea is to maximize value while minimizing waste, basically creating more value with fewer resources

**Learning** The acquisition of knowledge or skills through experience, study, or by being taught.

**Learning content management systems (LCMSs)** Software through which a technical framework is used to develop educational content and permit sharing and reusing content.

**Learning curve** When a new task is learned, productivity may decrease as a great deal of material is being learned. Later, when there is little new learning, productivity may increase greatly.

**Learning health system** A health system in which internal data and experience are systematically integrated with external evidence, and that knowledge is put into practice.

**Learning management systems (LMSs)** Web-based tool that assists the trainer by tracking grades and student access, presenting the content in a user-friendly manner, and collating statistics on use.

**Least harm** Ethical concept that applies to situations where two choices may both present necessary, justifiable harms. One should choose the situation that does the least amount of harm to the fewest number of people.

**Legacy systems** Older and out-of-date systems.

**Legal hold** An order typically issued by a court to lock or disengage any editing capabilities to a health record, whether paper or electronic, when there is concern that information relevant to a legal proceeding or an audit could be changed or destroyed.

**Legal system** The mechanism through which members of society settle disputes.

**Legislative branch** Government branch that enacts laws. It controls many activities related to industry, including the healthcare industry, through statutes.

**Length of stay (LOS)** The number of days a patient occupied a hospital bed.

**Lexicon,** The listings of words or expressions in a language (terminology) and information about the language such as definitions, related principles, and description of (grammatical) structure.

**Liabilities** Debts/amounts that are owed, often due to the acquisition of an asset.

**Libel** Defamation of character that is written.

**Licensure** Gives legal approval for a facility to operate or for a person to practice within his or her profession; Government regulation mandatory for hospitals and other healthcare organizations, depending on state law.

**Likert scale** A commonly used scale which allows respondents to record their level of agreement or disagreement along a range.

**Limited jurisdiction** When a trial court only has the authority to hear certain types of cases such as probate, domestic, juvenile, traffic, and small claims.

**Line authority** The right of managers to direct the activities of employees under their immediate control.

**Line plot** Used for two main purposes: (1) to present trends or patterns in the number of occurrences between groups, or (2) to present trends or patterns in the mean of a variable between groups.

**Liquidity** Refers to the ease with which assets can be turned into cash.

**Literature review** A systematic investigation of all the knowledge available about a topic from sources such as books, journal articles, theses, and dissertations.

**Litigation** The resolution of legal disputes in the court system.

**Living systematic reviews (LSR)** Dynamic reviews continually updated to incorporate new evidence as it emerges.

**Living will** A document executed by a competent adult, expressing the individual's wishes to limit treatment should the individual become afflicted with certain conditions (for example, a persistent vegetative state or a terminal condition) and no longer able to communicate on his or her own behalf.

**Local coverage determinations (LCDs)** Medicare Administrative Contractor (MAC) policies.

**Logical Observation Identifiers Names and Codes (LOINC)** The exchange standard for laboratory results.

**Logic bombs** Malware that will execute a program, or a string of code, when a certain event happens.

**Long-term care** Healthcare rendered in a non-acute-care facility to patients who require inpatient nursing and related services for over 30 consecutive days.

**Long-term care hospitals (LTCHs)** Hospitals having an average inpatient LOS greater than 25 days.

**Longitudinal health record** A record compiled about an individual that contains health records from various encounters and from numerous healthcare delivery settings.

**M-learning** Also known as mobile learning; an electronic learning mode in which content is typically delivered through the internet to computers, smartphones, or tablets, thereby expanding accessibility to a true anytime, anyplace level.

**Machine learning** "A process by which machines can be given the capability to learn about a given dataset without being explicitly programmed on what to learn" (NIH 2023).

**Major diagnostic categories (MDCs)** Categories based on body systems and including diseases and disorders relating to a particular system. However, some MDCs include disorders and diseases involving multiple organ systems (for example, burns). The number of MS-DRGs within a particular MDC varies.

**Malfeasance** Performance of a wrongful act that also may be unlawful.

**Malware** Any program that causes harm to systems by unauthorized access, unauthorized disclosure, destruction, or loss of integrity of any information.

**Managed care** A generic term for a healthcare reimbursement system that manages cost, quality, and access to services. Managed care refers to prepaid health plans that integrate the financial aspects and delivery of healthcare; A payment method in which the third-party payer has implemented some provisions to control the costs of healthcare while maintaining quality.

**Managed care organizations (MCOs)** Where healthcare organizations assume the financial risk and provide healthcare services for a defined population of patients.

**Management by objectives (MBO)** Technique in which clear target objectives can be stated and measured and can direct behavior.

**Managerial accounting** The development, implementation, and analysis of systems that track financial transactions for managerial control purposes; it includes both budget and cost analysis systems.

**MAP Keys** "The comprehensive revenue cycle strategy to *measure* performance, *apply* evidence-based improvement strategies, and *perform* to the highest standards to improve financial results and patient satisfaction" (HFMA n.d.).

**Mapping** The process of associating concepts from one coding system and defining their equivalence in accordance with a documented rationale and a given purpose.

**Maslow's Hierarchy of Needs** Developed by Abraham Maslow, a developmental view of needs that begins with physiological existence needs and progressed through safety, social belongingness, self-esteem, and finally self-actualization or creativity needs.

**Massed training** Training in one highly concentrated session.

**Master data management** Master data that an enterprise maintains about key business entities (such as customers, employees, or patients) and to reference data used to classify other data or identify allowable values for data such as codes for state abbreviations or products.

**Master patient index** A permanent database including patient-identifiable data for every patient ever admitted to or treated by the facility.

**Matching** Whenever possible, expenses are recorded in the same period as the associated revenue, thereby matching the expenses and revenues.

**Materiality** Refers to the thresholds below which items are not considered significant for reporting purposes.

**Maternal death** The death of any woman while pregnant or within 42 days of delivery from any cause related to, or aggravated by, pregnancy or its management, regardless of the duration of the pregnancy or the site of the death.

**Matrix organization** Arrangement where employees report to a functional manager from their original functional area to carry out their operational work. They may also report to a different manager, such as a project manager, who oversees their temporary project work outside of their operational duties.

**Maximization** Using unbundling and upcoding to increase reimbursement to the highest possible amount through coded data.

**Mean** The most common type of average, where the sum of all numbers in a group of data is divided by the number of items in that group of data.

**MEDCIN** A proprietary clinical terminology owned and maintained by Medicomp Systems.

**Median** The middle number in a set of scores, or the midpoint in a list of numbers or data.

**Mediation** When a dispute is taken to an objective third party to facilitate agreement between the disputing parties.

**Medicaid** A joint federal and state program that assists with medical costs for those with low income.

**Medical device** Any instrument, apparatus, implement, machine, appliance, implant, reagent for in vitro use, software, material or other similar or related article, intended by the manufacturer to be used, alone or in combination for a medical purpose.

**Medical identity theft** The inappropriate or unauthorized use of a person's identity to obtain medical goods or services or to falsify claims to fraudulently bill insurance companies.

**Medical Literature, Analysis, and Retrieval System Online (MEDLINE)** The best-known database from the National Library of Medicine. It includes bibliographic lists for publications in medicine, dentistry, nursing, pharmacy, allied health, and veterinary medicine. HIM professionals use MEDLINE to locate articles on HIM issues and articles on medical topics necessary to carry out quality improvement and medical research activities.

**Medical malpractice liability** Refers to instances where a civil claim for damages against a healthcare provider successfully proves the provider was negligent in their care of the patient leading to injury or death.

**Medical necessity** A determination that a service is reasonable and necessary for the related diagnosis or treatment of illness or injury.

**Medical staff** The aggregate of physicians and other approved practitioners granted permission by a healthcare organization's governing board to provide patient services in the organization within specific practice limits.

**Medical staff bylaws** Spell out specific qualifications that physicians must demonstrate before they can practice medicine in the hospital.

**Medical staff classification** Organization of physicians according to clinical assignment.

**Medical Subject Headings database (MeSH)** The NLM's controlled vocabulary thesaurus, which consists of terms naming descriptors in a hierarchical structure that permits searching at various levels of specificity.

**Medically needy option** Allows states to extend Medicaid eligibility to persons who would be eligible for Medicaid under one of the mandatory or optional groups except that their income and resources are above the eligibility level set by their state.

**Medically unlikely edits (MUEs)** A MUE identifies CPT and HCPCS codes reported with units greater than what has been deemed appropriate.

**Medicare** A federally funded program that helps pay the cost of providing healthcare services to those 65 years of age and older in addition to eligible individuals with disabilities.

**Medicare Administrative Contractor (MAC)** A private healthcare insurer awarded by Medicare for a geographic jurisdiction for multistate or regional contractor responsibilities to process Medicare Part A and Part B (A/B) medical claims.

**Medicare Advantage plan** A type of supplemental plan established by the Balanced Budget Act (BBA) of 1997, to expand the options for participation in private healthcare plans.

**Medicare Code Editor (MCE)** The inpatient code editor used to detect various claim errors.

**Medicare fee schedule (MFS)** The listing of allowed charges reimbursable to physicians under Medicare. Each year's MFS is published by CMS in the *Federal Register*.

**Medicare Prescription Drug, Improvement, and Modernization Act of 2003** Enacted to provide prescription drug coverage within the Medicare Program and to modernize the Medicare Program with additional options to better support Medicare beneficiaries.

**Medicare Provider Analysis and Review (MEDPAR)**  A file made up of acute-care hospital and skilled nursing facility (SNF) claims data for all Medicare claims.

**Medicare severity diagnosis-related groups (MS-DRGs)**  On October 1, 2007, the diagnosis-related groups (DRGs) system became known as this, better accounting for severity of illness and resource consumption.

**Medication administration records**  Records maintained by nursing staff for all patients, including medications given, time, form of administration, and dosage and strength.

**Medigap**  To fill gaps in Medicare coverage, most Medicare enrollees supplement their benefits with private insurance policies. These private policies are referred to as or supplemental insurance.

**Mentor**  A formalized arrangement in which an experienced worker meets with a trainee on a regular basis and often gives advice on personal career growth and development within the organization.

**Meta-analyses**  A specialized type of systematic review that introduces statistical techniques to combine summary-level information from at least two studies.

**Meta-syntheses**  Effectively address the challenge of synthesizing multiple qualitative studies. This approach allows researchers to collate and interpret qualitative findings across studies, leading to deeper theoretical understandings and insights that might not be apparent from individual studies alone.

**Metadata**  Electronic data about data that include information not previously available in paper documents, such as time stamps that show when and by whom a document or entry was created, accessed, or changed.

**mHealth**  Defined by HIMSS as "the generation, aggregation, and dissemination of health information through mobile and wireless devices" (HIMSS n.d.).

**Migration path**  A high-level outline of all components the organization has identified as required to achieve its goals. General statements of goals for each part of the timeline and the general nature of the applications (software), technology (computer systems), and operational elements (people, policy, and process) are documented.

**Minimum Data Set 3.0 (MDS)**  The minimum core of defined and categorized patient assessment data that serves as the basis for documentation and reimbursement in a SNF.

**Minimum necessary**  A standard that requires a covered entity or business associate make "reasonable efforts to limit protected health information to the minimum necessary to accomplish the intended purpose of the use, disclosure, or request" (HHS 2013, 78).

**Misdemeanor**  A less severe crime than a felony, subject to imprisonment for up to one year.

**Misfeasance**  Improper performance of a lawful act that causes injury to another.

**Mission statement**  A statement that sets forth the core purpose and philosophies of an organization or group.

**Mitigate the risk**  Refers to the process of reducing or eliminating the risk by implementing a control.

**Mixed methods research**  An approach that combines quantitative and qualitative techniques within a single study or across multiple complementary studies.

**Mode**  The value with the highest frequency of occurrence.

**Moral agent**  A person with decision-making responsibility for themselves or others.

**Moral courage**  Defined as the personal trait of individuals who act upon their ethical values to help others despite personal risk, adversity, and professional isolation and any consequences

**Moral dilemma**  A situation in which there is a decision to be made, but the right thing to do may be hard to choose or be unknown because any choice may violate a duty or standard.

**Moral distress**  Refers to the perception of dissonance between one's beliefs and values, standards, and issues they face at work.

**Morality**  General term used to describe norms, duties, manners, or customs that people use to distinguish between right and wrong; it conveys fundamental communal standards of conduct and character; In the context of research, there are two requirements: recognizing the autonomy of individuals to make their own decisions and providing additional protections for those with decreased autonomy (due to changes in their health capacity).

**Morbidity**  Being symptomatic of an illness or disease.

**Morphology**  A code that describes the characteristics of the tumor itself, including cell type and biologic activity.

**Mortality**  An incidence of death in a specific population.

**Motions for summary judgment**  When attorneys argue there are (or are not) any facts remaining in dispute and that plaintiff or defendant is (or is not) entitled to a judgment being entered without intervention by the trier of fact.

**Motivation**   The inner drive to accomplish a task.

**Multi-user virtual environment (MUVE)**   A computer-based virtual environment that can be accessed by multiple users simultaneously and can be used to simulate a work environment where users create avatars and interact with other users.

**Multihospital systems**   Include two or more hospitals owned, leased, sponsored, or contracted by a central organization.

**Multimedia**   When more than one unstructured data type is present in an information system, the data and system they represent are referred to as multimedia.

**Multivoting technique**   A variation of nominal group technique (NGT) that has the same purpose, to narrow and prioritize a group of ideas; rather than ranking each issue or idea, team members are asked to rate the issue using a distribution of points.

**Narrative**   A common format for procedure writing. The author details the processes of the procedure in a step-by-step descriptive method.

**National Academy of Medicine**   A branch of the National Academy of Sciences that exists "to advance science, inform policy, and catalyze action to achieve human health, equity, and well-being" (National Academy of Medicine n.d.).

**National Center for Health Statistics (NCHS)**   An agency that has responsibility for public health databases and that provides a database of statistical health information to guide public health actions and policymaking.

**National Committee for Quality Assurance (NCQA)**   A "private, not-for-profit organization dedicated to improving healthcare quality. Since its founding in 1990, NCQA has been a central figure in driving improvement throughout the healthcare system, helping to elevate the issue of healthcare quality to the top of the national agenda" (NCQA n.d.).

**National conversion factor (CF)**   Process that converts the Relative value units (RVUs) into payments.

**National Correct Coding Initiative (NCCI)**   Part of the IOCE. CMS developed the NCCI to promote correct coding methodologies and to control improper coding leading to inappropriate payment.

**National coverage determinations (NCDs)**   Medicare's national coverage policies.

**National Drug Codes (NDCs) Directory**   Developed by the Food and Drug Administration (FDA) to serve as a universal product identifier for human drugs.

**National Health Care Survey (NHCS)**   A collection of surveys that cover a broad spectrum of healthcare settings.

**National Labor Relations Act (Wagner Act) of 1935**   Federal pro-union legislation that provides, among other things, procedures for union representation and prohibits unfair labor practices by unions, such as coercing non-striking employees, and by employers, such as interference with the union selection process and discrimination against employees who support a union.

**National Library of Medicine (NLM)**   The world's largest medical library. It collects materials in all aspects of biomedicine and healthcare, and works on biomedical aspects of technology, the humanities, and the physical, life, and social sciences.

**National Practitioner Data Bank (NPDB)**   "An information clearinghouse…to collect and release certain information related to the professional competence and conduct of physicians, dentists, and, in some cases, other healthcare practitioners" (HHS 2018, A-2).

**National Vital Statistics System (NVSS)**   System used to collect the nation's vital statistics information; the data-sharing organization to which each state disseminates their vital statistics registry data.

**Natural language processing (NLP) technology**   A technology that converts human language (structured or unstructured) into data that can be translated then manipulated by computer systems.

**Naturalistic observation**   When researchers record observations that are unprompted and unaffected by their actions.

**Need-to-know principle**   Based on the minimum necessary standard; the least amount of information necessary to perform a task.

**Needs assessment**   Collecting and analyzing data about proposed programs, projects, and other activities or objects to determine what is required, lacking, or desired by an employee, group, or organization; An approach that focuses on three levels: the organization, the specific job tasks, and the individual employee. The outcome of the needs assessment is an understanding of where training is needed in the organization (entry-level, remedial, or management development), based on the firm's strategic mission and goals.

**Negligence**   Acting in an unreasonable manner or failing to act as a reasonably prudent person would in similar circumstances.

**Net assets**   The difference between assets and liabilities in a not-for-profit environment.

**Net autopsy rate**   Includes all of the deaths that occurred with inpatients, and indicates the proportion of those on which an autopsy was performed when the bodies of patients who were not available for autopsy are removed from the denominator.

**Net death rate**   A death rate adjusted so certain deaths are not counted against the hospital.

**Net income**   The arithmetic difference between total revenue and total expenses in a for-profit organization or excess of revenue over expense in a not-for-profit organization.

**Net loss**   When total expenses exceed total revenue, net income is a negative number.

**Net present value (NPV)**   The calculated present value of the future cash inflows compared to the initial investment.

**Network**   A group which comprises hospitals, physicians, and other providers and payers that collaborate to coordinate and deliver services to their community.

**Network model HMOs**   HMO contracts for services with two or more multispecialty group practices to provide medical services to members of the plan.

**Network providers**   Healthcare professionals who are members of a managed care network.

**Newborn death rate**   The number of newborns who died in comparison to the total number of newborns discharged, alive and dead.

**No Surprises Act (NSA)**   Enacted in 2022 to protect patients from being subjected to healthcare costs beyond their control when receiving out-of-network care.

**Nomenclature**   A recognized system of terms used in a science or an art that follows preestablished naming conventions.

**Nominal data**   Data expressed as categories that represent names of items, but do not have a natural order.

**Nominal group technique (NGT)**   A ranking process designed to reach consensus about an issue or an idea that the team considers most important.

**Non-economic compensatory (general) damages**   Damages that do not represent an objective monetary loss and, due to their incalculable nature, can be overrepresented by a plaintiff's attorney. These losses include pain and suffering, loss of enjoyment of life activities, and humiliation.

**Nonexempt employees**   Those who are covered by some or all of the FLSA provisions and who are paid an hourly wage.

**Nonfeasance**   Failure to perform an act that a person has a duty to perform and which a person of ordinary prudence would have done in similar circumstances.

**Nonmaleficence**   While beneficence requires providers to promote good, prevent harm, and remove harm, nonmaleficence requires them to refrain from actions that cause harm.

**Nonparticipant observation**   When researchers act as neutral observers who neither intentionally interact with nor affect the actions of the population being observed.

**Normal distribution**   The formal name of the distribution known as the bell-shaped curve. The shape of the normal distribution is symmetric around its mean and uniquely defined by its mean and standard deviation.

**Normalization**   Process that eliminates errors associated with updates, deletions, and data insertions into the database, reduces redundancy, and improves data quality.

**Nosocomial infection rates**   Hospital-acquired infection (HAI) rates that indicate the rate of infections acquired during a hospital stay.

**Not-for-profit healthcare organizations**   Use excess funds to improve their services and finance educational programs and community services.

**Not-for-profit organizations**   Organizations that are not owned but, instead, are held in trust for the benefit of the communities they serve.

**Notice of privacy practices**   Explain and give examples of the uses of the patient's health information for treatment, payment, and healthcare operations, and other disclosures for purposes established in the regulations.

**Notice of privacy practices (NPP)**   Notice which healthcare providers and health plans must give to patients to inform them of how they may use and share the patient's health information and how patients can exercise their health privacy rights

**Notifiable diseases**   Diseases a state must report to the CDC when the diseases are identified by hospitals or other healthcare facilities.

**Null hypothesis**   The status quo.

**Objective**   A statement of the result in measurable terms with time and cost limits, as applicable.

**Observational research** When researchers observe, record, and analyze behaviors and events.

**Observational study** An epidemiological study in which exposure and outcome for each individual in the study is observed.

**Occupational Safety and Health Act (OSHA) of 1970** Federal act created "to ensure safe and healthful working conditions for workers by setting and enforcing standards and providing training, outreach, education and assistance" (HHS 2018, A-2).

**Odds ratio** In a case-control study, the odds ratio compares the odds that the cases were exposed to the disease with the odds that the controls were exposed.

**Offer** When one party promises to either do something or not do something if the other party agrees to either do something or not do something

**Office for Human Research Protections (OHRP)** A federal agency that provides leadership and oversight on all matters related to the protection of human subjects participating in research conducted or supported by HHS.

**Office of Research Integrity (ORI)** The "role, mission, and structure of the ORI [are] focused on preventing research misconduct and promoting research integrity principally through oversight, education, and review of institutional findings and recommendations" (ORI n.d.a).

**Office of the Inspector General (OIG)** Agency that protects the integrity of Department of Health and Human Services (HHS) programs and operations, and the health and well-being of the people served.

**Offshoring** A type of outsourcing where a company's workforce is based overseas.

**OIG workplan** Sets forth various projects to be addressed during the fiscal year by the Office of Audit Services, Office of Evaluation and Inspections, Office of Investigations, and Office of Counsel to the Inspector General, including projects planned by CMS.

**Omnibus Budget Reconciliation Act (OBRA)** Mandated that CMS develop a prospective system for hospital-based outpatient services provided to Medicare beneficiaries.

**On-the-job training** A method of training in which the employee learns a task by performing it.

**Onboarding** A formal new employee orientation process that includes a series of activities designed to acclimate the new employee to the organization and job.

**One sample t-test** Used to compare a population to a standard value.

**One-on-one training** A training technique in which the employee learns by first observing a demonstration and then performing the task under supervision.

**Open systems** Systems affected by what is going on around them that must adjust as the environment changes.

**Open-record review** When qualitative analysis is done while the patient is in the facility or under active treatment; includes ongoing records review, point-of-care review, or continuous record review.

**Open-source technology** Open-source software products are applications whose source (human-readable) code is freely available to anyone who is interested in downloading the code. Advantages include its availability, its ability to be customized, and the collaborative nature of the product in which a community of developers and users can interact, review, and improve upon each other's ideas.

**Operation index** Similar to the disease index, except it is arranged in numerical order by the patients' procedure code(s), usually using ICD or Current Procedural Terminology (CPT) codes.

**Operational budget** Budget that allocates and controls resources in a manner consistent with the organization's goals and objectives.

**Operations** Daily activity that does not have a planned end date, the work is repeated routinely, and it changes only with the organization's objectives can no longer be met.

**Operations management** Theory developed after World War II; applies statistical, mathematical, and quantitative methods to decision-making in the business setting to better understand how products and services could be manufactured and delivered.

**Optical character recognition (OCR) technology** Technology that recognizes machine-generated characters (for example, preprinted numbers and letters) by interpreting the scanned, bitmapped shapes of the characters' images and then converting the characters into computer-processable codes.

**Ordinal data** Data where the categories have a natural order. Patient severity level, trauma center level, and trimester of gestation are all examples of ordinal data found in healthcare.

**Ordinary negligence** Failure to do what a reasonably prudent person would do, or doing something that a reasonably prudent person would not do, thus failing to exercise ordinary care.

**Organization development (OD)** The process in which an organization reflects on its own processes and consequently revises them for improved performance.

**Organizational chart** A chart that graphically represents the formal structure of an entity, often includes departmental subdivisions, and follows the scalar chain and unity of command.

**Organizational culture**  An organization's norms, beliefs, and values. It is what is felt by staff on any given day that is intangible but influences how an employee feels about their job and the environment in which they perform it.

**Organizational health literacy**  The degree to which organizations equitably enable individuals to find, understand, and use information and services to inform health-related decisions and actions for themselves and others.

**Organizational safeguards**  Practices, such as business associate agreements (BAAs) and other arrangements made to protect ePHI between organizations.

**Organizing**  The way in which the organization is designed and operated to attain the desired goals.

**Orientation**  A period of introduction to an organization's policies, practices, and procedures for a newly hired employee.

**Original jurisdiction**  The authority to first hear a case on a given matter.

**Out-group**  Those employees not included in the group that forms around the leader (in-group).

**Outcome and Assessment Information Set (OASIS-D)**  Developed by CMS and consisting of data elements that (1) represent core items for the comprehensive assessment of an adult home care patient and (2) form the basis for measuring patient outcomes for the purpose of outcome-based quality improvement (OBQI).

**Outcome evaluation**  Collecting and analyzing data at the end of an implementation or operating cycle to determine whether the program, project, or other activity or object has achieved its expected or intended impact, product, or other outcome (also known as summative evaluation).

**Outcomes and effectiveness research (OER)**  "Describes, interprets, and predicts the impact of healthcare interventions on endpoints that matter to patients, families and caregivers, providers, private and public payers and purchasers of healthcare, regulatory agencies, healthcare-accrediting organizations, and society generally" (NIH 2023).

**Outcomes research**  Assesses the quality and effectiveness of healthcare as measured by the attainment of a specified result or outcome, improved health, lowered morbidity or mortality, and improvement of abnormal states.

**Outpatient prospective payment system (OPPS)**  The Medicare prospective payment system used for hospital-based outpatient services and procedures, first implemented for services furnished on or after August 1, 2000.

**Outsourcing**  Arrangement wherein the organization contracts with an independent company with expertise in a specific job function. The outside company then assumes full responsibility for performing the function rather than just supplying staff.

**Outsourcing agencies**  A vendor partnership used to offload a portion of the work rather than being brought in to work directly with the project team.

**Overlap**  Occurs when a patient has more than one medical record number assigned across more than one database.

**Overlay**  Occurs when one patient record is overwritten with data from another patient's record.

**P-value**  The probability of making a type I error based on a particular set of data.

**Packaging**  When payment for that service is packaged into payment for other services and, therefore, there is no separate APC payment.

**Panel interview**  Process by which a team of people interview applicants at one time.

**Parallel work division**  The concurrent handling of tasks.

**Pareto chart**  Resembles a bar chart except the highest-ranking item is listed first, followed by the second highest, down to the lowest-ranked item.

**Participant observation**  When researchers are participants in the observed actions, activities, or processes. They can participate overtly (openly) or covertly (secretly).

**Partnership**  Structure in which individuals share in the responsibility for the business, and income still flows through the individuals' tax returns.

**Paternalism**  Term for interference with the actions and decision-making of others, when it is done for their benefit.

**Path–goal theory**  States that a person's ability to perform certain tasks is related to the direction and clarity available that lead to organizational goals.

**Patient activation measure (PAM)** Developed to predict the patient's level of engagement in healthcare, including the knowledge, beliefs, skills, and behaviors necessary to manage one's health.

**Patient-centered care** Relationship-based primary care with an orientation toward the whole person.

**Patient-centered medical home (PCMH)** A model that attempts to improve care outcomes and reduce care costs by reorganizing how primary care is delivered. There are five pillars to the PCMH model: a patient-centered orientation; comprehensive, team-based care; coordinated care; superb access to care; and a systems-based approach to quality and safety.

**Patient driven payment model (PDPM)** Developed to improve payment accuracy and appropriateness by focusing on the patient and their characteristics, rather than on the volume of services provided, to reduce administrative burden on providers, and to improve SNF payments to underserved beneficiaries.

**Patient engagement** "The desire and capability to actively choose to participate in care in a way uniquely appropriate to the individual, in cooperation with a healthcare provider or institution, for the purposes of maximizing outcomes or improving experiences of care" (Higgins et al. 2017).

**Patient-generated health data (PGHD)** "Health-related data created, recorded, or gathered by or from patients (or family members or other caregivers) to help address a health concern" (ONC n.d.).

**Patient-identifiable data** Every fact recorded in the record relating to a particular patient.

**Patient medical record information (PMRI)** Terminology for the adoption of uniform data standards for PMRI and electronic information exchange.

**Patient portals** Internet entryway that allows patients to pay their bills online and to securely view all or portions of their provider-based EHR, such as current medical conditions, immunization records, medications, allergies, and test results.

**Patient Protection and Affordable Care Act (ACA) of 2020** Enacted to reform healthcare. It was designed to increase the rate of health insurance coverage for Americans and reducing the overall costs of healthcare.

**Patient Self-Determination Act** Act that requires healthcare institutions that are Medicare or Medicaid providers to give adult patients information about advance directives; document in the health record whether patients have an advance directive or not; and treat patients equally despite the presence or absence of an advance directive.

**Payback period** The time required to recoup the cost of an investment.

**Payment status indicators (PSIs)** Indicators assigned to each HCPCS code and APCs, playing an important role in determining payment for services under the OPPS.

**Peer review** When a member of a profession assesses the work of colleagues within that same profession.

**Performance** The execution of a task.

**Performance improvement** The continuous study and adaptation of a healthcare organization's functions and processes to increase the likelihood of achieving desired outcomes.

**Performance measurement** The process of comparing the outcomes of an organization, work unit, or employee to preestablished performance standards.

**Performance measures** Sometimes referred to as *quality measure*, measure or quantify healthcare processes, outcomes, patient perceptions, and organizational structure and/or systems associated with the ability to provide high-quality healthcare and/or that relate to one or more quality goals for healthcare.

**Performance review** A system to periodically evaluate individual employees' performance.

**Personal health data** Facts maintained by an individual, often in a personal health record. Much of this data comes from various healthcare organizations that treat the patient, but some of the data may be compiled by the patient directly.

**Personal health literacy** The degree to which individuals have the ability to find, understand, and use information and services to inform health-related decisions and actions for themselves and others.

**Personal health records (PHRs)** An electronic or paper health record maintained and updated by an individual for himself or herself; a tool individuals can use to collect, track, and share past and current information about their health or the health of someone in their care.

**Persuasive authority** Although a precedent in one court system does not bind courts in other court systems, courts may use each other's precedents as, or guidance, in analyzing a specific legal problem.

**Petition for writ of certiorari** A request for the US Supreme Court to consider a case from a lower court. The court will either grant certiorari (that is, it will

**hear the case) or deny certiorari (that is, it declines to hear the case). Most requests are denied certiorari.

**Physical safeguards**  Surveillance cameras and identification badges and the like, to identify measures to protect information systems (ISs), buildings, and equipment from natural and environmental hazards.

**Physician champion**  Also known as the physician advisor; an individual who assists in communicating with and educating medical staff in areas such as documentation procedures for accurate billing and EHR procedures.

**Physician index**  A list of cases in order by physician name or physician identification number.

**Physician-patient privilege**  The information exchanged between patient and physician as part of the professional relationship is a confidential communication that the patient anticipates will be held in confidence, thus encouraging the patient to disclose all relevant information.

**Physiological signal processing systems**  Systems such as ECG and EEG, that store data based on the body's signals (such as heart activity and brain waves) and create output based on the lines plotted between the signals' points.

**Pie chart**  A circular chart used to present the count or proportion of subgroups to the whole.

**Piece-rate incentive**  A system in which workers received additional pay when they exceeded the standard output level for their task.

**Pilot study**  A trial run that allows researchers to work out the logistical details of their research plan and enhances the likelihood of the research's successful completion.

**Plaintext**  The original text that has not been altered.

**Plaintiff**  The party bringing an action or complaint in a civil case.

**Plan-Do-Check-Act (PDCA)**  A commonly used process in clinical quality management. PDCA is also referred to as the plan-do-study-act (PDSA) cycle, the Deming Wheel, or the Deming Cycle. PDCA is an ongoing process entailing "a systematic series of steps for gaining valuable learning and knowledge for the continual improvement of a product or process" (W. Edwards Deming Institute n.d.).

**Planning**  Determining what must be done and why when launching any organizational effort.

**Planning horizon**  Refers to both the scope of the system to be addressed and the number of years estimated for planning, acquiring, implementing, adopting, and optimizing use of the components identified.

**Playscript**  A format describing each player in a procedure, the action of the player, and the player's responsibility regarding the process from the start to completion of a specific task within the procedure.

**Point method**  A commonly used system that places weight (points) on each of the compensable factors in a job. The total points associated with a job establish its relative worth. Jobs that fall within a specific range of points fall into a grade associated with a specific wage or salary.

**Point of service (POS) plan**  Lets the beneficiary choose between the HMO or PPO model each time care is accessed. Subscribers must select a PCP from a network of participating physicians to coordinate their care but are allowed to obtain care from outside the network potentially at a higher cost.

**Point-of-care information systems**  Systems that allow healthcare providers to capture and retrieve data and information at the location where the healthcare service is performed.

**Point-of-service (POS) collection**  The collection of the portion of the bill that is the patient's responsibility to pay prior to the provision of service being rendered.

**Policy**  A directive statement that describes how a specific situation or process should be handled and reflects the organization's values and mission.

**Policy analysis**  Identifying options to meet goals and estimating the costs and consequences of each option prior to the implementation of any option

**Population health data**  Facts about the quality, cost, and risk associated with the health of a specific set of individuals.

**Population-based registry**  A registry gathering data from multiple facilities within a geographic area such as a state or region.

**Population-based statistics**  Statistics that track the mortality and morbidity of a population.

**Position (job) description**  Outlines the work to be performed by a specific employee or group of employees with the same responsibilities.

**Post-acute care**  Care that supports patients who require ongoing medical management or therapeutic, rehabilitative, or skilled nursing care.

**Potentially compensable event (PCE)**  Event that could result in a settlement or judgment against the organization, paid either through insurance or directly from the organization's funds.

**Preauthorization**  Also called *prior authorization*, occurs when the provider obtains permission to provide the service from the insurance carrier, usually to ensure the patient has the benefits available.

**Precertification**  When the insurance carrier must review the proposed service or procedure and approve it as medically necessary before payment will be granted to the provider.

**Precision medicine**  "Disease prevention and treatment for individual variability (e.g., genetic and lifestyle differences among patients)" (FDA 2022).

**Predictive modeling**  An application of data analytics in healthcare that applies statistical techniques to determine the likelihood of certain events occurring together.

**Preemption**  Gives federal law precedence over state law.

**Preferred provider organization (PPO)**  Represents contractual agreements between healthcare providers and a self-insured employer or a health insurance carrier; usually will pay for care delivered outside the network, but it may cost the individual more.

**Pregnancy Discrimination Act of 1978**  Federal legislation that prohibits discrimination against women affected by pregnancy, childbirth, or related medical conditions by requiring that affected women be treated the same as all other employees for employment-related purposes, including benefits.

**Prejudice**  The judgment of a person based on cultural elements without reviewing all the information.

**Premium**  A preestablished amount (usually monthly) paid by each covered individual or family to the insurance company, which sets aside the premiums from all the people covered by the plan in a special fund; Payments through which private commercial insurance plans are financed.

**Preponderance of the evidence**  When, in most civil cases, the plaintiff must prove his or her case by the standard of proof. This "more likely than not" standard means there is enough evidence to tip the scales, even slightly, in favor of the plaintiff's case. This is a substantially lower standard of proof than a criminal case.

**Present on admission (POA)**  A condition present at the time the order for inpatient admission occurs. Conditions that develop during an outpatient encounter, including in the emergency department, observation, or outpatient surgery, are considered POA.

**Prevalence**  The number of existing cases of a particular disease.

**Prevalence rates**  Proportion of persons with a certain disease to the number of persons in a population.

**Preventive control**  A front-end process that guides work in such a way that input and process variations are minimized.

**Preventive controls**  Front-end processes that guide work in such a way that input and process variations are minimized.

**Primary analysis**  Refers to analysis of original research data by the researchers who collected them.

**Primary care physician (PCP)**  Usually a family or general practice physician or an internal medicine specialist, and acts as a service gatekeeper to control the patient's access to specialty, surgical, and hospital care as well as expensive diagnostic services.

**Primary data source**  A "record that was developed by healthcare professionals in the process of providing care or services to a patient" (White 2023, 3).

**Primary keys**  The type of relationship and the unique identifier for each entity

**Primary sources**  The original works of the researchers who conducted the research study.

**Principal diagnosis**  The condition that, after study, is determined to have caused the patient's admission to the hospital for care. It determines the MDC assignment.

**Principal investigator (PI)**  The director of the research project who has full responsibility for all parts of the research conducted.

**Privacy**  Refers to freedom from unauthorized intrusion. In healthcare-related contexts it refers to the right of a patient to control disclosure of protected health information.

**Privacy Act of 1974**  An early piece of federal legislation that addressed the right to privacy. This act was written to give individuals some control over the large amounts of information collected about them by the federal government and its contractors.

**Privacy Rule**  The Standards for Privacy of Individually Identifiable Health Information, established to assure the protection of health information, with the goal to address the use and disclosure of PHI as well as standards for individuals' privacy rights to understand and control how their health information is used and shared, including rights to examine and obtain a copy of their health records as well as to request corrections.

**Private law**  Legislation involving the relationship between private individuals or entities, where the government is not a party.

**Privilege**   The nature of a relationship is confidential.

**Problem-oriented medical record (POMR)**   A patient record in which clinical problems are defined and documented individually.

**Problem statement**   A concise description of a research problem or an issue the researcher intends to address, or to resolve, and explains why the identified study is important

**Procedural justice**   Addresses the fairness of policies, processes, and strategies for setting priorities and resolving disputes.

**Procedure**   A document that describes how work is to be done and how policies are to be carried out.

**Procedure manual**   A compilation of all the procedures used in a specific unit, department, or organization.

**Process evaluation**   Monitoring programs, projects, and other activities or objects to check whether their development or implementation is proceeding as planned (also known as formative evaluation).

**Process improvement**   A series of actions taken to identify, analyze, and improve existing processes.

**Process innovations**   Enable firms to produce existing products or services more efficiently.

**Product liability**   The legal doctrine under which a manufacturer, seller, or supplier of a product may be liable to a buyer or other third party for injuries caused by a defective product.

**Productivity**   The level of measurable work expected for a specific function.

**Professionalism**   The knowledge, skills, and attitudes required to meet the expected standards of deliberate professional practice and excellence through lifelong learning.

**Profitability**   An organization's ability to increase in value.

**Program**   Several related projects, each contributing to the overall objectives of the program.

**Program management**   Used as another layer of management over projects where a program manager guides and coordinates the set of individual projects to ensure they produce deliverables that can be used by the other projects within the program.

**Programmed learning modules**   Training methods that lead learners through subject material presented in short sections, followed immediately by a series of questions that require a written response based on the section just presented. Answers are provided in the module for immediate feedback.

**Programs of All-Inclusive Care for the Elderly (PACE)**   A joint Medicare-Medicaid venture that provides an alternative to institutional care for individuals aged 55 or older who require a level of care usually provided at nursing facilities.

**Progress notes**   Chronological statements about the patient's response to treatment during their stay in the facility.

**Progressive discipline**   A process that begins with a verbal warning that may or may not be a part of the employee's file depending on organization policy and the severity and frequency of the offense. When the next offense occurs, the process progresses to a written reprimand with formal documentation of the problem and delineation of the steps needed to correct it. The next offense often results in suspension, with further related infractions resulting in dismissal.

**Project**   A temporary and unique instance of work involving specialized individuals working together to achieve a specific goal within resource and time limitations.

**Project budget**   Identifies the resources made available to the project and limits the amount of scope that can be delivered and the amount of time available to complete the project

**Project champion**   An executive in the organization who believes in the benefits of and advocates for the project.

**Project communication plan**   A plan specifying the types of communications needed at various stages of the project, who should deliver the communications, the medium for the communications, the communication undertaken, and any feedback or lessons learned from it.

**Project coordinator**   In a functional organization, facilitates resources and collaboration across the departments participating in a project.

**Project expediter**   In a weak matrix organization, this project role works directly with the functional staff rather than through the functional managers.

**Project failure**   Occurs when the entire scope identified is not delivered, all work is not completed before the targeted date, or all work cannot be completed while remaining within the defined resource budget.

**Project management**   "The application of knowledge, skills, tools, and techniques to project activities to meet the project requirements (PMI 2023, 2)"; An intentional effort to plan, organize, direct, and control the organization's resources toward achieving a specific short-term objective.

**Project management constraints**   Typically depicted as a triangle representing the three constraints (schedule, budget, and scope).

The triangle also represents the connectedness of the three constraints where each constraint is dependent upon the other two constraints.

**Project management life cycle** The collection of project phases.

**Project manager** An individual responsible for planning, organizing, directing, monitoring, and controlling the work from the beginning to the end of the project, keeping all stakeholders informed and engaged and ensuring the project is completed within the constraints of scope, schedule, and budget.

**Project plan** A tool that aids in carrying out a specific set of tasks that lead to the completion of a specific goal.

**Project portfolio management (PPM)** The method used to identify, select, and prioritize projects and programs in a manner to make best use of the limited resources.

**Project portfolio manager** Individual responsible for ensuring all projects and programs within the portfolio produce benefits to the organization.

**Project risk management** A process in an HIS project that identifies and reduces the possibility that a key step or series of steps may not be performed on time, where a component of the system may not work properly potentially delaying other aspects of the implementation or be costly to fix, and other risks.

**Project schedule** Defines target dates for when the scope must be completed and limits the amount of scope that can be completed within the time and given budget.

**Project scope** Determines the work to be completed.

**Project sponsor** The project owner who is a key decision maker for the project and responsible for ensuring the project deliverables effectively satisfy the needs of the organization.

**Project stakeholder** Anyone with an interest in the deliverables created as part of the project.

**Project team** Team consisting of individuals with knowledge or skills specific to the project needs.

**Projectized organization** In organizations designed around project work rather than operations, the operational department structures focused on a specialty or subspecialty are replaced by multidisciplinary project teams led by a project manager.

**Promotion** The upward progression of an employee in both job and salary. It can also mean a lateral move to a different position with similar job skills or a change within the same job because of completing higher education or credentialing requirements.

**Prosecutor** Also known as a prosecuting attorney, district or state attorney (depending on the state), or the US attorney (in the federal court system). The prosecutor determines sufficient evidence is present, and he or she files charges against the defendant on behalf of the government.

**Prospective payment system (PPS)** When the exact amount of the payment is determined before the service is delivered.

**Prospective study** Study designed to observe events that occur after the subjects have been identified.

**Protected health information (PHI)** Referred to as ePHI when it is in electronic form; individually identifiable health information held or transmitted by a covered entity or business associate.

**Proximate causation** That the breach was also the proximate or foreseeable cause of the harm.

**Public Company Accounting Oversight Board (PCAOB)** Board which oversees the audits of companies that are publicly traded.

**Public health** The area of healthcare dealing with the health of populations in geographic areas such as states or counties.

**Public health data** Facts used to prevent the spread of disease.

**Public law** Legislation involving the relationship between the government (at any level) and individuals or organizations.

**Punitive damages** Damages awarded beyond compensation for injury and intended to punish or deter wrongful conduct.

**Qualitative analysis** HIM personnel carefully review the quality and adequacy of record documentation to ensure it is in accordance with the policies, rules, and regulations established by the facility; the standards of licensing and accrediting bodies; and government requirements

**Qualitative approach** The interpretation of nonnumerical observations and seeking answers of "why" things happened.

**Qualitative standards** Specify the level of service expected from a function.

**Quality** "The degree to which health services for individuals and populations increase the likelihood of desired health outcomes and are consistent with current professional knowledge" (IOM 2001).

**Quality indicators** Standards against which actual care may be measured to identify a level of performance for that standard.

**Quality management** The evaluation of the quality of healthcare services and delivery using standards and guidelines developed by various entities, including the government and independent accreditation organizations.

**Quality professional** One who possesses a variety of knowledge and skills, including those related to data analytics and information management, quality and performance improvement, leadership, and patient safety and risk management.

**QualityNet** A CMS website that provides information about quality measurement and serves as the basis for communication between CMS, their contractors, and healthcare providers regarding quality data and metrics.

**Quantitative analysis** Often called discharge analysis; a review of the health record for completeness and accuracy.

**Quantitative approach** The explanation of phenomena by making predictions, collecting and analyzing evidence, testing alternative theories, and choosing the best theory.

**Quantitative standards** Specify the level of measurable work, or productivity, expected for a specific function.

**Query** A routine communication and education tool used to advocate for complete and compliant documentation.

**Query-based exchange** Used by providers to search and discover accessible clinical sources on a patient.

**Questionnaire surveys** Query members of a population by providing participants a means to record and submit their responses electronically or in print form.

**Qui tam relators** Those acting on behalf of the government, also known as whistleblowers.

**Radio frequency identification (RFID)** An automatic recognition technology that uses a device attached to an object to transmit data to a receiver and does not require direct contact.

**Random oval** A display like systematic ovals, but not as uniform, where the ovals are randomly filled in.

**Random sampling** The unbiased selection of subjects from the population of interest.

**Randomization** The arbitrary allocation of subjects between comparison groups.

**Randomized clinical trials (RCTs)** Trials in which participants are assigned to a treatment or a control group.

**Range** The difference between the minimum and maximum values.

**Ransomware** Programs that lock a device or files by deploying encryption technology that demands a ransom payment to restore access.

**RAT-STATS** A statistical package offered by the Office of the Inspector General (OIG). RAT-STATS can be used for both sample size determination and the generation of the random numbers required for sampling.

**Rate** A type of ratio where the two numbers are representing different things.

**Ratio** A comparison of two numbers of the same type of data.

**Ratio data** Naturally numeric data where zero has an interpretation and the values may be doubled or multiplied by a constant and still have meaning.

**Reasonable cause** An act or omission in which a covered entity or business associate knew, or by exercising reasonable diligence would have known, that the act or omission violated an administrative simplification provision, but in which the covered entity or business associate did not act with willful neglect.

**Recognized security practices** "The standards, guidelines, best practices, methodologies, procedures, and processes developed by the National Institute of Standards and Technology Act, the approaches promulgated under section 405(d) of the Cybersecurity Act of 2015, and other programs and processes that address cybersecurity and that are developed, recognized, or promulgated through regulations under other statutory authorities" (42 USC 17941).

**Record locator service (RLS)** The focal point for a query on a patient. An RLS provides the ability to identify where records are located based upon criteria such as a person ID and record data type, and provides functionality for the ongoing maintenance of this location information

**Record retention** Involves determining the schedule to be followed to protect and preserve active and inactive records.

**Recruitment** The process of finding, soliciting, and attracting new employees.

**Redundancy** The concept of building a backup computer system that is an exact version of the primary system and that can replace it in the event of a primary system failure.

**Reference checks** Background investigations conducted by the employer specifically to assess the applicants' compatibility with the position and to validate the accuracy of information the applicants provide on their application, resume, and during the interview.

**Reference terminology**   For clinical data, a set of concepts and relationships that provide a common consultation point for comparison and aggregation of data about the entire healthcare process, recorded by multiple individuals, systems, or institutions.

**Registry**   A collection of care information related to a specific disease, condition, or procedure that makes health record information available for analysis and comparison.

**Regulation**   A rule established by an administrative agency of a government after the passage of statutes.

**Reidentification**   Allowed if an organization that is deidentifying information wants to be able to reidentify the information, a specific code, or other means, to the data for future reidentification purposes. However, the specific code cannot be derived from any type of data elements that come from the patient's health information.

**Reinforcement**   A condition following a response that results in an increase in the strength of that response.

**Relational databases**   The most widely used in numerous industries, including healthcare. This model consists of a database with a set of formally described tables, related (linked) to each other by a shared reference

**Relationships**   Describe associations between entities and represented with diamonds.

**Relative risk (RR)**   The probability that an individual develops a disease over a specified period, if he or she did not die as a result of some other disease process during the same time period.

**Relative value units (RVUs)**   Used to calculate fee schedule amounts. RVUs are a measurement that represents the value of the work involved in providing a specific professional medical service in relation to the value of the work involved in providing other medical services.

**Reliability**   The consistency and stability of an instrument's measurements.

**Remittance advice (RA)**   After payers process claims, files are provided with final individual claim adjudication and payment information. The payment information can then be used to determine revenue audit and recovery efforts.

**Remote patient monitoring device**   A device that enables a healthcare provider to monitor and treat a patient from a remote location.

**Request for proposal (RFP)**   A solicitation to vendors that can include basic information about the healthcare organization, such as how many users will access the system, the timeline for implementation, and any special contractual issues to address.

**Requests for production**   Legal requests for documents from the opposing party.

**Required standards**   Mandatory standards an organization must implement as written by the HIPAA Security Rule.

**Requirements analysis**   The step that identifies, in detail, the precise requirements needed for both HIT (that is, hardware and software) and operational components (people, policy, and process) of the HIS to meet the goals specified in the strategic plan.

**Requirements document**   A detailed collection of expectations for the project output.

**Requirements specification**   A formal document detailing a list of functionalities that the system should be able to do, conveyed to vendors.

*Res ipsa loquitur*   Meaning, "the thing speaks for itself." Doctrine applied toward cases where the facts or circumstances allow for an inference of the defendant's negligence.

*Res judicata*   Doctrine that states that, once adjudicated, the same parties may not pursue the case again.

**Research**   A systematic process dedicated to discovering or formulating new knowledge about a topic; validating or assessing existing knowledge; or updating antiquated understanding.

**Research data**   Data that may be the same as administrative, clinical, or financial data, plus additional data associated with a specific research protocol.

**Research design**   Serves as the blueprint for a study, outlining the strategy to achieve the researchers' objectives, whether it is answering a question, addressing a problem, or generating new information.

**Research methodology**   The science of solving research problems by incorporating a set of procedures or strategies used by researchers to collect, analyze, and present data.

**Research methods**   The use of strategies, processes, or techniques to conduct research studies.

**Research protocols**   Sets of strict procedures that specify the language of informed consent, the types of subjects, the timing of treatments, the period of participation, and the evaluation of efficacy.

**Research question**   The central focus of the research asking about a particular issue within a topic a researcher wishes to study.

**Resident Assessment Instrument (RAI)** Developed by CMS to standardize the collection of SNF patient data, the RAI is composed of three components: the Minimum Data Set 3.0 (MDS), the Care Area Assessment (CAA) process, and the RAI utilization guidelines.

**Residual risk** Risks that remain even with the current safeguards and controls applied.

**Resource-based relative value scale (RBRVS)** In 1992, CMS implemented the system for physicians' services such as office visits covered under Medicare Part B. The system reimburses physicians according to a fee schedule based on predetermined values assigned to specific services.

**Respect** Being mindful of individual differences and cultural and ethnic diversity.

**Respite care** Any inpatient care provided to the hospice patient for the purpose of giving primary caregivers a break from their caregiving responsibilities.

*Respondeat superior* Meaning "let the master answer"; Doctrine in which employers may be held liable for any job-related acts of their employees or agents.

**Responsibility** An expectation that a person will perform tasks.

**Restitution** Monetary compensation or other actions stated to make the plaintiff as whole again as possible.

**Retail clinics** Treat non-life-threatening acute illnesses and offer routine wellness services such as vaccinations, sports physicals, and prescription refills.

**Retention** The ability to keep valuable employees from seeking employment elsewhere.

**Retrospective documentation** Refers to the addition of documentation related to clinical intervention after care has been given.

**Retrospective payment systems** When the exact amount of the payment is determined after the service has been delivered.

**Retrospective review** Review that occurs later after a patient has been discharged.

**Retrospective study** A study conducted by reviewing records from the past

**Return on investment (ROI)** Determines if the system has paid for itself, comparing the financial benefits to the total costs of the system; the increase in the value of an asset.

**Revenue** The compensation that is earned by providing goods and services to the client or patient and amounts received or earned from other sources.

**Revenue cycle** The sequence of processes to progress a patient account from creation to closing.

**Revenue cycle management (RCM)** The strategy implemented to direct administrative and clinical functions associated with capturing, monitoring, and collecting patient service revenue.

**Revenue principle** Principle that states that earnings resulting from activities and investments may only be recognized when they have been earned, can be measured, and have a reasonable expectation of being collected.

**Revenue projects** Projects that result in new or expanded products or services.

**Reverse mentoring** Process where the new employee mentors a senior person on subjects in which he or she may have more expertise, such as use of social media or digital technologies.

**Right to privacy** "The right to be let alone," including the rights of individuals to be free from surveillance and interference, as well as the right to keep one's information from being disclosed.

**Risk adjustment** In an accountable care organization (ACO) refers to the process of adjusting financial benchmarks or performance measures to account for the health status and demographic characteristics of the patient population. This ensures that providers are fairly evaluated, recognizing that patients with more complex health needs may require more resources and care.

**Risk analysis** A systemic process for reviewing all systems, applications, and processes to identify potential threats and vulnerabilities, document current controls, and understand the likelihood of the impact.

**Risk management** A comprehensive program of activities intended to minimize the potential for injuries to occur in a facility and to anticipate and respond to ensuring liability for those injuries that do occur.

**Role** A set of expectations about how a person is to behave from the perspective of oneself, peers, managers, staff, consumers (patients), and others (such as legislators).

**Role playing** An activity where learners are presented with a hypothetical situation they may encounter on the job, and they act out the response.

**Role theory** A prominent framework for examining behavior in the field of medical sociology for decades, applied in management to clarify the wide range of responsibilities held.

**Root cause analysis** An analysis of a sentinel event from all aspects (human, procedural, machinery, material) to identify how each contributed to the occurrence of the event and to develop new systems that will prevent recurrence.

**Rootkit** A type of malware that will remotely access or control a computer without being detected by users or security programs.

**Rules of engagement** Specify the way policy makers, data owners, data stewards, and other stakeholders interact with each other.

**Run chart** A chart that displays data points over time.

**RxNorm** A standardized nomenclature for clinical drugs that provides information on a drug's ingredients, strengths, and form in which it is to be administered or used.

**Safe harbor method** A method of deidentification that requires the covered entity or business associate to remove 18 data elements from the health information.

**Scalar chain** Also known as line of authority. Everyone from top to bottom knows who they report to and is clearly included in the chain of command.

**Scales** Progressive categories such as size, amount, importance, rank, or agreement.

**Scanning** Inserting paper into the optical scanner so that both the front and back of the forms are scanned at the same time.

**Scatter diagram** A data analysis tool used to plot points of two variables suspected of being related to each other in some way.

**Scatterplot** Displays the relationship between two quantitative variables using a best-fit line that represents the trend of the data.

**Scenarios** Stories describing the current and feasible future states of the business environment.

**Schema mapping** Process in which Entity relationship diagrams (ERDs) are converted into tables.

**Scientific management** An early effort to apply scientific principles and practices to business processes.

**Scope creep** When incremental and small changes in scope create significant changes and require more resources and time than originally planned.

**Scribe** An individual who performs data entry functions at the point of care.

**Secondary analysis** Involves using data originally collected by other researchers to address different questions.

**Secondary data sources** Created using the data from a primary data source.

**Secondary sources** Summaries of the original works.

**Secure information** Data considered unreadable, unusable, and indecipherable

**Secure messaging** Enables "a user to electronically send messages to, and receive messages from, a patient in a manner that ensures: (1) both the patient (or authorized representative) and EHR technology user are authenticated; and (2) the message content is encrypted and integrity-protected in accordance with the standard for encryption and hashing algorithms" (NIST 2013).

**Securities and Exchange Commission (SEC)** A federal agency that regulates public and some private transactions involving the ownership and debt of organizations.

**Security** The means used to control access and protect information from accidental or intentional disclosure to unauthorized persons and from unauthorized alteration, destruction, or loss.

**Security Rule** The purpose of the Security Standards for the Protection of Electronic Protected Health Information, or the privacy rule (45 CFR Part 160 and Subparts A and C of Part 164), is to operationalize the protections identified in the Privacy Rule by addressing the technical and nontechnical safeguards that covered entities must put in place to secure individuals' ePHI

**Semantic interoperability** When information being transmitted is understood.

**Sentinel event** An unexpected occurrence involving death or serious physical or psychological injury, or the risk thereof.

**Serial work division** The sequential handling of tasks.

**Servant leadership** A values-based leadership approach in which the leader's role is viewed as serving others.

**Service innovations** Create new market opportunities, and in many industries are the driving force behind growth and profitability.

**Service level agreements (SLAs)** Clear definitions of the work or services needed as well as the performance expectations in a contract for services. Details include price and payment terms, the reporting chain of command, terms for termination of the relationship, and privacy, security, and confidentiality expectations of the contracted staff.

**Settlements** Official agreements.

**Shift differential** A slightly higher hourly wage for employees who work less-desirable shifts (evening, night, or weekend).

**Shift rotation** Staff schedules change among morning, afternoon, and evening shifts.

**Simple linear regression (SLR)** Statistical inference that measures the strength of the relationship between two variables and estimates a functional relationship between them.

**Simple random sampling** When every member of the population has an equal probability of inclusion in the sample.

**Simulation** A form of training through an application that mimics work-related situations and imparts knowledge and skills as the user progresses.

**Simulation observation** When researchers stage events rather than allowing them to occur naturally.

**Single-blind studies** Randomized clinical trials (RCTs) in which the subject does not know the treatment.

**Situational theory of leadership** Based on the relationship between leaders and followers, it provides a framework to analyze each situation based on task behavior—(the amount of guidance and direction given by a leader) and relationship behavior (the amount of socioemotional support a leader provides). The leader's style should be adjusted to different situations and employees encountered.

**Six Sigma** A data-driven methodology for removing defects in any process.

**Skilled nursing facilities (SNFs)** Commonly called nursing homes, provide medical, nursing, and, in some cases, rehabilitative care around the clock. The majority of SNF residents are over age 65 and quite often are classified as the "frail elderly."

**Skilled nursing facility prospective payment system (SNF PPS)** A per diem reimbursement system for all costs (routine, ancillary, and capital) associated with covered SNF services furnished to Medicare Part A beneficiaries.

**Slander** Defamation of character that is spoken.

**Slicing and dicing** Refers to the process of taking what is known at the highest level of understanding and working downward to identify the underlying causes for the high-level observation.

**SMART goals** Statements that identify results that are Specific, Measurable, Achievable, Relevant, and Time-based.

**SOAP (subjective, objective, assessment, plan) note** A common method for recording progress notes that helps providers remember the specific and systematic decision-making process being documented.

**Social determinants of health** The conditions in which people are born, grow, work, live, and age, and the wider set of forces and systems shaping the conditions of daily life. These forces and systems include economic policies and systems, development agendas, social norms, social policies, and political systems.

**Social engineering** An attempt to trick someone into revealing information (for example, a password) that can be used to attack systems or networks or taking an action (for example, clicking a link or opening a document).

**Socialization** A period in which a new employee learns the values, behavior patterns, and expectations of the organization.

**Soft skills** Skills that contribute to an employee's career advancement and recognition beyond job knowledge. Soft skills include oral and written communication, critical thinking, organization, and others.

**Software as a Service (SaaS)** A subscription service to EHRs delivered over the cloud.

**Sole proprietorship** A venture with one owner in which all profits are considered the owner's personal income.

**Source systems** Information systems used to communicate data with multiple sources, whether within hospital departments or external to a physician practice.

**Spaced training** Training that occurs in several shorter sessions.

**Spaghetti diagram** A workflow diagram that helps visualize the flow of people, products, and process documents in a defined physical work area.

**Span of control** Each supervisor oversees a certain number of people.

**Spatial representations** Allow information to be viewed immediately, utilizing perceptual processes without needing to address the individual elements of the information separately or analytically.

**Special cause variation** A greater-than-expected variation.

**Specific performance** A contract action that arises when one party claims the other party failed to meet an obligation set forth in a valid contract.

**Speech recognition technology**   Software which translates speech to text.

**Spoliation**   "Intentional destruction, mutilation, alteration, or concealment of evidence" (Rinehart-Thompson 2023b, 63).

**Sponsor**   Often a high-level manager who approves and protects the idea, expedites testing and approval, and removes barriers within the organization.

**Staff authority**   Related to the expert knowledge of specialists in the organization and involves their ability or right to advise and recommend courses of action.

**Staff model HMO**   Directly employs physicians and other healthcare professionals to provide medical services to members, and members of the salaried medical staff are considered employees of the HMO rather than independent practitioners.

**Staging system**   A classification system that describes the extent of cancer within a patient.

**Stakeholder analysis**   A process that identifies and analyzes the attitudes or opinions of stakeholders.

**Stakeholders**   Defined as individuals within the company who have an interest in, or are affected by, the results of a project.

**Standard**   A performance criterion established by custom or authority for the purpose of assessing factors such as quality, productivity, and performance.

**Standard deviation**   The square root of the variance.

**Standard of care**   What an individual is expected to do or not do in each situation. In the healthcare context, the standard of care is the level of care that a reasonably prudent and similarly situated practitioner would have provided in similar circumstances.

**Standard of proof**   The requisite degree of belief to support the purported claims.

**Stare decisis**   A legal principle related to precedent which means "let the decision stand." It states that in lower court cases involving a fact pattern like that in a higher court within the same court system, the lower court is bound to apply the decision of the higher court.

**Stark Law**   Also known as the Physician Self-Referral Law. Prohibits a physician from referring certain health services to "an entity in which the physician (or member of immediate family) has an ownership or investment or with which the physician has a compensation arrangement, unless an exception applies" (CMS 2021, 9).

**Statement of cash flow**   A statement that details the reasons that cash changed from one balance sheet period to another.

**Statement of retained earnings**   A statement that expresses the change in retained earnings from the beginning of the balance sheet period to the end in a for-profit organization, while a statement of change in net assets is prepared in a not-for-profit organization.

**Statement of stockholder's equity**   Also called the statement of net assets; details the reasons for changes in each of the stockholder's equity accounts, including retained earnings.

**Statistics**   "A branch of mathematics concerned with collecting, organizing, summarizing, and analyzing data" (White 2023, 1).

**Statute of limitations**   If a lawsuit is not brought within a statutory time limit, the plaintiff is barred from pursuing the claim.

**Statutes**   Laws created by legislative bodies that set forth required actions.

**Statutory (legislative) law**   Written law established by federal and state legislatures, or municipalities (where the law is frequently called an ordinance).

**Steering committee**   A representative group of key stakeholders who provide advice and guidance.

**Stereotyping**   An assumption that everyone within a certain group is the same.

**Stewardship**   Data owners, data stewards, and data users all playing a role to maintain accuracy, security, and accessibility of data.

**Strategic goal**   A high-level set of key activities describing the actions needed to carry out each of the newly selected organizational strategies.

**Strategic management**   The process a leader and his or her leadership team uses for assessing a changing environment to create a vision of the future; determining how the organization fits into the future environment based on its mission and vision and gaining knowledge of its strengths, weaknesses, opportunities, and threats; and then setting in motion a strategic plan of action to position the organization accordingly.

**Strategic objectives**   Detailed steps to achieve the identified strategic goal and include specific timelines, resource allocation needs, and assignment of responsibility to the person(s) accountable for implementation of each strategic goal.

**Strategic plan**   A long-term plan, covering a period of at least three to five years, focused on the organization's mission, vision, and goals to help set the organization's direction.

**Strategic planning** A management tool used to develop a formalized roadmap that spells out where an organization is going over the next one to five years and describes how it can focus on its continuing mission and execute the chosen vision and strategy.

**Strategic profile** Identifies the existing key services or products of the department or organization, the nature of its customers and users, the nature of its industry and market segments, and the nature of its geographic markets.

**Strategic thinking** The thought process of an organization's leaders that helps them determine the vision for some point in the future and identify a strategy to achieve this vision.

**Strategy** The art and science of planning and marshaling resources for their most efficient and effective use to intentionally position and focus an organization for the future.

**Strategy map** A visual representation of the cause-and-effect relationships among the components of an organization's strategy.

**Stratified random sample** A sample selected by first dividing the population into subsets or strata, then selecting a simple random sample from each strata.

**Strict liability** Liability without fault, or error, wherein a person or entity is held liable for damages or loss resulting from acts or omissions regardless of whether there was fault.

**Stringent** A law is considered this if it prohibits or restricts use or disclosure in circumstances under which such use or disclosure would be permitted under federal law.

**Strong matrix organization** Similar to the balanced matrix but includes a department of project managers. In these organizations, project managers are not functional staff members assuming the role of project manager but rather project manager specialists reporting to a manager of project management.

**Structural metadata** Data that describes how the data for each data element are captured, processed, stored, and displayed.

**Structured data** Data that are organized and easily retrievable and interpreted by traditional databases and data models.

**Structured interview** Uses a set of standardized questions asked of all applicants.

**Structured Query Language (SQL)** The formal language used to retrieve information stored in relational databases.

**Subject matter jurisdiction** A legal doctrine that limits the types of cases, by subject, a court can decide.

**Subpoenas** Directives to attend or respond to legal proceedings

**Succession planning** A specific type of promotional plan in which senior-level position openings are anticipated and candidates are identified from within the organization.

**Summons** Also called a notice. An order by a court that requires an appearance or a written response, served along with the complaint to the defendant

**Sunsetting** The action taken by a vendor to no longer support ongoing maintenance or upgrades for a legacy system.

**Super users** Staff members who will ultimately be end users (those using the system for everyday tasks) who have agreed to help with the implementation, testing, training, and post go-live troubleshooting.

**Supreme court** A court at the highest level.

**Surgeon general** Officer appointed by the US president who provides leadership and authoritative, science-based recommendations about the public's health. The surgeon general has responsibility for the public health service (PHS) workforce.

**Surveys** A fundamental tool for systematically collecting data from a specific population or a subset of that population.

**Swimlane diagram** Diagram that shows an entire business process from beginning to end and highlights relevant variables (who, what, and when) while requiring little or no training to use and understand.

**SWOT analysis** Outlines the organization's strengths (S) and weaknesses (W), which are internal to the organization, and the opportunities (O) and threats (T) that are external to the organization.

**Symbolic representations** Require analytical processes where information is extracted from specific data values.

**Synchronously** Applies to web-based courses that can be delivered in real time to employees and trainers, interacting through chat rooms, whiteboards, or application sharing at a predetermined time with review of materials.

**System**  A set of components that work together to achieve a common purpose.

**System customization**  Process that includes loading data tables and master files (for example, files of all the names of staff members and their permissions for access to the system), adjusting decision support rules for transitioning, writing interfaces, customizing screens, and numerous other tasks that make the system work for the specific organization.

**System development life cycle (SDLC)**  The steps taken from an initial point of recognizing the need for a desired result, through the steps taken to ensure that all components needed for the system to achieve the desired result are addressed, to repeating this cycle whenever the system fails to produce the desired result.

**System integrator**  A best of fit vendor that acquires products and develops permanent interfaces between them, selling them then as a single technology offering.

**System optimization**  The activities that extend use of information systems beyond the basic functionality that characterizes adoption.

**Systematic ovals**  A graphical technique that displays stacked ovals with the height of the stack corresponding to the maximum of the scale.

**Systematic random sampling**  A method used to determine a simple random sample in which every N/nth record is selected from the population, with N being the number of units in the population and n the sample size.

**Systematic review**  A comprehensive review of the evidence on a clearly formulated question that uses systematic and explicit methods to identify, select, and critically appraise relevant published and unpublished research studies; to extract and analyze data from the studies included in the review; and to present integrated and synthesized information

**Systemized Nomenclature of Medicine Clinical Terminology (SNOMED CT)**  A comprehensive, multilingual, multi-hierarchical, concept-oriented clinical terminology owned, maintained, and distributed by the International Health Terminology Standards Development Organization (IHTSDO).

**Systems thinking**  Based on understanding that a system refers to the interconnections among many components that make up a whole.

**Systems view**  Considering all the components of a system when making any changes to improve its outcomes.

**Table**  A display that presents data organized in columns and rows.

**Tacit knowledge**  The actions, experiences, ideals, values, and emotions of an individual that tend to be highly personal and difficult to communicate.

**Tactical plan**  A short-term plan, focused on one component or project.

**Talent triangle**  Derived from the PMCD framework and representing the categorization of three areas of applied expertise project managers possess and must continually develop; they are ways of working, power skills, and business acumen.

**Task analysis**  A process to determine the specific skills required for the job.

**Tax Equity and Fiscal Responsibility Act of 1982 (TEFRA)**  TEFRA modified Medicare's retrospective reimbursement system for inpatient hospital stays by requiring implementation of the DRG PPS in 1983.

**Team building**  The process of organizing and acquainting team members to enhance the outcomes of collaborative work.

**Technical safeguards**  Things such as automatic log-off and unique user identification, to protect access and control of ePHI.

**Technical skills**  Ability to understand and master the technical information, methods, and equipment involved in a discipline.

**Telecommuting**  An option wherein employees work full- or part-time in their own homes.

**Telehealth**  "The use of electronic information and telecommunications technologies to support long-distance clinical healthcare, patient and professional health-related education, public health, and health administration" (HRSA 2022).

**Terminal-digit filing system**  Paper records are filed according to a three-part number made up of two-digit pairs.

**Termination**  Ending of a job.

**Terminology**  A set of terms representing a system of concepts of a particular subject or field.

**Terminology and classification management**  Consists of the processes for managing the breadth of healthcare terminologies, vocabularies, classification systems, and data sets an organization may use, and serves as a terminology authority for the enterprise.

**Text mining**  Describes the process of extracting and then quantifying and filtering free-text data.

**The Red Flags Rule** Set of Federal Trade Commission regulations that requires certain entities to develop and implement identity theft prevention programs.

**Theory X** Management theory that presumed workers inherently disliked work and would avoid it, had little ambition, and mostly wanted security; therefore, managerial direction and control were necessary.

**Theory Y** Management theory that assumed work was as natural as play, motivation could be both internally and externally driven, and under the right conditions people would seek responsibility and be creative.

**Theory Z** Approach based on the values of long-term employment, employee engagement and participation, and consensual decision-making.

**Thoughtflow** A process and its sequence when the process is largely conducted mentally.

**360-degree evaluation** A form of employee evaluation to which managers, peers, and staff contribute.

**Time and motion studies** Studies in which tasks were subdivided into their most basic movements. Detailed motions are timed to determine the most efficient way of carrying them out.

**Topography** A code that describes the site of origin of the neoplasm and uses the same three-character categories as in the neoplasm section of the second chapter of ICD-10.

**Tort** A civil, noncriminal wrong.

**Tort law** Law that encompasses actions brought when one party believes another party caused harm through wrongful conduct.

**Total margin ratio** Measurement of the overall profitability of an organization, which compares excess of revenue over expense by total revenue.

**Total quality management (TQM)** An approach that offers a way to build in high performance by maximizing employee potential and continuous improvement of processes.

**Total quality management (TQM) approach** Sought to overcome the limitations of MBO, criticizing the use of quotas because workers often spent too much time trying to look good or protect themselves by seeking short-term objectives and ignoring long-term and critical outcomes.

**Tracer methodology** "A process the Joint Commission surveyors use during the on-site survey to analyze an organization's systems, with particular attention to identified priority focus areas, by following individual patients through the organization's healthcare process in the sequence experienced by the patients; an evaluation that follows (traces) the hospital experiences of specific patients to assess the quality of patient care" (Joint Commission n.d.c).

**Train-the-trainer** Workshops conducted for instructors who may not have formal training experience. In these workshops the trainer—either a manager or employee—learns skills in communication and instruction to train others effectively on job tasks.

**Training** In traditional management theory, the process of providing entry-level skills required to begin a job for technical employees.

**Trait approach** Theory that gradually replaced the great person model, proposing leaders possessed a collection of traits or personal behaviors and attributes that distinguished them from non-leaders.

**Transfer the risk** Outsourcing or insuring against any potential loss to the organization.

**Transitions of care (ToC) initiative** One of the projects of the ONC Standards and Interoperability (S&I) Framework.

**Traumatic injury** A wound or other injury caused by an external physical force such as an automobile accident, a shooting, a stabbing, or a fall.

**Treatment** Also known as intervention; defined generically or broadly, beyond its usual meaning of therapy. It is the process in which the researcher manipulates the independent variables.

**Triangulation** The use of multiple sources or perspectives to investigate the same phenomenon.

**Trial court** Typically the lowest level of a state court system, where state civil and criminal cases are initiated, and has original jurisdiction.

**TRICARE** A federal healthcare program for active-duty members of the military and qualified family members.

**Trier of fact** A judge or jury.

**Triple Aim** Concept that indicates vast and systematic improvements are needed to improve experiences for patients in their pursuit of healthcare, enhance health among the population, and lower per capita costs.

**Triple constraint** Three constraints of project completion, including the schedule, budget, and scope.

**Trojan horses** Programs disguised as a normal program to trick users to download the file.

**Trust community**  A group of organizations that identified a set of mutual goals and dependencies that, through collaborative effort, led to mutual benefit.

**Turnover plan**  A plan that specifies how and when each part of an information system component is to be implemented for different users.

**Turnover strategy**  A type of staging that considers which users may be the easiest to train, which users are most interested in using the system, and which components are not dependent on other components not yet implemented.

**Two-factor authentication**  The most common multifactor authentication, which provides additional security to the authentication process as it requires one additional step to verify the user's identification.

**Type I error**  The probability of incorrectly rejecting the null hypothesis when it is true, given the values present in the sample.

**Type II error**  Occurs when the null hypothesis is not rejected when it is false

**Unbundling**  The reporting of multiple codes to describe a service or procedure when, according to coding conventions, one code would accurately describe the procedure.

**Unified Medical Language System (UMLS)**  A system that integrates biomedical concepts from various sources to show their relationships.

**Uniformed Services Employment and Reemployment Rights Act (USERRA) of 1994**  Federal legislation that prohibits discrimination against individuals because of their service in the uniformed services.

**Union**  Labor organizations that enter negotiations with employers on behalf of groups of employees who have elected to join the union.

**Unique identifier**  A combination of numbers or alphanumeric characters assigned to each patient of a specific healthcare organization, which is often called the health record number.

**Unit numbering system**  A number is assigned to a patient during the first encounter for care and kept for all subsequent encounters.

**Unit work division**  When different specialized tasks are performed at the same time.

**Unity of command**  Every employee receives direction and instructions from one boss.

**Unstructured data**  Data that do not have a predefined data model or are not stored in a traditional database structure.

**Upcoding**  Using diagnosis or procedure codes selected specifically because they result in higher payment from third-party payers.

**Usability**  The overall ability of a user to capture and retrieve data efficiently and effectively to achieve results from health information systems.

**Use**  The sharing, employment, application, utilization, examination, or analysis within a covered entity that creates and maintains the PHI.

**Use case analysis**  A technique to determine how users will interact with a system.

**User authentication**  The process where an end user logs into an electronic system using specific credentials defined by the organization.

**Users**  All internal and external stakeholders who are directly affected by the project deliverables.

**Utilitarianism**  Also known as the greatest happiness principle; proposes that to determine the greatest good we look to the consequences of action; that is, "actions are right in proportion as they tend to promote happiness, wrong as they tend to produce the reverse of happiness. By happiness is intended pleasure, and the absence of pain" (Mill 2007, 6).

**Utilization management (UM)**  A collection of systems and processes that ensures facilities and resources, both human and nonhuman, are used maximally and are consistent with patient care needs.

**Validity**  Whether a test or a measurement used in a study achieved what the researcher intended to measure.

**Value-based payments**  Any method of healthcare reimbursement that either financially incentivizes providers for good quality and outcomes or penalizes providers for inadequate quality and unfavorable outcomes.

**Value-based programs**  Programs based on data-driven metrics to measure both the quality and efficiency of a healthcare provider.

**Value-based purchasing**  To pay for care that rewards better value, patient outcomes, and innovation rather than just the volume of care provided.

**Values statement**  A statement that reflects the social and cultural beliefs an organization wishes to support among its members.

**Values-based leadership**  Refers to leadership behaviors that emphasize moral, authentic, and ethical orientations to how the organization and employees function.

**Variable costs**  Costs that are sensitive to volume.

**Variables**  The factors in correlational research and other research designs.

**Variance**  In sampling, refers to a measure of variability which is calculated as the average squared deviation from the mean; In accounting, the differences between budgeted and actual amounts; in project management, any deviation from the project's baseline expectations.

**Vector graphic data**  The data type used by physiological signal processing systems, referred to as signal tracing.

**Vertical dyad linkage (VDL)**  First formulated in 1975, to describe the single-person mentoring relationships that occur in organizations.

**Videoconferencing**  Training involving a computer monitor equipped with speakers, or a monitor and telephone, that enables learners to listen and respond to the same material presented by an instructor located at another site.

**Virtualization**  The emulation of one or more computers within a software platform that enables one physical computer to share resources across other computers.

**Virtue ethics**  In determining what is good or right in terms of conduct, this approach considers the character of the moral agent performing the action.

**Viruses**  Programs that search out other programs and infect them by embedding a copy of themselves.

**Vision**  A short description of an organization's ideal future state.

**Vision statement**  A statement that describes the ideal and desired future state toward which an organization is directed.

**Vital statistics**  Data on births, deaths, fetal deaths, marriages, and divorces.

**Volume logs**  Records used to document information about the volume of work units received and processed in a day by keeping track of the number of products produced or activities done.

**Vulnerable subject**  A subject with limited mental capacity or who is unable to freely volunteer.

**Waste**  Overutilization, underutilization, or misuse of resources.

**Waterfall method**  This sequential method of completing the project phases; the phases are structured so one phase begins at the end or near the end of the previous phase.

**Weak matrix organization**  Organization where the project manager role does not exist, but a project expediter role is used to work directly with the functional staff rather than through the functional managers.

**Web content management systems**  Systems that label and track the information placed on a website, so the information is easily located, modified, and reused.

**Web portal**  A single point of personalized access (an entryway) through which one can find and deliver information (content), applications, and services.

**Web services**  A platform for software applications (or services) whose basic communication mechanism is XML, the universal language of the web and the accepted format for data exchange over the internet.

**Webinars**  Seminars delivered through a web browser, either in real time or as a recorded broadcast.

**Whistleblowing**  Bringing lawsuits or alerting authorities based on knowledge of fraud

**Wikis**  A collection of user-modified web pages that together form a collaborative website.

**Willful neglect**  Conscious, intentional failure or reckless indifference to the obligation to comply with the administrative simplification provision violated.

**Wireless systems**  Systems that use wireless networks and wireless devices to access and transmit data in real time.

**Work breakdown structure (WBS)**  Diagram tool developed to summarize and illustrate the project work and is commonly used due to the analytical nature where the project is dissected into manageable components.

**Work distribution analysis**  A process for evaluating the types of work functions performed in a department, the amount of time given to those functions, who is performing each function, and the way work is distributed among the employees.

**Work distribution chart**  A chart initially completed by each employee that includes all responsible task content and hours or parts of hours spent on tasks gathered over a designated period.

**Work measurement**  The process of studying the amount of work accomplished and the amount of time it takes to accomplish it.

**Work sampling**  A technique of work measurement that involves using statistical probability (determined through random sample observations) to characterize the performance of the department and its functional work units.

**Worker immaturity–maturity** A concept that suggests job maturity (work-related ability) and psychological maturity (motivation related to work) of employees also influence the selection and effectiveness of the leadership style.

**Workers' Adjustment Retraining and Notification (WARN) Act** Requires organizations employing more than 100 people give the employees and the community a 60-day notice of its intent to close the business or to lay off 50 or more members of its workforce.

**Workflow** The sequence of steps in a process.

**Workers' Compensation** An insurance system operated by the individual states to provide covered workers with some protection against the costs of medical care and the loss of income resulting from work-related injuries and, in some cases, illnesses.

**Worms** Programs that reproduce on their own that have no need for a host application; they are self-contained programs.

**Zero-based budgets** Budgets that apply to organizations for which each budget cycle poses the opportunity to continue or discontinue services based on the availability of resources.

# Index

## A

AARP, 26
abbreviated injury scale (AIS), 126
absentee coverage, 658
abuse
    corporate compliance and, 221–229
    defined, 222
A&C (adults and children), 423, 424
acceptance
    of contract, 244
    risk, 277
acceptant functions, of change agents, 565
accession number, 124
accession registry, 124
accountability
    in data governance, 53, 55
    as recordkeeping principle, 44
accountable care organization (ACO), 22–23, 161, 163, 442
account follow-up, 194–195
accounting, 688–693
    authorities on, 689–690
    basics of, 694–706
    concepts and principles of, 688–689
    defined, 688
    management, 706–709
    managerial, 710
    organizational forms and, 690–692
    sources of financial data in, 692–693
    uses of financial data in, 693
accounting manager, 686
accounting of disclosures, 268
accounting rate of return (ARR), 717–718
accounting systems, 341
accounts payable, 696
accounts receivable, 694–695, 709
accounts receivable (A/R) days, 194
accreditation
    bodies for, 245–246, 300
    defined, 25
    health records and, 88, 246
    of hospitals, 5, 25, 63
    and quality management, 300
Accreditation Association for Ambulatory Health Care (AAAHC), 6, 300
Accredited Standards Committee (ASC), 113, 347
accrue, 700
accumulated depreciation, 715
accuracy rate, 662
acquisitions
    in capital budget, 715
    of health information systems, 379–382
acquittal, 239
activity-based budgets, 711
actors, in information blocking, 274
act step, in Deming Wheel, 308, 309
actual causation, 240
acute care
    disease index for, 123
    health records for, 63, 76
    in hospitals, 11–12
acute-care prospective payment system, 164, 165–166
A&D (admissions and discharges), 423
ADDIE model, 625–626
addressable standards, 262
adhesion contract, 244
adjudication, 239
administrative agencies, 236
administrative applications, 342
administrative branch, 235
administrative data, 389
administrative databases, 134–135
administrative information
    for CDI program evaluation, 214
    financial, 693
    in health record, 68–69
administrative law, 236
administrative management, 543–545
administrative metadata, 390–391
Administrative Procedure Act (1989), 236
administrative registries, 129
Administrative Requirements, of Privacy Rule, 262
administrative safeguards, 262
administrative services only (ASO) contract, 151
administrative staff, of hospitals, 13
administrative supervisor, 730
administrative support services, in hospitals, 16
administrative systems, 341–342
admissions. *See* registration
admit-discharge-transfer (ADT) messages, 355, 360
adopters, of innovations, 562–563
adoption
    defined, 387
    of health information systems, 387–388
adoption model for analytics maturity (AMAM), 388
adoption records, 254
adult day care programs, 21
adult learning strategies, 636–639
advance beneficiary notice of noncoverage (ABN), 181–182
advance directives, 68–69, 250, 764–766
Advance Notice of Proposed Rulemaking (ANPRM), 518
adverse determination, 185
adverse event, 305
aesthetics, at work, 654
affinity diagram, 674–675
Affordable Care Act (ACA) (2010). *See* Patient Protection and Affordable Care Act (ACA) (2010)
Age Discrimination in Employment Act (ADEA) (1967), 601–602
Agency for Healthcare Research and Quality (AHRQ), 311–313
    on care coordination, 315
    on consumer assessment of health plans, 400
    functions of, 137
    Healthcare Cost and Utilization Project of, 137, 312
    on health literacy, 403
    patient-centered care improvement guide by, 534
    quality indicators of, 312–313
    role of, 312
agency rules, 236
aggregate data, 122
agile approach, to project management, 725–726
Agile Certified Practitioner (PMP-ACP), 724
AIDS information, handling, 254
Alaska Natives, 27, 157
alcohol abuse, information about, handling, 253–254, 271–273
allied health professions, 6
allocation of overhead, 708–709
altruism, 759
ambulance fee schedule, 171
ambulatory care
    defined, 17
    freestanding ambulatory care centers for, 18–19
    health records for, 77
    health statistics on, 434
    home healthcare as, 19
    in hospitals, 12, 18
    organization of, 17–20
    private medical practices for, 18
    public health services for, 19
    voluntary agencies for, 19–20
ambulatory payment classification (APC), 169–170, 214

887

ambulatory surgery, 18, 19
ambulatory surgery center (ASC)
    defined, 170
    health records of, 77
    prospective payment system for, 170–171
American Academy of Professional Coders (AAPC), 209
American Association of Medical Record Librarians, 316
American Board of Quality Assurance and Utilization Review Physicians, 316
American Case Management Association (ACMA), 184
American College of Physicians, 5, 63
American College of Radiology (ACR), 300
American College of Surgeons (ACS)
    AHIMA created by, 316
    and cancer registries, 125
    formation of, 5, 296
    successor organization to, 63
American Dental Association (ADA), 103, 113
American Health Information Management Association (AHIMA)
    on career development, 646–647
    on clinical documentation integrity, 209, 212
    Code of Ethics of, 624, 758, 760–764, 766, 767
    creation of, 316
    on data backup plan, 279
    data dictionary guidelines by, 143
    data quality best practices by, 142
    data quality model of, 140, 141
    as not-for-profit organization, 691, 692
    Professional Ethics Committee of, 767
    Standards of Ethical Coding of, 761, 769
    vision of, 584, 585
American Hospital Association, 5, 63, 298, 316
American Indians, 27, 157
American Joint Replacement Registry, 129
American Medical Association (AMA)
    and CPT, 101–102
    establishment of, 4
    and Joint Commission on Accreditation of Hospitals, 5, 63
    on medical necessity, 181
American Medical Informatics Association (AMIA), 5, 139
American Osteopathic Association (AOA), 6
American Psychiatric Association (APA), 102
American Recovery and Reinvestment Act (ARRA) (2009), 112, 169, 246, 263, 326
American Red Cross, 691
American Society for Testing Materials (ASTM) International, 112, 113, 406

Americans with Disabilities Act (ADA) (1990), 602, 639, 647–648
American Trauma Society (ATS), 127
analysis statements, 702
analytics. *See* data analytics; healthcare data analytics
anatomic pathology, 15
ancillary systems, 342
ancillary units (services)
    census report used by, 425
    in health records, 73–74
    in hospitals, 16
anesthesia
    intraoperative, 74
    postoperative, 74
anesthesiology, in health records, 74
answer, in civil litigation, 238
antepartum record, 75
Anti-Kickback Statute (AKS), 229
antivirus software, 284
apology statutes, 243–244
appellate court, 237, 239
appendectomy, 12
application(s)
    administrative, 342
    for EHRs, 342–348
application, job, 608
application programming interface (API), 38
application service provider (ASP), 380
application software, 370
applied research, 486
*a priori*, 757
arbitration, 238, 619
architectural models, for health information exchange, 351–354
areas of excellence, 585
Aristotle, 756
Armed Forces Health Longitudinal Technology Application, 108
arraignment, 239
article, 510
artifacts, 46
artificial intelligence (AI)
    batch processing by, 38
    in business intelligence management, 48
    in clinical and biomedical research, 516
    in clinical documentation integrity, 115, 184, 220
    in data standardization, 115
    defined, 183
    in document creation, 81
    ethical use of, 32, 775–776
    healthcare uses of, 32, 328
    in literature review, 491
    in quality management, 315
    in revenue cycle management, 180, 183, 184, 186, 192, 193–194
    in training and development, 644–645
    and validity, 502
    in work safety programs, 603
assault, 241
assessment. *See also* needs assessment; quality assessment

consumer, of healthcare providers, 400–401
    of data quality, 41, 48
    environmental, in strategic planning, 579–583, 586, 595–596
    of in-service education, 635–636
    of mission statement, 580
    of on-the-job training programs, 632–633
    of risk, 276, 532–533, 582–583
assets, 694–696
    defined, 694
    examples of, 694–696
    net, 696–697, 702, 703
Association of Clinical Documentation Integrity Specialists (ACDIS), 209, 212, 217
Association of Credit and Collection Professionals (ACA) International, 195
Association of Records Management and Administrators International (ARMA International), 44, 56–57
assumption of risk, 243
asynchronous web-based courses, 644
attributable risk (AR), 533
attributes, 130
audiologists, 15
audit
    code compliance, 223, 225
    defined, 278
    external, 225, 227
    internal, 225, 227
    logs of, 278
    payment, 196–197
    revenue, 196–197
augmented intelligence, 32
augmented reality (AR), 509
aural learners, 638
Australian Institute of Health and Welfare, 129
authentication
    biometric, 281
    of health records, 82–83, 247
    two-factor, 281
    user, 280–281
authenticity, 247
authority
    binding, 235
    delegation of, 613–614
    in management, 544, 549, 550
    persuasive, 236
authorization
    compound, 267
    conditioned, 267–268
    defective, 267
    defined, 266
    for disclosure of substance abuse records, 272–273
    general, 272
    for giving orders, 71–72
    preauthorization, 180–181
    unconditioned, 267–268
    use and disclosure of patient information with, 266–268
    use and disclosure of patient information without, 268–269

autocoding, 330
autocratic leadership, 556
automated clinical care plans, 338
automated data collection, 138, 139
automated drug dispensing, 344
automatic recognition technologies, 333–334
autonomy
 in Belmont Report, 770
 and decision-making, 765, 766, 774
 defined, 759
 description of, 759
 in end-of-life care, 773
 in health information management, 760, 763, 765–766, 771
autopsy, reporting, in health record, 74
autopsy rates, 431–432
availability, as recordkeeping principle, 44
avatars, 642
average, 421, 449
average daily census, 424
average length of stay (ALOS), 11–12
 as aggregate data, 122
 calculating, 427
 in post-acute care, 20

## B

background checks, 609
Balanced Budget Act (BBA) (1997), 152, 172, 173
Balanced Budget Refinement Act (1999), 167, 173, 174
balanced matrix organizations, 730, 731
balanced scorecard (BSC), 551, 567, 596
Balanced Scorecard Collaborative, 589
balance sheet, 702, 703, 704
balancing measures, 311–312
barcode medication administration record (BCMAR), 371
bar-coding technology, 333, 343–344
Barnard, Chester, 544, 545
bar plot, 466, 470, 471, 472
basic interoperability, 104
basic research, 486
batch processing, 38
battery, 241
battery consent, 250
Baylor University Hospital, 7
BCMAR system, 343–344
bed capacity, 12
bed count, 426
bed turnover rate, 426–427
Beecher, Henry K., 517–518
behavioral description interview, 608
behavioral health information, as sensitive information, 253–254
behavioral health services
 health records for, 77
 long-term care in, 21–22
behavioral theories, of leadership, 556–557
Belmont Report: Ethical Principles and Guidelines for the Protection of Human Subjects of Research (HHS), 518, 769–770

benchmarks
 for clinical documentation integrity, 214–215
 for comparable performance, 663–664
 defined, 214
 external, 307
 internal, 307
 for quality management, 307
bench trial, 238
beneficence
 in AHIMA Code of Ethics, 763
 in Belmont Report, 770
 and decision-making, 765
 defined, 759
 description of, 759
 and health literacy, 774
Benefits Improvement Act (2000), 174
benefits program, 603, 614–615
benefits realization, for health information systems, 384–385
Benjamin, Regina, 399
bereavement counseling, 78
best-fit line, 475, 482
best of breed, 379
best of fit, 379
beyond a reasonable doubt, 239
bibliographic databases, 491
big data, 38
bill hold period, 187
billing
 consolidated, 172, 173
 double, 769
 system for, 192–194
binding authority, 235
bioethics, 756, 758–760
biomedical advances, in medicine, 9–10
biomedical research, 515–535
 artificial intelligence used in, 516
 comparative data in, 533–535
 conflict of interest in, 520–521
 defined, 516
 design types of, 528–532
 ethical treatment of human subjects in, 517–519, 769–770
 exempt, 521–522
 expedited, 522
 health information management in, 516, 526–533
 health records for, 65
 informed consent in, 523–524
 oversight of, 527–528
 privacy considerations in, 526–527
 protection of human subjects in, 519–524, 769–770
 recordkeeping and retention in, 523
 reporting problems in, 523
 risk assessment in, 532–533
 vulnerable subjects in, 525–526
biometric authentication, 281
biotechnology, 10
birth, in health records, 75
birth defect registries, 129
Bitcoin, 286
Blake, Robert, 557
Blanchard, Kenneth, 557–558

blanket authorization, 768
blended learning, 640
blockchain, 286
blogs, 644
Blue Button, 357
Blue Cross Blue Shield (BCBS), 26, 151
Blue Cross Blue Shield of Texas (BCBSTX), 188
blue ocean strategy, 587
board certification, for specialty physicians, 5
board of directors, 13, 552, 686
bookkeeping, double-entry, 700
boxplot, 474, 475
brainstorming, 674
branches of government, 235
breach
 of confidentiality, 254
 defined, 263
 of duty of care, 240, 243
 of warranty, 243
Breach Notification Rule, 263–264, 282
Breast Imaging Reporting and Data System Atlas (BI-RADS), 109, 111
bring your own device (BYOD), 286
budgets, 710–719
 capital, 715–719
 for clinical documentation integrity, 212–213
 components of, 712–713
 cycle of, 711–712
 defined, 711
 operational, 711–715
 of projects, 737, 743, 744, 747
 types of, 711
building blocks, for project managers, 738–739
buildings, as assets, 695
bundled payments, 162, 163
burden of proof, 241
bureaucracy, 542
business acumen, in PMI talent triangle, 740–741
business associate (BA)
 audit logs of, 278
 contingency plan of, 278–280
 defined, 261
 encryption used by, 282
 federal and state laws on, 274
 malicious software management by, 283
 Omnibus Rule on, 263, 264
 Privacy Rule on, 261–262, 269
 risk analysis and risk management by, 276–277
 Security Rule on, 262
business associate agreements (BAAs), 262
business case, 50
business continuity plan (BCP), 306
business intelligence (BI)
 defined, 47
 management of, 47–48
business office manager, 425
business process, 678, 680, 682
business process redesign (BPR), 678

business process reengineering (BPR), 547, 678–679
business record, 247
business records exception, 249
bylaws
  for health records, 64
  of medical staff, 14

## C

Camp Lejeune Family Member program, 156–157
Canadian Medical Association, 5
cancer
  hospitals for, 12
  prevalence of, 436, 437
  radiation therapy for, 15
  registry for, 124–126
  staging of, 125
Cancer Registries Amendment Act (1992), 124, 125
capital budgets, 715–719
capital projects, 716–719
capitation, 162
cardinality, 130, 131
cardiopulmonary resuscitation (CPR), 250
Care Area Assessment (CAA), 79, 171
care coordination, and quality management, 315
career plan, 646–647
CareQuality, 357
CARES Act (2020), 285
Caring Connections, 69
case-control studies, 530–531
case definition, 124
  for cancer registry, 124
  for diabetes registries, 127
  for immunization registries, 128–129
  for transplant registries, 128
  for trauma registries, 126
case finding, 124
  for cancer registry, 124
  for diabetes registries, 127
  for immunization registries, 128–129
  for transplant registries, 128
  for trauma registries, 126
case law. *See* common law
case management
  defined, 184
  and quality management, 314–315
  role of, 184–185
case mix, 212
case-mix analysis, 434–435
case-mix group (CMG), 173
case-mix group (CMG) relative weight, 174
case-mix index (CMI), 166, 186, 212, 434
case studies, 500
cash, as assets, 694
cash flow, statement of, 702
cash payment plans, 26
catalytic functions, of change agents, 565
categorical imperative, 757–758
categorical items, in research, 503
causal-comparative research, 492, 495–496

causal loop, 561
causation
  actual, 240
  product liability and, 243
  proximate, 240
census, inpatient, 422, 423–425
census reports, 424–425
census surveys, 498
Center for Program Integrity (CPI), 226
Centers for Disease Control and Prevention (CDC)
  and cancer registries, 124, 125
  and immunization registries, 129
  and long COVID registries, 129
  Morbidity and Mortality Weekly Report of, 419
  National Immunization Program of, 129
  statistics used by, 419, 436
Centers for Medicare and Medicaid Services (CMS)
  on accounting, 690
  as administrative agency, 236
  on background checks, 609
  on CDI training, 216
  Center for Program Integrity of, 226
  certifications by, 25
  on charge capture, 188
  on claims editing, 193
  on claims submission, 194
  on compliance programs, 221
  Conditions of Participation by, 69, 297
  Consumer Assessment of Healthcare Providers and Systems of, 400–401
  CPT codes adopted by, 101
  data standardization for, 112, 140–141
  EHR Incentive Programs of, 326, 401
  on health record retention, 88
  and health records, 63–64, 83
  on history and physical forms, 69–70
  on home health agencies, 172, 173
  on hospice care services, 78
  Hospital Compare by, 479
  on hospital-issued notice of noncoverage, 185
  Hospital Value-Based Purchasing Program of, 302, 401
  on ICD-10-CM, 97
  Inpatient Psychiatric Facility Quality Reporting Program of, 479–482
  on inpatient rehabilitation facilities, 173
  on long-term care, 79
  on order signatures, 72
  on organ transplantation, 75
  outpatient prospective payment system of, 169–170
  patient's rights statement and, 68
  peer review of, 23
  on performance measures, 306
  predictive modeling used by, 459
  on quality measures, 314
  QualityNet of, 445
  resource-based relative value scale system of, 168–169
  risk adjustment models of, 164, 460

  on sampling, 445–446
  on seclusion and restraint orders, 72
  Stark Law and, 229
  value-based programs by, 442
  on waste, 222
centralized model, for health information exchange, 351, 352
central purchasing systems, 698
central tendency measures, 449–450
certification
  board, for specialty physicians, 5
  for cancer registrars, 125–126
  for case managers, 184
  for clinical documentation integrity specialists, 209, 210
  defined, 25
  of electronic health records, 378
  for Medicare, 25
  precertification, 180–181
  for project management, 724
  for quality management, 316–317
  for risk management, 316
  for trauma registrars, 126–127
certification in health care quality and management (HCQM), 316
Certified Associate Project Management (CAPM), 724
certified nursing assistants (CNAs), 14
certified professional in healthcare quality (CPHQ), 316
certified professional in healthcare risk management (CPHRM), 316
champions, of innovations, 564
change
  benefits of, 748–749
  and communication, 593–594
  creating structure for, 592
  implementing, 594–596
  leadership and, 592–593, 595
  managing politics of, 592–593
  negotiating, 749
  sense of urgency and, 593
  strategic, 594–596
  systems approach to, 592
  to training model, 627
  types of, 748
  with vision, 584–585
change agent, 564, 565–566
change control, 393
change drivers, 542
change management, 564–570
  agents of, 564, 565–566
  cultural change and, 569
  defined, 304
  facilitation in, 567–569
  process of, 749–750
  and project management, 748–750
  and quality management, 304–305
  resistance in, 566–567
  response to, 569–570
  stages in, 568–569
change plans, 595
change program, 592–594
character, defamation of, 241–242
character recognition technologies, 333–334

charge capture, 186–188
charge code, 189
charge code description, 189
charge description master (CDM), 188–191, 461
charitable immunity, 243
charity care, 182
chart(s)
    control, 677–678
    for data visualization, 466, 468–471
    defined, 466
    flowchart, 661, 680, 681
    Gantt, 543, 544, 744, 746
    interpreting, 467
    line, 466
    organizational, 549, 550
    Pareto, 676
    pie, 467, 470, 471, 472
    purpose of, 466
    run, 677
    spatial representation in, 468
    work distribution, 656–657
chart conversion, 382
ChatGPT, 32
check sheet, 676
check step, in Deming Wheel, 308, 309
chief executive officer (CEO), 13, 552, 686
chief financial officer (CFO), 13, 372, 418, 552, 686
chief information officer (CIO), 13, 372–373, 552, 686
chief medical informatics officer (CMIO), 372
chief medical officer (CMO), 372, 552
chief nursing officer (CNO), 372, 552
chief operating officer (COO), 372, 552, 728
chief technology officer (CTO), 373
children, as vulnerable subjects in research, 525
Children of Women Vietnam Veterans Health Care Benefits Program, 157
Children's Health Insurance Program (CHIP), 155–156
Cigna, 775
cipher text, 282
circuit, 237
circuit courts, 237
Civilian Health and Medical Program of the Department of Veterans Affairs (CHAMPVA), 27, 156
civil law, 236–237
civil legal actions, 239–244
civil litigation, 237–239
Civil Monetary Penalties Law, 222, 223
civil monetary penalty (CMP), 264–265
Civil Rights Act (1964), 602, 647
Civil Rights Act (1991), 602, 647
claim(s)
    adjudication of, 194
    in civil litigation, 238
    clean, 194
    defined, 150
    editing, 193–194
    identifying fraudulent, 459
    preparation of, 192–193
    to private health insurance, 151
    submission of, 194
claims scrubber software, 193
classification systems
    code sets for, 96–103
    and data standardization, 112–115
    development of, 94–96
    management of, 49
    terminologies and, 104–111
classroom learning, 640–641, 643
clean claims, 194
clear trend (CT), 582–583
clinical, defined, 206
Clinical and Laboratory Standards Institute (CLSI), 113
Clinical Care Classification (CCC), 107
clinical classification, 94, 95
clinical coding, 185–186
clinical data
    defined, 389
    in health records, 69–75
clinical data analysts, 373
Clinical Data Interchange Standards Consortium (CDISC), 113
clinical data repository (CDR), 342, 345–346
clinical decision support (CDS) systems, 344–345, 494
clinical departmental systems, 342
Clinical Document Architecture (CDA), 112, 349, 361, 406
clinical documentation, 184
    assessing, 185–186
    for coded data, 207
    communication in, 184, 206
    ethical issues of, 768
    financial data in, 692
    importance of, 206
    and interoperability, 349
    quality management of, 308–309
    retrospective, 768
    specificity in, 211–212
clinical documentation integrity (CDI), 205–220
    alignment of, 209
    artificial intelligence and, 115, 184, 220
    benchmarks for, 214–215
    budget for, 212–213
    defined, 206
    ethical standards of, 209–210, 212
    goals of, 207–208
    operational considerations in, 208–215
    performance measures for improving, 214
    physician champions and, 209, 211, 213, 216
    physicians and, 208–209, 210–211, 213, 215–216
    query for, 210, 215–218
    record review in, 211–212
    scope of practice for, 213
    staff for, 208–210
    staff training for, 213
    stakeholders in, 207–208, 213
    technology considerations in, 218–220
Clinical Laboratory Improvement Amendments (CLIA), 300
Clinical LOINC, 106–107
clinical pathology, 15
clinical pathways, 314, 315, 338
clinical plagiarism, 247
clinical privileges, 14, 310
clinical quality management. *See* quality management
clinical research, 515–535
    artificial intelligence used in, 516
    comparative data in, 533–535
    conflict of interest in, 520–521
    defined, 516
    design types of, 528–532
    ethical treatment of human subjects in, 517–519, 769–770
    exempt, 521–522
    expedited, 522
    health information management in, 516, 526–533
    health records for, 65
    informed consent in, 523–524
    oversight of, 527–528
    privacy considerations in, 526–527
    protection of human subjects in, 519–524, 769–770
    recordkeeping and retention in, 523
    reporting problems in, 523
    risk assessment in, 532–533
    vulnerable subjects in, 525–526
clinical risks, 305
clinical supplies, 712–713
clinical support services, in hospitals, 16
clinical terminology, 95
clinical transformation, 388
clinical trials, 516, 528–529
clinical trials databases, 137
clinical vocabulary, 95
Clinician and Group Consumer Assessment of Healthcare Providers and Systems (CC-CAHPS), 401
clinician web portals, 335
closed adoptions, 254
closed-ended queries, 217, 219
closed-record review, 82
closed records, 82
closed system, 670
closing phase, in project management, 747–748
cloud-based technologies, 334–336
cloud computing, 48, 335
Cloudficient, 57
cluster sampling, 445
CMS-1450 (format), 193
CMS-1500 (format), 193
coaching, 632, 641
code of ethics, 754, 761–763
Code of Ethics (AHIMA), 624, 758, 760–764, 766, 767
Code of Federal Regulations (CFR), 236, 518, 519
coding
    in content analysis, 506
    ethical, 761, 769

coding compliance, 222–228
coding optimization, 225
coding systems. *See* classification systems
Codman, Ernest, 5
coefficient of determination, 455
coercive power, 550
cognitive complexity, 552
cohort studies, 531–532
collaboration, 593
Collaborative Institutional Training Institute (CITI), 521
collections, 194–195
co-located teams, 734
colors, at work, 654
command, unity of, 544, 549
commercial health insurance, 26, 150–151, 161
Commission for Case Manager Certification (CCMC), 184
Commission on Accreditation for Health Informatics and Information Management Education, 6
Commission on Accreditation of Rehabilitation Facilities (CARF), 6, 300
Common Agreement, 357
common cause variation, 671
Common Data Model (PCORnet), 133–134
common law, 235–236
Common Rule, 518
communication
 in case management, 185
 in change process, 593–594
 charge description master and, 191
 clinical documentation and, 184, 206
 content analysis of, 506
 in emergency mode operation plan, 279
 false, 241–242
 of health information, 403
 health records for, 65, 206
 HIPAA on, 76
 by HR, 611
 passive participant observation of, 500
 patient access team and, 180, 183
 in project management, 378
 project managers and, 728, 737, 747
 in query process, 215–218
 of standards, 663
communication disorders, 15
*Communication of Innovations* (Rogers and Shoemaker), 562
communication sciences, 15
community-based disease tracking, 436–437
community health centers, 22
comorbidities and complications (CCs), 165, 212
comorbidity, 165
comparative data, 533–535
comparative effectiveness research (CER), 494, 516, 534
comparative negligence, 243

compensable factor, 615
compensation surveys, 615
compensation systems, 603, 614–615
competition, determining impact of, 587
complaint, in civil litigation, 237, 238
complex adaptive systems, 560
complexity leadership, 560–561
compliance
 audits and reviews of, 223, 224
 coding, 222–228
 corporate, 221–229
 defined, 222
 developing plan for, 225–226
 institutional assurance of, 519–520
 legislation on, 222–223, 228–229
 with quality management, 317
 as recordkeeping principle, 44
 training for, 227–228
compliance projects, 723
complication, 165
complications and comorbidities (CCs), 165, 212
compound authorization, 267
compressed workweek, 658
compromise, in conflict management, 618
computer-assisted coding (CAC), 186, 219, 227, 330, 589
computer-based training (CBT), 628, 632, 642
computerized provider order entry (CPOE) system, 343, 371, 500
computer vision technology, 603
concepts, in SNOMED CT, 105
conceptual database design, 130, 131
conceptual skills, 552, 553
concurrent analysis (review), 82, 207, 208, 212, 218
conditioned authorization, 267–268
Conditions of Participation (CoP)
 healthcare organizations subject to, 297–298
 on health record management, 83–84
 on history and physical forms, 69
confidence interval, 444, 451–452
confidentiality
 Breach Notification Rule on, 264
 breach of, 254
 data security and, 139
 defined, 260, 761
 ethics of, 758, 761
 privilege and, 252
 of quality improvement activities, 255–256
 of reproductive health information, 270
 Security Rule on, 262
 social media and, 775
 of substance abuse patient records, 253–254
 utility and, 758
Confidentiality of Substance Use Disorder Patient Records, 253, 271–273
conflict management, 618–619
conflict of interest, in research, 520–521

confounding variables, 494
congestive heart failure (CHF), 446, 457–458
consent, 250
 as defense to tort, 243
 emergency, 250
 express, 250
 general, 250
 in health records, 68
 implied, 250
 informed, 250, 523–524
 voluntary, in research, 517
conservatism, 688, 689
consideration, 244
consistency, in accounting, 688, 689
consolidated billing, 172, 173
Consolidated Omnibus Budget Reconciliation Act (COBRA) (1985), 158, 229
constant comparative method, 506
constitutional law, 235
constructive confrontation, in conflict management, 618–619
construct validity, 502
consultants, 733–734
consultations, 73
Consumer and Patient Health Information Section (CAPHIS), 404
Consumer Assessment of Healthcare Providers and Systems (CAHPS), 400–401
consumer-directed healthcare, 29
consumer engagement. *See* patient engagement
consumer health informatics, 397–411
 defined, 399
 examples of, 397
 focus of, 397, 403
 future of, 411
 internet forums for, 404–405
 model of, 400
 patient activation measure for, 405
 and patient engagement, 399–401
 patient-generated health data in, 409–410
 patient portals for, 406
 personal health records for, 406–408
 precision medicine and, 410–411
 social determinants of health and, 402–403
 strategic plan for, 398
 telehealth for, 408–409
 websites for, 404
consumer-mediated exchange, 356–357
content analysis, 506
content management, 47, 331, 335, 336
content theory of motivation, 550
content validity, 502
contingency plan, 278–280, 305–306, 587
contingency theories, of leadership, 557–559
continuing education (CE), 624, 645–646
Continuity of Care Document (CCD), 112, 349
continuity of care record (CCR), 112, 406
continuous data, 443, 449–452

continuous quality improvement (CQI), 671–678
  defined, 671
  development of, 24
  leadership and, 671
  methods of, 672–674
  purpose of, 671
  tools for, 674–678
continuous speech input, 329–330
continuous variables, 449
continuum of care, 21, 22
contract(s)
  adhesion, 244
  defined, 244
  in health information exchange, 359
  laws on, 244
  negotiation of, for health information systems, 381–382
  for services, 660
contract management, 197–198
contractors, 734
contrary state laws, 274
contributory negligence, 243
control(s)
  in conflict management, 618
  corrective, 709
  detective, 709
  feedback, 666
  financial data for, 693
  internal, in accounting, 709
  performance, 665–666
  preventive, 666, 709
  in process improvement, 670
  in project management, 747
  span of, 549–550
  visual, 673
control chart, 677–678
control group, 495
controller, 686
controlling, by management, 551
controls, of data governance, 53
conversion factor (CF), 168
conviction, 236, 239
copayments, 19, 22, 152, 153–154
copy and paste, in EHRs, 66, 247, 249
*Core Competencies for Interprofessional Collaborative Practice* (IPEC), 6
Coronavirus Aid, Relief, and Economic Security (CARES) Act (2020), 285
corporate compliance, 221–229
corporate governance, 39
corporate integrity agreements (CIAs), 226
corporate negligence, 254
corporation, 690, 691
corrective action, 392–393
corrective action plan (CAP), 264, 265
corrective controls, 709
correlation, 455
correlational research, 492, 493
correlation coefficient, 455, 456
correlation matrix, 480
cost(s)
  defined, 688, 689
  direct, 706
  fixed, 707
  indirect, 706–707
  of projects, 737, 743, 744, 747
  semifixed, 707
  variable, 707
cost accounting, 706–707
cost allocation, 708–709
cost–benefit analysis, 715, 717
cost justification, 717
cost outlier, 166, 167, 170, 173, 174
cost reports, 707–709
counterclaim, 238
county public health databases, 135–136
court decisions, 235–236
courts of appeal, 237
court system, 237
covered entity (CE)
  audit logs of, 278
  contingency plan of, 278–280
  defined, 261
  encryption used by, 282
  federal and state laws on, 274
  malicious software management by, 283
  Omnibus Rule on, 263, 264
  Privacy Rule on, 261–262
  risk analysis and risk management by, 276–277
  Security Rule on, 262
  training by, 287, 289
  use and disclosure policies of, 266–270
cover letter, 608
COVID-19 pandemic
  and average length of stay in hospitals, 12
  clinical and biomedical research during, 516
  clinical trials during, 529
  human resources challenges during, 601
  leadership during, 555
  and long COVID registries, 129
  telehealth during, 163, 318, 339, 408
credentialing, 198, 310
credits, 700, 701
crime(s)
  defined, 236
  types of, 236–237
criminal law, 236–237
criminal negligence, 240
criminal proceedings, 239
critical access hospitals (CAHs), 167, 169
criticality analysis, 280
critical pathways. *See* clinical pathways
critics, of innovations, 564
crossclaim, 238
cross-footing financial reports, 709, 710
cross-functional data steward teams, 55
*Crossing the Quality Chasm: A New Health System for the 21st Century* (IOM), 299
cross-sectional studies, 530
cross-training, 632
cryptocurrency, 286
cryptographic key, 282
cultural awareness, 620
cultural change, leadership and, 569
cultural diversity, 771
cultural humility, 770–771
culturally and linguistically appropriate services (CLAS), 774
culture
  characteristics of, 770
  organizational, 304
Cures Act. *See* 21st Century Cures Act (2016)
Current Dental Terminology (CDT), 103
Current Procedural Terminology (CPT), 101–102
  charge capture and, 186, 188
  in charge description master, 189, 190
current ratio, 702–703
curriculum design, 626
customer data platform, 38
customer service, 199, 669
customer's role, in strategic planning, 588
cyberattacks, 252, 261, 275, 278, 283–284
cybernetic systems, 670
cybersecurity, 263, 275, 283–284, 286
cyclical staffing, 658

# D

daily census report, 425
daily inpatient census, 423
damages
  in civil litigation, 238
  punitive, 242
*Darling v. Charleston Community Memorial Hospital*, 243, 297
dashboard, 477–478
data
  aggregate, 122
  big, 38
  comparative, 533–535
  continuous, 443, 449–452
  discrete, 443
  financial, 389, 686, 692–693
  in hierarchy of data to wisdom, 41, 307–308
  information, knowledge, and wisdom (DIKW) hierarchy, 41, 307–308
  *vs.* information, 40, 43
  interval, 443
  loss of, 139
  master (*see* master data)
  in motion, 281
  nominal, 443
  ordinal, 443
  ownership of, 139–140
  patient-identifiable, 122, 123
  ratio, 443
  reference, 46–47
  at rest, 281
  structured, 47, 48, 329
  technologies supporting access to and flow of, 333–336
  technologies supporting capture of, 329–331
  unstructured, 47, 48, 329, 330
Data Administration Management Association (DAMA), 45–46
data administrators, 373

data analysis, in research, 506
data analytics. *See also* healthcare data analytics
  defined, 441
  maturity models of, 387–388
  predictive, 48
  for quality management, 317
data architecture, 46
data backup plan, 278–279
database(s)
  bibliographic, 491
  centralized, 351
  for electronic health records, 133, 345–346
  for healthcare, 134–138
  implementation of, 132–133
  management and design of, 130–134
  relational, 130
  secondary, processing and maintenance of, 138–140
  security and confidentiality issues with, 139
database administrators, 373
database management system (DBMS), 130, 132, 133, 142
data capture, 38, 329–331
data cleaning, 505
data collection
  automated, 138, 139
  for cancer registry, 124–125
  for diabetes registries, 127
  for immunization registries, 129
  instrument selection for, 502–503
  knowledge generated from, 307–308
  manual, 138
  methods of, 497–501
  procedures of, 503–505
  for quality reviews, 307
  reliability of, 502
  for research, 497–505
  security concerns about, 139
  for transplant registries, 128
  for trauma registries, 126
  trends in, 139–140
  validity of, 501–502
data complexity, 466, 477–478
data conversion, 382
data definition stewards, 55
data dictionaries
  defined, 38, 142
  development of, 143
  and interoperability, 38
  types of, 142
data exchange standards, 347
data formats, 329
data governance (DG)
  accountability in, 53, 55
  background of, 42
  components of, 52
  controls for, 53
  decision rights for, 53
  defined, 38, 40, 42
  domains of, 42, 45–49
  frameworks for, 42, 51–55
  in health information exchange, 360
  information governance compared to, 40–42
  key terms used in, 38–39
  mission statement of, 53
  participants in, 54–55
  policies of, 53–54
  processes of, 54
  program planning for, 49–51
  purpose of, 42
  rules of engagement of, 53
  steering committee for, 54
data governance office, 54–55
data interoperability, 38–39
data lake, 38
data life cycle, 45–46
data literacy, 467
data management, 121–143
data management domains, 42, 45–49
data mining, 458–461, 496
data modeling, 130, 133–134, 390
data privacy, 139
data production stewards, 55
data provenance, 368
data quality, 140–143
  assessment of, 41, 48
  data standardization for, 140–141
  discovery process for, 392
  management of, 48–49, 391–393
  of master data, 47, 55
  measurement of, 391
  requirements for, 142
data repository, 342, 345–346
data security
  defined, 47, 280, 761
  ethics of, 761
  framework for, 57
  management of, 47
  methods of, 280–284
  of registries, 139
data sources
  for health statistics, 419
  primary, 122, 419
  secondary, 122, 419
data stakeholders, 55
data standardization, 112–115, 140–141
data stewards, 55. *See also* stewardship
data type mismatch, 132
data usage stewards, 55
Data Use and Reciprocal Support Agreement (DURSA), 359
data visualization, 465–482
  charts for, 466, 468–471
  context of situation and, 469–470
  data complexity in, 477–478
  and decision-making, 467, 468
  defined, 466
  graphical perception in, 466–467
  presentation methods for, 470–476
  for quality reporting, 479–482
  tables for, 466, 468–471
  user experience of, 470
data warehouses, 133–134, 346
day health centers, 21
day hospitals, 22
days in accounts receivable ratio, 704–705
"day surgery." *See* ambulatory surgery
day treatment programs, 22
death, recording, in health records, 74, 75, 76
death rates, 429–431, 478
debits, 700, 701
debt, in accounting, 696
debt ratio, 705
debt resolution, 182
debt service, 702–705
decentralized model, for health information exchange, 351–352, 353
decisional activities, 553, 554
decision analysis, 587
decision-making
  autocratic-democratic continuum and, 556
  autonomy and, 759
  data visualization and, 467, 468
  ethical, 763–766
  health records for, 65
  paternalism and, 759
  strategic thinking and, 577
decision matrix, 757
decision rights, for data governance, 53
decision support, 391
decision trees, 459
Declaration of Helsinki, 517–518
decryption, 281–283
deductive reasoning, 487, 500
deemed status, 25, 246
defamation of character, 241–242
default-in states, 355
default judgment, 238
default-out states, 355
defendant, 237, 238, 239
Defense, Department of. *See* Department of Defense (DoD)
defenses to torts, 243
deferred future earnings (DFE), 758
Deficit Reduction Act (DRA) (2005), 166, 222, 223
define, measure, analyze, improve, and control (DMAIC), 673–674
degrees of freedom, 451–452
deidentification, 269
delegation
  defined, 613
  and employee empowerment, 613–614
  rules of, 613
delinquent health records, 83
Deming, W. Edwards, 546, 568
Deming's principles, 546
Deming Wheel, 308–309
democratic leadership, 556
demographic information, in health record, 68
denial(s)
  artificial intelligence used in, 775
  defined, 195
  management of, 195–196
dental terminology, 103
deontology
  in AHIMA Code of Ethics, 763, 766
  and decision-making, 765, 766

description of, 757–758
in health information management, 758, 760, 772
Department of Defense (DoD), 108, 156, 246
Department of Education, 639
Department of Health and Human Services (HHS)
   Belmont Report by, 518
   on clinical and biomedical research oversight, 527–528
   on cybersecurity, 275
   on human subjects in research, 518, 519–520
   on ICD-10-CM, 97
   Office of Minority Health of, 774
   Office of the Inspector General and, 221, 224–225
   and Omnibus Rule, 263
   on privacy, 246
   public health services by, 19
   responsibilities of, 9
   risk adjustment models of, 164
   and SNOMED CT, 105
   strategic plan of, 9
Department of Labor, 11, 157, 601–602, 620
Department of Veterans Affairs (VA)
   healthcare services provided by, 27, 156–157
   interviews by, 499
   licensure and, 25
   patient portal of, 406, 407
   and privacy rights, 246
   and SNOMED CT, 106
dependency, in health information systems, 375
dependent variables, 456, 495
depositions, 238
depreciation, 695–696, 715–716
descriptive metadata, 390
descriptive research, 492, 493
descriptive statistics, 419–421, 444–449, 453
design, research, 492–497, 528–532
designated record, 266
designated record set (DRS), 247
Designated Standard Maintenance Organization (DSMO), 113
destruction, of health records, 88–90
detective controls, 709
development, 623–648
   artificial intelligence in, 644–645
   defined, 624
   in-service education for, 633–636
   planning for, 625–627
   positioning employees for, 645–648
   special considerations for, 638–639
diabetes registries, 127
diagnosis index, 122, 123
diagnosis-related groups (DRGs), 164, 165–166, 187, 435
*Diagnostic and Statistical Manual of Mental Disorders (DSM)*, 95
*Diagnostic and Statistical Manual of Mental Disorders, Fifth Edition (DSM-5)*, 102
diagnostic and therapeutic orders, 70–72
diagnostic services
   in hospitals, 14–17
   for outpatients, 18
dietitian/dietary department, 425
Diffusion of Innovation Theory, 562–563
digital signature, 82–83, 247
digital surveys, 498
direct allocation, 708
direct costs, 706
directed exchange, 356
direct maternal death, 431
disabilities, and development, 639
Disability Assessment Schedule, 102
disaster plan. *See* contingency plan
disaster recovery plan, 279, 306
discharge
   continuing medication use after, 481–482
   defined, 422
   against medical advice, 241
discharge analysis, 81–82
discharged, not final billed (DNFB), 186, 460–461, 701
discharge data, 123, 135, 137
discharge orders, 72
discharge plans, 76
discharge summary, 75–76
disciplinary action, 617–618, 767
discipline
   defined, 542
   management as, 542–548
disclosure(s)
   in accounting, 688, 689
   accounting of, 268
   with authorization, 266–268
   defined, 266
   least harm concept and, 759
   objection to, 269–270
   patient identity management for, 270
   privacy and security and, 266–273
   of protected health information, 261–262, 266–273
   for reproductive health care, 270
   of substance abuse patient records, 253–254
   without authorization, 268–269
   wrongful, 254
discounts/discounting
   applying, 194
   on hospital bills, 182
   surgical procedures, 170
discovery
   in civil litigation, 238
   e-discovery, 251–252, 346
discovery process for data quality, 392
discrete data, 443
discrimination, 602, 647
disease index, 123
disposition
   of health records, 88
   as recordkeeping principle, 44
disproportionate share hospital (DSH), 166
distributed teams, 734
distribution department, 698
distributive justice, 759
district attorney, 239
district court, 237
diversity
   cultural, 771
   and development, 639
   ethical issues in, 770–771
diversity jurisdiction, 237
diversity training, 620, 624, 639
DMAIC methodology, 673–674
DNV, 300
*Dobbs v. Jackson Women's Health Organization*, 270
Doctor's Management Services (DMS), 283
documentation. *See* clinical documentation
doers (learning style), 638
domain coordinators, 55
domain stewards, 55
do-not-resuscitate (DNR) order, 72, 250
do step, in Deming Wheel, 308, 309
dot plot, 471, 481, 482
double billing, 769
double-blind studies, 528
double distribution, 708
double-entry bookkeeping, 700
Drucker, Peter, 546, 560
drugs (prescription)
   applications for managing, 343–344
   charge capture and, 187
   codes for, 103
   continuing use of, after discharge, 481–482
   standardized nomenclature for, 107–108
   variability of, 349
due diligence, 381
duplicates, in master patient index, 86
durable medical equipment (DME), 153
durable power of attorney for healthcare decisions, 69, 250
duty of care, 240, 243
dyadic relationship theory, 558–559

# E

early adopters, of innovations, 563
early majority, of innovations, 563
economically disadvantaged subjects, in research, 525
economic compensatory damages, 238
e-discovery, 251–252, 346
education. *See also* training
   of adult learners, 637–638
   for cancer registrars, 125–126
   for coding compliance, 227–228
   continuing, 624, 645–646
   in-service, 633–636
   interprofessional, 6, 304
   for trauma registrars, 126–127

Education, Department of. *See* Department of Education
educationally disadvantaged subjects, in research, 525
efficiency
  functional work environment and, 652–655
  in management, 542–543
eHealth Exchange, 356
85/15 rule, 546
e-learning, 642–643
electronic claims preparation, 193
electronic clinical quality measures (eCQM), 419
Electronic Discovery Reference Model (EDRM), 251
electronic document/content management (ED/CM) system, 331
electronic document management (EDM) systems, 331
electronic health information (EHI)
  defined, 247
  e-discovery of, 251–252, 346
electronic health records (EHRs), 62, 339–340
  access to, 66
  accuracy of, 62
  advantages of, 62
  amendments to, 82
  applications for, 342–348
  artificial intelligence systems and, 115
  audit log of, 278
  authentication of, 82–83, 247
  certification of, 378
  charge capture and, 187
  complexity of, 340
  content of, 339
  copy and paste in, 66, 247, 249
  correction of, 82
  databases for, 133, 345–346
  data standardization for, 112
  data warehouses for, 133–134
  defined, 62, 340
  destruction and transfer of, 88–90
  disclosures made from, 269
  e-discovery of, 251–252, 346
  effectiveness of, 62
  ethical issues related to, 771–773
  as evidence, 249–250
  functions of, 339, 366
  gaps in, 378–379
  HIPAA on, 261
  incentives to adopt, 326, 366, 401
  initial implementation of, 543, 544
  integrity of, 247
  interoperability and, 104, 340
  maturity models of, 387–388
  MEDCIN and, 108
  on outdated media, 90
  ownership of, 248
  personal health record and, 408
  in quality management, 315
  record completion process for, 82
  release of, 76
  retention of, 88
  retrieval of, 87–88
  source systems for, 341–342
  storage of, 87, 89, 346
  supporting infrastructure for, 345–348
  technologies of, 341–348
  terms of, 339–340
  transcription to, 80
  transitioning from paper to, 66–67, 81, 84
electronic medical record (EMR), 339, 340. *See also* electronic health records (EHRs)
electronic medication administration record (EMAR), 343–344
electronic protected health information (ePHI)
  data backup of, 278
  encryption and decryption of, 281–283
  HIPAA Privacy Rule on, 261, 262
  HIPAA Security Rule on, 250, 261, 262–263
  legal issues concerning exchange of, 355
  mobile health technology and, 286
  21st Century Cures Act on, 247, 273–274
electronic remittance advice (ERA), 196
electronic signature, 82–83, 247
electronic surveys, 498
emergency access, 280
emergency care/services
  census report used by, 425
  determining typical waiting time for, 444–445, 450–451
  health records for, 76–77
  in hospitals, 18
  legislation on, 229, 253
  patient registration during, 180
  point-of-service collection for, 182–183
emergency consent, 250
emergency department prevention quality indicators, 312, 313
Emergency Medical Treatment and Active Labor Act (EMTALA) (1986), 229, 253, 300
emergency mode operation plan, 279–280
emergency preparedness process. *See* contingency plan
emotional distress, infliction of, 242
emotional intelligence (EI), 552–553
employee(s). *See also* development; human resources management; medical staff; nurse(s); orientation of employees; physician(s); training; work
  background checks of, 609
  benefits of, 712
  compensation and benefits program for, 603, 614–615
  conflict management and, 618–619
  demographic trends of, 619–620
  disciplinary action against, 617–618
  empowerment of (*see* employee empowerment)
  equal opportunities of, 601–602
  exempt, 614
  financial personnel, 686
  float, 658
  grievance management and, 619
  health and safety program for, 603
  hiring, 609–610
  job evaluations of, 614
  and labor relations, 603–604, 605
  maintaining records of, 619
  nonexempt, 614
  nonphysician, 687
  performance counseling for, 617–618
  performance review of, 615–617
  promotion of, 607
  recruitment of, 607–610
  reference checks of, 609
  retention of, 610–611
  rights of, 602–603
  selection of, 608–609
  self-logging by, 664
  termination of, 618
employee empowerment
  defined, 611
  delegation and, 613–614
  by HR, 611–614
  management and, 544–545
  team building and, 612–613
employee handbook, 628
employer(s), rights of, 602–603
employer-based self-insurance, 7, 26, 151
employment-at-will, 602–603
empowerment. *See* employee empowerment
encounter, 434
encryption, 281–283, 406
end-of-life care
  ethical issues of, 765, 773
  Joint Commission on Accreditation of Hospitals on, 72
End-Stage Renal Disease Quality Incentive Program (ESRD QIP), 442
end users, 378
Enforcement Rule, of HIPAA, 264–265
English as second language, 639
enhanced security controls, 348
enterprise governance, 39, 57
enterprise master patient index (EMPI), 86, 334, 500
entity, 130, 688
entity relationship diagram (ERD), 130–132
entity relationship modeling, 130–132
environmental assessment, in strategic planning, 579–583, 586, 595–596
Environmental Protection Agency (EPA), 109, 110
environmental scan, 374
epidemiological studies, 529–530
epidemiology statistics, 436

Index  **897**

episode-of-care (EOC) reimbursement, 162–163, 166
e-prescribing, 343
equal employment opportunity (EEO), 601–602
Equal Employment Opportunity (EEO) Act (1972), 602
Equal Employment Opportunity Commission (EEOC), 602
Equal Pay Act (EPA) (1963), 603, 614
equipment
   as assets, 695–696
   and workspace design, 654
equity, 696–697, 770–771
ergonomics, 654–655
error
   and ethical lapse, 755
   liability without, 242
   standard, 451, 453
error rate, 662
E-Rx, 343
esprit de corps, 544
ethical lapse, 755, 767
ethics, 753–776
   of artificial intelligence use, 775–776
   breach of, 766–767
   in change process, 594
   in clinical documentation integrity, 209–210, 212
   code of, 754, 761–763
   of coding, 761, 769
   coding compliance and, 222, 227
   of confidentiality, 758, 761
   of data security, 761
   in decision-making, 763–766
   defined, 756
   of diversity, equity, and inclusion, 770–771
   of documentation, 768
   of electronic health records, 771–773
   of end-of-life care, 765, 773
   in health information management, 753–776
   of health literacy, 774
   in leadership, 559–560
   morality and, 754–755
   of privacy, 761, 768
   of public health information, 769
   of release of information, 768–769
   of research, 517–519, 769–770
   of sensitive health information, 769
   of social disparities, 773–774
   of social media use, 774–775
   theories, principles, and concepts of, 756–760
   Tuskegee Syphilis Study and, 518–519
   values and, 763, 770–771
ethics committee, 766–767
ethnic groups, in workforce, 620
ethnography, 500–501
European Committee for Standardization (CEN), 113
evaluation
   job, 615
   by management, 551
   of orientation program, 631

outcome, 494
process, 493–494
summative, 494
360-degree, 617
of training model, 626–627
evaluation research, 492, 493–494, 500
events
   adverse, 305
   sentinel, 305
evidence
   in civil litigation, 238
   health records as, 249–253
evidence-based clinical practice guideline, 314, 315
evidence-based management, 554
evidence-based practice, 313–314
excellence
   areas of, 585
   progression of, 756–757
   search for, 547–548
exchange relationship, 558
Exclusion Provisions, 223
exclusive provider organizations (EPOs), 160
execution phase, in project management, 747
executive dashboard, 551
executive data governance council, 54
executive managers, 551, 552
executive role, 544
exempt employees, 614
exempt research, 521–522
exit interviews, 611
expanded Likert scale, 504
expectancy theory, of motivation, 558
expected mortality rate, 460
expedited research, 522
expense projects, 723
expenses
   in accounting, 689, 697–699
   in budgets, 712–713
experimental (study) group, 495
experimental research, 492, 494–495
experimental studies, 529–530
expert determination method, 269
expert power, 550
explanation of benefits (EOB), 194
explanation of payment (EOP), 194
explicit knowledge, 307
exploratory research, 492
*ex post facto*, 495
express consent, 250
express warranty, 243
external assessment, in strategic planning, 582
external audit, 225, 227
external benchmarking, 307
external change agents, 565–566
external customers, 669
external environment, in process improvement, 670
external medical identity theft, 255
external stakeholders, 55
external validity, 501
extract, transform, and load (ETL) process, 38

extranets, 335
extrapolation method, 224

## F

facility-based registry, 124, 125, 126, 127
facility-specific systems, 138
factor comparison method, of job evaluation, 615
Fair Information Practice Principles (FIPPs), 350, 351
Fair Labor Standards Act (FLSA) (1938), 603, 614, 658
False Claims Act (1863), 222–223
false imprisonment, 241
Family Medical Leave Act (FMLA) (1993), 602
Fast Healthcare Interoperability Resources (FHIR), 107, 114, 349–350, 379–380, 406
favorable variances, 713, 714–715
Fayol, Henri, 543–544
Fayol's principles, 544
federal administrative agencies, 236
federal court decisions, 235
federal court system, 237
Federal Drug Administration (FDA), usability testing by, 348
federal health insurance, 26–27, 152–157
Federal Health IT Strategic Plan, 326, 327, 398
federal question jurisdiction, 237
*Federal Register*, 236
Federal Rules of Civil Procedure (FRCP), 251
Federal Rules of Evidence (FRE), 247, 249
Federal Trade Commission (FTC), 228, 255
federal workers' compensation funds, 157
federated model, for health information exchange, 351–352, 353
feedback
   on in-service education, 635
   leadership and, 561
   in management, 551
   in process improvement, 670
   on training, 627
feedback controls, 666
fee-for-service (FFS) reimbursement, 150, 153–154, 161–162
feelers (learning style), 638
felony, 237, 239
fetal autopsy rate, 432
fetal death rate, 430–431
fetal monitoring strips, 88
fetuses, as vulnerable subjects in research, 525
fiduciary duty, 254
filing equipment, for health records, 87
filing systems, for health records, 85
Final Rule, of Cures Act, 273–274
Financial Accounting Standards Board (FASB), 689–690
financial counselors, 182
financial data, 389, 686, 692–693

financial management, 685–719. See also accounting
  budgets in, 710–719
  health information management and, 686, 693, 697, 708, 711–713, 715
  internal controls for, 709
  personnel in, 686
  roles in, 686
financial risks, 305
financial systems, 341
financial transaction
  defined, 686
  example of, 701
  recording, 699–701
  sources of, 692–693
  statements of, 701–702
  steps in, 692
  tracking, 700–701
fingerprint scanning, 281
fiscal period, 711
fiscal year, 689
fishbone diagram, 675
501(c)(3), 692
501(c)(6), 691–692
five-point scale, 503, 504
five S's, 673
fixed budgets, 711
fixed costs, 707
flexible budgets, 711
flexible spending account (FSA), 151
Flexner, Abraham, 5
Flexner Report, 5
flextime, 658
float employees, 658
flowcharts, 661, 680, 681
flow sheets, for medication administration records, 73
focus groups, 499
Follett, Mary Parker, 545, 548
follow-up. See patient follow-up
Food and Drug Administration (FDA)
  on clinical trials, 528, 529
  and clinical trials databases, 137
  Device Classification Panels, 108, 110
  on human subjects in research, 519
  NDCs of, 103, 107
  on precision medicine, 410
Food and Drug Administration Modernization Act (1997), 137
footing financial reports, 709, 710
force-field analysis, 567, 676
forecasting, financial data for, 693
foreign keys, 132
foreword, of procedure manuals, 661
formats, procedure, 660–661
for-profit healthcare organizations, 12
for-profit organizations, 691
Foundation Component, of IDC-11, 98
*The Four Principles of Biomedical Ethics*, 758–760
frameworks
  for data governance, 42, 51–55
  for data quality, 141
  for data security, 57

defined, 39
for information governance, 43–44, 56–57
for justice, 759
Nationwide Privacy and Security Framework, 351
for process groups, 741, 742
Project Manager Competency Development, 738, 739
Framingham Study, 531
Franklin, Benjamin, 4
fraud. See also identity theft
  auditing, 223, 224, 227
  corporate compliance and, 221–229
  defined, 222, 242
  and exclusion from federal programs, 223
  legislation on, 222–223, 228–229
  proving, 242
  surveillance of, 226, 227
freedom, degrees of, 451–452
Freedom of Information Act (FOIA) (1967), 246
freestanding ambulatory care centers, 18–19
freestanding ambulatory surgery centers, 19
FUH-30, 481–482
full service contracts, 660
Functional Independence Assessment, 173
functional interoperability, 104
functional manager, 730
functional organization, 729–730

## G

Gantt, Henry, 543
Gantt chart, 543, 544, 744, 746
general acute-care hospitals, 12
general authorization, 272
general consent, 250
general damages, 238
generalizability, 486
general jurisdiction, 237
general ledger, 700–701
generally accepted accounting principles (GAAP), 690
generally accepted auditing standards (GAAS), 690
Generally Accepted Recordkeeping Principles (GARP), 44, 56–57
general rules, in procedure manuals, 661
generative AI, 32
Genetic Information Non-Discrimination Act (GINA) (2008), 254, 602
genetics, 411
geographic practice cost index (GPCI), 168
germ theory, 4
gesture recognition technology, 333
Global Assessment of Functioning (GAF), 102
Global Medical Device Nomenclature (GMDN), 108
global payment, 162–163

global surgery payment, 163
goals. See also objectives
  of clinical documentation integrity, 207–208
  comparing performance to, 668
  of health information systems, 373–374
  in management, 549
  of standards, 662
  strategic, 589–590, 592
  of training, 627
going concern, 688
go-live, 383–384
Good Clinical Practices module, 521
good faith estimates, 180
Good Samaritan statutes, 243
governance, 39. See also data governance (DG); information governance (IG)
  corporate, 39
  defined, 39, 372
  enterprise, 39, 57
  of health information systems, 372–373, 388–389
governance committees, 359
government
  branches of, 235
  right of, to access health records, 252–253
Government Accountability Office (GAO), 285
Government Accounting Standards Board (GASB), 690
governmental (sovereign) immunity, 243
government-owned hospitals, 12–13
government-sponsored reimbursement systems, 26–28, 152–157
G-Power, 446
grand jury, 239
graphical perception, 466
graphical user interfaces (GUIs), 133
graph type bar plot, 473–474
Great Depression, 7
great person theory, 556
Great Society, 7
Greenleaf, Robert, 560
grey literature, 490, 491
grievance, 619
grievance management, 619
grievance procedures, 619
gross autopsy rate, 432
gross death rate, 430
gross negligence, 240
grounded theory, 506
group discussions, 641
group model HMOs, 159
group-oriented behaviors, 551
guilty, pleading, 239

## H

hacking, 255, 278, 282
halfway houses, 22
handwritten signature, 247
happiness, 758
harassment, 602, 647
"hard coding," 186

harm
    intentional torts and, 241, 242
    negligence and, 240
    product liability and, 243
Hawthorne effect (observer effect), 545
Hay method, of job evaluation, 615
hazards, 305
Health and Human Services, Department of. *See* Department of Health and Human Services (HHS)
health and safety program, 603
healthcare civil actions, 239–244
Healthcare Common Procedure Coding System (HCPCS), 101
    ambulatory surgery center and, 171
    charge capture and, 186, 187, 188
    charge description master and, 189, 190
    payment status indicators and, 170
    relative value scale for, 168, 169
Healthcare Cost and Utilization Project (HCUP), 137, 312
healthcare data analytics, 441–462
    for continuous data, 449–452
    for correlation, 455
    for data mining, 458–461
    defined, 441
    descriptive statistics and, 444–449, 453
    in electronic health records, 345
    health information management and, 461–462
    impact of, 442
    inferential statistics and, 444–449, 450–452, 453–454
    for quality management, 317
    for rates and proportions, 453–454
    sampling for, 445–449
    for simple linear regression, 456–458
healthcare databases, 134–138
Healthcare Effectiveness Data and Information Set (HEDIS), 158–159
healthcare facilities, licensure of, 24–25
Health Care Financial Administration (HCFA), 25
Healthcare Financial Management Association (HFMA), 195, 199, 442
Health Care Financing Administration, 158
healthcare legislation, 7–9
Health Care Professionals Advisory Committee (HCPAC), 101
healthcare providers, consumer assessment of, 400–401
Health Care Quality Improvement Act (HCQIA) (1986), 8, 24, 135, 309
healthcare quality management. *See* quality management
Healthcare Research and Quality Act (1999), 312
health data
    defined, 368
    and governance plan, 388–389
    types of, 389–390
health data stewardship, 317

health equity, 32
Health Industry Business Communications Council (HIBCC), 113
health informatics, 326–327
health information
    defined, 368
    ongoing management of, 388–393
    types of, 389–390
Health Information Career Map, 647
health information exchange (HIE), 348–349
    defined, 348
    health information management in, 361–362
    implementation considerations of, 359–360
    initiatives of, 357–358
    interoperability challenges of, 349–350
    legal issues in, 284, 285, 355
    methodologies of, 355–357
    models for, 351–354
    privacy and security management in, 284–286
    stages of, 360–361
health information management (HIM)
    artificial intelligence used in, 220
    certifications for, 316
    charge capture in, 186–188
    and charge description master, 190
    in clinical and biomedical research, 516, 526–533
    clinical coding in, 185–186
    and confidentiality, 253, 254, 761
    and database implementation, 133
    data dictionary development in, 143
    data models used by, 133
    data standardization for, 112
    data visualization in, 466
    development of staff, 645
    e-discovery in, 251–252
    empowerment in, 612
    ethical issues in, 753–776
    and financial management, 686, 693, 697, 708, 711–713, 715
    healthcare data analytics and, 461–462
    health information exchange in, 361–362
    for health records, 63, 64, 66–67, 80–88
    in hospitals, 16
    and human resources management, 600, 601, 603, 604–614
    information sources of, 490, 491
    legal issues in, 245–248
    morality in, 754–755
    and privacy, 246, 255, 761
    and quality management, 316–317
    research by, 487, 493, 495, 500, 501
    responsibilities of, 66, 122
    and security, 255
    strategic management and, 577
    in strategic planning process, 373
    technical skills in, 553

    training and development of staff, 624, 633–634, 645–647
    and uncertainty, 583
    vision in, 584–585
    work distribution chart for, 657
    work schedule of, 658, 659
Health Information Management and Systems Society (HIMSS), 406, 410
Health Information Management Association of Australia (HIMAA), 498
health information systems (HISs), 365–393
    acquisitions of, 379–382
    adoption of, 387–388
    benefits realization for, 384–385
    case studies in, 500
    challenges of, 374
    chart conversion for, 382
    clinical transformation of, 388
    continued review and support of, 384–386
    contract negotiation for, 381–382
    data conversion for, 382
    data quality management in, 391–393
    defined, 366
    dependency in, 375
    document design for, 374–376
    enhancements to, 385–386
    environmental scan of, 374
    gaps in, 378–379
    goals of, 373–374
    go-live for, 383–384
    governance of, 372–373, 388–389
    historical overview of, 366
    implementation of, 382–384, 387
    implementation plans for, 375–376
    installation of, 382
    life cycle of, 366
    metadata of, 390–391
    migration path for, 374–376
    planning horizon for, 373
    policies and procedures of, 383
    process improvement for, 379
    project management in, 377–378
    replacements for, 386
    request for proposal for, 380–381
    requirements analysis for, 378–379
    requirements specification for, 379
    SMART goals of, 373–374
    strategic planning for, 370–376, 377
    system customization of, 382
    system development life cycle of, 369–370
    system maintenance for, 385
    system optimization for, 388
    systems view for, 367–369
    testing of, 383
    training for, 383
    upgrades to, 385
    use of, and quality management, 315
    vendor strategy for, 379–380
    workflow improvement for, 379, 382–383

health information technologies (HITs), 325–362. *See also* electronic health records (EHRs)
  defined, 368
  for EHRs, 341–348
  initiatives of, 327, 328
  legislation on, 326
  strategic plan framework of, 326, 327
  supporting access to and flow of data, 333–336
  supporting capture of data and formats, 329–331
  supporting diagnosis, treatment and care, 337–340
  trends in, 328
Health Information Technology for Economic and Clinical Health (HITECH) Act, 9, 112, 246, 263–265, 301, 326
health insurance, 28
  behavioral health services covered by, 22
  commercial, 26, 150–151, 161
  employer-based, 7, 26, 151
  federal, 26–27, 152–157
  Great Depression and, 7
  individual, 26
  managed care plans, 28
  medical necessity coverage issues, 181–182
  national, 7
  not-for-profit, 151
  private, 28, 151
  public, 28
  rising costs of, 28, 30
  verification of, 180
Health Insurance Portability and Accountability Act (HIPAA) (1996), 236, 260–265. *See also* Privacy Rule, of HIPAA; Security Rule, of HIPAA
  on audit logs and monitoring, 278
  breach notification in, 263–264, 282
  business associates in, 261
  and CDT, 103
  on claims preparation, 193
  and clinical coding, 185
  on coding compliance, 223
  on communication with patients, 76
  on conflict of interest in research, 521
  covered entities in, 261
  on data backups, 278
  on deidentification, 269
  on disclosure, 759
  on electronic remittance advice, 196
  on encryption, 281–282
  Enforcement Rule of, 264–265
  on fraud, 223, 226
  on health information exchange, 284, 285, 355
  on health records, 66, 68, 76, 77, 248, 261
  and HITECH Act, 263–265
  and ICD-10-CM, 97
  on malware, 283
  on mental health records, 77
  on mobile health technology, 286–287
  and NDCs, 103
  Omnibus Rule of, 263–265, 267, 282
  on outsourcing, 659
  on protected health information, 66, 68, 250, 261, 266, 270
  Right of Access Initiative of, 248
  on risk analysis and risk management, 276–277
  security regulations of, 139, 285
  and state laws, 274
  on substance abuse patient records, 271–273
  on training, 287–289
Health Level 7 (HL7)
  Clinical Document Architecture by, 406
  description of, 113, 347
  Fast Healthcare Interoperability Resources developed by, 114, 349, 379–380
  frameworks created by, 356
health literacy, 402–403, 774
Health Maintenance Organization Assistance Act (HMO Act) (1973), 158, 298
health maintenance organizations (HMOs), 28, 153, 159
  benefits of, 159, 298
  creation of, 298
  models of, 159
  POS plans compared to, 159–160
health plan contracts, 197–198
Health Professions Accreditors Collaborative (HPAC), 6
*Health Professions Education: A Bridge to Quality* (IOM), 304
health professions/professionals. *See also specific professions*
  defined, 11
  expansion of, 6
  interprofessional education for, 6
  licensing of, 4, 6
  training of, 4–5
health record(s). *See also* electronic health records (EHRs)
  access to, 248, 252–253
  accreditation and, 88, 246
  for acute care, 63, 76
  administrative information in, 68–69
  admissibility of, 249
  advance directives in, 68–69, 250
  for ambulatory care, 77
  amendments to, 82
  ancillary services in, 73–74
  authentication of, 82–83, 247
  autopsy recording in, 74
  for behavioral health services, 77
  as business record, 247
  bylaws for, 64
  clinical data in, 69–75
  for communication, 65, 206
  consent to treatment in, 68, 250
  consent to use or disclose in, 68
  consultations in, 73
  content management of, 80–84
  content of, 63, 68–79, 245–246, 247
  correction of, 82
  creation and identification of, 85–87
  death recorded in, 74, 75, 76
  for decision-making and communication, 65
  demographic information in, 68
  destruction and transfer of, 88–90
  diagnostic and therapeutic orders in, 70–72
  discharge orders in, 72
  discharge plans in, 76
  discharge summary in, 75–76
  DNR in, 72, 250
  documentation and maintenance standards for, 63–64
  document creation for, 80–81
  for emergency care, 76–77
  as evidence, 249–253
  evolution of, 62–67
  external records filed with, 76
  filing equipment for, 87
  filing systems for, 85
  format of, 72–73, 206, 245
  functions of, 64–66
  government right of access to, 252–253
  HIM for, 64
  HIPAA on, 66, 68, 76, 77, 248, 261
  historical overview of, 62–63, 296–297
  history and physical examination in, 69–70
  for home healthcare, 77–78
  hospice care in, 78
  incomplete record control for, 81–84
  internal standards for, 64
  inventory of, 89
  Joint Commission on Accreditation of Hospitals and, 63, 65, 246
  legal, 247, 355
  legal issues concerning, 65–66, 88, 89, 249–253
  licensure and, 64, 245
  life cycle of, 85–90
  longitudinal, 66
  long-term care in, 79
  for medical research, 65
  Medicare and, 63–64, 77, 248
  nurses and, 73
  obstetrics in, 75
  for ongoing care, 65
  for operational management, 65
  order signatures in, 72
  organ transplantation in, 74–75
  for outpatients, 77
  ownership of, 248
  paper-based, 62, 63, 66–67, 80–85, 87–90
  patient identity management and, 66, 85–87
  patient's rights statement in, 68
  as primary data source, 122
  progress notes in, 72
  property and valuables list in, 69

qualitative analysis of, 82
for quality documentation, 65, 66–67
quantitative analysis of, 81–82
rehabilitation services in, 78–79
for reimbursement, 65
restraint orders in, 72
retention of, 66, 88–90, 247–248
retrieval of, 83, 87–88
review of (see record review)
seclusion orders in, 72
serial-unit numbering system for, 85
SOAP note format in, 72–73
state licensure and, 64
storage of, 83, 87, 89
surgical services in, 74
templates for, 81, 84
transcription of, 80
unit numbering system for, 85
health record banking model, for health information exchange, 353–354
health record committee, 83
health reimbursement accounts (HRAs), 29–30, 151–152
Health Research Extension Act (1985), 527
Health Resources and Services Administration (HRSA), 498
health savings accounts (HSAs), 29, 151–152
health services research, 516
health services research databases, 137
health statistics, 417–438
on ambulatory care, 434
on case-mix index, 434–435
data sources for, 419
defined, 418
on public health and epidemiology, 436–437
related to clinical services and patient care, 429–433
related to volume of service, 423–427
on revenue cycle management, 434
terminology of, 422
use of, 418–419, 437–438
health technology assessment (HTA), 494
HealthyPeople 2030, 128, 402, 438
hearing loss, 15
hearsay, 249
heat map, 467
Hersey, Paul, 557–558
Hersey and Blanchard's situational theory, 557–558
Hierarchical Condition Categories (HCCs), 164
hierarchical regression model, 460
Hierarchy of Needs, 545
high-cost outlier, 173, 174
high-cost outlier adjustments, 174
highly sensitive information, handling, 253–254, 271–273
HIPAA. See Health Insurance Portability and Accountability Act (HIPAA) (1996)
Hippocratic tradition, 754, 756, 758
hiring, 609–610

histogram, 473, 476, 677
historical research, 492–493
history and physical examination (H&P)
components of, 69, 70, 71
in health records, 69–70
for obstetrics, 75
time frame of, 69–70
HITECH-HIPAA Omnibus Privacy Act, 263–265, 267, 282
HIV information, handling, 254
HMO. See health maintenance organizations (HMOs)
HMO point-of-service (HMO POS) plans, 154
holding, in common law, 235
home health agency (HHA), 153, 173
home healthcare, 19
health records for, 77–78
Medicare on, 19, 153, 172–173
prospective payment system for, 172–173
services in, 77–78
home health resource groups (HHRGs), 173
honesty, 757–758
horizontal bar plot, 470, 471
hospice
defined, 78
in health records, 78
long-term care in, 21
Medicare on, 78, 153
hospital(s)
accreditation of, 5, 25, 63
acute care in, 11–12
administrative staff of, 13
admission to, 11
ambulatory care in, 12, 18
ancillary units in, 16
average length of stay in, 11–12
bed capacity in, 12
board of directors for, 13
CEO of, 13
critical access, 167, 169
diagnostic services in, 14–17
emergency services in, 18
Great Depression and, 7
health statistics of, 423–433
history of, 4
inpatients in, 11, 422
integrated delivery system in, 22
licensure of, 25
medical staff of, 13–14
Medicare paying for care in, 153, 165–167
network of, 4
number of, 4
nurses in, 14
organization and operation of, 11–16
organ transplantation procedures in, 75
outpatients in, 12, 422, 434
ownership of, 12–13, 28
quality improvement programs in, 23–24
quality reporting by, 24

rural, 169
standardization of care in, 5–6
therapeutic services in, 14–17
types of, 12–13
hospital-acquired conditions (HACs), 166–167
Hospital Acquired Conditions (HAC) Reduction Program, 442
hospital-acquired infection (HAI) rates, 432
hospital autopsy rate, 432
hospital census, 422, 423–425
Hospital Compare, 479
Hospital Consumer Assessment of Healthcare Providers and Systems (HCAHPS), 401, 534
hospital death rate, 429
hospital infection rates, 432–433
hospital inpatient, 11, 422
Hospital Inpatient Quality Reporting Program, 24
hospital-issued notice of noncoverage (HINN), 182, 185
hospital newborn inpatient, 422
hospital outpatient, 12, 422
Hospital Readmission Reduction Program (HRRP), 442
Hospital Standardization Program, 5
Hospital Value-Based Purchasing Program, 302, 401, 442
House, Robert, 558
Huffman, Edna, 206
human capital risks, 305
human-computer interface (HCI), 347–348
Human Gene Nomenclature Committee (HGNC), 108, 110
Human Genome Project, 411
humanistic management, 545
human resources management, 599–620, 652
analysis in, 600–601
communication by, 611
and compensation systems, 603, 614–615
employee empowerment by, 611–614
employee records maintained by, 619
equal employment opportunity practices of, 601–602
and grievance management, 619
and health and safety program, 603
and health information management, 600, 601, 603, 604–614
historical overview of, 545
and labor relations, 603–604, 605
and performance management, 615–619
planning in, 600–601, 605–606
policies and procedures by, 607
position descriptions by, 606–607
recruitment by, 607–610
and rights of employees and employers, 602–603
roles of, 600–604
staffing by, 603
trends in, 619–620
workforce retention by, 610–611

human subjects, in research
   defined, 520
   ethical treatment of, 517–519, 769–770
   protection of, 519–524, 769–770
   vulnerable subjects, 525–526
*Human Subjects Research Protections: Enhancing Protections for Research Subjects and Reducing Burden, Delay, and Ambiguity for Investigators* (HHS), 518
humility, cultural, 770–771
hung jury, 239
hybrid model, for health information exchange, 352–353, 354
hybrid records, 62, 83, 84, 89
hypothesis, 491
hypothesis test, 444

# I

ICD. *See* International Classification of Diseases (ICD)
identity management, 334
identity theft
   defined, 228
   medical, 82, 228, 254–255
immunity, in torts, 243
immunization registries, 128–129
implant registries, 129
implementation plans, 375–376, 589–591
implied consent, 250
implied warranty, 243
IMRAD guideline, 510
incentive pay, 637
incidence, 532
incidence rate, 436
incident, 255
incident reports, 255–256, 305
inclusion, 770–771
income statement, 701–702, 703
incomplete record control, 81–84
independent practice association (IPA) model, 159
independent variables, 456, 494–495
index/indices, 123. *See also* master patient index (MPI)
   case-mix, 166, 186, 212, 434–435
   defined, 123
   for health records, 81
   issues with, 132–133
   of procedure manuals, 661
   as secondary data source, 122
Indian Health Service (IHS), 27, 157
indictment, 239
indirect costs, 706–707
indirect maternal death, 431
indirect medical education (IME), 166
indirect standardization, 460
individual health insurance, 26
individually identifiable health information, 261
inductive reasoning, 487, 500
industry experience, of project managers, 738
infection control, census report used for, 425

infection rates, 432
inferential statistics, 420, 444–449, 450–452, 453–454
infliction of emotional distress, 242
informatics, 326–328, 399. *See also* health information technologies (HITs)
information
   *vs.* data, 40, 43
   in hierarchy of data to wisdom, 41, 307–308
   release of, 253–254, 755, 768–769
   secure, 282
informational activities, 553, 554
information blocking, 273–274
information economics, 42–43
information governance (IG)
   background of, 42–45
   components of, 57
   data governance compared to, 40–42
   defined, 38, 40, 42
   domains of, 45–49
   frameworks for, 43–44, 56–57
   key terms used in, 38–39
   principles of, 44–45, 56
   program planning for, 49–51
   purpose of, 42
   quality management and, 317
Information Governance Maturity Model, 44, 56–57
Information Governance Principles for Healthcare, 44–45
information management (IM)
   defined, 42, 326
   program planning for, 49–51
information overload, 470
information power, 550
information security, 57
information system (IS)
   data quality requirements for, 142
   defined, 38, 136
   *vs.* health information systems, 366
   life cycle of, 366
information technology. *See* health information technologies (HITs)
informed consent, 250, 523–524
in-group, 558–559
initiation phase, in project management, 741–743
injunction, 244
injury
   defenses and, 243
   intentional torts and, 242
   negligence and, 240, 241
   product liability and, 243
injury severity score (ISS), 126
innovations, 562–564
   adopters of, 562–563
   factors of adoption of, 563–564
   management and, 562–564
   strategic, 588
innovators
   defined, 562
   roles of, 564
inpatient admission, 422
inpatient bed occupancy rate, 426

inpatient census, 422, 423–425
inpatient discharge, 422
Inpatient-Prospective Payment System (IPPS), 302, 442
inpatient psychiatric facilities (IPFs), 167, 479–482
Inpatient Psychiatric Facility Quality Reporting (IPFQR) Program, 479–482
inpatient quality indicators, 312, 313
inpatient rehabilitation facilities (IRFs), 173–174
inpatients, defined, 11, 422
inpatient service day (IPSD), 422, 423–424
input, in process improvement, 670
*In Search of Excellence* (Peters and Waterman), 547
in-service education, 633–636
installation
   defined, 382
   of health information systems, 382
Institute for Healthcare Improvement (IHI), 299, 400, 674
Institute of Electrical and Electronic Engineers (IEEE), 113
Institute of Medicine (IOM), 298–299
   on healthcare quality, 23
   on health literacy, 403
   on interprofessional education, 304
   on medical errors, 673
   on social determinants of health, 402
institutional assurance of compliance, 519–520
Institutional Review Board (IRB), 519–523, 526, 527, 769
instructor-directed training, 640–641
instruments, in research
   defined, 502
   features of, 503
   selection of, 502–503
insurance. *See* health insurance
insurance verification, 180
integrated delivery network/system (IDN/IDS), 4, 22–23, 160
Integrated Outpatient Code Editor (IOCE), 193
integrity
   of electronic health records, 247
   as recordkeeping principle, 44
intelligent character recognition (ICR) technology, 333
intelligent document recognition (IDR) technology, 334
intensive study courses, 641
intent, 241
intentional acts (threats), 306
intentional torts, 241–242
interactive learners, 638
interface
   defined, 379
   for health information systems, 379–380
   terminology, 104–105
interim periods, 711–712

internal assessment, in strategic planning, 580–582
internal benchmarking, 307
internal change agents, 565–566
internal controls, in accounting, 709
internal customers, 669
internal medical identity theft, 255
internal rate of return (IRR), 718–719
Internal Revenue Service (IRS), 690
internal self-audit, 226
internal stakeholders, 55
internal validity, 501
*International Classification of Diseases (ICD)*, 96, 123
*International Classification of Diseases, Eleventh Revision (ICD-11)*, 96, 97–98
*International Classification of Diseases, Ninth Revision, Clinical Modification (ICD-9-CM)*, 207
*International Classification of Diseases, Tenth Revision (ICD-10)*, 94–95
*International Classification of Diseases, Tenth Revision, Clinical Modification (ICD-10-CM)*, 97, 207, 216, 219, 227, 228
*International Classification of Diseases, Tenth Revision, Procedure Coding System (ICD-10-PCS)*, 98, 207, 212, 216, 219, 227
*International Classification of Diseases for Oncology, Third Edition (ICD-O-3)*, 98–100
International Classification of Health Interventions (ICHI), 103
*International Classification of Primary Care (ICPC-3)*, 102–103
*International Classification on Functioning, Disability, and Health (ICF)*, 100–101
International Health Terminology Standards Development Organization (IHTSDO), 105
International List of Causes of Death (WHO), 96
International Organization for Standardization (ISO), 113
Internet and American Life Project, 404
internet forums, for consumer health informatics, 404–405
Internet of Medical Things (IoMT), 338
interoperability, 349–350
    basic, 104
    CCC and, 107
    challenges of, 349–350
    commitment to, 350
    data, 38–39
    data standardization for, 112–114
    defined, 38–39, 104, 349
    and electronic health records, 104, 340
    functional, 104
    lack of, 339
    levels of, 104
    LOINC and, 107
    message format standards and, 347
    NDCs and, 103
    program for promoting, 344, 366, 401

    RxNorm and, 107
    semantic, 104, 347
    SNOMED CT and, 105
    technical, 347
    utility and, 758
Interoperability Standards Advisory (ISA), 112
interpersonal activities, 553, 554
interpersonal skills, 552–553, 735, 736
interprofessional education (IPE)
    defined, 6, 304
    for quality management, 304
Interprofessional Education Collaborative (IPEC), 6
interrater reliability, 502
interrogatories, 238
interval data, 443
intervention, in experimental research, 495
interventional radiologists, 15
interviews, 498–499, 608, 611
intranets, 335
intraoperative anesthesia, 74
intrarater reliability, 502
introduction, methods, results, and discussion (IMRAD) guideline, 510
invasion of privacy, 242
inventors, 564
inventory, as assets, 694
inventory slips, 699
investor-owned hospital chains, 28
invoices, 698–699
Iron Mountain, 44–45, 57
iterative approach, to project management, 725

## J

job classification method, 615
job descriptions, 606–607
job evaluations, 615
job procedure, 660–661
job ranking, 615
job requirements, 632
job rotation, 632
job sharing, 658–659
job specifications, 606
joinder, 238
Joint Commission on Accreditation of Hospitals, 72, 300
    on advance directives, 250
    on discharge summary, 76
    on end-of-life care, 72
    formation of, 5
    on giving orders, 71–72
    on health record retention, 88, 248
    on health records, 63, 65, 83, 246
    on history and physical forms, 70
    on open-record review, 82
    on operative reports, 74
    on order signatures, 72
    on organ transplantation, 74–75
    on patient identity management, 270
    peer review of, 23

    on performance measures, 307
    on research, 516, 534
    role of, 5, 63, 245
    on seclusion and restraint orders, 72
    on tracer methodology, 310
    voluntary programs of, 25
journal entry, in accounting, 700, 701
judge-make law. *See* common law
judicial branch, 235
judicial law. *See* common law
jurisdiction, 237
justice
    in AHIMA Code of Ethics, 763
    in Belmont Report, 770
    and decision-making, 766
    defined, 759
    description of, 759
    distributive, 759
    and health literacy, 774
    and morality, 755
    procedural, 759
just-in-time training, 638

## K

Kant, Immanuel, 757–758
Kantianism. *See* deontology
key indicators, 663
key performance indicators (KPIs), 199, 460–461, 551, 577
Kids' Inpatient Database, 137
kinesthetic learners, 638
knowledge
    explicit, 307
    generation of, in quality management, 307–308
    in hierarchy of data to wisdom, 41, 307–308
    learning curve and, 637
    process, 739
    tacit, 307
knowledge-based CDS systems, 344
knowledge discovery. *See* data mining
Kotter, John, 568–569
Kubler-Ross, Elizabeth, 568

## L

Lab LOINC, 106
Labor, Department of. *See* Department of Labor
labor and delivery record, 75
laboratory reports, 73, 74
laboratory results, LOINC codes for exchanging, 106–107
laboratory science, 15
Labor-Management Relations Act (1947), 604
Labor-Management Reporting and Disclosure Act (1959), 604
labor relations, 603–604, 605
laggards, of innovations, 563
Landrum-Griffin Act (1959), 604, 605
laparoscopic surgical techniques, 12
large-dollar purchases, 715
late majority, of innovations, 563

law. *See also* legal issues; legislation
  administrative, 236
  civil *vs.* criminal, 236–237
  common, 235–236
  constitutional, 235
  contract, 244
  *vs.* morality, 755
  public *vs.* private, 236
  regulatory, 246
  sources of, 235–236
  statutory, 236, 246
layoffs, 618
leader-member exchange (LMX), 558–559
leadership, 554
  and areas of excellence, 585
  autocratic, 556
  behavioral theories of, 556–557
  and change, 592–593, 595
  classical theories of, 555–556
  communication by, 594
  complexity, 560–561
  contingency theories of, 557–559
  and continuous quality
    improvement, 671
  during COVID-19 pandemic, 555
  cultural change and, 569
  defined, 303
  democratic, 556
  great person theory of, 556
  in management, 550–551, 565
  and quality management, 303–304
  situational theories of, 557–559
  strategic planning by, 579, 588
  strategic thinking by, 576, 577
  systems thinking in, 561
  trait approach to, 556
  trends in, 555–562
  values-based, 559–560
Lean (CQI method), 672–673
Lean Six Sigma, 674
learning
  blended, 640
  classroom, 640–641, 643
  defined, 636
  e-learning, 642–643
  machine, 38, 115, 220, 496, 644–645
  m-learning, 644
  strategies for, 636–639
  styles of, 638
learning content management systems
    (LCMSs), 644
learning curve, 637
learning health systems, 318–319,
    398, 399
learning management systems
    (LMSs), 626
least harm, 759
least squares line, 456–457
legacy systems, 66, 386
legal awareness, 620
legal health record (LHR), 247, 355
legal hold, 251–252
legal issues
  in consent and advance
    directives, 250

  government right to access health
    records, 252–253
  in health information exchange, 284,
    285, 355
  in health information management,
    245–248
  in health records, 65–66, 88, 89,
    249–253
  in medical identity theft, 254–255
  in privilege, 252
  in quality improvement activities,
    255–256
  in quality of care, 297
  in release of information, 253–254
legal risks, 305
legal structures, of organizations,
    690–692
legal system, 235
legislation
  on emergency care, 229, 253
  on equal employment opportunity,
    601–602
  on healthcare, 7–9
  on healthcare fraud and abuse,
    222–223, 228–229
  on health information
    technologies, 326
  on labor relations, 604, 605
  on malpractice, 24, 297
  on training, 647–648
legislative branch, 235
legislative law. *See* statutory law
length of stay (LOS), 427. *See also* average
    length of stay (ALOS)
Lewin, Kurt, 566, 567, 568
lexicon, 95
liability/liabilities
  in accounting, 696–697
  medical malpractice, 297
  product, 242–243
  strict, 242, 243
  training to avoid, 647
libel, 241
licensure. *See also* state licensure
  of healthcare facilities, 24–25
  for health professionals, 4, 6
  and health records, 64, 245
  on history and physical forms, 70
  of hospitals, 25
  for medical practices, 4
life cycle
  of data, 45–46
  of health information systems, 366
  of health records, 85–90
  of project management, 724–726,
    741–748
  of system development, 369–370
life expectancy, 32
light, at work, 654
Likert scale, 503, 504
Likert survey, 405
limited jurisdiction, 237
line authority, 549
line chart, 466
line plot, 471, 472–473, 474

liquidity, 702–705
literacy
  data, 467
  health, 402–403, 774
literature review, 490–491
litigation, 234, 237–239
living systematic review (LSR), 496
living will, 250, 764, 765, 767, 773
loans payable, 696
local coverage determinations
    (LCDs), 181
logical database design, 131, 132
Logical Observation Identifiers Names
    and Codes (LOINC), 106–107,
    112, 342
logic bombs (malware), 283
longitudinal health record, 66
long-term care (LTC), 20–22, 79
long-term care hospitals (LTCHs), 11–12,
    20, 174
lower control limit (LCL), 677
lying, 757–758

# M

machine learning, 38, 115, 220, 496,
    644–645
magnetic tapes, 88
major diagnostic categories (MDCs), 165
malfeasance, 240
malicious software management,
    283–284
malpractice, 24, 297
malware, 283–284
managed care
  capitated, 162
  defined, 28, 298
  reimbursement of, 28–30, 157–160
managed care organizations (MCOs),
    28–29
managed fee-for-service reimbursement,
    161–162
management. *See also specific types*
  activities of, 553–554
  of bureaucracy, 542
  controlling by, 551
  defined, 652
  as discipline, 542–548
  efficiency in, 542–543
  and employee empowerment, 544–545
  evaluating by, 551
  executive role in, 544
  innovations and, 562–564
  key functions of, 543–544, 548–554
  leadership in, 550–551, 565
  levels of, 551–552
  organizing by, 549–550
  planning by, 549
  principles of, 544, 546, 548–554
  skills of, 552–553
  socioeconomic approach to, 548
  trends in, 554, 555
management accounting, 706–709
management by objectives (MBO), 546
managerial accounting, 710
*Managing Transitions* (Bridges), 568

manmade threats, 306
manual, procedure, 661
manual data collection, 138
*Manual for Medical Records Librarians* (Huffman), 206, 207
manuscript, 510
MAP indicators, 442
MAP Keys, 199–200
map/mapping
   defined, 112
   schema, 130
   top-down process, 680–682
   value stream, 673
mark sense technology, 333
Martin, Franklin H., 5
Maslow, Abraham, 545
Maslow's Hierarchy of Needs, 545
massed training, 633
master data
   defined, 46
   management of, 46–47
   quality of, 47, 55
master patient index (MPI), 85–87, 360
   challenges of, 86
   content of, 86, 123
   enterprise, 86, 334
   in health information exchange, 360
   importance of, 123
   regional, 86
matching, in accounting, 688, 689
materiality, 688, 689, 714
maternal death rate, 431
matrix organization, 730–732
maturity models, 387–388
maximization, 225
Mayo, Elton, 545
Mayo Clinic, 404, 407–408
McGregor, Douglas, 545, 556
mean, 421, 449, 451–452
Meaningful Use incentive program, 772
measure, apply, perform (MAP) indicators, 442
MEDCIN, 108
medcont, 480–482
median, 421, 449
mediation, 238, 619
Medicaid, 7, 26, 154–155
   on advance directives, 250
   certification for, 25
   charge description master and, 189
   coding compliance and, 222
   creation of, 297
   eligibility for, 154, 155
   fraud in, 223
   government right to access health records in, 252–253
   Medicare certification and, 25
   notification of denial of care, 185
   reimbursement for, 27, 154–155
medical device, 10
Medical Dictionary for Regulatory Activities (MedDRA), 109
medical homes, patient-centered, 315, 401

medical identity theft, 82, 228–229, 254–255
medical laboratory science, 15
medical laboratory scientists (MLSs), 15
Medical Library Association, 404
Medical Literature, Analysis, and Retrieval System Online (MEDLINE), 137
medically needy option, 155
medically unlikely edits (MUEs), 193
medical malpractice liability, 297
medical necessity, 181–182
medical paternalism, 400
medical practice
   expansion of professions in, 6
   Great Depression and, 7
   licenses for, 4
   standardization of, 4–5
   training in, 4–5
medical research. *See* biomedical research; clinical research
medical scribes, 80
medical staff. *See also* nurse(s); physician(s); staffing
   authorized to give orders, 71–72
   bylaws of, 14
   classification of, 14
   for clinical documentation integrity, 208, 209, 210–211
   database of, 135
   defined, 310
   health records completed by, 83, 84
   of hospitals, 13–14
   interprofessional education of, 6, 304
Medical Subject Headings (MeSH) database, 114
medical transcriptionists, 80
Medicare, 7, 26, 63, 152–154
   on ACOs, 23, 163
   advance beneficiary notice of noncoverage to, 181–182
   on advance directives, 250
   on ambulance fee, 171
   on ambulatory surgery center, 170–171
   certification for, 25
   charge capture and, 188
   charge description master and, 189
   claims preparation for, 193
   claims submission to, 194
   coding compliance and, 222
   creation of, 297
   and deemed status, 246
   fraud in, 222, 223
   government right to access health records in, 252–253
   and health records, 63–64, 77, 248
   on home healthcare, 19, 153, 172–173
   on hospice care services, 78, 153
   on hospital care, 153, 165–167
   identifying fraudulent claims, 459
   Inpatient-Prospective Payment System of, 302
   on inpatient psychiatric facilities, 167
   on inpatient rehabilitation facilities, 173–174

   on long-term care hospitals, 20, 174
   on medical necessity, 181
   patient's rights statement and, 68
   prospective payment system of, 164–174, 312
   on rehabilitation services, 78–79
   reimbursement for, 26–27, 152–154, 164–174
   on respite care, 153
   on retail clinics, 19
   on SNF care, 153, 171–172
   value-based programs and, 442
   value-based purchasing and, 24
Medicare Access and CHIP Reauthorization Act (MACRA), 248
Medicare Administrative Contractor (MAC), 181
Medicare Advantage plan (Medicare Part C), 27, 152, 153–154
Medicare Claims Processing Manual, 188
Medicare Code Editor (MCE), 193
Medicare Conditions of Participation (Medicare CoP), 69, 236, 246, 297
Medicare Electronic Health Records Incentive Program, 419
Medicare fee schedule (MFS), 168
Medicare Modernization Act (MMA) (2003), 170
Medicare Part A, 26–27, 152–153, 171, 181
Medicare Part B, 26–27, 153, 154, 181
Medicare Part D, 27, 152
Medicare Prescription Drug, Improvement, and Modernization Act (2003), 24, 154, 301
Medicare Promoting Interoperability (PI) Program, 277, 326
Medicare Provider Analysis and Review (MED-PAR), 134–135
Medicare severity diagnosis-related groups (MS-DRGs), 165–168, 174, 435, 443, 447, 460–461
Medicare Shared Savings Program, 163
medication. *See* drugs (prescription)
medication administration records (MARs), 73
medication management applications, 343–344
medication reconciliation, 344
medication variability, 349
medicine, biomedical and technological advances in, 9–10
Medigap insurance, 152, 154
mental disorders, classification system for, 102
mental health records, 77
mentally disabled individuals, as vulnerable subjects in research, 525
mentoring, 632, 641
mergers, 569
Merit-Based Incentive Payment System (MIPS), 248, 277
message format standards, 347
meta-analysis, 490, 496

metadata
  administrative, 390–391
  defined, 46, 251
  descriptive, 390
  e-discovery of, 251
  of health information systems, 390–391
  management of, 46
  structural, 390
  types of, 46
meta-syntheses, 496–497
mHealth, 410
middle management, 551–552
migration path, 374–376
Minimum Data Set (MDS), 79, 171
minimum necessary standard, 261
minority groups, in workforce, 620
Mintzberg, Henry, 553, 554
misdemeanor, 237, 239
misfeasance, 240
mission, organizational, 303, 580
mission statement
  assessment of, 580
  of data governance, 53
  defined, 576
  of healthcare organizations, 303
  in management, 549
mitigation, risk, 277
mixed costs, 707
mixed methods research, 487
m-learning, 644
mobile application management (MAM), 287
mobile device management (MDM), 286–287
mobile health technology, 286–287
mobile learning, 644
mobile technology, 337–338
mode, 421, 449–450
Modified Adjusted Gross Income, 155
monitoring
  in project management, 747
  system logins, 278
moral agent, 755
moral courage, 755
moral dilemma, 755
moral distress, 755, 756
morality, 517, 754–755
Morbidity and Mortality Weekly Report (MMWR), 419
morbidity statistics, 96, 429
morphology codes, 100
mortality rate, 453, 460
mortality statistics, 96, 429
mortgage, 696
motions for summary judgment, 238
motivation, 545, 550, 558, 636–637
Mouton, Jane Srygley, 557
multi-factor authentication, 281
multihospital systems, 4
multimedia, 329
multiple imputation, 505
multiuser virtual environment (MUVE), 642
multivoting technique, 675

# N

NANDA International, 343
narrative formats, 661
National Academy of Medicine, 298
national administrative databases, 134–135
National Alliance for Health Information Technology (NAHIT), 340
National Ambulatory Medical Care Survey (NAMCS), 136
National Archives and Records Administration, 236
National Association for Healthcare Quality (NAHQ), 316
National Association for Home Care and Hospice, 77
National Business Ethics Survey, 559–560
National Cancer Institute (NCI) Thesaurus, 108, 109
National Center for Health Statistics (NCHS), 97, 135–136, 139
National Commission for the Protection of Human Subjects in Biomedical and Behavioral Research, 518–519
National Committee for Quality Assurance (NCQA), 158, 516, 533
National Committee on Vital and Health Statistics (NCVHS), 104
national conversion factor (CF), 168
National Coordinator for Health Information Technology, 114
National Correct Coding Initiative (NCCI), 193
National Council for Prescription Drug Programs (NCPDP), 113, 343
national coverage determinations (NCDs), 181
National Drug Codes (NDCs), 103, 107, 344
National Electronic Disease Surveillance System (NEDSS), 136
National Health and Nutrition Examination Survey, 136
National Health Care Survey (NHCS), 135–136
National Health Interview Survey, 129, 136
National Health Service (NHS), 40, 43–44
National Hospice and Palliative Care Organization, 69
National Hospital Ambulatory Medical Care Survey (NHAMCS), 136
National Hospital Care Survey (NHCS), 136
National Information Standards Organization (NISO), 113
National Inpatient Sample, 137
National Institute of Health (NIH), 137, 528
National Institute of Health (NIH) Revitalization Act (1993), 527
National Institute of Standards and Technology (NIST), 276, 279, 306
National Labor Relations Act (1935), 604

National Library of Medicine (NLM), 107, 112, 114–115, 137–138
National Notifiable Diseases Surveillance System (NVDSS), 436–437
National Patient-Centered Clinical Research Network (PCORnet), 133–134
National Post-Acute and Long-Term Care Study (NPALS), 136
National Practitioner Data Bank (NPDB), 24, 135, 310
National Program of Cancer Registries (NPCR), 124
National Provider Identifier (NPI) Registry, 129
national public health databases, 135–136
National Quality Forum, 307
National Quality Strategy in Person and Family-Centered Care, 535
National Sample Survey of Registered Nurses (NSSRN), 498
National Strategy for Quality Improvement of Healthcare (2016), 534
National Study of Long-Term Care Providers, 136
National Uniform Billing Committee (NUBC), 113, 193
National Uniform Claim Committee (NUCC), 113, 193
National Vaccine Advisory Committee, 129
National Vital Statistics System (NVSS), 436
National Voluntary Hospital Reporting Initiative, 442
Nationwide Ambulatory Surgery Sample, 137
Nationwide Emergency Department Sample, 137
Nationwide Interoperability Roadmap, 326
Nationwide Privacy and Security Framework, 351
Nationwide Readmissions Database, 137
native hypothesis, 444
naturalistic observation, 499
natural language processing (NLP), 115, 328, 330, 331, 347, 443, 603
natural threats, 306
NDCs. See National Drug Codes (NDCs)
needs assessment
  for employee orientation, 630
  for in-service education, 633
  for on-the-job training, 632
  for research design, 493
  for training model, 625, 626
need-to-know principle, 768
negative relationship among variables, 493
negative variances, 713
neglect, willful, 264
negligence, 240–241, 243, 254
net assets, 696–697, 702, 703
net autopsy rate, 432
net death rate, 430

net income, 701
net loss, 701
net present value (NPV), 718
network model HMOs, 159
network providers, 160
networks, of hospitals, 4
newborn(s), 424
newborn autopsy rate, 432
newborn death rate, 430
newborn inpatients, 422
*Nicomachean Ethics* (Aristotle), 756
Nightingale, Florence, 94
nomenclature, 94, 95
nominal data, 443
nominal group technique (NGT), 675
noncoverage
  advance beneficiary notice of, 181–182
  hospital-issued notice of, 182, 185
non-economic compensatory damages, 238
nonexempt employees, 614
nonfeasance, 240
nonmaleficence, 759
  in AHIMA Code of Ethics, 763
  and decision-making, 765
  defined, 759
  description of, 759
  and health literacy, 774
nonoperating revenue, 697
nonparticipant observation, 499
normal distribution, 452, 476
normalization, 132
North American Association of Central Cancer Registries (NAACCR), 125
nosocomial infection rates, 432
No Surprises Act (NSA) (2022), 180, 195
not-for-profit healthcare organizations, 12
not-for-profit health insurance, 151
not-for-profit organizations, 691–692
Notice of Confidentiality of Alcohol and Drug Abuse Patient Records, 273
notice of privacy practices (NPP), 68, 262
Notice of Proposed Rulemaking (NPRM), 265
notifiable diseases, 436
nuclear medicine, 15
null hypothesis, 444, 450–452, 453–454
numeric items, in research, 503
Nuremberg Code, 517–518
nurse(s)
  care provided by, 14
  and health records, 73
  in hospitals, 14
  responsibilities of, 14
  surveys of, 498
  types of, 14
nurse practitioners (NPs), 14
Nurses' Health Study, 530
Nursing Home Quality Initiative, 25
nursing homes. *See* skilled nursing facilities (SNFs)
nursing terminology, CCC system for, 107
nutritional care plans, 74

# O

objection to health information disclosure, 269–270
objectives. *See also* goals
  of in-service education, 634
  of projects, 722–723, 743, 751
  of standards, 662
  strategic, 589–590, 592
  of training, 626
obligations, and ethics, 763
Observational Medical Outcomes Partnership (OMOP), 133, 134
observational research, 499–500
observational studies, 529–530
observed mortality rate, 460
observer effect (Hawthorne effect), 545
observers (learning style), 638
obstetrics and gynecology, in health records, 75
occasion of service, 434
occupancy data, 425–426
Occupational Safety and Health Act (OSHA) (1970), 603, 647
Occupational Safety and Health Administration, 88
occupational therapists (OTs), 15–16
occupational therapy, 15–16, 172
occupational therapy assistants (OTAs), 16
odds ratio, 532–533
offer, 244
Office for Human Research Protections (OHRP), 518–520
Office of Civil Rights (OCR), 263, 264, 265, 283
Office of Disease Prevention and Health Promotion (ODPHP), 19
Office of Managed Care, 158
Office of Management and Budget (OMB), 518
Office of Minority Health (OMH), 774
Office of Research Integrity (ORI), 527
Office of Scientific Integrity (OSI), 527
Office of Scientific Review (OSIR), 527
Office of the Assistant Secretary for Health (OASH), 527
Office of the Inspector General (OIG), 221, 223–226, 446–447
Office of the National Coordinator (ONC)
  and Blue Button, 357
  and data standardization, 112
  and patient engagement, 397–398
  and risk analysis, 276
  Trusted Exchange Framework of, 357
  21st Century Cures Act by, 66, 76, 114, 273–274
Office of the Surgeon General of the United States, 19
Office of Workers' Compensation Programs (OWCP), 157
office supplies, 713
offshoring, 659

Ohio State University, 557
OIG workplan, 221, 225
older employees, 620
Omnibus Budget Reconciliation Act (1981), 158
Omnibus Budget Reconciliation Act (1986), 164
Omnibus Rule, 263–265, 267, 282
onboarding process, 628
oncology, classification system for, 98–100
one sample t-test, 450–451
ongoing care, health records for, 65
ongoing processes, 54
online resources, for patient engagement, 404–405
online transaction processing (OLTP), 345
on-on-one training, 632
on-the-job training, 631–633
open access (OA) publishing, 510
open-ended queries, 217, 219
open-record review, 82
open-source technology, 336
open systems, 670
operating revenue, 697
operation(s)
  defined, 722
  *vs.* project, 722–723
operational budgets, 711–715
operational islands, 737
operational management, health records for, 65
operational policies, in health information exchange, 359–360
operational risks, 305
operational stewards, 55
operation index, 123
operations improvement management, 583–584
operations management, 545
operative reports, 74
opportunities, in SWOT analysis, 581
optical character recognition (OCR) technology, 333
optimization, system, 388
oral presentation, of research, 509–510
order(s), 70–72
  authority to give, 71–72
  discharge, 72
  special types of, 72
  verbal, 71–72
order signatures, 72
ordinal data, 443
ordinary negligence, 240
organizational chart, 549, 550
organizational culture, 304
organizational experience, of project managers, 738–739
organizational forms/structures
  and accounting, 690–692
  and project management, 729–733
organizational health literacy, 403
organizational mission, 303, 580
organizational safeguards, 262
organizational vision, 303

organization development (OD), 545, 564–565
organization-wide data dictionary, 142
organizing
    by management, 549–550
    work, 655–661
organ procurement organizations (OPOs), 74–75
organ transplantation, in health records, 74–75
organ transplant registries, 127–128
orientation of employees
    checklist for, 628
    to department, 630
    evaluation of program for, 630–631
    by HR, 603
    individual, 630
    to organization, 628
original jurisdiction, 237
Ouchi, William, 547
Outcome and Assessment Information Set (OASIS), 78
Outcome and Assessment Information Set D (OASIS-D), 173
outcome evaluation, 494
outcome measures, 311–312
outcomes and effectiveness research (OER), 311–313
outcomes research, 533–535
out-group, 558–559
outlier. *See* cost outlier
outlier values, 449, 450, 475
outpatient(s)
    diagnostic and therapeutic services for, 18
    health records for, 77
    health statistics on, 434
    in hospitals, 12, 422
    surgical services for, 18, 19
outpatient code editor (OCE), 190
outpatient prospective payment system (OPPS), 169–170, 188, 442
output, in process improvement, 670
outsourcing, 659–660, 734
outsourcing agency, 734
ovals
    random, 469–470
    systematic, 469–470
overhead, 708–709
overlaps, in master patient index, 86
overlays, in master patient index, 86

# P

packaging, 170
panel interview, 608
paper-based health records, 62, 63, 66–67, 80–85, 87–90
paper-claim format, 193
parallel work division, 655
Pareto chart, 676
participant agreements, 359
participant observation, 500
partnership, 690, 691
part-time team members, 733
passive participant observation, 500

passphrases, 280–281
passwords, 82–83, 280–281
patch management process, 284
paternalism, 759
path-goal theory, 558
pathologists, 15
pathology
    anatomic, 15
    clinical, 15
pathology reports, 73, 74
PatientsLikeMe, 404
patient access
    components of, 180–183
    defined, 180
patient accounts, 692–693
patient accounts manager, 686
patient activation measure (PAM), 405
patient adjustment instrument (PAI), 173
patient advocacy movement, 298–299
patient advocacy services, in hospitals, 16
patient anti-dumping statute, 229
patient as consumer, 302
patient assessment, of healthcare providers, 400–401
patient authorization, 266–268
*Patient Care Partnership* (AHA), 298
patient care technicians (PCTs), 14
patient-centered medical homes (PCMH), 315, 401
Patient-Centered Outcomes Research Institute (PCORI), 516, 534–535
Patient-Centered Research Trust Fund, 534
Patient Driven Groupings Model (PDGM), 172–173
patient driven payment model (PDPM), 171–172
patient engagement, 397–411
    clinical outcomes of, 401
    consumer health informatics and, 399–401
    defined, 399
    focus of, 399, 400
    historical overview of, 400
    online resources for, 404–405
    patient-generated health data and, 409–410
    patient portals for, 406
    personal health records for, 406–408
    telehealth for, 408
patient financial services (PFS), 192, 194
patient financial services (PFS) systems, 341
patient follow-up
    for cancer registry, 125
    for diabetes registries, 127
    for immunization registries, 129
    for transplant registries, 128
    for trauma registries, 126
Patient Friendly Billing principles, 195
patient-generated health data (PGHD), 409–410
patient-identifiable data, 122, 123
patient identity management

and health records, 66, 85–87
    for use and disclosure of health information, 270
patient matching, 285
patient medical record information (PMRI), 105
patient portals, 335, 406
Patient Protection and Affordable Care Act (ACA) (2010), 7, 158, 301
    ACOs established by, 163
    and comparative effectiveness research, 494
    health insurance marketplace created by, 26, 28
    on Medicaid eligibility, 155
    PCORI established by, 534
    on rural hospitals, 169
    value-based purchasing in, 24
patient relations, 199
patient reported outcomes (PROs), 770
patient safety
    historical perspectives on, 296–299
    patient advocacy movement and, 298
patient safety indicators, 312, 313
patient safety risks, 305
*A Patient's Bill of Rights* (AHA), 298
Patient Self-Determination Act (1990), 250
Patient's rights statement, 68
patient web portal, 76
payback period, 717
payer relations, 197–198
payment audit, 196–197
payment posting, 194
payment recovery, 197
payment status indicators (PSIs), 170
payroll, 707, 709, 712–713, 715
PCORI. *See* Patient-Centered Outcomes Research Institute (PCORI)
Pearson's correlation coefficient, 455, 456
pediatric quality indicators, 312, 313
pediatrics, residential treatment centers for, 22
peer review
    changes in, 510
    defined, 309
    description of, 23
    in quality management, 309–310
    value of, 490
performance, defined, 296
performance controls, 665–666
performance counseling, 617–618
performance improvement (PI), 669–683
    benchmarks for, 214–215
    business process reengineering and, 678–679
    care coordination and, 315
    case management and, 314–315
    for clinical documentation integrity, 214
    clinical pathways and, 314
    continuous quality improvement and, 671–678
    defined, 296, 669
    evidence-based practice and, 313–314

information technology use and, 315
opportunities for, 669–670
principles of, 670
for revenue cycle management, 199–201
workflow analysis and process redesign and, 679–683
performance management, 615–619, 652
performance measures
of actual performance, 664
defined, 306, 665
for quality management, 306–307
for work, 665–668
performance review, 615–617
performance standards, for work, 662–664
permanent variances, 713, 714, 715
personal health data, 389
personal health literacy, 402–403
personal health record (PHR), 76, 406–408
personal protective equipment (PPE), 499
persuasive authority, 236
Peters, Tom, 547
petition for writ of certiorari, 237
pharmaceuticals. *See* drugs (prescription)
pharmacy/pharmacists, in hospitals, 16
phishing attacks, 283
physical database design, 131, 132, 133
physical examination. *See* history and physical examination (H&P)
physical safeguards, 262
physical therapist (PT), 16
physical therapist assistant (PTA), 16
physical therapy, 16, 172
physician(s)
ambulatory care provided by, 18
authorized to give orders, 71–72
and clinical documentation integrity, 208–209, 210–211, 213, 215–216
consultations with, 73
database of, 135
hospital admission privileges of, 11
peer review of, 309–310
specialty, 5
surveys of, 498
training of, 4–5
web portals of, 335
physician assistants (PAs), 5
physician champions, 209, 211, 213, 216
physician index, 123
physician-patient privilege, 252
Physician Self-Referral Law, 229
Physician Value-Based Modifier (PVBM), 442
physiological signal processing systems, 337
piece-rate incentive, 543
pie chart, 467, 470, 471, 472
pilot study, 505
plagiarism, 247
plaintext, 282
plaintiff, 237–238

plan-do-check-act (PDCA) cycle, 308–309
planning horizon, 373
plan/planning. *See also* strategic planning
business continuity, 306
contingency, 278–280, 305–306, 587
corrective action, 264, 265
data backup, 278–279
defined, 50
disaster recovery, 279, 306
discharge, 76
emergency mode operation, 279–280
ergonomic, 654
financial data for, 693
for governance, 49–51
human resources, 600–601
implementation, 375–376, 589–591
by management, 549
nutritional care, 74
point-of-service, 28, 159–160
project, 377
project communication, 378
project management, 743–744
special needs, 154
tactical, 370
for training, 625–627
turnover, 377
workspace, 652–654
plan step, in Deming Wheel, 308, 309
playscripts, 661
pleading guilty, 239
PMI talent triangle, 739–741
point method, of job evaluation, 615
point-of-care documentation applications, 342–343
point-of-care information systems, 337
point-of-service (POS) collection, 182–183
point-of-service (POS) plans, 28, 159–160
policy
defined, 607
by HR, 607
policy analysis, 494
politics, of change, 592–593
population-based registry, 124, 125, 126, 127
population-based statistics, 436
population health data, 389
Portfolio Management Professional (PfMP), 724
POS collection, 182–183
position (job) descriptions, 606–607
positive relationship among variables, 493
positive variances, 713
POS plans, 28, 159–160
post-acute care, 20
poster session, for research presentation, 508–509
postmortem examination. *See* autopsy
postoperative anesthesia, 74
postoperative infection rates, 433
postpartum record, 75

potentially compensable event (PCE), 256
power
in management, 550
types of, 550
power skills, in PMI talent triangle, 740
practice management system (PMS), 370
preauthorization, as patient access component, 180–181
precertification, as patient access component, 180–181
precision medicine, 410–411
predictive analytics, 48, 603
predictive modeling, 459
pre-emption, 248, 274
pre-encounter services, 183
Preferred Provider Health Care Act (1985), 158
preferred provider organizations (PPOs), 28, 153, 156, 159
pregnancy, in health records, 75
Pregnancy Discrimination Act (1978), 602
pregnant women, as vulnerable subjects in research, 525
prejudice, 771
preliminary research, 492
premiums, 151
prenatal record, 75
preponderance of the evidence, 238
preregistration, as patient access component, 180–182
prescription drugs. *See* drugs (prescription)
prescriptive analytics, 603
prescriptive functions, of change agents, 565
presentation, research, 508–510
present on admission (POA), 166–167
prevalence, 532
prevalence rate, 436
prevention quality indicators, 312, 313
preventive controls, 666, 709
primary analysis, 496
primary care, classification system for, 102–103
primary care medical homes, 315, 401
primary care physicians (PCPs)
for ambulatory care, 17–18
HMOs using, 159
POS plans using, 159–160
responsibilities of, 28
primary data source, 122, 419
primary keys, 132
primary sources, of literature review, 490
principal diagnosis, 165
principal investigator (PI), 524
principle functions, of change agents, 565
principlism, 758–760
print learners, 638
prisoners, as vulnerable subjects in research, 525

privacy
  in clinical and biomedical research, 526–527
  cloud computing and, 335
  data, 139
  defined, 260, 761
  disclosures and, 266–273
  ethics of, 761, 768
  in health information exchange, 284–286, 355
  invasion of, 242
  notice of practices of, 68, 262
  right to, 242, 246
  state laws on, 274–275
  workforce training for, 287–289
Privacy Act (1974), 246
Privacy Rule, of HIPAA, 246, 261–262
  Administrative Requirements of, 262
  on clinical and biomedical research, 525–526
  enforcement of, 264–265
  felony crimes in, 237
  on mental health records, 77
  on patient amendment requests, 66
  on patient identity management, 270
  proposed modifications of, 265
  on protected health information, 66, 68
  purposes of, 261
  sections of, 261–262
  on substance abuse patient records, 271, 273
  and training, 287–289
  on use and disclosure of patient information, 261–262, 266–269
private FFS plans, 153–154
private health insurance, 28, 151
private law, 236
private medical practice, for ambulatory care, 18
private ownership, 691
privilege, 252
proactive processes, 54
problem-oriented medical record (POMR), 73
problem statement, 488
procedural justice, 759
procedure(s)
  defined, 607
  by HR, 607
  of work, 660–661
procedure formats, 660–661
procedure manuals, 661
procedure writing guidelines, 660
processes
  of data governance, 54
  defined, 54
  ongoing, 54
  proactive, 54
  reactive, 54
  redesign of, 679–683
process evaluation, 493–494
process group framework, 741, 742
process improvement
  components of, 670

defined, 670
  for health information systems, 379
process innovations, 588
process knowledge, of project managers, 739
process measures, 311–312
process simulation software, 682
process theory of motivation, 550
production line, 655
productivity standards, 663
product liability, 242–243
professional behaviors, 739
Professional in Business Analysis (PMI-PBA), 724
professional review. *See* peer review
profitability, 705–706
program, defined, 751
Program for Evaluating Payment Patterns Electronic Report (PEPPER), 212
program management, 751
Program Management Professional (PgMP), 724
programmed learning modules, 637
Programs of All-Inclusive Care for the Elderly (PACE), 155
progress notes, 72
project
  champions of, 728
  characteristics of, 722
  costs of, 737, 743, 744, 747
  defined, 722–723
  failure of, 724, 726, 751
  objectives of, 722–723, 743, 751
  *vs.* operations, 722–723
  purpose of, 723
  resources of, 736, 743, 744
  schedule of, 727, 737, 743, 744
  scope of, 726–727, 736–737, 743
  selection of, 751
  sponsors of, 727–728
  users of, 728
project-based contracts, 660
project champions, 728
project communication plan, 378
project coordinator, 730
project expediter, 730
projectized organization, 731–732
project management, 721–752. *See also* project managers
  certifications for, 724
  and change management, 748–750
  constraints on, 726–727
  defined, 724
  development of, 543
  in health information exchange, 360
  in health information systems planning, 377–378
  life cycle of, 724–726, 741–748
  members in, 727–728
  methodologies of, 724–726
  organizational structures and, 729–733
  process of, 724, 725, 741–748
  teams in, 728, 732, 733–734

Project Management Body of Knowledge (PMBOK), 724
Project Management Institute (PMI), 724, 738, 741
Project Management Professional (PMP), 724
Project Manager Competency Development (PMCD), 738, 739
project managers, 735–741
  building blocks for, 738–739
  and change, 749
  and communication, 728, 737, 747
  competencies of, 737–739
  defined, 728
  in functional organizations, 730
  in matrix organizations, 730
  in projectized organizations, 732
  responsibilities of, 728, 735, 736–737
  roles of, 736–737
  skills of, 735–736
  successful, 728
  talent triangle of, 739–741
project performance, 739
project plan, 377
project portfolio management (PPM), 751–752
project portfolio manager, 751
project risk management, 378
project sponsors, 727–728
project stakeholders, 727–728
project teams, 728, 732, 733–734
Promoting Interoperability (PI) program, 344, 366, 401
promotion, 607, 646
property and valuables list, 69
proportions, 453–454
proprietary hospitals, 13
prosecutor, 239
prospective payment system (PPS), 161, 707
  for ambulance services, 171
  for ambulatory surgery center, 170–171
  for home healthcare, 172–173
  for inpatient psychiatric facilities, 167
  for inpatient rehabilitation facilities, 173–174
  for long-term care, 173–174
  of Medicare, 164–174, 312
  and outpatient prospective payment system, 169–170
  and resource-based relative value scale system, 168–169
  for skilled nursing facilities, 171–172
prospective studies, 532
protected health information (PHI)
  access to, 262
  Breach Notification Rule on, 263, 264, 282
  consent to use or disclose, 68
  HIPAA on, 66, 68, 250, 261–262, 266, 270
  mobile health technology and, 286
  patient identity management and, 270
  on patient portals, 406

uses and disclosures of, 261–262, 266–273
protection, as recordkeeping principle, 44
proximate causation, 240
psychiatric hospitals, 12
   long-term care in, 22
   prospective payment system for, 167
psychiatric records, 77
psychological needs, of employees, 545
publication, of research, 510
Public Company Accounting Oversight Board (PCAOB), 690
public health, 135
   ethical issues in, 769
   statistics on, 436–437
public health data, 389
public health databases, 135–136
public health insurance, 28
Public Health Service (PHS), 527
public health services, 19
public hospitals, 12–13
public law, 236
Public Law 89-97 (1965), 26
Public Law 98-21 (1982/1983), 8
public ownership, 691
pull system, 673
punitive damages, 238, 242
purchase orders, 698
purchase price, 695
purchasing, 697–699, 715
p-value, 444, 445, 475
PxDx system, 775

## Q

qualitative analysis
   of health records, 82
   in research, 506
qualitative analytical software, 506, 507
qualitative approach, 486–487
qualitative standards, 662
quality (healthcare)
   defined, 296
   factors influencing, 296, 299–302
   historical perspectives on, 296–299
   legal issues of, 297
   patients influencing, 302
   paying for, 302
quality assessment
   health records for, 65
   performance measures for, 306–307
quality improvement (QI), 23–24
   confidentiality of activities for, 255–256
   continuous, 24
quality indicators (QIs)
   of AHRQ, 312–313
   defined, 301
   reporting, 301
   and transparency, 302
quality management, 295–319
   accreditation and, 300
   business continuity plan in, 306
   care coordination and, 315
   case management and, 314–315
   certifications for, 316–317
   change management and, 304–305
   clinical pathways and, 314, 315
   compliance with, 317
   contingency plan in, 305–306
   defined, 296
   drivers of, 299–302
   evidence-based practice and, 313–314
   health data analytics for, 317
   health information management and, 316–317
   in health information systems, 391–393
   historical perspectives on, 296–299
   information governance and, 317
   information technology use and, 315
   interprofessional education for, 304
   knowledge generation in, 307–308
   leadership and, 303–304
   learning health systems and, 318–319
   legal issues of, 297
   organizational culture and, 304
   organizational influence on, 303–306
   outcomes and effectiveness research in, 311–313
   peer review in, 309–310
   performance measures for, 306–307
   plan-do-check-act (PDCA) cycle in, 308–309
   project managers and, 737
   quality indicators and, 301–302, 312–313
   quality measures for, 306–307, 311–312, 314
   reengineering compared to, 678
   regulatory requirements for, 300–301
   risk management and, 305
   social media and, 318
   stewardship and, 317
   telehealth services and, 318
   tools and processes of, 306–311
   tracer methodology in, 310–311
   transparency of, 301–302
   trends in, 318–319
   value-based care in, 302
quality measures, 306–307, 311–312, 314
QualityNet, 445
quality professional, 316
quality reporting, 24
   data visualization for, 479–482
   health records for, 65, 66–67
quantitative analysis, of health records, 81–82
quantitative approach, 486, 487
quantitative standards, 663
quasi-experimental research, 495
query-based exchange, 356
query/queries
   for clinical documentation integrity, 210, 215–218
   defined, 215–216
   documentation of, 218
   format of, 218
question, research, 488–489
questionnaire surveys, 498

Quintuple Aim, of Institute for Healthcare Improvement, 400
qui tam relators, 223

## R

radiation oncologists, 15
radiation therapy, 15
radio frequency identification (RFID) technology, 334
radiologists, 15
radiology, in hospitals, 15
radiology reports, 73–74
randomization, 495
randomized clinical trials (RCTs), 528
random ovals, 469–470
random sampling, 445, 495
range, 450
ransomware (malware), 283
Rapid Estimate of Adult Literacy in Medicine, 403
rapid reviews, 496
rate, 420–421, 453–454
ratio, 420, 702
ratio analysis, 702–706
ratio data, 443
RAT-STATS, 446–448
reactive processes, 54
real-time analytics, 460–461
reasonable cause, 264
reasoning
   deductive, 487, 500
   inductive, 487, 500
receiving documents, 698
recipients, of projects, 728
recognized security practices, 263
recordkeeping principles, 44
record locator service (RLS), 351–352, 360–361
record review
   in clinical documentation integrity, 211–212
   frequency and number of, 212
   open and closed, 82
recovery audit contractor (RAC), 212, 446
recovery houses, 22
recruitment, 607–610
Red Flags Rule, 228
redundancy, 346
reengineering, 547, 678–679
*Reengineering the Corporation* (Hammer and Champy), 547
reference checks, 609
reference data, 46–47
reference terminology, 104
referent power, 550
Regenstrief Institute, 106
regional master patient index (RMPI), 86
registered dietitians (RDs), 16
registered health information administrator (RHIA), 316
registered health information technician (RHIT), 316, 487
registered nurses (RNs), 14
registration
   common errors with, 182
   as patient access component, 182–183

registries, 124–129
    for administrative purposes, 129
    for birth defects, 129
    for cancer, 124–126
    defined, 124
    for diabetes, 127
    for immunization, 128–129
    for implants, 129
    importance of, 129
    for long COVID, 129
    patient-identifiable data in, 122
    as secondary data source, 122
    for transplant, 127–128
    for trauma, 126–127
    vendor systems *vs.* facility-specific systems, 138
regression, simple linear, 456–458
regulations
    administrative agencies developing, 235, 236
    examples of, 300–301
    in procedure manuals, 661
regulatory agencies, 236
regulatory law, 246
regulatory risks, 305
rehabilitation hospitals, 12, 20, 173–174
rehabilitation services, 78–79
reidentification, 269
reimbursement, 26–30, 149–175
    audit for, 224
    data standardization for, 112
    financial data for, 693
    government-sponsored systems of, 26–28, 152–157
    health records for, 65
    for managed care, 28–30, 157–160
    for Medicare, 26–27, 152–154, 164–174
    methodologies of, 161–164
    for quality of care, 302
    systems of, 150–160
    for telehealth, 163, 318
    third-party, 26, 150–151, 161, 162
reinforcement, 637
relational databases, 130
relationships, 130–132
relative risk (RR), 532
relative value units (RVUs), 168
release of information (ROI), 253–254, 755, 768–769
reliability
    in accounting, 688, 689
    in employee testing, 608
    in research, 502
remittance advice (RA), 196
remittance management, 196
remote patient monitoring device, 318
reporting
    in electronic health records, 345
    research results, 507–508
reproductive health care, use and disclosure of health information for, 270
request for production, 238
request for proposal (RFP), 359, 380–381
required standards, 262

requirements analysis, for health information systems, 378–379
requirements document, 743
requirements matrix, 743, 744
requirements specification, for health information systems, 379
research. *See also* biomedical research; clinical research
    applied, 486
    basic, 486
    causal-comparative, 492, 495–496
    comparative effectiveness, 494
    correlational, 492, 493
    data analysis in, 506
    data collection for, 497–505
    defined, 486
    descriptive, 492, 493
    design of, 492–497, 528–532
    ethical issues in, 517–519, 769
    evaluation, 492, 493–494, 500
    experimental, 492, 494–495
    historical, 492–493
    literature review for, 490–491
    methodology of, 486–487
    methods of, 485–510
    mixed methods, 487
    observational, 499–500
    outcomes, 533–535
    preliminary, 492
    primary analysis in, 496
    problem statement in, 488–489
    process of, 488–510
    question, 488–489
    secondary analysis in, 496–497
    sharing results of, 507–510
research data, 389
research findings, 507–508
research protocols, 528
Resident Assessment Instrument (RAI), 79, 171
residential care facilities, long-term care in, 21
residential recovery houses, 22
residential treatment centers, for pediatrics, 22
residual risk, 277
residual uncertainty (RU), 582–583
*res ipsa loquitur*, 241, 243
resistance to change, 566–567
*res judicata*, 239
resource(s)
    human (*see* human resources management)
    online, for patient engagement, 404–405
    of project, 736, 743, 744
resource-based relative value scale system (RBRVS), 168–169
Resource Utilization Group, Version IV (RUG-IV), 171
respiratory therapists (RTs), 16
respiratory therapy, 16
respite care, 153
*respondent superior*, 254
response bias, 505

response rate, to surveys, 505
response time, 662
responsibility, 613
restitution, 238
restraint orders, 72
results management, 342
resume, 607–608
resuscitative services, 72
retail clinics, 19
retained earnings, 702
retention
    of health records, 66, 88–90
    as recordkeeping principle, 44
    of workforce, 610–611
retina scan technology, 281
retrieval of health records, 83, 87–88
retrospective documentation, 768
retrospective payment systems, 161, 165
retrospective review, 207, 211, 212
retrospective studies, 530–531, 532
return on investment (ROI)
    benefits realization and, 385
    in budgets, 718
    calculating, 718
    defined, 705, 718
    formula of, 705
    of new technologies, 603
    work division patterns and, 655–656
revenue
    in accounting, 688, 689, 697
    in budgets, 712
    categories of, 697
    sources of, 697
revenue audit, 196–197
revenue code, 189
revenue cycle, 178
revenue cycle management (RCM), 177–201
    back-end process of, 192–197
    defined, 178
    front-end process of, 179–183
    middle process of, 184–191
    performance measures in, 199–201
    statistics in, 434
    support services for, 197–199
revenue integrity, 187
Revenue Principle, 689
revenue projects, 723
revenue recovery, 197
reverse mentoring, 632
reward power, 550
right to privacy, 242, 246
risk(s)
    accepting, 277
    analysis of, 276–277
    assessing, 276, 532–533, 582–583
    assumption of, 243
    attributable risk, 533
    managing (*see* risk management)
    mitigating, 277
    relative, 532
    residual, 277
    transfer of, 277
    types of, 305
risk-adjusted quality indicators, 460

risk adjustment models, 161, 164, 460
risk management, 276–277
    certifications in, 316
    components of, 277
    defined, 305
    project risk management, 378
    and quality management, 305
    and strategic planning, 582–583
Risk Management Professional (PMI-RMP), 724
risk standardized mortality rate (RSMR), 460
role(s)
    defined, 553
    of managers, 553–554
role-based access, 262
role playing, 632
role theory, 553
Roosevelt, Franklin D., 7
root cause analysis, 305, 673
rootkit (malware), 283
R Statistical Software, 479
rules, in procedure manuals, 661
rules of engagement, 53
run chart, 677
rural hospitals, 169
RxNorm, 107–108

## S

safe harbor method, 269
Safe Harbor Regulations, 229
safety. *See* patient safety
sampling
    in experimental research, 495
    for healthcare data analytics, 445–449
    impact of, 445–446
    tools for, 446–449
    types of, 445
sandbox, for system testing, 360
Sarbanes-Oxley Act (2002), 690
scalar chain, 544, 549
scales, 503, 504
scanning, of health records, 81, 88, 89, 90
scatterplot, 467, 475–476, 676–677
scenarios, 586–587
scheduling
    as patient access component, 180
    projects, 727, 737, 743, 744
    work, 657–660
Scheduling Professional (PMI-SP), 724
schema mapping, 130
Schmidt, Warren, 556
scientific innovations, 9–10
scientific management, 542–543
scope, of project, 726–727, 736–737, 743
scope creep, 750
scoping reviews, 496
scribes, 80, 378
scrubber software, 193
Scrum method, 726
seclusion orders, 72
secondary analysis, 496–497
secondary databases, 138–140
secondary data source, 122, 419
secondary sources, of literature review, 490

secure information, 282
secure messaging, 406
Securities and Exchange Commission (SEC), 690
security
    audit logs and monitoring for, 278
    and authentication of health records, 82–83
    awareness of, 288
    cloud computing and, 335
    confidentiality and, 139
    contingency plan for, 278–280
    cybersecurity, 263, 275, 283, 286
    data security (*see* data security)
    defined, 260
    disclosures and, 266–273
    effective program for, 275–284
    enhanced, 348
    framework for, 57
    in health information exchange, 284–286, 355
    health information management and, 255
    HIPAA on, 246
    recognized practices of, 263
    risk analysis and risk management for, 276–277
    state laws on, 274–275
    workforce training for, 287–289
Security Rule, of HIPAA, 261, 262–263
    on audit logs, 278
    on contingency plan, 278, 280
    on data security, 280
    on encryption, 282
    enforcement of, 264–265
    proposed modifications of, 265
    on protected health information, 250
    purpose of, 262
    on risk analysis and risk management, 276, 277
    safeguards of, 262
    standards in, 262–263
    and training, 287–289
self-insurance, employer-based, 7, 26, 151
self-logging, by employees, 664
self-paced training, 641–642
semantic differential scales, 503, 504
semantic interoperability, 104, 347
semifixed costs, 707
seminars, 641
semistructured questions, 503
sensitive information, handling, 253–254, 271–273, 769
sensitivity analysis, 587
sensitivity awareness, 620
sentencing, in criminal proceedings, 239
sentinel event, 305
Sequoia Project, 357
serial-unit numbering system, 85
serial work division, 655
servant leadership, 560
service innovations, 588
service level agreements (SLAs), 660
settlements, in civil litigation, 238
shift differential, 658

shift rotation, 658
shipping documents, 698
Shoemaker, Floyd, 562
Short Assessment of Health Literacy – Spanish and English (SAHL–S&E), 403
short-stay outlier, 174
side-by-side bar plot, 471
signatures
    electronic, 82–83, 247
    handwritten, 247
    order, 72
significance, 508
simple linear regression (SLR), 456–458
simple object access protocols (SOAP), 336
simple random sampling, 445
simulation observation, 499
simulation training, 642
simultaneous equations method, 708
single-blind studies, 528
situational theories, of leadership, 557–559
Six Sigma, 673–674
skilled nursing facilities (SNFs)
    health records of, 79
    long-term care in, 20, 21, 79
    Medicare paying for care in, 153, 171–172
    post-acute care in, 20
    prospective payment system for, 171–172
    quality initiative for, 25
skin cancer, 124
slander, 241
slicing and dicing, 478
SMART goals, 373–374
smart peripherals, 342
SNFs. *See* skilled nursing facilities (SNFs)
SNODENT, 109
SNOMED CT, 104, 105–106, 112
SOAP note format, 72–73
Social and Rehabilitation Service, 25
social determinants of health (SDOH), 402–403, 773–774
social disparities, 773–774
social engineering, 283
socialization, 628
social media
    ethical use of, 774–775
    and quality management, 318
    research presentation on, 509
social networks, 644
social orientation, 551
Social Security Act (1935), 8, 25, 26, 154, 223, 297
Social Security Administration, 25
Social Security Death Index, 125
social services, 425
social workers, in hospitals, 16
socioeconomic approach to management (SEAM), 548
soft skills, 646
Software as a Service (SaaS), 87, 346
software criticality analysis, 280

sole proprietorship, 690, 691
sort, straighten, scrub, standardize, and sustain (five Ss), 673
sound, at work, 654
source systems, for electronic health records, 341–342
spaced training, 633
spaghetti diagram, 652, 653, 680
span of control, 549–550
spatial representation, 468
special cause variation, 671
special damages, 238
special needs plan, 154
specialty clinical systems, 342
specialty hospitals, 12
specialty physicians, 5
specific performance, 244
speech-language pathologists (SLPs), 15
speech language pathology, 172
speech recognition technology, 80, 329–330
Spina Bifida Health Care Benefits, 157
spoilation, 252
sponsors
    of innovations, 564
    of projects, 727–728
spread measures, 450
SQL, 132, 133
stable monetary unit, 688
stacked bar plot, 466–467, 471
staff authority, 549
staffing, 603. *See also* medical staff
staff model HMOs, 159
staging system, for cancer, 125
stakeholders
    in clinical documentation integrity process, 207–208, 213
    communication with, 593–594
    in data governance, 55
    external, 55
    internal, 55
    project, 727–728
    in strategic planning, 579
standard(s)
    communicating, 663
    comparing performance to, 668
    defined, 662
    developing, 663–664
    effective, 662
    and performance, 662–664
    in process improvement, 670
    types of, 662–663
standard deviation, 450
standard error, 451, 453
standardization
    of hospital care, 5–6
    of medical practice, 4–5
standardized mortality rate (SMR), 460
standard of care, 240
standard of proof, 238
Standards and Interoperability Framework (S&I), 112
Standards of Ethical Coding (AHIMA), 761, 769
*stare decisis*, 236

Stark Law (1989), 229
state administrative databases, 135
state ambulatory surgery databases, 137
state attorney, 239
state constitutions, 235
state court decisions, 235
state court system, 237
state emergency department databases, 137
State Inpatient Database, 137
state licensure
    on giving orders, 71
    of healthcare facilities, 24–25
    and health records, 64, 245
    on history and physical forms, 70
statement of cash flow, 702
statement of retained earnings, 702
statement of stockholder's equity, 702
statements, in accounting, 699, 701–702, 703
state public health databases, 135–136
Statewide Planning and Research Cooperative System (SPARCS), 135
state workers' compensation funds, 157
statistical process control (SPC) chart, 677
statistical significance, 508
statistics. *See also* health statistics
    basic calculations for, 420–421
    community-based, 436–437
    defined, 418
    descriptive, 419–421, 444–449, 453
    inferential, 420, 444–449, 450–452, 453–454
    population-based, 436
    vital, 136–137
statute of limitations, 243
statutes, 235
statutory law, 236, 246
steering committee
    for data governance, 54
    defined, 377
step-down allocation, 708
step mixed costs, 707
stereotyping, 771
stewardship
    for data governance, 55
    quality management and, 317
stockholder's equity, statement of, 702
storage
    backup, 279, 346
    of health records, 83, 87, 89, 346
storytelling, 586
strategic change, 594–596
strategic findings, 588
strategic goals, 589–590, 592
strategic innovation, 588
strategic management, 575–596
    concepts in, 577
    defined, 576
    phases of, 580–590
    skills of, 577–578
strategic objectives, 589–590, 592
strategic planning
    change program and, 592–594

    for consumer health informatics, 398
    customer's role in, 588
    defined, 370, 576
    elements of, 578–579
    environmental assessment in, 579–583, 586, 595–596
    execution of, 377–386
    formulation of, 549
    for health information systems, 370–376, 377
    historical overview of, 576
    for information management, 49–50
    phases of, 579–590
    vision in, 576–577, 584–585
strategic profile, 580–582, 587–588
strategic risks, 305
strategic thinking
    competencies of, 577
    concepts in, 577
    defined, 576
    techniques and tools for, 586–587
strategy
    defined, 576, 583
    formulating, 585–588
strategy map, 596
stratified random sample, 445
strengths, in SWOT analysis, 581
stress exposure training (SET), 499–500
strict liability, 242, 243
stringent state laws, 274
strong matrix organization, 730, 732
structural alignment, 132
structural measures, 312
structural metadata, 390
structured data, 47, 48, 329
structured interview, 498, 608
Structured Product Labeling (SPL), 107
structured query language (SQL), 132, 133
structured questions, 503
study group, 495
subjective, objective, assessment, plan (SOAP) note format, 72–73
subject matter jurisdiction, 237
subject matter managers, 55
subpoenas, 238
substance abuse
    behavioral health services for, 22
    information about, handling, 253–254, 271–273
Substance Registry System (SRS), 109, 110
succession planning, 646
summary judgment, 238
summative evaluation, 494
summons, 237, 238
sunsetting, 386
super users, 378
supervisory management, 551
supplemental medical insurance (SMI), 152
supplies, 698, 699, 700–701, 712–713, 714
supplies inventory, 699
support software, 346–347
supreme court (state), 237

Supreme Court of the United States, 237
surgeon general, 19
surgery/surgical services
   ambulatory (*see* ambulatory surgery; ambulatory surgery center)
   in health records, 74
   historical perspectives on, 296
   laparoscopic, 12
surgical assistants (SAs), 5
surveys, 498, 504, 505, 615
swimlane diagram, 682
SWOT analysis, 580–582
symbolic representation, 468
symbol recognition technologies, 333–334
synchronous web-based courses, 644
syphilis study, 518–519
systematic ovals, 469–470
systematic random sampling, 445
systematic review, 496
Systematized Nomenclature for Dentistry (SNODENT), 109
Systematized Nomenclature of Medicine-Clinical Terms (SNOMED CT), 104, 105–106, 112
system customization, 382
system development life cycle (SDLC), 369–370
system integrator, 380
system optimization, 388
systems thinking, in leadership, 561
systems view, 367–369
System Usability Scale (SUS), 502

# T

table(s)
   for data visualization, 466, 468–471
   defined, 466
   interpreting, 467
   purpose of, 466
   symbolic representation in, 468
table of contents, of procedure manuals, 661
tacit knowledge, 307
tactical plan, 370
tactile learners, 638
Taft-Hartley Act (1947), 604, 605
talent triangle, 739–741
Tannenbaum, Robert, 556
task analysis, 630
task-by-time chart, 543
task-oriented behaviors, 550–551
Tax Cuts and Jobs Act (2017), 7
Tax Equity and Fiscal Responsibility Act (TEFRA) (1982), 158, 165
tax status, 692
tax year, 689
Taylor, Frederick W., 542–543
team, project, 728, 732, 733–734
team building, 612–613, 628
technical interoperability, 347
technical/manmade threats, 306
technical safeguards, 262
technical skills, 553, 735

technological advances. *See also* artificial intelligence (AI); health information technologies (HITs)
   augmented intelligence, 32
   blockchain, 286
   in clinical documentation integrity, 218–220
   in compliance programs, 223–224
   in health information exchange, 359
   and health record retention, 248
   in medicine, 9–10
   mobile health technology, 286–287
   new, in hospitals, 166
   in quality management, 315
   research on, 494
   in security, 280–284
   special payments for, 170
   speech recognition technology, 80, 329–330
technology risks, 305
telecommuting, 654, 659
telehealth
   challenges of, 339
   during COVID-19 pandemic, 163, 318, 339, 408
   defined, 408–409
   and patient engagement, 408–409
   quality management and, 318
   reimbursement for, 163, 318
   technologies used in, 338–339
templates, for health records, 81, 84
Temporary Assistance for Needy Families, 155
temporary contracts, 660
temporary variances, 713, 714
termination of employees, 618
terminology
   and classification systems, 104–111
   clinical, 95
   defined, 95
   of health statistics, 422
   interface, 104–105
   management of, 49
   reference, 104
text mining, 330
theory functions, of change agents, 565
Theory X, 545, 556
Theory Y, 545, 556
Theory Z, 547
therapeutic orders. *See* diagnostic and therapeutic orders
therapeutic services
   in hospitals, 14–17
   for outpatients, 18
thinkers (learning style), 638
third-party reimbursement, 26, 150–151, 161, 162
thoughtflow, 383
threats
   as assault, 241
   in contingency plan, 306
   in SWOT analysis, 581
3D bar plot, 467
360-degree evaluation, 617
three-point scale, 504

time and motion studies, 543
time period, in accounting, 688–689
title, of procedure manuals, 661
Title VII, of Civil Rights Act (1964), 602, 647
Title XIX of Society Security Act Amendments, 297
*To Err Is Human: Building a Safer Health System* (IOM), 299
top-down process map, 680–682
top management, 551, 552
topography codes, 100
tort(s), 240–244
   apology statutes and, 243–244
   categories of, 240–243
   defenses to, 243
   defined, 240
   laws on, 240
   reform laws on, 238
total length of stay, 427
total margin ratio, 705–706
total quality management (TQM), 546–547, 672
tracer methodology, 310–311
traditional fee-for-service reimbursement, 161
training, 623–648
   and adult learning strategies, 636–639
   artificial intelligence in, 644–645
   for clinical documentation integrity, 213
   for coding compliance, 227–228
   computer-based, 628, 632, 642
   curriculum of, 626
   defined, 624
   delivery methods of, 626, 640–644
   diversity, 620, 624, 639
   elements of, 627–636
   for emergencies, 280
   evaluation of, 626–627
   feedback on, 627
   goal of, 627
   of health information management staff, 624, 633–634, 645–647
   for health information systems, 383
   history of, in medical practice, 4–5
   in-service education for, 633–636
   instructor-directed, 640–641
   just-in-time, 638
   legislation on, 647–648
   making changes to, 627
   massed, 633
   needs assessment for, 625, 626
   objectives of, 626
   on-the-job, 631–633
   orientation program in, 627–631
   planning for, 625–627
   for privacy and security, 287–289
   for quality management, 304
   self-paced, 641–642
   spaced, 633
train-the-trainer, 626
trait approach, 556
transcription, of health records, 80

## Index

transfer
    of health records, 88–89
    risk, 277
transgender patients, 771
transitions of care (ToC) initiative, 112
transparency
    in health and safety programs, 603
    in quality management, 301–302
    as recordkeeping principle, 44
transplant registries, 127–128
trauma care, in hospitals, 18
trauma registries, 126–127
traumatic injury, 126
treatment
    in experimental research, 495
    payments, or healthcare operations (TPO), 262, 268, 274
trial court, 237, 239
triangulation, 500
TRICARE, 27, 152, 156
TRICARE Prime, 156
TRICARE Select, 156
trier of fact, 238
tri-factor authentication, 281
Triple Aim, of Institute for Healthcare Improvement, 299, 400
triple constraint, 727
Trojan horses (malware), 283
trust community, 359
Trusted Exchange Framework, 357
Trusted Exchange Framework and Common Agreement (TEFCA), 357, 358
t-test, 450–451
turnaround time, 662
turnover plan, 377
turnover strategy, 377
Tuskegee Syphilis Study, 518–519
21st Century Cures Act (2016), 66, 76, 114, 247, 273–274, 517
two-factor authentication, 281
two-point scale, 504
type I error, 444–445, 450, 452, 453
type II error, 444

## U

UB-04 (format), 193
unbundling, 222, 223, 225
uncertainty, 582–583
unconditioned authorization, 267–268
unfavorable variances, 713, 714–715
Unified Medical Language System (UMLS), 106, 112, 114–115, 137–138
Uniformed Services Employment and Reemployment Rights Act (USERRA) (1994), 602
Uniform Hospital Discharge Data (UHDDS), 135
unions, 604
unique identifier, 68
United Network for Organ Sharing, 75
United States Core Data for Interoperability (USCDI), 113, 114
unit numbering system, 85
unit work division, 656
unity of command, 544, 549
universal description, discovery, and integration (UDDI), 336
Universal Medical Device Nomenclature System (UMDNS), 108
University of Michigan, 557
"unknown that is knowable" (UK), 582–583
unstructured data, 47, 48, 329, 330
unstructured interview, 499
unstructured questions, 503
upcoding, 212, 223, 225
upper control limit (UCL), 677
urgency, sense of, 593
usability, 347–348
US Census, 619–620
US Constitution, 235
use, of health information
    with authorization, 266–268
    consent to, 68
    defined, 266
    objection to, 269–270
    patient identity management for, 270
    Privacy Rule on, 261–262, 266–269
    for reproductive health care, 270
    without authorization, 268–269
use case analysis, 682–683
user(s)
    of health information systems, 378
    of projects, 728
user access rights, 133
user authentication, 280–281
User Centered Design (UCD), 347
user identification (ID), 280
US healthcare delivery system, 3–32
    federal legislation and, 7–9
    forces affecting, 23–25
    future of, 30–32
    growth of, 4
    legal issues of, 297
    as part of GDP, 4
    quality of care in, 297–299
    reimbursement in, 26–30, 149–175
    rising costs of, 28, 30, 301
    social determinants of health and, 402, 774
    in 20th century, 7–9, 297–299
US Public Health Services Syphilis Study, 518–519
utilitarianism, 758, 763, 766, 772
utilization controls, 162
utilization management (UM), 185, 208
utilization review (UR) coordinator, 425

## V

vacation staffing, 658
validity
    in employee testing, 608
    in research, 501–502
value-based care (VBC), 24, 302, 366
value-based payments/purchases, 24, 302, 401
value-based programs, 442
Value Modifier (VM) Program, 442
values, and ethics, 763, 770–771
values-based leadership, 559–560
values statement, 549
value stream mapping, 673
variable(s)
    in causal-comparative research, 495
    confounding, 494
    continuous, 449
    in correlational research, 493
    defined, 493
    dependent, 456, 495
    in experimental research, 494–495
    independent, 456, 494–495
    relationship among, 480–482, 493
variable costs, 707
variance
    in budget, 712, 713
    explanation of, 713–715
    identification of, 713
    in project management, 727
variance analysis, 666, 713
variation
    common cause, 671
    special cause, 671
vector graphic data, 337
vendor partners, 733–734
vendor strategy, 379–380
vendor systems, 138
verbal frequency scale, 504
verbal orders, 71–72
verdict, 238, 239
vertical bar plot, 470, 471
vertical dyad linkage (VDL), 558
Veterans Affairs, Department of. *See* Department of Veterans Affairs (VA)
Veterans Health Administration (VHA), 27, 152, 156–157
videoconferencing, 509, 643
virtualization, 346
virtual private network (VPN), 355
virtual reality (VR) module, 499–500
virtual sandbox, for system testing, 360
virtue ethics, 756–757, 763
viruses (malware), 283
vision
    assessment of, 580
    in change management, 569
    characteristics of, 584
    defined, 576
    organizational, 303
    in strategic planning, 576–577, 584–585
vision statement, 549, 584
visual controls, 673
visual learners, 638
vital statistics, 136–137
vocabulary, clinical, 95
voice recognition, 281
volume logs, 664
voluntary agencies, for ambulatory care, 19–20
voluntary consent, in research, 517
voluntary hospitals, 13
vulnerable subjects, in research, 525–526

## W

Wagner Act (1935), 604, 605
warranty
   breach of, 243
   express, 243
   implied, 243
waste, 222
waterfall method, of project management, 724–725
Waterman, Robert, 547
ways of working, in PMI talent triangle, 739–740
weak matrix organization, 730, 731
weaknesses, in SWOT analysis, 581
web-based courses, 643–644
web content management systems, 336
Weber, Max, 542
web forums, 404–405
webinars, 642
web portals, 76, 335, 406
web services, 336
web services description language (WSDL), 336
Western medicine, 4–6
whistleblowing, 223, 225, 227
wikis, 644
willful neglect, 264
wireless systems, 338
wireless technology, 337–338
wireless workstations on wheels (WOWs), 344
wisdom, in hierarchy of data to wisdom, 41, 307–308
women, in workforce, 619–620

work
   aesthetics at, 654
   design and process improvement of, 651–683
   distribution analysis for, 656–657
   division patterns for, 655–656
   ergonomics at, 654–655
   functional environment for, 652–655
   organizing, 655–661
   performance improvement for, 669–683
   performance measures for, 665–668
   performance standards for, 662–664
   procedures of, 660–661
   scheduling, 657–660
work breakdown structure (WBS), 744, 745
work distribution analysis, 656–657
work distribution chart, 656–657
worker immaturity–maturity, 557–558
Workers' Adjustment Retraining and Notification (WARN) Act (1988), 618
Workers' compensation, 27–28, 157
workflow
   departmental, 652, 653
   improvement of, for health information systems, 379, 382–383
workflow analysis, 679–683
workforce retention, 610–611
work measurement, 664
work sampling, 664
workshops, 641
workspace, 652–654
World Health Organization (WHO)
   Disability Assessment Schedule of, 102
   on hospital-acquired infection rates, 433
   ICD-10-CM by, 97
   ICD-11 by, 97, 98
   ICD by, 96
   ICD-O-3 by, 98, 100
   ICF by, 100, 101
   on interprofessional education, 6
   on social determinants of health, 402, 773
World Medical Association, 517
World Organization of Family Doctors (WONCA), 103
World Organization of Family Doctors (WONCA) International Classification Committee (WICC), 103
World Privacy Forum (WPF), 254
worms (malware), 283
writing guidelines, 660
wrongful disclosure, 254

## X

XML, 336

## Y

Yale University, 165

## Z

zero-based budgets, 711
z-test, 454